Effusion,
  chylous, 263
  pericardial, 131
  pleural, 259
Electrocution/electric shock, 135
Electrolyte maintenance and
  abnormalities, 37
Emetics, list of and recommended
  doses, 219
End-tidal carbon dioxide monitoring
  (capnometry), 52
Endotracheal intubation, 494
Enema, administration, 219
Epididymitis, infectious, 143
Epistaxis, 269
Esophageal foreign body, 160

F

Feline lower urinary tract disorders
  (FLUTD), 289
Flail chest, 264
Fluid deficits, calculation of, 43
Fluid requirements, maintenance, 43
Fluid therapy, 43
  colloid, 45
  crystalloid, 43
  rates of administration, 47
Foreign body
  airway, 257
  ear, 133
  esophageal, 160
  gastric, 161
  large intestinal, 164
  ocular, 200
  oral cavity, 158
  rectum and anus, 165
  small intestinal, 162
Fractures,
  and musculoskeletal trauma, 154
  initial management, 155
  os penis, 144
  rib, 264
Frostbite, 146

G

Gastric dilatation-volvulus (GDV), 165
Gastritis, acute, 171
Gastroenteritis, hemorrhagic, 173
Gastrointestinal emergencies, 158
Gila monster bite, 153
Glaucoma, acute, 203

H

Head injuries, 185
Heartworm caval syndrome, 130
Heat-induced illness (hyperthermia,
  heat stroke), 147
Hemorrhagic gastroenteritis, 173

Hemostasis, c
Hemothorax,
Hepatic failur
Hernia,
  diaphragmat
  strangulated, 170
High-rise syndrome, 158
Hypercalcemia, 181
Hyperkalemia, 39
Hypernatremia, 41
Hyperosmolar non-ketotic diabetes, 180
Hypertension,
  drugs used to treat, 177
  systemic, 176
Hyperthermia
  heat-induced illness, heat
    stroke, 147
  malignant, 148
Hypocalcemia, 181
Hypoglycemia, 180
Hypokalemia, 40
Hyponatremia, 41
Hypotension, perianesthetic, 98
Hypothermia, 147
Hypovolemic shock, 276
Hypoxia, 48

I-K

Intestinal obstruction,
  large, 169
  small, 162
Intubation, endotracheal, 494
Intussusception, acute, 165

L

Laparotomy, exploratory, 92
Large intestinal obstruction, 169
Laryngeal collapse, 256
Laryngeal paralysis, 255
Lavage, orogastric, 47
Ligamentous injuries, 157

M-N

Malignant hyperthermia, 148
Mesenteric volvulus, 168
Metabolic acidosis, 36
Metabolic alkalosis, 35
Metabolic emergencies, 178
Metritis, acute, 138
Mexican bearded lizard bite, 153
Musculoskeletal trauma, 154
Neurologic emergencies, 185

O

Obstipation, 169
Obstruction,
  biliary, 87
  large intestinal, 169

organ system obstruction caused by neoplasia, 170, 208
  small intestinal, 162
  upper airway, 254
  urinary tract, 289
Ocular emergencies, 196
  chemical injuries, 198
  cornea
    abrasions, 199
    penetrating injury, 200
  foreign body, 200
  glaucoma, acute, 203
  hyphema, 201
  lacerations
    conjunctival, 198
    lid, 197
  proptosis, 202
  subconjunctival hemorrhage, 198
  sudden loss of vision, 196
Oncologic emergencies, 205
  chemotherapy-related toxicities, 210
  neoplasia causing organ system obstruction, 208
  paraneoplastic syndromes, 205
Oral cavity, 158
Orchitis, infectious, 143
Orogastric lavage, 47
  Venomous creature bites, 149
Oxygen,
  nasal and nasopharygeal, 50
  supplementation, 48
  therapy, 49

P

Pain,
  management, 73
  acute abdominal, 86
  recognition and assessment, 71
Pancreatitis, 173
Paraneoplastic syndromes, 205
Paraphimosis, 144
Penile fracture, 144
Penile laceration, 144
Perforation, bowel, 170
Pericardial effusion, 131
Pericardiocentesis, 132
Peritoneal lavage, diagnostic, 93
Pleural effusions, analysis of, 261
Pneumonia, aspiration, 267
Pneumothorax, 258
Poisons and toxins, 212
Potassium supplementation, 40
Pregnancy, termination, 140
Prolapse
  rectal, 171
  urethral, 145
  uterine, 136
  vaginal, 138

Proptosis, 202
Prostatitis, acute, 143
Puerperal tetany (eclampsia), 181
Pulmonary contusion, 266
Pulmonary edema, 267
Pulmonary thromboembolism, 268
Pulse oximetry, 51
Pyometra, 136
Pyothorax, 260

R

Radiation injury, 112
Rapidly decompensating patient, 5
Rectal prolapse, 171
Renal failure, acute intrinsic, 288
Renal perfusion, maintenance of, 223
Respiratory emergencies, 253
Resuscitative measures, 114
Rib fracture and management of flail chest, 264
Rodenticide toxicity, Vitamin K antagonist, 106

S

Scrotal dermatitis, 142
Scrotal hernia, 142
Scrotal trauma, 141
Seizures, 194
Shock, 275
  anaphylactic (anaphylactoid), 94
  cardiogenic, 277
  electric, 135
  hypovoplemic, 276
  "Rule of Twenty," management of shock patient, 277
  septic, 276
Skeletal trauma, 154
Smoke inhalation, 269
Snake bites
  Coral snake envenomation, 151
  Non-poisonous, 149
  Pit viper envenomation, 149
Soft tissue injuries, acute superficial, 275
Spider bites
  black widow, 152
  brown spider, 152
Spinal cord injuries, 188
Systemic hypertension, 176
Systemic thromboembolism, 285

T

Tachycardia, 98
  Drugs and doses used for treatment, 281
Testicular torsion, 143
Thermal injury, 108
Thoracocentesis, 52

Thoracostomy, 53
Thrombocytopathia, 106
Thromboembolism,
  pulmonary, 268
  systemic, 285
Thyrotoxicosis, 184
Toad toxicosis (*Bufo* species), 153
Toxicities,
  chemotherapy-related, 210
  specific toxins, emergency
    treatment of, 214
  supportive and symptomatic care, 223
Toxicology resources, 212
Toxins,
  clearance of, 222
  treatment of specific, 224
Tracheal collapse, 256
Tracheostomy, 55
Transfusion therapy,
  dose and administration rates, 29
  in cats, 31
  in dogs, 30
  indications for, 26
  reactions, 31
Triage, 3

U
Urethral prolapse, 145
Urinary tract emergencies, 287
Uroabdomen, 290
Urohydropulsion, 57
Urticaria, 95
Uterine prolapse, 136
Uterine rupture, 138
Uterine torsion, 140

V
Vaginal prolapse, 138
Vascular access techniques, 58
Vascular surgical cut-down technique, 68
Ventilation, mechanical, 50
Volvulus/torsion, small intestinal
  mesenteric, 168

W
Wounds,
  classification and management, 272
  closed, 9
  open contaminated and infected, 8
  open, healing, 9
  superficial soft tissue, 275

Kirk and Bistner's

HANDBOOK OF

VETERINARY PROCEDURES AND EMERGENCY TREATMENT

Kirk and Bistner's

HANDBOOK OF

VETERINARY PROCEDURES AND EMERGENCY TREATMENT

EIGHTH EDITION

Richard B. Ford, DVM, MS

Professor of Medicine
Department of Clinical Sciences
College of Veterinary Medicine
North Carolina State University
Raleigh, North Carolina
Diplomate, American College of Veterinary Internal Medicine
Diplomate (Honorary), American College of Preventive Medicine

Elisa M. Mazzaferro, MS, DVM, PhD

Diplomate, American College of Veterinary Emergency and Critical Care
Director of Emergency Services
Wheat Ridge Veterinary Specialists
Wheat Ridge, Colorado

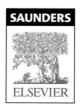

SAUNDERS

ELSEVIER

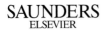

11830 Westline Industrial Drive
St. Louis, Missouri 63146

KIRK AND BISTNER'S HANDBOOK OF VETERINARY
PROCEDURES AND EMERGENCY TREATMENT

ISBN-13: 978-0-7216-0138-0
ISBN-10: 0-7216-0138-3

Copyright © 2006, Elsevier Inc.

Notice

Knowledge and best practice in this field are constantly changing. As new research and experience broaden our knowledge, changes in practice, treatment and drug therapy may become necessary or appropriate. Readers are advised to check the most current information provided (i) on procedures featured or (ii) by the manufacturer of each product to be administered, to verify the recommended dose or formula, the method and duration of administration, and contraindications. It is the responsibility of the practitioner, relying on their own experience and knowledge of the patient, to make diagnoses, to determine dosages and the best treatment for each individual patient, and to take all appropriate safety precautions. To the fullest extent of the law, neither the Publisher nor the Authors assumes any liability for any injury and/or damage to persons or property arising out or related to any use of the material contained in this book.

The Publisher

Previous editions copyrighted 2000, 1995, 1990, 1985, 1981, 1975, 1969

ISBN-13: 978-0-7216-0138-0
ISBN-10: 0-7216-0138-3

Publishing Director: *Linda Duncan*
Editor: *Anthony J. Winkel*
Associate Developmental Editor: *Heather Fogt*
Publishing Services Manager: *Melissa Lastarria*
Project Manager: *Rich Barber*
Design Manager: *Bill Drone*

Printed in the United States

Last digit is the print number: 9 8 7 6 5 4 3 2 1

Working together to grow
libraries in developing countries
www.elsevier.com | www.bookaid.org | www.sabre.org

ELSEVIER   BOOK AID International   Sabre Foundation

In veterinary medicine, there are perhaps no individuals more worthy of recognition than the veterinarians and veterinary technicians who have committed time and effort to sustaining the health of companion animal patients. With advances in disease prevention, diagnostic testing, treatment protocols, and critical care continuing to increase exponentially, the challenge for all of us is to maintain currency in the practice of small animal medicine and surgery. The 8th edition of Kirk and Bistner's Handbook of Veterinary Procedures and Emergency Treatment *is therefore dedicated to all who strive to bring the very best care to the patients we are entitled to treat.*

No dedication would be complete without recognizing the sustaining contributions that Drs. Bob Kirk and Steve Bistner have made to veterinary medicine. The first edition of this text, published in 1969, and the seven editions that follow, are remarkable testimony to all that these two individuals have given our profession. We have all benefited from their work. It has been my distinct honor to have worked with you both!

Richard B. Ford

Thanks, Mom, for not making me put down the ants. Your constant guidance, motivation, and support have allowed me to become the person I am today. Love, Elisa

Elisa M. Mazzaferro

Preface

In the Preface to the first edition of the *Handbook of Veterinary Procedures and Emergency Treatment*, published in 1969, Dr. Kirk and Dr. Bistner described the format of that book as being divided into six sections, "each emphasizing a facet of early examination, clinical methods, or emergency care."

Today, 37 years later, those original objectives remain unchanged. What has changed, however, are the numerous advances in clinical diagnostic and therapeutic capabilities in companion animal medicine. It's the volume of new information, combined with the level of expectation of our clientele today, which presents the most demanding challenges in producing the eighth edition of what has become known as the *"Emergency Handbook."*

WHAT'S INSIDE

Neither the original format of the book nor the objectives have changed. The content and utility of the book, however, are significantly different. **Section 1**, Emergency Care, is completely updated and reorganized to facilitate rapid access to diagnostic and treatment recommendations for emergency and critical care patients. Included are major subsections on Prehospital Management, Initial Emergency Triage and Management, Emergency Procedures, and the expanded Emergency Management of Specific Conditions. A QUICK REFERENCE Index has been added to enhance rapid access to any of the 170+ emergency and critical care topics in this section. New to this edition is a special subsection on Pain contributed by three of the leading authors on pain diagnosis and management.

Sections 2 through 5 focus on patient evaluation, problem assessment, and diagnostics. Each of these four sections addresses specific aspects of the patient's clinical presentation. **Section 2** focuses on the initial examination and has been expanded to include templates for medical record entries and plans for advanced diagnostics. **Section 3** is a problem-based approach to differential diagnoses and is redesigned such that the patient's problem is represented from the client's perspective—the same way problems are presented in clinical practice.

Section 4 has been revised to specifically address both routine *and* advanced diagnostic, as well as therapeutic, procedures. Advanced procedures are now presented in an organ-system format to enhance access to current diagnostic procedures that may be needed when evaluating complex cases.

Section 5, now entitled Laboratory Diagnosis and Test Protocols, has been completely rewritten. Considerable effort has gone into developing a reference section on laboratory testing that will have immediate application in the clinical setting. The majority of this section is a succinct, highly structured reference for performing routine and advanced diagnostic testing in cats and dogs. Each test represented includes information on patient preparation, the test protocol, type of sample to collect versus type of sample to submit, interpretation of test results, and more. We have not found any other reference in the veterinary literature that is comparable to this section.

The most noteworthy addition to **Section 6,** Charts and Tables, is Table 6-26, Common Drug Indications and Dosages, completely updated and expanded to include not only drug names (generic and proprietary) and dosages, but also specific conditions for which administration is indicated. For drugs having two or more indications, dosages for each indication are called out. Additionally, drugs most likely to be used in the management of critical and emergency patients are called out specifically with an eye-catching icon.

The eighth edition of the *Handbook of Veterinary Procedures and Emergency Treatment* represents the most comprehensive update in several years. True to the purpose of the first edition of this book, it has been designed to support the day-to-day clinical decision-making challenges faced by practicing veterinarians.

Richard B. Ford
Elisa M. Mazzaferro
2006

Contents

SECTION 1

Emergency Care, 1

SECTION 2

Patient Evaluation and Organ System Examination, 293

SECTION 3

Clinical Signs, 387

SECTION 4

Diagnostic and Therapeutic Procedures, 449

SECTION 5

Laboratory Diagnosis and Test Protocols, 573

SECTION 6

Charts and Tables, 643

Emergency Hotlines, 644
Dog Breeds Recognized by the American Kennel Club (AKC), 645
Cat Breeds Recognized by the Cat Fanciers'
    Association (CFA), 647
Useful Information for Rodents and Rabbits, 648
Determination of the Sex of Mature and Immature Rodents and
    Rabbits, 650
Blood Values and Serum Chemical Constituents for Rodents and
    Rabbits, 651
Ferrets—Physiologic, Anatomic, and Reproductive Data, 652
Hematologic Values for Normal Ferrets, 652
Serum Chemistry Values for Normal Ferrets, 653
Electrocardiographic Data for Normal Ferrets, 653

Conversion of Body Weight in Kilograms to Body Surface Area in
  Meters Squared for Dogs, 654
Conversion of Body Weight in Kilograms to Body Surface Area in
  Meters Squared for Cats, 654
French Scale Conversion Table, 655
International System of Units (SI) Conversion Guide, 656
Units of Length, Volume, and Mass in the Metric System, 659
Annualized Vaccination Protocols and Criteria Defining Risk for the
  Dog and Cat, 660
Types of Vaccines Licensed for Use in Dogs in the United States, 661
Types of Vaccines Licensed for Use in Cats in the United States, 662
Annualized Vaccination Protocol for Dogs at Moderate Risk, 663
Annualized Vaccination Protocol for Dogs at Low Risk, 665
Annualized Vaccination Protocol for Dogs at High Risk, 667
Annualized Vaccination Protocol for Cats at Moderate Risk, 669
Annualized Vaccination Protocol for Cats at Low Risk, 670
Annualized Vaccination Protocol for Cats at High Risk, 671
Compendium of Animal Rabies Prevention and Control, 2005,
  National Association Of State Public Health Veterinarians, Inc.
  (NASPHV), 674
Prescription Writing Reference...Do's and Don'ts, 684
Common Drug Indications and Dosages, 685

Kirk and Bistner's

HANDBOOK OF

VETERINARY PROCEDURES AND EMERGENCY TREATMENT

Prehospital Management of the Injured Animal, *2*
  Survey of the Scene, *2*
  Initial Examination, *2*
  Preparation for Transport, *3*
Initial Emergency Examination, Management, and Triage, *3*
  Primary Survey and Emergency Resuscitation Measures, *3*
  Ancillary Diagnostic Evaluation, *5*
  Summary of Patient Status, *5*
  The Rapidly Decompensating Patient, *5*
Emergency Diagnostic and Therapeutic Procedures, *6*
  Abdominal Paracentesis and Diagnostic Peritoneal Lavage, *6*
  Bandaging and Splinting Techniques, *8*
  Blood Component Therapy, *21*
  Central Venous Pressure Measurement, *33*
  Fluid Therapy, *34*
  Orogastric Lavage, *47*
  Oxygen Supplementation, *48*
  Pulse Oximetry, *51*
  Capnometry (End-Tidal Carbon Dioxide Monitoring), *52*
  Thoracocentesis, *52*
  Tracheostomy, *55*
  Urohydropulsion, *57*
  Vascular Access Techniques, *58*
Pain: Assessment, Prevention, and Management, *69*
  Physiologic Impact of Untreated Pain, *70*
  Recognition and Assessment of Pain, *71*
  Acute Pain Management for Emergent, Critical/Intensive Care and Trauma Patients, *73*
  Pharmacologic Means to Analgesia: Major Analgesics, *73*
  Analgesia: Minor Analgesics, *77*
  Adjunctive Analgesic Drugs, *77*
  Local and Regional Techniques for the Emergent Patient, *78*
Emergency Management of Specific Conditions, *81*
  Acute Condition in the Abdomen, *81*
  Anaphylactic (Anaphylactoid) Shock, *94*
  Angioneurotic Edema and Urticaria, *95*
  Anesthetic Complications and Emergencies, *96*
  Bleeding Disorders, *100*
  Burns, *108*
  Cardiac Emergencies, *113*
  Ear Emergencies, *133*
  Electrocution/Electric Shock, *135*
  Emergencies of the Female Reproductive Tract and Genitalia, *136*
  Emergencies of the Male Genitalia and Reproductive Tract, *141*
  Environmental and Household Emergencies, *146*
  Fractures and Musculoskeletal Trauma, *154*
  Gastrointestinal Emergencies, *158*
  Hypertension: Systemic, *176*

Metabolic Emergencies, *178*
Neurologic Emergencies, *185*
Ocular Emergencies, *196*
Oncologic Emergencies, *205*
Poisons and Toxins, *212*
Respiratory Emergencies, *253*
Pulmonary Diseases, *265*
Superficial Soft Tissue Injuries, *271*
Shock, *275*
Management of Shock Patient, *277*
Thromboembolism: Systemic, *285*
Urinary Tract Emergencies, *287*

PREHOSPITAL MANAGEMENT OF THE INJURED ANIMAL

SURVEY OF THE SCENE

1. CALL FOR HELP! At the accident scene, it usually takes more than one person to assist the animal and prevent injury to the animal and human bystanders.
2. If an accident has occurred in a traffic zone, alert oncoming traffic of the injured animal in the road. Make sure you have a piece of clothing or other object to alert oncoming traffic. Do not become injured yourself because oncoming traffic cannot see or identify you.
3. If the animal is conscious, prevent yourself from becoming injured while moving the animal to a safe location. Use a belt, rope, or piece of long cloth to make a muzzle to secure around the animal's mouth and head. If this is not possible, cover the animal's head with a towel, blanket, or coat before moving it.
4. If the animal is unconscious or is unconscious and immobile, move it to a safe location with a back support device that can be made from a box, door, flat board, blanket, or sheet.

INITIAL EXAMINATION

1. Is there a patent airway? If airway noises are present or the animal is stuporous, gently and carefully extend the head and neck. If possible, extend the tongue. Wipe mucus, blood, or vomitus from the mouth. In unconscious animals, maintain head and neck stability.
2. Look for signs of breathing. If there is no evidence of breathing or the gum color is blue, begin mouth-to-nose breathing. Encircle the muzzle area with your hands to pinch down on the gums, and blow into the nose 15 to 20 times per minute.
3. Is there evidence of cardiac function? Check for a palpable pulse on the hind legs or for an apex beat over the sternum. If no signs of cardiac function are found, begin external cardiac compressions at 80 to 120 times per minute.
4. Is there any hemorrhage? Use a clean cloth, towel, paper towel, or disposable diaper or feminine hygiene product to cover the wound. Apply firm pressure to slow hemorrhage and prevent further blood loss. Do not use a tourniquet because this can cause further damage. Apply pressure, and as blood seeps through the first layer of bandage material, place a second layer over the top.
5. Cover any external wounds. Use a clean bandage material soaked in warm water, and transport the animal to the nearest veterinary emergency facility. Address penetrating wounds to the abdomen and thorax immediately.
6. Are there any obvious fractures present? Immobilize fractures with homemade splints made of newspaper, broom handles, or sticks. Muzzle the awake animal before

attempting to place any splints. If a splint cannot be attached safely, place the animal on a towel or blanket and transport the animal to the nearest veterinary emergency facility.
7. Are there any burns? Place wet, cool towels over the burned area and remove as the compress warms to body temperature.
8. Wrap the patient to conserve heat. If the animal is shivering or in shock, wrap it in a blanket, towel, or coat and transport it to the nearest veterinary emergency facility.
9. Is the animal suffering from heat-induced illness (heat stroke)? Cool the animal with room-temperature wet towels (NOT COLD) and transport it to the nearest veterinary emergency facility.

PREPARATION FOR TRANSPORT

1. Call ahead! Let the facility know that you are coming. Be prepared by having emergency numbers and locations available. The police or sheriff's department may be able to aid in locating the nearest veterinary emergency facility.
2. Line upholstery with plastic bags or sheeting to prevent soilage, when possible.
3. Move the injured patient carefully. Use the same approach as moving the animal from the pavement.
4. DRIVE SAFELY. Do not turn one accident into two. Ideally, have a bystander or friend or family member drive while another person stays in the backseat with the animal.

INITIAL EMERGENCY EXAMINATION, MANAGEMENT, AND TRIAGE

Examination of the acutely injured animal that is unconscious, in shock, or suffering from acute hemorrhage or respiratory distress must proceed simultaneously with immediate aggressive lifesaving treatment. Because there often is no time for detailed history taking, diagnosis is largely based on the physical examination findings and simple diagnostic tests. Triage is the art and practice of being able to assess patients rapidly and sort them according to the urgency of treatment required. Immediate recognition and prompt treatment potentially can be lifesaving.

PRIMARY SURVEY AND EMERGENCY RESUSCITATION MEASURES

Perform a brief but thorough systematic examination of the animal, noting the most important ABCs of any emergent patient.

A = AIRWAY

Is the airway patent? Pull the patient's tongue forward and remove any debris obstructing the airway. Suction and a laryngoscope may be necessary. If necessary, intubate or place a transtracheal oxygen source. An emergency tracheostomy may be necessary if upper airway obstruction is present and cannot be resolved immediately with the foregoing measures.

B = BREATHING

Is the animal breathing? If the animal is not breathing, immediately intubate the animal and start artificial ventilations with a supplemental oxygen source (see Cardiac Arrest and Cardiopulmonary Cerebral Resuscitation).

If the animal is breathing, what is the respiratory rate and pattern? Is the respiratory rate normal, increased, or decreased? Is the respiratory pattern normal, or is the breathing rapid and shallow, or slow and deep with inspiratory distress? Are the respiratory noises normal, or is there a high-pitched stridor on inspiration characteristic of an upper airway obstruction? Does the animal have its head extended and elbows abducted away from the body with orthopnea? Do the commissures of the mouth move with inhalation and exhalation? Is there evidence of expiratory distress with an abdominal push upon exhalation? Note the lateral chest wall. Do the ribs move out and in with inhalation and exhalation, or is there paradoxical chest wall motion in an area that moves in during inhalation and out during exhalation, suggestive of a flail chest? Is there any subcutaneous emphysema that suggests airway injury?

Auscultate the thorax *bilaterally.* Are the breath sounds normal? Do they sound harsh with crackles because of pneumonia, pulmonary edema, or pulmonary contusions? Are the lung sounds muffled because of pleural effusion or pneumothorax? Are there inspiratory wheezes in a cat with bronchitis (asthma)? What is the mucous membrane color? Is it pink and normal, or is it pale or cyanotic? Palpate the neck, lateral thorax and dorsal cervical region to check for tracheal displacement, subcutaneous emphysema, or rib factures.

C = Circulation

What is the circulatory status? What is the patient's heart rate and rhythm? Can you hear the heart, or is it muffled because of hypovolemia, pleural or pericardial effusion, pneumothorax, or diaphragmatic hernia? Palpate the pulses. Is the pulse quality strong and regular and synchronous with each heartbeat, or are there thready, dropped pulses? What are the patient's electrocardiogram (ECG) rhythm and blood pressure?

Is there arterial hemorrhage? Note whether there is any bleeding present. Use caution if there is any blood on the fur. Wear gloves. The blood may be from the patient, and gloves will help prevent further contamination of any wounds; or the blood may be from a good Samaritan bystander. If external wounds are present, note their character and condition. Place a pressure bandage on any arterial bleeding or external wounds to prevent further hemorrhage or contamination with nosocomial organisms.

Establish large-bore vascular or intraosseous access (See VASCULAR ACCESS TECHNIQUES). If hypovolemic or hemorrhagic shock is present, institute immediate fluid resuscitation measures. Start with one fourth of a calculated shock dose of crystalloid fluids (0.25 × [90 mL/kg/hour for dogs]; 0.25 × [44 mL/kg/hour for cats]), and reassess perfusion parameters of heart rate, capillary refill time, and blood pressure. If pulmonary contusions are suspected, use of a colloid such as hetastarch at 5 mL/kg in incremental boluses can improve perfusion with a smaller volume of fluid. In cases of head trauma, hypertonic (7%) sodium chloride (saline) can be administered (4 mL/kg IV bolus) with hetastarch or Dextran-70 (10 mL/kg). Acute abdominal hemorrhage caused by trauma can be tamponaded with an abdominal compression bandage.

After the immediate ABCs, proceed then with the rest of the physical examination and treatment by using the mnemonic A CRASH PLAN.

A = Airway

C and R = Cardiovascular and Respiratory

A = Abdomen

Palpate the patient's abdomen. Is there any pain or are there any penetrating injuries present? Look at the patient's umbilicus. Reddening around the umbilicus can suggest intraabdominal hemorrhage. Is there a fluid wave or mass palpable? Examine the inguinal, caudal, thoracic, and paralumbar regions. Clip the fur to examine the patient for bruising or penetrating wounds. Percuss and auscultate the abdomen for borborygmi.

S = Spine

Palpate the animal's spine for symmetry. Is there any pain or obvious swelling or fracture present? Perform a neurologic examination from C1 to the last caudal vertebra.

H = Head

Examine the eyes, ears, mouth, teeth, nose, and all cranial nerves. Stain the eyes with fluorescence dye to examine for corneal ulcers in any case of head trauma. Is there anisocoria or Horner syndrome present?

P = Pelvis

Perform a rectal examination. Palpate for fractures or hemorrhage. Examine the perineal and rectal areas. Examine the external genitalia.

L = Limbs

Examine the pectoral and pelvic extremities. Are there any obvious open or closed fractures? Quickly splint the limbs to prevent further damage and help control pain. Examine the skin, muscles, and tendons.

A = Arteries

Palpate the peripheral arteries for pulses. Use a Doppler piezoelectric crystal to aid in finding a pulse if thromboembolic disease is present. Measure the patient's blood pressure.

N = Nerves

From afar, note the level of consciousness, behavior, and posture. Note respiratory rate, pattern, and effort. Is the patient conscious, or is the patient obtunded or comatose? Are the pupils symmetric and responsive to light, or is there anisocoria present? Does the patient display any abnormal postures such as Schiff-Sherington (extended rigid forelimbs, flaccid paralysis of the hind limbs) that may signify severe spinal shock or a severed spinal cord? Examine the peripheral nerves for motor and sensory input and output to the limbs and tail.

ANCILLARY DIAGNOSTIC EVALUATION

Hemodynamic techniques: Perform electrocardiography, direct or indirect blood pressure monitoring, and pulse oximetry in any critically ill traumatized patient.

Imaging techniques: Obtain radiographs of the thorax and abdomen in any animal that has sustained a traumatic injury once the patient is more stable and can tolerate positioning for the procedures. Survey radiographs may reveal pneumothorax, pulmonary contusions, diaphragmatic hernia, pleural or abdominal effusion, or pneumoperitoneum.

Laboratory testing: Immediate diagnostic testing should include a hematocrit, total solids, glucose, blood urea nitrogen (BUN)/azostick, and urine specific gravity. Ancillary diagnostic tests that can be performed soon thereafter include a complete blood count and peripheral blood smear to evaluate platelet count and red and white blood cell morphology. Also consider arterial blood gas and electrolytes, coagulation parameters (activated clotting time [ACT], prothrombin time [PT], activated partial thromboplastin time [APTT]), serum biochemistry profile, serum lactate, and urinalysis.

Invasive testing: Invasive diagnostic techniques that may need to be performed include thoracocentesis, abdominal paracentesis, and diagnostic peritoneal lavage.

SUMMARY OF PATIENT STATUS

After completing the initial physical examination, answer the following questions: What supportive care is required at this time? Are additional diagnostic procedures needed? If so, which procedures, and is the patient stable enough to tolerate those procedures without further stress? Should an additional period of observation be instituted before further definitive treatment plans are undertaken? Is immediate surgical intervention necessary? Is additional supportive care required before surgery? What anesthetic risks are evident?

THE RAPIDLY DECOMPENSATING PATIENT

Animals that do not respond to initial resuscitation usually have severe ongoing or preexisting physiologic disturbances that contribute to severe cardiovascular and metabolic instability. A patient that does not respond to or responds to and then stops responding to

---

BOX 1-1   CLINICAL SIGNS OF DECOMPENSATION

Weak or poor peripheral pulse quality
Cool peripheral extremities
Cyanosis or muddy-colored (gray) mucous membranes
Pale mucous membranes
Prolonged capillary refill time
Increased or decreased body temperature
Decreased renal output in a euvolemic patient
Inappropriate mentation or confusion
Depression
Tachycardia or bradycardia
Declining hematocrit
Distended, painful abdomen
Cardiac dysrhythmia
Abnormal respiratory pattern
Respiratory difficulty or distress
Gastrointestinal blood loss via hematemesis or in feces

BOX 1-2   CAUSES OF ACUTE DECOMPENSATION

Acute renal failure
Acute respiratory distress syndrome
Bowel and gastric rupture
Cardiac dysrhythmia
Central nervous system edema and hemorrhage, and brainstem herniation
Coagulopathies including disseminated intravascular coagulation
Internal hemorrhage
Multiple organ dysfunction syndrome
Pneumothorax
Pulmonary contusions
Pulmonary thromboembolism
Sepsis or septic shock
Systemic inflammatory response syndrome
Urinary bladder rupture

---

initial resuscitation efforts should alert the clinician that decompensation is occurring (Boxes 1-1 and 1-2).

Additional Reading

Ettinger SJ, Feldman EC, editors: Critical care. In *Textbook of veterinary internal medicine,* ed 6, St Louis, 2005, Elsevier-Saunders.

Mathews KA: *Veterinary emergency and critical care manual,* Guelph, Ontario, Canada, 1996, Lifelearn.

Wingfield WE: Decision making in veterinary emergency medicine. In Wingfield WE, editor: *Veterinary emergency secrets,* ed 2, Philadelphia, 2001, Hanley & Belfus.

Wingfield WE: Treatment priorities in trauma. In Wingfield WE, editor: *Veterinary emergency secrets,* ed 2, Philadelphia, 2001, Hanley & Belfus.

EMERGENCY DIAGNOSTIC AND THERAPEUTIC PROCEDURES

ABDOMINAL PARACENTESIS AND DIAGNOSTIC PERITONEAL LAVAGE

Abdominocentesis (abdominal paracentesis) refers to puncture into the peritoneal cavity for the purpose of fluid collection. Abdominal paracentesis is a sensitive technique for fluid collection as long as more than 6 mL/kg of fluid is present within the abdominal cavity.

In the event that you suspect peritonitis and have a negative tap with abdominal paracentesis, a diagnostic peritoneal lavage can be performed.

To perform abdominal paracentesis, follow this procedure:

1. Place the patient in left lateral recumbency and clip a 4- to 6-inch square with the umbilicus in the center.
2. Aseptically scrub the clipped area with antimicrobial scrub solution.
3. Wearing gloves, insert a 22- or 20-gauge needle or over-the-needle catheter in four quadrants: cranial and to the right, cranial and to the left, caudal and to the right, and caudal and to the left of the umbilicus. As you insert the needle or catheter, gently twist the needle to push any abdominal organs away from the tip of the needle. Local anesthesia typically is not required for this procedure, although a light sedative or analgesic may be necessary if severe abdominal pain is present. In some cases, fluid will flow freely from one or more of the needles. If not, gently aspirate with a 3- to 6-mL syringe or aspirate with the patient in a standing position. Avoid changing positions with needles in place because iatrogenic puncture of intraabdominal organs may occur.
4. Save any fluid collected in sterile red- and lavender-topped tubes for cytologic and biochemical analyses and bacterial culture. Monitor hemorrhagic fluid carefully for the presence of clots. Normally, hemorrhagic effusions rapidly become defibrinated and do not clot. Clot formation can occur in the presence of ongoing active hemorrhage or may be due to the iatrogenic puncture of organs such as the spleen or liver.

If abdominal paracentesis is negative, a diagnostic peritoneal lavage can be performed. Peritoneal dialysis kits are commercially available but are fairly expensive and often impractical.

To perform a diagnostic peritoneal lavage, follow this procedure:

1. Clip and aseptically scrub the ventral abdomen as described previously.
2. Wearing sterile gloves, cut multiple side ports in a 16- or 18-gauge over-the needle catheter. Use care to not cut more than 50% of the circumference of the catheter, or else the catheter will become weakened and potentially can break off in the patient's abdomen.
3. Insert the catheter into the peritoneal cavity caudal and to the right of the umbilicus, directing the catheter dorsally and caudally.
4. Infuse 10 to 20 mL of sterile lactated Ringer's solution or 0.9% saline solution that has been warmed to the patient's body temperature. During the instillation of fluid into the peritoneal cavity, watch closely for signs of respiratory distress because an increase in intraabdominal pressure can impair diaphragmatic excursions and respiratory function.
5. Remove the catheter.
6. In ambulatory patients, walk the patient around while massaging the abdomen to distribute the fluid throughout the abdominal cavity. In nonambulatory patients, gently roll the patient from side to side.
7. Next, aseptically scrub the patient's ventral abdomen again, and perform an abdominal paracentesis as described previously. Save collected fluid for culture and cytologic analyses; however, biochemical analyses may be artifactually decreased because of dilution. Remember that you likely will retrieve only a small portion of the fluid that you instilled.

Additional Reading

Bjorling DE, Latimer KA, Rawlings CA, et al: Diagnostic peritoneal lavage before and after abdominal surgery in dogs, *Am J Vet Res* 44(5):816-820, 1983.

Crowe DT: Abdominocentesis and diagnostic peritoneal lavage in small animals, *Mod Vet Pract* 13:877-882, 1984.

Crowe DT: Diagnostic abdominal paracentesis techniques: clinical evaluation in 129 dogs and cats, *J Am Anim Hosp Assoc* 20:223-230, 1984.

Walters JM: Abdominal paracentesis and diagnostic peritoneal lavage, *Clin Tech Small Anim Pract* 18(1):32-38, 2003.

1

BANDAGING AND SPLINTING TECHNIQUES

In general bandages can be applied to open or closed wounds. Bandaging is used for six general wound types: open contaminated or infected wounds, open wound in the repair stage of healing, a closed wound, a wound in need of a pressure bandage, a wound in need of pressure relief, and a wound in need of immobilization. Box 1-3 lists various functions of bandages.

The materials and methods of bandaging depend on the type of injury, the need for pressure and immobilization, the need to prevent pressure, and the stage of healing. In general, bandage material has three component layers. If pressure relief or immobilization is required, splint material also may be incorporated into the bandage. The contact layer is the layer of bandage material that actually is adjacent to the wound itself. The secondary or intermediary layer is placed over the contact (primary) layer. Finally, the outer tertiary layer covers the bandage and is exposed to the outside.

Open Contaminated and Infected Wounds

Open contaminated or infected wounds often have large amounts of necrotic tissue and foreign debris and emit copious quantities of exudate. The contact layer used in an open contaminated or infected wound should be wide-mesh gauze sponges with no cotton filling. The sponges can be left dry if the wound has minimal exudate but should be moistened with sterile 0.9% saline or lactated Ringer's solution if the wound has high-viscosity exudate. Topical ointments may be applied (silver sulfadiazine, chlorhexidine ointment) if necessary. The intermediate layer should be thick absorbent wrapping material, covered by an outer layer of porous tape: Elastikon (Johnson & Johnson Medical, Arlington, Texas), or Vetrap (3M, St. Paul, Minnesota). Change the bandages at least once daily or more frequently if strike-through of exudate occurs through the bandage.

To place a wet-to-dry bandage over a wound, first place the contact layer over the wound. Next, place strips of adhesive tape to the patient's paw on either side, if possible. The strips (stirrups) will be used to hold the bandage in place and prevent it from slipping down the limb. Wrap the intermediate layer over the contact layer. Turn the adhesive strips around so that the adhesive layer can be secured to the intermediary layer in place. Wrap the final, or tertiary layer over the bandage.

The function of a wet-to-dry bandage is to help debride a wound. The moistened gauze dries and is pulled off the wound at each bandage change. Dry necrotic tissue and debris that is adhered to the gauze is pulled off with it. In addition, the moistened material dilutes the wound exudates and enhances its absorption into the gauze contact layer. If large amounts of exudate come from the wound, the contact layer and intermediate layer absorb the exudate, wicking the material away from the wound. Finally, delivery of medications into the wound can occur to promote the development of healthy granulation tissue.

BOX 1-3 FUNCTIONS OF BANDAGES AND SPLINTS	
Exert pressure	Protect a wound from environmental bacteria
Obliterate dead space	Protect the environment from wound blood,
Reduce edema	exudate, and bacteria
Minimize hemorrhage	Immobilize a wound and support underlying
Prevent pressure on wounds	osseous structures
Decubitus ulcers	Minimize patient discomfort
Pack a wound	Serve as a vehicle for antiseptics and antibiotics
Wet-to-dry bandages for deep shearing	Serve as an indicator of wound secretions
injuries	Provide an aesthetic appearance
Absorb exudate and debride a wound	
Wet-to-dry bandages	

OPEN WOUND IN REPAIR STAGE OF HEALING

Early repair

During the early stage of repair, granulation tissue, some exudate, and minor epithelialization is observed. Place a nonadherent bandage with some antibacterial properties (petroleum or nitrofurazone-impregnated gauze) or absorbent material (foam sponge, hydrogel, or hydrocolloid dressing) in direct contact with the wound to minimize disruption of the granulation tissue bed. Next, place an absorbent intermediate layer, followed by a porous outer layer, as previously described. Granulation tissue can grow through gauze mesh or adhere to foam sponges and can be ripped away at the time of bandage removal. Hemorrhage and disruption of the granulation tissue bed can occur.

Late repair

Later in the repair process, granulation tissue can exude sanguineous drainage and have some epithelialization. A late nonadherent bandage is required. The contact layer should be some form of nonadherent dressing, foam sponge, hydrogel, or hydrocolloid substance. The intermediate layer and outer layers should be absorbent material and porous tape, respectively. With nonadherent dressings, wounds with viscous exudates may not be absorbed well. This may be advantageous and enhance epithelialization, provided that complications do not occur. Infection, exuberant granulation tissue, or adherence of absorbent materials to the wound may occur and delay the healing process.

MOIST HEALING

Moist healing is a newer concept of wound management in which wound exudates are allowed to stay in contact with the wound. In the absence of infection a moist wound heals faster and has enzymatic activity as a result of macrophage and polymorphonuclear cell breakdown. Enzymatic degradation or "autolytic debridement" of the wound occurs. Moist wounds tend to promote neutrophil and macrophage chemotaxis and bacterial phagocytosis better than use of wet-to-dry bandages. A potential complication and disadvantage of moist healing, however, is the development of bacterial colonization, folliculitis, and trauma to wound edges that can occur because of the continuously moist environment.

Use surfactant-type solutions (Constant Clens; Kendall, Mansfield, Massachusetts) for initial wound cleansing and debridement. Use occlusive dressings for rapid enzymatic debridement with bactericidal properties to aid in wound healing. Bandage wet necrotic wounds with a dressing premoistened with hypertonic saline (Curasalt [Kendall], 20% saline) to clean and debride the wounds. Hypertonic saline functions to desiccate necrotic tissue and bacteria to debride the infected wound. Remove and replace the hypertonic saline bandage every 24 to 48 hours. Next, place gauze impregnated with antibacterial agents (Kerlix AMD [Kendall]) over the wound in the bandage layer to act as a barrier to bacterial colonization.

If the wound is initially dry or has minimal exudate and is not obviously contaminated or infected, place amorphous gels of water, glycerin, and a polymer (Curafil [Kendall]) over the wound to promote moisture and proteolytic healing. Discontinue moisture gels such as Curafil once the dry wound has become moist.

Finally, the final stage of moist healing helps to promote the development of a healthy granulation tissue bed. Use calcium alginate dressings (Curasorb or Curasorb Zn with zinc [Kendall]) in noninfected wounds with a moderate amount of drainage. Alginate gels promote rapid development of a granulation tissue bed and epithelialization.

Foam dressings also can be applied to exudative wounds after a healthy granulation bed has formed. Change foam dressings at least once every 4 to 7 days.

CLOSED WOUNDS

Wounds with no drainage

For closed wounds without any drainage, such as a laceration that has been repaired surgically, a simple bandage with a nonadherent contact layer (Telfa pad [Kendall], for example), intermediate layer of absorbent material, and an outer porous layer (Elastikon, Vetrap) can be placed to prevent wound contamination during healing. The nonadherent pad will not stick to the wound and cause patient discomfort. Because there usually is minimal drainage from the wound, the function of the intermediate layer is more protective than absorptive. Any small amount will be absorbed into the intermediate layer of the bandage. It is important in any bandage to place the tape strips or "stirrups" on the patient's limb and then overlap in the bandage, to prevent the bandage from slipping. Place the intermediate and tertiary layers loosely around the limb, starting distally and working proximally, with some overlap with each consecutive layer. This method prevents excessive pressure and potential to impair venous drainage. Leave the toenails of the third and fourth digits exposed, whenever possible, to allow daily examination of the bandage to determine whether the bandage is impairing venous drainage. If the bandage is too tight and constricting or impeding vascular flow, the toes will become swollen and spread apart. When placed and maintained properly (e.g., the bandage does not get wet), there usually are relatively few complications observed with this type of bandage.

Open Wounds

Wounds with drainage

In some cases, it is necessary to cover a wound in which a Penrose drain has been placed to allow drainage. In many cases, there is a considerable amount of drainage from the drain and underlying soft tissues. The function of the bandage is to help obliterate dead space created by the wound itself, absorb the fluid that drains from the wound and that will contaminate the environment, and prevent external wicking of material from the external environment into the wound. When the bandage is removed, the clinician can examine the amount and type of material that has drained from the wound in order to determine when the drain should be removed.

When placing a bandage over a draining wound, the contact layer should be a commercially available nonadherent dressing and several layers of absorbent wide-mesh gauze placed directly over the drain at the distal end of the incision. Overlay the layers of gauze with a thick layer of absorbent intermediate dressing to absorb fluid that drains from the wound. If the gauze and intermediate layers are not thick or absorbent enough, there is a potential for the drainage fluid to reach the outer layer of the bandage and provide a source of wicking of bacteria from the external environment into the wound, leading to infection.

Wounds in Need of a Pressure Bandage

Minor hemorrhage

Some wounds such as lacerations have minor bleeding or hemorrhage that require an immediate bandage until definitive care can be provided. To create a pressure bandage, place a nonadherent dressing immediately in contact with the wound, followed by a thick layer of absorbent material, topped by a layer of elastic bandage material such as Elastikon or Vetrap. Unlike the bandage for a closed wound, the top tertiary outer layer should be wrapped with some tension and even pressure around the limb, starting from the distal extremity (toes) and working proximally. The pressure bandage serves to control hemorrhage but should not be left on for long periods. Pressure bandages that have been left on for too long can impair nerve function and lead to tissue necrosis and slough. Therefore, pressure bandages should be used in the hospital only, so that the patient can be observed closely. If hemorrhage through the bandage occurs, place another bandage over the first until the wound can be repaired definitively. Removal of the first bandage will only disrupt any clot that has formed and cause additional hemorrhage to occur.

Initial fracture immobilization

Fractures require immediate immobilization to prevent additional patient discomfort and further trauma to the soft tissues of the affected limb. As with all bandages, a contact layer, intermediate layer, and outer layer should be used. Place the contact layer in accordance with any type of wound present. The intermediate layer should be thick absorbent material, followed by a top layer of elastic bandage material. An example is to place a Telfa pad over a wound in an open distal radius-ulna fracture, followed by a thick layer of cotton gauze cast padding, followed by an elastic layer of Kling (Johnson & Johnson Medical, Arlington, Texas), pulling each layer tightly over the previous layer with some overlap until the resultant bandage can be "thumped" with the clinician's thumb and forefinger and sound like a ripe watermelon. The bandage should be smooth with consecutive layers of even pressure on the limb, starting distally and working proximally. Leave the toenails of the third and fourth digits exposed to monitor for impaired venous drainage that would suggest that the bandage is too tight and needs to be replaced. Finally, place a top layer of Vetrap or Elastikon over the intermediary layer to protect it from becoming contaminated. If the bandage is used with a compound or open fracture, drainage may be impaired and actually lead to enhanced risk of wound infection. Bandages placed for initial fracture immobilization are temporary until definitive fracture repair can be performed once the patient's cardiovascular and respiratory status are stable.

Exuberant granulation tissue

Wounds with exuberant granulation tissue must be handled carefully so as to not disrupt the healing process but to keep an overabundance of tissue from forming that will impair epithelialization. To bandage a wound with exuberant granulation tissue, place a corticosteroid-containing ointment on the wound, followed by a nonadherent contact layer. The corticosteroid will help control the exuberant growth of granulation tissue. Next, carefully wrap an absorbent material over the contact layer, followed by careful placement of and overlay of elastic bandage material to place some pressure on the wound. Leave the toenails of the third and fourth digits exposed so that circulation can be monitored several times daily. Bandages that are too tight must be removed immediately to prevent damage to neuronal tissue and impaired vascularization, tissue necrosis, and slough. Because wound drainage may be impaired, there is a risk of infection.

Obliteration of dead space

Gaping wounds or those that have undermined in between layers of subcutaneous tissue and fascia should be bandaged with a pressure bandage to help obliterate dead space and prevent seroma formation. An example of a wound that may require this type of bandage is removal of an infiltrative lipoma on the lateral or ventral thorax. Use caution when placing pressure bandages around the thorax or cervical region because bandages placed too tightly may impair adequate ventilation. To place a pressure bandage and obliterate dead space, place a nonadherent contact layer over the wound. Usually, a drain is placed in the wound, so place a large amount of wide-mesh gauze at the distal end of the drain to absorb any wound exudate or drainage. Place several layers of absorbent material over the site to further absorb any drainage. Place a layer of elastic cotton such as Kling carefully but firmly over the dead space to cause enough pressure to control drainage. Place at least two fingers in between the animal's thorax and the bandage to ensure that the bandage is not too tight. In many cases, the bandage should be placed once the animal has recovered from surgery and is able to stand. If the bandage is placed while the animal is still anesthetized and recumbent, there is a tendency for the bandage to be too tight. Finally, the tertiary layer should be an elastic material such as Elastikon or Vetrap.

WOUNDS IN NEED OF PRESSURE RELIEF

Many wounds require a pressure relief bandage to prevent contact with the external environment. Wounds that may require pressure relief for healing include decubitus ulcers, pressure bandage or cast ulcers, impending ulcer areas (such as the ileum or ischium of recumbent or cachexic patients), and surgical repair sites of ulcerated areas. Pressure relief bandages can be of two basic varieties: modified doughnut bandage and doughnut-shaped bandage.

1

Modified doughnut bandage

A modified doughnut bandage should be placed over bony prominences on the limbs when there are early signs of pressure such as hyperemia, to prevent further injury. To place a modified doughnut bandage, cast padding material, thick wrapping material, and porous adhesive or loose elastic tape are required. Because this type of bandage becomes compressed after two to three bandage changes, it must be replaced frequently.

To place a modified doughnut bandage, follow this procedure (Figure 1-1):
1. Make several layers of cast padding, and fold them over together, making a 3 × 3-inch pad.
2. Fold the pad over on itself, and cut a slit in the center. Form this slit into a hole.
3. Place the hole in the cast padding over the bony prominence.
4. Wrap bandaging material over the pad.
5. Place tapes over the wrapping material, with overlap of the tape strips, to secure it in place.
6. Alternatively, place several loose stay sutures percutaneously in the skin surrounding the bony prominence, and secure the doughnut in place with umbilical tape woven through the stay sutures and over the doughnut.

Doughnut-shaped bandage

Like the modified doughnut-shaped bandage, a doughnut-shaped bandage is used over bony prominences to help prevent excessive pressure over the area. The bandage commonly is used over bony prominences on the distal limbs, such as the lateral malleolus, when more padding is indicated than is provided with a modified doughnut-shaped bandage. To make a doughnut-shaped bandage, use a hand towel or length of stockinet bandage material, tape, cotton gauze, elastic bandage material, or suture with umbilical tape. As the bandage becomes compressed or soiled, change it to prevent further damage to the underlying tissues.

To create a doughnut-shaped bandage, follow this procedure (Figures 1-2 and 1-3):
1. Roll a hand towel tightly and wrap tape around it to create a circle with a hole in the center. Alternatively, take a length of stockinet bandage material and roll it as you would a sock, creating a padded circle with a hole in the center. Make sure that the hole in the center is large enough to fit around the surgical repair site or ulcer.
2. Place the hole in the center over the ulcer or surgical repair site.
3. Secure the roll in place with strips of tape and cotton and then elastic bandage material. Alternatively, place loose loops of suture through the skin adjacent and around the wound. Secure the doughnut in place with umbilical tape secured through the suture loops and over the bandage. The wound in the center can be observed and treated through the hole in the center, if necessary.

WOUNDS IN NEED OF IMMOBILIZATION

External pin splints

An external pin splint is required when fractures or luxations are associated with open wounds. In some cases, it may be difficult to bandage under the bars of the pin splint in such a way that the bandage is in contact with the wound. To create padding around the pins, fit foam rubber sponges to lie securely under and around the pins. Place bandage layers around the external fixator apparatus in layers to decrease contamination of the wound from the external environment and to absorb fluid that drains from the wound (Figures 1-4 to 1-6).

Cup or clamshell splints

A cup splint is indicated when bandaging pad wounds to decrease pressure on the footpad and prevent spreading of the footpads when the dog or cat places the paw down. If the toes spread, spreading of the footpad can delay or impair wound healing. The splint functions to place the paw in a more vertical direction so that the patient bears weight on the toe tips and not directly on the pads during the healing process.

Text continued on p. 18

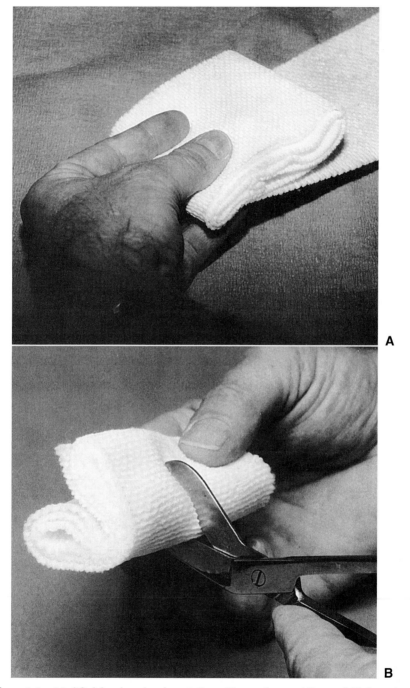

Figure 1-1: Modified doughnut bandage. **A,** Several layers of cast padding are folded together. **B,** The pad is folded on itself and a slit is cut in its center.

Continued

1

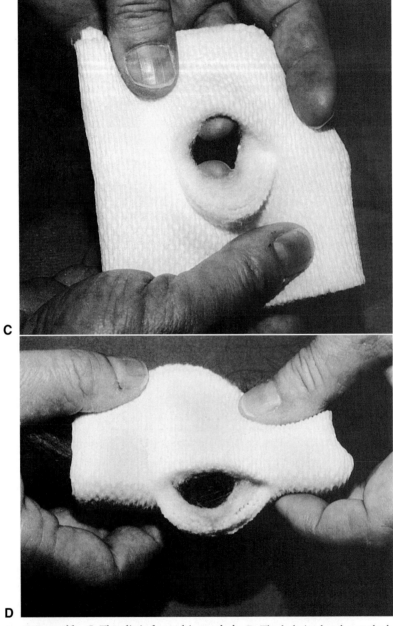

C

D

Figure 1-1, cont'd   C, The slit is formed into a hole. **D,** The hole is placed over the bony prominence.
(From Swaim SF, Henderson RA: *Small animal wound management.* 2nd Edition. Williams & Wilkins, Media, Pa, 1997.)

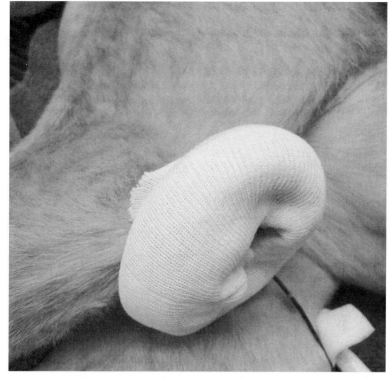

Figure 1-2: Doughnut-shaped bandage created from stockinet bandage material over the olecranon.

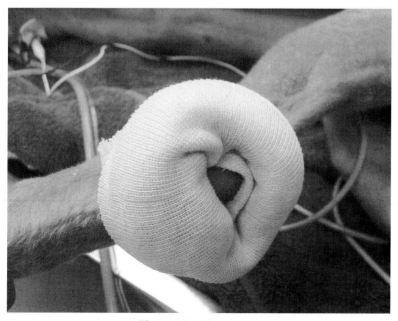

Figure 1-3: The tarsus.

Continued

1

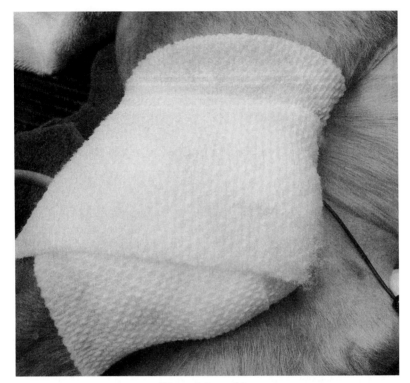

Figure 1-3, cont'd.

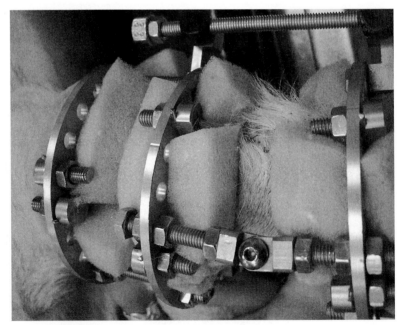

Figure 1-4:   Foam rubber pads are placed under and around the pins of the external fixator, adjacent to the wound.

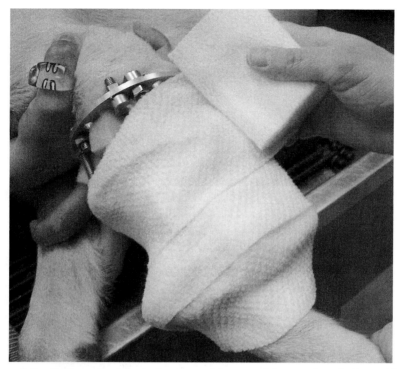

Figure 1-5: Cotton cast padding is placed around the external fixator to keep the foam rubber and contact layer securely in place.

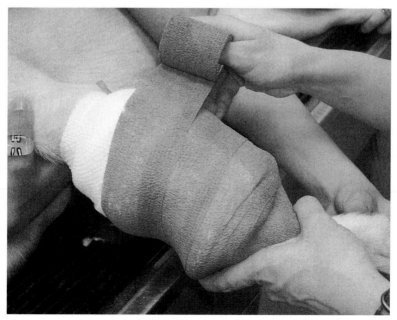

Figure 1-6: Vetrap is placed over the intermediate layer to prevent contamination from the external environment.

1

To create a cup or clamshell splint, follow this procedure (Figures 1-7 to 1-11):
1. Place a nonadherent contact layer directly over the wound.
2. Place stirrups of tape in contact with the skin of the dog, to be placed over the intermediate layer and prevent the bandage from slipping.
3. Place a fairly thick layer of absorbent intermediate bandage material over the contact layer such that the bandage is well-padded. Pull the tape stirrups and secure them to the intermediate layer.
4. Place a length of cast material that has been rolled to the appropriate length, such that the cast material is cupped around the patient's paw, and lies adjacent to the caudal aspect of the limb to the level of the carpus or tarsus. In the case of a clamshell splint, place a layer of cast material on the cranial and caudal aspect of the paw and conform it in place.

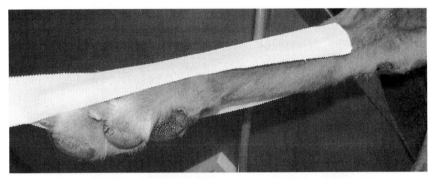

Figure 1-7: Tape stirrups in place.

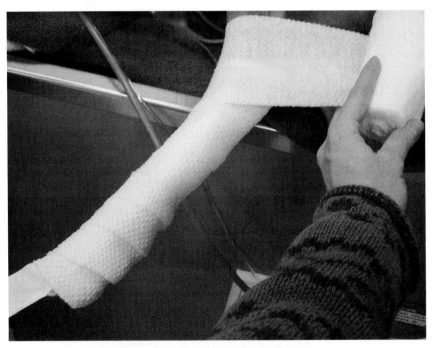

Figure 1-8: Layer of absorbent roll cotton.

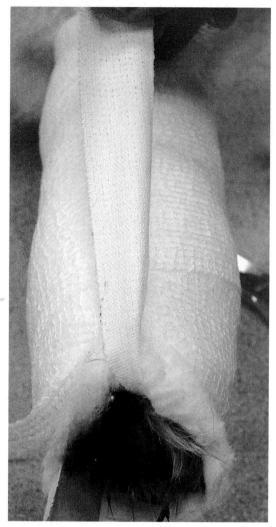

Figure 1-9: Secure tape stirrups to intermediate layer to prevent bandage from slipping.

5. Take the length of cast padding and soak it in warm water after it has been rolled to the appropriate length. Wring out the pad, and secure/conform it to the caudal (or cranial and caudal, in the case of a clamshell splint) aspect of the distal limb and paw.
6. Secure the cast material in place with a layer of elastic cotton gauze (Kling).
7. Secure the bandage in place with a snug layer of Elastikon or Vetrap.

Lateral or caudal splints

Short or long splints made of cast material can be incorporated into a soft padded bandage to provide extra support of a limb above and below a fracture site. For a caudal or lateral splint to be effective, it must be incorporated for at least one joint above any fracture site to prevent a fulcrum effect and further disruption or damage to underlying soft tissue structures. A short lateral or caudal splint is used for fractures and luxations of the distal metacarpus, metatarsus, carpus, and tarsus.

1

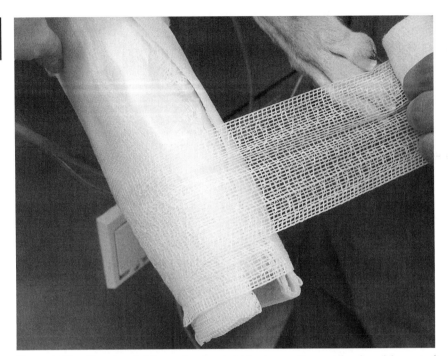

Figure 1-10: Place clamshell layer of cast material in place on the cranial and caudal aspect of the limb.

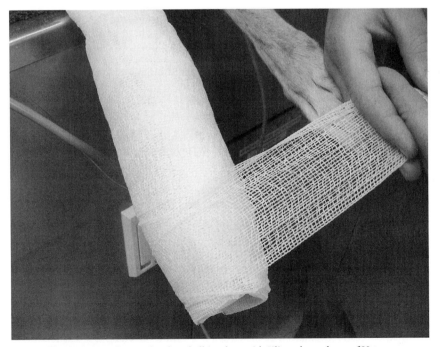

Figure 1-11: Secure the clamshell in place with Kling, then a layer of Vetrap.

To place a short lateral or caudal splint, follow this procedure:
1. Secure a contact layer as determined by the presence or absence of any wound in the area.
2. Place tape stirrups on the distal extremity to be secured later to the intermediate bandage layer and to prevent slipping of the bandage distally.
3. Place layers of roll cotton from the toes to the level of the mid tibia/fibula or mid radius/ulna. Place the layers with even tension, with some overlap of each consecutive layer, moving distally to proximally on the limb.
4. Secure the short caudal or lateral splint and conform it to the distal extremity to the level of the toes and proximally to the level of the mid tibia/fibula or mid radius/ulna.
5. Secure the lateral or caudal splint to the limb with another outer layer of elastic cotton (Kling).
6. Cover the entire bandage and splint with an outer tertiary layer of Vetrap or Elastikon. Make sure that the toenails of the third and fourth digits remain visible to allow daily evaluation of circulation.

Long lateral or caudal splints are used to immobilize fractures of the tibia/fibula and radius/ulna. The splints are fashioned as directed for short splints but extend proximally to the level of the axilla and inguinal regions to immobilize above the fracture site.

Spica splint

A spica splint is used to immobilize the humerus and elbow and shoulder joints in the case of luxation or fracture. To place a spica splint, follow this procedure:
1. Place a contact layer if any wounds are present.
2. Place tape stirrups to the distal limb to attach to the intermediate layer and prevent slipping of the bandage distally.
3. Place layers of conforming cotton gauze circumferentially and overlapping, moving up the limb from distal to proximal.
4. Incorporate the leg bandage into a layer of cotton bandage that is secured over the thorax.
5. Secure the cotton in place with a layer of snug elastic cotton material such as Kling. Make sure that the bandage is not so tight that breathing is impaired.
6. Place splint material on the lateral aspect of the limb, extending the material from the level of the toes proximally over the entire limb and extending proximally to over the scapula and dorsal midline.
7. After rolling the splint to an appropriate length and width, moisten the splint material in warm water to allow it to set and harden.
8. Replace the splint and conform it to the bandage over the patient's body.
9. Secure the splint in place with another layer of cotton Kling.
10. Wrap the entire bandage in place with a layer of tertiary bandage material such as Elastikon or Vetrap.

Additional Reading

Piermattei DL, Flo GL: *Brinker, Piermattei, and Flo's handbook of small animal orthopedics and fracture management*, ed 3, Philadelphia, 1997, WB Saunders.

BLOOD COMPONENT THERAPY

COLLECTION AND ADMINISTRATION

Blood component therapy involves the separation of blood into its cellular and fluid components and infusing the components specific for each patient's needs. Blood component therapy is the mainstay of initial and ongoing management of hematologic emergencies and can provide support of the critically ill patient until the underlying disease process is controlled. The separation of blood into red blood cells, plasma, cryoprecipitate, and platelet-rich products allows for more specific replacement of the animal's deficit(s),

---

BOX 1-4   APPROACH TO BLOOD COMPONENT THERAPY

RED BLOOD CELL SUPPORT
- Packed cell volume drops rapidly to less than 20% in the dog and less than 12% to 15% in the cat
- Acute loss of more than 30% of blood volume (30 mL/kg in dog, 20 mL/kg in cat)
- Clinical signs of lethargy, collapse, hypotension, tachycardia, tachypnea (acute or chronic blood loss)
- Ongoing hemorrhage is present
- Poor response to crystalloid and colloid infusion

PLATELET SUPPORT
- Life-threatening hemorrhage caused by thrombocytopenia or thrombocytopathia
- Surgical intervention is necessary in a patient with severe thrombocytopenia or thrombocytopathia

PLASMA SUPPORT
- Life-threatening hemorrhage with decreased coagulation factor activity
- Severe inflammation (pancreatitis, systemic inflammatory response syndrome)
- Replenish antithrombin (disseminated intravascular coagulation, protein-losing enteropathy or nephropathy)
- Surgery is necessary in a patient with decreased coagulation factor activity
- Severe hypoproteinemia is present; to partially replenish albumin, globulin, and clotting factors

---

decreases the risks of transfusion reactions, and allows for more efficient use of donor blood. Box 1-4 lists indications for transfusion of red blood cells, platelet-rich plasma, fresh frozen or fresh plasma, and cryoprecipitate.

BLOOD TYPES AND ANTIGENICITY

Cell membrane receptors on the surface of red blood cells (RBCs) serve the purpose of self-recognition versus non–self-recognition during states of health. The presence or absence of various glycoprotein and glycolipid moieties on the RBC surface helps to define blood groups or "types" within a species. In dogs, six cell surface dog erythrocyte antigens (DEAs, 1.1, 1.2, 3, 4, 5, and 7) have been identified. Dogs that are negative for DEA 1.1, 1.2, and 7 but positive for DEA 1.4 are known as universal donors and have type A-negative blood. Dog erythrocyte antigens 1.1 and 1.2 are the most immunogenic RBC antigens known in canine transfusion medicine. Transfusion of DEA 1.1- or 1.2-positive blood to a DEA 1.1- and 1.2-negative dog can result in immediate hemolysis or a delayed-type hypersensitivity reaction. Additionally, viability of DEA 1.1- and 1.2-positive cells in a DEA 1.1- and 1.2-negative recipient is short-lived, ultimately defeating the long-term goal of increasing oxygen delivery in the recipient.

Like dogs, feline blood groups are defined by specific carbohydrate moieties attached to lipids (glycolipids) and proteins (glycoproteins) on the RBC surface. Three blood types (A, B, and AB) have been identified in cats. Type A is the most common blood type in cats. Type B is relatively uncommon and occurs in Abyssinian, Persian, Devon Rex, and British Shorthair cats but can be found in domestic shorthair and longhair cats as well. Type A is completely dominant over type B by simple mendelian genetics. Type AB is a rare blood type that has been identified infrequently in domestic short-haired cats, Birman, Abyssinian, Somali, British Shorthair, Scottish Fold, and Norwegian Forest Cats. Unlike dogs, cats possess naturally occurring antibodies against other feline blood types. The presence of naturally occurring autoantibodies is of paramount importance, necessitating blood typing with or without crossmatch before any feline transfusion, because hemolytic transfusion reactions potentially can be fatal, even with no prior sensitization or blood transfusion. Type B cats possess large quantities of anti-A antibodies, primarily of the immunoglobulin M (IgM) subclass. Type A blood infused into a type B cat will be destroyed within minutes to hours, and as little as 1 mL of incompatible blood can cause a life-threatening reaction.

Type A cats typically possess weak anti-B antibodies of IgG and IgM subtypes. Transfusion of type B blood into a type A cat will result in milder clinical signs of reaction and a markedly decreased survival half-life of the infused RBCs to just 2 days. Because type AB cats possess both moieties on their cell surface, they lack naturally occurring alloantibodies; transfusion of type A blood into a type AB cat can be performed safely if a type AB donor is not available. The life span of an RBC from a type-specific transfusion into a cat is approximately 33 days.

BLOOD DONORS PROGRAMS

Each clinic must weigh the cost-benefit ratio, the need for blood products, and the overall quantity of blood products in the practice when deciding which option works best for the staff, clientele, and patient needs. Busy hospitals requiring large quantities of blood products at regular intervals may elect to keep an in-house colony of donor dogs and cats. Maintenance of a closed donor colony may be impractical because of the economics of feeding and housing the animals and using cage space that can be used for other patients. Additionally, care of the animals—including frequent health examinations, blood testing (complete blood count, biochemistry panels, heartworm tests), and daily care—are labor intensive for veterinarian and support staff alike. Other options include using staff- or client-owned animals as donors. This practice eliminates the expense of housing donors within the clinic and the labor required for daily care. Donor animals can be used as needed or can have scheduled collections to replenish the stock of blood products. The final option, which may be more practical for clinics with an infrequent need for blood products, is to purchase blood components from a commercial blood bank (Table 1-1).

Blood donors should receive annual physical examinations and general health screens, including a complete blood count, serum biochemistry panel, and occult heartworm antigen test. Canine donors also should be screened initially for Lyme disease, *Babesia,* Rocky Mountain spotted fever *(Rickettsia rickettsii), Ehrlichia,* and *Brucella.* The prevalence of *Babesia* spp. in the racing Greyhound industry in Florida, Arizona, and Colorado is high (estimated to be 30% to 50%). Dogs ideally should weigh greater than 50 lb (27 kg), be between 1 and 8 years of age, have a packed cell volume (PCV) of at least 40%, be spayed

TABLE 1-1 List of Veterinary Blood Banks		
Name/Address	Telephone number	Web site
Animal Blood Bank P.O. Box 1118 Dixon, CA 95620	800-243-5759 (800-2HELPK9)	www.animalbloodbank.com/
Eastern Veterinary Blood Bank 844 Ritchie Highway Suite 204 Severna Park, MD 21146	800-949-EVBB (800-949-3822)	www.evbb.com
Hemopet Blood Bank Office 11330 Markon Drive Garden Grove, CA 92841	714-891-2022	www.itsfortheanimals.com/HEMOPET.HTM
Midwest Animal Blood Services 4983 Bird Drive Stockbridge, MI 49285	877-517-MABS (877-517-6227)	www.midwestabs.com

and/or nulliparous, and have never received a transfusion. A healthy donor safely can donate 10 to 20 mL/kg of whole blood every 3 to 4 weeks if necessary.

Feline blood donors ideally should weigh greater than 8 lb, be between 1 and 8 years of age, be nulliparous and/or spayed, and have never received a transfusion. Additionally, donor cats should be screened for feline leukemia virus, feline immunodeficiency virus, *Hemobartonella, Mycoplasma haemofelis* and feline infectious peritonitis before donations and should have a minimally acceptable PCV of 30%, although between 35% and 40% is preferred. Whole blood and plasma from donors that previously have been pregnant or received a transfusion should not be used because of the risk of previous exposure to foreign RBC antigens and the development of antibodies.

BLOOD COLLECTION AND HANDLING

Any blood collection should be performed in a manner that is the least stressful for the donor animal. Physical examination and determination of PCV and total solids should be performed before any donation. Blood can be obtained from a jugular vein or femoral artery. However, because of the risk of lacerating the femoral artery, with subsequent hemorrhage or development of compartmental syndrome, I strongly advocate using the jugular vein as the primary site of blood collection in dogs and cats. Carefully clip the fur over the jugular vein, avoiding skin abrasions. Place dogs in lateral recumbancy; however, sternal recumbancy or sitting on the floor are also acceptable methods. Aseptically scrub the area over the clipped jugular vein with iodine or chlorhexidine wipes, alternating with alcohol or sterile saline. Blood can be collected from an open or closed system. Closed-system collection is preferred because it decreases the potential for contamination of the blood product and facilitates processing of blood components. Alternatively, an open system can be used if the blood is going to be transfused within 24 hours. Gently insert a 16-gauge needle into the jugular vein. Place the collection system on a scale on the floor and zero the scale. Then remove the hemostat placed on the collection tubing and allow the blood to flow by gravity. Canine units should be approximately 450 mL, which translates to 450 g on the tared scale, because 1 mL weighs approximately 1 g. Although a volume of 450 mL can be obtained every 21 days, if necessary, from a healthy canine donor, less frequent donation of every 3 months is preferred.

Alternatively, feline blood collection often requires the use of sedation, unless a multi-access port has been implanted surgically. All donor cats should have a physical examination and determination of PCV and total solids performed before sedation and subsequent blood donation. Clip the fur over the jugular vein and aseptically prepare the site as described previously. Insert a 19-gauge butterfly catheter into the jugular vein and aspirate blood with gentle pressure to avoid venous collapse. The butterfly catheter is attached to a three-way stopcock and 60-mL syringe into which 7 mL of citrate phosphate dextrose adenine anticoagulant has been placed. In most cases, a total volume of 53 mL of blood is obtained. The blood can be transfused immediately or placed into a small sterile collection bag that contains 0.14 mL of citrate phosphate dextrose adenine anticoagulant per milliliter of whole blood. No more than 11 to 15 mL/kg should be obtained at any given time from a feline donor (Box 1-5).

BOX 1-5 SUPPLIES NEEDED FOR BLOOD COLLECTION AND PROCESSING	
CANINE	**FELINE**
Blood donor collection bag	60-mL syringe
Sealing clips	Three-way stopcock
Pliers or tube stripper (optional)	7 mL citrate phosphate dextrose adenine
Guarded hemostat	anticoagulant solution
Plasma press	Ketamine
	Diazepam

Blood Component Processing and Storage

Production of blood component therapy has become more commonplace in human and veterinary medicine. Component therapy involves the separation of whole blood into its cellular and plasma components and then administration of specific components to a recipient based on each patient's individual needs. Preparation of fresh frozen plasma, frozen plasma, cryoprecipitate, and cryopoor plasma requires the use of a refrigerated centrifuge. Floor and tabletop models are currently available for purchase. In many cases, purchase of a refrigerated centrifuge is impractical because of the expense and the space required for its storage. A veterinary community potentially can pool resources for the cost of the equipment and house the unit at a centrally located facility, such as a local emergency hospital. Alternatively, human hospitals or blood banks may provide separation services for a nominal fee. Investigation of guidelines in your area may provide a means of creating blood components from your donors for use in your practice.

Once obtained, blood should be stripped from the collection tubing, and the line sealed using a thermal seal or aluminum clips. The bag should be labeled clearly with donor name, donor blood type, date of collection, PCV or donor at time of collection, and date of expiration. If the blood is not going to be used immediately or prepared for platelet-rich plasma, the unit should be refrigerated. The unit then can be spun at 4000 to 5000 times gravity for 5 minutes to separate the RBCs from plasma components. Use of a plasma extractor will facilitate flow of plasma into designated satellite bags for further storage.

Fresh frozen plasma, cryoprecipitate, and cryopoor plasma should be frozen within 8 hours of collection to ensure preservation of labile clotting factors, including factors V and VIII and von Willebrand's factor (vWF). Fresh frozen plasma has a shelf life of 1 year past the date of collection. Before freezing, place an elastic band around the bag to crimp the bag during the freezing process. The elastic band is removed once the unit is frozen. In case of an inadvertent or unobserved power failure, the crimp in the unit provides a quality control measure that inadvertent thawing has not occurred. Partial thawing and differential centrifugation of fresh frozen plasma allows preparation of cryoprecipitate and cryopoor plasma. Following 1 year, or if a unit of plasma has been prepared after 8 hours of collection, frozen plasma results. Frozen plasma contains all of the vitamin K–dependent coagulation factors (II, VII, IX, X), immunoglobulins, and albumin but is relatively devoid of the labile clotting factors. Frozen plasma has a shelf life of 5 years after the original date of collection or 4 years after expiration of a unit of fresh frozen plasma. Packed RBCs should be stored at 1 to 6° C immediately after collection and processing. Packed RBCs and frozen plasma also can be prepared in the absence of a refrigerated centrifuge by storing the unit of whole blood upright in a refrigerator at 1 to 6° C for 12 to 24 hours until the RBCs have separated out. The plasma can be drawn off into a second storage bag and frozen as frozen plasma. Because of the delay in processing, the resultant plasma does not contain the labile clotting factors. Fresh frozen plasma, frozen plasma, cryoprecipitate, and cryopoor plasma should be stored at −20° C until use (Table 1-2). The products should be thawed in tepid water until no crystals are observed. No plasma product should be heated to greater than 37° C because protein denaturation can occur.

Crossmatch procedure

Before administering blood products, find out the donor and recipient's blood types and perform a crossmatch procedure as time allows. At minimum, a blood type should be performed before administration. Rapid blood typing cards are available for use in dogs and cats (Rapid Vet-H; DMS Laboratories, Flemington, New Jersey). A crossmatch procedure simulates in vitro the response of a recipient to donor plasma and RBC antigens. The crossmatch procedure is performed to decrease the risk of transfusion reactions in patients that have been sensitized previously, that have naturally occurring alloantibodies, or in situations of neonatal isoerythrolysis. Other indications for crossmatching include decreasing the risk of sensitizing a patient if more than one transfusion is anticipated. Crossmatching can be divided into major and minor categories. The major crossmatch mixes the donor's

TABLE 1-2 Storage of Blood Components

Component	Anticoagulant	Shelf life	Comments
Whole blood (WB)	Heparin 625 IU/ 250 mL WB	37 days, 4° C	No preservation, coagulation factor inhibition
	ACD, 10 mL/ 60 mL WB	24 hours, 4° C	ACD rarely used
	CPDA-1, 1 mL/ 7 mL WB	21 days, 4° C	Will maintain 75% PTV
	AS-1	35 days, 4° C	
Packed RBCs	CPDA-1	20 days, 4° C	Will maintain 75% PTV
	AS-1	37 days, 4° C	
Platelet-rich plasma	CPDA-1	3-5 days, 23° C 2 hours, 4° C	Needs constant agitation
Fresh frozen plasma	CPDA-1	1 year, −30° C 3 months, −18° C	Frozen <6 hours after collection of blood; all coagulation factors present
Plasma/cryopoor plasma	CPDA-1	5 years, −30° C	Does not contain factors V and VIII
Cryoprecipitate	CPDA-1	1 year, −30° C	High concentration of vWF, factor VIII, and fibrinogen

ACD, Acid citrate dextrose; *AS,* additive solution; *CPDA-1,* citrate phosphate dextrose adenine; *PTV,* posttransfusion viability; *RBCs,* red blood cells; *vWF,* von Willebrand's factor; *WB,* whole blood.

RBCs with recipient's plasma, thus testing whether the recipient contains antibodies against donor RBCs. A minor crossmatch mixes donor plasma with recipient RBCs, testing for the unlikely occurrence that the donor serum contains antibodies directed against recipient RBCs. Box 1-6 gives a complete step-by-step description of major and minor crossmatch procedures. The crossmatch procedures do not check for other sources of immediate hypersensitivity transfusion reactions, including white blood cell and platelets.

INDICATIONS FOR TRANSFUSION THERAPY

There are many indications for administering transfusions of whole blood and component blood products. Take a stepwise approach for every patient that may require a transfusion. If a patient is at risk for blood loss or is anemic, consider a transfusion. Make a decision on the type of transfusion therapy appropriate for each particular patient. Once a decision is made about which components need to be administered, calculate a volume to be delivered. Exercise caution when administering larger volumes to small patients or those with cardiac insufficiency, because volume overload potentially can occur. If RBC products are to be administered, a minimum of a blood type should be performed before giving type-specific blood. The gold standard is to perform a crossmatch for each unit administered to decrease the risk of a transfusion reaction or sensitizing the patient to foreign RBC antigens. In patients with severe hemorrhage when there is not enough time even for performing a blood type, universal blood (DEA 1.1-, 1.2-, and 1.7-negative) or Oxyglobin (Biopure, Cambridge, Massachusetts) can be administered.

A common misconception is that administration of whole blood or packed RBCs should occur when patient PCV decreases to a certain number. In fact, no absolute "transfusion trigger" number actually exists. Administer a transfusion whenever a patient demonstrates clinical signs of anemia, including lethargy, anorexia, weakness, tachycardia, and/or tachypnea

---

BOX 1-6   PROTOCOL FOR PERFORMING MAJOR AND MINOR CROSSMATCH

Supplies needed: 0.9% physiologic saline in wash bottle
    3-mL test tubes
    Pasteur pipettes
    Centrifuge
    Agglutination viewer lamp

1. Label test tubes as follows:
RC	Recipient control
RR	Recipient RBCs
RP	Recipient plasma
DB	Donor whole blood*
DC	Donor control*
DR	Donor whole blood*
DP	Donor plasma*
Ma	Major crossmatch*
Mi	Minor crossmatch*

2. Obtain a crossmatch segment from blood bank refrigerator for each donor to be cross-matched, or use an EDTA tube of donor's blood. MAKE SURE TUBES ARE LABELED PROPERLY.
3. Collect 2 mL of blood from recipient and place in an EDTA tube. Centrifuge blood for 5 minutes.
4. Extract blood from donor tubing. Centrifuge blood for 5 minutes. Use a separate pipette for each transfer because cross-contamination can occur.
5. Pipette plasma off of donor and recipient cells and place in tubes labeled DP and RP, respectively.
6. Place 125 μL of donor and recipient cells in tubes labeled DR and RR, respectively.
7. Add 2.5 mL 0.9% sodium chloride solution from wash bottle to each red blood cell (RBC) tube, using some force to cause cells to mix.
8. Centrifuge RBC suspension for 2 minutes.
9. Discard supernatant and resuspend RBCs with 0.9% sodium chloride from wash bottle.
10. Repeat steps 8 and 9 for a total of three washes.
11. Place 2 drops of donor RBC suspension and 2 drops of recipient plasma in tube labeled Ma (this is the major crossmatch).
12. Place 2 drops of donor plasma and 2 drops recipient RBC suspension in tube labeled Mi (this is the minor crossmatch).
13. Prepare control tubes by placing 2 drops donor plasma with 2 drops donor RBC suspension (this is the donor control); and place 2 drops recipient plasma with 2 drops recipient RBC suspension (this is the recipient control).
14. Incubate major and minor crossmatches and control tubes at room temperature for 15 minutes.
15. Centrifuge all tubes for 1 minute.
16. Read tubes using an agglutination viewer.
17. Check for agglutination and/or hemolysis.
18. Score agglutination with the following scoring scale:
    4+ One solid clump of cells
    3+ Several large clumps of cells
    2+ Medium-sized clumps of cells with a clear background
    1+ Hemolysis, no clumping of cells
    NEG = Negative for hemolysis; negative for clumping of red blood cells

*Indicates that this must be done for each donor being tested.

(Table 1-3). Indications for fresh whole blood transfusion include disorders of hemostasis and coagulopathies including disseminated intravascular coagulation, von Willebrand's disease, and hemophilia. Fresh whole blood and platelet-rich plasma also can be administered in cases of severe thrombocytopenia and thrombocytopathia. Stored whole blood and packed RBCs can be administered in patients with anemia. If PCV drops to below 10% or if rapid hemorrhage causes the PCV to drop below 20% in the dog or less than 12% to

1

TABLE 1-3 Indications for Administration of Blood Products

Blood products	Indications
Fresh whole blood	Coagulopathy with active hemorrhage (disseminated intravascular coagulation, thrombocytopenia; massive acute hemorrhage; no stored blood available)
Stored whole blood	Massive acute or ongoing hemorrhage; hypovolemic shock caused by hemorrhage that is unresponsive to conventional crystalloid and colloid fluid therapy; unavailability of equipment required to prepare blood components
Packed red blood cells	Nonregenerative anemia, immune-mediated hemolytic anemia, correction of anemia before surgery, acute or chronic blood loss
Fresh frozen plasma	Factor depletion associated with active hemorrhage (congenital: von Willebrand's factor, hemophilia A, hemophilia B; acquired: vitamin K antagonist, rodenticide intoxication, DIC); acute or chronic hypoproteinemia (burns, wound exudates, body cavity effusion; hepatic, renal, or gastrointestinal loss); colostrum replacement in neonates
Frozen plasma (contains stable clotting factors)	Acute plasma or protein loss; chronic hypoproteinemia; colostrum replacement in neonates; hemophilia B and selected clotting factor deficiencies
Platelet-rich plasma*	Thrombocytopenia with active hemorrhage (immune-mediated thrombocytopenia, DIC); platelet function abnormality (congenital: thrombasthenia in Bassett hounds; acquired: NSAIDs, other drugs)
Cryoprecipitate (concentration of factor VIII, von Willebrand's factor, and fibrinogen)	Congenital factor deficiencies (routine or before surgery): hemophilia A, hemophilia B, von Willebrand's disease, hypofibrinogenemia; acquired factor deficiencies

*Must be purchased because logistically one cannot obtain enough blood simultaneously to provide a significant amount of platelets; platelets infused have a very short (<2 hours) half-life.
DIC, Disseminated intravascular coagulation; NSAIDs, nonsteroidal antiinflammatory drugs.

15% in the cat, a transfusion is advocated. Consider fresh frozen plasma or cryoprecipitate administration in cases of coagulopathy, including von Willebrand's disease, rodenticide intoxication with depletion of activated vitamin K–dependent coagulation factors, and hemophilia or in cases of severe hypoproteinemia with albumin concentrations less than 2.0 g/dL. Frozen plasma also will suffice in cases of severe hypoproteinemia, warfarin-like compound intoxication, and factor IX deficiency (hemophilia B).

CONSIDERATIONS FOR ADMINISTRATION OF BLOOD COMPONENT THERAPY

When considering the type of blood component product required for transfusion, one should answer a number of questions to decrease the risk of a transfusion reaction and to decrease the risk for rejection or destruction of the component that has been infused. First, knowledge of a patient's blood type is essential. Whenever possible, type-specific RBCs should be administered. If an animal has received prior transfusion(s), the risk of a transfusion reaction or rejection is increased because of the development of antibodies directed against glycoprotein moieties on the surface of RBCs. If a prior transfusion has taken place, the patient's blood (RBCs and plasma) must be crossmatched with the donor blood (RBCs and plasma) to make sure that no incompatibility exists. In dogs, if neither blood typing nor crossmatch procedure is available, or if the emergent situation requires that a transfusion be administered before a blood type or crossmatch can be performed, blood from a

TABLE 1-4 **Blood Component Dose and Administration Rates**

Component	Dose	Administration rate	
		Normovolemia	Hypovolemia
Whole blood	20 mL/kg will increase volume by 10%	Max rate: 22 mL/kg/ 24 hours	Max: 22 mL/kg/ hour
Packed red blood cells	10 mL/kg will increase volume by 10%		Critically ill patients (e.g., cardiac failure or renal failure): 3-4 mL/kg/hour
Fresh frozen plasma	10 mL/kg body mass (repeat in 2-3 days or in 3-5 days or until bleeding stops); monitor ACT, APTT, and PT before and 1 hour after transfusion	4-10 mL/minute or use rates as for whole blood (infuse within 4-6 hours)	
Cryoprecipitate	General: 1 unit/10 kg/12 hours or until bleeding stops Hemophilia A: 12-20 units factor VIII/kg; 1 unit of cryoprecipitate contains approximately 125 units of factor VIII	4-10 mL/minute or use rates as for whole blood (infuse within 4-6 hours)	
Platelet-rich plasma	1 unit/10 kg (1 unit of platelet-rich plasma will increase platelet count 1 hour after transfusion by 10,000/μl)	2 mL/minute Check platelet count before and 1 hour after transfusion	

ACT, Activated clotting time; *APTT,* activated partial thromboplastin time; *PT,* prothrombin time.

universal donor (e.g., DEA 1.1-, 1.2-, and 1.7-negative) should be administered whenever possible. Because there is no universal donor in the cat and because cats possess naturally occurring alloantibodies, all cat blood should be typed and crossmatched before any transfusion. If fresh whole blood is not available, a hemoglobin-based oxygen carrier (Oxyglobin, 2 to 7 mL/kg IV) can be administered until blood products become available.

TRANSFUSION OF BLOOD COMPONENT PRODUCTS

Table 1-4 indicates blood component dose and administration rates.

Red blood cell component therapy

Blood products should be warmed slowly to 37° C before administering them to the patient. Blood warmer units are available for use in veterinary medicine to facilitate rapid transfusion without decreasing patient body temperature (Thermal Angel; Enstill Medical Technologies, Inc., Dallas, Texas). Red blood cell and plasma products should be administered in a blood administration set containing a 170-μm in-line filter. Smaller in-line filters (20 μm) also can be used in cases in which extremely small volumes are to be administered. Blood products should be administered over a period of 4 hours, whenever possible, according to guidelines set by the American Association of Blood Banks.

The volume of blood components required to achieve a specific increment in the patient's PCV depends largely on whether whole blood or packed RBCs are transfused and whether there is ongoing hemorrhage or RBC destruction. Because the PCV of packed RBCs is unusually high (80% for Greyhound blood), a smaller total volume is required than whole blood to achieve a comparable increase in the patient's PCV. In general, 10 mL/kg of packed RBCs or 20 mL/kg whole blood will raise the recipient's PCV by 10%. The "Rule of Ones" states that 1 mL per 1 lb of whole blood will raise the PCV by 1%. If the patient's PCV does not raise by the amount anticipated by the foregoing calculation(s), causes of ongoing hemorrhage or destruction should be considered. The goal of red blood component therapy is to raise the PCV to 25% to 30% in dogs and 15% to 20% in cats.

If an animal is hypovolemic and whole blood is administered, the fluid is redistributed into the extravascular compartment within 24 hours of transfusion. This will result in a secondary rise in the PCV 24 hours after the transfusion in addition to the initial rise 1 to 2 hours after the RBC transfusion is complete.

Use of fresh frozen plasma

The volume of plasma transfused depends largely on the patient's need. In general, plasma transfusion should not exceed more than 22 mL/kg during a 24-hour period for normovolemic animals. Thaw plasma at room temperature, or place it in a ziplock freezer bag and run under cool (not warm) water until thawed. Then administer the plasma through a blood administration set that contains an in-line blood filter or through a standard drip-type administration set with a detachable in-line blood administration filter. The average rate of plasma infusion in a normovolemic patient should not exceed 22 mL/kg/hour. In acute need situations, plasma can be delivered at rates up to 5 to 6 mL/kg/minute. For patients with cardiac insufficiency or other circulatory problems, plasma infusion rates should not exceed 5 mL/kg/hour. Plasma or other blood products should not be mixed with or used in the same infusion line as calcium-containing fluids, including lactated Ringer's solution, calcium chloride, or calcium gluconate. The safest fluid to mix with any blood product is 0.9% sodium chloride.

Administer fresh frozen plasma, frozen plasma, and cryoprecipitate at a volume of 10 mL/kg until bleeding is controlled or source of ongoing albumin loss ceases. The goal of plasma transfusion therapy is to raise the albumin to a minimum of 2.0 g/dL or until bleeding stops as in the case of coagulopathies. Monitor the patient to ensure that bleeding has stopped, coagulation profiles (ACT, APTT, and PT) have normalized, hypovolemia has stabilized, and/or total protein is normalizing, which are indications for discontinuing ongoing transfusion therapy.

Use of plasma cryoprecipitate

Plasma cryoprecipitate can be purchased or manufactured through the partial thawing and then centrifugation of fresh frozen plasma. Cryoprecipitate contains concentrated quantities of vWF, factor VIII, and fibrinogen and is indicated in severe forms of von Willebrand's disease and hemophilia A (factor VIII deficiency).

Platelet-rich plasma

Platelet-rich plasma must be purchased from a commercial source. One unit of fresh whole blood contains 2000 to 5000 platelets. The viability of the platelets contained in the fresh whole blood is short-lived, just 1 to 2 hours after transfusion into the recipient. Because platelet-rich plasma is difficult to obtain, animals with severe thrombocytopenia or thrombocytopathia should be treated with immunomodulating therapies and the administration of fresh frozen plasma.

Transfusion in Dogs

In dogs, blood and plasma transfusions can be administered intravenously or intraosseously. The cephalic, lateral saphenous, medial saphenous, and jugular veins are used most commonly. Fill the recipient set so that the blood in the drip chamber covers the filter (normal 170-μm filter). With small amounts of blood (50 mL) or critically ill patients, use a 40-μm filter. Avoid latex filters for plasma and cryoprecipitate administration. Blood can be administered at variable rates, but the routine figure of 4 to 5 mL/minute often is used. Normovolemic animals can receive blood at 22 mL/kg/day. Dogs in heart failure should receive infusions at no more than 4 mL/kg/hour. Volume is given as needed. To calculate the approximate volume of blood needed to raise hematocrit levels, use the following formula for the dog:

$$\text{Anticoagulated blood volume (mL)}$$
$$= \text{Body mass (kg)} \times 90 \times \frac{\text{PCV desired} - \text{PCV of recipient}}{\text{PCV of donor in anticoagulant}}$$

An alternative formula is the following:

$$2.2 \times \text{Recipient body mass (kg)} \times 30 \text{ (dog)} \times \frac{\text{PCV desired} - \text{PCV of recipient}}{\text{PCV of donor in anticoagulant}}$$

Surgical emergencies and shock may require several times this volume within a short period. If greater than 25% of the patient's blood volume is lost, supplementation with colloids, crystalloids, and blood products is indicated for fluid replacement. One volume of whole blood achieves the same increase in plasma as two to three volumes of plasma. If the patient's blood type is unknown and type A-negative whole blood is not available, any dog blood can be administered to a dog in acute need if the dog has never had a transfusion before. If mismatched blood is given, the patient will become sensitized, and after 5 days, destruction of the donor RBCs will begin. In addition, any subsequent mismatched transfusions may cause an immediate reaction (usually mild) and rapid destruction of the transfused RBCs.

The clinical signs of a transfusion reaction typically only are seen when type A blood is administered to a type A-negative recipient that has been sensitized previously. Incompatible blood transfusions to breeding females can result in isoimmunization and in hemolytic disease in the puppies. The A-negative bitch that receives a transfusion with A-positive and that produces a litter from an A-positive stud can have puppies with neonatal isoerythrolysis.

TRANSFUSION IN CATS

Cats with severe anemia in need of a blood transfusion are typically extremely depressed, lethargic, and anorexic. The stress of restraint and handling can push these critically ill patients over the edge and cause them to die. Extreme gentleness and care are mandatory in restraint and handling. The critically ill cat should be cradled in a towel or blanket. Supplemental flow-by or mask oxygen should be administered, whenever possible, although it may not be clinically helpful until oxygen-carrying capacity is replenished with infusion of RBCs or hemoglobin.

Blood can be administered by way of cephalic, medial saphenous, or the jugular vein. Intramedullary infusion is also possible, if vascular access cannot be accomplished. The average 2- to 4-kg cat can accept 40 to 60 mL of whole blood injected intravenously over a period of 30 to 60 minutes. Administer filtered blood at a rate of 5 to 10 mL/kg/hour. The following formula can be used to estimate the volume of blood required for transfusion in a cat:

$$\text{Anticoagulated blood volume (mL)}$$
$$= \text{Body mass (kg)} \times 70 \times \frac{\text{PCV desired} - \text{PCV of recipient}}{\text{PCV of donor in anticoagulant}}$$

TRANSFUSION REACTIONS

The exact overall incidence and clinical significance of transfusion reactions in veterinary medicine are unknown. Several studies have been performed that document the incidence of transfusion reactions in dogs and cats. Overall, the incidence of transfusion reactions in dogs and cats is 2.5% and 2%, respectively. Transfusion reactions can be immune-mediated and non–immune-mediated and can happen immediately or can be delayed until after a transfusion. Acute reactions usually occur within minutes to hours of the onset of transfusion but may occur up to 48 hours after the transfusion has been stopped. Acute immunologic reactions include hemolysis and acute hypersensitivity including RBCs, platelets, and leukocytes. Signs of a delayed immunologic reaction include hemolysis, purpura, immunosuppression, and neonatal isoerythrolysis. Acute nonimmunologic reactions include donor cell hemolysis before onset of transfusion, circulatory volume overload, bacterial contamination, citrate toxicity with clinical signs of hypocalcemia, coagulopathies, hyperammonemia, hypothermia, air embolism, acidosis, and pulmonary microembolism. Delayed nonimmunologic reactions include the transmission and development of infectious diseases and hemosiderosis. Clinical signs of a transfusion reaction typically depend on the amount of blood transfused, the type and amount of antibody involved in the reaction, and whether the recipient has had previous sensitization.

Monitoring the patient carefully during the transfusion period is essential in recognizing early signs of a transfusion reaction, including those that may become life threatening. A general guideline for patient monitoring is first to start the transfusion slowly during the first 15 minutes. Monitor temperature, pulse, and respiration every 15 minutes for the first hour, 1 hour after the end of the transfusion, and every 12 hours minimally thereafter. Also obtain a PCV immediately before the transfusion, 1 hour after the transfusion has been stopped, and every 12 hours thereafter. Monitor coagulation parameters such as an ACT and platelet count at least daily in patients requiring transfusion therapy.

The most common documented clinical signs of a transfusion reaction include pyrexia, urticaria, salivation/ptyalism, nausea, chills, and vomiting. Other clinical signs of a transfusion reaction may include tachycardia, tremors, collapse, dyspnea, weakness, hypotension, collapse, and seizures. Severe intravascular hemolytic reactions may occur within minutes of the start of the transfusion, causing hemoglobinemia, hemoglobinuria, disseminated intravascular coagulation, and clinical signs of shock. Extravascular hemolytic reactions typically occur later and will result in hyperbilirubinemia and bilirubinuria.

Pretreatment of patients to help decrease the risk of a transfusion reaction remains controversial, and in most cases, pretreatment with glucocorticoids and antihistamines is ineffective at preventing intravascular hemolysis and other reactions should they occur. The most important component of preventing a transfusion reaction is to screen each recipient carefully and process the donor component therapy carefully before the administration of any blood products. Treatment of a transfusion reaction depends on its severity. In all cases, stop the transfusion immediately when clinical signs of a reaction occur. In most cases, discontinuation of the transfusion and administration of drugs to stop the hypersensitivity reaction will be sufficient. Once the medications have taken effect, restart the transfusion slowly and monitor the patient carefully for further signs of reaction. In more severe cases in which a patient's cardiovascular or respiratory system become compromised and hypotension, tachycardia, or tachypnea occurs, immediately discontinue the transfusion and administer diphenhydramine (1 mg/kg IM), dexamethasone-sodium phosphate (0.25 to 0.5 mg/kg IV), and epinephrine to the patient. The patient should have a urinary catheter and central venous catheter placed for measurement of urine output and central venous pressures. Aggressive fluid therapy may be necessary to avoid renal insufficiency or renal damage associated with severe intravascular hemolysis. Overhydration with subsequent pulmonary edema generally can be managed with supplemental oxygen administration and intravenous or intramuscular administration of furosemide (2 to 4 mg/kg). Plasma products with or without heparin can be administered for disseminated intravascular coagulation.

Hemoglobin-based oxygen carriers

Hemoglobin-based oxygen carriers (HBOCs) are currently in the forefront of veterinary and human transfusion medicine. Stroma-free purified bovine hemoglobin is currently available for use in dogs and cats when fresh or stored red blood products are unavailable.

The HBOCs can be stored at room temperature and have a relatively long shelf life compared with red blood component products. The HBOCs function to carry oxygen through the blood and can diffuse oxygen past areas of poor tissue perfusion. An additional characteristic of HBOCs is as a potent colloid, serving to maintain fluid within the vascular space. For this reason, HBOCs must be used with caution in euvolemic patients and patients with cardiovascular insufficiency.

Additional Reading

Day TK: Current development and use of hemoglobin based oxygen carrier solutions, *J Vet Emerg Crit Care* 13(2):77-93, 2003.

Gibson GR, Callan MB, Hoffman V, et al: Use of a hemoglobin-based oxygen-carrying solution in cats: 72 cases (1998-2000), *J Am Vet Med Assoc* 221:96-102, 2002.

Hale AS: Canine blood groups and their importance in veterinary transfusion medicine, *Vet Clin North Am Small Anim Pract* 25(6):1323-1332, 1995.

Harrell KA, Kristensen AT: Canine transfusion reactions and their management, *Vet Clin North Am Small Anim Pract* 25(6):1333-1361, 1995.

Jutkowitz LA, Rozanski EA, Moreau JA, et al: Massive transfusion in dogs: 15 cases (1997-2001), *J Am Vet Med Assoc* 220:1664-1669, 2002.

Kirby R: Transfusion therapy in emergency and critical care medicine, *Vet Clin North Am Small Anim Pract* 25:1365-1386, 1995.

Kristensen AT, Feldman BF: General principles of small animal blood component administration, *Vet Clin North Am Small Anim Pract* 25(6):1277-1290, 1995.

Muir WW, Wellman ML: Hemoglobin solutions and tissue oxygenation, *J Vet Intern Med* 17(2):127-135, 2003.

Schneider A: Blood components: collection, processing and storage, *Vet Clin North Am Small Anim Pract* 25(6):1245-1261, 1995.

Waddell LS, Holt DE, Hughes D, et al: The effect of storage on ammonia concentrations in canine packed red blood cells, *J Vet Emerg Crit Care* 11(1):23-26, 2001.

CENTRAL VENOUS PRESSURE MEASUREMENT

Central venous pressure (CVP) measures the hydrostatic pressure in the anterior vena cava and is influenced by vascular fluid volume, vascular tone, function of the right side of the heart, and changes in intrathoracic pressure during the respiratory cycle. The CVP is not a true measure of blood volume but is used to gauge fluid therapy as a method of determining how effectively the heart can pump the fluid that is being delivered to it. Thus the CVP reflects the interaction of the vascular fluid volume, vascular tone, and cardiac function. Measure CVP in any patient with acute circulatory failure, large volume fluid diuresis (i.e., toxin or oliguric or anuric renal failure), fluid in-and-out monitoring, and cardiac dysfunction. The placement of central venous catheters and thus CVP measurements is contraindicated in patients with known coagulopathies including hypercoagulable states.

To perform CVP monitoring, place a central venous catheter in the right or left jugular vein. In cats and small dogs, however, a long catheter placed in the lateral or medial saphenous vein can be used for trends in CVP monitoring. First, assemble the equipment necessary for jugular catheter (see Vascular Access Techniques for how to place a jugular or saphenous long catheter) and CVP monitoring (Box 1-7). After placing the jugular catheter, take a lateral thoracic radiograph to ensure that the tip of the catheter sits just outside of the right atrium for proper CVP measurements (see Figure 1-13).

BOX 1-7   SUPPLIES NEEDED FOR CENTRAL VENOUS PRESSURE MONITORING

- Two lengths of intravenous extension tubing
- Three-way stopcock
- Heparinized 0.9% saline solution
- 20-mL syringe
- Manometer or ruler (centimeter)

To establish an intravenous catheter for CVP, follow this procedure:

1. Assemble the CVP setup such that the male end of a length of sterile intravenous catheter extension tubing is inserted into the T port of the jugular or medial/lateral saphenous catheter. Make sure to flush the length of tubing with sterile saline before connecting it to the patient to avoid iatrogenic air embolism.
2. Next, insert the male end of a three-way stopcock into the female end of the extension tubing.
3. Attach a 20-mL syringe filled with heparinized sterile 0.9% saline to one of the female ports of the three-way stopcock and either a manometer or a second length of intravenous extension tubing attached to a metric ruler.
4. Lay the patient in lateral or sternal recumbancy.
5. Turn the stopcock OFF to the manometer/ruler and ON to the patient. Infuse a small amount of heparinized saline through the catheter to flush the catheter.
6. Next, turn the stopcock OFF to the patient and ON to the manometer. Gently flush the manometer or length of extension tubing with heparinized saline from the syringe. Use care not to agitate the fluid and create air bubbles within the line or manometer that will artifactually change the CVP measured.
7. Next, lower the 0 cm point on the manometer or ruler to the level of the patient's manubrium (if the patient is in lateral recumbancy) or the point of the elbow (if the patient is in sternal recumbancy).
8. Turn the stopcock OFF to the syringe, and allow the fluid column to equilibrate with the patient's intravascular volume. Once the fluid column stops falling and the level rises and falls with the patient's heartbeat, measure the number adjacent to the bottom of the meniscus of the fluid column. This is the CVP in centimeters of water (see Figure 1-4).
9. Repeat the measurement several times with the patient in the same position to make sure that none of the values has been increased or decreased artifactually in error. Alternately, attach the central catheter to a pressure transducer and perform electronic monitoring of CVP.

There is no absolute value for normal CVP. The normal CVP for small animal patients is 0 to 5 cm H_2O. Values less than zero are associated with absolute or relative hypovolemia. Values of 5 to 10 cm H_2O are borderline hypervolemia, and values greater than 10 cm H_2O suggest intravascular volume overload. Values greater than 15 cm H_2O may be correlated with congestive heart failure and the development of pulmonary edema. In individual patients, the trend in change in CVP is more important than absolute values. As a rule of thumb, when using CVP measurements to gauge fluid therapy and avoid vascular and pulmonary overload, the CVP should not increase by more than 5 cm H_2O in any 24-hour period. If an abrupt increase in CVP is found, repeat the measurement to make sure that the elevated value was not obtained in error. If the value truly has increased dramatically, temporarily discontinue fluid therapy and consider administration of a diuretic.

Additional Reading

DeLaforcade AM, Rozanski EA: Central venous pressure and arterial blood pressure measurements, *Vet Clin North Am Small Anim Pract* 31(6):1163-1174, 2001.

Gookin JL, Atkins CE: Evaluation of the effects of pleural effusion on the central venous pressure in cats, *J Vet Intern Med* 13(6):561-563, 1999.

Oakley RE, Olivier B, Eyster GE, et al: Experimental evaluation of central venous pressure monitoring in the dog, *J Am Anim Hosp Assoc* 33:77-82, 1997.

Waddell LS: Direct blood pressure monitoring, *Clin Tech Small Anim Pract* 15(3):111-118, 2000.

FLUID THERAPY

The diagnosis of intracellular fluid deficit is difficult and is based more on the presence of hypernatremia or hyperosmolality than on clinical signs. An intracellular fluid deficit is expected when free water loss by insensible losses and vomiting, diarrhea, or urine is not matched by free water intake. Consideration of the location of the patient's fluid deficit,

TABLE 1-5 **Correlation of Clinical Signs with Estimated Percent Dehydration**

Clinical signs of interstitial dehydration	Percent (%) deficit
History of vomiting and diarrhea, no visible clinical signs of deficit	4%
Dry mucous membranes, mild skin tenting	5%
Increased skin tenting, dry mucous membranes, mild tachycardia, normal pulse*	7%
Increased skin tenting, dry mucous membranes, tachycardia, weak pulse pressure	10%
Increased skin tenting, dry corneas, dry mucous membranes, elevated or decreased heart rate, poor pulse quality, altered level of consciousness*	12%

*Note: These measures are largely subjective because patients with severe weight loss and loss of subcutaneous fat and very young and very old animals may have increased skin tenting or sunken eyes even in the absence of dehydration.

degree and type of acid-base and electrolyte disorders, and the presence of any ongoing fluid losses should dictate and help guide each patient's individualized fluid therapy plan (Table 1-5).

ACID-BASE PHYSIOLOGY

Normal pH in dogs and cats ranges from 7.30 to 7.45. The three major mechanisms that maintain blood pH within a normal physiologic range include buffering systems, respiratory mechanisms that alter carbon dioxide, and renal (metabolic) mechanisms that retain or excrete hydrogen and bicarbonate ions. The metabolic contribution to acid-base balance can be estimated by measuring total carbon dioxide and pH or by calculating the bicarbonate or base deficit/excess values. Hydrogen and bicarbonate ions have an important influence on normal structure and function of cellular proteins. Treat acidemia if the bicarbonate is less than 12 mEq/L, if the pH is less than 7.2, or if the base deficit is less than −10 mEq/L. Normal bicarbonate concentration is 18 to 26 mEq/L in dogs and 17 to 23 mEq/L in cats (Boxes 1-8 and 1-9).

BOX 1-8   DIFFERENTIAL DIAGNOSES FOR METABOLIC ALKALOSIS

CHLORIDE RESPONSIVE
Vomiting of stomach contents
Diuretic therapy
Posthypercapnia

CHLORIDE RESISTANT
Primary hyperaldosteronism
Hyperadrenocorticism

ALKALI ADMINISTRATION
Oral administration of sodium bicarbonate or other organic anions (e.g., lactate, citrate, gluconate, and acetate)
Oral administration of cation exchange resin with nonabsorbable alkali (e.g., phosphorus binder)

MISCELLANEOUS
Refeeding after fasting
High-dose penicillin
Severe potassium or magnesium deficiency

Modified from DiBartola SP: *Fluid, electrolyte and acid-base disorders in small animal practice*, St Louis, 2005, Saunders.

1

BOX 1-9   DIFFERENTIAL DIAGNOSES FOR METABOLIC ACIDOSIS

INCREASED ANION GAP (NORMOCHLOREMIC)
Ethylene glycol intoxication
Salicylate intoxication
Other rare intoxications (e.g., paraldehyde or methanol)
Diabetic ketoacidosis[*]
Uremic acidosis[†]
Lactic acidosis

NORMAL ANION GAP (HYPERCHLOREMIC)
Diarrhea
Renal tubular acidosis
Carbonic anhydrase inhibitors (e.g., acetazolamide)
Ammonium chloride
Cationic amino acids (e.g., lysine, arginine, and histidine)
Posthypocapnic metabolic acidosis
Dilutional acidosis (e.g., rapid administration of 0.9% saline)
Hypoadrenocorticism[‡]

Modified from DiBartola SP: *Fluid, electrolyte and acid-base disorders in small animal practice,* St Louis, 2005, Saunders.
[*]Patients with diabetic ketoacidosis may have some component of hyperchloremic metabolic acidosis along with increased anion gap acidosis.
[†]The metabolic acidosis early in renal failure may be hyperchloremic and later may convert to typical increased anion gap acidosis.
[‡]Patients with hypoadrenocorticism typically have hypochloremia because of impaired water excretion, absence of aldosterone, impaired renal function, and lactic acidosis. These factors prevent manifestation of hyperchloremia.

The respiratory system further contributes to acid-base status by changes in the elimination of carbon dioxide. Hyperventilation decreases the blood PCO_2 and causes a respiratory alkalosis. Hypoventilation increases the blood PCO_2 and causes a respiratory acidosis. Depending on the altitude, the PCO_2 in dogs can range from 32 to 44 mm Hg. In cats, normal is 28 to 32 mm Hg. Venous PCO_2 values are 33 to 50 mm Hg in dogs and 33 to 45 mm Hg in cats.

Use a systematic approach whenever attempting to interpret a patient's acid-base status. Ideally, obtain an arterial blood sample so that you can monitor the patient's oxygenation and ventilation. Once an arterial blood sample has been obtained, follow these steps:

1. Determine whether the blood sample is arterial or venous by looking at the oxygen saturation (SaO_2). The SaO_2 should be greater than 90% if the sample is truly arterial, although it can be as low as 80% if a patient has severe hypoxemia.
2. Consider the patient's pH. If the pH is outside of the normal range, an acid-base disturbance is present. If the pH is within the normal range, an acid-base disturbance may or may not be present. If the pH is low, the patient is acidotic. If the pH is high, the patient is alkalotic.
3. Next, look at the base excess or deficit. If the base excess is increased, the patient has higher than normal bicarbonate. If there is a base deficit, the patient may have a low bicarbonate or increase in unmeasured anions (e.g., lactic acid or ketoacids).
4. Next, look at the bicarbonate. If the pH is low AND the bicarbonate is low, the patient has a metabolic acidosis. If the pH is high AND the bicarbonate is elevated, the patient has a metabolic alkalosis.
5. Next, look at the $PaCO_2$. If the patient's pH is low and the $PaCO_2$ is elevated, the patient has a respiratory acidosis. If the patient's pH is high and the $PaCO_2$ is low, the patient has a respiratory alkalosis.
6. Finally, if you are interested in the patient's oxygenation, look at the PaO_2. Normal PaO_2 is greater than 80 mm Hg.

TABLE 1-6 Compensatory Renal and Respiratory Responses in Patients with Primary Acid-Base Disorders

Disorder	Primary change	Compensatory response
Metabolic acidosis	$\downarrow HCO_3^-$	0.7 mm Hg decrement in P_{CO_2} for each 1 mEq/L decrement in HCO_3^-
Metabolic alkalosis	$\uparrow HCO_3^-$	0.7 mm Hg increment in P_{CO_2} for each 1 mEq/L increment in HCO_3^-
Acute respiratory acidosis	$\uparrow P_{CO_2}$	1.5 mEq/L increment in HCO_3^- for each 10 mm Hg increment in P_{CO_2}
Chronic respiratory acidosis	$\uparrow P_{CO_2}$	3.5 mEq/L increment in HCO_3^- for each 10 mm Hg increment in P_{CO_2}
Acute respiratory alkalosis	$\downarrow P_{CO_2}$	2.5 mEq/L decrement in HCO_3^- for each 10 mm Hg decrement in P_{CO_2}
Chronic respiratory alkalosis	$\downarrow P_{CO_2}$	5.5 mEq/L decrement in HCO_3^- for each 10 mm Hg decrement in P_{CO_2}

From DiBartola SP: *Fluid, electrolyte and acid-base disorders in small animal practice,* St Louis, 2005, Saunders.

TABLE 1-7 Acid-Base Values in Acute Uncompensated Disturbances

Disturbance	pH	Pa_{CO_2}	Sodium bicarbonate
Metabolic acidosis	$\downarrow$	—	$\downarrow$
Metabolic alkalosis	$\uparrow$	—	$\uparrow$
Respiratory acidosis	$\downarrow$	$\downarrow$	—
Respiratory alkalosis	$\uparrow$	$\downarrow$	—

7. Next, you must determine whether the disorders present are primary disorders or an expected compensation for disorders in the opposing system. For example, is the patient retaining bicarbonate (metabolic alkalosis) because of carbon dioxide retention (respiratory acidosis)? Use the chart in Table 1-6 to evaluate whether the appropriate degree of compensation is occurring. If the adaptive response falls within the expected range, a *simple* acid-base disorder is present. If the response falls outside of the expected range, a *mixed* acid-base disorder is likely present.
8. Finally, you must determine whether the patient's acid-base disturbance is compatible with the history and physical examination findings. If the acid-base disturbance does not fit with the patient's history and physical examination abnormalities, question the results of the blood gas analyses and possibly repeat them.

The most desirable method of assessing the acid-base status of an animal is with a blood gas analyzer. Arterial samples are preferred over venous samples, with heparin used as an anticoagulant (Table 1-7).

ELECTROLYTE MAINTENANCE AND ABNORMALITIES

Potassium

Potassium primarily is located in the intracellular fluid compartment. Serum potassium is regulated by the actions of the sodium-potassium-adenosinetriphosphatase pump on cellular membranes, including those of the renal tubular epithelium. Inorganic metabolic acidosis artifactually can raise serum potassium levels because of redistribution of extracellular potassium in exchange for intracellular hydrogen ion movement in an attempt to correct serum pH.

Potassium is one of the major players in the maintenance of resting membrane potentials of excitable tissue, including neurons and cardiac myocytes. Changes in serum potassium can affect cardiac conduction adversely. Hyperkalemia lowers the resting membrane potential and makes cardiac cells, particularly those of the atria, more susceptible to depolarization. Characteristic signs of severe hyperkalemia that can be observed on an ECG rhythm strip include an absence of P waves, widened QRS complexes, and tall tented or spiked T waves. Further increases in serum potassium can be associated with bradycardia, ventricular fibrillation, and cardiac asystole (death). Treatment of hyperkalemia consists of administration of insulin (0.25 to 0.5 units/kg, IV regular insulin) and dextrose (1 g dextrose per unit of insulin administered, followed by 2.5% dextrose IV CRI to prevent hypoglycemia), calcium (2 to 10 mL of 10% calcium gluconate administered IV slowly to effect), or sodium bicarbonate (1 mEq/kg, IV slowly). Insulin plus dextrose and bicarbonate therapy help drive the potassium intracellularly, whereas calcium antagonizes the effect of hyperkalemia on the myocardial cells. All of the treatments work within minutes, although the effects are relatively short-lived (20 minutes to 1 hour) unless the cause of the hyperkalemia is identified and treated appropriately (Box 1-10). Dilution of serum potassium also results from restoring intravascular fluid volume and correcting metabolic acidosis, in most cases. Treatment with a fluid that does not contain potassium (preferably 0.9% sodium chloride) is recommended.

Hypokalemia elevates the resting membrane potential and results in cellular hyperpolarization. Hypokalemia may be associated with ventricular dysrhythmias, but the ECG changes are not as characteristic as those observed with hyperkalemia. Causes of hypokalemia include renal losses, anorexia, gastrointestinal loss (vomiting, diarrhea), intravenous fluid diuresis, loop diuretics, and postobstructive diuresis (Box 1-11). If the serum potassium concentration is known, potassium supplementation in the form of potassium chloride or potassium phosphate can be added to the patient's intravenous fluids. Correct serum potassium levels less than 3.0 mEq/L or greater than 6.0 mEq/L. Potassium rates should not exceed 0.5 mEq/kg/hour (Table 1-8).

Bicarbonate concentration

Metabolic acidosis from bicarbonate depletion often corrects itself with volume restoration in most small animal patients. Patients with moderate to severe metabolic acidosis may benefit from bicarbonate supplementation therapy. The metabolic contribution to acid-base balance is identified by measuring the total carbon dioxide concentration or calculating the bicarbonate concentration. If these measurements are not available, the degree of expected metabolic acidosis can be estimated subjectively by the severity of underlying disease that often contributes to metabolic acidosis: hypovolemic or traumatic shock, septic shock, diabetic ketoacidosis, or oliguric/anuric renal failure. If the metabolic acidosis is estimated to be mild, moderate, or severe, add sodium bicarbonate at 1, 3, and 5 mEq/kg body mass, respectively. Patients with diabetic ketoacidosis may not require bicarbonate administration once volume replacement and perfusion is restored, and the ketoacids are metabolized to bicarbonate. If the bicarbonate measurement of base deficit is known, the following formula can be used as a gauge for bicarbonate supplementation:

$$\text{Base deficit} \times 0.3 = \text{Body mass (kg)} = \text{mEq Bicarbonate to administer}$$

Osmolality

Osmolality is measured by freezing point depression or a vapor pressure osmometer, or it may be calculated by the following formula:

$$mOsm/kg = 2[(Na^+) + (K^+)] + BUN/2.8 + Glucose/18$$

where sodium and potassium are measured in milliequivalents, and BUN and glucose are measured in milligrams per deciliter. Osmolalities less than 260 mOsm/kg or greater

BOX 1-10 DIFFERENTIAL DIAGNOSES FOR HYPERKALEMIA

PSEUDOHYPERKALEMIA
Thrombocytosis
Hemolysis

INCREASED INTAKE
Unlikely to cause hyperkalemia in presence of normal renal function unless iatrogenic (e.g., continuous infusion of potassium-containing fluids at an excessively rapid rate)

TRANSLOCATION (INTRACELLULAR FLUID TRANSFER TO EXTRACELLULAR FLUID)
Acute mineral acidosis (e.g., hydrochloric acid or ammonium chloride)
Insulin deficiency (e.g., diabetic ketoacidosis)
Acute tumor lysis syndrome
Reperfusion of extremities after aortic thromboembolism in cats with cardiomyopathy
Hyperkalemic periodic paralysis (one case report in a pit bull)
Mild hyperkalemia after exercise in dogs with induced hypothyroidism
Infusion of lysine or arginine in total parenteral nutrition solutions

DRUGS
Nonspecific β-blockers (e.g., propranolol)*
Cardiac glycosides (e.g., digoxin)*

DECREASED URINARY EXCRETION
Urethral obstruction
Ruptured bladder
Anuric or oliguric renal failure
Hypoadrenocorticism
Selected gastrointestinal disease (e.g., trichuriasis, salmonellosis, or perforated duodenal ulcer)
Late pregnancy in Greyhound dogs (mechanism unknown but affected dogs had gastrointestinal fluid loss)
Chylothorax with repeated pleural fluid drainage
Hyporeninemic hypoaldosteronism†

DRUGS
Angiotensin-converting enzyme inhibitors (e.g., enalapril)*
Angiotensin receptor blockers (e.g., losartan)*
Cyclosporine and tacrolimus*
Potassium-sparing diuretics (e.g., spironolactone, amiloride, and triamterene)*
Nonsteroidal antiinflammatory drugs*
Heparin*
Trimethoprim*

From DiBartola SP: *Fluid, electrolyte and acid-base disorders in small animal practice*, St Louis, 2005, Saunders.
*Likely to cause hyperkalemia only in conjunction with other contributing factors (e.g., other drugs, decreased renal function, or concurrent administration of potassium supplements).
†Not well documented in veterinary medicine.

than 360 mOsm/kg are serious enough to warrant therapy. The difference between the measured osmolality and the calculated osmolality (the osmolal gap) should be less than 10 mOsm/kg. If the osmolal gap is greater than 20 mOsm/kg, consider the presence of unmeasured anions such as ethylene glycol metabolites.

Sodium

The volume of extracellular fluid is determined by the total body sodium content, whereas the osmolality and sodium concentration are determined by water balance. Serum sodium concentration is an indication of the amount of sodium relative to water in the extracellular fluid and provides no direct information about the total body sodium content.

1

BOX 1-11   DIFFERENTIAL DIAGNOSES FOR HYPOKALEMIA

DECREASED INTAKE
Alone unlikely to cause hypokalemia unless diet is aberrant
Administration of potassium-free (e.g., 0.9% sodium chloride or 5% dextrose in water) or potassium-deficient fluids (e.g., lactated Ringer's solution over several days)
Bentonite clay ingestion (e.g., cat litter)

TRANSLOCATION (EXTRACELLULAR FLUID TRANSFER TO INTRACELLULAR FLUID)
Alkalemia
Insulin/glucose-containing fluids
Catecholamines
Hypothermia
Hypokalemic periodic paralysis (Burmese cats)
Albuterol overdosage

INCREASED LOSS
Gastrointestinal (FE_K less than 4% to 6%)
  Vomiting of stomach contents
  Diarrhea
Urinary (fractional excretion of potassium [FE_K] greater than 4% to 6%)
  Chronic renal failure in cats
  Diet-induced hypokalemic nephropathy in cats
  Distal (type I) renal tubular acidosis
  Proximal (type II) renal tubular acidosis after sodium bicarbonate treatment
  Postobstructive diuresis
  Dialysis
  Mineralocorticoid excess
    Hyperadrenocorticism
    Primary hyperaldosteronism (adenoma, adenocarcinoma, hyperplasia)

DRUGS
Loop diuretics (e.g., furosemide and ethacrynic acid)
Thiazide diuretics (e.g., chlorothiazide and hydrochlorothiazide)
Amphotericin B
Penicillins
Unknown mechanism
Rattlesnake envenomation

From DiBartola SP: *Fluid, electrolyte and acid-base disorders in small animal practice,* St Louis, 2005, Saunders.

TABLE 1-8   Guidelines for Routine Intravenous Potassium Supplementation in Dogs and Cats

Serum potassium (mEq/L)	Potassium chloride to add to 250 mL of fluid (mEq)	Potassium chloride to add to 1 L of fluid (mEq)	Maximal fluid rate (mL/kg/hour)*
<2.0[†]	20	80	6
2.1-2.5	15	60	8
2.6-3.0	10	40	12
3.1-3.5	7	28	18
3.6-5.0	5	20	25

*Maximal rate of potassium supplementation should not exceed 0.5 mEq/kg/hour.
[†]If refractory hypokalemia is present, supplement magnesium at 0.75 mEq/kg/day for 24 hours.

Patients with hyponatremia or hypernatremia may have decreased, normal, or increased total body sodium content (Boxes 1-12 and 1-13). An increased serum sodium concentration implies hyperosmolality, whereas a decrease in serum sodium concentration usually, but not always, implies hypoosmolality. The severity of clinical signs of hypernatremia and hyponatremia is related primarily to the rapidity of the onset of the change rather than to the magnitude of the associated plasma hyperosmolality or hypoosmolality. Clinical signs of neurologic disturbances include disorientation, ataxia, and seizures, and coma may occur at serum sodium concentrations less than 120 mEq/L or greater than 170 mEq/L in dogs.

BOX 1-12 DIFFERENTIAL DIAGNOSES FOR HYPONATREMIA

WITH NORMAL PLASMA OSMOLALITY
Hyperlipemia
Hyperproteinemia

WITH HIGH PLASMA OSMOLALITY
Hyperglycemia
Mannitol infusion

WITH LOW PLASMA OSMOLALITY
And hypervolemia
  Severe liver disease
  Congestive heart failure
  Nephrotic syndrome
  Advanced renal failure
And normovolemia
  Psychogenic polydipsia
  Syndrome of inappropriate antidiuretic
    hormone secretion

Antidiuretic drugs
Myxedema coma of hypothyroidism
Hypotonic fluid infusion
And hypovolemia
  Gastrointestinal loss
    Vomiting
    Diarrhea
  Third-space loss
    Pancreatitis
    Peritonitis
    Uroabdomen
    Pleural effusion (e.g., chylothorax)
    Peritoneal effusion
  Cutaneous loss
    Burns
  Hypoadrenocorticism
  Diuretic administration

From DiBartola SP: *Fluid, electrolyte and acid-base disorders in small animal practice,* St Louis, 2005, Saunders.

BOX 1-13 DIFFERENTIAL DIAGNOSES FOR HYPERNATREMIA

PURE WATER DEFICIT
Primary hypodipsia (e.g., in Miniature
  schnauzers)
Diabetes insipidus
  Central
  Nephrogenic
High environmental temperature
Fever
Inadequate access to water

HYPOTONIC FLUID LOSS
Extrarenal
  Gastrointestinal
    Vomiting
    Diarrhea
    Small intestinal obstruction
  Third-space loss
    Peritonitis
    Pancreatitis
  Cutaneous
    Burns

Renal
  Osmotic diuresis
    Diabetes mellitus
    Mannitol infusion
  Chemical diuretics
  Chronic renal failure
  Nonoliguric acute renal failure
  Postobstructive diuresis

IMPERMEANT SOLUTE GAIN
Salt poisoning
Hypertonic fluid administration
  Hypertonic saline
  Sodium bicarbonate
  Parenteral nutrition
  Sodium phosphate enema
Hyperaldosteronism
Hyperadrenocorticism

From DiBartola SP: *Fluid, electrolyte and acid-base disorders in small animal practice,* St Louis, 2005, Saunders.

Therapy of hypernatremia or hyponatremia with fluid containing low or higher concentrations of sodium should proceed with caution, for rapid changes (decreases or increases) of serum sodium and osmolality can cause rapid changes in the intracellular and extracellular fluid flux, leading to intracellular dehydration or edema, even though the serum sodium has not been returned to normal. A rule of thumb is to not raise or lower the serum sodium by more than 15 mEq/L during any one 24-hour period. Restoration of the serum sodium concentration over a period of 48 to 72 hours is better. In almost all circumstances, an animal will correct its sodium balance with simple fluid restoration. If severe hypernatremia exists that suggests a free water deficit, however, the free water deficit should be calculated from the following formula:

$$\text{Free water deficit} = 0.4 \times \text{Body mass (kg)} \times \{[(\text{Plasma sodium})/140] - 1\}$$

Hypernatremia can be corrected slowly with 0.45% sodium chloride plus 2.5% dextrose, 5% dextrose in water, or lactated Ringer's solution (sodium content: 130 mEq/L). Correct hyponatremia initially with 0.9% sodium chloride.

Anion gap

Sodium is balanced predominantly by chloride and bicarbonate. The difference between these concentrations, $(\text{Na}^+) - [(\text{Cl}^-) + (\text{HCO}_3^-)]$, has been called the *anion gap*. The normal anion gap is between 12 and 25 mEq/L. When the anion gap exceeds 25, consider the possibility of an accumulation of unmeasured anions (e.g., lactate, ketoacids, phosphate, sulfate, ethylene glycol metabolites, and salicylate). Abnormalities in the anion gap may be helpful in determining the cause of metabolic acidosis (Boxes 1-14 and 1-15).

ONCOTIC PRESSURE

The colloid oncotic pressure of blood is associated primarily with large-molecular-weight colloidal substances in circulation. The major player in maintaining intravascular and interstitial oncotic pressure, the water-retaining property of each fluid compartment, is albumin. Albumin contributes roughly 80% to the colloidal oncotic pressure of blood. The majority of albumin is located within the interstitial space. Hypoalbuminemia can result from increased loss in the form of protein-losing enteropathy or nephropathy and wound exudates, or it may be due to lack of hepatic albumin synthesis. Serum albumin pools are

---

BOX 1-14   DECREASED ANION GAP

- Myeloma (immunoglobulin G)
- Hypoalbuminemia
- Dilutional from crystalloid fluid administration
- Potassium bromide therapy
- Pseudohyponatremia

BOX 1-15   INCREASED ANION GAP

- Follow the mnemonic A MUD PILE:
- Aspirin (salicylates)
- Methanol
- Uremia
- Diabetic ketoacidosis
- Phosphate, Paraldehyde
- Indomethacin
- Lactic acidosis
- Ethylene glycol intoxication

in a constant flux with interstitial albumin. Once interstitial albumin pools become depleted from replenishing serum albumin, serum albumin levels can continue to decrease, which can lead to a decrease in colloidal oncotic pressure. Serum albumin less than 2.0 g/dL has been associated with inadequate intravascular fluid retention and the development of peripheral edema and third spacing of fluid. Oncotic pressure can be restored with the use of artificial or synthetic colloids or natural colloids (see Colloids).

MAINTENANCE FLUID REQUIREMENTS

Maintenance fluid requirements have been extrapolated from the formulas used to calculate a patient's daily metabolic energy requirements because it takes 1 mL of water to metabolize 1 Kcal of energy (Table 1-9). The patient's daily metabolic water (fluid) requirements can be calculated by the following formula:

$$\text{Fluid (mL)} = [30 \times \text{Body mass (kg)}] + 70$$

Administration of an isotonic crystalloid fluid for maintenance requirements often can produce iatrogenic hypokalemia. In most cases, supplemental potassium must be added to prevent hypokalemia resulting from inappetance, kalliuresis, and supplementation with isotonic crystalloid fluids.

CALCULATION OF FLUID DEFICITS AND ONGOING LOSSES

The most reliable method of determining the degree of fluid deficit is by weighing the animal and calculating acute weight loss. Acute weight loss in a patient with volume loss in the form of vomiting, feces, wound exudates, and urine is due to fluid loss and not loss of muscle or fat. Lean body mass normally is not gained or lost rapidly enough to cause major changes in body weight. One milliliter of water weighs approximately 1 g. This fact allows calculation of the patient's fluid deficit, if ongoing losses can be measured. When a patient first presents, however, the body weight before a fluid deficit has occurred rarely is known. Instead, one must rely on subjective measures of dehydration to estimate the patient's percent dehydration and to calculate the volume of fluid required to rehydrate the patient over the next 24 hours. To calculate the volume deficit, use the following formula:

$$\text{Body mass (kg)} \times (\% \text{ dehydration}) \times 1000 = \text{Fluid deficit (mL)}$$

The patient's fluid deficit must be added to the daily maintenance fluid requirements and administered over a 24-hour period. Ongoing losses can be determined by measuring urine output, weighing the patient at least 2 to 3 times a day, and measuring the volume or weight of vomitus or diarrhea.

CRYSTALLOID AND COLLOID FLUIDS

Crystalloid fluids

A crystalloid fluid contains crystals of salts with a composition similar to that of the extracellular fluid space and can be used to maintain daily fluid requirements and replace fluid deficits or ongoing fluid losses (Table 1-10). Metabolic, acid-base, and electrolyte imbalances also can be treated with isotonic fluids with or without supplemental electrolytes and buffers. Depending on the patient's clinical condition, choose the specific isotonic crystalloid fluid to replace and maintain the patient's acid-base and electrolyte status (Table 1-11). Crystalloid fluids are readily available, are relatively inexpensive, and can be administered safely in large volumes to patients with no preexisting cardiac or renal disease or cerebral edema. Following infusion, approximately 80% of the volume of a crystalloid fluid infused will redistribute to the interstitial fluid compartment. As such, crystalloid fluids alone are ineffective for ongoing intravascular volume depletion when given as a bolus. The crystalloid fluid bolus must be followed by a constant rate infusion, taking into consideration the patient's daily maintenance fluid requirements and ongoing fluid losses. Administration of a large volume of crystalloid fluids can cause dilutional anemia and coagulopathies.

TABLE 1-9   Approximate Daily Energy and Water Requirements of Dogs and Cats Based on Body Mass*

Body mass (kg)	Total energy (Kcal) per day	Total water (mL) per hour
1	100	4.2
2	130	5.4
3	160	6.7
4	190	7.9
5	220	9.2
6	250	10.4
7	280	11.7
8	310	12.9
9	340	14.2
10	370	15.4
11	400	16.7
12	430	17.9
13	460	19.2
14	490	20.4
15	520	21.7
16	550	22.9
17	580	24.2
18	610	25.4
19	640	26.7
20	670	27.9
21	700	29.2
22	730	30.4
23	760	31.7
24	790	32.9
25	820	34.2
26	850	35.4
27	880	36.7
28	910	37.9
29	940	39.2
30	970	40.4
35	1120	46.7
40	1270	52.9
45	1420	59.2
50	1570	65.4
55	1720	71.7
60	1870	77.9
65	2020	84.2
70	2170	90.4
75	2320	96.7
80	2470	102.9
85	2620	109.2
90	2770	115.4
95	2920	121.7
100	3070	127.9

*$30 \times BW_{kg} + 70 = Kcal/day = mL/day$. Note: This formula will slightly underestimate the requirements for patients that are less than 2 kg and will slightly overestimate the requirements for patients greater than 70 kg.

TABLE 1-10 Electrolyte Composition (mEq/L) of Commonly Used Isotonic and Hypotonic Crystalloid Fluids

	0.9% Saline	0.45% NaCl	Lactated Ringer's	Normosol-R
Sodium	154	77	130	140
Chloride	154	77	109	98
Potassium	0	0	4	5
Calcium	0	0	3	0
Magnesium	0	0	0	3
pH	7.386	5.7	6.7	7.4
Buffer	None	None	Lactate 28	Acetate 27 Gluconate 23

TABLE 1-11 Indications for Use of Specific Crystalloid Fluids in Specific Disease Processes

Crystalloid fluid	Indications
Lactated Ringer's solution	Hypocalcemia, to replace dehydration deficit, metabolic acidosis, use as a maintenance fluid, renal failure
Plasmalyte-M and Normosol-R*	To replace dehydration deficit, metabolic acidosis, hypomagnesemia Use as a maintenance fluid, renal failure
0.45% sodium chloride + 2.5% dextrose	Cardiac disease, hepatic failure, hypernatremia
5% dextrose in water	Cardiac disease, hepatic failure, hypernatremia
0.9% sodium chloride	Conditions associated with hypercalcemia and hyperkalemia (e.g., hypoadrenocorticism, vitamin D toxicity, renal failure, and various neoplasias)

*Abbott Laboratories, Abbott Park, Illinois.

Obtain the patient's hematocrit before fluid infusion and regularly during the course of fluid therapy, particularly in patients with preexisting anemia or hypoproteinemia.

Colloids

A colloid is a large-molecular-weight particle that acts as an effective volume expander by drawing fluid from the interstitial fluid compartment into the intravascular space. When administered with a crystalloid, a colloid serves to hold or retain the crystalloid fluid within the vascular space for a longer time than if the crystalloid fluid were administered alone. Because of this property, colloids can promote better tissue perfusion at lower infusion volumes and equivalent colloid oncotic pressures and mean blood pressures than crystalloids. Administer the synthetic colloids in incremental boluses of 5 to 10 mL/kg over 5 to 15 minutes during the treatment of hypotension. When synthetic colloids are administered for maintenance of colloidal oncotic pressure in hypoalbuminemic/hypoproteinemic patients, the recommended dose is 20 to 30 mL/kg/day as a constant rate infusion. Because colloids retain fluid in the vascular space, the volume of crystalloid fluid infused (maintenance + deficit + ongoing losses) should be decreased by 25% to 50% to avoid vascular volume overload.

Two major classes of colloids exist: natural and synthetic. Natural colloids (whole blood, packed RBCs, plasma) are discussed elsewhere in this text. Concentrated human albumin is a natural purified colloid that recently has become more popular in the treatment of advanced hypoalbuminemia and hypoproteinemia and will be discussed here. Synthetic colloids are starch polymers and include dextrans and hetastarch.

Concentrated human albumin is available as a 5% or 25% solution. The 5% solution has an osmolality similar to that of serum (308 mOsm/L), whereas the 25% solution is hyperoncotic (1500 mOsm/L). A 25% albumin solution draws fluid from the interstitial space into the intravascular space. Concentrated albumin solutions often are used to restore circulating volume when synthetic colloids are not available. Albumin not only is important at maintaining the colloidal oncotic pressure of blood but also serves as a valuable free-radical scavenger and carrier of drugs and hormones necessary for normal tissue function and healing. Albumin levels less than 2.0 g/dL have been associated with increased morbidity and mortality. Concentrated human albumin solutions can be administered as an effective method of restoring interstitial and serum albumin concentrations in situations of acute and chronic hypoalbuminemia. Albumin (25%) is available in 50- and 100-mL vials and is more cost-efficient as an albumin replacement than procurement and administration of fresh frozen plasma. Recommended albumin infusion rates are 2 to 5 mL/kg over 4 hours, after pretreatment with diphenhydramine. Although concentrated human albumin is structurally similar to canine albumin, closely monitor the patient for signs of allergic reaction during and after the infusion.

Dextran-70 is a synthetic high-molecular-weight polysaccharide (sucrose polymer) with a molecular weight of 70,000 D. Particles less than 50,000 D, are cleared rapidly by the kidneys, whereas larger particles are cleared more slowly by the hepatic reticuloendothelial system. Dextran-70 can coat platelets and inhibit platelet function and so must be used with caution in patients with known coagulopathies. The total daily dosage should not exceed 40 mL/kg/day.

Hetastarch (hydroxyethyl starch) is a large-molecular-weight amylopectin polymer, has molecules with a molecular weight that exceeds 100,000 D, and has an average half-life of 24 to 36 hours in circulation. Hetastarch can bind with vWF and cause prolongation of the ACT and APTT; however, it does not cause a coagulopathy. Recommended rates of hetastarch infusion are 5- to 10-mL incremental boluses for the treatment of hypotension and 20 to 30 mL/kg/day as a constant rate infusion for maintenance of colloidal oncotic pressure.

IMPLEMENTING THE FLUID THERAPY PLAN

Many are the acceptable ways to administer the fluids prescribed for each patient based on the degree of dehydration, estimation of ongoing losses, ability to tolerate oral fluid, and metabolic, acid-base, and electrolyte derangements. Administer the fluids in a manner that is best for the patient and most appropriate for the practice.

To determine the rate of intravenous fluid infusion, take the total volume of fluids that have been prescribed and divide the total volume by the total number of hours in a day that intravenous fluids can be delivered safely and monitored. The safest and most accurate way to deliver intravenous fluids, particularly in extremely small animals or those with congestive heart failure, is through an intravenous fluid pump. Fluid should not be administered intravenously if the patient cannot be monitored to make sure that the fluids are being delivered at a safe rate and that the fluid line has not become disconnected.

Supplement fluids over as many hours as possible to allow the patient as much time as possible to redistribute and fully utilize the fluids administered. Fluids administered too quickly can cause a diuresis to occur, such that the majority of the fluids administered will be excreted in the urine. If time is limited or if extra time is needed for safe administration of fluids, consider using a combination of intravenously and subcutaneously administered fluids. Intravenous is the preferred route of administration of fluids in any patient with dehydration and hypovolemia. As intravascular volume depletion occurs, reflex peripheral vasoconstriction occurs to restore core perfusion. The subcutaneous tissue are not perfused well and therefore fluids administered subcutaneously will not be absorbed well into the interstitial and intravascular spaces. Subcutaneously administered fluids can be absorbed slowly and delivered effectively in the management of mild interstitial dehydration and in the treatment of renal insufficiency. Subcutaneously administered fluids should never take the place of intravenously administered fluids in a hypovolemic patient or one with severe interstitial dehydration.

Intramedullary (intraosseous) infusion works well in small patients in which vascular access cannot be established. Shock doses of fluids and other substances, including blood products, can be administered under pressure through an intraosseous cannula. Because of the inherent discomfort and risk of osteomyelitis with intraosseous infusion, establish vascular access as soon as possible.

RATES OF ADMINISTRATION

The safest and most efficient method of intravenous fluid infusion is through a fluid pump. In cases in which a fluid pump is unavailable, infusion by gravity feed is the next option. Infusion sets from various manufacturers have calibrated drip chambers such that a specific number of drops will equal 1 mL of fluid. Fluid rates can be calculated based on the number of drops that fall into the drip chamber per minute:

$$\frac{\text{Fluid volume to be infused (mL)}}{\text{Number of hours available}} = \text{mL/hour}$$

Many pediatric drip sets deliver 60 drops/mL, such that milliliters/hour equals drops/minute. Carefully record fluid orders so that the volume to be administered is recorded as milliliters/hour, milliliters/day, and drops/minute. This will allow personnel to detect major discrepancies and calculation errors more readily. The volume actually delivered should be recorded in the record by nursing personnel. All additives should be listed clearly on the bottle on a piece of adhesive tape or a special label manufactured for this purpose. A strip of adhesive tape also can be attached to the bottle and marked appropriately to provide a quick visualization of the estimate of volume delivered.

Additional Reading

Greco DS: The distribution of body water and general approach to the patient, *Vet Clin North Am* 28(3):473-482, 1998.
Kirby R, Rudloff E: The critical need for colloids: maintaining fluid balance, *Compend Contin Educ Pract Vet* 19(6):705-716, 1997.
Mathews KA: The various types of parenteral fluids and their indications, *Vet Clin North Am Small Anim Pract* 28(3):483-513, 1998.
Mazzaferro EM, Rudloff E, Kirby R: The role of albumin in health and disease, *J Vet Emerg Crit Care* 12(2):113-124, 2002.
Moore LE: Fluid therapy in the hypoproteinemic patient, *Vet Clin North Am Small Anim Pract* 28(3):709-715, 1998.
Otto CM, McCall-Kauffman G, Crowe DT: Intraosseous infusion of fluids and therapeutics, *Compend Contin Educ Pract Vet* 11:421-430, 1989.
Rozanski E, Rondeau M: Choosing fluids in traumatic hypovolemic shock: the role of crystalloids, colloids and hypertonic saline, *J Am Anim Hosp Assoc* 38(6):499-501, 2002.
Rudloff E, Kirby R: Colloid and crystalloid resuscitation, *Vet Clin North Am Small Anim Pract* 31(6):1207-1229, 2001.

OROGASTRIC LAVAGE

Orogastric lavage is indicated for gastric decontamination of most types of toxins, for elimination of food during food bloat, and for gastric decompression during surgery for gastric dilatation-volvulus syndrome (GDV). Equipment needed to perform an orogastric lavage includes a large-bore flexible orogastric lavage tube, permanent marker or white tape, lubricating jelly, warm water, two large buckets, a roll of 2-inch white tape, and a manual lavage pump.

To perform the orogastric lavage, follow this procedure:

1. Place all animals under general anesthesia with a cuffed endotracheal tube in place to protect the airway and prevent aspiration of gastric contents into the lungs.
2. Place a roll of 2-inch white tape into the animal's mouth, and secure the tape around the muzzle. You will insert the tube through the hole in the center of the roll of tape.
3. Next, place the distal end of the tube at the level of the last rib, directly adjacent to the animal's thorax and abdomen. Measure the length of the tube from the most distal end to the point where it comes out of the mouth, and label this location on the tube with a permanent marker or piece of white tape.
4. Lubricate the distal portion of the tube, and gently insert it through the roll of tape in the animal's mouth.
5. Gently push the tube down the esophagus. Palpate the tube within the esophagus. Two tubes should be palpable, the orogastric tube, and the patient's trachea. Push the tube down into the stomach. You can verify location by blowing into the proximal end of the tube and simultaneously auscultating the stomach for borborygmi.
6. Insert the manual pump to the proximal end of the tube, and instill the warm water. Alternate instilling water with removal of fluid and gastric debris by gravity. Repeat the process until the efflux fluid is clear of any debris.
7. Save fluid from the gastric efflux fluid for toxicologic analyses.

Additional Reading

Hackett TB: Emergency approach to intoxications, *Clin Tech Small Anim Pract* 15(2):82-87, 2000.

OXYGEN SUPPLEMENTATION

Hypoxia, or inadequate tissue oxygenation, is the primary reason for supplemental oxygen therapy. Major causes of hypoxia include hypoventilation, ventilation-perfusion mismatch, physiologic or right-to-left cardiac shunt, diffusion impairment, and decreased fraction of inspired oxygen (Table 1-12). Inadequate tissue perfusion caused by low cardiac output or vascular obstruction also can result in circulatory hypoxia. Finally, histiocytic hypoxia results from inability of cells to use oxygen that is delivered to them. This form of hypoxia can be observed with various toxin ingestions (bromethalin, cyanide) and in septic shock.

TABLE 1-12 Types of Hypoxia and Response to Oxygen Supplementation

Type of hypoxia	Cause	Response to oxygen
Hypoxic hypoxia		
Alveolar hypoventilation	Central nervous system disease, drugs, rib fractures, thoracic cage damage, pneumothorax, pleural effusion	Responsive
Arteriovenous (physiologic) shunt	Pneumonia, atelectasis	Partially responsive
Diffusion impairment	Pneumonia, pulmonary edema, fibrosis, emphysema	Responsive
Decreased F_{IO_2}	Smoke inhalation, altitude	Responsive
Histiocytic hypoxia	Septic shock, toxins	Not very responsive
Circulatory hypoxia	Low cardiac output, vascular obstruction	Responsive

A patient's oxygenation status can be monitored invasively by drawing of arterial blood gas samples or noninvasively through pulse oximetry, in most cases (see Acid-Base Physiology and Pulse Oximetry). Inspired air at sea level has a P_{O_2} of 150 mm Hg. As the air travels through the upper respiratory system to the level of the alveolus, the P_{O_2} drops to 100 mm Hg. Tissue oxygen saturation in a normal healthy animal is 95 mm Hg. After oxygen has been delivered to the tissues, the oxygen left in the venous system (P_{VO_2}) is approximately 40 mm Hg.

Normally, oxygen diffuses across the alveolar capillary membrane and binds reversibly with hemoglobin in RBCs. A small amount of oxygen is carried in an unbound diffusible form in the plasma. When an animal has an adequate amount of hemoglobin and hemoglobin becomes fully saturated while breathing room air, supplemental oxygen administration will only increase the S_{aO_2} a small amount. The unbound form of oxygen dissolved in plasma will increase. If, however, inadequate hemoglobin saturation is obtained by breathing room air, as in a case of pneumonia or pulmonary edema, for example, breathing a higher fraction of inspired oxygen (F_{IO_2}) will improve bound and unbound hemoglobin levels. The formula for calculating oxygen content of arterial blood is as follows:

$$C_{aO_2} = (1.34 \times [Hb] \times S_{aO_2}) + (0.003 \times P_{aO_2})$$

where C_{aO_2} is the arterial oxygen content, 1.34 is the amount of oxygen that can be carried by hemoglobin (Hb), S_{aO_2} is the hemoglobin saturation, and 0.003 $\times P_{aO_2}$ is the amount of oxygen dissolved (unbound) in plasma.

Dissolved oxygen actually contributes little to the total amount of oxygen carried in the arterial blood, and the majority depends on the amount or availability of hemoglobin and the ability of the body (pH and respiratory status) to saturate the hemoglobin at the level of the alveoli.

INDICATIONS FOR OXYGEN THERAPY

Oxygen therapy is indicated whenever hypoxia is present. The underlying cause of the hypoxia also must be identified and treated, for chronic, lifelong oxygen therapy is rarely feasible in veterinary patients. If hemoglobin levels are low due to anemia, oxygen supplementation must occur along with RBC transfusions to increase hemoglobin mass. Whenever possible, use arterial blood gas analyses or pulse oximetry to gauge a patient's response to oxygen therapy and to determine when an animal can be weaned from supplemental oxygen.

The goal of oxygen therapy is to increase the amount of oxygen bound to hemoglobin in arterial blood. Oxygen supplementation can be by hood, oxygen cage or tent, nasal or nasopharyngeal catheter, or tracheal tube. In rare cases, administration of oxygen with mechanical ventilation may be indicated.

Administration of supplemental oxygen to patients with chronic hypoxia is sometimes necessary but also dangerous. With chronic hypoxia the patient develops a chronic respiratory acidosis (elevated P_{aCO_2}) and depends almost entirely on the hypoxic ventilatory drive to breathe. Administration of supplemental oxygen increases P_{aO_2} and may inhibit the central respiratory drive, leading to hypoventilation and possibly respiratory arrest. Therefore, closely monitor animals with chronic hypoxia that are treated with supplemental oxygen.

OXYGEN HOOD

Oxygen hoods can be purchased from commercial sources or can be manufactured in the hospital using a rigid Elizabethan collar, tape, and plastic wrap. To make an oxygen hood, place several lengths of plastic wrap over the front of the Elizabethan collar and tape them in place. Leave the ventral third of the collar open to allow moisture and heat to dissipate and carbon dioxide to be eliminated. Place a length of flexible oxygen tubing under the patient's collar into the front of the hood, and run humidified oxygen at a rate of 50 to 100 mL/kg/minute. Animals may become overheated with an oxygen hood in place.

Carefully monitor the patient's temperature so that iatrogenic hyperthermia does not occur.

OXYGEN CAGE

Commercially available plexiglass oxygen cages can be purchased from a variety of manufacturers. The best units include a mechanical thermostatically controlled compressor cooling unit, a circulatory fan, nebulizers or humidifiers to moisten the air, and a carbon dioxide absorber. Alternately, a pediatric (infant) incubator can be purchased from hospital supply sources, and humidified oxygen can be run into the cage at 2 to 10 L/minute (depending on the size of the cage). High flow rates may be required to eliminate nitrogen and carbon dioxide from the cage. In most cases, the FIO_2 inside the cage reaches 40% to 50% using this technique. Disadvantages of using an oxygen cage are high consumption/use of oxygen, rapid decrease in the FIO_2 within the cage whenever the cage must be opened for patient treatments, lack of immediate access to the patient, and potential for iatrogenic hyperthermia.

NASAL OR NASOPHARYNGEAL OXYGEN

One of the most common methods for oxygen supplementation in dogs is nasal or nasopharyngeal oxygen catheters:
1. To place a nasal or nasopharyngeal catheter, obtain a red rubber catheter (8F to 12F, depending on the size of the patient).
    a. For nasal oxygen supplementation, measure the distal tip of the catheter from the medial canthus of the eye to the tip of the nose.
    b. For nasopharyngeal oxygen supplementation, measure the catheter from the ramus of the mandible to the tip of the nose.
2. Mark the tube length at the tip of the nose with a permanent marker.
3. Instill topical anesthetic such as proparacaine (0.5%) or lidocaine (2%) into the nostril before placement.
4. Place a stay suture adjacent to (lateral aspect) the nostril while the topical anesthetic is taking effect.
5. Lubricate the tip of the tube with sterile lubricant.
6. Gently insert the tube into the ventral medial aspect of the nostril to the level made with the permanent marker. If you are inserting the tube into the nasopharynx, push the nasal meatus dorsally while simultaneously pushing the lateral aspect of the nostril medially to direct the tube into the ventral nasal meatus and avoid the cribriform plate.
7. Once the tube has been inserted to the appropriate length, hold the tube in place with your fingers adjacent to the nostril, and suture the tube to the stay suture. If the tube is removed, you can cut the suture around the tube and leave the stay suture in place for later use, if necessary.
8. Suture or staple the rest of the tube dorsally over the nose and in between the eyes to the top of the head, or laterally along the zygomatic arch.
9. Attach the tube to a length of flexible oxygen tubing, and provide humidified oxygen at 50 to 100 mL/kg/minute.
10. Secure an Elizabethan collar around the patient's head to prevent the patient from scratching at the tube and removing it.

MECHANICAL VENTILATION

The Rule of 60s states that if a patient's PaO_2 is less than 60 mm Hg, or if the $PaCO_2$ is 60 mm Hg, mechanical ventilation should be considered. For mechanical ventilation, anesthetize the patient and intubate the patient with an endotracheal tube. Alternately, a temporary tracheostomy can be performed and the patient can be maintained on a plane of light to heavy sedation and ventilated through the tracheostomy site. This method, although technically more invasive initially, allows the patient to be awake despite requiring mechanical ventilation.

Additional Reading

Camp-Palau MA, Marks SL, Cornick JL: Small animal oxygen therapy, *Compend Contin Educ Pract Vet* 21(7):587-597, 1999.

Drobatz K, Hackner S, Powell S: Oxygen supplementation. In Bonagura JD, editor: *Current veterinary therapy XII. Small animal practice*, Philadelphia, 1995, WB Saunders.

Dunphy EA, Mann FA, Dodam JR, et al: Comparison of unilateral versus bilateral nasal catheters for oxygen administration in dogs, *J Vet Emerg Crit Care* 12(4):245-251, 2002.

Marks SL: Nasal oxygen insufflation, *J Am Anim Hosp Assoc* 35(5):366-367, 1999.

PULSE OXIMETRY

A noninvasive means of determining oxygenation is through the use of pulse oximetry. A pulse oximeter uses different wavelengths of light to distinguish characteristic differences in the properties of the different molecules in a fluid or gas mixture, in this case, oxygenated (oxyhemoglobin) and deoxygenated hemoglobin (deoxyhemoglobin) in pulsatile blood. The process is termed *pulse oximetry*.

Oxyhemoglobin and deoxyhemoglobin are different molecules that absorb and reflect different wavelengths of light. Oxyhemoglobin absorbs light in the infrared spectrum, allowing wavelengths of light in the red spectrum to transmit through it. Conversely, deoxyhemoglobin absorbs wavelengths of the red spectrum and allows wavelengths in the infrared spectrum to transmit through the molecule. The spectrophotometer in the pulse oximeter transmits light in the red (660 nanometers) and infrared (920 nanometers) spectra. The different wavelengths of light are transmitted across a pulsatile vascular bed and are detected by a photodetector on the other side. The photodetector processes the amount of light of varying wavelengths that reaches it, then transmits an electrical current to a processor that calculates the difference in the amount of light originally transmitted and the amount of light of similar wavelength that actually reaches the photodetector. The difference in each reflects the amount of light absorbed in the pulsatile blood and can be used to calculate the amount or ratio of oxyhemoglobin to deoxyhemoglobin in circulation, or the functional hemoglobin saturation by the formula:

$$Sao_2 = HbO_2/HbO_2 + Hb$$

where *HbO$_2$* is oxygenated hemoglobin, and *Hb* is deoxygenated hemoglobin. Four molecules of oxygen reversibly bind to hemoglobin for transport to the tissues. Carbon monoxide similarly binds to hemoglobin and forms carboxyhemoglobin, a molecule that is detected similarly as oxygenated hemoglobin. Thus Sao$_2$ as detected by a pulse oximeter is not reliable if carboxyhemoglobin is present.

In most cases, pulse oximetry or Sao$_2$ corresponds reliably to the oxyhemoglobin dissociation curve. Oxygen saturation greater than 90% corresponds to a Pao$_2$ greater than 60 mm Hg. Above this value, large changes in Pao$_2$ are reflected in relatively small changes in Sao$_2$, making pulse oximetry a relatively insensitive method of determining oxygenation status when Pao$_2$ is normal.

Because pulse oximetry measures oxygenated versus nonoxygenated hemoglobin in pulsatile blood flow, it is fairly unreliable when severe vasoconstriction, hypothermia, shivering or trembling, or excessive patient movement are present. Additionally, increased ambient lighting and the presence of methemoglobin or carboxyhemoglobin also can cause artifactual changes in the Sao$_2$, and thus the measurement is not reliable or accurate. Most pulse oximeters also display a waveform and the patient's heart rate. If the photodetector does not detect a good quality signal, the waveform will not be normal, and the heart rate displayed on the monitor will not correlate with the patient's actual heart rate.

1

CAPNOMETRY (END-TIDAL CARBON DIOXIDE MONITORING)

The efficiency of ventilation is evaluated using the $PaCO_2$ value on an arterial blood gas sample. Alternatively, a noninvasive method to determine end-tidal carbon dioxide is through use of a capnograph. The science of capnometry uses a spectrophotometer to measure carbon dioxide levels in exhaled gas. The capnometer is placed in the expiratory limb of an anesthetic circuit. A sample of exhaled gas is aliquoted from the breath, and an infrared light source is passed across the sample. A photodetector on the other side of the sample flow measures the amount or concentration of carbon dioxide in the sample of expired gas. The calculated value is displayed as end-tidal carbon dioxide. This value also can be displayed as a waveform.

When placed in graphic form, a waveform known as a capnograph is displayed throughout the ventilatory cycle. Normally, at the onset of exhalation, the gas exhaled into the expiratory limb of the tubing comes from the upper airway or physiologic dead space and contains relatively little carbon dioxide. As exhalation continues, a steep uphill slope occurs as more carbon dioxide is exhaled from the bronchial tree. Near the end of exhalation, the capnogram reaches a plateau, which most accurately reflects the carbon dioxide level at the level of the alveolus. Because carbon dioxide diffuses across the alveolar basement membrane so rapidly, this reflects arterial carbon dioxide levels. If a plateau is not reached and notching of the waveform occurs, check the system for leaks. If the baseline waveform does not reach zero, the patient may be rebreathing carbon dioxide or may be tachypneic, causing physiologic positive end-expiratory pressure. The soda-sorb in the system should be replaced if it has expired. Conversely, low end-tidal carbon dioxide may be associated with a decrease in perfusion or blood flow. Decreased perfusion can be associated with low end-tidal carbon dioxide values, particularly during cardiopulmonary cerebral resuscitation. End-tidal carbon dioxide levels are one of the most accurate predictors of the efficacy of cardiopulmonary cerebral resuscitation and patient outcome. Additionally, the difference between arterial carbon dioxide levels ($PaCO_2$) and end-tidal carbon dioxide can be used to calculate dead-space ventilation. Increases in the difference also occur with poor lung perfusion and pulmonary diffusion impairment.

Additional Reading

Day TK: Blood gas analysis, *Vet Clin North Am Small Anim Pract* 32:1031-1048, 2002.
Hackett TB: Pulse oximetry and end-tidal carbon dioxide monitoring, *Vet Clin North Am Small Anim Pract* 32:1021-1029, 2002.
Hendricks JC, King LG: Practicality, usefulness, and limits of pulse oximetry in critical small animal patients, *J Vet Emerg Crit Care* 3:5-12, 1993.
Marino PL: Oximetry and capnography. In *The ICU book,* ed 2, Baltimore, 1998, Williams & Wilkins.
Proulx J: Respiratory monitoring: arterial blood gas analysis, pulse oximetry, and end-tidal carbon dioxide analysis, *Clin Tech Small Anim Pract* 14:227-230, 1999.
Wright B, Hellyer PW: Respiratory monitoring during anesthesia: pulse oximetry and capnography, *Compend Contin Educ Pract Vet* 18:1083-1097, 1996.

THORACOCENTESIS

Thoracocentesis refers to the aspiration of fluid or air from within the pleural space. Thoracocentesis may be diagnostic to determine whether air or fluid is present and to characterize the nature of the fluid obtained. Thoracocentesis also can be therapeutic when removing large volumes of air or fluid to allow pulmonary reexpansion and correction of hypoxemia and orthopnea.

To perform thoracocentesis, follow this procedure:

1. First, assemble the equipment necessary (Box 1-16).
2. Next, clip a 10-cm square in the center of the patient's thorax on both sides.
3. Aseptically scrub the clipped area.
4. Ideally, thoracocentesis should be performed within the seventh to ninth intercostal space. Rather than count rib spaces in an emergent situation, visualize the thoracic

---

BOX 1-16   EQUIPMENT REQUIRED FOR THORACOCENTESIS

- 22- to 20-inch over-the-needle catheters or hypodermic needles
- 60-mL catheter-tipped syringe
- Intravenous extension tubing
- Three-way stopcock
- Clippers
- Antimicrobial scrub
- Latex gloves

---

cage as a box, and the clipped area as a box within the box. You will insert your needle or catheter in the center of the box and then direct the bevel of the needle dorsally or ventrally to penetrate pockets of fluid or air present.

5. Attach the needle or catheter hub to the length of intravenous extension tubing. Attach the female port of the intravenous extension tubing to the male port of the three-way stopcock. Attach the male port of the 60-mL syringe to one of the female ports of the three-way stopcock. The apparatus is now assembled for use.
6. Insert the needle through the intercostal space such that the bevel of the needle initially is directed downward.
7. Next, push down on the hub of the needle such that the needle becomes parallel with the thoracic wall. By moving the hub of the needle in a clockwise or counterclockwise manner, the bevel of the needle will move within the thoracic cavity to penetrate pockets of air or fluid. In general, air is located dorsally and fluid is located more ventrally, although this does not always occur.
8. Aspirate air or fluid. Save any fluid obtained for cytologic and biochemical analyses and bacterial culture and susceptibility testing. In cases of pneumothorax, if the thoracocentesis needs to be repeated more than 3 times, consider using a thoracostomy tube.

THORACOSTOMY TUBE

Place a thoracostomy tube in cases of pneumothorax whenever negative suction cannot be obtained or repeated accumulation of air requires multiple thoracocentesis procedures. Thoracostomy tubes also can be placed to drain rapidly accumulating pleural effusion and for the medical management of pyothorax. Before attempting thoracostomy tube placement, make sure that all necessary supplies are assembled (Box 1-17; Table 1-13).

To place a thoracostomy tube, follow this procedure:

1. Lay the patient in lateral recumbency.
2. Clip the patient's entire lateral thorax.
3. Aseptically scrub the lateral thorax.
4. Palpate the tenth intercostal space.
5. Have an assistant pull the patient's skin cranially and ventrally toward the point of the elbow. This will facilitate creating a subcutaneous tunnel around the thoracostomy tube.
6. Draw up 2 mg/kg 2% lidocaine (1 mg/kg for cats) along with a small amount of sodium bicarbonate to take away some of the sting.
7. Insert the needle at the dorsal aspect of the tenth intercostal space and to the seventh intercostal space. Inject the lidocaine into the seventh intercostal space at the point where the trocarized thoracic drainage catheter will penetrate into the thoracic cavity. Slowly infuse the lidocaine as you withdraw the needle to create an anesthetized tunnel through which to insert the catheter.
8. While the local anesthetic is taking effect, remove the trocar from the catheter and cut the proximal end of the catheter with a Mayo scissors to facilitate adaptation with the Christmas tree adapter.

1

BOX 1-17   SUPPLIES REQUIRED FOR PLACEMENT OF A THORACOSTOMY TUBE

- Argyle trocar thoracic drainage catheter
- Three-way stopcock
- 22-gauge orthopedic wire
- No. 10 scalpel blade
- Needle holder (sterile)
- Sterile huck towels
- Thumb forceps (sterile)
- 2-0 to 0 nonabsorbable suture
- Gauze 4 × 4-inch squares (sterile)
- Clippers
- Clear adhesive antimicrobial barrier drape
- Christmas tree adapter
- Intravenous extension tubing
- Mayo scissors (sterile)
- Scalpel handle (sterile)
- 2% lidocaine
- Towel clamps
- 25-gauge hypodermic needle
- 3- to 6-mL syringe
- Cotton roll gauze
- Elastikon
- Sterile gloves

TABLE 1-13   Size of Dog or Cat and Appropriate Chest Catheter Size

Dog/Cat size	Catheter
<7 kg	14-16 F
7-15 kg	18-22 F
16-30 kg	22-28 F
>30 kg	28-36 F

---

9. Attach the Christmas tree adapter to the three-way stopcock and the three-way stopcock to a length of intravenous extension tubing and the 60-mL syringe so that the apparatus can be attached immediately to the thoracostomy tube after placement.
10. Aseptically scrub the lateral thorax a second time and then drape it with sterile huck towels secured with towel clamps.
11. Wearing sterile gloves, make a small stab incision at the dorsal aspect of the tenth intercostal space.
12. Insert the trocar back into the thoracostomy drainage tube. Insert the trocar and tube into the incision. Tunnel the tube cranially for approximately 3 intercostal spaces while an assistant simultaneously pulls the skin cranially and ventrally toward the point of the elbow.
13. At the seventh intercostal space, direct the trocar and catheter perpendicular to the thorax. Grasp the catheter apparatus at the base adjacent to the thorax to prevent the trocar from going too far into the thorax.
14. Place the palm of your dominant hand over the end of the trocar, and push the trocar and catheter into the thoracic cavity, throwing your weight into the placement in a swift motion, not by banging the butt of your hand on the end of the stylette. For small individuals, standing on a stool, or kneeling over the patient on the triage table can create leverage and make this process easier. The tube will enter the thorax with a pop.
15. Gently push the catheter off of the stylette, and remove the stylette.
16. Immediately attach the Christmas tree adapter and have an assistant start to withdraw air or fluid while you secure the tube in place.
17. First, place a horizontal mattress suture around the tube to cinch the skin securely to the tube. Use care to not penetrate the tube with your needle and suture.
18. Next, place a purse-string suture around the tube at the tube entrance site. Leave the ends of the suture long, so that you can create a finger-trap suture to the tube, holding the tube in place.

19. Place a large square of antimicrobial-impregnated adhesive tape over the tube for further security and sterility.
20. If antimicrobial adhesive is not available, place a gauze pad 4 × 4 inches square over the tube, and then wrap the tube to the thorax with cotton roll gauze and Elastikon adhesive tape.
21. Draw the location of the tube on the bandage to prevent cutting it with subsequent bandage changes.

An alternate technique to use if a trocar thoracic drainage catheter is not available is the following:

1. Prepare the lateral thorax and infuse local lidocaine anesthetic as listed before.
2. Make a small stab incision with a No. 10 scalpel blade, as listed before.
3. Obtain the appropriately sized red rubber catheter and cut multiple side ports in the distal end of the catheter, taking care to not cut more than 50% of the circumference of the diameter of the tube.
4. Insert a rigid, long urinary catheter into the red rubber catheter to make the catheter more rigid during insertion into the pleural space.
5. Grasp the distal end of the catheter(s) in the teeth of a large Carmalt. Tunnel a Metzenbaum scissors under the skin to the seventh intercostal space and make a puncture through the intercostal space.
6. Remove the Metzenbaum scissors, and then tunnel the Carmalt and red rubber tube under the skin to the hole created in the seventh intercostal space with the Metzenbaum scissors.
7. Insert the tips of the Carmalt and the red rubber catheter through the hole, and then open the teeth of the Carmalt.
8. Push the red rubber catheter cranially into the pleural cavity.
9. Remove the Carmalt and the rigid urinary catheter, and immediately attach the suction apparatus. Secure the red rubber catheter in place as listed before.

Additional Reading

Mazzaferro EM: Pulmonary injury secondary to trauma. In Wingfield WE, Raffe MR, editors: *The veterinary ICU book,* Jackson, Wyo, 2002, Teton NewMedia.

Tseng LW, Waddell LS: Approach to the patient in respiratory distress, *Clin Tech Small Anim Pract* 15(2):53-62, 2000.

TRACHEOSTOMY

Placement of a temporary tracheostomy can be lifesaving to relieve upper respiratory tract obstruction, to facilitate removal of airway secretions, to decrease dead space ventilation, to provide a route of inhalant anesthesia during maxillofacial surgery, and to facilitate mechanical ventilation.

In an emergent situation in which asphyxiation is imminent and endotracheal intubation is not possible, any cutting instrument placed into the trachea distal to the point of obstruction can be used. To perform a slash tracheostomy, quickly clip the fur and scrub the skin over the third tracheal ring. Make a small cut in the trachea with a No. 11 scalpel blade, and insert a firm tube, such as a syringe casing. Alternately, insertion of a 22-gauge needle attached to intravenous extension tubing and adapted with a 1-mL syringe case to attach to a humidified oxygen source also temporarily can relieve obstruction until a temporary tracheostomy can be performed.

In less emergent situations, place the patient under general anesthesia and intubate the patient. Assemble all the equipment necessary before starting the temporary tracheostomy procedure (Box 1-18).

To perform a tracheostomy, follow this procedure:

1. Place the patient in dorsal recumbency.
2. Clip the ventral cervical region from the level of the ramus of the mandible caudally to the thoracic inlet and dorsally to midline.

1

BOX 1-18 SUPPLIES REQUIRED FOR A TRACHEOSTOMY	
• Sterile huck towels • Towel clamps • Antimicrobial scrub • No. 10 scalpel blade • Curved mosquito hemostats • Metzenbaum scissors • Thumb forceps	• 3-0 to 2-0 nonabsorbable suture material • Needle holders • Shiley low-pressure cuff tracheostomy tube OR endotracheal tube that has been cut and adapted to create a tracheostomy tube • Umbilical tape

3. Aseptically scrub the clipped area, and then drape with sterile huck towels secured with towel clamps.
4. Make a 3-cm ventral midline skin incision over the third to sixth tracheal rings, perpendicular to the trachea.
5. Bluntly dissect through the sternohyoid muscles to the level of the trachea.
6. Carefully pick up the fascia overlying the trachea and cut it away with a Metzenbaum scissors.
7. Place two stay sutures through/around adjacent tracheal rings.
8. Incise in between trachea rings with a No. 11 scalpel blade. Take care to not cut more than 50% of the circumference of the trachea.
9. Using the stay sutures, pull the edges of the tracheal incision apart, and insert the tracheostomy tube. The Shiley tube contains an internal obturator to facilitate placement into the tracheal lumen. Remove the obturator, and then insert the inner cannula, which can be removed for cleaning as needed.
10. Once the tube is in place, secure the tube around the neck with a length of sterile umbilical tape.

TRACHEOSTOMY TUBE CARE

Postoperative care of the tracheostomy tube is as important as the procedure itself. Because the tracheostomy tube essentially bypasses the protective effects of the upper respiratory system, one of the most important aspects of tracheostomy tube care and maintenance is to maintain sterility at all times. Any oxygen source should be humidified with sterile water or saline to prevent drying of the respiratory mucosa. If supplemental oxygen is not required, instill 2 to 3 mL of sterile saline every 1 to 2 hours to moisten the mucosa. Wearing sterile gloves, remove the internal tube and place it in a sterile bowl filled with sterile hydrogen peroxide and to be cleaned every 4 hours (or more frequently as necessary). If a Shiley tube is not available, apply suction to the internal lumen of the tracheostomy tube every 1 to 2 hours (or more frequently as needed) with a sterile 12F red rubber catheter attached to a vacuum pump to remove any mucus or other debris that potentially could plug the tube. Unless the patient demonstrates clinical signs of fever or infection, the prophylactic use of antibiotics is discouraged because of the risk of causing a resistant infection. After the temporary tracheostomy is no longer necessary, remove the tube and sutures, and leave the wound to heal by second intention. Primary closure of the wounds could predispose the patient to subcutaneous emphysema and infection.

Additional Reading

Baker GD: Trans-tracheal oxygen therapy in dogs with severe respiratory compromise due to tick (*I. holocyclus*) toxicity, *Aust Vet Pract* 34(2):83, 2004.

Colley P, Huber M, Henderson R: Tracheostomy techniques and management, *Compend Contin Educ Pract Vet* 21(1):44-53, 1999.

Hedlund CS: Surgery of the upper respiratory system. In Fossum TW, editor: *Small animal surgery*, St Louis, 2002, Mosby.

Hedlund CS: Tracheostomies in the management of canine and feline upper respiratory disease, *Vet Clin North Am Small Anim Pract* 24(5):873-886, 1994.

UROHYDROPULSION

Urohydropulsion is a therapeutic procedure for removal of uroliths from the urethra of the male dog. The technique works best if the animal is heavily sedated or is placed under general anesthesia (Figure 1-12).

To perform urohydropulsion, follow this procedure:

1. Place the animal in lateral recumbency.
2. Clip the fur from the distal portion of the prepuce.
3. Aseptically scrub the prepuce and flush the prepuce with 12 to 20 mL of antimicrobial flush solution.
4. Have an assistant who is wearing gloves retract the penis from the prepuce.
5. While wearing sterile gloves, lubricate the tip of a rigid urinary catheter as for urethral catheterization.
6. Gently insert the tip of the catheter into the urethra until you meet the resistance of the obstruction.
7. Pinch the tip of the penis around the catheter.
8. Have an assistant insert a gloved lubricated finger into the patient's rectum and press ventrally on the floor of the rectum to obstruct the pelvic urethra.
9. Attach a 60-mL syringe filled with sterile saline into proximal tip of the catheter.
10. Quickly inject fluid into the catheter and alternate compression and relaxation on the pelvic urethra such that the urethra dilates and suddenly releases the pressure, causing dislodgement of the stone. Small stones may be ejected from the tip of the urethra, whereas larger stones may be retropulsed back into the urinary bladder to be removed surgically at a later time.

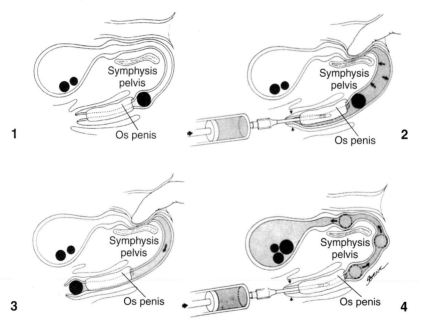

Figure 1-12: Removal of urethrolith in a male dog by urohydropropulsion: *1,* Urethrolith originating from the urinary bladder has lodged behind the os penis. *2,* Dilation of the urethral lumen is achieved by injecting fluid with pressure. Digital pressure applied to the external urethral orifice and the pelvic urethra has created a closed system. *3,* Sudden release of digital pressure at the external urethral orifice and subsequent movement of fluid and urethrolith toward the external urethral orifice. *4,* Sudden release of digital pressure at the pelvic urethra and subsequent movement of fluid and urethrolith toward the urinary bladder.

(From Osborne CA, Finco DR: Canine and Feline Nephrology and Urology. Williams and Wilkins, Baltimore, 1995.)

Additional Reading

Osborne CA, Finco DR: *Canine and feline nephrology and urology,* Baltimore, 1995, Williams & Wilkins.

VASCULAR ACCESS TECHNIQUES

The type of catheter that you choose for vascular access depends largely on the size and species of the patient, the fragility of the vessels to be catheterized, the proposed length of time that the catheter will be in place, the type and viscosity of the fluid or drug to be administered, the rate of fluid flow desired, and whether multiple repeated blood samples will be required (Table 1-14).

A variety of over-the-needle, through-the-needle, and over-the-wire catheters are available for placement in a variety of vessels, including the jugular, cephalic, accessory cephalic, medial saphenous, lateral saphenous, dorsal pedal artery, and femoral artery.

One of the most important aspects of proper catheter placement and maintenance is to maintain cleanliness at all times. The patient's urine, feces, saliva, and vomit are common sources of contamination of the catheter site. Before placing a peripheral or central catheter in any patient, consider the patient's physical status including whether vomiting, diarrhea, excessive urination, or seizures. In a patient with an oral mass that is drooling excessively or a patient that is vomiting, peripheral cephalic catheterization may not be the most appropriate, to prevent contamination. Conversely, in a patient with excessive urination or diarrhea, a lateral or medial saphenous catheter is likely to become contaminated quickly.

Whenever one places or handles a catheter or intravenous infusion line, the person should wash the hands carefully and wear gloves to prevent contamination of the intravenous catheter and fluid lines. One of the most common sources of catheter contamination in veterinary hospitals is through caretakers' hands. In emergent situations, placement of a catheter may be necessary under less than ideal circumstances. Remove those catheters as soon as the patient is more stable, and place a second catheter using aseptic techniques.

In general, once the location of the catheter has been decided, set up all equipment necessary for catheter placement before starting to handle and restrain the patient. Box 1-19 lists the equipment needed for most types of catheter placement.

TABLE 1-14 Catheter Sizes for Vascular Access

	Cephalic or tarsal vein (catheter gauge)	Jugular (catheter gauge)
Cat or small dog	20-24	16-18
Medium-sized dog	18-22	16-18
Large dog	14-20	14-18

BOX 1-19 EQUIPMENT NECESSARY FOR INTRAVENOUS CATHETER PLACEMENT

- Antimicrobial ointment
- Antimicrobial scrub
- Cotton ball
- Electric clippers and No. 40 blade
- Gauze, 4 × 4-inch squares
- Heparinized saline flush
- Intravenous catheter
- 1/2- and 1-inch white adhesive tape
- Male adapter or T port flushed with heparinized saline

After setting up all of the supplies needed, clip the fur over the site of catheter placement. Make sure to clip all excess fur and long feathers away from the catheter site, to prevent contamination. For catheter placement in limbs, clip the fur circumferentially around the site of catheter placement to facilitate adherence of the tape to the limb and to facilitate catheter removal with minimal discomfort at a later date. Next, aseptically scrub the catheter site with an antimicrobial scrub solution such as Hibiclens. The site is now ready for catheter insertion.

Central Venous Catheters

Consider using a central venous catheter whenever multiple repeated blood samples will need to be collected from a patient during the hospital stay. Central venous catheters also can be used for CVP measurement, administration of hyperoncotic solutions such as parenteral nutrition, and administration of crystalloid and colloid fluids, anesthesia, and other injectable drugs (Figures 1-13 and 1-14).

Percutaneous through-the-needle jugular catheter placement

To place a jugular central venous catheter, place the patient in lateral recumbency and extend the head and neck such that the jugular furrow is straight. Clip the fur from the ramus of the mandible caudally to the thoracic inlet and dorsally and ventrally to midline. Wipe the clipped area with gauze 4 × 4-inch squares to remove any loose fur and other debris. Aseptically scrub the clipped area with an antimicrobial cleanser.

Venocaths (Abbott Laboratories) are a through-the-needle catheter that is contained within a sterile sleeve for placement. Alternately, other over-the-wire central venous catheters can be placed by the Seldinger technique. Sterility must be maintained at all times, regardless of the type of catheter placed.

Wearing sterile gloves, drape the site of catheter placement with sterile drapes, and occlude the jugular vein at the level of the thoracic inlet. Pull the clear ring and wings of

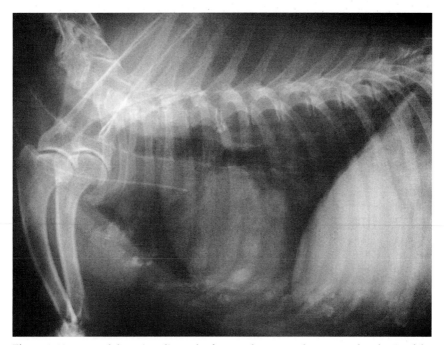

Figure 1-13:   Lateral thoracic radiograph of a central venous catheter. Note that the tip of the catheter is inserted in its proper location, just outside of the right atrium.

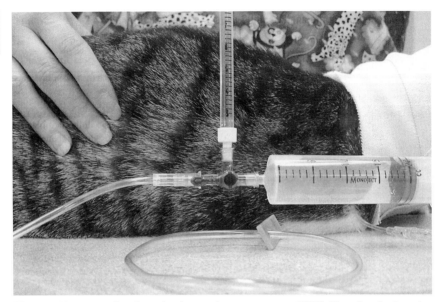

Figure 1-14: Measuring the patient's central venous pressure (CVP). Note that the 0 marker on the manometer is at the patient's manubrium.

the catheter cover down toward the catheter itself to expose the needle. Remove the guard off of the needle. Lift the skin over the proposed site of catheter insertion and insert the needle under the skin, with the bevel of the needle facing up. Next, reocclude the vessel and pull the skin tight over the vessel to prevent movement of the vessel as you attempt to insert the needle. In some cases, it may be difficult actually to see the vessel in obese patients. If you cannot visualize or palpate the needle, gently bounce the needle over the vessel with the bevel up. The vessel will bounce in place slightly, allowing a brief moment of visualization to facilitate catheter placement. Once the vessel has been isolated and visualized, insert the needle into the vessel at a 15- to 30-degree angle. Watch closely for a flash of blood in the catheter. When blood is observed, insert the needle a small distance farther, and then push the catheter and stylette into the vessel for the entire length, until the catheter and stylette can be secured in the catheter hub. If the catheter cannot be inserted fully into the vessel for its entire length, the tip of the needle may not be within the entire lumen, the catheter may be directed perivascularly, and the catheter may be caught at the thoracic flexure and may be moving into one of the tributaries that feeds the forelimb. Extend the patient's head and neck, and lift the forelimb up to help facilitate placement. Do not force the catheter in because the catheter potentially can form a knot and will need to be removed surgically. Remove the needle from the vessel, and have an assistant place several 4 × 4-inch gauze squares over the site of catheter placement with some pressure to control hemorrhage. Secure the catheter hub into the needle guard, and remove the stylette from the catheter. Immediately insert a 3- to 6-mL syringe of heparinized saline and flush the catheter and draw back. If you are in the correct place, you will be able to draw blood from the catheter.

To secure the catheter in place, tear a length of 1-inch white tape that will wrap around the patient's neck. Pull a small length of the catheter out of the jugular vein to make a semicircle. The semicircle should be approximately ½ inch in diameter. Let the length of catheter lie on the skin, and then place 4 × 4-inch gauze squares impregnated with antimicrobial ointment over the site of catheter insertion. Secure the proximal end of white tape around the white and blue pieces of the catheter, and wrap the tape around the patient's neck so that the tape adheres to the skin and fur. Repeat the process by securing the gauze to the skin with two additional lengths of white tape, starting to secure the gauze in place by first wrapping the tape dorsally over the patient's neck, rather than under the patient's neck. In between each piece of tape and bandage layer, make sure that the catheter flushes and draws back freely, or else occlusion can occur. Gently wrap layers of cotton roll gauze, Kling, and Elastikon or Vetrap over the catheter. Secure a male adapter or T port that has been flushed with heparinized saline, and then label the catheter with the size and length of catheter, date of catheter placement, and initials of the person who placed the catheter. The catheter is ready for use. Monitor the catheter site daily for erythema, drainage, vessel thickening, or pain upon infusion. If any of these signs occur, or if the patient develops a fever of unknown origin, remove the catheter, culture the catheter tip aseptically, and replace the catheter in a different location. As long as the catheter is functional without complications, the catheter can remain in place.

Percutaneous over-the-wire jugular catheter placement (Seldinger technique)

Central catheters also can be placed via the Seldinger or over-the-wire technique. A number of companies manufacture kits that contain the supplies necessary for over-the-wire catheter placement. Each kit minimally should contain an over-the-needle catheter to place into the vessel, a long wire to insert through the original catheter placed, a vascular dilator to dilate the hole in the vessel created by the first catheter, and a long catheter to place into the vessel over the wire. Additional accessories can include a paper drape, sterile gauze, a scalpel blade, local anesthetic, 22-gauge needles, and 3- or 6-mL syringes.

Restrain the patient and prepare the jugular furrow aseptically as for the percutaneous through-the-needle catheter placement. The person placing the catheter should wear sterile gloves throughout the process to maintain sterility. Pick up the skin over the site of catheter placement, and insert a small bleb of local anesthetic through the skin. The local anesthetic should not be injected into the underlying vessel (Figure 1-15). Make a small

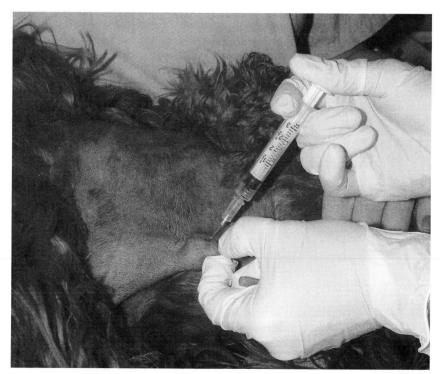

Figure 1-15: Infusion of local anesthetic. Before making a nick incision through the skin, insert a bleb of lidocaine over the proposed site of catheter insertion. Pick up the skin to avoid intravenous injection of the anesthetic.

nick into the skin through the local anesthetic with a No. 10 or No. 11 scalpel blade. Use care to avoid lacerating the underlying vessel. Next, occlude the jugular vein as previously described, and insert the over-the-needle catheter into the vessel. Watch for a flash of blood in the catheter hub. Remove the stylette from the catheter. Next, insert the long wire into the catheter and into the vessel (Figures 1-16 and 1-17). Never let go of the wire. Remove the catheter, and place the vascular dilator over the wire and into the vessel (Figure 1-18). Gently twist to place the dilator into the vessel a short distance, creating a larger hole in the vessel. The vessel will bleed more after creating a larger hole. Remove the vascular dilator, and leave the wire in place within the vessel. Insert the long catheter over the wire into the vessel (Figure 1-19). Push the catheter into the vessel to the catheter hub (Figure 1-20). Slowly thread the wire through a proximal port in the catheter. Once the catheter is in place, remove the wire, and suture the catheter in place to the skin with nonabsorbable suture. Cover the catheter site with sterile gauze and antimicrobial ointment, cotton roll bandaging material, gauze, and Kling or Vetrap. Flush the catheter with heparinized saline solution, and then use the catheter for infusion of parenteral nutrition, blood products, crystalloid and colloid fluids, medications, and frequent blood sample collection. Examine the catheter site daily for evidence of infection or thrombophlebitis. The catheter can remain in place as long as it functions and no complications occur.

PERIPHERAL ARTERIAL AND VENOUS CATHETER PLACEMENT

Cephalic catheterization

Place the patient in sternal recumbency as for cephalic venipuncture. Clip the antebrachium circumferentially, and wipe the area clean of any loose fur and debris (Figure 1-21). Aseptically scrub the clipped area, and have an assistant occlude the cephalic vein at the crook of the elbow. The person placing the catheter should grasp the distal carpus with the nondominant hand and insert the over-the-needle catheter into the vessel at a 15- to 30-degree angle (Figure 1-22). Watch for a flash of blood in the catheter hub, and then gently push the

Text continued on p. 66.

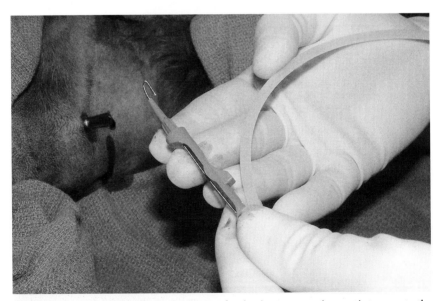

Figure 1-16:   The J-Wire. The J-wire is curved at its tip to prevent iatrogenic trauma to the vessel and the heart. Pull the J-wire back so that the curve straightens out, and then insert the J-wire into the vessel.

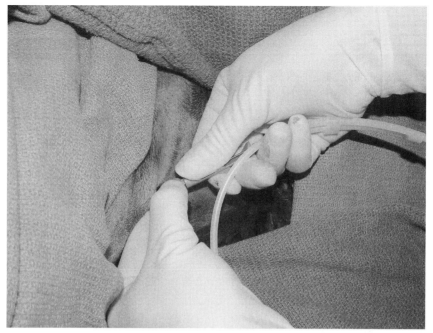

Figure 1-17:   Feeding the J-wire through the catheter. Insert the J-wire through the over-the-needle catheter into the vessel and then remove the over-the-needle catheter, leaving the J-wire in place. Never let go of the J-wire!

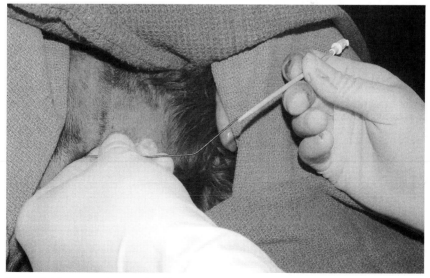

Figure 1-18:   Insert the vascular dilator over the wire into the vessel with a twisting motion, to enlarge the hole in the vessel for ease of catheter placement later.

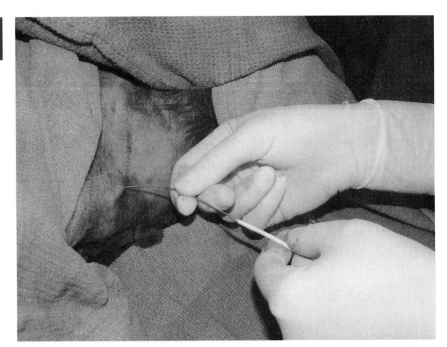

Figure 1-19: Feed the multi-lumen catheter over the wire that has already been inserted into the patient's vessel. Remember to never let go of the wire. The wire will eventually emerge from an open port in the proximal portion of the catheter, allowing its removal after the catheter has been seated in the vessel.

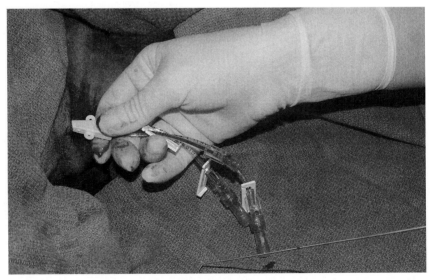

Figure 1-20: Catheter in vessel. The catheter is now seated in the patient's jugular vein, where it can be secured to the skin with nonabsorbable suture and then bandaged.

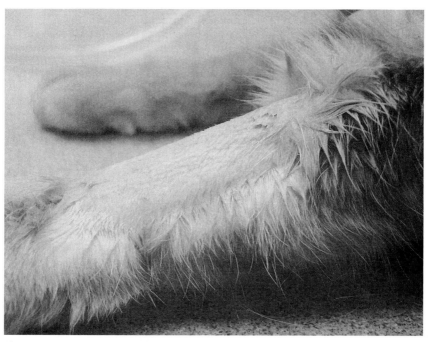

Figure 1-21: Clip the patient's antebrachium circumferentially to allow proper placement of the cephalic intravenous catheter.

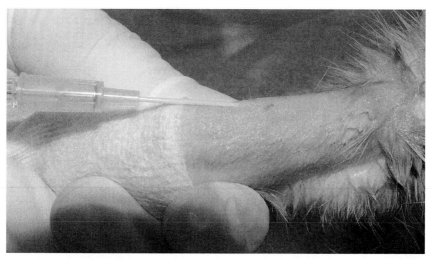

Figure 1-22: Insert the catheter through the skin into the vessel, watching for a flash of blood in the catheter hub.

catheter off of the stylette (Figure 1-23). Have the assistant occlude the vessel over the catheter to prevent backflow. Flush the catheter with heparinized saline solution. Make sure that the skin and catheter hub are clean and dry to ensure that the tape adheres to the catheter hub and skin. Secure a length of ½-inch white tape tightly around the catheter and then around the limb. Make sure that the catheter hub does not "spin" in the tape, or else the catheter will fall out. Next, secure a second length of 1-inch adhesive tape under the catheter and around the limb and catheter hub (Figure 1-24). This piece of tape helps to stabilize the catheter in place. Finally, place a flushed T port or male adapter in the catheter hub and secure to the limb with white tape. Make sure that the tape is adhered to the skin

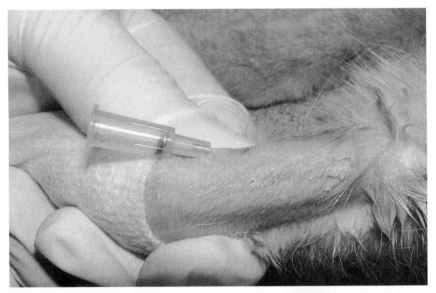

Figure 1-23:   Blood in the catheter hub.

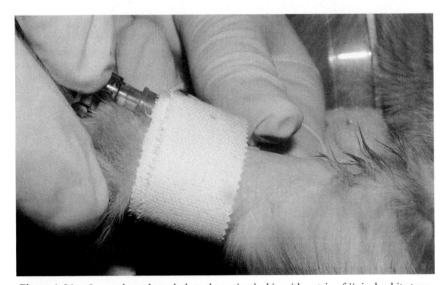

Figure 1-24:   Secure the catheter hub to the patient's skin with a strip of ½-inch white tape.

securely, but not so tightly as to impede venous outflow (Figure 1-25). The catheter site can be covered with a cotton ball impregnated with antimicrobial ointment and layers of bandage material. Label all catheters with the date of placement, the type and gauge of catheter inserted, and the initials of the person who placed the catheter.

Percutaneous femoral artery catheterization

The femoral artery can be catheterized for placement of an indwelling arterial catheter. Indwelling arterial catheters can be used for continuous invasive arterial blood pressure monitoring and for procurement of arterial blood samples. Place the patient in lateral recumbancy, and tape the down leg in an extended position. Clip the fur over the femoral artery and aseptically scrub the clipped area. Palpate the femoral artery as it courses distally on the medial surface of the femur and anterior to the pectineus muscle. Make a small nick incision over the proposed site of catheter placement using the bevel of an 18-gauge needle. Place a long over-the-needle catheter through the nick in the skin and direct it toward the palpable pulse. Place the tip of the catheter so that the needle tip rests in the subcutaneous tissue between the artery and the palpating index finger. Advance the needle steeply at a 30-degree angle to secure the superficial wall of the vessel and then the deep wall of the vessel. The spontaneous flow of blood in the catheter hub ensures that the catheter is

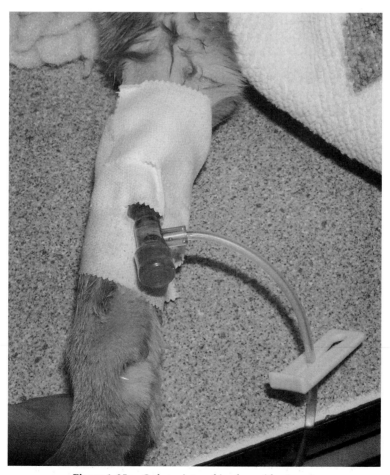

Figure 1-25:   Catheter is taped in place with a t-port.

situated in the lumen of the artery. Feed the catheter off of the stylette, and cover the hub with a catheter cap. Flush the catheter with sterile heparinized saline solution, and then secure it in place. Some persons simply tape the catheter in place with pieces of ½- and 1-inch adhesive tape. Others use a "butterfly" piece of tape around the catheter hub and suture or glue the tape to the adjacent skin for added security.

Percutaneous dorsal pedal artery catheterization

The dorsal pedal artery commonly is used for catheter placement. To place a dorsal pedal arterial catheter, place the patient in lateral recumbency. Clip the fur over the dorsal pedal artery, and then aseptically scrub the clipped area. Tape the distal limb so that the leg is twisted slightly medially for better exposure of the vessel, or the person placing the arterial catheter can manipulate the limb into the appropriate position. Palpate the dorsal pedal pulse as it courses dorsally over the tarsus. Place an over-the-needle catheter percutaneously at a 15- to 30-degree angle, threading the tip of the needle carefully toward the pulse. Advance the needle in short, blunt movements, and watch the catheter hub closely for a flash of pulsating blood that signifies penetration into the lumen of the artery. Then thread the catheter off of the stylette, and cover the catheter hub with a catheter cap. Secure the catheter in place with lengths of ½- and 1-inch adhesive tape as with any other intravenous catheter, and then flush it with heparinized saline solution every 2 to 4 hours.

Surgical cutdown for arterial and venous catheter placement

Any vessel that can be catheterized percutaneously also can be catheterized with surgical cutdown. Restrain the patient and clip and aseptically scrub the limb or jugular vein as for a percutaneous catheterization procedure. Block the area for catheter placement with a local anesthetic before cutting the skin over the vessel with a No. 11 scalpel blade. While wearing sterile gloves, pick up the skin and incise the skin over the vessel. Direct the sharp edge of the blade upward to avoid lacerating the underlying vessel. Using blunt dissection, push the underlying subcutaneous fat and perivascular fascia away from the vessel with a mosquito hemostat. Make sure that all tissue is removed from the vessel. Using the mosquito hemostat, place two stay sutures of absorbable suture under the vessel. Elevate the vessel until it is parallel with the incision, and gently insert the catheter and stylette into the vessel. Secure the stay sutures loosely around the catheter. Suture the skin over the catheter site with nonabsorbable suture, and then tape and bandage the catheter in place as for percutaneous placement. Remove catheters placed surgically as soon as possible and exchange them for a percutaneously placed catheter to avoid infection and thrombophlebitis.

MAINTENANCE OF INDWELLING ARTERIAL AND VENOUS CATHETERS

The most important aspect of catheter maintenance is to maintain cleanliness and sterility at all times. An indwelling catheter can remain in place for as long as it is functional and no complications occur. Change the bandage whenever it becomes wet or soiled to prevent wicking of bacteria and debris from the environment into the vessel. Check the bandages and catheter sites at least once a day for signs of thrombophlebitis: erythema, vessel hardening or ropiness, pain upon injection or infusion, and discharge. Also closely examine the tissue around and proximal and distal to the catheter. Swelling of the paw can signify that the catheter tape and bandage are too tight and are occluding venous outflow. Swelling above the catheter site is characteristic of perivascular leakage of fluid and may signify that the catheter is no longer within the lumen of the vessel.

Remove the catheter if it is no longer functional, if there is pain or resistance upon infusion, if there is unexplained fever or leukocytosis, or if there is evidence of cellulitis, thrombophlebitis, or catheter-related bacteremia or septicemia. Aseptically culture the tip of the indwelling catheter for bacteria. Animals should wear Elizabethan collars or other forms of restraint if they lick or chew at the catheter or bandage.

Catheter patency may be maintained with constant fluid infusion or by intermittent flushing with heparinized saline (1000 units of unfractionated heparin per 250 to 500 mL

1

of saline) every 6 hours. Flush arterial catheters more frequently (every 2 hours). Disconnect intravenous connections only when absolutely necessary. Wear gloves whenever handling the catheter or connections. Label all fluid lines and elevate them off of the floor to prevent contamination. Date each fluid line and replace it once every 24 to 36 hours.

INTRAOSSEOUS CATHETER PLACEMENT

If an intravenous catheter cannot be placed because of small patient size, hypovolemia, hypothermia, or severe hypotension, needles can be placed into the marrow cavity of the femur, humerus, and tibia for intraosseous infusion of fluids, drugs, and blood products. This technique is particularly useful in small kittens and puppies and in exotic species. Contraindications to intraosseous infusion is in avian species (which have air in their bones), fractures, and sepsis, because osteomyelitis can develop. An intraosseous catheter is relatively easy to place and maintain but can cause patient discomfort and so should be changed to an intravenous catheter as soon as vascular access becomes possible.

To place an intraosseous catheter, clip and aseptically scrub the fur over the proposed site of catheter placement. The easiest place for intraosseous placement is in the intertrochanteric fossa of the femur. Inject a small amount of a local anesthetic through the skin and into the periosteum where the trocar or needle will be inserted. Place the patient in lateral recumbency, and grasp the leg in between your fingers, with the stifle braced against the palm of your hand. Push the stifle toward the abdomen (medially) to abduct the proximal femur away from the body. This will shift the sciatic nerve out of the way of catheter placement. Insert the tip of the needle through the skin and into the intertrochanteric fossa. Gently push with a simultaneous twisting motion, pushing the needle parallel with the shaft of the femur, toward your palm. You may feel a pop or decreased resistance as the needle enters the marrow cavity. Gently flush the needle with heparinized saline. If the needle is plugged with bone debris, remove the needle and replace it with a fresh needle of the same type and size in the hole that you have created. A spinal needle with an internal stylette also can be placed. The stylette will prevent the needle from becoming clogged with bone debris during insertion. Secure the hub of the needle with a butterfly length of white adhesive tape and then suture it to the skin to keep the catheter in place. The catheter is now ready for use. The patient should wear an Elizabethan collar to prevent disruption or removal of the catheter. The intraosseous catheter can be maintained as any peripheral catheter, with frequent flushing and daily evaluation of the catheter site.

Additional Reading

Beal MW, Hughes D: Vascular access: theory and techniques in the small animal emergency patient, *Clin Tech Small Anim Pract* 15(2):101-109, 2000.

Hansen BD: Technical aspects of fluid therapy. In DiBartola S, editor: *Fluid therapy in small animal practice,* Philadelphia, 2000, WB Saunders.

Otto CM, Kaufman GM, Crowe DT: Intraosseous infusion of fluids and therapeutics, *Compend Contin Educ Pract Vet* 11:421-430, 1989.

Shaw S, Walshaw S: *Manual of clinical procedures in the dog, cat, and rabbit,* ed 2, Philadelphia, 1997, Lippincott-Raven.

PAIN: ASSESSMENT, PREVENTION, AND MANAGEMENT*

The definition of pain has been debated philosophically over the ages and has changed as knowledge has increased. Pain is defined as an unpleasant sensory or emotional experience associated with actual or perceived tissue damage. Until recognition of a noxious stimulus occurs in the cerebral cortex, no response or adaptation results. Rational management of pain requires an understanding of the underlying mechanisms involved in pain and an appreciation of how analgesic agents interact to disrupt pain mechanisms.

*Contributed by A. Looney, B. Hansen, and E. Hardie.

BOX 1-20 CATEGORIES AND CAUSES OF PAIN IN DOGS AND CATS	
ACUTE PAIN	**CHRONIC PAIN**
Trauma	Arthritis
Thermal burn	Cancer
Postoperative	Neurologic: diabetes mellitus
Musculoskeletal	Musculoskeletal
Visceral/pleural	Sympathetic dystrophies

Multiple factors and causes produce pain in human beings and domestic animal species. The causes of pain, psychological and physical, may derive from many different mechanisms within emergency medicine, among them trauma, infectious disease, neglect, environmental stress, surgery, and acute decompensation of chronic medical conditions. The two major classes of pain are acute and chronic pain. Box 1-20 gives specific categories and causes of pain.

The pain sensing and response system can be divided into the following categories: *nociceptors,* which detect and filter the intensity of the noxious stimuli; *primary afferent nerves,* which transmit impulses to the central nervous system (CNS); *ascending tracts,* which are part of the dorsal horn and the spinal cord that conveys stimuli to higher centers in the brain; *higher centers,* which are involved in pain discrimination, some memory, and motor control; and *modulating* or *descending systems,* which are a means of processing, memorizing, and modifying incoming impulses. Current analgesic therapies may inhibit afferent nociceptive transmission within the brain and spinal cord; directly interrupt neural impulse conduction through the dorsal horn, primary afferent nerves, or dorsal root ganglion; or prevent the nociceptor sensitization that accompanies initial pain and inflammation. The physiologic aspects of pain are believed to be produced by the transmission, transduction, and integration of initial nerve endings, peripheral neuronal input, and ascending afferent nerves via the thalamus to the cerebral cortex. Ascending afferent nerves to the limbic system are believed to be responsible for the emotional aspects of pain.

There are several classification schemes for different types of pain. *Acute pain,* such as that which results from trauma, surgery, or infectious agents, is abrupt in onset, relatively short in duration, and may be alleviated easily by analgesics. In contrast, *chronic pain* is a long-standing physical disorder or emotional distress that is slow in onset and difficult to treat. Both types of pain can be classified further based on site of origin. *Somatic pain* arises from superficial skin, subcutaneous tissue, body wall, or appendages. *Visceral pain* arises from abdominal or thoracic viscera and primarily is associated with serosal irritation. *Analgesia,* then, is the loss of pain WITHOUT the loss of consciousness. This is in contrast to *anesthesia,* which is the loss of sensation in the whole body or a part of the body WITH the loss of consciousness or at least depression of the CNS.

PHYSIOLOGIC IMPACT OF UNTREATED PAIN

Untreated pain causes immediate changes in the neurohormonal axis, which in turn causes restlessness, agitation, increased heart and respiratory rates, fever, and blood pressure fluctuations, all of which are detrimental to the healing of the animal. A catabolic state is created as a result of increased secretion of catabolic hormones and decreased secretion of anabolic hormones. The net effect the majority of neurohormonal changes produce is an increase in the secretion of catabolic hormones. Hyperglycemia is produced and may persist because of production of glucagon and relative lack of insulin. Lipolytic activity is stimulated by cortisol, catecholamines, and growth hormone. Cardiorespiratory effects of pain include increased cardiac output, vasoconstriction, hypoxemia, and hyperventilation. Protein catabolism is a common occurrence and major concern regarding healing. Pain associated with inflammation causes increase in tissue and blood levels of prostaglandins

1

and cytokines, both of which promote protein catabolism indirectly by increasing the energy expenditure of the body.

Powerful evidence indicates that local anesthetic, sympathetic agonist, and opioid neural blockade may produce a modification of the responses to these physiologic changes. Variable reduction in plasma cortisol, growth hormone, antidiuretic hormone, β-endorphin, aldosterone, epinephrine, norepinephrine, and renin is based on the anesthetic technique and the drugs selected. Prophylactic administration of analgesics blunts the response before it occurs; analgesics administered following perception or pain are not as effective, and higher doses are generally necessary to achieve an equivalent level of analgesia.

RECOGNITION AND ASSESSMENT OF PAIN

Effective pain control can be achieved only when the signs of pain can be assessed effectively, reliably, and regularly. The experience of pain is unique to each individual, which makes pain assessment difficult, especially in traumatized and critical patients. Most attempts to assess clinical pain use behavioral observations and interactive variables in addition to assessment of physiologic responses such as heart rate and respiratory rate, blood pressure, and temperature. But many factors can influence the processing and outward projection of pain, including altered environments, species differences, within-species variations (age, breed, sex), and the type, severity, and chronicity of pain.

Within-species differences (age, breed, and sex) further complicate the pain assessment. Most notable is that different breeds of dogs act differently when confronted with pain or fear. Labrador Retrievers tend to be stoic, whereas Greyhounds and teacup breeds tend to react with a heightened state of arousal around even the simplest of procedures (e.g., subcutaneous injections and nail trims). The individual character and temperament of the animal further influences its response. Pediatric and neonatal animals seem to have a lower threshold for pain and anxiety than older animals. In any species, the duration and type of pain make it more (acute) or less (chronic) likely to be expressed or exhibited outwardly. Unfamiliarity with normal behaviors typical of a particular species or breed makes recognition of their painful behaviors and responses impossible.

The definition and recognition of pain in an individual animal is challenging. Because of all the differences discussed, there is no straight line from *insult*, albeit actual or perceived, to *degree* of pain experienced. Nor is there a formula for treating "X" type of pain with "Y" type of analgesic. A goal of analgesia is to treat all animals with analgesic drugs and modalities as PREEMPTIVELY as possible and using a multimodal approach. Use analgesic treatment as a tool for diagnosis of pain in the event that recognition of these phenomena is difficult for the patient. In other words, with countless drugs and treatment modalities available, analgesic administration should NEVER be withheld in an animal, even if pain is questionable.

Pain Assessment in Dogs and Cats

It is important to remember that no behavior or physiologic variable in and of itself is pathognomonic for pain. Interactive and unprovoked (noninteractive) behavior assessments and trending of physiologic data are useful to determine the pain in an individual animal. This is known as *pain scoring*. Baseline observations, especially those observations from someone who has known the animal well, can be helpful to serial behavior and pain assessments. Pain scoring systems have been developed and are reviewed elsewhere; the purposes of these systems are to evaluate and to help guide diagnostic and analgesic treatments (Table 1-15). Regardless of the scale or method used to assess pain, the caregiver must recognize the limitations of the scale. If in doubt of whether pain is present or not, analgesic therapy should be used as a diagnostic tool.

Behavioral Signs of Acute Pain

Classic behaviors associated with pain in dogs and cats include abnormal postures, gaits, movements, and behaviors (Boxes 1-21 and 1-22). Stoicism is the apparent apathy and

TABLE 1-15 Pain Scale

Number	Description
1	No pain
2	Mild pain
3	Moderate pain
4	Severe pain
5	Excruciating pain

BOX 1-21 BEHAVIORAL SIGNS ASSOCIATED WITH PAIN IN DOGS AND CATS

ABNORMAL POSTURES
Hunched-up
Prayer position
Inability to lie down
Muscle atrophy (chronic)
Reluctance to move
Low tail carriage

ABNORMAL GAITS
Stiffness
Non–weight bearing
Limping
Pacing versus trotting
Abnormal nail wear

ABNORMAL MOVEMENTS
Thrashing
Restlessness
Circling

ABNORMAL BEHAVIORS
Focusing on area of pain (licking or chewing)
Inappetence
Lack of grooming
Abnormal urination or defecation
Stoicism
Aggression
Yawning
Hiding
Vocalizations
Whimper
Screaming/crying

BOX 1-22 PHYSIOLOGIC SIGNS OF PAIN

- Acute pain
- Allodynia
- Blepharospasm
- Bradycardia
- Bruxism
- Cardiac dysrhythmias
- Hyperesthesia
- Incontinence
- Mydriasis
- Panting
- Ptyalism
- Tachycardia
- Tachypnea

---

indifference in the presence of pain and is perhaps the No. 1 sign of ineffective pain relief or persistent pain in many animals, because so many display apathy and classically normal physiologic parameters even in the face of severe distress, overt suffering, or blatant trauma and illness. The *absence of normal behaviors* is also a clinical sign of pain, even when abnormal behaviors are not observed.

SIGNS OF CHRONIC PAIN IN CATS AND DOGS

Acute pain results in many of the aforementioned behavioral and physiologic signs, but chronic pain in small animals is an entirely different and distinct entity. Chronic pain is often present in the absence of obvious tissue pathology and changes in physical demeanor.

1

Again, the severity of the pain may not correlate with the severity of any pathologic condition that may or may not be present. Chronic pain, especially if insidious in onset (cancer, dental, or degenerative pain), may well go unnoticed in dogs and cats, even by family members or intermittent caregivers. Inappetance, lack of activity, panting in a species classically designed to be nose breathers, decreased interest in surroundings, different activity patterns, and abnormal postures are just a few signs of chronic pain in cats and dogs. Cats are a species that in particular are exemplary in their abilities to hide chronic pain. They will exhibit marked familial withdrawal, finding secluded areas where they may remain for days to weeks when they experience acute and chronic pain.

ACUTE PAIN MANAGEMENT FOR EMERGENT, CRITICAL/INTENSIVE CARE AND TRAUMA PATIENTS

When deciding on a pain management protocol for a patient, always perform a thorough physical examination and include a pain score assessment before injury and pain has occurred, whenever possible. Form a problem list to guide your choice of anesthesia and analgesia. For example, using a nonsteroidal antiinflammatory drug (NSAID) in an animal with renal failure would not be wise. Remember to account for current medications that the patient may be taking that may augment or interfere with the analgesic or anesthetic drugs. Use multimodal techniques and regional therapy and drugs to target pain at different sites before it occurs. Once a strategy is decided upon, frequently reassess the patient and tailor the protocol to meet each patient's response and needs.

METHODS TO REDUCE PAIN

Drug therapy (in particular, opioids with or without α_2-agonists) is a cornerstone for acute pain treatment and surgical preemptive pain prevention. However, local anesthetics delivered epidurally, via perineural or plexus injection, intraarticular or trigger point injection, are also effective analgesics for acute and chronic forms of pain and inflammation. The NSAIDs that classically have been reserved for treatment of more chronic or persistent pain states now are being used regularly for treatment of acute and perioperative pain once blood pressure, coagulation, and gastrointestinal parameters have been normalized.

PHARMACOLOGIC MEANS TO ANALGESIA: MAJOR ANALGESICS

OPIOIDS

An opioid is any natural or synthetic drug that is derived from the poppy, which interacts with opiate receptors identified on cell membranes. The drugs from this class constitute the most effective means of controlling acute, perioperative, and chronic pain in human and veterinary medicine (Table 1-16). Their physiologic effects result from the interaction with one or more of at least five endogenous opioid receptors (μ, σ, δ, ϵ, and κ). μ-Receptor agonists are noted for their ability to produce profound analgesia with mild sedation. These drugs diminish "wind-up," the hyperexcitable state resulting from an afferent volley of nociceptive impulses. They elevate the pain threshold and are used preemptively to prevent acute pain.

As a class, opioids cause CNS depression with their intense analgesia. Dose-related respiratory depression reflects diminished response to carbon dioxide levels. Cardiac depression is secondary only to bradycardia and is more likely with certain opioids such as morphine and oxymorphone. Narcotics produce few if any clinically significant cardiovascular effects in dogs and cats; they are considered cardiac soothing or sparing. Because opioids increase intracranial and intraocular pressure, use them more cautiously in patients with severe cranial trauma and or ocular lesions. Opioids directly stimulate the chemoreceptor trigger zone and may cause nausea and vomiting. Most opioids depress the cough reflex via a central mechanism; this may be helpful in patients recovering from endotracheal intubation irritation. A key characteristic of opioids that makes them desirable for use in emergency and critical care situations is their reversibility. Antagonists block or

1

TABLE 1-16 Drugs Used in Pain Management

Drug	Agonist effects	Dose	Cardiovascular effects	Disadvantage/ Side effects
Fentanyl	Pure μ	2 μg/kg IV bolus 2-8 μg/kg/hour CRI 10-20 μg/kg/hour CRI (inotropic)	Minimal	Hypoventilation at high doses
Buprenorphine	Partial agonist	0.005-0.03 mg/kg q8h IM, IV, SQ; can be placed topically on oral mucosa in cats	Minimal	Partial agonist activity, so not as potent as pure μ-agonists
Butorphanol	Agonist/ antagonist	0.2-1.0 mg/kg q2-4h IM, IV, SQ	Minimal	Poor analgesic, adequate sedative if used in combination with an anxiolytic; extremely short duration of action; ceiling effect—more is not better
Codeine	Pure agonist	1-4 mg/kg PO q6h (dogs)	Minimal	Constipation, dysphoria
Morphine	Pure agonist	0.1-0.5 mg/kg q4-8h IM, IV, SQ 0.05-0.1 mg/kg/hour IV CRI	Minimal, can cause histamine release and hypotension if IV is high dose	
Oxymorphone	Pure agonist	0.02-0.1 mg/kg q4-12h IM, IV, SQ	Minimal	Noise hypersensitivity, dysphoria, panting when given IV
Hydromor- phone	Pure agonist	0.02-0.2 mg/kg q4-12h IM, IV, SQ	Minimal	Panting during IV, vomiting; hyperthermia in cats

reverse the effect of agonists by combining with receptors and producing minimal or no effects. Administer all reversal agents, such as naloxone and naltrexone, slowly if given intravenously and to effect.

α₂-AGONISTS

As a class of drugs, α_2-agonists warrant special attention because most members of the group possess potent analgesic power at doses that are capable of causing sedation, CNS depression, cardiovascular depression, and even general anesthetic states. Originally developed for antihypertensive use, α_2-agonists quickly have attained sedative analgesic status in veterinary medicine (Table 1-17). Like the opioids, α_2-agonists produce their effects by aggravating α-adrenergic receptors in the CNS and periphery.

1

TABLE 1-17 α₂-Agonists Used for Analgesia and Sedation

Drug	Dose	Effects	Proposed uses
Xylazine	0.05-0.1 mg/kg IV	Short duration Profound cardiovascular depression Vomiting, chemoreceptor trigger zone stimulation Bradycardia, vasoconstriction Second-degree atrioventricular block Reversible with yohimbine	Microdose to decrease dysphoria and anxiety Short-duration procedures in HEALTHY dogs
Medetomidine	0.001-0.005 mg/kg IV, IM q4-6h (dog) 0.01-0.03 mg/kg IV, IM q4-6h (cat) 1-3 μg/kg/hour	Longer duration Cardiovascular depression Vasoconstriction Bradycardia, second-degree atrioventricular block Reversible with atipamezole (Antesedan) Vomiting, chemoreceptor trigger zone stimulation	Microdose to decrease dysphoria and anxiety Augment analgesia in orthopedic procedures Short-duration procedures in HEALTHY dogs

NONSTEROIDAL ANTIINFLAMMATORY DRUGS

Nonsteroidal antiinflammatory drugs, which classically have been used to treat chronic pain and inflammation, as well as cardiovascular diseases, have taken on a new role in the treatment of perioperative and acute pain. Recently, the development of potent oral and parenteral forms of these drugs has compared favorably with and sometimes superiorly to the use of opioids for treatment of acute inflammation and pain (Table 1-18). Nonsteroidal drugs can be used alone, but their best use is that of providing synergistic analgesia with different classes of analgesics (narcotics) or modalities (local, regional and epidural analgesia, physical therapy, acupuncture).

Most NSAIDS act by cyclooxygenase (aka prostaglandin synthetase) inhibition, an enzyme that catalyzes the incorporation of molecular oxygen into arachidonic acid to produce mediators of inflammation. There are at least a few forms of cyclooxygenase,

TABLE 1-18 Nonsteroidal Antiinflammatory Drugs and Dosages

Drug	Dose
Carprofen	2-4 mg/kg PO, IM, SQ, IV q12-24h
Etodolac (EtoGesic)	10-15 mg/kg q24h (dogs only)
Ketoprofen (cat)	0.5-1.0 mg/kg IM, SQ, IV, PO q12h (dogs); q48-72h (cats)
Meloxicam	0.1-0.2 mg/kg PO q24h (dogs); q48-72h (cats)
Piroxicam	0.3 mg/kg PO q48h (dogs and cats)
Ketorolac	0.25-0.5 mg/kg IM, SQ, IV q12h (dogs only)
Deracoxib (Deramaxx)	3-4 mg/kg PO q24h (dogs)
Acetaminophen	10-15 mg/kg PO q6-8h (dogs only)
Aspirin (dog)	10 mg/kg PO q12h
Aspirin (cat)	10 mg/kg PO q48-72h

among them cyclooxygenase-1 (COX-1), the major constitutive enzyme primarily involved in normal physiologic functions, and COX-2, the enzyme responsible for most of the hyperalgesia and pain responses experienced after tissue injury or trauma. Some NSAIDS inhibit cyclooxygenase and lipoxygenase activity. Most of the currently available oral and parenteral NSAIDS for small animal medicine and surgery target the cyclooxygenase pathways predominantly, although one (tepoxalin) is thought to inhibit both pathways. Inhibition of COX-1 and COX-2 can inhibit the protective effects and impair platelet aggregation and lead to gastrointestinal ulceration.

There are definite contraindications and relative contraindications for the use of NSAIDs. Nonsteroidal antiinflammatory drugs should not be administered to patients with renal or hepatic insufficiency, dehydration, hypotension or conditions that are associated with low circulating volume (congestive heart failure, *unregulated anesthesia*, shock), or evidence of ulcerative gastrointestinal disease. TRAUMA PATIENTS should be stabilized completely regarding vascular volume, tone, and pressure before the use of NSAIDs. Patients receiving concurrent administration of other NSAIDs or corticosteroids, or those considered to be cushingoid, should be evaluated carefully for an adequate "washout" period (time of clearance of drug from the system) before use of an NSAID or before switching NSAIDs. Patients with coagulopathies, particularly those that are caused by platelet number or function defects or those caused by factor deficiencies, and patients with severe, uncontrolled asthma or other bronchial disease are probably not the patients in which to use NSAIDs. Other advice is that NSAIDs not be administered to pregnant patients or to females attempting to become pregnant because COX-2 induction is necessary for ovulation and subsequent implantation of the embryo. The administration of NSAIDs should be considered ONLY in the well-hydrated, normotensive dog or cat with normal renal or hepatic function, with no hemostatic abnormalities, and no concurrent steroid administration.

Nonsteroidal antiinflammatory drugs can be used in many settings of acute and chronic pain and inflammation. Among these are the use in well-stabilized musculoskeletal trauma and surgical pain, osteoarthritis management, meningitis, mastitis, animal bite and other wound healing, mammary or transitional cell carcinoma, epithelial (dental, oral, urethral) inflammation, ophthalmologic procedures, and dermatologic or otic disease. Whereas opioids seem to have an immediate analgesic effect when administered, most NSAIDS will take up to 30 minutes for their effect to be recognized. As such, most perioperative or acute NSAIDs use is PART of a balanced pain management scheme, one that uses narcotics and local anesthetic techniques. Nonsteroidal antiinflammatory drugs are devoid of many of the side effects of narcotic administration; namely, decreased gastrointestinal motility, altered sensorium, nausea/vomition, and sedation. Nonsteroidal antiinflammatory drugs are also devoid of many of the side effects of steroid administration; namely, suppression of the pituitary adrenal axis.

Nonsteroidal antiinflammatory drugs in cats

The toxic effects of salicylates in cats are well documented. Cats are susceptible because of slow clearance and dose-dependent elimination because of deficient glucuronidation in this species. Because of this, the dose and the dosing interval of most commonly used NSAIDs need to be altered in order for these drugs to be used. Cats that have been given canine doses of NSAIDs (twice daily or even once daily repetitively) may show hyperthermia, hemorrhagic or ulcerative gastritis, kidney and liver injury, hyperthermia, respiratory alkalosis, and metabolic acidosis. Acute and chronic toxicities of NSAIDs have been reported in cats, especially after repeat once daily dosing. Ketoprofen, flunixin, aspirin, carprofen, and meloxicam have been administered safely to cats, although like most antibiotics and other medications, they are not approved and licensed for use in cats. An important note, though, is that dosing intervals ranging from 48 to 96 hours have been used, and antithrombotic effects often can be achieved at much lower doses than those required to treat fevers and inflammation. I recommend the use of no loading doses, minimum 48-hour dosing intervals, and assurance of adequate circulating blood volume, blood pressure, and renal function.

Because many of the NSAIDs are used off-label in cats, it is imperative that the clinician carefully calculate the dose, modify the dosing interval, and communicate this information to the client before dispensing the drug. Even drugs that come in liquid form (meloxicam), if administered to cats via box-labeled directions used for dogs, will be given in near toxic doses. To worsen the misunderstanding about dosages for cats, drops from manufacturer's bottles often are calibrated drops; when these same liquids are transferred into pharmacy syringes for drop administration, the calibration of course is lost, and the animal potentially is overdosed. A more accurate method of dispensing and administering oral NSAIDs in cats is to calculate the dose in milligrams and determine the exact number of milliliters to administer, rather than use the drop method.

ANALGESIA: MINOR ANALGESICS

Ketamine classically was considered a dissociative anesthetic, but it also has potent activity as an *N*-methyl-D-aspartate (NMDA) receptor antagonist. This receptor located in the CNS mediates windup and central sensitization (a pathway from acute to chronic pain). Blockade of this receptor with microdoses of ketamine results in the ability to provide body surface, somatic, and skin analgesia with potentially lower doses of opioids and α-agonists. Loading doses of 0.5 to 2 mg/kg are used intravenously with continuous rate infusions of 2 to 20 μg/kg/minute. In and of itself, this drug possesses little to no analgesic ability and indeed in high doses alone often can aggravate, sensitize, or excite the animal in subacute or acute pain.

Amantadine is another NMDA blocker that has been used for its antiviral and Parkinson's stabilizing effects. Amantadine has been used for neuropathic pain in human beings but is only available in an oral form. Suggested starting doses for cats and dogs range from 3 to 10 mg/kg PO daily. When the drug is given orally and intravenously, patients are unlikely to develop behavioral or cardiorespiratory effects with ketamine or amantadine.

Tramadol is an analgesic that possesses weak opioid μ-agonist activity and norepinephrine and serotonin reuptake inhibition. Tramadol is useful for mild to moderate pain in small animals. Although the parent compound has very weak opioid activity, the metabolites have excellent binding affinity for the μ-receptor. Tramadol has been used for perisurgical pain control when given orally in cats and dogs at a dose of 1 to 10 mg/kg PO sid to bid. Cats appear to require only once daily dosing. Regardless of its affinity for the opioid receptors, the true mechanism of action of tramadol in companion animals remains largely unknown.

Gabapentin is a synthetic analog of γ-aminobutyric acid (GABA). Originally introduced as an antiepileptic drug, the mechanism of action of gabapentin remains somewhat unclear in veterinary medicine. The drug is among a number of commonly used antiepileptic medications used to treat central pain in human beings. The rationale for use is the ability of the drugs to suppress discharge in pathologically altered neurons. Gabapentin does this through calcium channel modulation without binding to glutamate receptors. Chronic, burning, neuropathic, and lancinating pain in small animals responds well to 1 to 10 mg/kg PO daily.

ADJUNCTIVE ANALGESIC DRUGS

Local anesthetic agents are the major class used as a peripheral-acting analgesic (Table 1-19). Local anesthetics block the transmission of pain impulses at the peripheral nerve nociceptor regions. Local anesthetics may be used to block peripheral nerves or inhibit nerve "zones" using regional techniques. Although all local anesthetics are capable of providing pain relief, agents with a longer duration of action are preferred for pain management purposes. Bupivacaine is an example of a long-acting local anesthetic drug that is used along with lidocaine for long-acting pain relief. A single dose of bupivacaine injected at a local site will provide local anesthesia and analgesia for 6 to 10 hours.

TABLE 1-19 Analgesics

Drug	Dose	Use
Amantadine	3 mg/kg, PO q24h (dogs and cats)	Chronic pain
Dextromethorphan	1-2 mg/kg PO q6-8h (dogs and cats)	Prevent windup
Gabapentin	1.25-10 mg/kg PO q24h (dogs and cats)	Chronic pain
Tramadol	1-10 mg/kg PO q8-24h	Acute and chronic pain

TABLE 1-20 Commonly Used Analgesic Assistance Drugs

Drug	Dose
Acepromazine	0.01-0.03 mg/kg IV, IM, SQ q8-24 hours 0.2-0.5 mg/kg PO q12-24h
Diazepam	0.5-1.0 mg/kg IV in cats and dogs, followed by 0.1-0.2 mg/kg/hour IV CRI
Midazolam	0.3-0.5 mg/kg IV, IM, SQ in cats and dogs, followed by 0.05 mg/kg/hour IV CRI

Combination Approach: Mix with one another and give as a constant rate infusion at 10 mL/kg/hour

Drug	Dose	CRI dose provided
Morphine	5 mg in 500 mL	0.1 mg/kg/hour
Lidocaine	150 mg	3 mg/kg/hour
Ketamine	100 mg	2 mg/kg/hour

When lidocaine is administered as an intravenous constant rate infusion (50 to 75 μg/kg/minute in dogs, 1 to 10 μg/kg/minute in cats) is effective in the treatment of chronic neuropathic pain and periosteal and peritoneal pain (e.g., pancreatitis). Mexiletine, an oral sodium channel blocker, can be used as an alternative to injectable lidocaine for provision of background analgesia.

ANXIOLYTICS AND SEDATIVES

Many drugs (Table 1-20) are used in combination with opioids, α_2-agonists, and ketamine to provide anxiolysis and sedation.

LOCAL AND REGIONAL TECHNIQUES FOR THE EMERGENT PATIENT

Injection of local anesthetic solution into the connective tissue surrounding a particular nerve produces loss of sensation (sensory blockade) and/or paralysis (motor nerve blockade) in the region supplied by the nerve. Local anesthetics also may be administered epidurally, intrathoracically, intraperitoneally, and intraarticularly. Lidocaine and bupivacaine are the most commonly administered local anesthetics. Lidocaine provides for quick, short-acting sensory and motor impairment. Bupivacaine provides for later-onset, longer-lasting desensitization without motor impairment. Combinations of the two agents diluted with saline are used frequently to provide for quick-onset analgesia that lasts between 4 and 6 hours in most patients. Adding narcotic and/or α_2 agent often maximizes the analgesia and increases the pain-free interval to 8 to 18 hours. Epinephrine and preservative-free solutions are recommended. Precision placement of anesthetic close to nerves, roots, or plexuses is improved with the use of a stimulating nerve locator. Cats seem to be more sensitive to the effects of local anesthetics; as such the lower ends of most dosing ranges are used for blockades in this species.

Unlike most instances of general anesthesia, during which the animal is rendered unconscious and nerve transmission is decreased by virtue of CNS depression, local and regional techniques block the initiation of noxious signals, thereby effectively preventing pain from entering the CNS. This is an effective means of not only preventing initial pain but also reducing the changes that take place in the dorsal horn of the spinal cord, spinothalamic tracts, limbic and reticular activating centers, and cortex. Frequently, the neurohormonal response that is stimulated in pain and stress is blunted as well. Overall, the patient has fewer local and systemic adverse effects of pain, disease processes are minimized, chronic pain states are unlikely, and outcome is improved. Regional techniques are best used as part of an analgesic regimen that consists of their continuous administration, narcotics, α-agonists, anxiolytics, and good nursing.

TOPICAL AND INFILTRATIVE BLOCKADE

Lidocaine can be added to sterile lubricant in a one-to-one concentration to provide decreased sensation for urinary catheterization, nasal catheter insertion, minor road burn analgesia, and pyotraumatic dermatitis analgesia. Proparacaine is a topical anesthetic useful for corneal or scleral injuries. Local anesthetics can be used to infiltrate areas of damage or surgery by using long-term continuous drainage catheters and small, portable infusion pumps. This is an effective means of providing days of analgesia for massive surgical or traumatic soft tissue injury. Even without the catheter, incisional or regional soft tissue blocking using a combination of 1 to 2 mg/kg lidocaine and 0.5 to 2 mg/kg bupivacaine diluted with equal volume of saline and 1:9 with sodium bicarbonate is effective for infiltrating large areas of injury.

CRANIAL NERVE BLOCKADE

Administration of local anesthetic drugs around the infraorbital, maxillary, ophthalmic mental, and alveolar nerves can provide excellent analgesia for dental, orofacial, and ophthalmic trauma and surgical procedures. Each nerve may be desensitized by injecting 0.1 to 0.3 mL of a 2% lidocaine hydrochloride solution and 0.1 to 0.3 mL of 0.5% bupivacaine solution using a 1.2- to 2.5-cm, 22- to 25-gauge needle. Precise placement perineurally versus intraneurally (neuroma formation common) is enhanced by using catheters in the foramen versus needle administration. Always perform aspiration before administration to rule out intravascular injection of agents.

INTRAPLEURAL BLOCKADE

This block is used to provide analgesia for thoracic, lower cervical, cranial abdominal, and diaphragmatic pain. Following aseptic preparation, place a small through-the-needle (20- to 22-gauge) catheter in the thoracic cavity between the seventh and ninth intercostal space on the midlateral aspect of the thorax. Aseptically mix a 0.5 to 1 mg/kg lidocaine and a 0.2 to 0.5 mg/kg bupivacaine dose with volume of saline equal to the volume of bupivacaine, and slowly inject it over a period of 2 to 5 minutes following aspiration to ensure that no intravascular injection occurs. Depending on where the lesion is, position the patient to allow the intrapleural infusion to "coat" the area. Most effective is positioning the patient in dorsal recumbency for several minutes following the block to make sure local anesthetic occupies the paravertebral gutters and hence the spinal nerve roots. The block should be repeated every 3 hours in dogs and every 8 to 12 hours in cats. Secure the catheter to the skin surface for repetitive administration.

BRACHIAL PLEXUS BLOCKADE

Administration of local anesthetic around the brachial plexus provides excellent analgesia for forelimb surgery, particularly that distal to the shoulder, and amputations. Nerve locator–guided techniques are much more accurate and successful than blind placement of local anesthetic; however, even the latter is useful.

To administer a brachial plexus blockade, follow this procedure:
1. Aseptically prepare a small area of skin over the point of the shoulder.
2. Insert a 22-gauge, 1½- to 3-inch spinal needle medial to the shoulder joint, axial to the lesser tubercle, and advance it caudally, medial to the body of the scapula, and toward the costochondral junction of the first rib. Aspirate first before injection to make sure that intravenous injection does not occur.
3. Inject one third of the volume of local anesthetic mix, and then slowly withdraw the needle and fan dorsally and ventrally while infusing the remaining fluid.
4. Local anesthetic doses are similar to those for intrapleural blockade.

EPIDURAL ANESTHESIA AND ANALGESIA

Epidural analgesia refers to the injection of an opioid, a phencyclidine, an α-agonist, or an NSAID into the epidural space. Epidural anesthesia refers to the injection of a local anesthetic. In most patients a combination of the two is used. Epidural analgesia and anesthesia are used for a variety of acute and chronic surgical pain or traumatically induced pain in the pelvis, tail, perineum, hind limbs, abdomen, and thorax (Table 1-21). Procedures in which epidural analgesia and anesthesia are useful include forelimb and hind limb amputation, tail or perineal procedures, cesarean sections, diaphragmatic hernia repair, pancreatitis, peritonitis, and intervertebral disk disease. Epidural blocks performed using opioids or bupivacaine will not result in hind limb paresis or decreased urinary or anal tone (incontinence), unlike lidocaine or mepivicaine epidural blocks. Morphine is one of the most useful opioids for administration in the epidural space because of its slow systemic absorption. Epidural catheters used for the instillation of drugs through constant rate infusion or intermittent injection can be placed in dogs and cats. Routinely placed at the lumbosacral junction, these catheters are used with cocktails including preservative-free morphine, bupivacaine, medetomidine, and ketamine. Extremely effective for preventing windup pain in the peritoneal cavity or caudal half of the body, the catheters may be maintained if placed aseptically for 7 to 14 days.

To provide epidural analgesia or anesthesia, follow this procedure:
1. Position the animal in lateral or sternal recumbency.
2. Clip and aseptically scrub over the lumbosacral site.
3. Palpate the craniodorsal-most extent of the wings of the ileum bilaterally and draw an imaginary line through them to envision the spine of L7 located immediately behind the imaginary line.
4. Advance a 20- to 22-gauge, 1½- to 3-inch spinal or epidural needle through the skin just caudal to the spine of L7.
5. The needle will lose resistance as it is introduced into the epidural space. Drop saline into the hub of the needle, and the saline will be pulled into the epidural space as the needle enters.

TABLE 1-21   Drugs to Use for Epidural Anesthesia

Drug	Dose
Bupivacaine 0.25%*	0.1-0.3 mg/kg (1 mL/5 kg epidural q4-6h (canine only, not recommended for cats)
Morphine (Duramorph)*,†	0.05-0.1 mg/kg spinal q8h

*Preservative-free solutions should be used, with filtered needles or in-line filters if an epidural catheter with constant rate infusion is used.
†Can be diluted to a total volume of 0.1 to 0.15 mL/kg with sterile saline if advancement of the solution into the thoracic area is desired (forelimb amputation, thoracostomy, diaphragmatic hernia repair).

Intercostal Nerve Blocks

Discrete intercostal nerve blocks can provide effective analgesia for traumatic or postsurgical pain. Identify the area of the injury, and infiltrate three segments on either side of the injury with analgesic.

To perform an intercostal nerve block, follow this procedure:
1. Clip and aseptically scrub the dorsal and ventral third of the chest wall.
2. Palpate the intercostal space as far dorsally as possible.
3. Use a 25-gauge, 0.625-inch needle at the caudolateral aspect of the affected rib segments and those cranial and caudal.
4. Direct the tip of the needle caudally such that the tip of the needle "drops" off of the caudal rib. (This places the needle tip in proximity to the neuromuscular bundle that contains the intercostal nerve that runs in a groove on the caudomedial surface of the rib.)
5. Aspirate to confirm that the drug will not go intravenously.
6. Inject while slowly withdrawing the needle. Inject 0.5 to 1.0 mL at each site, depending on the size of the animal.

Additional Reading

Gaynor JS, Muir WW: *Handbook of veterinary pain management,* St Louis, 2003, Mosby, 2003.
Melzack R, Wall PD: *Handbook of pain management, a clinical companion to Wall and Melzack's textbook of pain,* Edinburgh, 2003, Churchill Livingstone.
Muir WW, Hubbell JAE, Skarda RT, et al: *Handbook of veterinary anesthesia,* ed 3, St Louis, 2000, Mosby.

EMERGENCY MANAGEMENT OF SPECIFIC CONDITIONS

ACUTE CONDITION IN THE ABDOMEN

An acute condition in the abdomen is defined as the sudden onset of abdominal discomfort or pain caused by a variety of conditions involving intraabdominal organs. Many animals have the primary complaint of lethargy, anorexia, ptyalism, vomiting, retching, diarrhea, hematochezia, crying out, moaning, or abnormal postures. Abnormal postures can include generalized rigidity, walking tenderly or as if "on eggshells," or a prayer position in which the front limbs are lowered to the ground while the hind end remains standing. In some cases, it may be difficult initially to distinguish between true abdominal pain or referred pain from intervertebral disk disease. Rapid progression and decompensation of the patient's cardiovascular status can lead to stupor, coma, and death in the most extreme cases, making rapid assessment, treatment, and definitive care extremely challenging.

Signalment and History

Often the patient's signalment and history can increase the index of suspicion for a particular disease process. A thorough history often is overlooked or postponed in the initial stages of resuscitation of the patient with acute abdominal pain. Often, asking the same question in a variety of methods can elicit an answer from the client that may lead to the source of the problem and the reason for acute abdominal pain. Important questions to ask the client include the following:
- What is your chief complaint or reason that you brought your animal in on emergency?
- When did the signs first start, or when was your animal last normal?
- Do you think that the signs have been the same, better, or getting worse?
- Does your animal have any ongoing or past medical problems?
- Have similar signs occurred in the past?
- Does your animal have access to any known toxins, or does he or she run loose unattended?

- Has your animal ingested any garbage, compost, or table scraps recently?
- Are there any other animals in your household, and are they acting sick or normal?
- Has your animal been vaccinated recently?
- Has there been any change in your pet's appetite?
- Have you noticed any weight loss or weight gain?
- Have you noticed any increase or decrease in water consumption or urination?
- Does your animal chew on bones or toys?
- Have you noticed any toys, socks, underwear, or other items missing from your household?
- Is there a possibility of any trauma including being hit by a car or kicked by a larger animal or person?
- Have you noticed a change in your pet's defecation habits?
- Have you seen any vomiting or diarrhea?
- What does the vomitus or diarrhea look like?
- Is the vomitus in relation to eating?
- Is there any blood or mucus in the vomitus or diarrhea?
- When was the last time your animal vomited or had diarrhea?
- When your animal vomits, does it actively retch with abdominal contractions, or is it more passive like regurgitation?
- What is the color of the feces? Is it black or red?
- Does the vomit smell malodorous like feces?

IMMEDIATE ACTION

As with any other emergency, the clinician must follow the ABCs of therapy, treating the most life-threatening problems first. First, perform a perfunctory physical examination. Examination of the abdomen ideally should be performed last, in case inciting a painful stimulus precludes you from evaluating other organ systems more thoroughly. Briefly observe the patient from a distance. Are there any abnormal postures? Is there respiratory distress? Is the animal ambulatory, and if so, do you observe any gait abnormalities? Do you observe any ptyalism or attempts to vomit? Auscultate the patient's thorax for crackles that may signify aspiration pneumonia resulting from vomiting. Examine the patient's mucous membrane color and capillary refill time, heart rate, heart rhythm, and pulse quality. Many patients in pain have tachycardia that may or may not be accompanied by dysrhythmias. If a patient's heart rate is inappropriately bradycardic, consider hypoadrenocorticism, whipworm infestation, or urinary obstruction or trauma as a cause of hyperkalemia. Assess the patient's hydration status by evaluating skin turgor, mucous membrane dryness, and whether the eyes appear sunken in their orbits. A brief neurologic examination should consist of whether the patient is actively having a seizure, or whether mental dullness, stupor, coma, or nystagmus are present. Posture and spinal reflexes can assist in making a diagnosis of intervertebral disk disease versus abdominal pain. Perform a rectal examination to evaluate for the presence of hematochezia or melena.

Finally, examination of the abdomen should proceed first with superficial and then deeper palpation. Visually inspect the abdomen for the presence of external masses, bruising, or penetrating injuries. Reddish discoloration of the periumbilical area often is associated with the presence of intraabdominal hemorrhage. It may be necessary to shave the fur to inspect the skin and underlying structures visually for bruising and ecchymoses. Auscultate the abdomen for the presence or absence of borborygmi to characterize gut sounds. Next, perform percussion and ballottement to evaluate for the presence of a gas-distended viscus or peritoneal effusion. Finally, perform first superficial and then deep palpation of all quadrants of the abdomen, noting abnormal enlargement, masses, or whether focal pain is elicited in any one area. Once the physical examination has been performed, implement initial therapy in the form of analgesia, fluid resuscitation, and antibiotics.

TREATMENT

Treatment for any patient with an acute condition in the abdomen and shock is to treat the underlying cause, maintain tissue oxygen delivery, and prevent end-organ damage and failure. A more complete description of shock and oxygen delivery is given in the section on shock.

ANALGESIA

The administration of analgesic agents to any patient with acute abdominal pain is one of the most important therapies in the initial stages of case management. Table 1-22 lists analgesic drugs for use in the patient with an acute condition in abdomen. Table 1-23 lists analgesic and anxiolytic drugs to avoid in the patient with an acute condition in abdomen.

TABLE 1-22 Analgesic Agents for Use in Dogs and Cats with Acute Abdominal Pain

Drug	Dose
Butorphanol	0.1-0.2 mg/kg IV (dogs and cats); 0.2-0.4 mg/kg SQ or IM (dogs and cats)
Buprenorphine	0.005-0.02 mg/kg IV, IM, SQ q6-12h (dogs) 0.005-0.01 mg/kg IV, IM, SQ, q6-12h (cats) (Also can be placed in the mouth for buccal absorption in cats)
Fentanyl	2 µg/kg IV bolus, followed by 3-7 µg/kg/hour CRI (dogs and cats)
Hydromorphone	0.1-0.2 mg/kg SQ, IM, IV (dogs and cats)
Lidocaine	1-2 mg/kg IV slowly over 2-5 minutes, then 30-50 µg/kg/minute CRI
Morphine	0.5-1.0 mg/kg SQ, IM; 0.1 mg/kg/hour CRI (dogs) 0.25-0.5 mg/kg SQ, IM; 0.05 mg/kg/hour CRI (cats)

TABLE 1-23 Analgesic and Anxiolytic Agents That Are Contraindicated and Should Be Avoided in the Patient with Acute Abdominal Pain

Drug	Potential risks
α-*Antagonists* Acepromazine Chlorpromazine	α-Receptor antagonist, hypotension
α₂-*Agonists* Xylazine Medetomidine	α2-agonist, peripheral vasoconstriction, dose-dependent decrease in cardiac output, hypotension
Antiprostaglandins Aspirin Flunixin meglumine Indomethacin Phenylbutazone Ibuprofen Carprofen Ketoprofen Aminopyrine Flufenamic acid	Decreased renal and gastrointestinal perfusion, gastrointestinal ulceration
Glucocorticoids Dexamethasone Dexamethasone sodium phosphate Hydrocortisone sodium phosphate Prednisone Prednisolone sodium phosphate Methylprednisolone sodium succinate	Decreased renal and gastrointestinal perfusion, gastrointestinal ulceration

FLUID RESUSCITATION

Many patients with acute abdominal pain are clinically dehydrated or are in hypovolemic shock because of hemorrhage. Careful titration of intravenous crystalloid and colloid fluids including blood products is necessary based on the patient's perfusion parameters including heart rate, capillary refill time, blood pressure, urine output, and PCV. Fluid therapy also should be based on the most likely differential diagnoses, with specific fluid types administered according to the primary disease process. In dogs, a shock volume of fluids is calculated based on the total blood volume of 90 mL/kg/hour. In cats, shock fluid rate is based on plasma volume of 44 mL/kg/hour. In most cases, any crystalloid fluid can be administered at an initial volume of one fourth of a calculated shock dose and then titrated according to whether the patient's cardiovascular status responds favorably or not. In cases of an acute condition in the abdomen from known or suspected hypoadrenocorticism, severe whipworm infestation, or urinary tract obstruction or rupture, 0.9% sodium chloride fluid without added potassium is the fluid of choice. When hemorrhage is present, the administration of whole blood or packed RBCs may be indicated if the patient has clinical signs of anemia and shows clinical signs of lethargy, tachypnea, and weakness. Fresh frozen plasma is indicated in cases of hemorrhage resulting from vitamin K antagonist rodenticide intoxication or hepatic failure or in cases of suspected disseminated intravascular coagulation (DIC). A more thorough description of fluid therapy is given under the sections on shock and fluid therapy.

ANTIBIOTICS

The empiric use of broad-spectrum antibiotics is warranted in cases of suspected sepsis or peritonitis as a cause of acute abdominal pain. Ampicillin sulbactam (22 mg/kg IV q6-8h) and enrofloxacin (10 mg/kg once daily) are the combination treatment of choice to cover gram-negative, gram-positive, aerobic, and anaerobic infections. Alternative therapies include a second-generation cephalosporin such as cefotetan (30 mg/kg IV tid) or cefoxitin (22 mg/kg IV tid) or added anaerobic coverage with metronidazole (10 to 20 mg/kg IV tid).

OXYGEN SUPPLEMENTATION

Tissue oxygen delivery depends on a number of factors, including arterial oxygen content and cardiac output. If an animal has had vomiting and subsequent aspiration pneumonitis, treatment of hypoxemia with supplemental oxygen in the form of nasal, nasopharyngeal, hood, or transtracheal oxygen administration is important (see Oxygen Supplementation under Emergency Diagnostic and Therapeutic Procedures).

DIAGNOSTIC PROCEDURES

Complete blood count

Perform a complete blood count in all cases of acute abdominal pain to determine if life-threatening infection or coagulopathy including DIC is present. In cases of sepsis, infection, or severe nonseptic inflammation, the white blood cell count may be normal, elevated, or low. Examine a peripheral blood smear for the presence of toxic neutrophils, eosinophils, atypical lymphocytes, nucleated RBCs, platelet estimate, anisocytosis, and blood parasites. A falling PCV in the face of RBC transfusion suggests ongoing hemorrhage.

Biochemistry panel

Perform a biochemistry panel to evaluate organ system function. Azotemia with elevated BUN and creatinine may be associated with prerenal dehydration, impaired renal function, or postrenal obstruction or leakage. The BUN also can be elevated when gastrointestinal hemorrhage is present. Serum amylase may be elevated with decreased renal function or in cases of pancreatitis. A normal serum amylase, however, does not rule out pancreatitis as a source of abdominal pain. Serum lipase may be elevated with gastrointestinal inflammation or pancreatitis. Like amylase, a normal serum lipase does not rule out pancreatitis. Total bilirubin, alkaline phosphatase, and alanine transaminase may be elevated with primary cholestatic or hepatocellular diseases or may be due to extrahepatic causes including sepsis.

Urinalysis

Obtain a urinalysis via cystocentesis whenever possible, except in cases of suspected pyometra or transitional cell carcinoma. Azotemia in the presence of a nonconcentrated (isosthenuric or hyposthenuric) urine suggests primary renal disease. Secondary causes of apparent renal azotemia and lack of concentrating ability also occur in cases of hypo-adrenocorticism and gram-negative sepsis. Renal tubular casts may be present in cases of acute renal ischemia or toxic insult to the kidneys. Bacteriuria and pyuria may be present with infection and inflammation. When a urinalysis is obtained via free catch or urethral catheterization, the presence of bacteriuria or pyuria also may be associated with pyometra, vaginitis, or prostatitis/prostatic abscess.

Lactate

Serum lactate is a biochemical indicator of decreased organ perfusion, decreased oxygen delivery or extraction, and end-organ anaerobic glycolysis. Elevated serum lactate greater than 6 mmol/L has been associated with increased morbidity and need for gastric resection in cases of GDV and increased patient morbidity and mortality in other disease processes. Rising serum lactate in the face of adequate fluid resuscitation is a negative prognostic sign.

Abdominal radiographs

Obtain abdominal radiographs as one of the first diagnostic tests when deciding whether to pursue medical or surgical management. The presence of GDV, linear foreign body, pneumoperitoneum, pyometra, or splenic torsion warrants immediate surgical intervention. If a loss of abdominal detail occurs because of peritoneal effusion, perform additional diagnostic tests including abdominal paracentesis (abdominocentesis) and abdominal ultrasound to determine the cause of the peritoneal effusion.

Abdominal ultrasound

Abdominal ultrasonography is often useful in place of or in addition to abdominal radiographs. The sensitivity of abdominal ultrasonography is largely operator dependent. Indications for immediate surgical intervention include loss of blood flow to an organ, linear bunching or placation of the intestinal tract, intussusception, pancreatic phlegmon or abscess, a fluid-filled uterus suggestive of pyometra, gastrointestinal obstruction, intra-luminal gastrointestinal foreign body, dilated bile duct, or gallbladder mucocele, or gas within the wall of the stomach or gallbladder (emphysematous cholecystitis). The presence of peritoneal fluid alone does not warrant immediate surgical intervention without cytologic and biochemical evaluation of the fluid present.

Abdominocentesis

See also Abdominal Paracentesis and Diagnostic Peritoneal Lavage.

Abdominal paracentesis (abdominocentesis) often is the deciding factor in whether to perform immediate surgery. Abdominocentesis is a sensitive technique for detecting peritoneal effusion when more than 6 mL/kg of fluid is present within the abdominal cavity. Abdominal effusion collected should be saved for bacterial culture and evaluated biochemically and cytologically based on your index of suspicion of the primary disease process. If creatinine, urea nitrogen (BUN) or potassium is elevated compared with that of serum, uroabdomen is present. Elevated abdominal fluid lipase or amylase compared with serum supports a diagnosis of pancreatitis. Elevated lactate compared with serum lactate or an abdominal fluid glucose less than 50 mg/dL is highly sensitive and specific for bacterial/septic peritonitis. The presence of bile pigment or bacteria is supportive of bile and septic peritonitis, respectively. Free fibers in abdominal fluid along with clinical signs of abdominal pain strongly support gastrointestinal perforation, and immediate surgical exploration is required.

Text continued on p. 93

TABLE 1-24   Conditions That Can Cause Clinical Signs of Acute Abdominal Pain

The following are clinical conditions, patient signalment, common history, physical examination, and characteristic findings of various diagnostic tests. A blank column next to a condition indicates no specific signalment, history, physical examination, or diagnostic test characteristic for a particular disease process.

Condition	Signalment	History/Chief complaint	Physical examination findings
Abdominal wall			
Hernia	Any	History of trauma, vomiting Abdominal wall swelling Pain, lethargy, anorexia	Abdominal wall swelling, fever, pain
Abscess	Any	Anorexia, pain, lethargy Abdominal wall swelling	Abdominal wall swelling, fever, pain
Blunt trauma	Any	History of trauma, lethargy, pain, inappetance	Pain, hematoma or ecchymosis, periumbilical redness/hemorrhage
Gastrointestinal			
Diaphragmatic hernia	Any	History of trauma, vomiting, lethargy, anorexia, respiratory difficulty	Cyanosis, respiratory difficulty, abdominal pain
Gastroenteritis bacterial	Any	Vomiting, diarrhea, history of toxin or garbage ingestion	Abdominal pain, increased borborygmi vomiting, diarrhea, hematochezia
Parvovirus/Panleukopenia	Young puppy Young kitten	Inadequate vaccination, vomiting, diarrhea, anorexia, lethargy	Dehydration, vomiting, diarrhea, lethargy
Parasitic	Any	Vomiting, diarrhea, history of worms in feces	Ileus, increased or decreased borborygmi
Metabolic/ hypoadrenocorticism	Any, young female, specific breed predisposition	Waxing and waning, lethargy, vomiting, diarrhea, weakness, anorexia, weight loss, stress	Muscle atrophy, dehydration, melena, hematochezia, inappropriate bradycardia
Toxin	Any	History of toxin or garbage exposure	Abdominal pain, lethargy
Gastric dilatation	Any	History of garbage or food exposure	Distended abdomen, ptyalism
Gastric dilatation-volvulus	Large breed or deep- chested dog; can occur in any breed	History of unproductive retching	Distended painful tympanic abdomen, cyanosis, respiratory difficulty, ptyalism, retching or unproductive vomiting

Condition	Age	History	Physical examination
Gastric ulcer	Any	Hematemesis, coffee ground vomitus, lethargy, anorexia, melena	Abdominal pain, melena
Cecal inversion			
Colonic ulcer/perforation	Any	Vomiting, hematochezia, dyschezia, lethargy	Hematochezia, abdominal pain
Linear foreign body	Any	Vomiting, history of exposure to string, thread, ribbon	Abdominal pain, clumped intestines on palpation, string under tongue
Luminal foreign body	Any	History of vomiting, inappetance, history of eating foreign object(s)	Abdominal pain, palpate abdominal mass
Intestinal/ulcer perforation	Any	Vomiting, anorexia, lethargy	Abdominal pain, fever, lethargy, dehydration, palpable mass effect
Intussusception	Any, primarily young dogs/cats	Vomiting, diarrhea, lethargy	Abdominal pain, fever, palpable abdominal mass ("sausage")
Obstipation	Older	Vomiting, straining to defecate, crying out in pain, anorexia	Palpable mass effect, dry feces on rectal examination
Vascular ischemia/bowel compromise	Any	Vomiting, diarrhea, hematochezia, anorexia, abdominal pain	Abdominal pain, fever, palpable fluid wave, hematochezia with luminal tissue on rectal examination
Liver and gallbladder			
Cholangiohepatitis/hepatitis	Any	Anorexia, vomiting, pain, lethargy, icterus	Dehydration, painful abdomen, vomitus, icterus
Cholecystitis/Emphysematous cholecystitis/gallbladder mucocoele	Any	Anorexia, vomiting, pain, lethargy	Dehydration, painful abdomen, vomitus, icterus, fever
Biliary rupture/bile peritonitis	Any	History of trauma, pain, lethargy, vomiting, anorexia	Dehydration, painful abdomen, vomitus, icterus, fever
Biliary obstruction	Any	Anorexia, vomiting, pain, lethargy	Dehydration, painful abdomen, vomitus, fever
Hepatic abscess	Any	Anorexia, vomiting, pain, lethargy	Dehydration, painful abdomen, vomitus, fever
Hepatic torsion	Any	Anorexia, vomiting, pain, lethargy	Dehydration, painful abdomen, vomitus, fever
Hepatic neoplasia	Any/older animals	Anorexia, vomiting, pain, lethargy	Painful abdomen, vomitus, fever, dehydration, seizures
			Painful abdomen, vomitus, fever, dehydration, seizures

Continued

1

TABLE 1-24 Conditions That Can Cause Clinical Signs of Acute Abdominal Pain—cont'd

Condition	Signalment	History/Chief complaint	Physical examination findings
Pancreas			
Pancreatitis	Any, some breed Predisposition	Anorexia, vomiting, pain, lethargy; History of eating fatty meal	Dehydration, abdominal pain, vomitus, alopecia, palpable abdominal mass
Pancreatic abscess			
Pancreatic pseudocyst or mucocoele			
Pancreatic neoplasia	Any, older animals	Anorexia, vomiting, pain, lethargy, weight loss, truncal alopecia	Dehydration, abdominal pain, vomitus, alopecia, palpable abdominal mass
Spleen			
Splenic torsion	Any	Acute pain, vomiting, lethargy	Pale mm, decompensatory shock, palpable abdominal mass and splenomegaly, abdominal pain
Splenic mass	Any/older animals	Acute pain, lethargy, collapse	Pale mm, decompensatory shock, premature ventricular contractions on ECG, anemia
Splenic infarction	Any	Acute pain, lethargy, collapse	Fever, abdominal pain, splenomegaly
Traumatic splenic laceration	Any	History of trauma	Abdominal pain, ballotable fluid wave, anemia, compensatory or decompensatory shock
Genitourinary			
Mastitis	Female	History of lactation	Abdominal pain, fever, lethargy, anorexia painful swollen sometimes abscessed mammary glands, discolored milk
Penis fracture	Male dogs	History of trauma, history of traumatic breeding	Painful abdomen and penis
Paraphimosis	Male dogs	Persistent erection	Swollen penis outside of prepuce
Prostate			
Prostatitis	Male dogs	Straining to defecate	Painful enlarged prostate on rectal palpation, fever
Prostatic abscess	Older male dogs	Straining to defecate, pain, lethargy	Painful enlarged prostate on rectal palpation
Prostatic neoplasia	Older male dogs	Straining to defecate	Enlarged prostate on rectal examination
Renal acute nephritis	Any	Lethargy, vomiting, anorexia	Painful abdomen, dehydration, fever
Pyelonephritis	Any	Lethargy, PU/PD, vomiting, anorexia	Painful abdomen, fever
Renal neoplasia	Any, older	Anorexia, vomiting, lethargy, weight loss	Painful abdomen, fever, cachexia, palpable abdominal mass
Renal abscess	Any	Anorexia, vomiting, lethargy, weight loss	Painful abdomen, fever, cachexia, palpable abdominal mass
Renal infarct/thrombus	Any	Lethargy, PU/PD, vomiting	Painful abdomen, fever

Condition	Signalment	History	Physical Findings
Renolithiasis	Any	Lethargy, PU/PD, vomiting	Painful abdomen, fever
Ureteral obstruction	Any	Lethargy, PU/PD, vomiting	Painful abdomen, fever, dehydration
Ureteral rupture	Any	Lethargy, PU/PD, vomiting	Painful abdomen, fever, dehydration
Urethral obstruction	Any	Lethargy, PU/PD, vomiting, straining to urinate	Painful abdomen, dehydration, vomitus, painful distended nonexpressible urinary bladder
Urethral tear/rupture	Any	Lethargy, PU/PD, vomiting, history of trauma	Painful abdomen, dehydration, vomitus, fever
Urinary bladder neoplasia	Any, older animals	Stranguria, hematuria, weight loss, pollakiuria	Thickened urethra may be palpable on rectal examination
Testicles			
Testicular torsion	Intact male dogs	Pain, chewing or looking at back end	Swollen painful testicle, fever
Uterus and Ovaries			
Uterine torsion	Intact gravid females	Acute collapse, vaginal discharge, history of breeding	Decompensatory shock, vaginal discharge
Pyometra	Intact females	Recent heat cycle, PU/PD, vomiting, diarrhea, lethargy, vaginal discharge	Dehydration, soft tissue mass in caudal abdomen, vaginal discharge, fever
Uterine rupture	Intact gravid females	History of recent whelping/queening, lethargy, acute collapse	Abdominal pain, vaginal discharge, decompensatory shock
Other			
Discospondylitis	Any	History of pain, lethargy, anorexia	Painful spine, fever
Envenomation			
Black widow spider	Any	History of possible exposure, pain, acute collapse, vomiting	Recumbency, muscle fasciculations, pain, vomiting, fever, collapse
Brown recluse	Any	History of possible exposure, pain, necrotizing bulls-eye ulcer formation	Ulcer, pain, fever, granulomatous lesion
Intervertebral disk disease	Any	Acute paresis or paralysis	Paresis or paralysis, spinal pain
Meningitis	Any	Acute pain, lethargy, anorexia	Fever, extreme pain
Myositis	Any	Acute pain, lethargy, anorexia	Fever, extreme pain
Neoplasia	Any	Acute pain, lethargy, anorexia, collapse	Decompensatory shock, palpable abdominal mass
Peritonitis	Any	Vomiting, anorexia, lethargy, pain, history of trauma or penetrating abdominal injury	Pain, fever, palpable foreign object
Sublumbar or retroperitoneal abscess	Any	Pain, anorexia, lethargy	Pain, lethargy, dehydration, fever

Continued

1

TABLE 1-24 **Conditions That Can Cause Clinical Signs of Acute Abdominal Pain—cont'd**

Diagnostic tests	Treatment
Lack of contiguity of body wall Soft tissue density or abdominal contents SQ on RADS	Surgical (immediate)
Lack of contiguity of body wall Soft tissue density or abdominal contents SQ on RADS; inflammatory cells and bacteria on aspirate	Surgical (immediate)
Hemoabdomen on abdominocentesis or DPL	Medical
Radiographic evidence of abdominal organs in thorax, may require contrast celiotomy	Medical unless stomach is in thorax
Ileus on radiographs, white blood cells in feces	Medical
Parvovirus CITE test positive on feces leuko-/neutropenia	Medical
Parasite oocysts or parasites in feces	Medical
Atrial standstill on EGG, hyperkalemia, hyponatremia, hypocholesterolemia, hypoglycemia, hyperphosphatemia, azotemia, normal WBC and differential positive ethylene glycol	Medical
Calcium oxalate dihydrate crystals U/A "halo sign" = hyperechoic renal cortex on U/S	Medical
Soft tissue density/food with gastric dilation on radiographs	Medical
Dorsal and cranial displacement of pylorus with dilation of gastric fundus on right lateral radiograph, premature ventricular contractions on ECG, elevated lactate	Surgical (Immediate)
Regenerative anemia, melena, loss of abdominal detail on radiographs if perforation present	Medical unless perforation present
Loss of detail on radiographs if perforation and peritonitis present	Medical unless perforation present
C-shaped abnormal gas pattern with plication on radiographs	Surgical (Immediate)
Dilation of bowel cranial to foreign object, radiopaque object in stomach or intestines, hypochloremic metabolic acidosis on bloodwork if pyloric outflow obstruction is present	Surgical (Immediate)
Elevated or decreased WBC; foreign material, WBCs and bacteria on abdominal fluid, elevated lactate and decreased glucose on abdominal fluid	Medical unless perforation present
Target shaped soft tissue density on abdominal U/S, soft tissue density with gas dilation cranially on abdominal radiographs	Surgical (Immediate): medical management of primary cause
Colonic distension with hard feces on radiographs	Medical
Increased or decreased WBC, septic abdominal effusion	Surgical (Immediate)
Elevated T Bili, ALT, Alk Phos, and WBC hypoechoic hepatic parenchyma on ultrasound hepatomegaly	Medical after biopsy
Elevated T Bili, ALT, Alk Phos, and WBC hyperechoic foci in gallbladder or sludge on U/S, free gas in wall of gall bladder	Surgical (Immediate)
Abdominal effusion, bile pigment in effusion	Surgical (Immediate)
Elevated T Bili, Alk Phos, ALT	Surgical (Immediate)
Elevated or decreased WBC, elevated T Bili, Alk Phos and ALT, free gas in hepatic parenchyma on RADS, hypoechoic mass with hyperechoic material in hepatic parenchyma on U/S	Surgical (Immediate)
Heteroechoic liver with hyperechoic center on ultrasound	Surgical (Immediate)
Mixed echogenic mass on ultrasound, soft tissue mass density on radiographs, elevated alk phos, ALT, T Bili, hypoglycemia	Surgical (Immediate or delayed)

T A B L E 1 - 2 4 Conditions That Can Cause Clinical Signs of Acute Abdominal Pain—cont'd

Diagnostic tests	Treatment
Elevated T Bili, Alk Phos, ALT, amylase and/or lipase, elevated or decreased WBC, hypocalcemia, focal loss of detail in right cranial quadrant on radiographs hypo- to hyperechoic pancreas with hyperechoic peri-pancreatic fat on ultrasound, abdominal and/or pleural effusion on radiographs and ultrasound	Medical in most cases unless abscess or phlegmon is present
Pancreatic soft tissue mass effect on radiographs and ultrasound, elevated amylase and lipase, hypoglycemia, elevated serum insulin	Surgical if mass identified, otherwise medical management of hypoglycemia
Splenomegaly on radiographs, hyperechoic spleen with no blood flow on ultrasound	Surgical (Immediate)
Soft tissue mass effect and loss of abdominal detail on radiographs, cavitated mass with abdominal effusion on U/S	Surgical (Immediate)
Hyperechoic spleen with no blood flow on abdominal U/S, abdominal effusion, thrombocytopenia	Surgical (Immediate)
Loss of abdominal detail on radiographs, peritoneal effusion on U/S, hemoabdomen on abdominocentesis	Medical unless refractory hypotension
Diagnosis based primarily on clinical signs	Medical
Fracture of the os penis on radiographs	Largely medical unless urethral tear
Diagnosis based primarily on clinical signs	Medical, although prepuce may need to be incised to allow replacement of penis into sheath
Prostatomegaly on radiographs and ultrasound hypoechoic prostate on U/S, pyuria and bacteriuria and U/A	Medical
Prostatomegaly on radiographs and ultrasound hypo- to hyperechoic prostate on U/S, bacteriuria and pyuria on U/A	Surgical (Delayed)
Prostatomegaly on radiographs and ultrasound, prostatic mineralization on radiographs and ultrasound	Medical/Surgical
Hypoechoic kidneys on U/S, pyuria on U/A, elevated WBC, azotemia	Medical
Pyuria, bacteriuria on U/A	Medical
Pyelectasia in abdominal U/S, azotemia Renomegaly on radiographs, azotemia	Surgical (Immediate)
Renal mass on U/S, renomegaly on radiographs	Surgical (Immediate)
Renal mass on U/S, azotemia, lack of renal blood flow on U/S	Surgical (Delayed)
Calculi in renal pelvis on radiographs and ultrasound, azotemia	Medical unless both kidneys affected
Ureteral calculi on radiographs and ultrasound, hydronephrosis, azotemia	Medical unless both kidneys affected
Ureteral calculi on radiographs and ultrasound, hydronephrosis, fluid or soft tissue density on U/S, azotemia	Surgical (Delayed until electrolyte stabilization)
Diagnosis largely based on physical examination findings	Medical unless cannot pass urethral catheter

Continued

TABLE 1-24 Conditions That Can Cause Clinical Signs of Acute Abdominal Pain—cont'd

Diagnostic tests	Treatment
Azotemia, no peritoneal effusion, lack of urine output or outflow with ureteral catheterization, double contrast cystourethrogram indicated	Surgical (Delayed until electrolyte stabilization)
Transitional cellular casts on U/A, hematuria, mass effect or thickened irregular urethra on ultrasound or cystourethrogram	Surgical and medical management
Hypoechoic swollen testicle on testicular ultrasound	Surgical (Immediate)
Fluid or gas-filled tubular structure on abdominal ultrasound or abdominal radiographs	Surgical (Immediate)
Soft tissue tubular structure on radiographs, fluid-filled uterus on ultrasound, azotemia, isosthenuria, elevated T Bili, ALT and Alk Phos	Surgical (Immediate)
Pneumoperitoneum on radiographs, abdominal effusion, degenerative neutrophils and bacteria on abdominal fluid cytology	Surgical (Immediate)
Elevated WBC, increased density to bony endplates on radiographs	Medical
Hypocalcemia, markedly elevated CK	Medical
Diagnosis of exclusion	Medical
Decreased intervertebral disk space on radiographs, evidence of disk herniation and cord compression with myelogram or MRI	Surgical (Immediate)
Elevated protein and neutrophils on CSF analysis	Medical
Muscle biopsy	Medical
Mass effect and loss of abdominal detail on radiographs, mass and peritoneal effusion on ultrasound, anemia	Surgical (Immediate)
Degenerative neutrophils, plant material, bile pigment, or bacteria on abdominal fluid cytology; peritoneal effusion on U/S, loss of abdominal detail on radiographs, elevated or decreased WBC	Surgical (Immediate)
Elevated or decreased WBC, retroperitoneal mass effect on radiographs or ultrasound	Surgical (Immediate)

BOX 1-23   INDICATIONS TO PERFORM EXPLORATORY LAPAROTOMY

- Penetrating abdominal injury
- Presence of bacterial on abdominal fluid
- Presence of greater than 500 µL of white blood cells in lavage fluid effluent, particularly if degenerative neutrophils are present
- Presence of food or plant material in lavage fluid
- Presence of creatinine, blood urea nitrogen, potassium, or lactate in abdominal fluid greater than that in peripheral blood
- Presence of glucose in abdominal fluid less than 50 mg/dL or less than that of peripheral blood
- Presence of bilirubin in lavage fluid
- Pneumoperitoneum on radiographs
- Continued evidence of peritoneal irritation

Diagnostic peritoneal lavage

In the event of a negative abdominocentesis, but peritoneal effusion or bile or gastrointestinal perforation are suspected, perform a diagnostic peritoneal lavage. Peritoneal dialysis kits are commercially available but are often expensive and impractical (see p. 6).

MANAGEMENT

Animals that have acute abdominal pain can be divided into three broad categories, depending on the primary cause of pain and the initial definitive treatment (Table 1-24). Some diseases warrant a nonsurgical, medical approach to case management. Other conditions require immediate surgery following rapid stabilization. Other conditions initially can be managed medically until the patient is hemodynamically more stable and then may or may not require surgical intervention at a later time. Specific management of each disease entity is listed under its own subheading.

Exploratory laparotomy/celiotomy

Box 1-23 lists specific indications for exploratory laparotomy. The best means to explore the abdominal cavity accurately and thoroughly is to open the abdomen on midline from the level of the xyphoid process caudally to the pubis for full exposure and then to evaluate all organs in every quadrant in a systematic manner. Address specific problems such as gastric or splenic torsion, enteroplication, and foreign body removal, and then copiously lavage the abdomen with warmed sterile saline solution. Suction the saline solution thoroughly from the peritoneal cavity so as to not impair macrophage function. In cases of septic peritonitis, the abdomen may be left open, or a drain may be placed for further suction and lavage. The routine use of antibiotics in irrigation solutions is contraindicated because the antibiotics can irritate the peritoneum and delay healing. When the abdominal cavity is left open, secure sterile laparotomy towels and water-impermeable dressings over the abdominal wound with umbilical tape, and then change these daily or as strike-through occurs. Open abdomen cases are often effusive and require meticulous evaluation and management of electrolyte imbalances and hypoalbuminemia. The abdomen can be closed and/or the abdominal drain removed when the volume of the effusion decreases, when bacteria are no longer present, and when the neutrophils become more healthy in appearance.

Additional Reading

Bischoff MG: Radiographic techniques and interpretation of the acute abdomen, *Clin Tech Small Anim Pract* 18(1):7-19, 2003.

Bonczynski JJ, Ludwig LL, Barton LJ, et al: Comparison of peritoneal fluid and peripheral blood pH, bicarbonate, glucose, and lactate as a diagnostic tool for septic peritonitis in dogs and cats, *Vet Surg* 32(2):161-166, 2003.

Connally HE: Cytology and fluid analysis of the acute abdomen, *Clin Tech Small Anim Pract* 18(1):39-44, 2003.

Cruz-Arambulo R, Wrigley R: Ultrasonography of the acute abdomen, *Clin Tech Small Anim Pract* 18(1):20-31, 2003.

Herren V, Edwards L, Mazzaferro EM: Acute abdomen: diagnosis, *Compend Contin Educ Pract Vet* 26(5):350-363, 2004.

Hofmeister EH: Anesthesia for the acute abdomen patient, *Clin Tech Small Anim Pract* 18(1):45-52, 2003.

Mann FA: Acute abdomen: evaluation and emergency treatment. In Bonagura JD, editor: *Kirk's current veterinary therapy XIII,* Philadelphia, 2002, WB Saunders.

Mazzaferro EM: *Triage and approach to the acute abdomen, Clin Tech Small Anim Pract* 18(1):1-6, 2003.

Mueller MG, Ludwig LL, Barton LJ: Use of closed-suction drains to treat generalized peritonitis in dogs and cats: 40 cases (1997-1999), *J Am Vet Med Assoc* 219(6):789-794, 2001.

Schmiedt C, Tobias KM, Otto CM: Evaluation of abdominal fluid: peripheral blood creatinine and potassium ratios for diagnosis of uroperitoneum in dogs, *J Vet Emerg Crit Care* 11(4):275-280, 2001.

Walters JM: Abdominal paracentesis and diagnostic peritoneal lavage, *Clin Tech Small Anim Pract* 18(1):32-38, 2003.

ANAPHYLACTIC (ANAPHYLACTOID) SHOCK

Anaphylactic shock occurs as an immediate hypersensitivity reaction to a variety of inciting stimuli (Box 1-24). In animals, the most naturally occurring anaphylactic reaction results from wasp or bee stings. Most other reactions occur as a result of an abnormal sensitivity to items used in making medical diagnoses or treatment.

During an anaphylactic reaction, activation of C5a and the complement system results in vascular smooth muscle dilation and the release of a cascade of inflammatory mediators, including histamine, slow-reacting substance of anaphylaxis, serotonin, heparin, acetylcholine, and bradykinin.

Clinical signs associated with anaphylaxis differ between dogs and cats. In dogs, clinical signs may include restlessness, vomiting, diarrhea, hematochezia, circulatory collapse, coma, and death. In cats, clinical signs often are associated with respiratory system abnormalities. Clinical signs may include ptyalism, pruritus, vomiting, incoordination, bronchoconstriction, pulmonary edema and hemorrhage, laryngeal edema, collapse, and death.

IMMEDIATE ACTION/TREATMENT

The most important steps to remember in any emergency is to follow the ABCs of *Airway*, *Breathing*, and *Circulation*. First, establish an airway through endotracheal intubation or emergency tracheostomy, if necessary. Concurrently, an assistant should establish vascular or intraosseous access to administer drugs and fluids (Box 1-25).

DIFFERENTIAL DIAGNOSIS

Differential diagnoses to consider for anaphylactic shock include the following:
Any cause of vomiting, diarrhea
Toxin
Internal hemorrhage
Congestive heart failure

BOX 1-24   INCITING ALLERGENS THAT CAN CAUSE ANAPHYLACTOID REACTIONS, ANGIONEUROTIC EDEMA, OR URTICARIA

- Adrenocorticotropic hormone
- Antihistamines/antitoxins (foreign serums)
- Benzocaine
- Chloramphenicol
- Erythromycin
- Food
- Heparin
- Hypersensitization and skin testing
- Insect stings
- Insulin
- Iodinated contrast media
- Lidocaine
- Oxytocin
- Penicillin
- Penicillinase
- Procaine
- Salicylates
- Streptomycin
- Tetracaine
- Tetracycline
- Tranquilizers
- Vaccines
- Vancomycin
- Vitamins

BOX 1-25   IMMEDIATE TREATMENT OF ANAPHYLACTIC SHOCK

1. Administer epinephrine (0.01 mL/kg 1:1000 epinephrine IV or IO). If vascular access cannot be established, administer the epinephrine intramuscularly (0.2 to 0.5 mL/kg). Repeat epinephrine dose in 10 to 15 minutes if clinical signs are not resolving.
2. Start intravenous crystalloid fluids (Normosol-R, PlasmaLyte-M, lactated Ringer's solution) at one fourth of a calculated shock dose (90 mL/kg/hour in dogs, 44 mL/kg/hour in cats).
3. Administer a short-acting steroid (dexamethasone sodium phosphate [Dex-SP], 0.25 to 1.0 mg/kg IV).
4. Administer antihistamines. Administer diphenhydramine (0.5 mg/kg IM). Administer famotidine (0.5 to 1.0 mg/kg IV).

Lower airway disease
Upper airway obstruction

MANAGEMENT

The patient should be hospitalized until complete resolution of clinical signs. After initial stabilization and treatment, it is important to maintain vascular access and continue intravenous fluid therapy until the patient is no longer hypotensive, and vomiting and diarrhea have resolved. In cases of fulminant pulmonary hemorrhage and edema, administer supplemental oxygen until the patient is no longer hypoxemic or orthopneic on room air. Normalize and maintain blood pressure using positive inotropes (dobutamine, 3-10 μg/kg/minute CRI) or pressors (dopamine, 3 to 10 μg/kg/minute IV CRI; SEE SHOCK). If blood-tinged vomitus or diarrhea has been observed, administer antibiotics to decrease the risk of bacterial translocation and sepsis (cefoxitin, 22 mg/kg IV tid; metronidazole, 10 mg/kg IV tid). Also consider using gastroprotectant drugs (famotidine, 0.5 to 1.0 mg/kg IV; ranitidine, 0.5 to 2.0 mg/kg PO, IV, IM bid; sucralfate, 0.25 to 1.0 g PO tid; omeprazole, 0.7 to 1.0 mg/kg PO sid).

ANGIONEUROTIC EDEMA AND URTICARIA

A second and less serious form of allergic reaction is manifested as angioneurotic edema and urticaria. In most cases, clinical signs develop within 20 minutes of an inciting allergen. Although this type of reaction causes patient discomfort, it rarely poses a life-threatening problem. Most animals have mild to severe swelling of the maxilla and periorbital regions. The facial edema also may be accompanied by mild to severe generalized urticaria. Some animals may paw at their face, rub at their eyes, or have vomiting or diarrhea.

IMMEDIATE ACTION/TREATMENT

The treatment for angioneurotic edema involves suppressing the immune response by administration of short-acting glucocorticoid drugs and blocking the actions of histamine by the synergistic use of histamine$_1$ and histamine$_2$ receptor blockers (Box 1-26).

DIFFERENTIAL DIAGNOSIS

In some cases, the inciting cause is a known recent vaccination or insect sting. Many times, however, the inciting cause is not known and is likely an exposure to a stinging insect or arachnid. Differential diagnoses for acute facial swelling and/or urticaria include acetaminophen toxicity (cats), anterior caval syndrome, lymphadenitis, vasculitis, hypoalbuminemia, and contact dermatitis.

MANAGEMENT

Observe animals that have presented for angioneurotic edema for a minimum of 20 to 30 minutes after injection of the short-acting glucocorticoids and antihistamines. Monitor blood pressure to make sure that the patient does not have concurrent anaphylaxis and hypotension. After partial or complete resolution of clinical signs, the animal can be discharged to its owner for observation. In dogs, mild vomiting or diarrhea may occur within 1 to 2 days after this type of reaction. Wherever possible, exposure to the inciting allergen should be avoided.

BOX 1-26   IMMUNE RESPONSE SUPPRESSION AGENTS FOR ANGIONEUROTIC EDEMA

- Administer short-acting glucocorticoid:
- Dexamethasone sodium phosphate (Dex-SP), 0.25 to 1.0 mg/kg IV, SQ, IM
- Administer antihistamines:
- Diphenhydramine, 0.5 to 1.0 mg/kg IM, SQ
- Famotidine, 0.5 to 1.0 mg/kg IV, SQ, IM

Additional Reading

Cohen R: Systemic anaphylaxis. In Bonagura J, editor: *Current veterinary therapy XII. Small animal practice*, Philadelphia, 1995, WB Saunders.

Friberg CA, Lewis DT: Insect hypersensitivity in small animals, *Compend Contin Educ Pract Vet* 20(10):1121-1131, 1998.

Meyer EK: Vaccine-associated adverse events, *Vet Clin North Am Small Anim Pract* 31(3): 493-514, 2001.

Noble SJ, Armstrong PJ: Bee sting envenomation resulting in secondary immune-mediated hemolytic anemia in two dogs, *J Am Vet Med Assoc* 214(7):1026-1027, 1999.

Plunkett SJ: Anaphylaxis to ophthalmic medication in a cat, *J Vet Emerg Crit Care* 10(3):169-171, 2000.

Waddell LS, Drobatz KJ: Massive envenomation by *Vespula* spp in two dogs, *J Vet Emerg Crit Care* 9(2):67-71, 1999.

ANESTHETIC COMPLICATIONS AND EMERGENCIES

Complications observed while a patient is under anesthesia can be divided into two broad categories: (1) those related to equipment malfunction or human error and (2) the patient's physiologic response to the cardiorespiratory effects of the anesthetic drugs. Careful observation of the patient and familiarity with anesthetic equipment, drug protocols, and monitoring equipment is necessary for the safest anesthesia to occur. Despite this, however, anesthetic-related complications are frequent and need to be recognized and treated appropriately.

THE RESPIRATORY SYSTEM

Many anesthetic drugs have a dose-dependent depressive effect on the respiratory system and cause a decrease in respiratory rate and tidal volume, leading to hypoventilation. Respiratory rate alone is not a reliable indicator of the patient's oxygenation and ventilatory status. The respiratory tidal volume can be measured with a Wright's respirometer. Perform pulse oximetry and capnography as noninvasive measures of the patient's oxygenation and ventilation.

Ventilation can be impaired as a result of anesthetic drugs, patient position, pneumothorax, pleural effusion (chylothorax, hemothorax, pyothorax), equipment malfunction, rebreathing of carbon dioxide, thoracic wall injury, or alveolar fluid (pulmonary edema, hemorrhage, or pneumonia). Problems such as a diaphragmatic hernia, GDV, or gravid uterus can impede diaphragmatic excursions once the patient is placed on its back and can lead to impaired ventilation. The work of breathing also may be increased because of increased resistance of the anesthesia circuit and increased dead space ventilation. This is particularly important in small toy breeds.

Clinical signs of inadequate ventilation and respiratory complications include abnormal respiratory pattern, sudden changes in heart rate, cardiac dysrhythmias, cyanosis, and cardiopulmonary arrest. End-tidal carbon dioxide, or capnography, gives a graphic display of adequacy of ventilation. Rapid decreases in end-tidal carbon dioxide can be caused by disconnection or obstruction of the patient's endotracheal tube or poor perfusion, namely, cardiopulmonary arrest (see Capnometry [End-Tidal Carbon Dioxide Monitoring]).

Postoperatively, hypoventilation can occur because of the residual effects of the anesthetic drugs, hypothermia, overventilation during intraoperative support, surgical techniques that compromise ventilation (thoracotomy, cervical disk surgery, atlantooccipital stabilization), postoperative bandaging of the abdomen or thorax, ventilatory muscle fatigue, or injury to the CNS.

CARDIOVASCULAR SYSTEM

Cardiac output is a function of heart rate and stroke volume. Factors that influence stroke volume include vascular and cardiac preload, cardiac afterload, and cardiac contractility. The patient's cardiac output can be affected adversely by the negative inotropic and chronotropic and vasodilatory effects of anesthetic drugs, all leading to hypotension.

1

Bradycardia, tachycardia, cardiac dysrhythmias, and vascular dilation can lead to hypotension and inadequate organ perfusion. Table 1-25 lists the normal heart rate and blood pressure in dogs and cats.

Bradycardia

Bradycardia is defined as a heart rate below normal values. Many anesthetic drugs can cause bradycardia. Causes of bradycardia include the use of narcotics or α_2-agonist drugs, deep plane of anesthesia, increased vagal tone, hypothermia, and hypoxia. Table 1-26 lists the causes of bradycardia and the necessary immediate action or treatment.

Tachycardia

Tachycardia is defined as a heart rate above normal values. Common causes of tachycardia include vasodilation, drugs, inadequate anesthetic depth and perceived pain, hypercapnia, hypoxemia, hypotension, shock, or hyperthermia. Table 1-27 lists the causes and immediate action or treatment for tachycardia.

Hypotension

Hypotension is defined as physiologically low blood pressure (mean arterial pressure less than 65 mm Hg). A mean arterial blood pressure less than 60 mm Hg can result in inadequate tissue perfusion and oxygen delivery. The coronary arteries are perfused during diastole. Inadequate diastolic blood pressure, less than 40 mm Hg, can cause decreased coronary artery perfusion and myocardial hypoxemia that can predispose the heart to dysrhythmias. Causes of perianesthetic hypotension include peripheral vasodilation by anesthetic drugs, bradycardia or tachyarrhythmias, hypothermia, inadequate cardiac preload from vasodilation or hemorrhage, decreased venous return from patient position or surgical manipulation of viscera, and decreased cardiac contractility. Table 1-28 lists possible causes of hypotension and immediate actions to take.

TABLE 1-25   Normal Parameters for Heart Rate and Blood Pressure in Dogs and Cats

Species	Normal heart rate (beats/minute)	Normal blood pressure (mm Hg)		
		Systolic	Diastolic	Mean
Dogs (large)	60-100	100-160	60-90	80-120
Dogs (medium)	80-120			
Dogs (small)	90-140			
Cats	140-200	100-160	60-90	80-120

TABLE 1-26   Causes and Treatment of Bradycardia

Cause	Immediate action
Anesthetic drug:	
Opioid	Reverse effects with naloxone.
α_2-Agonist	Reverse effects with yohimbine or atipamezole.
Deep anesthesia	Decrease vaporizer setting.
Increased vagal tone	Administer a parasympatholytic (atropine or glycopyrrolate).
Hypothermia	Provide ambient rewarming.
Hypoxia	Provide supplemental oxygen.

TABLE 1-27   Causes and Treatment of Tachycardia

Cause	Immediate action
Vagolytic drugs	
Atropine	Allow time for the drug to wear off.
Glycopyrrolate	Allow time for the drug to wear off.
Sympathomimetic drugs	
Epinephrine	Allow time for the drug to wear off; administer a β-blocker; turn off infusion.
Isoproterenol	Administer a β-blocker.
Dopamine	Turn off infusion; administer a β-blocker.
Ketamine	Allow time for drug to wear off.
Inadequate anesthetic depth	Increase anesthetic depth.
Hypercapnia	Increase ventilation (assisted ventilation).
Hypoxemia	Increase gas flow and oxygenation.
Hypotension	Decrease anesthetic depth; administer an intravenous crystalloid or colloid bolus, positive inotrope drug, positive chronotrope drug, or pressor.
Hyperthermia	Apply ambient or active cooling measures; administer dantrolene sodium if malignant hyperthermia is suspected.

TABLE 1-28   Causes and Treatment of Perianesthetic Hypotension

Cause	Immediate action
Hypothermia	Provide ambient rewarming.
Hypocalcemia*	Administer calcium chloride (10 mg/kg IV) or calcium gluconate (23 mg/kg).
Increased anesthetic	Decrease vaporizer setting/anesthetic depth. Reverse with opioids or α_2-agonists.
Vasodilation	Administer an intravenous crystalloid bolus (10 mL/kg). Administer an intravenous colloid bolus (5 mL/kg). Administer a pressor (epinephrine, phenylephrine).
Negative inotropy	Decrease anesthetic depth. Administer ephedrine (0.1-0.25 mg/kg IV). Administer dobutamine (2-20 μg/kg IV CRI). Administer dopamine (2-10 μg/kg/minute). Administer norepinephrine (0.05-0.4 μg/kg/minute IV CRI). Administer epinephrine (0.05-0.4 μg/kg/minute IV CRI).
Bradycardia	Administer atropine (0.01-0.04 mg/kg IV or SQ). Administer glycopyrrolate (0.005-0.02 mg/kg IV, SQ).

*Hypocalcemia caused by chelation from EDTA with multiple blood product transfusion (cats are particularly susceptible).

Cardiac dysrhythmias

Electrocardiogram monitoring is useful for the early detection of cardiac dysrhythmias during the perianesthetic period. Clinical signs of cardiac dysrhythmias include irregular pulse rate or pressure, abnormal or irregular heart sounds, pallor, cyanosis, hypotension, and an abnormal ECG tracing. Remember that the single best method of detecting cardiac dysrhythmias is with your fingertips (palpate a pulse or apex heartbeat) and ears (auscultate the heart). Confirm the dysrhythmia by auscultating the heart rate and rhythm, identify the P waves and the QRS complexes, and evaluate the relationship between the P waves and QRS complexes. Is there a P wave for every QRS, and a QRS for every P wave? During anesthesia, fluid, acid-base, and electrolyte imbalances can predispose the patient to dysrhythmias. Sympathetic and parasympathetic stimulation, including the time of intubation, can predispose the patient to dysrhythmias. If the patient's plane of anesthesia is too light, perception of pain can cause catecholamine release, sensitizing the myocardium to ectopic beats. Atrioventricular blockade can be induced with the administration of α_2-agonist medications, including xylazine and medetomidine. Thiobarbiturates (thiopental) can induce ventricular ectopy and bigeminy. Although these dysrhythmias may not be harmful in the awake patient, anesthetized patients are at a particular risk of dysrhythmia-induced hypotension. Carefully monitor and treat all dysrhythmias (see Cardiac Dysrhythmias). Box 1-27 lists steps to take to prevent perianesthetic dysrhythmias.

DEPTH EVALUATION AND HUMAN ERROR

Awakening during anesthesia can occur and can be caused by equipment failure and simply, although no one likes to admit it, human error. Table 1-29 lists causes of arousal during anesthesia and appropriate immediate actions.

BOX 1-27   STEPS TO PREVENT PERIANESTHETIC DYSRHYTHMIAS

- Stabilize acid-base and electrolyte balance before anesthetic induction, whenever possible.
- Rehydrate patient before anesthetic induction.
- Select anesthetic agents appropriate for the particular patient.
- Be aware of the effects of the drugs on the myocardium.
- Ensure adequate anesthetic depth and oxygenation before anesthetic induction.
- Ensure ventilatory support during anesthesia.
- Monitor heart rate, rhythm, blood pressure, pulse oximetry, and capnometry during anesthesia.
- Ensure adequate anesthetic depth before surgical stimulation.
- Avoid surgical manipulation to the heart or great vessels, whenever possible.
- Avoid changes in perianesthetic depth.
- Avoid hypothermia.

T A B L E   1 - 2 9   Causes and Treatment of Arousal during Anesthesia

Cause	Immediate action
Postinduction hypoventilation	Increase ventilatory rate and volume.
Too low an inspired gas flow	Increase anesthetic gas flow.
Fresh gas flow too low	Increase fresh gas flow.
Equipment malfunction in machine or vaporizer	Change anesthetic machines.
Esophageal intubation	Reintubate into trachea, and check placement with capnometry or laryngoscope.
Undersized endotracheal tube with leaks	Replace with appropriate sized endotracheal tube.
Inadequate endotracheal cuff inflation	Inflate endotracheal cuff appropriately to decrease leaks.
Surgical stimulus	Increase depth of anesthesia.
Conditions that mimic anesthetic arousal (e.g., malignant hyperthermia)	Awaken patient, and administer dantrolene sodium.

1

POSTANESTHETIC COMPLICATIONS

Delayed recovery can be caused by a number of factors, including excessive anesthetic depth, hypothermia, residual action of narcotics or tranquilizers, delayed metabolism of anesthetic drugs, hypoglycemia, hypocalcemia, hemorrhage, and breed or animal predisposition. Careful monitoring of the patient's blood pressure, acid-base and electrolyte status, anesthetic depth, PCV, and vascular volume intraoperatively and taking care with supportive measures to prevent abnormalities can hasten anesthetic recovery and avoid postoperative complications.

Additional Reading

Gaynor JS, Muir WW: *Handbook of veterinary pain management,* St Louis, 2003, Mosby.

Mazzaferro EM, Wagner AE: Hypotension during anesthesia in dogs and cats: recognition, causes, and treatment, *Compend Contin Educ Pract Vet* 23(8):728-737, 2001.

Melzack R, Wall PD: *Handbook of pain management: a clinical companion to Wall and Melzack's textbook of pain,* Edinburgh, 2003, Churchill Livingstone.

Muir WW, Hubbell JAE, Skarda RT, et al: *Handbook of veterinary anesthesia,* ed 3, St Louis, 2000, Mosby.

Thurmon JC, Tranquilli WJ, Benson GJ: *Lumb and Jones' veterinary anesthesia,* ed 3, Philadelphia, 1996, Lippincott Williams & Wilkins.

BLEEDING DISORDERS

The presentation of a patient with a bleeding disorder often is a diagnostic challenge for the veterinary practitioner (Boxes 1-28 and 1-29). In general, abnormal bleeding can be caused by five major categories: (1) vascular trauma, (2) defective production of hemostatic factors, (3) dilution of hemostatic factors, (4) use or toxicity of systemic anticoagulants, and (5) DIC. A clotting disorder should be suspected in any patient with a history of

---

BOX 1-28   CAUSES OF DEFECTIVE PRIMARY HEMOSTASIS

THROMBOCYTOPENIA
Impaired or defective thrombopoiesis
  Immune-mediated destruction
  Myelophthisis
  Drug-induced
Decreased platelet life span in circulation
  Antibody-mediated platelet destruction
  Consumption in disseminated intravascular
    coagulopathy

THROMBOCYTOPATHIA
Congenital illness
  Von Willebrand's disease
  Other hereditary thrombocytopathies

Systemic illness
  Uremia
  Pancreatitis
  Ehrlichiosis
  Dysproteinemias
  Myeloproliferative and myelodysplastic
    disorders
  Disseminated intravascular coagulation
Antiplatelet drugs
  Aspirin

BOX 1-29   CAUSES OF DEFECTIVE SECONDARY HEMOSTASIS

Clotting factor deficiency
Decreased production
  Hereditary causes
  Chronic hepatic insufficiency/failure
  Vitamin K antagonist rodenticides
Increased consumption
  Disseminated intravascular coagulation
  Hemangiosarcoma

Circulating inhibitors of coagulation
Heparin
Fibrin degradation products

development of spontaneous deep hematomas, unusually prolonged bleeding after traumatic injury, bleeding at multiple sites throughout the body involving multiple organ systems, delayed onset of severe hemorrhage after bleeding, and an inability on the practitioner's part to find an organic cause of bleeding. The signalment, history, clinical signs, and results of coagulation often can aid in making a rapid diagnosis of the primary cause of the disorder and in the selection of appropriate case management. When taking a history, ask the following important questions:
- What is the nature of the bleeding?
- What sites are affected?
- How long has the bleeding been going on?
- Has your animal had any previous or similar episodes?
- Is there any possibility of any toxin exposure?
- If so, when and how much did your animal consume?
- Is there any possibility of trauma?
- Does your animal run loose outdoors unattended?
- Have you ever traveled, and if so, where?
- Has your animal been on any medications recently or currently?
- Has your animal been vaccinated recently?
- Have any known relatives of your animal had any bleeding disorders?
- Are there any other abnormal signs that you have seen?

Abnormalities found on physical examination may aid in determining whether the hemorrhage is localized or generalized (i.e., bleeding from a venipuncture site versus bleeding diathesis). Note whether the clinical signs are associated with a platelet problem and superficial hemorrhage or whether deep bleeding can be associated with abnormalities of the coagulation cascade. Also, make an attempt to identify any concurrent illness that can predispose the patient to a bleeding disorder (i.e., pancreatitis, snakebite, sepsis, immune-mediated hemolytic anemia, or severe trauma and crush or burn injury).

Abnormalities associated with coagulopathies include petechiae and ecchymoses, epistaxis, gingival bleeding, hematuria, hemarthrosis, melena, and hemorrhagic cavity (pleural and peritoneal or retroperitoneal) effusions.

SPECIFIC COAGULOPATHIES

Disseminated intravascular coagulation (DIC)

Disseminated intravascular coagulation is a complex syndrome that results from the inappropriate activation of the clotting cascade, leading to disruption of the normal balance between thrombosis and fibrinolysis. The formation of diffuse microthrombi with concurrent consumption of platelets and activated clotting factors leads to end-organ thrombosis with various degrees of clinical hemorrhage. In animals, DIC always results from some other pathologic process, including various forms of neoplasia, crush and heat-induced injury, sepsis, inflammation, and immune-mediated disorders (Box 1-30). The pathophysiologic mechanisms involved in DIC include vascular endothelial damage, activation and consumption of platelets, release of tissue procoagulants, and consumption of endogenous anticoagulants.

Diagnosis of disseminated intravascular coagulation

Because DIC always results from some other disease process, diagnosis of DIC is based on a number of criteria when evaluating various coagulation tests, peripheral blood smears, platelet count, and end products of thrombosis and fibrinolysis.

There is no one definitive criterion for the diagnosis of DIC (Box 1-31). Thrombocytopenia occurs as platelets are consumed during thrombosis. It is important to remember that trends in decline in platelet numbers are just as important as thrombocytopenia when making the diagnosis. In some cases the platelet count still may be within the normal reference range but has significantly decreased in the last 24 hours. Early in DIC the procoagulant cascade dominates, with hypercoagulability. Activated clotting time, APTT, and PT may be rapid and shorter than normal. In most cases, we do not recognize the

---

BOX 1-30   DISORDERS ASSOCIATED WITH DISSEMINATED INTRAVASCULAR COAGULATION IN THE DOG

Neoplasia
  Hemangiosarcoma
  Lymphoma
Inflammation
  Pancreatitis
  Heat-induced injury
  Gastric dilatation-volvulus
  Mesenteric torsion
Sepsis
  Gram-negative and gram-positive sepsis
  Septic peritonitis
  Gangrenous mastitis
  Pyothorax

Heartworm disease
Immune-mediated disease
  Immune-mediated hemolytic anemia
Trauma
  Crush injury
  Burn injury
Snake envenomation

BOX 1-31   LABORATORY FINDINGS ASSOCIATED WITH A DIAGNOSIS OF DISSEMINATED INTRAVASCULAR COAGULATION*

- Red blood cell fragments
- Thrombocytopenia
- Rapid or prolonged activated partial thromboplastin time
- Rapid or prolonged prothrombin time
- Rapid or prolonged activated clotting time
- Hypofibrinogenemia
- Positive fibrin degradation products without concurrent hepatic disease
- Decrease in antithrombin concentration
- Positive D-dimer test

*More than one of the above criteria should be present to aid in the diagnosis of disseminated intravascular coagulation.

---

hypercoagulable state in our critically ill patients. Later in DIC, as platelets and activated clotting factors become consumed, the ACT, APTT, and PT become prolonged. Antithrombin, a natural anticoagulant, also becomes consumed, and antithrombin levels decline. Antithrombin levels can be measured at commercial laboratories and in some large veterinary institutions. The end products of thrombosis and subsequent fibrinolysis also can be measured. Fibrinogen levels may decline, although this test is not sensitive or specific for DIC. Fibrin degradation (split) products also become elevated. Fibrin degradation products are normally cleared by the liver, and these also become elevated in cases of hepatic failure because of lack of clearance. More recently, cageside D-dimer tests have become available to measure the breakdown product of cross-linked fibrin as a more sensitive and specific monitor of DIC.

Management of disseminated intravascular coagulation

Management of DIC first involves treating the primary underlying cause. By the time DIC becomes evident, rapid and aggressive treatment is necessary. If you are suspicious of DIC in any patient with a disease known to incite DIC, then ideally, you should begin treatment BEFORE the hemostatic abnormalities start to occur for the best possible prognosis. Treatment involves replacement of clotting factors and antithrombin and prevention of further clot formation. To replenish clotting factors and antithrombin, administer fresh whole blood or fresh frozen plasma. Heparin requires antithrombin as a cofactor to inactivate thrombin and other activated coagulation factors. Administer heparin (50 to 100 units/kg SQ q6-8h of unfractionated heparin; or fractionated enoxaparin [Lovenox], 1 mg/kg SQ bid). Aspirin (5 mg/kg PO bid in dogs; every third day in cats) also can be administered to prevent platelet adhesion. Management of DIC also involves the rule of twenty monitoring and case management to maintain end-organ perfusion and oxygen delivery (see the Rule of 20).

CONGENITAL DEFECTS OF HEMOSTASIS

Factor VIII deficiency (hemophilia A)

Hemophilia A is a sex-liked recessive trait that is carried by females and manifested in males. Female hemophiliacs can occur when a hemophiliac male is bred with a carrier female. Hemophilia A has been reported in cats and a number of dog breeds, including Miniature Schnauzer, Saint Bernard, Miniature Poodle, Shetland Sheepdog, English and Irish Setters, Labrador Retriever, German shepherd, Collie, Weimaraner, Greyhound, Chihuahua, English bulldog, Samoyed, and Vizsla. Mild to moderate internal or external bleeding can occur. Clinical signs of umbilical cord bleeding can become apparent in some animals shortly after weaning. Gingival hemorrhage, hemarthrosis, gastrointestinal hemorrhage, and hematomas may occur. Clotting profiles in animals with factor VIII deficiency include prolonged APTT and ACT. The PT and buccal mucosa bleeding time are normal. Affected animals have low factor VIII activity but normal to high levels of factor VIII–related antigen. Carrier females can be detected by low (30% to 60% of normal) factor VIII activity and normal to elevated levels of factor VII–related antigen.

Von Willebrand's disease

Von Willebrand's disease is a deficiency or defect in von Willebrand's protein. A number of variants of the disease have been described: Von Willebrand's disease type I is associated with a defect in factor VIIR/protein concentration, and von Willebrand's disease type II is associated with a defect in VIIIR:vWF. Type I von Willebrand's disease is most common in veterinary medicine. Von Willebrand's disease has been identified in more than 29 breeds of dogs, with an incidence that varies from 10% to 60% depending on the breed of origin. Affected breeds include Doberman Pinchers, German Shepherd Dogs, Scottish Terriers and standard Manchester Terriers, Golden Retrievers, Chesapeake Bay Retrievers, Miniature Schnauzers, and Pembroke Welsh Corgis. Two forms of genetic expression occur: (1) autosomal recessive disease in which homozygous von Willebrand's disease individuals have a bleeding disorder, whereas heterozygous individuals carry the trait but are clinically normal. The second variant of genetic expression involves an autosomal dominant disease with incomplete expression such that heterozygous individuals are affected carriers and homozygous individuals are severely affected. Von Willebrand's disease has high morbidity, but fortunately a low mortality. Dogs with 30% or less than normal vWF tend to hemorrhage. Platelet counts are normal, but bleeding times can be prolonged. The APTT can be slightly prolonged when factor VIII is less than 50% of normal. Routine screening tests are nondiagnostic for this disease, although in a predisposed breed with a normal platelet count, a prolonged buccal mucosa bleeding time strongly supports a diagnosis of von Willebrand's disease. Documentation of clinical bleeding with low or undetectable levels of factor VIII antigen or platelet-related activities of vWF support a diagnosis of von Willebrand's disease. Recessive animals have zero vWF:antigen (a subunit of factor III); heterozygotes have 15% to 60% of normal. In the incompletely dominant form, levels of vWF antigen are reduced (less than 7% to 60%). Clinical signs in affected animals include epistaxis, hematuria, diarrhea with melena, penile bleeding, lameness, hemarthrosis, hematoma formation, and excessive bleeding with routine procedures such as nail trimming, ear cropping, tail docking, surgical procedures (spay, neuter), and lacerations. Estrous and postpartum bleeding may be prolonged. A DNA test to detect carriers of the vWF gene is available through VetGen (Ann Arbor, Michigan) and Michigan State University. Patients with von Willebrand's disease should avoid drugs known to affect platelet function adversely (sulfonamide, ampicillin, chloramphenicol, antihistamines, theophylline, phenothiazine tranquilizers, heparin, and estrogen).

Factor IX (Christmas factor) deficiency (hemophilia B)

Hemophilia B is an X-linked recessive trait that occurs with less frequency that hemophilia A. The disease has been reported in Scottish Terriers, Shetland and Old English Sheepdogs, Saint Bernards, Cocker Spaniels, Alaskan Malamutes, Labrador Retrievers, Bichon Frises, Airdale Terriers, and British Shorthair cats. Carrier females have low (40% to 60% of normal) factor IX activity. Clinical signs are more severe than for hemophilia A.

Factor VII deficiency

Congenital deficiencies of factor VII have been reported as an autosomal, incompletely dominant characteristic in Beagles. Heterozygotes have 50% factor VII deficiency. Bleeding tends to be mild. The PT is prolonged in affected individuals.

Factor X deficiency

Factor X deficiency has been documented in Cocker Spaniels and resembles fading-puppy syndrome in newborn dogs. Internal or umbilical bleeding can occur, and affected dogs typically die. Bleeding may be mild in adult dogs. In severe cases, factor X levels are reduced to 20% of normal; in mild cases, factor X levels are 20% to 70% of normal.

Factor XII (Hageman factor) deficiency

Factor XII deficiency has been documented as an inherited autosomal recessive trait in domestic cats. Heterozygotes can be detected because they have a partial deficiency (50% of normal) of factor XII. Homozygote cats have less than 2% factor XII activity. Deficiency of Hageman factor usually does not result in bleeding or other disorders.

Factor XI deficiency

Factor XI deficiency is an autosomal disease that has been documented in Kerry Blue Terriers, Great Pyrenees, and English Springer Spaniels. In affected individuals, protracted bleeding may be observed. Homozygotes have low factor XI activity (< 20% of normal), and heterozygotes have 40% to 60% of normal.

Management of congenital defects of hemostasis

The management of congenital defects of hemostasis typically involves replenishing the clotting factor that is present. Usually, this can be accomplished in the form of fresh frozen plasma transfusion (20 mL/kg). If anemia is present because of severe hemorrhage, fresh whole blood or packed RBCs also can be administered. Recent research has investigated the use of recombinant gene therapy in the treatment of specific factor deficiencies in dogs; however, the therapy is not yet available for use in clinical practice.

In cases of von Willebrand's disease, administration of fresh frozen plasma (10 to 20 mL/kg) or cryoprecipitate (1 unit/10 kg body mass) provides vWF, factor VIII, and fibrinogen. Doses can be repeated until hemorrhage ceases. 1-Desamino-8-D-arginine vasopressin (DDAVP) also can be administered (1 µg/kg SC or IV diluted in 0.9% saline given over 10 to 20 minutes) to the donor and patient to increase the release of stored vWF from endothelial cells. A fresh whole blood transfusion can be obtained from the donor and immediately administered to the patient, or spun down and the fresh plasma administered if RBCs are not needed. Administer a dose of DDAVP to any affected dog before initiating any elective surgical procedures. A supply of fresh frozen plasma and RBCs should be on hand, should uncontrolled hemorrhage occur.

ACQUIRED DISORDERS OF HEMOSTASIS

Platelets are essential to normal blood coagulation. After a vessel is damaged, release of vasoactive amines causes vasoconstriction and sluggish flow of blood in an attempt to squelch hemorrhage. Platelets become activated by platelet activating factor, and attach to the damaged vascular endothelium. Normal platelet adhesion depends on mediators such as calcium, fibrinogen, vWF:antigen, and a portion of factor VIII. After adhesion, the platelets undergo primary aggregation and release a variety of chemical mediators including adenosine diphosphate, prostaglandins, serotonin, epinephrine, thromboplastin, and thromboxane A that promote secondary aggregation and contraction. Platelet abnormalities can include decreased platelet production (thrombocytopenia), decreased platelet function (thrombocytopathia), increased platelet destruction, increased platelet consumption, and platelet sequestration.

Thrombocytopathia

Thrombocytopathia refers to platelet function abnormalities. Alterations in platelet function can affect platelet adhesion, aggregation, or release of vasoactive substances that help form a stable clot (Box 1-32). In von Willebrand's disease there is a deficiency in vWF:antigen that results in altered platelet adhesion. Vascular purpuras are reported and have been seen in collagen abnormalities such as Ehlers-Danlos syndrome, which can be inherited as an autosomal dominant trait with complete penetrance and has been recognized in German Shepherd Dogs, Dachshunds, Saint Bernards, and Labrador Retrievers.

Thrombasthenic thrombopathia is a hereditary autosomal dominant abnormality that has been described in Otterhounds, Foxhounds and Scottish Terriers. In this condition, platelets do not aggregate normally in response to adenosine diphosphate and thrombin stimulation.

Evaluation of platelet function is based on a total platelet count, buccal mucosa bleeding time, and thromboelastography. Platelet function defects (thrombocytopenia and thrombocytopathia) can affect both sexes. Clinical signs can resemble von Willebrand's disease. In most cases, buccal mucosa bleeding time will be prolonged, but platelet count and clotting tests will be normal.

BOX 1-32   CAUSES OF THROMBOCYTOPATHIA

DRUGS
Aspirin or other nonsteroidal antiinflammatory drugs
Heparin
Phenothiazine tranquilizers
Cephalosporin

SYSTEMIC DISORDERS
Uremia
Liver disease

HEMATOLOGIC DISORDERS
Antiplatelet antibody production
Myeloproliferative disorders
Dysproteinemia
von Willebrand's disease defects

INHERITED
Thrombasthenic thrombopathia of Otterhounds
Glanzmann's thrombasthenia of Great Pyrenees
Thrombopathia of Bassett Hound and American Eskimo Dog (Spitz)
Cyclic hematopoiesis of the gray Collie
Platelet storage pool disease of American Cocker Spaniel

Thrombocytopenia

Platelet count can be decreased because of problems with production, increased consumption, sequestration, or destruction. Causes of accelerated platelet destruction are typically immune-mediated autoantibodies, drug antibodies, infection, and isoimmune destruction. Consumption and sequestration usually are caused by DIC, vasculitis, microangiopathic hemolytic anemia, severe vascular injury, hemolytic uremic syndrome, and gram-negative septicemia. Primary thrombocytopenia with no known cause has been called *idiopathic thrombocytic purpura*. In approximately 80% of the cases, thrombocytopenia is associated with immune-mediated destruction caused by immune-mediated hemolytic anemia, systemic lupus erythematosus, rheumatoid arthritis, DIC, and diseases that affect the bone marrow. In systemic lupus erythematosus, 20% to 30% of the affected dogs have concurrent idiopathic thrombocytic purpura. When immune-mediated hemolytic anemia and idiopathic thrombocytic purpura are present in the same patient, the disease is called *Evans syndrome*. PF-3 is a non–complement-fixing antibody that is produced in the spleen and affects peripheral and bone marrow platelets and megakaryocytes. Antibodies directed against platelets are usually of the IgG subtype in animals. Antiplatelet antibodies can be measured by a PF-3 release test. Platelet counts with immune-mediated destruction typically are less than 50,000 platelets/µL. Infectious causes of thrombocytopenia include *Ehrlichia canis, Anaplasma phagocytophilum* (formerly, *Ehrlichia equi*), and *Rickettsia rickettsii* (Rocky Mountain spotted fever). Primary immune-mediated thrombocytopenia has an unknown cause and most frequently is seen in middle- to older-aged female dogs. Breed predispositions include Cocker Spaniels, German Shepherd Dogs, Poodles (toy, miniature, standard), and Old English Sheepdogs.

Thrombocytopenia usually is manifested as petechiae, ecchymoses of skin and mucous membranes, hyphema, gingival and conjunctival bleeding, hematuria, melena, and epistaxis. To make a diagnosis of idiopathic thrombocytic purpura, measure the severity of thrombocytopenia (< 50,000 platelets/µL), analyze the peripheral blood smear for evidence of platelet fragmentation or microthrombocytosis, normal to increased numbers of megakaryocytes in the bone marrow, detection of antiplatelet antibody, increased platelet counts after starting glucocorticoid therapy, and elimination of other causes of thrombocytopenia. If tick-borne illnesses are suspected, antibody titers for *E. canis, A. phagocytophilum* (formerly *E. equi*), and *R. rickettsii* should be performed.

Treatment of immune-mediated thrombocytopenia involves suppression of the immune system to stop the immune-mediated destruction and to stimulate platelet release from the bone marrow. Traditionally, the gold standard to suppress the immune system is to use glucocorticoids (prednisone or prednisolone, 2 to 4 mg/kg PO bid divided, OR dexamethasone, 0.1 to 0.3 mg/kg IV or PO q12h). More recently human serum immunoglobulin (IgG) also has been used (0.2 to 0.5 g/kg IV in saline over 8 hours; pretreat with 1 mg/kg diphenhydramine 15 minutes before starting infusion). Vincristine (0.5 mg/m^2 IV once) can stimulate the release of platelets from the bone marrow if megakaryocytic precursors are present; however, the platelets released may be immature and potentially nonfunctional. Treatment with fresh whole blood or packed RBCs is appropriate if anemia is present; however, unless specific platelet-rich plasma has been purchased from a blood bank, fresh whole blood contains relatively few platelets, which are short-lived (2 hours) and will not effectively raise the platelet count at all. Finally, long-term therapy is usually in the form of azathioprine (2 mg/kg PO once daily, tapered to 1 mg/kg daily to every other day after 1 week) and cyclosporine (10 to 25 mg/kg PO divided). If a tick-borne illness is suspected, administer doxycycline (5 to 10 mg/kg PO bid) for 4 weeks or if titers come back negative.

Thrombocytopenia also can occur in the cat. Causes for thrombocytopenia in cats include infections (29%), neoplasia (20%), cardiac disease (7%), primary immune-mediated disease (2%), and unknown causes (20%). In one study of cats with feline leukemia and myeloproliferative disease, 44% of cases had thrombocytopenia.

Vitamin K antagonist rodenticide intoxication

Warfarin and coumarin derivatives are the major class of rodenticides used in the United States. Vitamin K antagonist rodenticides inhibit the epoxidase reaction and deplete active vitamin K, causing a depletion of vitamin K–dependent coagulation factors (II, VII, IX, X) within 24 hours to 1 week of ingestion, depending on the ingested dose. Affected animals can spontaneously hemorrhage anywhere in the body. Clinical signs can include hemoptysis, respiratory difficulty, cough, gingival bleeding, epistaxis, hematuria, hyphema, conjunctival bleeding, petechiae and ecchymoses, cavity hemorrhage (pleural, peritoneal, retroperitoneal) with acute weakness, lethargy or collapse, hemarthrosis with lameness, deep muscle bleeds, and intracranial or spinal cord hemorrhage. Diagnosis of vitamin K antagonism includes prolonged PT. A PIVKA (protein induced by vitamin K absence or antagonism) test also can be performed, if possible.

TABLE 1-30 **Clinical Interpretation of Laboratory Test Results for Coagulation Profiles**

Disorder	BMBT	ACT	PT	APTT	Platelets	Fibrinogen	FDPs	D-dimers
Thrombocytopenia	↑	N	N	N	↓	N	N	N
Thrombocytopathia	↑	N	N	N	N	N	N	N
Von Willebrand's disease	↑	↑/N	N	↑/N	N	N	N	N
Hemophilias	N	↑	N	↑	N	N	N	N
Warfarin toxicity	N	↑	↑	↑	N/↓	N/↓	N/↑	N
Disseminated intravascular coagulopathy	↑	↑	↑	↑	↓	N/↓	↑	↑

ACT, Activated clotting time; *APTT,* activated partial thromboplastin time; *BMBT,* buccal mucosa bleeding time; *FDP,* fibrin degradation products; *N,* normal; *PT,* prothrombin time.

Treatment of vitamin K antagonist rodenticide intoxication and other causes of vitamin K deficiency involves supplementation with vitamin K_1 (phytonadione, 5 mg/kg SQ once with 25-gauge needle in multiple sites, and then 2.5 mg/kg PO bid to tid for 30 days). Never administer injections of vitamin K intramuscularly, because of the risk of causing deep muscle hematomas, or intravenously, because of the risk of anaphylaxis. The PT should be rechecked 2 days after the last vitamin K capsule is administered, for some of the second-generation warfarin derivates are fat-soluble, and treatment may be required for an additional 2 weeks.

Table 1-30 summarizes criteria for interpreting coagulation profiles.

Additional Reading

Bateman SW, Mathews KA, Abrams-Ogg ACG: Disseminated intravascular coagulation in dogs: a review of the literature, *J Vet Emerg Crit Care* 8:29-45, 1998.

Bateman SW, Mathews KA, Abrams-Ogg AC, et al: Diagnosis of disseminated intravascular coagulation in dogs admitted to an intensive care unit, *J Am Vet Med Assoc* 215(6):798-804, 1999.

Bateman SW, Mathews KA, Abrams-Ogg ACG, et al: Evaluation of point-of-care tests for diagnosis of disseminated intravascular coagulation in dogs admitted to an intensive care unit, *J Am Vet Med Assoc* 215:805-810, 1999.

Couto CG: Spontaneous bleeding disorders. In Bonagura JD, editor: *Current veterinary therapy XII. Small animal practice,* Philadelphia, 1995, WB Saunders.

Feldman B, Kirby R, Caldin M: Recognition and treatment of disseminated intravascular coagulation. In Bonagura JD, editor: *Kirk's current veterinary therapy XIII,* Philadelphia, 2000, WB Saunders.

Hackner S: Approach to the diagnosis of bleeding disorders, *Compend Contin Educ Pract Vet* 17:331, 1995.

Honeckman A, Knapp D, Reagan W: Diagnosis of canine immune-mediated hematologic disease, *Compend Contin Educ Pract Vet* 18:113, 1996.

Lisciandro SC, Hoenhaus A, Brooks M: Coagulation abnormalities in 22 cats with naturally occurring liver disease, *J Vet Intern Med* 12:71-75, 1998.

Mischke R, Grebe S, Jacobs C, et al: Amidolytic heparin activity and values for several hemostatic variables after repeated subcutaneous administration of high dose low molecular weight heparin in healthy dogs, *Am J Vet Res* 62(4):595-598, 2001.

Peterson J, Couto G, Wellman M: Hemostatic disorders in cats: a retrospective study and review of the literature, *J Vet Intern Med* 9:298-303, 1995.

Stokol T, Brooks MB, Erb HN, et al: D-dimer concentrations in healthy dogs and dogs with disseminated intravascular coagulation, *Am J Vet Res* 61:393-398, 2001.

1

BURNS

THERMAL INJURY

Thermal burns are fortunately a relatively infrequent occurrence in veterinary patients. Box 1-33 lists various causes of malicious and accidental burns. The location of the burn is also important in assessing its severity and potential to lose function. Burns on the perineum, feet, face, and ears are considered to be the most severe because of loss of function and severe pain. Often the severity of thermal injury is difficult to assess in animals because hair coat potentially can mask clinical signs and because the thermal injury can continue after the animal has been removed from the heat source. The skin cools slowly and warms slowly, considerations that become important when initiating therapy for burns. The severity of thermal injury is associated with the temperature to which the animal is exposed, the duration of contact, and the ability of the tissue to dissipate heat. The tissue closest to the heat source undergoes necrosis and has decreased blood flow.

The severity of thermal burn injury is associated directly with the temperature to which the animal is exposed, the percentage of total body surface area affected, the thickness of injured tissue, and whether underlying complications with other body systems occur. Prognosis largely depends on the total body surface area affected (Table 1-31).

Superficial partial thickness, or first-degree, burns offer the most favorable prognosis. The affected epidermis initially appears erythematous and then quickly desquamates within 3 to 6 days. In most cases, fur grows back without leaving a scar. Deep partial thickness, or second-degree, burns involve the epidermis and dermis and are associated with subcutaneous edema, inflammation, and pain. Deep partial thickness burns heal from deeper adnexal tissues and from the wound edges and are associated with an increased chance of scarring and depigmentation. The most severe type is known as full thickness, or third-degree, burns, in which thermal injury destroys the entire thickness of the skin and forms an eschar. Thrombosis of superficial and deeper skin vasculature and gangrene occurs. Treatment involves sequential wound debridement. Healing occurs by second intention and reepithelialization or by wound reconstruction. In most cases, scarring is extensive in affected areas.

Burns greater than 20% of total body surface area will have systemic effects, including impaired cardiovascular function, pulmonary dysfunction, and impaired immune function. Burned tissue, with capillary damage, has increased permeability. The release of inflammatory cytokines, oxygen-derived free radical species, prostaglandins, leukotrienes,

---

BOX 1-33   CAUSES OF THERMAL INJURY

- Automobile engines
- Automobile exhaust systems
- Boiling water
- Cooking oil (hot)
- Electric heating pads
- Hair dryers
- Heat lamps
- Heat packs
- Improperly grounded electrosurgical units
- Semiliquids (i.e., hot tar)
- Solar exposure
- Steam
- Stove

TABLE 1-31   Percent Burn Estimation: Rule of Nines

Body region	Percent of body surface area
Head	9%
Torso	18%
Forelimb (per limb)	9%
Hind limb (per limb)	18%

histamine, serotonin, and kinins results in increased vascular permeability and leakage of plasma proteins into the interstitium and extravascular space.

Immediate action/treatment

At the time of presentation, first examine the patient and ascertain whether airway obstruction, impaired ventilatory function, circulatory shock, or pain are present. If necessary, establish an airway with endotracheal intubation or emergency tracheostomy. Next, cool the burned area(s) with topical cool water. Use care to avoid overcooling and iatrogenic hypothermia. The best approach is to cool only one portion of the patient's body at a time, then dry, and repeat the process for all affected areas to avoid overcooling and iatrogenic hypothermia. Establish vascular access and administer appropriate and judicious analgesic drugs and intravenous fluid therapy. Whenever possible, avoid placing a catheter through an area of burned or damaged skin. In the early stages of burn injury, shock doses of intravenous crystalloid fluids usually are not required. Later, however, as severe tissue exudation occurs, protein and fluid losses can become extensive, requiring aggressive crystalloid and colloid support to treat hypovolemia and hypoproteinemia. Flush the eyes with sterile saline and examine behind the third eyelids for any particulate matter. Stain the corneas to make sure that superficial corneal burns are not present. Treat superficial corneal burns with triple antibiotic ophthalmic ointment.

Next, assess the total body surface area affected, as this will gauge prognosis. Depending on the extent of the damage, decide whether the burn is superficial and local therapy is indicated or whether more severe injuries exist that may involve systemic therapy or possibly euthanasia.

Differential diagnosis

In most cases the diagnoses of thermal burns are based on a clinical history of being in a house fire, clothes dryer, or under a heating lamp. Too frequently, however, thermal burns become apparent days after an elective surgical procedure in which the patient was placed on a faulty heating pad rather than a circulating warm water or warm air blanket. Superficial burns appear as singed fur with desquamating, easily epilated hair. This condition also can resemble a superficial or deeper dermatophytosis if history is unknown. Other differential diagnoses include immune-mediated vasculitis or erythema multiforme. Unless the superficial dermis is blistered, it may be difficult to distinguish between a thermal burn, chemical burn, or electrical burn if the trauma went unnoticed.

Management

Management of burn injury largely depends on the depth of injury and the total body surface area affected. Partial thickness burns and those affecting less than 15% of the total body surface area will require support in the form of antibiotic ointment and systemic analgesic drugs.

Burns affecting greater than 15% of total body surface area or deep thickness burns require more aggressive therapy. Central venous catheters can be placed to administer crystalloid and colloid fluids, parenteral nutrition if necessary, antibiotics, and analgesic drugs. Monitor perfusion parameters closely, including heart rate, blood pressure, capillary refill time, and urine output. Respiratory function can be impaired because of concurrent smoke inhalation, thermal damage to the upper airways and alveoli, and carboxyhemoglobin or methemoglobin intoxication. Respiratory function also can be impaired because of burn injury to the skin around the thoracic cage. Thoracic radiographs may reveal patchy interstitial to alveolar infiltrates associated with pulmonary edema, pneumonia, and atelectasis. Bronchoscopy often reveals edema, inflammation, particulate matter, and ulceration of the tracheobronchial tree. In some cases, upper airway inflammation is so severe that an emergency tracheostomy must be performed to treat airway obstruction. Administer supplemental humidified oxygen at 50 to 100 mL/kg/minute via endotracheal tube, tracheostomy, nasal or intratracheal tube, or hood oxygen if respiratory function and hypoxemia are present. Perform blood work including a hematocrit, albumin, BUN, creatinine, and glucose at the time of presentation. Monitor serum electrolytes, albumin, and colloid oncotic pressure closely because derangements can be severe as burns become exudative.

The goal of fluid therapy in the burn patient is to establish and maintain intravascular and interstitial fluid volume, normalize electrolyte and acid-base status, and maintain serum albumin and oncotic pressure. In the first 24 hours following burn injury, direct fluid therapy to maintaining the patient's metabolic fluid requirements. Crystalloid fluids in the form of Normosol-R, Plasmalyte-M, or lactated Ringer's solution can be administered according to the patient's electrolyte and acid-base status (see Fluid Therapy). Monitor urine output, and keep it at 1 to 2 mL/kg/hour. Avoid overhydration in the early stages of burn injury. In affected burn patients, calculate the amount of fluid that should be administered over a 24-hour period from the formula $1 - 4$ mL/kg $\times$ percent total body surface area. Administer half of this calculated dose over the first 8 hours and then the remaining half over the next 16 hours. In cats, administer only 50% to 75% of this calculated volume. To administer this volume and also avoid fluid overload is often difficult in critically ill patients with pulmonary involvement associated with smoke inhalation injury. Avoid colloids in the first 6 hours after burn injury. Monitor the patient closely for serous nasal discharge, chemosis, and rales that may signify pulmonary edema.

As burns become exudative, weigh the patient at least twice daily. Infused fluid should equal fluid output in the form of urine and wound exudates. Acute weight loss signifies acute fluid loss and that crystalloid fluid infusion should be more aggressive. Ideally, keep the patient's serum albumin equal to or greater than 2.0 g/dL and total protein between 4.0 and 6.5 g/dL using a combination of fresh frozen plasma or concentrated human albumin. Adjunct colloidal support can be provided with synthetic colloids including hetastarch or HBOCs. Keep serum potassium within 3.5 to 4.5 mEq/L using potassium chloride or potassium phosphate supplementation. If potassium supplementation exceeds 80 to 100 mEq/L and the patient continues to have severe refractory hypokalemia, administer magnesium chloride (0.75 mEq/kg/day) to enhance potassium retention. If anemia occurs, administer packed RBCs or whole blood (see Blood Component Therapy).

Lavage wounds daily with lactated Ringer's solution or 0.9% sodium chloride solution. Place wet-to-dry bandages or bandages soaked in silver sulfadiazine or nitrofurazone ointment over the wounds. Depending on the thickness of the burn, epilation and eschar formation and separation may take 2 to 10 days. At each bandage change, debride devitalized tissue to normal tissue. Perform staged partial or total escharectomy, and leave the wound to heal by second intention or by reconstruction using skin advancement flaps or grafts. Maintain meticulous sterility at all times, given that burn patients are at high risk for infection. Administer broad-spectrum antibiotics including cefazolin and enrofloxacin. Perform wound culture if a resistant bacterial infection is suspected.

ELECTRICAL INJURY

The most common cause of electrical injury is associated with an animal chewing on low-voltage alternating current electrical cords in the household. Damage is caused by the current flowing through the path of least resistance, causing heat and thrombosis of vessels and neurons. In some cases, the owner witnesses the event. In other cases, the owner presents the patient because of vague nonspecific signs, and characteristic abnormalities on physical examination support a diagnosis of electrocution. Burns on the face, paws, commissures of the mouth, tongue, and soft palate may be present. Electrocution causes a massive release of catecholamines and can predispose the patient to noncardiogenic pulmonary edema within 36 hours of the incident. Clinical signs may be isolated to the pulmonary system, including orthopnea, pulmonary crackles, and cyanosis.

Immediate action

Assess the patient's lips, tongue, soft palate, gingivae, and commissures of the mouth. Early after electrocution, the wound may appear small and white, black, or yellow. Later, the wound may become larger as tissue sloughs because of damaged vascular supply. Assess the patient's respiratory status. Auscultate the lungs to determine whether pulmonary crackles are present. If the patient is stable, thoracic radiographs may demonstrate an interstitial to alveolar lung pattern in the dorsocaudal lung fields. Measure the patient's heart rate, blood pressure, oxygenation as determined by pulse oximetry or arterial blood gas and urine output. Immediate treatment consists of judicious use of analgesics for the burn injury, antibiotics (cefazolin, 22 mg/kg q8h; cephalexin, 22 mg/kg q8h), and humidified supplemental oxygen (50 to 100 mL/kg/minute). Direct fluid therapy at providing the patient's metabolic fluid requirements. Because of the risk of development of noncardiogenic pulmonary edema, avoid overzealous administration of crystalloid fluids.

Differential diagnosis

Differential diagnoses for the patient with electrical burn injury and electrocution include chemical or thermal burn, immune-mediated glossitis, cardiogenic pulmonary edema, and pneumonia.

Management

Management of the patient with electrical burn injury and electrocution primarily involves the administration of analgesic agents, supplemental humidified oxygen, and topical treatment of electrical burns. The noncardiogenic pulmonary edema is typically unresponsive to diuretics (i.e., furosemide), bronchodilators (i.e., aminophylline), and splanchnic vascular dilators (i.e., low-dose morphine). The use of glucocorticoids has no proven benefit and may impair respiratory immune function and is therefore contraindicated. Oral burns may require debridement and advancement flaps if large defects or oronasal fistulas develop. If oral injury is severe, place an esophagostomy or percutaneous gastrostomy tube to ensure adequate nutrition during the healing process. If an animal survives the initial electrocution, prognosis is generally favorable with aggressive supportive care.

CHEMICAL INJURY

Chemical burns are associated with a number of inciting causes, including oxidizing agents, reducing agents, corrosive chemicals, protoplasmic poisons, desiccants, and vesicants. The treatment for chemical burns differs slightly from that for thermal burns, so it remains important to investigate the cause of the burn when providing initial treatment, whenever possible. At the scene, advise the owner to wrap the patient in a clean towel for transport. Chilling can be avoided by then wrapping the patient in a second or third blanket. Placement of ointments by well-doers should be avoided. Encourage immediate transport to the nearest triage facility.

Immediate action/treatment

The first and foremost consideration when treating a patient with chemical burn is to remove the animal from the inciting cause or offending agent. Make no attempt to neutralize alkaline or acid substances because the procedure potentially could cause an exothermic reaction, leading to thermal injury in addition to the chemical injury.

Remove collars or leashes that may act as tourniquets or constricting devices. Flush affected areas with copious amounts of cool water for several minutes, not cooling more than 10% to 20% of the body at any one time to prevent iatrogenic hypothermia. Support breathing by extending the patient's head and neck.

Carefully clip the fur over affected areas for further evaluation of the extent of the injury. Lavage exposed eyes with sterile saline, and stain the cornea to evaluate for any corneal burns. Debride any wounds carefully, knowing that the full extent of the wound may not manifest itself for several days. Then cover the wounds with antibiotic burn ointment such as silver sulfadiazine and an occlusive dressing.

Differential diagnosis

Without a history of exposure, the differential diagnosis for any chemical burn includes thermal burn, necrotizing vasculitis, erythema multiforme, or superficial or deep pyoderma.

Management

Contact local or national animal poison control regarding whether to attempt neutralization. Perform daily bandage changes with staged debridement as the full extent of the wound manifests itself. Place antimicrobial ointment and silver sulfadiazine ointment over the wound to prevent infection. The routine use of antibiotics may promote the development of a resistant bacterial infection. First-generation cephalosporin can be administered. If a more serious infection develops, perform culture and susceptibility testing to direct appropriate antibiotic therapy. The wound can heal by second intention or may require reconstructive repair for definitive closure.

RADIATION INJURY

The primary cause of radiation injury in small animal patients is radiation therapy for neoplastic conditions. The goal of radiation therapy is to kill neoplastic cells. An unfortunate side effect is damage to adjacent normal tissue that results in necrosis, fibrosis, and impaired circulation to the affected area. Radiation burns result in dermatitis, mucositis, impaired surgical wound healing, and chronic nonhealing wounds. In many cases, the degree of secondary radiation injury to normal tissue can be prevented or decreased with careful radiation planning and mapping of the radiation field, such that radiation exposure to normal tissue is limited to the smallest extent possible. With the advent of three-dimensional imaging modalities such as computed tomography (CT) and magnetic resonance imaging (MRI), this has become more routine in veterinary oncology to date.

Radiation injury can be early and appear at the later stage of the course of radiation therapy. Late effects can be delayed and occur 6 months to years after treatment. The degree of radiation injury is categorized based on the depth of tissue affected. First-degree changes cause cutaneous erythema. Second-degree changes cause superficial desquamation. Third-degree changes cause deeper moist desquamation, and fourth-degree changes are associated with complete dermal destruction and ulceration. During the early stages of radiation injury, affected tissues may appear erythematous and edematous. Wound exudates may be moist, or the skin may appear dry and scaly with desquamation or ulceration. Later, the area may scar and depigment or may have induration, atrophy, telangiectasia, keratosis, and decreased adnexal structures.

Immediate action/treatment

Treatment for radiation dermatitis is to irrigate the area with warmed saline and to protect the area from self-mutilation. No-bite, or Elizabethan, collars or loose clothing can be used to protect the area for patient-induced injury. Mucositis can be treated with topical green tea baths and the administration of an oral solution of L-glutamine powder (4 g/m^2). Local irrigation of xylocaine or lidocaine viscous jelly can be used in dogs but should be avoided in cats because of the risk of inducing hemolytic anemia and neurotoxicity. Topical and systemic antibiotics (cephalexin, 22 mg/kg PO tid) also can be administered. Avoid antibiotics that can be sensitized by radiation (i.e., metronidazole).

Differential diagnosis

Because most radiation burns are associated with a known exposure to radiation therapy, the cause of the patient's injury usually is known. If an animal presents to you with a scar, however, differential diagnoses may include nasal planum solar dermatitis, pemphigus foliaceus, discoid lupus, superficial necrolytic dermatitis, superficial or deep pyoderma, chemical burn, or thermal burn.

Management

Treatment of radiation injury involves making the patient as comfortable as possible with analgesic drugs, prevention of self-mutilation, and staged debridement techniques. Wounds can heal by second intention or may require reconstructive surgery.

Additional Reading

Adamiak Z, Brzeski W, Nowicki M: Burn wound management with hydrocolloid dressings in dogs, *Aust Vet Pract* 32(4):171-172, 2002.

Aragon CL, Harvey SE, Allen SW, et al: Partial thickness skin grafting for large thermal wounds in dogs, *Compend Contin Educ Pract Vet* 26(3):200-212, 2004.

Dernell WS, Wheaton LG: Surgical management of radiation injury: part I, *Compend Contin Educ Pract Vet* 17:181, 1995.

Dernell WS, Wheaton LG: Surgical management of radiation injury: part II, *Compend Contin Educ Pract Vet* 17:499, 1995.

Papazoglou LG, Kazakos G, Moustardas N: Thermal burns in 2 dogs associated with inadequate grounding of electrosurgical unit patient plates, *Aust Vet Pract* 21(2):67-70, 2001.

Pope ER, Payne JT: Pathophysiology and treatment of thermal burns. In Harari J, editor: *Surgical complications and wound healing in small animal practice*, Philadelphia, 1993, WB Saunders.

Singh A, Cullen DL, Grahn BH: Alkali burns to the right eye, *Can Vet J* 45(9):777-778, 2004.

CARDIAC EMERGENCIES

CARDIAC ARREST AND CARDIOPULMONARY CEREBRAL RESUSCITATION

Cardiopulmonary arrest is the abrupt cessation of spontaneous and effective ventilation and perfusion. Cardiac arrest must be treated rapidly and aggressively for any chance of success. The goal of cardiopulmonary cerebral resuscitation (CPCR) is to perform effective thoracic compressions such that an adequate amount of oxygen is delivered to the brain and other vital tissues. At the time of admission into the hospital, all patients, regardless of their disease process, should have a plan in the event that cardiopulmonary arrest occurs. Do the owners want to proceed with CPCR? Should you proceed with intubation, cardiac compressions and drugs, or do the owners want you to perform open-chest CPCR?

One of the most important aspects of cardiopulmonary resuscitation is to anticipate whether a patient is rapidly decompensating and likely to arrest and to be prepared at all times. Stock a crash cart at all times with the equipment and drugs necessary in the event that cardiopulmonary resuscitation is required (Box 1-34).

By having routine drills in the hospital on cadavers or stuffed animals, your emergency team can become efficient at performing the responsibilities and jobs required for successful CPCR. The staff should know how to recognize impending signs of a decompensating patient, clinical signs of cardiac arrest, how to call for an emergency in the hospital, how to intubate patients, and how to start cardiac compressions, hook up an ECG, and draw up the drugs required for various arrhythmias.

Conditions that predispose a patient to cardiopulmonary arrest include vagal stimulation, cellular hypoxia, septicemia, endotoxemia, severe acid-base and electrolyte derangements, prolonged seizures, pneumonia, pleural or pericardial effusion, severe multisystemic trauma, electrical shock, urinary obstruction or damage, acute respiratory

---

BOX 1-34   ITEMS TO STOCK IN THE CRASH CART

- Laryngoscope (various size blades)
- Endotracheal tubes (various sizes)
- Cotton roll gauze to tie in endotracheal tube
- Stylette for intubation
- Rigid catheter (tomcat and long urinary) to assist with intubation and endotracheal drug administration
- 3-, 6-, and 12-mL syringes, taken out of case and attached to 22-gauge needles
- 22-gauge needles
- Ambubag and oxygen source
- Electrocardiogram monitor
- Epinephrine
- Atropine
- Naloxone
- Calcium gluconate or calcium chloride
- Magnesium chloride
- Amiodarone
- 0.9% saline
- 50% dextrose
- Laceration pack for slash tracheostomy
- Intravenous catheters
- 1-inch white tape
- Emergency drug table with dose and volume and route of administration for various size animals

distress syndrome (ARDS), and anesthetic agents. The acute onset of bradycardia, change in mucous membrane color and capillary refill time, change in respiratory pattern, and change in mentation are signs of possible deterioration and impending cardiopulmonary arrest.

The diagnosis of cardiopulmonary arrest is based on the absence of effective ventilation, severe cyanosis, absence of a palpable pulse or apex heartbeat, absence of heart sounds, and ECG evidence of asystole or other nonperfusing rhythm such as electrical-mechanical dissociation (aka pulseless electrical activity) or ventricular fibrillation.

Immediate action/treatment

Cardiopulmonary cerebral resuscitation

The goals of CPCR are to obtain airway access, provide artificial ventilation and supplemental oxygen, implement cardiac compressions and cardiovascular support, recognize and treat dysrhythmias and arrhythmias, and provide stabilization and treatment for cardiovascular, pulmonary, and cerebral function in the event of a successful resuscitation. Even with aggressive treatment and management, the overall success of CPCR is less than 5% in critically ill or traumatized patients and 20% to 30% in anesthetized patients.

Basic life support

Basic life support involves rapid intubation to gain airway access, artificial ventilation, and cardiac compressions to promote blood flow and delivery of oxygen to the brain and other important tissues (Figure 1-26). Perform the ABCs or CABs of CPCR, where *A* is airway, *B* is breathing, and *C* is compression and circulation. Recently, the paradigm has shifted to CABs. While a team member is grabbing an endotracheal tube, clearing the airway of foreign debris, and establishing airway access through endotracheal intubation, a second person starts external cardiac compressions to deliver oxygen that is in the bloodstream to the vital organs. The patient should be positioned in dorsal (> 7 kg) or lateral (< 7 kg) recumbency for external cardiac compressions. Approximately 80 to 120 external compressions should be performed over the patient's sternum. A team member should palpate for a peripheral pulse to determine whether cardiac compressions are actually effective. If a peripheral pulse cannot be palpated for every chest compression, change the patient's position and have a larger individual perform compressions, or initiate open-chest cardiac resuscitation. Once the patient is intubated, tie in the endotracheal tube and attach it to an oxygen source (anesthetic machine or mechanical ventilator or Ambu bag) for artificial ventilation. The oxygen flow rate should be 150 mL/kg/minute. Give two long breaths, and then 12 to 16 breaths per minute. Simultaneous ventilation with thoracic compression increases the pressure difference in the thorax and allows more forward flow of oxygenated blood through the great vessels into the periphery. If possible, a third team member can initiate interposed abdominal compressions, compressing the abdomen when the thoracic cage is relaxed, to improve forward flow. If only one person is available to perform the thoracic compressions and ventilation, give two breaths for every 15 compressions (i.e., 15 thoracic compressions followed by two long breaths, and then start thoracic compressions again). The Jen Chung maneuver can be performed by placing a 25- to 22-gauge hypodermic needle through the skin of the nasal philtrum and twisting the needle into the periosteum to stimulate respirations. This maneuver appears to work better in cats than dogs at return to spontaneous respiration.

Advanced life support

Advanced life support during CPCR involves ECG, pulse oximetry and capnometry monitoring, administration of drugs, and the administration of intravenous fluids (in select cases). Most of the drugs used during CPCR can be administered directly into the lungs from the endotracheal tube (intratracheal tube). Therefore, only in select instances is it necessary to establish vascular or intraosseous access during CPCR (Figure 1-27). If an animal experiences cardiopulmonary arrest because of extreme hemorrhage or hypovolemia,

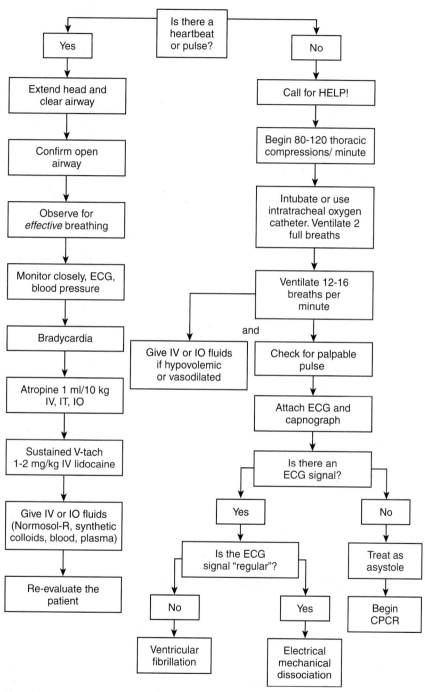

Figure 1-26:   Basic cardiopulmonary life support. *ECG,* Electrocardiogram; *CPCR,* cardiopulmonary cerebral resuscitation.

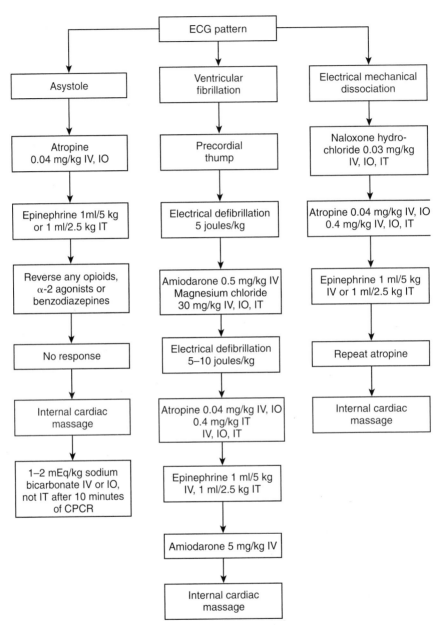

Figure 1-27:   Advanced cardiopulmonary life support

inappropriate vasodilation caused by sepsis or systemic inflammation, or vasodilation resulting from anesthesia, the administration of shock volumes (90 mL/kg/hour in dogs and 44 mL/kg/hour in cats) is appropriate. If a patient is euvolemic and experiences cardiopulmonary arrest, however, an increase in circulating fluid volume actually can impair coronary artery perfusion by increasing diastolic arterial blood pressure and is therefore contraindicated. Place a capnograph on the end or side of the endotracheal tube to measure end-tidal carbon dioxide.

RECOGNITION AND TREATMENT OF COMMON NONPERFUSING CARDIAC RHYTHMS DURING CPCR

Asystole: "He's flatlined"

Asystole is one of the most common rhythm disturbances that causes cardiac arrest in small animal patients. One of the most important things to do when the ECG looks like asystole is to make sure that the ECG monitor is working properly and that all ECG leads are attached properly to the patient. If asystole is truly present, reverse any opiate, α_2-agonist, or benzodiazepine drugs with their appropriate reversal agents. Low-dose epinephrine (0.02 to 0.04 mg/kg diluted with 5 mL sterile saline) can be administered directly into the endotracheal tube via a rigid or red rubber catheter. If vascular access is available, epinephrine (0.02 to 0.04 mg/kg) can be administered intravenously. No drug should ever be administered directly into the heart by intracardiac injection. Unless the heart is in the veterinarian's hand during open-chest CPCR, intracardiac injection is risky and potentially could lacerate a coronary artery or cause the myocardium to become more irritable and refractory to other therapies, if a drug is delivered into the myocardium and not into the ventricle. For these reasons, intracardiac injections are contraindicated.

Administer atropine (0.4 mg/kg IV, IO, or 0.4 mg/kg IT) immediately after the epinephrine. Atropine, a vagolytic drug, serves to decrease tonic vagal inhibition of the sinoatrial and atrioventricular node and increase heart rate. Administer atropine and epinephrine every 2 to 5 minutes during asystole while cardiac compressions, interposed abdominal compressions, and artificial ventilation are continued. Although discontinuation of thoracic compressions can decrease the chance of success during CPCR, you must intermittently evaluate the ECG monitor for any rhythm change that may require different drug therapies. If the cardiac arrest was not witnessed or more than 2 to 5 minutes have passed without successful return to a perfusing rhythm, perform open-chest CPCR, if the client wishes. Administer sodium bicarbonate (1 to 2 mEq/kg IV) every 10 to 15 minutes during CPCR. Sodium bicarbonate is the only drug used in CPCR that SHOULD NOT be administered intratracheally because of inactivation of pulmonary surfactant.

Electrical-mechanical dissociation

Electrical-mechanical dissociation also is known as pulseless electrical activity and is an electrical rhythm that may look wide and bizarre and irregular with no associated mechanical contraction of the ventricles. The rhythm can appear different from patient to patient. Electrical-mechanical dissociation is one of the more common nonperfusing rhythms observed during cardiopulmonary arrest in small animal patients (Figure 1-28).

When electrical-mechanical dissociation is identified, first confirm the rhythm and proceed with CPCR as previously described. Electrical-mechanical dissociation is thought to be associated with high doses of endogenous endorphins and high vagal tone. The treatment of choice for electrical-mechanical dissociation is high-dose atropine (4 mg/kg IV, IT [10 times the normal dose]) and naloxone hydrochloride (0.03 mg/kg IV, IO, IT). Administer epinephrine (0.02 to 0.04 mg/kg diluted in 5 mL sterile 0.9% saline IT). If the rhythm does not change within 2 minutes, consider open-chest cardiac massage.

Ventricular fibrillation

Ventricular fibrillation can be coarse (Figure 1-29). Patients with coarse ventricular fibrillation are easier to defibrillate than those with fine defibrillation. If ventricular fibrillation is identified, initiate CPCR as described previously (Figure 1-30). If an electrical defibrillator is available, administer 5 J/kg of direct current externally. When a patient in cardiopulmonary arrest is attached to ECG leads, it is important to use contact electrode paste, water-soluble gel such as KY jelly, or water, rather than any form of alcohol. Electrical defibrillation of a patient who has alcohol on the ECG leads can lead to fire and thermal burns. Reverse any opioid, α_2-agonist, and phenothiazine drugs that have been administered to the patient. If fine ventricular fibrillation is identified, administer epinephrine

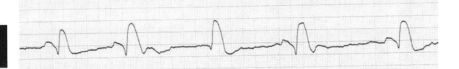

Figure 1-28: Electrical-mechanical dissociation (EMD), also known as pulseless electrical activity (PEA). The complexes often appear wide and bizarre without a palpable apex beat or functional contraction of the heart. This is just one example of EMD, as many shapes and complexes may be observed.

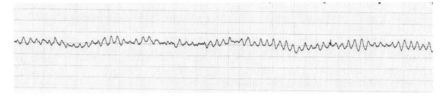

Figure 1-29: Rhythm strip of ventricular fibrillation.

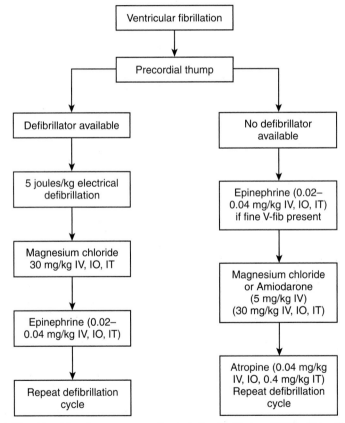

Figure 1-30: Algorithm for treatment of ventricular fibrillation (V-fib). This algorithm is organized according to whether an electrical defibrillator is available. After each intervention step, the ECG should be reevaluated and the next step initiated if V-fib is still seen. If a new arrhythmia develops, the appropriate therapy for that rhythm should be inititated. If a sinus rhythm is seen with a palpable apex beat, postresuscitation measures should be implemented.

BOX 1-35   INDICATIONS FOR IMMEDIATE OPEN-CHEST CARDIOPULMONARY CEREBRAL RESUSCITATION

- Pleural effusion
- Pneumothorax
- Rib fractures or flail chest
- Pericardial effusion
- Diaphragmatic hernia
- Obesity
- More than 5 minutes has passed since cardiopulmonary arrest

---

(0.02 to 0.04 mg/kg in 5 mL sterile 0.9% saline IT) to attempt to convert fine ventricular fibrillation to coarse ventricular fibrillation. After administration of epinephrine, repeat electrical defibrillation. If an electrical defibrillator is not available, chemical defibrillator drugs can be used. First, administer magnesium chloride (30 mg/kg IV or IT). Even if an electrical defibrillator is available, magnesium chloride can increase the success of converting ventricular fibrillation to asystole or some other rhythm during CPCR. Amiodarone (5 mg/kg IV, IO, IT) also can be used to convert ventricular fibrillation. If drug therapy and external thoracic compressions are ineffective after 2 minutes, consider open-chest CPCR.

Open-chest cardiopulmonary cerebral resuscitation

Perform open-chest CPCR immediately if a pathologic condition exists that prevents enough of a change in intrathoracic pressure that closed-chest CPCR will not be effective in promoting forward blood flow (Box 1-35).

To perform open-chest CPCR, place the patient in right lateral recumbency. Clip a wide strip of fur over the left fifth to seventh intercostal space and quickly aseptically scrub over the clipped area. Using a No. 10 scalpel blade, incise over the fifth intercostal space through the skin and subcutaneous tissue to the level of the intercostal muscles. With a Mayo scissors, make a blunt stab incision through the intercostal muscles in the left sixth intercostal space. Make sure that the person who is breathing for the patient deflates the lungs as you make the stab incision to avoid iatrogenic lung puncture. After the stab incision, open the tips of the Mayo scissors and quickly open the muscle dorsally and ventrally to the sternum with a sliding motion. Avoid the internal thoracic artery at the sternum and the intercostal arteries at the caudal aspect of each rib. Cut the rib adjacent to the sternum and push it behind the rib in front of and at the caudal aspect of the incision to allow more room and better visualization if a rib spreading retractor is not available. Visualize the heart in the pericardial sac. Visualize the phrenic nerve, and incise the pericardium just ventral to the phrenic nerve. Make sure to not cut the phrenic nerve. Grasp the heart in your hand(s) and gently squeeze it from apex to base, allowing time for the ventricle to fill before the next "contraction." If the heart does not seem to be filling, administer fluids intravenously or directly into the right atrium. The descending aorta can be cross-clamped with a Rummel tourniquet or red rubber catheter to improve perfusion to the brain and heart.

Management

Postresuscitation care and monitoring (prolonged life support)

Postresuscitation care involves careful monitoring and management of the adverse effects of hypoxia and reperfusion injury on the brain and other vital organs. The first 4 hours after an arrest are most critical, because this is the time period in which an animal is most likely to rearrest unless the underlying cause of the initial arrest has been determine and treated (Table 1-32). Until an animal is adequately ventilating on its own, artificial ventilation by manual bagging or attaching the patient to a mechanical ventilator with supplemental oxygen must continue. The efficacy of oxygenation and ventilation can be monitored using a Wright's respirometer, pulse oximetry, capnometry, and arterial blood

1

TABLE 1-32 Drugs Used in Advanced and Prolonged Life Support	
Drug	Dose
Advanced life support	
Atropine	0.04 mg/kg IV, IO; 0.4 mg/kg IT
Amiodarone	5 mg/kg IV, IO, IT
Epinephrine	0.02-0.04 mg/kg IV, IO, IT
Isoproterenol	0.04-0.08 µg/kg/minute IV CRI for third-degree atrioventricular block
Magnesium chloride	30 mg/kg IV, IO, IT
Naloxone	0.03 mg/kg IV, IO, IT
Sodium bicarbonate	1-2 mEq/kg IV, IO; NEVER administer intratracheally
Postresuscitation/Prolonged life support	
Furosemide	1 mg/kg IV
Lidocaine	1-2 mg/kg IV, followed by 50-100 µg/kg/minute CRI
Mannitol	0.51 g/kg IV

gas analyses (see also Pulse Oximetry and Capnometry [End-Tidal Carbon Dioxide Monitoring]). Once an animal is extubated, administer supplemental oxygen (50 to 100 mL/kg/minute) (see Oxygen Supplementation).

The brain is sensitive to ischemia and reperfusion injury. The effects of cellular hypoxia and reperfusion include the development of oxygen-derived free radical species that contribute to cerebral edema. Administer mannitol (0.5 to 1 g/kg IV over 5 to 10 minutes), followed by furosemide (1 mg/kg IV) 20 minutes later, to all patients that have experienced cardiopulmonary arrest and have had successful resuscitation. Mannitol and furosemide work synergistically to decrease cerebral edema formation and scavenge oxygen-derived free radical species.

The combination of cardiac arrest, myocardial ischemia and acidosis, and external or internal cardiac compressions often make the myocardium irritable and predisposed to dysrhythmias following successful CPCR. Start lidocaine (1 to 2 mg/kg IV, followed by 50 to 100 µg/kg/minute IV CRI) in all patients following successful resuscitative efforts. Monitor the ECG continuously for the presence of cardiac dysrhythmias and recurrence of nonperfusing rhythms. Perform direct or indirect blood pressure monitoring. If a patient's systolic blood pressure is less than 80 mm Hg, diastolic pressure is less than 40 mm Hg, or mean arterial blood pressure is less than 60 mm Hg, administer positive inotropic drugs (dobutamine, 1 to 20 µg/kg/minute) and pressor agents (epinephrine, 0.02 to 0.04 mg/kg IV, IO, IT) to improve cardiac contractility, cardiac output, and core organ perfusion.

The kidneys are sensitive to decreased perfusion and cellular hypoxia. Place a urinary catheter and monitor urine output. In a euvolemic patient, normal urine output should be no less than 1 to 2 mL/kg/hour. If urine output is low, administer low-dose dopamine (3 to 5 µg/kg/minute IV CRI) in an attempt to dilate afferent renal vessels and improve renal perfusion.

Maintain acid-base and electrolyte status within normal reference ranges. Monitor serum lactate as a rough indicator of organ perfusion and cellular oxygen extraction. The presence of elevated or rising serum lactate in the face of aggressive cardiorespiratory and cerebral support makes prognosis less favorable.

Additional Reading

Cole SG, Otto CM, Hughes D: Cardiopulmonary cerebral resuscitation: a clinical practice review part I, *J Vet Emerg Crit Care* 12(4):261-267, 2002.

Cole SG, Otto CM, Hughes D: Cardiopulmonary cerebral resuscitation: a clinical practice review part II, *J Vet Emerg Crit Care* 13(1):13-23, 2003.

Crowe DT: Clinic and staff readiness: the key to successful outcomes in emergency care, *Vet Med* 98(9):760-776, 2003.

Hackett TB: Cardiopulmonary cerebral resuscitation, *Vet Clin North Am Small Anim Pract* 31(6):1253-1264, 2001.

Haldane S, Marks SL: Cardiopulmonary cerebral resuscitation: emergency drugs and post-resuscitative care, *Compend Contin Educ Pract Vet* 26(10):791-799, 2004.

Haldane S, Marks SL: Cardiopulmonary cerebral resuscitation: techniques, *Compend Contin Educ Pract Vet* 26(10):780-790, 2004.

Johnson T: Use of vasopressin in cardiopulmonary arrest: controversies and promise, *Compend Contin Educ Pract Vet* 25(6):448-451, 2003.

Kruse-Elliott KT: Cardiopulmonary resuscitation: strategies for maximizing success, *Vet Med* 96(1):51-58, 2001.

Lehman TL, Manning AM: Post-arrest syndrome and the respiratory and cardiovascular systems in post-arrest patients, *Compend Contin Educ Pract Vet* 25(7):492-502, 2003.

Lehman TL, Manning AM: Renal, central nervous and gastrointestinal systems in post-arrest patients, *Compend Contin Educ Pract Vet* 25(7): 504-512, 2003.

Rieser T: Cardiopulmonary resuscitation, *Clin Tech Small Anim Pract* 15(2):76-81, 2000.

Waldrop JE, Rozanski EA, Swanke Ed, et al: Causes of cardiopulmonary arrest, resuscitation management, and functional outcome in dogs and cats surviving cardiopulmonary arrest, *J Vet Emerg Crit Care* 14(1):22-29, 2004.

Wingfield WE: Cardiopulmonary arrest. In Wingfield WE, Raffee MR, editors: *The veterinary ICU book,* Jackson, Wyo, 2001, Teton NewMedia.

Wingfield WE: Cardiopulmonary arrest and resuscitation in small animals. In Wingfield WE, editor: *Veterinary emergency medicine secrets,* ed 2, Philadelphia, 2001, Hanley & Belfus.

CARDIAC DYSRHYTHMIAS REQUIRING EMERGENCY MANAGEMENT

Cardiac dysrhythmias can encompass a wide range of clinical syndromes that vary in their clinical significance and signs, depending on the rate and frequency and whether coexisting cardiac disease is present. Ventricular and supraventricular dysrhythmias can occur because of primary myocardial disease or some other, secondary underlying disease process, including thoracic trauma, sepsis, systemic inflammatory response syndrome, pancreatitis, GDV, splenic disease, hypoxia, uremia, and acid-base and electrolyte disturbances. Common cardiac causes of dysrhythmias include dilative cardiomyopathy, end-stage degenerative valvular disease, infectious endocarditis, myocarditis, and cardiac neoplasia. In the cat, hypertrophy, restrictive, and unclassified cardiomyopathies and hyperthyroidism are the most common causes of dysrhythmias. In addition to structural cardiac or systemic disease, dysrhythmias can occur as an adverse effect of some drugs, including digoxin, dobutamine, aminophylline, and anesthetic agents.

Immediate action

Immediate action depends largely on recognition of the primary or secondary cause of the dysrhythmia and treating the dysrhythmia and underlying cause.

Differential diagnosis

Diagnosis of cardiac dysrhythmias is based on physical examination findings of abnormal thoracic/cardiac auscultation, the presence of abnormal pulse rhythm and quality, and recognition of ECG abnormalities. The ECG is critical to the accurate diagnosis of dysrhythmias.

Ventricular dysrhythmias

Ventricular dysrhythmias arise from ectopic foci in the ventricles that cause the wave of depolarization to spread from cell to cell rather than spread through fast-conducting tissue. This causes the QRS complex to appear wide and bizarre, unless the ectopic focus originates close to the atrioventricular node high in the ventricle. Other ECG features of ventricular dysrhythmias include a T wave polarity that is opposite to the QRS complex and nonrelated P waves. Ventricular dysrhythmias may manifest as isolated ventricular premature complexes, couplets, or triplets; bigeminy; or ventricular tachycardia. Relatively slow ventricular tachycardia is known as an idioventricular rhythm and is not as

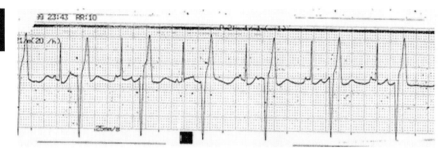

Figure 1-31: Unifocal premature ventricular complexes (PVCs). All the PVCs are the same shape and size and originate from the same ectopic focus in the ventricle. Note that this rhythm is actually an example of ventricular bigeminy.

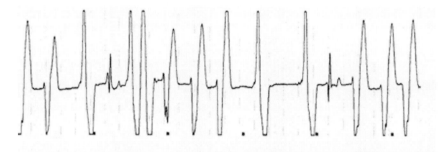

Figure 1-32: Multifocal premature ventricular complexes (PVCs). Note that the complexes change shape, size, and orientation, indicating multiple ectopic foci within the ventricle.

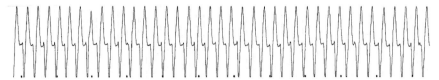

Figure 1-33:   Sustained ventricular tachycardia.

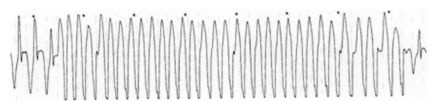

Figure 1-34:   An example of R-on-T phenomenon. Note that there is no return to baseline or isoelectric shelf in between the T wave of one complex and the R wave of the next complex. This rhythm can be very dangerous and can lead to ventricular fibrillation.

hemodynamically significant as faster ventricular tachycardia. Idioventricular rhythm usually is less than 130 beats per minute and may alternate spontaneously with sinus arrhythmias (Figures 1-31 to 1-34).

Supraventricular dysrhythmias

Supraventricular dysrhythmias arise from ectopic foci in the atria and are commonly associated with atrial dilatation and structural heart disease such as advanced acquired or congenital heart disease, cardiomyopathies, cardiac neoplasia, or advanced heartworm disease. Occasionally, supraventricular dysrhythmias may be associated with respiratory or other systemic illness. Sustained supraventricular tachycardia in the absence of underlying structural heart or systemic disease is disturbing and should alert the clinician that an accessory pathway conduction disturbance may be present, particularly in Labrador Retrievers.

Supraventricular dysrhythmias can manifest as isolated premature complexes (atrial premature complexes or contractions), sustained or paroxysmal supraventricular tachycardia (atrial tachycardia), or atrial fibrillation or flutter. In the dog, atrial fibrillation most commonly is associated with dilative cardiomyopathy. Rarely and primarily in giant breed dogs, lone atrial fibrillation can occur with no underlying heart disease. Atrial fibrillation and the resultant sustained elevation in ventricular rate are presumed to progress to dilative cardiomyopathy in such breeds. By comparison, atrial fibrillation is relatively uncommon in cats because of the small size of their atria but is associated most commonly with hypertrophic and restrictive cardiomyopathy.

The ECG is critical to the diagnosis of a supraventricular dysrhythmia. The ECG usually demonstrates a normal appearance to the QRS complex unless aberrant conduction occurs in the ventricles, in which case the QRS can be wide but still originate from above the atrioventricular node. In most cases of a supraventricular dysrhythmia, some evidence of atrial activity including P waves, atrial flutter, or atrial fibrillation is apparent. In some cases, it may be difficult to diagnose the exact rhythm without slowing the rate down mechanically or through pharmacologic intervention. Once a rhythm diagnosis is made, appropriate treatment strategies can be implemented (Figures 1-35 and 1-36).

Management

Ventricular dysrhythmias

Treatment of ventricular dysrhythmias largely depends on the number of ectopic foci discharging, the rate and character of the dysrhythmia, and whether the presence of the abnormal beats is of adverse hemodynamic consequence, including risk of sudden death. Many ventricular dysrhythmias, including slow idioventricular rhythms, ventricular bigeminy, or intermittent ventricular premature complexes, do not warrant antiarrhythmic

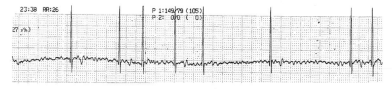

Figure 1-35: Atrial fibrillation.

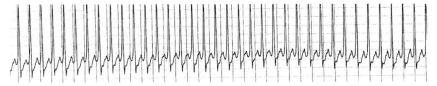

Figure 1-36: Supraventricular tachycardia.

TABLE 1-33   Oral Management of Ventricular Dysrhythmias in Dogs

Drug	Dose
Procainamide	10-20 mg/kg PO q6-8h
Tocainide*	10-20 mg/kg PO q8h
Sotalol	40-120 mg per dog q12h (start low, then titrate up to effect)
Mexiletine	5-8 mg/kg PO q8h
Atenolol	0.25-1.0 mg/kg PO q12-24h (start low, titrate upward to effect)

*Do not use for longer than 2 weeks because of idiosyncratic blindness.

therapy unless the patient is hypotensive and the dysrhythmia is thought to be contributing to the hypotension. In such cases, correction of the underlying disease process including hypoxia, pain, or anxiety often alleviates or decreases the incidence of the dysrhythmia.

More serious ventricular dysrhythmias that warrant antiarrhythmic therapy (Table 1-33) include sustained ventricular tachycardia (>160 beats/minute in dogs; >220 beats/minute in cats), multifocal ventricular premature complexes originating from more than one place in the ventricles, and the presence of R-on-T phenomena where the T wave of the preceding complex is superimposed on the QRS of the next complex with no return to isoelectric shelf in between complexes. Treat these ventricular dysrhythmias immediately and aggressively. In dogs, the mainstay of emergency treatment for ventricular dysrhythmias is lidocaine therapy. Administer lidocaine (1 to 2 mg/kg IV bolus) over a period of 5 minutes to prevent the adverse side effects of seizures or vomiting. The bolus can be repeated an additional 3 times (total dose 8 mg/kg) over 15 minutes, or the patient can be placed on a constant rate infusion (50 to 100 μg/kg/minute) if control of ventricular tachycardia is accomplished. Also correct the patient's magnesium and potassium deficiencies to maximize the success of lidocaine therapy in the treatment of ventricular tachycardia. Procainamide (4 mg/kg IV slowly over 3 to 5 minutes) also can be used to control ventricular tachycardia. If procainamide is successful at controlling ventricular tachycardia, administer it as a constant rate infusion (25 to 40 μg/kg/minute). Side effects of procainamide include vomiting, diarrhea, and hypotension.

Chronic oral therapy may or may not be necessary in the treatment of acute ventricular tachycardia. The decision to continue antiarrhythmic therapy depends on the underlying disease process and the expectation of persistent arrhythmogenesis of the underlying disease process. Oral antiarrhythmic therapy is warranted in cases in which a serious ventricular dysrhythmia is recognized but the animal does not require hospitalization, such as the syncopal Boxer with intermittent ventricular dysrhythmias and no evidence of structural heart disease. It deserves emphasis that asymptomatic, low-grade ventricular dysrhythmias probably do not require treatment. If maintenance therapy for ventricular dysrhythmias is needed, use an oral drug based on the underlying disease process, clinical familiarity, class of drug, dosing frequency, owner compliance, concurrent medications, cost, and potential adverse side effects.

Treatment of ventricular dysrhythmias in cats

In the cat the mainstay of antiarrhythmic therapy is the use of a β-adrenergic antagonist. In the acute management of ventricular dysrhythmias in cases of hypertrophic, restrictive, or unclassified cardiomyopathies, consider using injectable esmolol (0.05 to 1.0 mg/kg IV slowly to effect) or propranolol (0.02 to 0.06 mg/kg IV slowly to effect), particularly if the dysrhythmia results from hyperthyroidism. For chronic oral ventricular antiarrhythmic therapy in cats, propranolol (2.5 to 5.0 mg PO per cat q8h) or atenolol (6.25 to 12.5 mg PO per cat q12-24h) can be used.

Supraventricular dysrhythmias

The decision to treat supraventricular dysrhythmias depends on the ventricular rate and the hemodynamic consequences of the dysrhythmia. For intermittent isolated atrial

T A B L E   1 - 3 4   Parenteral and Oral Management of Supraventricular Dysrhythmias

Drug	Dose
Parenteral	
Esmolol	50-100 μg/kg IV bolus, 50-200 μg/kg/minute IV CRI
Propranolol	0.04-0.1 mg/kg IV slowly to effect
Diltiazem	0.1-0.25 mg/kg IV slowly to effect, then 2-6 μg/kg/minute CRI
Digoxin	0.0025 mg/kg bolus IV; can be repeated every hour up to 0.01 mg/kg maximum dose
Oral	
Digoxin	0.005-0.01 mg/kg PO bid; animal >15 kg, 0.22 mg/m² PO bid
Diltiazem	0.5 mg/kg PO bid
Diltiazem (Dilacor-XR)	1.5-6 mg/kg q12-24h (dog); cat, 30-60 mg PO q12-24h
Atenolol	0.25-1 mg/kg q12-24h; cat, 6.25 mg PO q12-24h
Propranolol	0.1-0.2 mg/kg PO q8h, titrated up to a maximum of 0.5 mg/kg PO q8h; cat, 2.5-10 mg/kg PO q8h
Amiodarone	10 mg/kg PO q12h for 7 days, then 5 mg/kg PO q24h (maintenance)

premature contractions, couplets, and triplets, usually no treatment is required. When the ventricular rate exceeds 180 beats/minute, diastolic filling time is shortened, causing the heart to not fill adequately. The consequence is decreased cardiac output and decreased coronary artery perfusion. The goal of therapy is rhythm control or, in most cases, rate control. In cases of atrial fibrillation and congestive heart failure, conversion to a normal sinus rhythm rarely can be achieved, although electrocardioversion or pharmacoconversion can be attempted.

In the dog a vagal maneuver can be attempted by pressing on the eyeballs or massaging the carotid body. For sustained supraventricular tachycardia, diltiazem (0.25 mg/kg IV), esmolol (0.05 to 0.1, titrated upward to a cumulative dose of 0.5 mg/kg IV), or propranolol (0.04 to 0.1 mg/kg IV slowly to effect) can be administered in an attempt to slow the ventricular rate in emergent situations. Administer oral diltiazem (0.5 mg/kg PO q8h), diltiazem (Dilacor-XR) (1.5 to 6 mg/kg PO q12-24h), propranolol (0.1 to 0.2 mg/kg tid, titrated up to a maximum of 0.5 mg/kg PO q8h), atenolol (0.25 to 1 mg/kg q12-24h), or digoxin (0.005 to 0.01 mg/kg bid or 0.22 mg/m² for dogs greater than 15 kg).

In the cat a vagal maneuver can be attempted by ocular or carotid massage. (Diltiazem [Dilacor] 30 to 60 PO q12-24h), propranolol (2.5 to 10 mg/kg q12-24h), or atenolol (6.25 mg q12-24h) also can be administered. If structural heart disease is present, treat pulmonary edema and start angiotensin-converting enzyme inhibitor therapy. Table 1-34 summarizes the drugs used in the management of supraventricular dysrhythmias.

BRADYARRHYTHMIAS

Severe bradycardia often results from systemic disease, drug therapy, anesthetic agents, or hypothermia and thus rarely requires specific therapy except to treat or reverse the underlying mechanisms promoting bradycardia. Hemodynamically significant bradyarrhythmias that must be treated include atrial standstill, atrioventricular block, and sick sinus syndrome.

Atrial standstill

Atrial standstill most commonly is associated with hyperkalemia and is seen most often in urinary obstruction, renal failure, urinary trauma with uroabdomen, and hypoadrenocorticism. Characteristic ECG abnormalities observed in atrial standstill are an absence of P waves, widened QRS complexes, and tall spiked T waves (Figure 1-37).

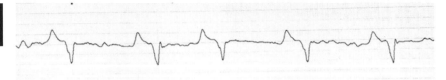

Figure 1-37: An example of atrial standstill caused by hyperkalemia in a blocked tomcat. Note that there are no P waves and that the ventricular QRS complexes are widened and blunted.

The treatment for hyperkalemia-induced atrial standstill is to correct the underlying cause and to drive potassium intracellularly and protect the myocardium from the adverse effects of hyperkalemia. Regular insulin (0.25 to 0.5 units/kg IV) followed by dextrose (1 g/unit insulin IV, followed by 2.5% dextrose CRI to prevent hypoglycemia) or sodium bicarbonate (1 mEq/kg IV) can be administered to drive potassium intracellularly. Calcium gluconate (0.5 mL/kg of 20% solution IV over 5 minutes) also can be administered as a cardioprotective drug until the cause of hyperkalemia has been identified and resolved. Also administer sodium chloride fluids (0.9% sodium chloride IV) to promote kaliuresis.

Less commonly, atrial standstill is associated with atrial cardiomyopathy or silent atrium syndrome. Persistent atrial standstill has been recognized without electrolyte abnormalities in the English Springer Spaniel and the Siamese cat. Short-term therapy for persistent atrial standstill includes atropine (0.04 mg/kg SQ) until definitive treatment by implantation of a cardiac pacemaker can be performed.

Third-degree atrioventricular block

Complete or third-degree atrioventricular block or high-grade symptomatic second-degree atrioventricular block can be hemodynamically significant when ventricular rates are less than 60 beats/minute in the dog. Classic clinical signs include weakness, exercise intolerance, lethargy, anorexia, syncope, and occasionally seizures. Advanced atrioventricular block usually is caused by advanced idiopathic degeneration of the atrioventricular node. Less commonly, atrioventricular block has been associated with digoxin toxicity, magnesium oversupplementation, cardiomyopathy, endocarditis, or infectious myocarditis (Lyme disease). An accurate diagnosis is made based on the ECG findings of nonconducted P waves with ventricular escape beats. First- and second-degree atrioventricular block may not be hemodynamically significant and therefore may not require therapy.

Initially treat third-degree (complete) or symptomatic high-grade second-degree atrioventricular block (<60 beats/minute) with atropine (0.04 mg/kg SQ or IM). Perform a follow-up ECG in 15 to 20 minutes. Atropine is rarely successful in treating complete atrioventricular block. Also attempt treatment with isoproterenol (0.04 to 0.08 µg/kg/minute IV CRI or 0.4 mg in 250 mL 5% dextrose in water IV slowly), a pure β-agonist. Definitive treatment requires permanent pacemaker implantation. Consultation with a veterinary cardiologist who implants pacemakers is suggested. Never attempt to convert or treat the observed ventricular escape beats with lidocaine (Figure 1-38).

Sick sinus syndrome

Sick sinus syndrome most commonly is recognized in the Miniature Schnauzer, although any dog can be affected. Sick sinus syndrome usually results from idiopathic degeneration of the sinus node in the dog. In the cat, sinus node degeneration usually is associated with cardiomyopathy. Dysfunction of the sinus node may manifest as marked bradycardia with periods of sinus arrest followed by junctional or ventricular escape complexes. A variant of sick sinus syndrome is the presence of severe bradycardia followed by periods of supraventricular tachycardia, often termed *bradycardia-tachycardia syndrome.* The most common clinical signs are syncope, exercise intolerance, and lethargy.

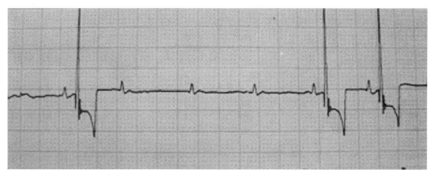

Figure 1-38: Example of third-degree atrioventricular block. Note that there does not appear to be conductance of any of the p-waves, leading to intermittent narrow complex ventricular escape beats.

Treatment of sick sinus syndrome involves permanent pacemaker implantation by a veterinary cardiologist. Less severe cases of sick sinus syndrome can be managed medically, at least short-term, with atropine (0.04 mg/kg IM) or probanthine (0.5 to 1.5 mg/kg PO q8h).

Additional Reading

Abbott JA: Beta-blockage in the management of systolic dysfunction, *Vet Clin North Am Small Anim Pract* 34(5):1157-1170, 2004.

Geltzer ARM, Kraus MS: Management of atrial fibrillation, *Vet Clin North Am Small Anim Pract* 34(5):1127-1144, 2004.

Kittleson MD, Kienle RD: Diagnosis and treatment of arrhythmias. In *Small animal cardiovascular medicine,* St Louis, 1999, Mosby.

O'Grady MR, O'Sullivan ML: Dilated cardiomyopathy: an update, *Vet Clin North Am Small Anim Pract* 34(5):1187-1207, 2004.

Wright KN: Interventional catheterization for tachyarrhythmias, *Vet Clin North Am Small Anim Pract* 34(5):1171-1185, 2004.

Congestive Heart Failure in Dogs and Cats

Presentation in the dog

The majority of animals that present with congestive heart failure (CHF) are older animals that have some acquired heart disease that develops later in life. Congenital defects are rarer than acquired heart disease. The most common congenital defect observed in dogs and in some cats is a patent ductus arteriosus.

The most common acquired cardiac disease in dogs is chronic valvular disease, or endocardiosis (mitral valve endocardiosis). In endocardiosis, the atrioventricular valves chronically lose the ability to close effectively, causing abnormalities in blood flow, including regurgitation during ventricular systole. In most cases, disease progression is chronic and slow, although acute exacerbations and onset of clinical signs can be associated with stress, rupture of a chordae tendinae, or ingestion of a high-salt meal. Mitral valve disease tends to affect older toy breeds such as miniature Poodles, Chihuahuas, and younger Cavalier King Charles Spaniels.

The second most common cause of acquired heart disease is dilated cardiomyopathy, which is a disease of primary myocardial failure. In dilated cardiomyopathy the muscular wall of the heart becomes thin and weak as the myocardium dilates, causing a decrease in contractility and cardiac output. Secondary mitral and tricuspid valvular insufficiency may result from chronic stretching of the valve annulus. This type of heart disease typically is associated with giant breed dogs including Irish Wolfhounds, English Mastiffs, Great Danes, Boxers, and Doberman Pinschers. A rare form of the disease has been documented in young Labrador Retrievers. Acute exacerbation of dilated cardiomyopathy may be related to the development of a dysrhythmia, including atrial fibrillation.

1

Presentation in the cat

In cats, hypertrophic cardiomyopathy is the most common form of acquired cardiac disease observed. Congestive heart failure resulting from hypertrophic cardiomyopathy can occur in animals as young as 6 to 10 months of age. Hypertrophic cardiomyopathy is characterized by stiff, noncompliant ventricles that do not relax during diastole, causing an increase in left atrial pressures and left atrial enlargement. Other cardiomyopathies, including unclassified, restrictive, and dilated, are less common but also can occur in the cat. Cats often develop acute exacerbation of clinical signs because of stress or arterial embolization.

Immediate action/treatment

The rapid diagnosis of CHF often is made on owner history, signalment, and physical examination findings (Box 1-36).

Typical physical examination findings include a cardiac murmur or gallop dysrhythmia, abnormal breath sounds, respiratory difficulty and orthopnea, tachycardia, weak pulse quality, cool peripheral extremities, and pale or cyanotic mucous membrane. Initiate immediate treatment based on physical examination findings and index of suspicion. In some cases, it is difficult to distinguish between CHF and feline lower airway disease (asthma) without performing thoracic radiographs. Let the animal rest and become stabilized before attempting any stressful procedures, including thoracic radiographs.

Immediate treatment consists of administering supplemental oxygen, decreasing circulating fluid volume with furosemide, dilating pulmonary and splanchnic capacitance vessels with topical nitroglycerine and morphine, and alleviating patient anxiety and stress (Box 1-37).

Differential diagnosis

Primary differential diagnoses are made based primarily on the patient's breed, age, clinical signs, history, and physical examination abnormalities. The most common differential diagnoses in a patient with CHF are cardiac abnormalities and respiratory disease (chronic bronchitis [asthma], pulmonary hypertension, cor pulmonale, neoplasia).

Postpone diagnostic tests in any patient with suspected CHF until the immediate treatments have taken effect and the patient is cardiovascularly more stable. In most cases, lateral and dorsoventral thoracic radiographs are one of the most important diagnostic tools in helping make a diagnosis of CHF. Increased perihilar interstitial to alveolar infiltrates are characteristic of pulmonary edema. Left atrial enlargement may be observed as a "backpack" sign at the caudal cardiac waist. Cardiomegaly of the right or left side also may

---

BOX 1-36   COMMON PRESENTING COMPLAINTS BY OWNERS OF PATIENTS WITH CONGESTIVE HEART FAILURE

- Lethargy
- Weakness
- Cough
- Respiratory difficulty
- Exercise intolerance
- Inappetance
- Weight loss
- Abdominal distention
- Syncope

BOX 1-37   IMMEDIATE MANAGEMENT OF CONGESTIVE HEART FAILURE

- Supplemental oxygen at 50 to 100 mL/kg/minute to supply 40% to 50% oxygen
- Furosemide, 4 to 8 mg/kg IV, IM, every 30 minutes until the patient urinates and body weight decreases by 7%
- Nitroglycerine ointment ($1/4$ to 1 inch topically) every 8 hours
- Morphine, 0.025 to 0.05 mg/kg IV (dog only)

> **BOX 1-38   VERTEBRAL HEART SUM TO DETERMINE CARDIOMEGALY**
>
> The vertebral heart sum can be calculated by performing the following steps:
> 1. Measure the long axis of the heart from the apex to the carina on the lateral view and mark the distance on a sheet of paper.
> 2. Measure the length of the long axis of the heart in terms of vertebral bodies, starting by counting caudally from the fourth thoracic vertebra; count the number of vertebrae that are covered by the length of the long axis of the heart.
> 3. Measure the short axis of the heart at the caudal vena cava, perpendicular to the long axis of the heart.
> 4. Count the number of thoracic vertebrae covered by the short axis of the heart, starting at T4.
> 5. Add the two numbers together to yield the vertebral heart sum; a vertebral heart sum greater than 10.5 is consistent with cardiomegaly.

be present in cases of valvular insufficiency. In cats, increased sternal contact and a classic valentine-shaped heart may be observed in cases of hypertrophic cardiomyopathy. Perform a vertebral heart score (sum) to measure cardiac size and determine whether cardiomegaly is present (Box 1-38).

Also obtain arterial blood pressure and ECG readings to determine whether hypotension and dysrhythmias are present. Atrial fibrillation, ventricular premature contractions, and supraventricular tachycardia are common rhythm disturbances that can affect cardiac output adversely and influence treatment choices.

The echocardiogram is a useful noninvasive and nonstressful method to determine the degree of cardiac disease present. The echocardiogram is largely user-dependent. The quality of the study is based on the experience of the operator and the quality of the ultrasound machine. Echocardiography can be a useful tool in making a diagnosis of pericardial effusion, dilated or hypertrophic cardiomyopathy, cardiac neoplasia, and endocarditis.

Management of congestive heart failure in dogs and cats

The medical management of CHF is designed to improve cardiac output and relieve clinical signs. The immediate goal of therapy is to reduce abnormal fluid accumulation and provide adequate cardiac output by increasing contractility, decreasing preload and ventricular afterload, and/or normalizing cardiac dysrhythmias. Strict cage rest is of utmost importance when managing a patient with CHF.

After initial administration of furosemide, morphine, oxygen, and nitroglycerine paste, clinical signs of respiratory distress should show improvement within 30 minutes. If no improvement is observed, administer repeated doses of furosemide. Reevaluate severe cases that are refractory to this standard treatment protocol. Vasodilation should be the next step in the management of refractory cases, provided that a normal blood pressure is present. Sodium nitroprusside is a potent balanced vasodilator that should be administered (1 to 10 μg/kg/minute IV CRI), taking care to monitor blood pressure continuously because severe vasodilation and hypotension can occur. The goal of nitroprusside therapy is to maintain a mean arterial blood pressure of 60 mm Hg. Sodium nitroprusside should not be considered in cases of refractory CHF with severe hypotension.

For more long-term management of CHF, the use of angiotensin-converting enzyme (ACE) inhibitors including enalapril (0.5 mg/kg PO q12-24h), benazepril (0.5 mg/kg PO q24h), and lisinopril (0.5 mg/kg PO q24h) have become the mainstay of therapy to reduce sodium and fluid retention and decrease afterload. Start angiotensin-converting enzyme inhibition as soon as a patient is able to tolerate oral medications.

Dobutamine (2.5 to 10 μg/kg/minute CRI diluted in 5% dextrose in water) can be administered to improve cardiac contractility, particularly in cases of dilated cardiomyopathy. At low doses, dobutamine, primarily a β-adrenergic agonist, will improve cardiac output with minimal effects on heart rate. Dobutamine must be given as a constant rate infusion with careful, continuous ECG monitoring. Despite minimal effects on heart rate, sinus tachycardia or ventricular dysrhythmias may develop during infusion. Cats are more sensitive to the effects of dobutamine than dogs. Monitor carefully for seizures and facial twitching.

Digoxin is a cardiac glycoside that acts as a positive inotrope and negative chronotrope in the long-term management of CHF. Digoxin has a long (24 hours in dogs, and 60 hours in cats) half-life and so has minimal use in the emergency management of CHF. In chronic management of CHF resulting from dilated cardiomyopathy or advanced mitral disease, however, digoxin is extremely useful. Oral digitalization protocols have been developed but are risky in that dysrhythmias and severe gastrointestinal side effects can occur.

Cats with CHF often have fulminant pulmonary edema, pleural effusion, arterial thromboembolism, or some combination of all three. If the pleural effusion is significant, perform therapeutic thoracocentesis to relieve pulmonary atelectasis and improve oxygenation. Once the diagnosis and initial management of CHF has been made, formulate a plan for continued management and monitoring. Tailor the therapeutic plan to the patient based on the cause of the CHF, the presence of concurrent diseases, and response to therapy. An important and often overlooked part of the successful emergency management of CHF is the open communication with the owner regarding the owner's emotional and financial commitment for immediate and long-term management to ensure appropriate quality of life for each patient.

Additional Reading

Abbott JA: Dilated cardiomyopathy. In Wingfield WE, editor: *Veterinary emergency medicine secrets,* Philadelphia, 2001, Hanley & Belfus.

Abbott JA: Feline myocardial disease. In Wingfield WE, editor: *Veterinary emergency medicine secrets,* Philadelphia, 2001, Hanley & Belfus.

Borgarelli M, Tarducci A, Tidholm A, et al: Canine idiopathic dilated cardiomyopathy. 2. Pathophysiology and treatment, *Vet J* 162(3):182-195, 2001.

Buston R: Treatment of congestive heart failure, *J Small Anim Pract* 44(11):516, 2003.

Fuentes VL: Use of pimobendan in the management of heart failure, *Vet Clin North Am Small Anim Pract* 34(5):1145-1155, 2004.

Goodwin JK, Strickland K: The emergency management of dogs and cats with congestive heart failure, *Vet Med* 93(9):818-822, 1998.

Goodwin JK, Strickland KN: Managing arrhythmias in dogs and cats with congestive heart failure, *Vet Med* 93(9):823-829, 1998.

Laste NJ: Cardiovascular pharmacotherapy, *Vet Clin North Am Small Anim* 31(6):1231-1252, 2001.

Martin M: Treatment of congestive heart failure as a neuroendocrine disorder, *J Small Anim Pract* 44(4):154-160, 2003.

Sisson D, Kittleson MD: Management of heart failure: principles of treatment, therapeutic strategies, and pharmacology. In Fox PR, Sisson D, Moise NS, editors: *Textbook of canine and feline cardiology,* ed 2, Philadelphia, 1999, WB Saunders.

Ware WA, Bonagura JD: Pulmonary edema. In Fox PR, Sisson D, Moise NS, editors: *Textbook of canine and feline cardiology,* ed 2, Philadelphia, 1999, WB Saunders.

CANINE CAVAL SYNDROME OF HEARTWORM DISEASE

Caval syndrome resulting from severe heartworm disease is caused by the rapid maturation of a large quantity of adult worms in the right atrium and cranial and caudal venae cavae. Most cases of caval syndrome occur in regions of the world where heartworm disease is highly endemic and dogs spend a large portion of time living outdoors. Caval syndrome is recognized by the following clinical signs and results of biochemical analyses: acute renal and hepatic failure, enlarged right atrium and posterior vena cava, ascites, hemoglobinuria, anemia, acute collapse, respiratory distress, DIC, jugular pulses, circulating microfilariae, and sometimes tricuspid insufficiency.

Immediate action

Immediate action in cases of caval syndrome in dogs involves immediate stabilization of the cardiovascular and respiratory systems with supplemental oxygen, furosemide (4 mg/kg IV), and careful crystalloid fluid infusion.

Diagnosis

Diagnosis of caval syndrome is based on clinical signs of cardiogenic shock with right ventricular heart failure, intravascular hemolysis, and renal and hepatic failure. Thoracic radiographs reveal cardiomegaly of the right side and enlarged tortuous pulmonary arteries. A right axis deviation may be seen on ECG tracings. Clinicopathologic changes observed include azotemia, inflammatory leukogram, regenerative anemia, eosinophilia, elevated hepatocellular enzyme activities, hemoglobinuria, and proteinuria. Circulating microfilariae may be observed on peripheral blood smears or in the buffy coat of microhematocrit tubes. Heart worm antigen tests will be strongly positive. Echocardiographic changes include visualization of a large number of heartworms in the right atrium, pulmonary arteries, and vena cava, tricuspid insufficiency, and right atrial and ventricular enlargement.

Management

Treatment involves surgical removal of as many of the adult heartworms as possible from the right jugular vein and right atrium. Glucocorticosteroids are recommended to decrease inflammation and microangiopathic disease associated with heartworm infection. For more long-term management, administer adulticide therapy several weeks following surgery, followed by routine microfilaricide therapy and then prophylaxis.

Additional Reading

Calvert CA, Rawlings CA, McCall JW: Canine heartworm disease. In Fox PR, Sisson D, Moise NS, editors: *Textbook of canine and feline cardiology,* ed 2, Philadelphia, 1999, WB Saunders.

Hidaka Y, Hagio M, Morakami T, et al: Three dogs under 2 years of age with heartworm caval syndrome, *J Vet Med Sci* 65(10):1147-1149, 2003.

Kitagawa H, Kitoh K, Ohba Y, et al: Comparison of laboratory results before and after surgical removal of heartworms in dogs with vena caval syndrome, *J Am Vet Med Assoc* 213(8):1134-1136, 1998.

Kuntz CA, Smith-Carr S, Huber M, et al: Use of a modified surgical approach to the right atrium for retrieval of heartworms in a dog, *J Am Vet Med Assoc* 208(5):692-604, 1996.

PERICARDIAL EFFUSION AND PERICARDIOCENTESIS

Pericardial effusion often develops as a consequence of neoplasia in the older dog and cat. The most common types of neoplasia that affect the heart and pericardium include hemangiosarcoma, chemodectoma, mesothelioma, and metastatic neoplasia. More rarely, other causes of pericardial effusion include benign idiopathic pericardial effusion, coagulopathy, left atrial rupture in dogs with chronic mitral valvular insufficiency, infection, or pericardial cysts. Regardless of the cause of the effusion, the development of pericardial tamponade adversely affects cardiac output.

Cardiac output is a function of heart rate and stroke volume. Stroke volume depends on cardiac preload. The presence of pericardial effusion can impede venous return to the heart and thus adversely affect preload. In addition, as preload decreases, heart rate reflexively increases in an attempt to maintain normal cardiac output. As heart rate increases more than 160 beats/minute, diastolic filling is impaired further, and cardiac output further declines. Animals with pericardial effusion often demonstrate the classic signs of hypovolemic or cardiogenic shock: anorexia, weakness, lethargy, cyanosis, cool peripheral extremities, tachycardia, weak thready pulses, hypotension, and collapse. Physical examination abnormalities may include muffled heart sounds, thready femoral pulses, pulsus paradoxus, jugular venous distention, weakness, tachycardia, cyanosis, and tachypnea. Electrocardiogram findings may include low amplitude QRS complexes (<0.5 mV), sinus tachycardia, ventricular dysrhythmias, or electrical alternans (Figure 1-39). Thoracic radiographs often demonstrate a globoid cardiac silhouette, although the cardiac silhouette rarely may appear normal with concurrent clinical signs of cardiogenic shock in cases of acute hemorrhage. In such cases the removal of even small amounts of pericardial effusion by pericardiocentesis can increase cardiac output exponentially and alleviate clinical signs (Table 1-35). Unless an animal is dying before your eyes, ideally perform an echocardiogram to attempt to

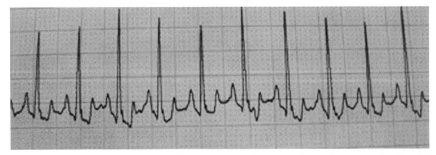

Figure 1-39: An example of electrical alternans. This rhythm is observed in cases of pericardial effusion, as the heart swings to and fro within the fluid, toward and away from the electrical axis.

TABLE 1-35   Differential Diagnosis of Pericardial Effusion

Type of pericardial effusion	Cause	Characteristic features
Hemorrhagic	Heart base tumors Hemangiosarcoma Metastatic neoplasia Benign idiopathic pericardial effusion Physical trauma Left atrial rupture	Usually brachycephalic breeds; >8 years old; blood usually nonclotting Large breed dogs Middle-aged large breed dogs Cardiac puncture Small breeds, >8 years of age; chronic valvular disease
Transudate	Coagulopathy Congestive heart failure Hypoproteinemia Following peritoneo-pericardial diaphragmatic hernia	Radiograph or echocardiogram will usually demonstrate lesion
Exudate	Infectious pericarditis Suppurative pericarditis	Exudate in distemper, leptospirosis, and systemic fungal infection Foreign body or hematologic spread of inflammatory process

determine whether a right atrial, right auricular, or heart base mass is present before pericardiocentesis.

Pericardiocentesis

Before attempting pericardiocentesis, assemble all of the required supplies (Box 1-39).

To perform pericardiocentesis, follow this procedure:

1. Place the patient in sternal or lateral recumbency.
2. Attach ECG leads to monitor the patient for dysrhythmias during the procedure.
3. Clip a 6-cm square caudal to the right elbow over the fifth to seventh intercostal space.
4. Aseptically scrub the clipped area, and infuse 1 to 2 mg/kg of 2% lidocaine mixed with a small amount of sodium bicarbonate just dorsal to the sternum at the sixth intercostal space. Bury the needle to the hub, and inject the lidocaine as you withdraw the needle.

BOX 1-39   SUPPLIES REQUIRED FOR PERICARDIOCENTESIS

- 2% lidocaine
- 3-mL syringe
- 25-gauge needle
- No. 11 scalpel blade
- 14- to 16-gauge Abbott-T catheter or Turkel thoracic drainage catheter
- Intravenous extension tubing
- Three-way stopcock
- 60-mL syringe
- Red- and lavender-topped tubes
- Collection bowl
- Clippers
- Antimicrobial scrub

---

5. While the local anesthetic is taking effect, assemble the intravenous extension tubing, three-way stopcock, and 60-mL syringe.
6. Wearing sterile gloves, make a small nick incision in the skin to decrease drag on the needle and catheter during insertion.
7. Slowly insert the needle and catheter, watching for a flash of blood in the hub of the needle, and simultaneously watching for cardiac dysrhythmias on the ECG monitor.
8. Once a flash of blood is observed in the hub of the needle, advance the catheter off of the stylette further into the pericardial sac, and remove the stylette.
9. Attach the length of intravenous extension tubing to the catheter, and have an assistant withdraw the fluid slowly.
10. Place a small amount of fluid in a red-topped tube, and watch for clots. Clot formation could signify that you have penetrated the right ventricle inadvertently or that active hemorrhage is occurring. Withdraw as much of the fluid as possible, and then remove the catheter. Monitor the patient closely for fluid reaccumulation and recurrence of clinical signs of cardiogenic shock.

Additional Reading

Less RD, Bright JM, Orton EC: Intrapericardial cyst causing cardiac tamponade in a cat, *J Am Anim Hosp Assoc* 36(2):115-119, 2000.

MacGregor JM, Rozanski EA, McCarthy RJ, et al: Cholesterol-based pericardial effusion and aortic thromboembolism in a 9-year-old mixed breed dog with hypothyroidism, *J Vet Intern Med* 18(3):354-358, 2004.

Machida N, Tanaka R, Takemura N, et al: Development of pericardial mesothelioma in a golden retriever with a long-term history of idiopathic pericardial haemorrhagic effusion, *J Comp Pathol* 131(2-3):166-175, 2004.

Shubitz LF, Matz ME, Noon TH, et al: Constrictive pericarditis secondary to *Coccidioides immitis* infection in a dog, *J Am Vet Med Assoc* 218(4):537-540, 2001.

Stafford Johnson M, Martin M, Binn S, et al: A retrospective study of clinical findings, treatment and outcome in 143 dogs with pericardial effusion, *J Anim Pract* 45(11):546-552, 2004.

Zoia A, Hughes D, Connolly DJ: Pericardial effusion and cardiac tamponade in a cat with extranodal lymphoma, *J Small Anim Pract* 45(9):467-471, 2004.

EAR EMERGENCIES

FOREIGN BODIES

Foreign bodies within the ear canal (e.g., foxtails) can present as emergencies because of acute inflammation and pressure necrosis of the tissue of the external auditory meatus causing pain and discomfort. Clinical signs may be limited to incessant head shaking or scratching of the ear canal.

Immediate action/treatment

Complete examination of the ear canal and removal of any foreign body often requires administration of a short-acting anesthetic agent. Once the animal has been restrained sufficiently and placed under anesthesia, carefully examine the ear canal and remove any foreign material with an alligator forceps. Stimulation of the ear canal can cause awakening and shaking of the head. Use care to not perforate the tympanum or cause trauma to the ear canal with the forceps. Heat-fix any purulent material within the ear canal and examine it cytologically for bacteria or fungal organisms. Gently irrigate the ear canal with warm sterile saline to remove excessive debris and exudates. Use care to avoid excessive pressure (>50 mm Hg) to avoid iatrogenic damage to the tympanic membrane.

Management

After removal of all debris and detritus, gently wipe the internal and external ear canal with a sterile gauze. Place a topical antimicrobial-antifungal-steroid ointment such as Otomax in the ear every 8 to 12 hours. If pain and discomfort is severe, systemically effective opioids or NSAIDs may be required.

OTITIS EXTERNA

Otitis externa is a common emergency that causes excessive head shaking, scratching, and purulent malodorous aural discharge.

Immediate action/treatment

Clean the ear canal with an irrigating solution such as Epiotic and wipe it clean of debris. Perform a complete aural examination to determine whether a foreign body or tumor is present and whether the tympanic membrane is intact. Heat-fix any discharge and examine it cytologically for bacteria and fungal organisms. Following careful cleansing, instill a topical antibiotic-antifungal-steroid ointment.

Management

In severe cases in which the ear canal has scarred and closed down with chronicity, consider administering systemically effective antibiotics (cephalexin, 22 mg/kg PO tid) and antifungal agents (ketoconazole, 10 mg/kg PO q12h) instead of topical therapy. Systemically effective steroids (prednisone or prednisolone, 0.5 mg/kg PO q12h) may be indicated in cases of severe inflammation to decrease pruritus and patient discomfort.

OTITIS INTERNA

Presentation of a patient with otitis interna often is characterized by torticollis, head tilt, nystagmus, circling to the affected side, or rolling. Fever, pain, vomiting, and severe depression may accompany clinical signs. Most cases of severe otitis interna are accompanied by severe otitis media. Both conditions must be treated simultaneously. The most common causes of otitis interna are *Staphylococcus aureus, Pseudomonas, Escherichia coli,* or *Proteus* spp. Otitis interna can develop by infection spreading across the tympanic membrane, through the eustachian tubes, or by hematogenous spread from the blood supply to the middle ear. In most cases of otitis media, the tympanic membrane is ruptured.

Immediate action

Perform a culture and susceptibility test of the debris behind the tympanic membrane and within the aural canal. Carefully clean the external ear canal. Medicate with a topical combination antibiotic, antifungal, and antibiotic ointment. Administer high-dose antibiotics (cephalexin, 22 mg/kg PO q8h, or enrofloxacin, 10 to 20 mg/kg PO q24h).

Management

If the tympanic membrane is not ruptured but appears swollen and erythematous, a myringotomy may need to be performed. If clinical signs of otitis media persist despite topical and systemic therapy, radiographic or CT/MRI examination of the tympanic bullae may be required.

AURAL HEMATOMA

Chronic shaking of the head and ears or aural trauma (bite wounds) causes disruption of the blood vessels and leads to the development of unilateral or bilateral aural hematomas.

Aural hematomas are clinically significant because they cause patient discomfort and are often due to the presence of some other underlying problem such as otitis externa, atopy, or aural foreign bodies. Acute swelling of the external ear pinna with fluid is characteristic of an aural hematoma. In some cases, swelling can be so severe that the hematoma breaks open, bathing the patient and external living environment in blood.

Immediate action

When a patient has an aural hematoma, investigate the underlying cause. Perform a complete aural examination to determine whether an aural foreign body, otitis externa, or atopy are present. Carefully examine and gently clean the inner ear canal. Treat underlying causes.

Management

Management of an aural hematoma involves draining the hemorrhagic fluid from the aural tissue and tacking the skin down in multiple places to prevent reaccumulation of fluid until the secondary cause is resolved. Many techniques have been described to surgically tack down the skin overlying the hematoma. After the animal has been placed under general anesthesia, lance the hematoma down the middle with a scalpel blade and remove the fluid and blood clot. Tack down the skin with multiple through-and-through interrupted or mattress sutures through the ear. Some clinicians prefer to suture through and attach a sponge or length of x-ray film to the front and back of the ear for stabilization and support. More recently, a laser can be used to drill holes in the hematoma and tack the skin down in multiple areas. Compress the ear against the head with a compression bandage, whenever possible, for 5 to 7 days after the initial surgery, and then recheck the ear. The patient must wear an Elizabethan collar until the surgical wound and hematoma heal to prevent self-mutilation. Also systemically treat underlying causative factors such as otitis externa with antibiotics, antifungals, and steroids as indicated. Investigate and treat other underlying causes such as hypothyroidism or allergies.

Additional Reading

Bass M: Symposium on otitis externa in dogs, *Vet Med* 99(3):252, 2004.

Dye TL, Teague HD, Ostwald DO, et al: Evaluation of a technique using the carbon dioxide laser for the treatment of aural hematomas, *J Am Anim Hosp Assoc* 38(4):385-390, 2002.

Gotthelf LN: Diagnosis and treatment of otitis media in dogs and cats, *Vet Clin North Am Small Anim* 34(2):469-487, 2004.

Lanz OI, Wood BC: Surgery of the ear and pinna, *Vet Clin North Am Small Anim Pract* 34(2): 567-599, 2004.

Murphy KM: A review of the techniques for the investigation of otitis externa and otitis media in dogs and cats, *Clin Tech Small Anim Pract* 16(4):236-241, 2001.

ELECTROCUTION/ELECTRIC SHOCK

Electrocution usually is observed in young animals after they have chewed on an electric cord. Other causes of electrocution include use of defective electrical equipment or being struck by lightning. Electric current passing through the body can produce severe dysrhythmias, including supraventricular or ventricular tachycardia and first- and third-degree atrioventricular block. The electric current also can produce tissue destruction from heat and electrothermal burns. Electrocution also commonly results in noncardiogenic pulmonary edema caused by massive catecholamine release and increase in pulmonary vascular pressures during the event. Ventricular fibrillation can occur, although that depends on the intensity and path of the electrical current and duration of contact.

Clinical signs of electrocution include acute onset of respiratory distress with moist rales, and localized necrosis or thermal burns of the lips and tongue. Often the skin at the commissures of the mouth appears white or yellow and firm to the touch. Muscle fasciculations, loss of consciousness, and ventricular fibrillation may occur. Thoracic radiographs often reveal an increased interstitial to alveolar lung pattern in the dorsocaudal lung fields.

Noncardiogenic pulmonary edema can develop up to 24 to 36 hours after the initial incident. The first 24 hours are most critical for the patient, and then prognosis improves.

The most important aspect in the treatment of the patient with noncardiogenic
pulmonary edema is to minimize stress and to provide supplemental oxygen, with positive
pressure ventilation, when necessary. Although treatment with vasodilators (low-dose
morphine) and diuretics (furosemide) can be attempted, noncardiogenic pulmonary
edema is typically resistant to vasodilator and diuretic therapy. Positive inotropes and pressor drugs may be necessary to treat shock and hypotension. Opioid drugs (morphine,
hydromorphone, oxymorphone) may be useful in controlling anxiety until the pulmonary
edema resolves. Administer broad-spectrum antibiotics (cefazolin; amoxicillin and clavulanic acid [Clavamox]) to treat thermal burns. Use analgesic drugs to control patient
discomfort. If thermal burns are extensive and prohibit adequate food intake, place a feeding tube as soon as the patient's cardiovascular and respiratory function are stable and the
patient can tolerate anesthesia.

EMERGENCIES OF THE FEMALE REPRODUCTIVE TRACT AND GENITALIA

UTERINE PROLAPSE

Prolapse of the uterus occurs in the immediate postparturient period in the bitch and
queen. Excessive straining during or after parturition causes the uterus to prolapse caudally
through the vagina and vulva. Immediate intervention is necessary. Examine the bitch or
queen for a retained fetus. Treatment consists of general anesthesia to replace the prolapsed
tissue. If the uterus is edematous, physical replacement may be difficult or impossible.
Application of a hypertonic solution such as hypertonic (7%) saline or dextrose (50%)
to the exposed endometrium can help shrink the tissue. That, combined with gentle
massage to stimulate uterine contraction and involution and lubrication with sterile lubricating jelly, can aid in replacement of the organ into its proper place. To ensure proper
placement in the abdominal cavity and to prevent recurrence, perform an exploratory
laparotomy and hysteropexy. Postoperatively, administer oxytocin (5 to 20 units IM) to
cause uterine contraction. If the uterus contracts, it is usually not necessary to suture the
vulva. Administer antibiotics postoperatively. Recurrence is uncommon, even with subsequent pregnancies.

If the tissue is damaged or too edematous to replace or if the tissue is devitalized, traumatized or necrotic, perform an ovariohysterectomy. In some instances, replacement of the
damaged tissue is not necessary before removal.

PYOMETRA

Pyometra occurs in dogs and cats. The disease process occurs as a result of infection overlying cystic endometrial hyperplasia under the constant influence of progesterone. During
the 2-month luteal phase after estrus or following copulation, artificial insemination, or
administration of hormones (particularly estradiol or progesterone), the myometrium
becomes relaxed and favors a quiescent environment for bacterial proliferation.

Clinical signs of pyometra are associated with the presence of bacterial endotoxin and
sepsis. Early, affected animals become lethargic and anorectic. Polyuria with secondary
polydipsia is often present because of the influence of bacterial endotoxin on renal tubular
concentration. If the cervix is open, purulent or mucoid vaginal discharge may be observed.
Later in the course of pyometra, vomiting, diarrhea, and progressive debilitation resulting
from sepsis occur. Diagnosis is based on clinical signs in an intact queen or bitch and radiographic or ultrasonographic evidence of a fluid-filled tubular density in the ventrocaudal
abdomen, adjacent to the urinary bladder (Figures 1-40 and 1-41).

Treatment of open and closed pyometra is correction of fluid and electrolyte abnormalities, administration of broad-spectrum antibiotics, and ovariohysterectomy. Close pyometra is a life-threatening septic condition. Open pyometra also can become life-threatening
and so should be treated aggressively. In closed pyometra, conservative medical therapy is
not advised. Administration of prostaglandins and oxytocin do not reliably cause the cervix

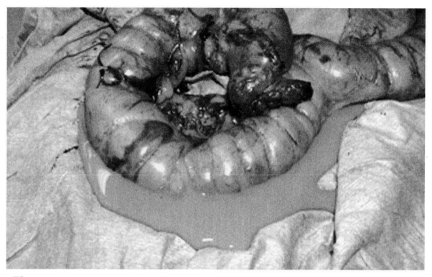

Figure 1-40:   An example of a large pus-filled uterus after emergency ovariohysterectomy.

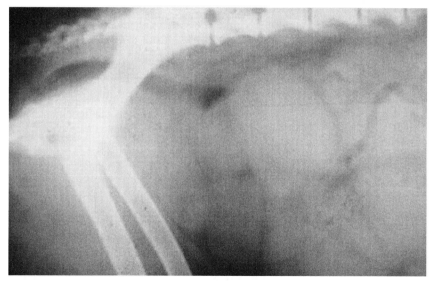

Figure 1-41:   Abdominal radiograph of a pyometra. Note the fluid-filled soft tissue density in the caudal abdomen.

to open and can result in ascending infection from the uterus into the abdomen or uterine rupture, both of which can result in severe peritonitis.

For animals with an open pyometra, ovariohysterectomy is the most reliable treatment for chronic cystic endometrial hyperplasia. Although less successful than ovariohysterectomy, medical therapy may be attempted in breeding bitches as an alternative to surgery. The most widely used medical therapy in the breeding queen and bitch is administration of prostaglandin $F_{2\alpha}$. This drug has not been approved for use in the queen or bitch in the United States. To proceed with medical management of pyometra, first determine the size of the uterus. Start the patient on antibiotic therapy (ampicillin, 22 mg/kg IV q6h, or enrofloxacin, 10 mg/kg PO q24h). Administer the prostaglandin $F_{2\alpha}$ (250 µg/kg SQ q24h) for 2 to 7 days until the size of the uterus approaches normal. Measure serum progesterone concentrations if the bitch is in diestrus. As the corpus luteum degrades under the influence of prostaglandin $F_{2\alpha}$, serum progesterone levels will decline.

Prostaglandin $F_{2\alpha}$ is an abortifacient and thus should not be administered to the pregnant bitch or queen. Clinical signs of a reaction to prostaglandin $F_{2\alpha}$ can occur within 5 to 60 minutes in the bitch and can last for as long as 20 minutes. Clinical signs of a reaction include restlessness, hypersalivation, panting, vomiting, defecation, abdominal pain, fever, and vocalization. In a very ill animal, death can occur. The efficacy of prostaglandin $F_{2\alpha}$ is limited and may require more than one treatment. The bitch should be bred on the next heat cycle and then spayed because progressive cystic endometrial hyperplasia will continue to occur.

ACUTE METRITIS

Acute metritis is an acute bacterial infection of the uterus that typically occurs within 1 to 2 weeks after parturition. The most common organism observed in metritis is *E. coli* ascending from the vulva and vaginal vault. Sepsis can progress rapidly. Clinical signs of acute metritis include inability to nurse puppies, anorexia, lethargy, foul-smelling purulent-sanguineous vaginal discharge, vomiting, or acute collapse.

Physical examination may reveal fever, dehydration, and a turgid distended uterus. Septic inflammation will be observed on vaginal cytologic examination. An enlarged uterus can be observed with abdominal radiographs and ultrasonography.

Treatment of acute metritis is directed at restoring hydration status with intravenous fluids and treating the infection with antibiotics. Because the primary cause of metritis is *E. coli* infection, start enrofloxacin (10 mg/kg IV or PO once daily) therapy. As soon as the patient's cardiovascular status is stable enough for anesthesia, perform an ovariohysterectomy. If the patient is not critical and is a valuable breeding bitch, medical therapy can be attempted. Medical management of acute bacterial metritis includes administration of oxytocin (5 to 10 units q3h for three treatments) or administration of prostaglandin $F_{2\alpha}$ (250 µg/kg/day for 2 to 5 days) to evacuate the uterine exudate and increase uterine blood flow. Either drug should be used concurrently with antibiotics.

UTERINE RUPTURE

Rupture of the gravid uterus is rare in cats and dogs but has been reported. Uterine rupture may occur as a consequence of parturition or result from blunt abdominal trauma. Feti expelled into the abdominal cavity may be resorbed but more commonly cause the development of peritonitis. If fetal circulation is not disrupted, the fetus actually may live to term. Uterine rupture is an acute surgical emergency. An ovariohysterectomy with removal of the extrauterine puppies and membranes is recommended. If only one horn of the uterus is affected, a unilateral ovariohysterectomy can be performed to salvage the remaining unaffected puppies and preserve the breeding potential for the valuable bitch. If uterine rupture occurs because of pyometra, peritonitis is likely, and copious peritoneal lavage should be performed at the time of surgery. The patient should be placed on 7 to 14 days of antibiotic therapy (amoxicillin or amoxicillin and clavulanic acid [Clavamox] with enrofloxacin).

VAGINAL PROLAPSE

Vaginal prolapse occurs from excessive proliferation and hyperplasia of vaginal tissue while under the influence of estrogen during proestrus (Figure 1-42). The hyperplastic tissue usually recedes during diestrus but reappears with subsequent heat cycles. Vaginal prolapse can be confused with vaginal neoplasia. The former condition occurs primarily in younger animals, whereas the latter condition occurs primarily in older animals. Treatment for vaginal hyperplasia or prolapse generally is not required if the tissue remains within the vagina. The proliferation can lead to dysuria or anuria, however. In some cases, the tissue becomes

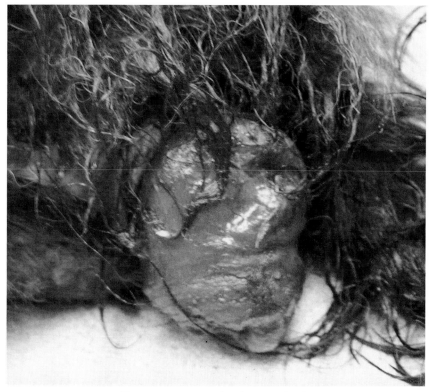

Figure 1-42:   Vaginal prolapse in a bitch.

dried out and devitalized or becomes traumatized by the animal. Such extreme cases warrant immediate surgical intervention. The treatment for vaginal prolapse consists of ovariohysterectomy to remove the influence of estrogen, placement of an indwelling urinary catheter if the patient is dysuric, and protection of the hyperplastic tissue until it recedes on its own. Although surgical resection of the hyperplastic tissue has been recommended, excessive hemorrhage after removal can occur, and so the procedure should not be attempted. The patient should wear an Elizabethan collar at all times to prevent self-mutilation. Administer broad-spectrum antibiotics for a minimum of 7 to 14 days or until the hyperplastic tissue recedes. Keep the tissue clean with saline solution.

EMERGENCIES OF PREGNANCY AND PARTURITION

Dystocia

Dystocia, or difficult birth, can occur in the dog and cat but is more common in the dog. A diagnosis of dystocia is made based on the time of onset of visible labor and the time in which the last puppy or no puppy has been born, the intensity and timing of contractions, the timing of when the amniotic membranes first appear, the condition of the bitch, and the timing of gestation. Causes of dystocia can be maternal or fetal and include primary or secondary uterine inertia, narrowing of the pelvic canal, hypocalcemia, psychological disturbances, or uterine torsion. Maternal-fetal disproportion, or large fetus size in relation to the bitch or queen, also can result in dystocia (Box 1-40).

Obtain an abdominal radiograph for all cases of suspected dystocia at the time of presentation to determine the size of the fetus, presentation of the fetus (Both anterior or posterior presentation can be normal in the bitch or queen, but fetal malpositioning can

1

BOX 1-40   DIAGNOSTIC CRITERIA FOR DYSTOCIA

- Fetus lodged in birth canal
- Presence of vaginal stricture or band of tissue preventing normal delivery
- Prolonged gestation (>70 days)
- Drop in rectal temperature (<100° F) with no evidence of labor
- Green vaginal discharge and no evidence of delivery of fetus
- No puppies delivered after 2 to 3 hours of a visible amniotic sac
- Strong contractions with no puppy or kitten delivered after 30 minutes
- Weak, infrequent contractions with no puppy delivered in 4 hours from onset of labor
- More than 2 hours have passed with no evidence of further contraction or delivery of a puppy
- Signs of systemic illness or pain: depression, weakness, sepsis

---

cause dystocia), and whether there is radiographic evidence of a uterine rupture or torsion. If maternal-fetal disproportion, uterine torsion, or uterine rupture is observed, take the patient immediately to surgery. If the puppies or kittens are in a normal position for birth, medical management can be attempted.

Clip the perineum and aseptically scrub it. Wearing sterile gloves, insert a lubricated finger into the vagina and palpate the cervix. Massage (or "feather") the dorsal wall of the vagina to stimulate contractions. Place an intravenous catheter, and administer oxytocin (2 to 20 units IM), repeating up to 3 times at 30-minute intervals. In some cases, hypoglycemia or hypocalcemia can contribute to uterine inertia. Administration of a calcium-containing solution (lactated Ringer's solution) with 2.5% dextrose is advised. Alternately, administer 10% calcium gluconate (100 mg/5 kg IV slowly). If labor has not progressed after 1 hour, immediately perform a cesarean section.

Uterine torsion

Uterine torsion is an uncommon emergency seen in the gravid and nongravid uterus and has been reported in dogs and cats. The onset of clinical signs of abdominal pain and straining as if to whelp/queen or defecate is usually acute and constitutes a surgical emergency. In some cases, there may have been a history of delivery of a live or dead fetus. Vaginal discharge may or may not be present. Radiographs or ultrasound examination reveal a fluid-filled or air-filled tubular density in the ventral abdomen. Treatment consists of placing an intravenous catheter, stabilizing the patient's cardiovascular status with intravenous fluids and sometimes blood products, and performing an immediate ovariohysterectomy. If there are viable feti, the uterus should be delivered *en mass* and the puppies or kittens delivered.

Spontaneous abortion

The expulsion of one or more fetus before term is known as spontaneous abortion. In dogs and cats, it is possible to expel or abort one or more fetuses and still carry viable fetuses to term and deliver normally. Clinical signs of spontaneous abortion include vaginal discharge and abdominal contractions. In some cases, the fetus is found, or there may be evidence of fetal membranes or remnants. Causes of spontaneous abortion in dogs include *Brucella canis,* herpesvirus, coronavirus, and toxoplasmosis. In cats, herpesvirus, coronavirus, and feline leukemia virus can cause spontaneous abortion. In both species, trauma, hormonal factors, environmental pathogens, drugs, and fetal factors also can result in spontaneous abortion.

Pregnancy termination in the bitch and queen

The safest method of pregnancy termination in the bitch or queen is by performing an ovariohysterectomy. Oral diethylstilbesterol is not an effective mechanism of pregnancy termination in the bitch. A so-called mismating shot, an injection of estradiol cypionate (0.02 mg/lb IM) is effective at causing termination of an early pregnancy but can be associated with severe side effects, including bone marrow suppression and pyometra. Estradiol cypionate is not approved for use in the bitch or queen and is not recommended.

Prostaglandin $F_{2\alpha}$ is a natural abortifacient in the bitch if treatment is started within 5 days of cytologic evidence of diestrus (noncornified epithelium on a vaginal smear). The prostaglandin $F_{2\alpha}$ causes lysis of the corpora lutea and a rapid decline in progesterone concentration. The prostaglandin $F_{2\alpha}$ is administered for a total of eight injections (250 µg/kg q12h for 4 days), along with atropine (100 to 500 µg/kg SQ). Side effects can occur within 5 to 40 minutes of injection and include restlessness, panting, salivation, abdominal pain, urination, vomiting, and diarrhea. Walking the patient for 20 to 30 minutes after each treatment sometimes decreases the intensity of the reactions.

Bitches in the first half of the pregnancy often resorb the embryos. If prostaglandin $F_{2\alpha}$ is administered in the second half of the pregnancy, the fetuses are aborted within 5 to 7 days of treatment. Measure serum progesterone concentrations at the end of treatment to ensure complete lysis of the corpus luteum. Prostaglandin $F_{2\alpha}$ is not approved for pregnancy termination in the bitch.

In cats, prostaglandin $F_{2\alpha}$ can terminate pregnancy after day 4 of gestation. Prostaglandin $F_{2\alpha}$ should be used only in healthy queens (100 to 250 µg/kg SQ q24h for 2 days). Side effects in the queen are similar to those observed in the bitch but typically have a shorter duration (2 to 20 minutes). Prostaglandin $F_{2\alpha}$ is not approved for use in cats in the United States. The use of prostaglandin $F_{2\alpha}$ does not preclude breeding and pregnancy at a later date.

Additional Reading

Biddle D, Macintire DK: Obstetrical emergencies, *Clin Tech Small Anim Pract* 15(2):88-93, 2000.

Drobatz KJ, Mandell DC, Neath P: Urinary bladder herniation thru a vaginal tear in a Rottweiler with dystocia, *J Vet Emerg Crit Care* 10(3):173-175, 2000.

Greenberg D, Yates D: What is your diagnosis? Vaginal hyperplasia, *J Small Anim Pract* 43(9):381, 406, 2002.

Hayes G: Asymptomatic uterine rupture in a bitch, *Vet Rec* 154(14):438-439, 2004.

Jutkowitz LA: Reproductive emergencies, *Vet Clin North Am Small Anim* 35:397-420, 2005.

Lucas X, Agut A, Ramis G, et al: Uterine rupture in a cat, *Vet Rec* 152(10):301-302, 2003.

Misumi K, Fujiki M, Miura N, et al: Uterine torsion in two non-gravid bitches, *J Small Anim Pract* 41(10):468-471, 2000.

Ridyard AE, Welsh EA, Gunn-Moore DA: Successful treatment of uterine torsion in a cat with severe metabolic and haemostatic complications, *J Feline Med Surg* 2(2):115-119, 2000.

EMERGENCIES OF THE MALE GENITALIA AND REPRODUCTIVE TRACT

Figure 1-43 illustrates conditions of the male genitalia and reproductive tract that require emergent care.

SCROTAL TRAUMA

In the dog and cat the majority of injuries to the scrotum are associated with animal fights or shearing and abrasive injuries sustained in accidents involving automobiles. Scrotal injuries should be categorized as superficial or penetrating.

Treatment of superficial injuries to the scrotum includes cleaning the wound with dilute antimicrobial cleanser and drying it. Administer antiinflammatory doses of steroids (prednisolone, 0.5 to 1.0 mg/kg PO q12-24h) or NSAIDs (carprofen, 2.2 mg/kg PO q12h in dogs) for the first several days after scrotal injury to prevent or treat edema. Administer topical antibiotic ointment until the wound heals. In most cases, place an Elizabethan collar to prevent self-mutilation. Prognosis is generally favorable; however, semen quality may be affected for months after injury because of scrotal swelling and increased scrotal temperature.

Penetrating injuries to the scrotum are more serious and are associated with severe swelling and infection. Surgically explore and debride penetrating scrotal wounds. Administer systemically effective antibiotics and analgesics. In extreme cases, particularly those that involve the testicle, consider castration and scrotal ablation.

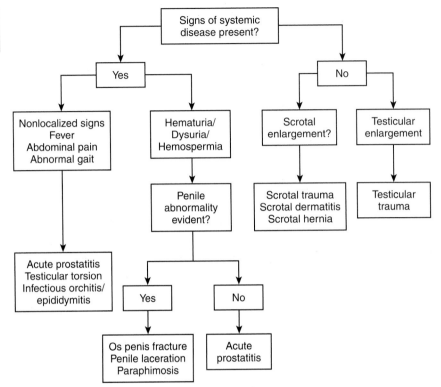

Figure 1-43:   Emergencies of the male genitalia and reproductive tract.

ACUTE SCROTAL DERMATITIS

Scrotal dermatitis is common in intact male dogs and can be associated with direct physical injury, self-infliction from licking, chemical irritation, burns, or contact dermatitis. In affected animals, the scrotum can become extremely inflamed, swollen, and painful. If left untreated, pyogranulomatous dermatitis can develop.

Make an attempt to determine whether an underlying systemic illness is present that could predispose the animal to scrotal dermatitis. Widespread vasculitis with scrotal edema, pain, fever, and dermatitis has been associated with *Rickettsia rickettsii* (Rocky Mountain spotted fever) infection. *Brucella canis* also has been associated with scrotal irritation and dermatitis. If scrotal dermatitis follows from an infectious cause, empiric use of glucocorticosteroids potentially can make the condition worse by suppressing immune function. Empiric treatment with antibiotics also potentially can confound making an accurate diagnosis.

Treatment of scrotal dermatitis is to eliminate predisposing causes, if possible. Place an Elizabethan collar at all times to prevent self-mutilation. Bathe the scrotum with a mild antimicrobial soap and dry it to remove any offending chemical irritants. Topical medications including tar shampoo, tetracaine, neomycin, and petroleum can cause further irritation and are contraindicated. Use oral or parenteral administration of glucocorticosteroids or NSAIDs to control discomfort and inflammation.

SCROTAL HERNIA

Scrotal hernias occur when the contents of the abdomen (intestines, fat, mesentery, omentum) protrude through the inguinal ring into the scrotal sac. Like inguinal hernias, scrotal hernias are surgical emergencies only if intestinal incarceration or vascular obstruction occurs. Differential diagnoses for scrotal hernias include epididymitis, orchitis, testicular torsion, and testicular neoplasia.

Definitive therapy for a scrotal hernia involves exploratory laparotomy and surgical reduction of the contents of the hernia, surgical correction of the rent in the inguinal ring, and castration.

TESTICULAR TRAUMA

Trauma to the epididymis or testicle can cause testicular pain and swelling of one or both testes. Treat penetrating trauma to the testicle by castration to prevent infection and self-mutilation. Administer oral antibiotics (amoxicillin or amoxicillin-clavulanate) for 7 to 10 days after the injury. Nonpenetrating injuries to the scrotum and testicle rarely may cause acute testicular hemorrhage or hydrocele formation. Palpation of the affected area often reveals a peritesticular, soft, compliant area. Treatment consists of cool compresses on the scrotum and testicle and administration of antiinflammatory doses of glucocorticosteroids or NSAIDs. If the swelling does not resolve spontaneously in 5 to 7 days, consider surgical exploration and drainage. Increased scrotal temperature and testicular inflammation can affect semen quality for months after the initial incident.

TESTICULAR TORSION

Testicular torsion, or torsion of the spermatic cord, causes rotation of the testicle, ultimately causing obstruction to venous drainage. Testicular torsion often is associated with a neoplastic mass of a retained testicle within the abdomen but also can be observed with nonneoplastic testes located within the scrotum. The predominant clinical signs are pain, stiff stilted gait, and the presence of an abnormally swollen testicle (if located within the scrotum). If an intraabdominal testicular torsion is present, pain, lethargy, anorexia, and vomiting can occur (see Acute Condition in the Abdomen). An intraabdominal mass may be palpable. Perform an abdominal or testicular ultrasound, preferably with color flow Doppler to evaluate perfusion to the testicle. Treatment involves surgical removal of the involved testes.

INFECTIOUS ORCHITIS AND EPIDIDYMITIS

Bacterial infections of the testicle or epididymis most commonly are caused by ascending infections of the normal bacterial flora of the prepuce or urethra. Common inhabitants include *Escherichia coli, Staphylococcus aureus, Streptococcus* spp., and *Mycobacterium canis. Brucella canis* and *R. rickettsii* are also capable of causing orchitis and epididymitis in the dog. Clinical signs of orchitis or epididymitis include testicular enlargement, stiff stilted gait, and reluctance to walk. Physical examination often reveals a fever and self-induced trauma to the scrotum from licking or chewing at the inflamed area. Collect a semen sample by ejaculation, and culture it to identify the causative organism. Alternately, collect samples by needle aspiration of the affected organ(s) and test serologically for *B. canis*.

Treatment of infectious orchitis involves a minimum of 3 to 4 weeks of specific anti-microbial therapy, based on culture and susceptibility testing, whenever possible. If a bacterial culture cannot be obtained, initiate fluoroquinolone therapy (enrofloxacin, 10 mg/kg PO q24h). Doxycycline (5 mg/kg PO bid for 7 days) has been shown to suppress but not eradicate *B. canis* infection. Testicular inflammation and increased temperature can affect sperm quality for months after infection.

ACUTE PROSTATITIS

The most common causes of acute prostatitis are associated with acute bacterial infection (*E. coli, Proteus* spp., *Pseudomonas* spp., and *Mycoplasma* spp.). Less common causes include fungal infection *(Blastomyces dermatitidis)* or anaerobic bacterial infection.

Acute prostatitis is characterized by fever, caudal abdominal pain, lethargy, anorexia, blood in the ejaculate, hematuria, dyschezia, and occasionally stranguria or dysuria. The patient often appears painful and depressed and may be dehydrated on physical examination.

Symmetric or asymmetric prostatomegaly and prostate pain may be evident on rectal palpation. In severely affected dogs, clinical signs of tachycardia, hyperemic or injected mucous membranes, bounding pulses, lethargy, dehydration, and fever may be present because of sepsis. Death can occur within 2 days if a prostatic abscess ruptures.

Diagnosis of acute prostatitis is confirmed based on the presenting clinical signs, neutrophilic leukocytosis (with or without a left shift), and positive urine culture results. Prostatic samples may be obtained from the prostatic portion of the ejaculate, prostatic massage, urethral discharge, urine, or (less commonly) prostatic aspirate. Although semen samples can yield positive bacterial cultures, dogs with acute prostatitis are often unwilling to ejaculate. Radiography may reveal an enlarged prostate, but this alone does not confirm the diagnosis of prostatitis. An abdominal ultrasound often reveals prostatic abscessation and allows for the collection of samples from the affected area(s) via prostatic aspirate. Aspiration of the affected tissue potentially can wick infection into periprostatic tracks. Cytologic examination of the patient's ejaculate or prostatic wash from a dog with acute prostatitis reveals numerous inflammatory cells and may contain bacterial organisms.

The treatment of a patient with acute prostatitis is directed at correcting dysuria and constipation associated with prostatic enlargement. Enrofloxaxin (10 mg/kg PO sid) can penetrate the inflamed prostatic tissue and is effective in treating gram-negative and *Mycoplasma* spp. infections. Ciprofloxacin does not appear to penetrate prostatic tissue as readily. Alternatives to enrofloxacin therapy are trimethoprim-sulfamethoxazole (30 mg/kg PO q12h) or chloramphenicol (25-50 mg/kg PO q8h) for a minimum of 2 to 3 weeks. Castration is recommended because benign prostatic hyperplasia may be a predisposing factor in the development of acute prostatitis. Do not perform castration until the patient has been on antibiotic therapy for a minimum of 7 days, to prevent the surgical complication of schirrous cords. Finasteride (Proscar, 1 mg/kg PO q24h), an antiandrogen 5α-reductase inhibitor, may help reduce the size of prostatic tissue until the effects of castration are observed. If a prostatic abscess is present, perform marsupialization, surgical drainage, or ultrasonographic drainage. Surgical therapy is associated with a large incidence of complications, including incontinence, chronic drainage from fistulas and stomas, septic shock, and death.

Os Penis Fracture

Fracture of the os penis is an uncommon condition encountered in male dogs. Os penis fractures can occur with minimal soft tissue damage but cause hematuria and dysuria. On physical examination, urethral obstruction and crepitus in the penis are found. A lateral abdominal radiograph is usually sufficient to document the fracture. Treatment consists of conservative therapy, in most cases, and consists primarily of analgesia administration. If the urethra also is damaged, place a urethral catheter for 5 to 7 days to allow the urethral mucosa to heal. Fractures of the os penis that are comminuted or severe enough to cause urethral obstruction require open reduction and fixation, partial penile amputation, or antescrotal (prescrotal) urethrostomy.

Laceration

Lacerations of the penis cause significant bleeding because of the extensive vascular supply to the penis. Dogs and cats tend to lick penile lacerations and prevent adequate clot formation. Sedation or general anesthesia often is required to evaluate and treat the laceration. After sedation or general anesthesia, place a urinary catheter and examine the penis under a stream of cold water. Small lacerations can be managed with cold compresses and one to several absorbable sutures. Extensive suturing usually is not required. Prevent erection by isolating the patient from females in estrus or allowing excitement or excessive activity. Place an Elizabethan collar to prevent self-mutilation. Initiate systemic antibiotic therapy to prevent infection.

Paraphimosis

The inability to withdraw the penis into the prepuce in male dogs or cats is known as paraphimosis. Paraphimosis usually develops following an erection in young male dogs and in older dogs after coitus. Mucosal edema, hemorrhage, self-mutilation, and necrosis requir-ing penile amputation can occur if left untreated. Treatment consists of applying cold water to the penis and reducing edema with application of an osmotic substance such as sugar. Examine the base of the penis for hair rings that can prevent retraction of the penis into the prepuce. Rinse the penis carefully with cold water and lubricate it with sterile lubricant and replace it into the prepuce. If the penis cannot be reduced easily into the prepuce, anes-thetize the patient and make a small incision at the lateral aspect of the preputial opening. Replace the penis and close the incision with absorbable suture. Place a purse-string suture and leave it in place for several days to prevent recurrence. Instill topical antimicrobial oint-ment with steroids into the prepuce several times a day. In severe cases, a urinary catheter may need to be placed to prevent urethral obstruction, until penile swelling and edema resolve. Place an Elizabethan collar to prevent excessive licking during the healing process.

URETHRAL PROLAPSE

Prolapse of the distal urethra is a condition usually confined to intact male English Bulldogs, although isolated incidences also have been reported in Yorkshire and Boston Terriers. The exact cause of this condition is unknown but usually is associated with a condition that causes increased intraabdominal pressure or urethral straining, including sexual excitement, coughing, vomiting, obstructed airway or brachycephalic airway syndrome, urethral calculi, genitourinary tract infection, and masturbation.

The urethral prolapse usually appears as a mushroom-tip congested, irritated mass at the end of the penis that may or may not bleed (Figure 1-44). In some cases, bleeding occurs or worsens with sexual excitement. Clinical signs associated with the prolapsed

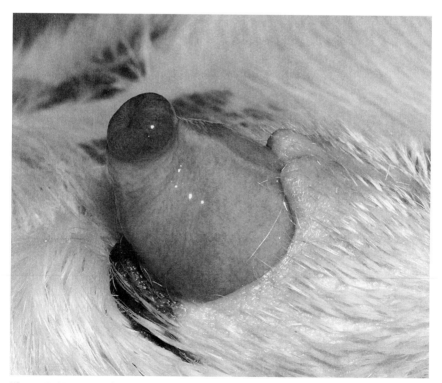

Figure 1-44: Example of urethral prolapse. This condition is most commonly observed in intact male Bulldogs, although it has been associated with neoplasia and urethral calculi in other breeds.

urethra include excessive licking of the prepuce, stranguria, and preputial bleeding. Once the mass is observed, other differential diagnoses include transmissible venereal tumor, urethral polyp, trauma, urethritis, and neoplasia. In most cases, however, the prolapse occurs in intact young dogs, making neoplastic conditions less likely.

Treatment for urethral prolapse should occur at the time of diagnosis to prevent self-induced trauma and infection. Immediate therapy includes manual reduction of the prolapsed tissue and placement of a purse-string suture around an indwelling urinary catheter. The purse-string suture can remain in place for up to 5 days until definitive repair. Until the time of surgery, place an Elizabethan collar on the patient to prevent self-mutilation. Several forms of surgical correction have been described. In some cases, surgical resection of the prolapsed tissue with apposition of the urethral and penile mucosa can be attempted. More recently, a technique involving placement of several mattress sutures to reduce and secure the prolapsed tissue has been described. Recurrence of prolapse can occur with either technique, particularly if the inciting event recurs. Because there may be a genetic predisposition in this breed and because the prolapse can recur with sexual excitement, neutering should strongly be recommended.

Additional Reading

Boland LE, Hardie RJ, Gregory SP, et al: Ultrasound-guided percutaneous drainage as the primary treatment for prostatic abscesses and cysts in dogs, *J Am Anim Hosp Assoc* 39(2): 151-159, 2003.

Gobello C, Corrada Y: Noninfectious prostatic diseases in dogs, *Compend Contin Educ Pract Vet* 24(2):99-107, 2002.

Hecht S, King R, Tidwell AS, et al: Ultrasound diagnosis: intraabdominal torsion of a non-neoplastic testicle in a cryptorchid dog, *Vet Radiol Ultrasound* 45(1):58-61, 2004.

Kirsch JA, Hauptman JG, Walshaw R: A urethropexy technique for surgical treatment of urethral prolapse in the male dog, *J Am Anim Hosp Assoc* 38:381-384, 2002.

Kutzler MA, Yeager A: Prostatic diseases. In Ettinger S, Feldman EC, editors: *Textbook of veterinary internal medicine*, ed 6, Philadelphia, 2005, WB Saunders.

L'Abee-Lung TM, Heiene R, Friis NF, et al: *Mycoplasma canis* and urogenital disease in dogs in Norway, *Vet Rec* 153(8):231-235, 2003.

Ober CP, Spaulding K, Breitschwerdt EB, et al: Orchitis in two dogs with Rocky Mountain spotted fever, *Vet Radiol Ultrasound* 45(5);458-465, 2004.

ENVIRONMENTAL AND HOUSEHOLD EMERGENCIES

FROSTBITE

Local freezing or frostbite most commonly affects the peripheral tissues of the ears, tail, paws, and genitalia that are sparsely covered with fur, are poorly vascularized, and may have been traumatized previously by cold. Clinical signs of frostbite are paleness and appearance of a blanched pink to white discoloration to the skin. The skin also may appear black and necrotic.

Immediate action

Immediate treatment consists of slowly rewarming the affected area with moist heat at 29.5° C (85° F) or by immersion in warm water baths. Analgesics may be required to alleviate patient discomfort. Carefully dry the injured areas and protect them from further trauma.

Management

The use of prophylactic antibiotics is controversial because it can promote resistant bacterial infection. Use of antibiotics should be based on the presence of infection. Treatments that are ineffective and may be harmful include rubbing the affected areas, pressure bandages, and ointments. Corticosteroids can decrease cellular immunity and promote infection and are therefore contraindicated. Many frostbitten areas that appear nonviable can regain function gradually. Use care when removing areas of necrotic tissue. Affected areas may take several days to a week before fully manifesting areas of demarcation between healthy viable and necrotic nonviable tissue.

HYPOTHERMIA

Chilling of the entire body from exposure or immersion in extremely cold water results in a decrease in core body temperature and physiologic processes that become irreversible when the body temperature falls below 24° C (75° F). Mild hypothermia can be 32° to 37° C, moderate hypothermia from 28° to 32° C, and severe hypothermia below 28° C. The duration of exposure and the general condition of the animal influences its ability to survive.

Clinical signs and consequences associated with hypothermia include shivering, vasoconstriction, mental depression, hypotension, sinus bradycardia, hypoventilation with decreased respiratory rate, increased blood viscosity, muscle stiffness, atrial and ventricular irritability, decreased level of consciousness, decreased oxygen consumption, metabolic (lactic) acidosis, respiratory acidosis, and coagulopathies including DIC.

Immediate action

If the animal is breathing, administer warm, humidified oxygen at 4 to 10 breaths per minute. If the animal is not breathing or is severely hypoventilating, endotracheal intubation with mechanical ventilation may be necessary. Place an intravenous catheter and infuse warmed crystalloid fluids. If the blood glucose is less than 60 mg/dL, add supplemental dextrose (2.5%) to the crystalloid fluids. Monitor the core body temperature and ECG closely. Rewarming should occur in the form of external circulating warm water blankets, radiant heat, and circulating warm air blankets (Bair Hugger). *Never* use a heating pad, to avoid iatrogenic thermal burn injury. Severe hypothermia may require core rewarming in the form of intraperitoneal fluids (10 to 20 mL/kg of lactated Ringer's solution warmed to 39.4° C [103° F]). Place a temporary peritoneal dialysis catheter, and repeat the dialysis every 30 minutes until the patient's body temperature reaches 36.6° to 37.7° C (98° to 100° F).

Management

The body temperature should rise slowly, ideally no more than 1° F per hour. Because the response of the body to drugs is unpredictable, avoid administering drugs whenever possible, until the body temperature returns to normal. Complications observed during rewarming include DIC, cardiac dysrhythmias including cardiac arrest, pneumonia, pulmonary edema, CNS edema, ARDS, and renal failure.

HYPERTHERMIA AND HEAT-INDUCED ILLNESS (HEAT STROKE)

Heat stroke and heat-induced illness in dogs can be associated with excessive exertion, exposure to high environmental temperatures, stress, and other factors that cause an inability to dissipate heat. Brachycephalic breeds, obesity, laryngeal paralysis, and older animals with cardiovascular disease can be particularly affected. Hyperthermia is defined as a rectal temperature of 41° to 43° C (105° to 110° F). Clinical signs of hyperthermia include congested hyperemic mucous membranes, tachycardia, and panting. More severe clinical signs include collapse (heat prostration), ataxia, vomiting, diarrhea, hypersalivation, muscle tremors, loss of consciousness, and seizures. Heat-induced illness can affect all major organ systems in the body because of denaturation of cellular proteins and enzyme activities, inappropriate shunting of blood, hypotension, decreased oxygen delivery, and lactic acidosis. Cardiac dysrhythmias, interstitial and intracellular dehydration, intravascular hypovolemia, central nervous dysfunction, slough of gastrointestinal mucosa, oliguria, and coagulopathies can be seen as organ function declines. Excessive panting can result in respiratory alkalosis. Poor tissue perfusion results in a metabolic acidosis. Loss of water in excess of solutes such as sodium and chloride can lead to a free water deficit and severe hypernatremia. A marked increase in PCV occurs because of the free water loss. Severe abnormalities in electrolytes and pH can lead to cerebral edema and death.

Immediate action

Treatment goals for the patient with heat-induced illness are to lower the core body temperature and support cardiovascular, respiratory, renal, gastrointestinal, neurologic, and hepatic functions. At the scene the veterinarian or caretaker can spray the animal with tepid (NOT COLD) water. Immersion in cold water or ice baths is absolutely contraindicated. Cold water and ice will cause extreme peripheral vasoconstriction, inhibiting the patient's ability to dissipate heat through conductive and convective cooling mechanisms. As a result, core body temperature will continue to rise despite the good intentions of well-doers at the scene. Animals that present to the veterinarian that have been cooled to the point of hypothermia have a worse prognosis. Once the animal has presented to the veterinarian, the goal is to cool the animal's body temperature with towels soaked in tepid water, cool intravenous fluids, and fans until the temperature has decreased to 103° F. Organ system monitoring and support is based on the severity and duration of the heat stroke and the ability of the body to compensate and respond to treatment.

Management

Management of the patient with heat-induced illness involves prompt aggressive cooling without being overzealous and creating iatrogenic hypothermia. Administer cool intravenous crystalloid fluids to replenish volume and interstitial hydration and correct the patient's acid-base and electrolyte abnormalities. Management consists of rule of twenty monitoring (See Rule of 20), taking care to evaluate, restore, and maintain a normal cardiac rhythm, blood pressure, urine output, and mentation. Administer antibiotics if there are any signs of gastrointestinal bleeding that will predispose the patient to bacterial translocation. Monitor baseline chemistry tests including a complete blood count, biochemical panel, platelet count, coagulation tests, and urinalysis. Treat coagulopathies including DIC aggressively and promptly (see also Disseminated Intravascular Coagulation). Severe changes in mentation including stupor or coma worsen a patient's prognosis. Following initial therapy, monitor the patient for a minimum of 24 to 48 hours for secondary organ damage, including renal failure, myoglobinuria, cerebral edema, and DIC. Dogs that are going to die of heat-induced illness usually die within the first 24 hours. Animals that survive longer than 24 hours have a more favorable prognosis.

Additional Reading

Ahn A: Approach to the hypothermic patient. In Bonagura JD, editor: *Current veterinary therapy XII. Small animal practice,* Philadelphia, 1995, WB Saunders.

Dhupa N: Hypothermia in dogs and cats, *Compend Contin Educ Pract Vet* 17:61, 1995.

Drobatz KJ, Macintire DK: Heat-induced illness in dogs: 42 cases (1976-1993), *J Am Vet Med Assoc* 209:1894, 1996.

Garcia-Lacaze M, Kirby R, Rudloff E: Peritoneal dialysis: not just for renal failure, *Compend Contin Educ Pract Vet* 24(10):758-771, 2002.

Hackett TB: Heat stroke. In Wingfield WE, editor: *Veterinary emergency medicine secrets,* ed 2, Philadelphia, 2001, Hanley & Belfus.

Oncken AK, Kirby R, Rudloff E: Hypothermia in critically ill dogs and cats, *Compend Contin Educ Pract Vet* 23(6):506-520, 2001.

Walton RS: Hypothermia. In Wingfield WE, editor: *Veterinary emergency medicine secrets,* ed 2, Philadelphia, 2001, Hanley & Belfus.

MALIGNANT HYPERTHERMIA

Malignant hyperthermia is a syndrome that involves impaired muscular calcium metabolism. Malignant hyperthermia has been recognized as a consequence of exertion in Labrador Retrievers and in sensitized animals placed under anesthesia. Clinical signs of malignant hyperthermia are severe muscle spasm or fasciculation, unstable blood pressure, metabolic or respiratory acidosis, and a rapidly increased end-tidal carbon dioxide under anesthesia. The patient's temperature often rises above 42° C. Cellular death can result if the malignant hyperthermia is not recognized and treated rapidly.

1

Immediate action/treatment

Immediate treatment consists of cooling the patient with cooling measures as for hyperthermia and heat-induced illness (see the previous discussion), and eliminating the cause (i.e., exertion, anesthesia, or neuromuscular blockers such as succinylcholine). If the patient is under general anesthesia, hyperventilate the patient to help eliminate carbon dioxide and respiratory acidosis. Administer dantrolene sodium (1 to 2 mg/kg IV) to stabilize the sarcoplasmic reticulum and decrease its permeability to calcium.

Management

Animals with malignant hyperthermia should avoid any predisposing factors, including exertion, hyperthermia, and anesthesia. After an episode of malignant hyperthermia, administer crystalloid fluids intravenously to aid in the elimination of myoglobin. Monitor renal function closely for myoglobinuria and pigment damage to the renal tubular epithelium. Monitor and correct acid-base and electrolyte changes.

Additional Reading

Walters JM: Hyperthermia. In Wingfield WE, editor: *The veterinary ICU book,* Jackson, Wyo, 2001, Teton Newmedia.

SNAKEBITE: NONPOISONOUS

Sometimes it is difficult to assess whether an animal has been bitten by a poisonous or nonpoisonous snake. In Colorado, the bull snake closely resembles the prairie rattlesnake. Both snakes make similar noise and can be alarming if noticed on a hike or in the backyard. Whenever possible, identify the offending reptile but NEVER RISK BEING BITTEN. Know what types of venomous creatures are in the geographic area of the practice.

If an animal has been bitten by a nonpoisonous snake, usually the bite marks are small with multiple small tooth punctures, and the bite is relatively nonpainful. Usually local reaction is negligible. However, large boas or pythons also can inflict large crushing injuries that can cause severe trauma, including bony fractures.

Treatment for a nonpoisonous snakebite involves clipping the bite wound and carefully cleaning the area with antimicrobial scrub solution. Broad-spectrum antibiotics (e.g., amoxicillin-clavulanate, 16.25 mg/kg PO q12h) are indicated because of the extensive bacterial flora in the mouths of snakes. Monitor all snakebite victims for a minimum of 8 hours after the incident, particularly when the species of the offending reptile is in question. If clinical signs of envenomation occur, modify the patient's treatment appropriately and aggressively.

SNAKEBITE: POISONOUS

The two major groups of venomous snakes in North America are the pit viper and the coral snake. All venomous snakes are dangerous. The severity of any given bite depends on the toxicity of the venom, the amount of venom injected, the site of envenomation, the size of the animal bitten, and the time from bite/envenomation to seeking appropriate medical intervention.

PIT VIPER ENVENOMATION

The majority of reptile envenomations in the United States are inflicted by pit vipers, including the water moccasin (cottonmouth), copperhead, and numerous species of rattlesnakes. Pit vipers are characterized by a deep pit located between the eye and nostril, elliptic pupils, and retractable front fangs (Figure 1-45).

Localized clinical signs of pit viper envenomation may include the presence of bleeding puncture wounds, local edema close to puncture wounds, immediate severe pain or collapse, edema, petechiae, and ecchymosis with subsequent tissue necrosis. Systemic signs of pit viper envenomation may include hypotension, shock, coagulopathies, lethargy, weakness, muscle fasciculations, lymphangitis, rhabdomyolysis, and neurologic signs including respiratory depression and seizures. Neurologic signs largely are associated with envenomation

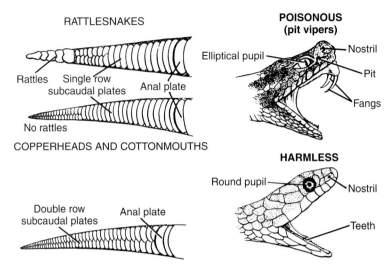

Figure 1-45: Characteristics of poisonous snakes.
(From Parrish HM, Carr CA: Bites by copperheads *(Ancistrodon contortrix)* in the United States. JAMA 201:927, 1967.)

by the Mojave and canebrake rattlesnakes, although a potent neurotoxin, Mojave toxin A, also has been identified in other subspecies of rattlesnake.

Clinical signs of envenomation may take several hours to appear. Hospitalize all suspected victims and monitor them for a minimum of 24 hours. The severity of envenomation cannot be judged solely on the basis of local tissue reaction. First aid measures by animal caretakers do little to prevent further envenomation. The most important aspect of initiating therapy is to transport the animal to the nearest veterinary emergency facility.

Immediate action

To determine whether an animal has been envenomated by a pit viper, examine a peripheral blood smear for the presence of echinocytes. Echinocytes will appear within 15 minutes of envenomation and may disappear within 48 hours. Other treatment should be initiated as rapidly and aggressively as possible, although controversy exists whether some therapies are warranted. The mainstay of therapy is to improve tissue perfusion with intravenous crystalloid fluids, prevent pain with judicious use of analgesic drugs, and when necessary, reverse or negate the effects of the venom with antivenin. Because pit viper venom consists of multiple fractions, treat each envenomation as a complex poisoning.

Obtain vascular access and administer intravenous crystalloid fluids (one fourth of a calculated shock dose) according to the patient's perfusion parameters of heart rate, blood pressure, and capillary refill time (see also Shock and Fluid Therapy). Opioid analgesics are potent and should be administered at the time of presentation. (See also Pharmacologic Means to Analgesia: Major Analgesics).

Diphenhydramine (0.5 to 1 mg/kg IM or IV) also can be administered to decrease the effects of histamine. Famotidine, a histamine$_1$ receptor antagonist, also can be administered (0.5 to 1 mg/kg IV) to work synergistically with diphenhydramine. Although antihistamines have no effect on the venom per se, they may have an effect on the tissue reaction to the venom and may prevent an adverse reaction to antivenin. The use of glucocorticosteroids is controversial. Glucocorticosteroids (dexamethasone sodium phosphate [Dex-SP], 0.25 to 0.5 mg/kg IV) may stabilize cellular membranes and inhibit phospholipase, an active component of some pit viper toxins.

Polyvalent antivenin is necessary in many cases of pit viper envenomation, except in most cases of prairie rattlesnake *(Crotalus viridis viridis)* envenomation in Colorado.

A recent study demonstrated no difference in outcome with or without the use of antivenin in cases of prairie rattlesnake envenomation. Clinically, however, patients that receive antivenin are more comfortable and leave the hospital sooner than those that do not receive antivenin. The exact dose of antivenin is unknown in small animal patients. Administer a dose of at least 1 vial of antivenin to neutralize circulating venom. Mix antivenin with a swirling, rather than a shaking motion, to prevent foaming. Mix the antivenin with a 250-mL bag of 0.9% saline, and then administer it slowly over a period of 4 hours. Pretreat animals with diphenhydramine (0.5 to 1 mg/kg IM) before the administration of antivenin, and then monitor the animal closely for clinical signs of angioneurotic edema, urticaria, tachyarrhythmias, vomiting, diarrhea, and weakness during the infusion. Administration of antivenin into the bite site is relatively contraindicated and ineffective because uptake is delayed, and systemic effects are the more life-threatening.

Management

Management of pit viper envenomation largely involves maintenance of normal tissue perfusion with intravenous fluids, decreasing patient discomfort with analgesia, and negating circulating venom with antivenin. Hydrotherapy to the affected bite site with tepid water is often soothing to the patient. The empiric use of antibiotics is controversial but is recommended because of the favorable environment created by a snakebite (i.e., impregnation of superficial gram-positive bacteria and gram-negative bacteria from the mouth of the snake into a site of edematous necrotic tissue). Administer amoxicillin-clavulanate (16.25 mg/kg PO q12h, or cephalexin, 22 mg/kg PO q8h). Also consider administration of NSAIDs (carprofen, 2.2 mg/kg PO q12h). Monitor the patient closely for signs of local tissue necrosis and the development of thrombocytopenia and coagulopathies including DIC (see Management of Disseminated Intravascular Coagulation). Treat coagulopathies aggressively to prevent end-organ damage.

CORAL SNAKE ENVENOMATION

Coral snakes are characterized by brightly colored bands encircling the body, with red and black separated by yellow. "Red on black, friend of Jack; red on yellow, kill a fellow." Types of coral snakes include the Eastern coral, Texas coral, and Sonoran coral snakes. Clinical signs of coral snake envenomation may include small puncture wounds, transient initial pain, muscle fasciculations, weakness, difficulty swallowing/dysphagia, ascending lower motor neuron paralysis, miotic pinpoint pupils, bulbar paralysis, respiratory collapse, and severe hemolysis. Clinical signs may be delayed for as long as 18 hours after the initial bite.

Immediate therapy

Immediate treatment with antivenin is necessary in cases of coral snake envenomation before the clinical signs become apparent, whenever possible. Support respiration during paralysis with mechanical ventilation. Secure the patient's airway with a cuffed endotracheal tube to prevent aspiration pneumonia.

Management

Clinical signs will progress rapidly once they develop. Rapid administration with antivenin is the mainstay of therapy in suspected coral snake envenomation. Respiratory and cardiovascular support should occur with mechanical ventilation and intravenous crystalloid fluids. Keep the patient warm and dry in a quiet place. Turn the patient every 4 to 6 hours to prevent atelectasis and decubitus ulcer formation. Maintain cleanliness using a urinary catheter and closed urinary collection system. Perform passive range of motion and deep muscle massage to prevent disuse atrophy of limb muscles and function. Treat aspiration pneumonia aggressively with broad-spectrum antibiotics (ampicillin, 22 mg/kg IV q6h, with enrofloxacin, 10 mg/kg IV q24h, and then change to oral once tolerated and the patient is able to swallow) for 2 weeks past the resolution of radiographic signs of pneumonia, intravenous fluids, and nebulization with sterile saline and coupage chest physiotherapy. Several weeks may elapse before a complete recovery.

Additional Reading

Brown DE, Meyer DJ, Wingfield WE, et al: Echinocytosis associated with rattlesnake envenoma-
tion in dogs, Vet Pathol 31:654-657, 1996.
Fogel JE: Pit viper envenomation in dogs, Stand Care Emerg Crit Care Med 6(8):1-5, 2004.
Hackett TB, Wingfield WE, Mazzaferro EM, et al: Clinical findings associated with prairie
rattlesnake bites in dogs: 100 cases (1989-1998), J Am Vet Med Assoc 220(11):1675-1680, 2002.
Kremer KA, Schaer M: Coral snake *(Micrarus fulvias fulvias)* envenomation in five dogs: present
and earlier findings, J Vet Emerg Crit Care 5(1):9-15, 1995.
Peterson P: Treating pit viper bites, Vet Med 93(10):885-890, 1998.

BLACK WIDOW SPIDER BITE

The adult black widow spider (*Latrodectus* spp.) can be recognized by a red to orange hour-glass-shaped marking on the underside of a globous, shiny, black abdomen. The immature female can be recognized by a colorful pattern of red, brown, and beige on the dorsal surface of the abdomen. Adult and immature females are equally capable of envenomation. The male is unable to penetrate the skin because of its small size. Black widow spiders are found throughout the United States and Canada. Black widow spider venom is neurotoxic and acts presynaptically, releasing large amounts of acetylcholine and norepinephrine. There appears to be a seasonal variation in the potency of the venom, lowest in the spring and highest in the fall. In dogs, envenomation results in hyperesthesia, muscle fascicula-tions, and hypertension. Muscle rigidity without tenderness is characteristic. Affected animals may demonstrate clinical signs of acute abdominal pain. Tonic-clonic convulsions may occur but are rare. In cats, paralytic signs predominate and appear early as a ascend-ing lower motor neuron paralysis. Increased salivation, vomiting, and diarrhea may occur. Serum biochemistry profiles often reveal significant elevations in creatine kinase and hypocalcemia. Myoglobinemia and myoglobinuria can occur because of extreme muscle damage.

Management

Management of black widow spider envenomation should be aggressive in the cat and dog, particularly when the exposure is known. In many cases, however, the diagnosis is made based on clinical signs, biochemical abnormalities, and lack of other apparent cause. Antivenin (one vial) is available and should be administered after pretreatment with diphenhy-dramine. If antivenin is unavailable, administer a slow infusion of calcium-containing fluid such as lactated Ringer's solution with calcium gluconate while carefully monitoring the patient's ECG.

BROWN SPIDER BITE

Fiddleback, brown recluse, Arizona brown, *Loxosceles* spp.

The small brown nonaggressive spider is characterized by a violin-shaped marking on the cephalothorax. The neck of the violin points toward the abdomen. Brown spiders are found primarily in the southern half of the United States but have been documented as far north as Michigan. The venom of the brown spider has a potent dermatonecrolytic effect and starts with a classic bull's-eye lesion. The lesion then develops into an indolent ulcer into dependent tissues promoted by complement fixation and influx of neutrophils into the affected area. The ulcer can take months to heal and often leaves a disfiguring scar. Systemic reactions are rare but can include hemolysis, fever, thrombocytopenia, weakness, and joint pain. Fatalities are possible.

Management

Immediate management of an animal with brown spider envenomation is difficult because there is no specific antidote and because clinical signs may be delayed until necrosis of the skin and underlying tissues becomes apparent through the patient's fur 7 to 14 days after the initial bite. Dapsone has been recommended at a dose of 1 mg/kg for 14 days. Surgical excision of the ulcer may be helpful if performed in the early stages of wound appearance.

Glucocorticosteroids may be of some benefit if used within 48 hours of the bite. The ulcer should be left to heal by second intention. Deep ulcers should be treated with antibiotics.

Additional Reading

Forrester MB, Stanley SK: Black widow spider and brown recluse spider bites in Texas from 1998-2002, Vet Hum *Toxicol* 45(5):270-273, 2003.

Twedt DC, Cuddon PA, Horn TW: Black widow spider envenomation in a cat, J Vet Intern Med 13(6):63-616, 1999.

OTHER POISONOUS CREATURES

Bufo species toxicosis

Bufo toad species (*B. marinus,* aka cane toad, marine toad, giant toad; and the Colorado River toad or Sonoran desert toad *B. alvarius*) can be associated with severe cardiac and neurotoxicity if an animal licks its skin. The severity of toxicity depends largely on the size of the dog. Toxins in the cane toad, *B. marinus,* include catecholamines and vasoactive substances (epinephrine, norepinephrine, serotonin, dopamine) and bufo toxins (bufagins, bufotoxin, and bufotenine), the mechanism of which is similar to cardiac glycosides. Clinical signs can range from ptyalism, weakness, ataxia, extensor rigidity, opisthotonus, and collapse to seizures. Clinical signs associated with *B. alvarius* toxicity are limited largely to cardiac dysrhythmias, ataxia, and salivation.

Immediate action

The animal should have its mouth rinsed out thoroughly with tap water even before presentation to the veterinarian. If the animal is unconscious or actively seizing and cannot protect its airway, flushing the mouth is contraindicated. Once an animal presents to the veterinarian, the veterinarian should place an intravenous catheter and monitor the patient's ECG and blood pressure. Attempt seizure control with diazepam (0.5 mg/kg IV) or pentobarbital (2 to 8 mg/kg IV to effect). Ventricular dysrhythmias can be controlled first with esmolol (0.1 mg/kg). If esmolol is ineffective, administer a longer-acting parenteral β-antagonist such as propranolol (0.05 mg/kg IV). Ventricular tachycardia also can be treated with lidocaine (1 to 2 mg/kg IV, followed by 50 to 100 μg/kg/minute IV CRI).

Management

Case management largely depends on supportive care and treating clinical signs as they occur. Monitor baseline acid-base and electrolyte balance because severe metabolic acidosis may occur that should be treated with intravenous fluids and sodium bicarbonate (0.25 to 1 mEq/kg IV). Monitor ECG, blood pressure, and mentation changes closely. Control seizures and cardiac dysrhythmias.

Additional Reading

Eubig PA: *Bufo* species intoxication: big toad, big problem, Vet Med 96(8)594-599, 2001.

Roberts BF, Aronson MG, Moses BL, et al: *Bufo marinus* intoxication in dogs: 94 cases (1997-1998), J Am Vet Med Assoc 216(12):1941-1944, 2000.

Gila monster *(Heloderma suspectum)* and Mexican bearded lizard *(Heloderma horridum)* bites

Lizards of the family Hemodermatidae are the only two poisonous lizards in the world. They are found in the Southwestern United States and Mexico. The venom glands are located on either side of the lower jaw. Because these lizards are typically lethargic and nonaggressive, bite wounds are rare. The lizards have grooved teeth that introduce the venom with a chewing motion as the lizard holds tenaciously to the victim. The majority of affected dogs are bitten on the upper lip, which is very painful.

Management

There are no proven first aid measures for bites from Gila monsters or Mexican bearded lizards. The lizard can be disengaged by inserting a prying instrument in between the jaws and pushing at the back of the mouth. The teeth of the lizard are brittle and break off in the wound. Topical irrigation with lidocaine and probing with a needle will aid in finding and removing the teeth from the victim. Bite wounds will bleed excessively. Irrigate wounds with sterile saline or lactated Ringer's solution, and place compression on the affected area until bleeding ceases. Monitor the patient for hypotension. Establish intravenous access, and administer intravenous fluids according to the patient's perfusion parameters. Antibiotic therapy is indicated because of the bacteria in the lizard's mouth. Because no antidote is available, treatment is supportive according to patient signs.

FRACTURES AND MUSCULOSKELETAL TRAUMA

The majority of musculoskeletal emergencies are the result of external trauma, most commonly from motor vehicle accidents. Blunt trauma invokes injury to multiple organ systems as a rule, rather than an exception. Because of this, massive musculoskeletal injuries are assigned a relatively low priority during the initial triage and treatment of a traumatized animal. Perform a rapid primary survey and institute any lifesaving emergency therapies. Adhere to A CRASH PLAN or the ABCs of resuscitation (see Initial Emergency Examination, Management, and Triage).

Although musculoskeletal injuries are assigned a relatively lower priority, the degree of recovery from these injuries and financial obligation for fracture repair sometimes becomes a critical factor in a client's decision whether to pursue further therapy. One of the most important deciding factors is the long-term prognosis for the patient to have a good quality of life following fracture repair.

The initial management of musculoskeletal injuries is important in ensuring the best chance for maximal recovery with minimal complications after definitive surgical fracture repair. This is particularly important for open fractures, spinal cord compromise, multiple fractures, open joints, articular fractures, physeal fractures, and concomitant ligamentous or neurologic compromise (Box 1-41).

IMMEDIATE ACTION

Immediately after the initial primary survey of a patient, perform a more thorough examination, including an orthopedic examination. Multiple injuries often are observed in the patient that falls from height (e.g., "high-rise syndrome"), motor vehicle accidents, gunshot wounds, and encounters with other animals (e.g., "big-dog-little-dog"). Address the most life threatening injuries, and palliate musculoskeletal injuries until more definitive repair can be attempted when the patient is more stable.

In animals with the history of potential for multiple injuries, search thoroughly and meticulously for areas of injury to the spinal column, extremities, and for small puncture wounds. Helpful signs that can provide a clue as to an underlying injury include swelling,

---

BOX 1-41 CLASSIFICATION OF SKELETAL TRAUMA

GROUP I: CRITICAL
Immediate therapy needed within a few hours
Examples: Compressive skull fractures, spine fracture or luxation/subluxation, open fractures or luxations

GROUP II: SEMICRITICAL
Early treatment within 2 to 5 days
If definitive repair is not attempted within 2 to 5 days, complications including delayed healing and poor long-term results may occur.
Examples: Articular fractures, physeal fractures, joint luxation/subluxation, slipped capital epiphysis

GROUP III: NONCRITICAL
Delayed treatment (within several days)
Scapular and pelvic fractures, greenstick fractures, closed long bone fractures

bruising, abnormal motion, and crepitus (caused by subcutaneous emphysema or bony fracture). If the patient is alert, look for areas of tenderness or pain. In unconscious or depressed patients, reexamine the patient after the patient becomes more mentally alert. Injuries often are missed during the initial examination in obtunded patients because of the early response and attenuation of pain. Unconscious or immobile patients must have radiographic examination of the spinal column following stabilization and support. Palpate the skull carefully for obvious depressions or crepitus that may be associated with a skull fracture. Localization of the injury can be determined by motion in abnormal locations, swelling caused by hemorrhage or edema, pain during gentle movement or palpation, deformity, angular change, or a significant increase or decrease in normal range of motion of bones and joints. Perform a rectal examination in all cases to palpate for pelvic fractures and displacement.

Once the diagnosis of a fracture or luxation has been confirmed, look for any evidence of skin lacerations or punctures near the fracture site. In long-haired breeds, clipping the fur near the fracture site often is necessary to perform a thorough examination of the area. If any wounds are found, the fracture is classified as an open fracture until proven otherwise. In some cases, the open fracture is obvious, with a large section of bone fragment protruding through the skin. In other cases, the puncture wound may be subtle, with only a small amount of blood or pinpoint hole in the skin surface. Characteristics observed with open fractures include bone penetration, fat droplets or marrow elements in blood coming from the wound, subcutaneous emphysema on radiographs, and lacerations in the area of a fracture. Protect the patient from further injury or contamination of wounds. Excessive palpation to intentionally produce crepitus is inappropriate because it causes severe patient discomfort and has the potential to cause severe soft tissue and neurologic injury at the fracture site. Sedation and analgesia aids in making the examination more comfortable for the patient and allows localization of the injury and comparison with the opposite extremity. Higher-quality radiographs can be performed to determine the extent of the injury when the animal is sedated adequately and pain is controlled.

INITIAL FRACTURE MANAGEMENT

Sedate the patient judiciously with analgesic drugs. Opioid drugs work well for orthopedic pain, produce minimal cardiorespiratory depression, and can be reversed with naloxone if necessary. Handle the fracture site gently to avoid causing further pain and soft tissue injury at the fracture site. Rough or careless handling of a fracture site can cause a closed fracture to penetrate through the skin and become an open fracture. Cover open fractures immediately to prevent contamination of the fracture with nosocomial infection from the hospital. Administer a first-generation cephalosporin (cephalexin, 22 mg/kg PO q8h, or cefazolin, 22 mg/kg IV q8h). The bandage also serves to control hemorrhage and prevent desiccation of the bones and surrounding soft tissue structures. Leave the initial bandages in place until the patient's cardiorespiratory status has been determined to be stable and more definitive wound management can occur in a clean, preferably sterile location.

Examine the neurologic status and cardiovascular status of the limb before and after treatment. Determine the vascular status of the limb by checking the color and temperature of the limb, the state of distal pulses, and the degree of bleeding from a cut nail bed. In patients with severe cardiovascular compromise and hypotension caused by hemorrhagic shock, the viability of the limb may be in question until the cardiovascular status and blood pressure are normalized. Reduction of the fracture or straightening of gross deformities may return normal vascularity to the limb. When checking neurologic status, examine for motor and sensory function to the limb. Swelling may increase pressure on the nerves as they run through osteofascial compartments, resulting in decreased sensory or motor function, or neurapraxia. Diminished function often returns to normal once the swelling subsides. Serial physical examinations in the patient and response to initial stabilization therapy can lead to a higher index of suspicion that more occult injuries are present, such as a diaphragmatic hernia, perforated bowel, lacerated liver or spleen, or uroabdomen.

To prevent ongoing trauma, reduce any fracture and then stabilize the site above and below the fracture. A modified Robert Jones splint or bandage often works well for fractures involving the distal extremities. Fractures of the humerus or femur are difficult to immobilize without the use of spica or over-the-hip coaptation splints to prevent mobility. Inappropriate bandaging of humerus or femur fractures can result in a fulcrum effect and worsen the soft tissue and neurologic injuries.

Further displacement of vertebral bodies or luxations can cause cord compression or laceration such that return to function becomes impossible. Immediately place any patient with a suspected spinal injury on a flat surface, and tape down the animal to prevent further movement until the spine has been cleared by a minimum or two orthogonal radiographic views (lateral and ventrodorsal views performed as a cross-table x-ray technique).

OPEN MUSCULOSKELETAL INJURY

Wounds associated with musculoskeletal trauma are common and include injury to the bones, joints, tendons, and surrounding musculature (Box 1-42). Major problems associated with these cases are the presence of soft tissue trauma that makes wound closure hazardous or impossible, because of the risk of infection. Chronic deep infection of traumatized wounds can cause delayed healing and sequestrum to develop, particularly if there is avascular bone or cartilage within the wound.

In the early management of an open fracture, the areas should be splinted without pulling any exposed bone back into the soft tissue. The wound should not be probed or soaked, as nosocomial bacteria and other external contaminants can be introduced into the wound, leading to severe infection. Because of the risk of actually causing infection, probing, flushing, or replacing tissues back into the wound should be performed at the time of formal debridement when the patient is physiologically stable. Immediate bactericidal antibiotic therapy with a first-generation cephalosporin should be started immediately to obtain adequate concentrations of antibiotics at the fracture site. The duration of antibiotic therapy should ideally be limited to 2–3 days to prevent the risk of superinfection.

Treatment

Treatment of open musculoskeletal injury involves three considerations: initial inspection and wound debridement, stabilization and repair, and wound bandaging.

BOX 1-42   CLASSIFICATION OF OPEN WOUNDS BY DEGREE OF SOFT TISSUE INJURY

TYPE I WOUND
Minimal soft tissue trauma and devitalization
When associated with a fracture, wound is created from the inside out by penetration of bone fragments through the skin or from a low-energy gunshot.
Simple or comminuted fracture pattern
Good stability of the two main bone segments
Treatment and prognosis are good and similar to those of a closed injury if wound is debrided and stabilized within 6 to 8 hours.

TYPE II WOUND
Moderate soft tissue contusion and devitalization
When associated with a fracture, wound is created from the outside in.
Major deep injury with considerable soft tissue stripping from bone and muscle damage
Simple or comminuted fracture pattern
Prognosis is good if wound is debrided within 6 hours of injury and provided rigid stabilization with a bone plate or external fixator.

TYPE III WOUND
Results from major external force
Severe damage and necrosis of skin, subcutaneous tissue, muscle, nerve, bone, tendon, and arteries
Soft tissue damage may vary from crush injury to shearing injury associated with bite wounds or low-speed automobile accidents.
Requires immediate and delayed sequential debridement and rigid external fixation
Can require prolonged healing times
Guarded prognosis

Initial inspection and wound debridement include the following steps:

1. After the patient's cardiovascular status has been stabilized and it has been determined that it can withstand anesthesia, place the animal under general anesthesia and remove the temporary splint.
2. Keeping the wound covered, shave the surrounding fur.
3. Remove the covering and then place sterile lubricant jelly over the wound. Shave the fur to the edges of the wound margin.
4. Wash away any entrapped fur and the lubricant jelly.
5. Complete an antiseptic scrub of the surrounding skin.
6. If the wound is a small puncture (e.g., gunshot pellets or bites), probe the wound with a sterile hemostat. Do a thorough debridement if tissues deep to the hole are cavitated. If not deep, create a hole for drainage.
7. Flush the wound with a physiologic solution (lactated Ringer's solution is preferred).
8. Debride the wound from outward to inward. Cut away damaged areas of skin and deeper tissues to open up underlying cavitations and tissue injury.
9. Continuously irrigate with warm physiologic solution (lactated Ringer's solution is preferred). The stream must be strong enough to flush debris out of the bottom of the wound. To accomplish this, attach a 20-gauge needle to a 35-mL syringe (will deliver 7 psi). Excise any obviously devitalized tissue.
10. Do not remove any bone fragments that are firmly attached to soft tissue. Do not cut into healthy soft tissue to find bullet or bone fragments, unless the bullet can cause injury to joints or nerve tissue.
11. Do a primary repair of tendons and nerves if the wound is type I and recent (within 8 hours of the initial injury). If the wound is too severe or if there is obvious infection, tag the ends of the tendons and nerves for later repair.

It is best to stabilize and repair open fractures as soon as the patient's cardiovascular and respiratory status can tolerate general anesthesia, provided that adequate stabilization is possible. If this is not possible because of the level of experience of the surgeon or the lack of necessary equipment, it is best to perform wound management and place a temporary splint until definitive repair can be performed.

Wound bandaging is discussed in the section on Bandaging Techniques.

Articular Cartilage Injury

Structural injuries to the joints are common and can involve both ligaments and articular cartilage injuries. Cartilage does not heal well; therefore, injuries involving articular cartilage can lead to a significant loss of function and degenerative joint disease (osteoarthritis). Cartilage injuries that are superficial evoke a short-lived enzymatic and metabolic response that does not stimulate enough cellular growth to repair the defect. Superficial lesions remain as defects but do not progress to chondromalacia or osteoarthritis. Deep cartilage lacerations that extend to subchondral bone produce an exuberant healing response from the cells of the underlying cartilage. In many cases, this material undergoes degeneration and leads to osteoarthritis. Impact injuries to surface cartilage can cause chondrocyte and underlying bone injury. These lesions rapidly progress to osteoarthritis; however, they may be totally or partially reversible.

Ligamentous Injuries

Treatment of grade I injuries requires short-term coaptation splints and has a good prognosis. Grade II injuries require surgical treatment with a suture stent and consistent postoperative coaptation splints to heal and maintain good function. Healing of grade III injuries often is a problem, and suture stents or surgical reapproximation may be indicated. Failure to immobilize joints that are frequently flexed (elbow and stifle) can result in late complications of ligament repair. Ligamentous injuries of joints, particularly the collateral ligaments of the stifle, elbow, and hock, and carpal hyperextension injuries are commonly missed and may require surgical fixation, including arthrodesis (Box 1-43).

1

BOX 1-43   CLASSIFICATION OF LIGAMENTOUS INJURIES

Grade I sprain: Rupture of a portion of the ligament with minimal lengthening. Preservation of anatomical and mechanical integrity.
Grade II sprain: A portion of the ruptured ligament is stretched. Ligament is longer but still intact.
Grade III sprain: Complete ligament disruption

FRACTURES IN THE IMMATURE ANIMAL

Fractures in immature animals differ from those in adults in that young puppies and kittens have a great ability to remodel bone. Remodeling is dependent on the age of the patient and the location of the fracture. The younger the puppy or kitten and the closer the fracture to the epiphysis or growth plate, the greater the potential for remodeling and the development of angular limb deformities. Remodeling occurs more effectively in long-limbed breeds of dogs than in short-limbed breeds. Fractures through the growth plate of immature animals may potentially cause angular limb deformities, joint dislocations or incongruity, and osteoarthritis. This form of injury is commonly observed in the distal ulnar growth plate and the proximal and distal radial growth plates.

HIGH-RISE SYNDROME

High-rise syndrome in cats is seen in cats that fall from a height usually greater than 30 feet. It occurs most frequently in high-rise buildings in urban areas where cats lie on window ledges and suddenly fall out the window. The most common lesions observed in cats that fall from heights are thoracic injuries (rib and sternal fractures, pneumothorax, and pulmonary contusions) and facial and oral trauma (lip avulsions, mandibular symphyseal fractures, fractures of the hard palate, and maxillary fractures). Limb and spinal cord fractures and luxations, radius and ulna fractures, abdominal trauma, urinary tract trauma, and diaphragmatic hernias are also common. The injuries sustained are often found in combination, rather than as an isolated injury of one area of the body.

Follow the mnemonic A CRASH PLAN when managing a cat suffering from high-rise syndrome, treating the animal immediately for shock. Following cardiovascular and respiratory stabilization, evaluate thoracic and abdominal radiographs, including those of the spine. Evaluate the bladder closely, making sure that the cat is able to urinate effectively. Examine the hard palate, maxilla, and mandibular symphysis for fractures. Palpate the pelvis and carefully manipulate all limbs to examine for fractures or ligamentous injuries. Finally, perform a complete neurologic examination. Patients that fall less than five stories often have a more guarded prognosis than patients that fall from higher levels.

Additional Reading

Aron DN: Emergency management of the musculoskeletal trauma patient. In: Emergency medicine and critical care in practice. Veterinary Learning Systems, Trenton, NJ, 1992,.
Gordon LE, Thacher C, Kapatkin A: High-rise syndrome in dogs: 81 cases. JAVMA 202(1): 118-122, 1993.
Papazoglou LG, Galatos AD, Patsikas MN, et al: High-rise syndrome in cats: 207 cases (1988-1998) Aust Vet Pract 31(3):98-102, 2001.
Vnuk D, Pirkic B, Maticic D, et al: Feline high-rise syndrome: 119 cases (1998-2001), J Feline Med Surg 6(5):301-312, 2004.

GASTROINTESTINAL EMERGENCIES

ORAL CAVITY

Sometimes the owner witnesses the ingestion of a foreign body during play, such as throwing a stick or fetching a ball. Cats tend to play with string or thread that becomes caught around the base of the tongue. In many cases, however, ingestion of the foreign object is not witnessed, and diagnosis is made based on clinical signs and physical examination.

Foreign bodies lodged in the oral cavity often cause irritation and discomfort, including difficulty breathing and difficulty swallowing. Often, an animal paws at its mouth in an attempt to dislodge a stick or bones wedged across the roof of the mouth. Irritation, inability to close the mouth, and blockage of the orpharynx can result in excessive drooling. The saliva may appear blood-tinged due to concurrent soft tissue trauma (Figs 1-46 and 1-47).

Obstruction of the glottis by a foreign body (e.g., tennis ball or toy) can result in cyanosis secondary to an obstructed airway and hypoxemia. In many cases, the object is small enough to enter the larynx but too large to be expelled. If a foreign object is lodged in the mouth for more than several days, halitosis and purulent discharge may be present.

Many animals are anxious at the time of presentation and may require sedation or a light plane of anesthesia to remove the foreign object. The animal may bite personnel and may have bitten the owner during his or her attempt to remove the object from the mouth en route to the hospital. Propofol (47 mg/kg IV) or a combination of propofol with diazepam (0.5-1 mg/kg IV) is an excellent combination for a light plane of anesthesia. Exercise caution when anesthetizing a patient with a ball lodged in the airway, as further compromise of respiratory function may occur and cause worsening of the hypoxemia.

Before inducing anesthesia, assemble all supplies necessary to remove the object. Make sure that rigid towel clamps, sponge forceps, and bone forceps are on hand, because the foreign object is often very slippery with saliva. Hemostats and carmalts may slip and not be useful in the removal of the foreign object.

Place a peripheral intravenous catheter to secure vascular access prior to anesthetic induction. Have available the supplies necessary for an emergency tracheostomy, if the foreign object cannot be removed by usual methods. Induce a light plane of anesthesia and then grasp the object with the sponge forceps or towel clamps, and extract. Monitor the cardiorespiratory status of the animal at all times during the extraction process. If you are

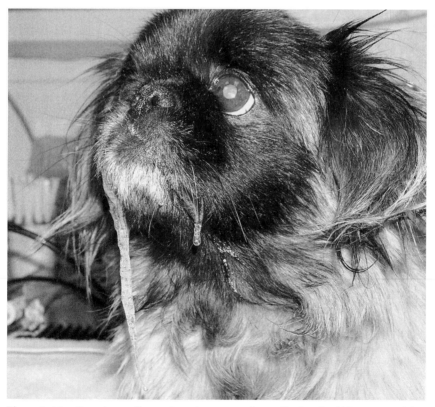

Figure 1-46: Excessive ptyalism and gagging or excessive swallowing should increase suspicion of the presence of an esophageal or pharyngeal foreign body.

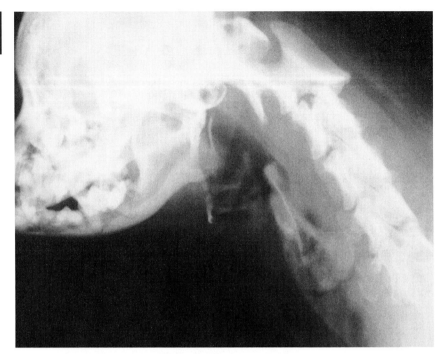

Figure 1-47:   Radiograph of a chicken bone lodged in the patient's pharynx.

unable to remove the object, and if severe respiratory distress, including cyanosis, bradycardia, or ventricular dysrhythmias, develop, perform a tracheostomy distal to the site of obstruction.

Once the foreign body has been removed, administer supplemental flow-by oxygen until the animal awakens. If laryngeal edema or stridor on inspiration is present, administer a dose of dexamethasone sodium phosphate (0.25 mg/kg IV, IM, SQ) to decrease inflammation. The patient should be carefully monitored for 24 hours, because noncardiogenic pulmonary edema can develop secondary to airway obstruction.

Esophageal Foreign Bodies

Esophageal foreign bodies pose a serious medical emergency. It is helpful if the owner witnessed ingestion of the object and noted rapid onset of clinical signs. In many cases, however, ingestion is not witnessed, and the diagnosis must be made based on clinical signs, thoracic radiographs, and results of a barium swallow. The most common clinical signs are excessive salivation with drooling, gulping, and regurgitation after eating. Many animals will make repeated swallowing motions. Some animals exhibit a rigid "sawhorse" stance, with reluctance to move immediately after foreign body ingestion and esophageal entrapment.

After completing a physical examination, evaluate cervical and thoracic radiographs to determine the location of the esophageal obstruction. Esophageal foreign objects are lodged most commonly at the base of the heart, the carina, or just orad to the lower esophageal sphincter. If the object has been lodged for several days, pleural effusion and pneumomediastinum may be present secondary to esophageal perforation. Endoscopy is useful for both diagnosis and removal of the foreign object; however, it is invasive and requires general anesthesia (Fig. 1-48).

Remove foreign objects lodged in the esophagus with a rigid or flexible endoscope after the patient has been placed under general anesthesia. Evaluate the integrity of the esophagus both before and after removal of the material because focal perforation or pressure

1

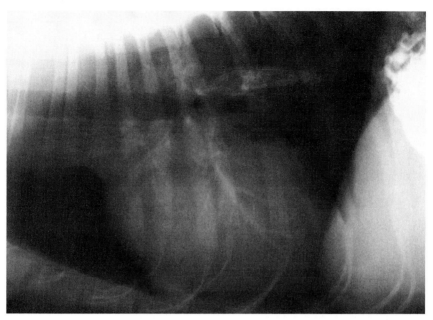

Figure 1-48:   Example of an esophageal foreign body. Common locations are the carina and thoracic inlet.

necrosis can be present. Necrosis of the mucosa and submucosa of the esophagus often leads to stricture formation or perforation.

Attempt to retrieve the object with a flexible fiberoptic endoscope if available. Rigid tube endoscopy can also be performed. In many cases, smooth objects that cannot be easily grasped can be pushed into the stomach and allowed to dissolve or may be removed by gastrotomy. If the foreign body is firmly lodged in the esophagus and cannot be pulled or pushed into the stomach, or if perforation has already occurred, the prognosis for return to function without strictures is not favorable. In such cases, referral to a surgical specialist is recommended for esophagostomy or esophageal resection.

After removal of the object, carefully examine the esophagus and then administer gastroprotectant agents (famotidine, 0.5 mg/kg PO bid; sucralfate slurry, 0.5-1.0 g/dog) for a minimum of 5 to 7 days. To rest the esophagus, the patient should receive nothing per os (NPO) for 24 to 48 hours. If esophageal irritation or erosion is moderate to severe, a percutaneous gastrotomy tube should be placed for feeding until the esophagus heals. Perform repeat endoscopy every 7 days to evaluate the healing process and to determine whether stricture formation is occurring.

STOMACH

Persistent vomiting immediately or soon after eating is often associated with a gastric foreign body. In some cases, the owner knows that the patient has ingested a foreign body of some kind. In other cases, continued vomiting despite lack of response to conservative treatment (NPO, antiemetics, gastroprotectant drugs) prompts further diagnostic procedures, including abdominal radiographs and bloodwork. Obstruction to gastric outflow and vomiting of hydrochloric acid often cause a hypochloremic metabolic acidosis. Radiopaque gastric foreign bodies may be observed on plain films. Radiolucent cloth material may require a barium series to delineate the shape and location of the foreign body (Fig. 1-49).

Treatment consists of removal with flexible endoscopy or a simple gastrotomy. Most animals with uncomplicated gastric foreign bodies are relatively healthy, but any metabolic and electrolyte abnormalities should be corrected prior to anesthesia and surgery.

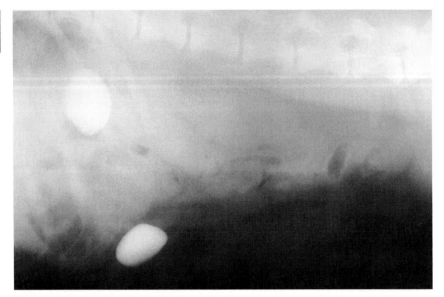

Figure 1-49: Lateral abdominal radiograph with two radiopaque densities within the lumen of the small intestine, consistent with rocks.

SMALL INTESTINAL OBSTRUCTION

Small intestinal obstruction can be caused by foreign bodies, tumors, intussusception, volvulus, or strangulation within hernias. Regardless of the cause, clinical signs of small intestinal obstruction depend on the location and degree of obstruction, and whether the bowel has perforated. Clinical signs associated with a high small intestinal obstruction are usually more severe and more rapid in onset compared with partial or complete obstruction of the jejunum or ileum. Complete obstructions that allow no fluid or chyme to pass are worse than partial obstructions, which can cause intermittent clinical signs interspersed with periods of normality (Table 1-36).

The most common clinical signs associated with a complete small intestinal obstruction are anorexia, vomiting, lethargy, depression, dehydration, and sometimes abdominal pain. Early clinical signs may be limited to anorexia and depression, making a diagnosis challenging unless the owner has a suspicion that the animal ingested some kind of foreign object. Obstructions cranial to the common bile duct and pancreatic papillae lead to vomiting of gastric contents, namely hydrochloric acid, and a hypochloremic metabolic alkalosis. Obstructions caudal to the common bile duct and pancreatic papillae result in loss of other electrolytes and sometimes mixed acid-base disorders.

TABLE 1-36   Localizing Signs for Patients with Bowel Obstruction

Condition	Onset	Progression of vomiting	Frequency	Volume of vomit	Tenesmus	Abdominal distention
High small bowel	Rapid	Rapid	Frequent	Large volume	Absent	Absent
Low small bowel	Slower	Slower	Less frequent	Small volume	Diarrhea	Present
Large bowel	Subacute to chronic	Slow	Occasional	Scant	Often with diarrhea	Present

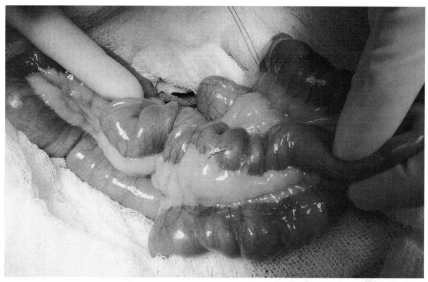

Figure 1-50: Intraoperative photograph depicting plication of the jejunum by a linear foreign body.

Eventually, all animals with small intestinal obstruction vomit and have fluid loss into dilated segments of bowel, leading to dehydration and electrolyte abnormalities. Increased luminal pressure causes decreased lymphatic drainage and bowel edema. The bowel wall eventually becomes ischemic and may rupture.

Linear foreign bodies should be suspected in any vomiting patient, particularly cats. String or thread often is looped around the base of the tongue and can be visualized in many cases by a thorough oral examination. To look properly under the tongue, grasp the top of the animal's head with one hand, and pull the lower jaw open with the index finger of the opposite hand while pushing up the thumb simultaneously on the tongue in between the intermandibular space. Thread and string can be observed lying along the ventral aspect of the tongue. In some cases, if a linear foreign body is lodged very caudally, it cannot be visualized without heavy sedation or anesthesia.

Linear foreign bodies eventually cause bowel obstruction and perforation of the intestines along the mesenteric border. The foreign material (e.g., string, thread, cloth, pantyhose) becomes lodged proximally, and the intestines become plicated as the body attempts to push the material caudally through the intestines (Fig. 1-50). Continued peristalsis eventually causes a sawing motion of the material and perforation of the mesenteric border of the intestines. Once peritonitis occurs, the prognosis is less favorable unless prompt and aggressive treatment is initiated.

Reevaluate any patient that does not respond to conservative symptomatic therapy, performing a complete blood count, serum biochemical panel (including electrolytes), and abdominal radiographs. Intestinal masses may be palpable on physical examination and are often associated with signs of discomfort or pain when palpating over the mass. Radiography and abdominal ultrasound are the most useful diagnostic aids. Plain radiographs may be diagnostic when the foreign object is radiodense or there is characteristic dilation or plication of bowel loops. As a rule of thumb, the width of a loop of small bowel should be no larger than twice the width of a rib. Diagnosis of small intestinal obstruction or ileus can be based on the appearance of stacking loops of dilated bowel. Comparison of the width of the bowel with the width of a rib is often performed. With mild dilation, the bowel width is three to four times the rib width; with extensive dilation, five to six times the rib width (Fig.1-51). In cases of linear foreign bodies, C-areas

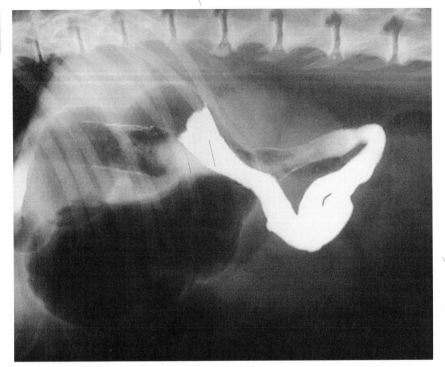

Figure 1-51:   After 60 minutes, the barium has stopped moving and has reached a blunt, intra-luminal intestinal foreign body. Note that barium appears wedge-shaped or square at the site of the foreign body.

(comma-shaped areas) of gas trapped in the plicated bowel will appear stacked on one another. Blunt, wedge-shaped areas of gas or square linear areas of gas adjacent to a distended bowel loop are characteristic of a foreign body lodged in the intestine. Contrast radiography is indicated when confirmation of the suspected diagnosis is necessary and ultrasonography is not available. Contrast material may outline the object or abruptly stop orad to the obstruction.

The definitive treatment of any type of small intestinal foreign body is surgical removal. Linear foreign bodies sometimes pass, but they should never be left untreated in a patient that is demonstrating clinical signs of inappetence, vomiting, lethargy, and dehydration. The timing of surgery is critical because the risk of intestinal perforation increases with time. Prior to surgery, correct any acid-base and electrolyte abnormalities with intravenous fluid therapy. Administer broad-spectrum antibiotics. Perform an enterotomy or intestinal resection and anastomosis as soon as possible once the patient's acid-base and electrolyte status have been corrected.

LARGE INTESTINAL FOREIGN BODIES

Clinical signs of a foreign body in the large bowel are usually nonexistent. In most cases, if a foreign object has passed successfully through the small bowel, it will pass through the large bowel without incident unless bowel perforation and peritonitis occur. Penetrating foreign bodies such as needles often cause localized or generalized peritonitis, abdominal pain, and fever. Hematochezia may be present if the foreign object causes abrasion of the rectal mucosa.

Symptomatic patients should have abdominal radiographs performed. Colonoscopy or exploratory laparotomy should be performed if survey radiographs are suggestive of a large intestinal obstruction or perforation. In most cases, large intestinal foreign bodies will pass without incident. Surgery is required to treat perforations, peritonitis, or abscesses.

1

Rectum and Anus

Foreign bodies in the rectum and anus often are the result of ingestion of bones, wood material, needles, and thread, or malicious external insertion. Often the material can pass through the entire gastrointestinal tract and then get stuck in the anal ring. Clinical signs include hematochezia and dyschezia with straining to defecate. Diagnosis is made by visual examination of the item in the anus, or by careful digital palpation after heavy sedation or short-acting general anesthesia. Radiography is helpful in locating needles that have penetrated the rectum and lodged in the perirectal or perinatal tissues. Treatment consists of careful removal of the needle digitally or surgically.

Acute Intussusception

Intussusception is the acute invagination of one segment of bowel (the *intussusceptum*) into another (the *intussuscipiens*). The proximal segment always invaginates into the distal segment of bowel. Intussusception most commonly occurs in puppies and kittens less than 1 year of age but can occur in an animal of any age with hypermotility of the small bowel, gastrointestinal parasites, and severe viral or bacterial enteritis. Intussusception occurs primarily in the small bowel in the jejunum, ileum, and ileocolic junction.

Clinical signs include vomiting, abdominal discomfort, and hemorrhagic diarrhea. Usually, hemorrhagic diarrhea is the first noticeable sign, and in puppies, may be due to parvoviral enteritis, with secondary intussusception. Usually, the obstruction is partial with mild clinical signs. More serious clinical signs develop as the obstruction becomes more complete. Differential diagnoses include hemorrhagic gastroenteritis, parvoviral enteritis, gastrointestinal parasites, intestinal foreign body, bacterial enteritis, and other causes of vomiting and diarrhea.

The diagnosis of intussusception is often made based on palpation of a sausage-shaped firm, tubular structure in the abdomen accompanied by clinical signs and abdominal pain. Plain radiographs may demonstrate segmental or generalized dilated segments of bowel, depending on the duration of the problem. Ultrasonographs of the palpable mass resemble the layers of an onion, with hyperechoic intestinal walls separated by less echogenic edema.

Treatment consists of correction of the patient's acid-base and electrolyte abnormalities with intravenous fluids and surgical reduction or removal of the intussusception with resection and anastomosis. Although enteroplication has been suggested, the technique has fallen out of favor because of the increased risk of later obstruction. The primary cause of intestinal inflammation and hypermotility must be identified and corrected.

Gastric Dilatation-Volvulus

Gastric dilatation can occur with or without volvulus in the dog. Gastric dilatation-volvulus (GDV) occurs primarily in large- and giant-breed dogs with deep chests, such as the Great Dane, Labrador Retriever, Saint Bernard, German Shepherd Dog, Gordon and Irish Setters, Standard Poodle, Bernese Mountain Dog, and Bassett Hound. The risk of GDV increases with age; however, it can be seen in dogs as young as 4 months. Deep, narrow-chested breeds are more likely to develop GDV than dogs with broader chests. The overall mortality for surgically treated gastric dilatation-volvulus ranges from 10% to 18%, with most deaths occurring in patients that required splenectomy and partial gastrectomy.

Clinical signs of GDV include abdominal distention, unproductive vomiting or retching, lethargy, weakness, sometimes straining to defecate, and collapse. The owner may think that the animal is vomiting productively because of the white foamy froth (saliva) that is not able to pass into the twisted stomach. In some cases, there is a history of the dog's being fed a large meal or consuming a large quantity of water prior to the onset of clinical signs. Instruct the owner of any patient with a predisposition for and clinical signs of GDV to transport the animal to the nearest veterinary facility immediately.

Physical examination often reveals a distended abdomen with a tympanic area on auscultation. In dogs with very deep chests, it may be difficult to appreciate abdominal distention if the stomach is tucked up under the rib cage. Depending on the stage of shock, the patient may have sinus tachycardia with bounding pulses, cardiac dysrhythmias with pulse deficits, or bradycardia. The mucous membranes may appear red and injected or pale with a prolonged capillary refill time. The patient may appear anxious and attempt to retch unproductively. If the patient is nonambulatory at the time of presentation, the prognosis is more guarded.

The definitive diagnosis of GDV is based on clinical signs, physical examination findings, and radiographic appearance of gas distention of the gastric fundus with dorsocranial displacement of the pylorus and duodenum (the so-called "Double-Bubble" or "Popeye arm" sign) (Fig.1-52). In simple gastric dilatation without volvulus, there is gas distention of the stomach with anatomy appearing normal on radiography. With "food bloat," or gastric distention from overconsumption of food, ingesta is visible in the distended stomach (Fig. 1-53).

As soon as a patient presents with a possible GDV, place a large-bore intravenous catheter in the cephalic vein(s) and assess the patient's ECG, blood pressure, heart rate, capillary refill time, and respiratory function. Obtain blood samples for a complete blood count, serum biochemistry profile, immediate lactate measurement, and coagulation tests *before* taking any radiographs. Rapidly infuse a colloid (hetastarch or Oxyglobin, 5 mL/kg IV bolus) along with shock volumes of a crystalloid fluid (up to 90 mL/kg/hour) (see section on Shock). Monitor perfusion parameters (heart rate, blood pressure, capillary refill time, and ECG) and titrate fluid therapy according to the patient's response. The use of short-acting glucocorticosteroids is controversial. Glucocorticosteroids may help stabilize cellular membranes and decrease the mechanisms of ischemia-reperfusion injury, but no detailed studies have proved them to be beneficial versus not using glucocorticosteroids in the patient with GDV.

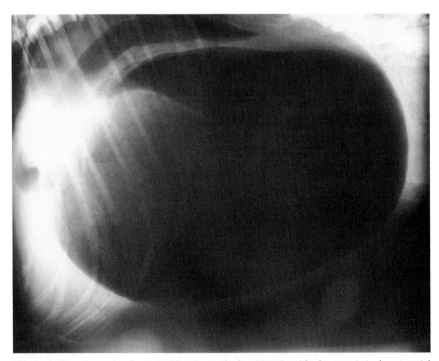

Figure 1-52:   Example of gastric dilatation-volvulus (GDV), with characteristic dorsocranial displacement of the pylorus and proximal duodenum and gas distention of the gastric fundus. Always obtain a right lateral radiograph if the presence of GDV is suspected.

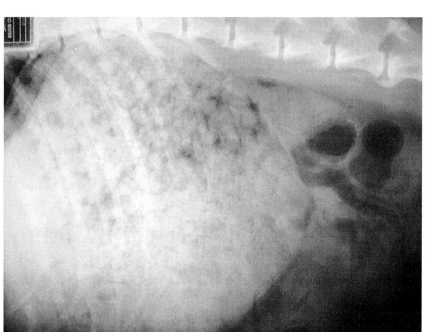

1

Figure 1-53: Example of "food bloat" with severe gastric distention caused by overconsumption of food. In rare cases, this can lead to decreased gastric perfusion, necrosis of the gastric wall, and perforation even without volvulus.

Attempt gastric decompression, either with placement of an orogastric tube or by trocharization. To place an orogastric tube, position the distal end of the tube at the level of the patient's last rib (Fig. 1-54) and place it adjacent to the animal's thorax; then put a piece of tape around the tube where it comes out of the mouth, once it is in place. Put a roll of 2-inch tape in the patient's mouth behind the canine teeth and then secure the roll in place by taping the mouth closed around the roll of tape. Lubricate the tube with lubricating jelly and slowly insert the tube through the center of the roll of tape into the stomach. The passing of the tube does not rule out volvulus.

In some cases, the front legs of the patient need to be elevated, and the caudal aspect of the patient lowered (front legs standing on a table with back legs on the ground) to allow gravity to pull the stomach down to allow the tube to pass. Once the tube has been passed, air within the stomach is relieved, and the stomach can be lavaged. The presence of gastric mucosa or blood in the efflux from the tube makes the prognosis more guarded.

If an orogastric tube cannot be passed, clip and aseptically scrub the patient's lateral abdomen and then insert 16-gauge over-the-needle catheter. "Pinging" the animal's side with simultaneous auscultation allows determination of the location that is most tympanic—that is, the proper location for catheter insertion.

Once intravenous fluids have been started in the animal, take a *right lateral abdominal radiograph* to document GDV. If no volvulus is present, the owner may elect for more conservative care, and the animal should be monitored in the hospital for a minimum of 24 hours. Because some cases of GDV intermittently twist and untwist, the owner should be cautioned that although the stomach is not twisted at that moment, a volvulus can occur at any time. If radiographs demonstrate food bloat, induce emesis (apomorphine, 0.04 mg/kg IV) or perform orogastric lavage under general anesthesia. Documentation of gastric dilatation-volvulus constitutes a surgical emergency.

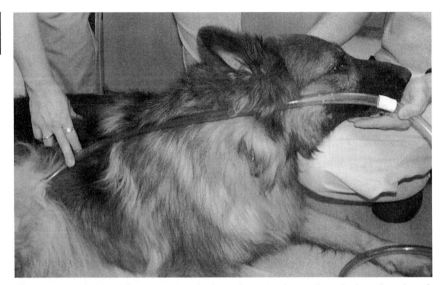

Figure 1-54:   Measure the orogastric tube from the patient's mouth to the last rib and mark the tube to prevent pushing it in too far.

Following diagnosis of GDV, continue administration of intravenous fluids. Serum lactate measurements greater than 6.0 mmol/L are associated with an increased risk of gastric necrosis, requirement for partial gastrectomy, and increased mortality. Administer fresh frozen plasma (20 mL/kg) to patients with thrombocytopenia or prolonged PT, activated partial thromboplastin time (APTT), or activated clotting time (ACT). Cardiac dysrhythmias, particularly ventricular dysrhythmias, are common in cases of GDV and are thought to occur secondary to ischemia and proinflammatory cytokines released during volvulus and reperfusion. Lidocaine (1-2 mg/kg followed by 50 mcg/kg/minute IV CRI) can be used to treat cardiac dysrhythmias preemptively that are associated with ischemia-reperfusion injury, or administration can be started when ventricular dysrhythmias are present. Correct any electrolyte abnormalities, including hypokalemia and hypomagnesemia. The use of nonsteroidal antiinflammatory drugs (flunixin meglumine, carprofen, ketoprofen) that can potentially decrease renal perfusion and predispose to gastric ulcers is *absolutely contraindicated*. Administer analgesic drugs (fentanyl, 2 µ/kg IV bolus, followed by 3-20 µ/kg/hour IV CRI; or hydromorphone, 0.1 mg/kg IV) before anesthetic induction. After carrying out a balanced anesthesia protocol, the patient should be taken immediately to surgery for gastric derotation and gastropexy.

Postoperatively, assess the patient's ECG, blood pressure, platelet count, coagulation parameters, and gastric function (see section on Rule of Twenty). If no resection is required, the animal can be given small amounts of water beginning 12 hours after surgery. Depending on the severity of the patient's condition, small amounts of a bland diet can be offered 12 to 24 hours postoperatively. Continute supportive care with analgesia and crystalloid fluids until the patient is able to tolerate oral analgesic drugs (tramadol, 1-3 mg/kg PO q8-12h). Once the patient is ambulatory and able to eat and drink on its own, it can be released from the hospital; instruct the owner to feed the animal multiple small meals throughout the day for the first week.

SMALL INTESTINAL MESENTERIC VOLVULUS/TORSION

When the intestines twist around the root of the mesentery, a small intestinal or mesenteric volvulus occurs. The problem is most common in the young German Shepherd Dog,

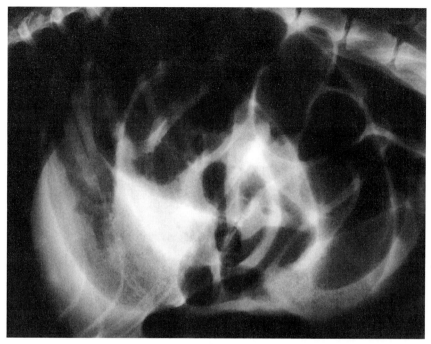

Figure 1-55: Severe generalized distention of the small intestine, characteristic of a mesenteric volvulus. This consistutes an immediate surgical emergency, and the prognosis is often poor. This condition is most common in young German Shepherd Dogs, but can be observed in any breed.

although it has been observed in other large and giant breeds. Predisposing factors include pancreatic atrophy, gastrointestinal disease, trauma, and splenectomy.

Clinical signs of mesenteric volvulus include vomiting, hemorrhagic diarrhea, bowel distention, acute onset of clinical signs of shock, abdominal pain, brick-red mucous membranes (septicemia), and sudden death.

Diagnosis is based on an index of suspicion and the presence of clinical signs in a predisposed breed. Plain radiographs often reveal grossly distended loops of bowel in a palisade gas pattern. In some dogs, multiple, tear-drop–shaped, gas-filled loops appear to rise from a focal point in the abdomen. Usually, massive distention of the entire small bowel is observed (Fig. 1-55). The presence of pneumoperitoneum or lack of abdominal detail secondary to the presence of abdominal fluid is characteristic of bowel perforation and peritonitis.

In a patient with mesenteric volvulus, immediate aggressive action is necessary for the animal to have any chance of survival. Treatment consists of massive volumes of IV crystalloid and colloid fluids (see section on IV Therapy), broad-spectrum antibiotics (ampicillin, 22 mg/kg IV qid, with enrofloxacin, 10 mg/kg IV once daily), and surgical correction of the bowel. Because of the massive release of proinflammatory cytokines, bacterial translocation, and ischemia, treatment for shock is of paramount importance (see sections on Rule of Twenty and Shock). Prognosis for any patient with mesenteric volvulus is poor.

LARGE INTESTINAL OBSTRUCTION

Obstipation

Obstipation (obstructive constipation) is most common in the older cat. In cases of simple constipation, rehydrating the animal with intravenous fluids and stool softeners is often sufficient for it to regain the ability to have a bowel movement. Obstipation, however, is caused by adynamic ileus of the large bowel that eventually leads to megacolon. Affected cats usually are anorectic, lethargic, and extremely dehydrated. Treatment consists of rehydration with intravenous crystalloid fluids, correction of electrolyte abnormalities, enemas, and promotility agents such as cisapride (0.5 mg/kg PO q8-24h). The use of phosphate enemas in cats is absolutely contraindicated because of the risk of causing acute, fatal hyperphosphatemia. In many cases, the patient should be placed under general anesthesia and manual deobstipation is performed with warm water soapy enemas and a gloved finger to relieve and disimpact the rectum. Stool softeners such as lactulose and docusate stool sofener (DSS) may also be used. Predisposing causes of obstipation such as narrowing of the pelvic canal, perineal hernia, and tumors should be ruled out.

TUMORS OF THE GASTROINTESTINAL TRACT

Adenocarcinoma

Adenocarcinoma is the most common neoplasm of the gastrointestinal tract that causes partial to complete obstruction. Adenocarcinomas tend to be annular and constricting, and they may cause progressive obstruction of the lumen of the small or large bowel. Siamese cats tend to have adenocarcinomas in the small intestine, whereas in dogs, the tumor tends to occur in the large intestine.

Clinical signs of adenocarcinoma are both acute and chronic and consist of anorexia, weight loss, and progressive vomiting that occur over weeks to months. Effusion may be present if metastasis to peritoneal surfaces has occurred.

Diagnosis is based on clinical signs and physical examination findings of a palpable abdominal mass, radiographic evidence of an abdominal mass and small or large intestinal obstruction, or ultrasonographic evidence of an intestinal mass.

Treatment consists of surgical resection of the affected bowel segment. The prognosis for long-term survival (10-12 months) is good if the mass is completely resected and if other clinical signs of cachexia or metastasis are observed at the time of diagnosis. Median survival is 15 to 30 weeks if metastasis to lymph nodes, liver, or the peritoneum are absent at the time of diagnosis. In dogs, the prognosis is more guarded.

Leiomyoma and Leiomyosarcoma

Leiomyoma and leiomyosarcoma are tumors that can cause partial or complete obstruction of the bowel. Clinical signs are often referred to progressive anemia, including weakness, lethargy, inappetence, and melena. Hypoglycemia can be observed as a paraneoplastic syndrome, or due to sepsis and peritonitis secondary to bowel perforation. Leiomyomas are most commonly observed at the ceco-colic junction or in the cecum. Surgical resection and anastomosis is usually curative, and has a favorable prognosis.

STRANGULATED HERNIAS

Incarceration of a loop of bowel into congenital or acquired defects in the body wall can cause small bowel obstruction. Pregnant females and young animals with congenital hernias are most at risk. Rarely, older animals with perineal hernias and animals of any age with traumatic hernias can be affected. Clinical signs are consistent with a small intestinal obstruction: anorexia, vomiting, lethargy, abdominal pain, and weakness. Diagnosis is often made based on physical examination of a reducible or nonreducible mass in the body wall. Hernias whose contents are reducible are usually asymptomatic. Treatment consists of supportive care and rehydration, administration of broad-spectrum antibiotics, and surgical correction of the body wall hernia. In some cases, intestinal resection and anastomosis of the affected area is necessary when bowel ischemia occurs.

BOWEL PERFORATION

The potential for bowel perforation should be suspected whenever there is any penetrating injury (knife, gunshot wound, bite wound, stick impalement) of the abdomen. Injuries that result in bowel ischemia and rupture can also occur secondary to nonpenetrating blunt trauma or shear forces (e.g., big dog–little dog/cat). Perforation of the stomach and small and large intestines can occur with use of nonsteroidal antiinflammatory drugs.

Diagnosis of bowel perforation first depends on the alertness to the possibility that the bowel may have been perforated or penetrated. As a general rule, all penetrating injuries of the abdomen should be investigated by exploratory laparotomy. Diagnostic peritoneal lavage (DPL) can be performed; however, early after penetrating injury of the bowel, DPL may be negative or nondiagnostic until peritonitis develops. Whenever any patient with blunt or penetrating abdominal trauma does not respond to initial fluid therapy, or responds and then deteriorates, the index of suspicion for bowel injury should be raised. The findings of pneumoperitoneum on abdominal radiographs or of intracellular bacteria, extracellular bacteria, bile pigment, bowel contents, and cloudy appearance of fluid obtained by abdominocentesis or diagnostic peritoneal lavage fluid (see sections on Abdominocentesis and Diagnostic Peritoneal Lavage) warrant immediate surgical exploration.

Treatment largely consists of stabilizing the patient's cardiovascular and electrolyte status with intravenous fluids, administration of broad-spectrum antibiotics, and definitive surgical exploration and repair of injured structures.

RECTAL PROLAPSE

Prolapse of the rectum is observed most frequently secondary to parasitism and gastrointestinal viral infections in young puppies and kittens with chronic diarrhea. Older animals with rectal prolapse often have an underlying problem such as a tumor or mucosal lesion that causes straining and dyschezia. The diagnosis of a rectal prolapse is made based on physical examination findings. The diagnosis of rectal prolapse is sometimes difficult to distinguish from small intestinal intussusception. In rare cases, the intussusception can invaginate through the large bowel, rectum, and anus. The two entities are distinguished from one another by inserting a lubricated thermometer or blunt probe into the cul-de-sac formed by the junction of the prolapsed mucosa and mucocutaneous junction at the anal ring. Inability to insert the probe or thermometer indicates that the rectal mucosa is prolapsed. Passage of the probe signifies that the prolapsed segment is actually the intussusceptum.

Treatment can be performed easily if the prolapse is acute and the rectal mucosa is not too irritated or edematous. The presence of severely necrotic tissue warrants surgical intervention. To reduce an acute rectal prolapse, after placing the patient under general anesthesia, lubricate the prolapsed tissue and gently push it back into the rectum, using a lubricated syringe or syringe casing. Apply a loose purse-string suture, leaving it in place for a minimum of 48 hours. De-worm the patient and administer stool softeners. If a rectal prolapse cannot be reduced, or if the tissue is nonviable, surgical intervention is warranted.

In patients in which viable tissue does not stay reduced with a purse-string suture, a colopexy can be performed during a laparotomy. First, place tension on the colon to reduce the prolapse, and then suture the colon to the peritoneum of the lateral abdominal wall with two to three rows of 2-0 or 3-0 monofilament suture material. If the prolapsed tissue is nonviable, it must be amputated. Place four stay sutures at 90-degree intervals through the wall of the prolapse at the mucocutaneous junction. Resect the prolapse distal to the stay sutures and then reestablish the rectal continuity by suturing the seromuscular layers together in one circumferential line and the mucosal layers together in the other. Replace the suture incision into the anal canal. Following surgery, de-worm the patient and administer a stool softener and analgesic drugs. Avoid using thermometers or other probes in the immediate postoperative period because they may disrupt suture lines.

ACUTE GASTRITIS

Acute gastritis may be associated with a variety of clinical conditions, including oral hemorrhage, ingestion of highly fermentable nondigestable foods or garbage, toxins, foreign bodies, renal or hepatic failure, inflammatory bowel disease, and bacterial and viral infections. Diarrhea often accompanies or follows acute gastritis. Hemorrhagic gastroenteritis often occurs as a shock-like syndrome with a rapidly rising hematocrit level. Clinical signs of gastritis include depression, lethargy, anterior abdominal pain, excessive water consumption, vomiting, and dehydration. Differential diagnosis of acute gastritis includes pancreatitis, hepatic or renal failure, gastrointestinal obstruction, and toxicities (Box 1-44).

The diagnosis is often a diagnosis of exclusion of other causes (see preceding text). A careful and thorough examination of the vomitus may be helpful in arriving at a diagnosis. A complete blood count, serum biochemistry profile including amylase and lipase, parvovirus test (in young puppies), fecal flotation and cytology, abdominal radiographs (plain and/or contrast studies), and abdominal ultrasound may be warranted to rule out other causes of acute vomiting.

While diagnostic tests are being performed, treatment consists of withholding all food and water for a minimum of 24 hours. After calculating the patient's degree of dehydration, administer a balanced crystalloid fluid to normalize acid-base and electrolyte status. Control vomiting with antiemetics such as metoclopramide, prochlorperazine, chlorpromazine, dolasetron, and ondansetron (Table 1-37). If vomiting is accompanied by diarrhea, administer broad-spectrum antibiotics (cefazolin, 22 mg/kg IV q8h, with metronidazole, 10 mg/kg IV q8h; or ampicillin, 22 mg/kg IV q6h, with enrofloxacin, 10 mg/kg IV q24h) to decrease the risk of bacterial translocation and bacteremia/septicemia. Although antacids (famotidine, ranitidine, cimetidine) do not have a direct antiemetic effect, their use can decrease gastric acidity and esophageal irritation during vomiting. If gastritis is secondary to uremia or nonsteroidal antiinflammatory drug use, administer gastroprotectant and antiemetic drugs (ranitidine, 1 mg/kg PO q12h; sucralfate, 0.25-1 g/dog PO q8h; or omeprazole (0.5-1 mg/kg PO Q24h) to decrease acid secretion and coat areas of gastric ulceration (Table 1-37). Once food and water can be tolerated, the patient can be placed on an oral diet and medications, and intravenous fluids can be discontinued.

BOX 1-44   CAUSES OF ACUTE GASTRITIS

- Bacterial toxin
- Brain lesion
- Dietary indiscretion
- Drugs
- Food allergy
- Hepatic failure
- Infectious disease
- Renal failure
- Stress
- Toxic chemicals
- Trauma

TABLE 1-37   Antiemetic Drugs and Dosages

Drugs (Proprietary name)	Suggested dosages*
Phenothiazines	
Chlorpromazine (Thorazine)	0.2-0.5 mg/kg IM q8h, 0.05 mg/kg IV q4h, 1.0 mg/kg per rectum q8h (dog)
Prochlorperazine (Compazine)	0.1 mg/kg IM q6h, 0.5 mg/kg IV, IM q8h
Serotonin antagonists	
Dolasetron (Anzemet)	0.1-0.3 mg/kg IV q24h
Ondansetron (Zofran)	0.6-1.0 mg/kg IV q12h
Others	
Metoclopramide (Reglan)†	0.2-0.5 mg/kg SQ q8h, 1.0-2.0 mg/kg/day IV, 3 mg/kg IM q8h (dog)

*All doses apply to dogs and cats unless otherwise noted.
†Do not use until a gastrointestinal obstruction has been ruled out.

Hemorrhagic Gastroenteritis

Hemorrhagic gastroenteritis (HGE) is an acute onset of severe hemorrhagic vomiting and diarrhea most commonly observed in young small-breed dogs (e.g., Poodles, Miniature Dachshunds, Miniature Schnauzers) 2 to 4 years of age. Clinical signs develop rapidly and include vomiting and fetid diarrhea with hemorrhage, often strawberry jam–like in appearance. The hematocrit can rise from 55% to 75%. Often, the animal is extremely hypovolemic but has no apparent signs of abdominal pain. There is no known cause of HGE, although *Clostridium perfringens*, *Escherichia coli*, *Campylobacter*, and viral infections have been suggested but not consistently confirmed. Other differential diagnoses of of hematemesis and hemorrhagic diarrhea include coronavirus, parvovirus, vascular stasis, sepsis, hepatic cirrhosis with portal hypertension, and other causes of severe shock.

Immediate treatment consists of placement of a large-bore intravenous catheter and replenishment of intravascular fluid volume with crystalloid fluids (up to 90 mL/kg/hour), while carefully monitoring the patient's hematocrit and total protein.

Administer broad-spectrum antibiotics (ampicillin, 22 mg/kg IV q6h, and enrofloxacin 10 mg/kg IV q24h) because of the high risk of bacterial translocation and sepsis. Control vomiting with antiemetic drugs. Monitor the patient's platelet count and coagulation tests for impending disseminated intravascular coagulation (DIC), and administer fresh frozen plasma and heparin, as needed (see section on Disseminated Intravascular Coagulation). When vomiting has ceased for 24 hours, offer the animal small amounts of water, and then a bland diet (e.g., boiled chicken and rice or boiled ground beef and rice mixed with low-fat cottage cheese).

Pancreatitis

Pancreatitis occurs most frequently in dogs but can occur in cats as well. In dogs, the onset of pancreatitis is sometimes preceded by ingestion of a fatty meal or the administration of drugs (e.g., potassium bromide or glucocorticoids). Glucocorticoids can increase the viscosity of pancreatic secretions and induce ductal proliferation, resulting in narrowing and obstruction of the lumen of the pancreatic duct. Pancreatitis can also occur following blunt or penetrating abdominal trauma, high duodenal obstruction causing outflow obstruction of the pancreatic papilla, pancreatic ischemia, duodenal reflux, biliary disease, and hyperadrenocorticism.

In cats, acute necrotizing pancreatitis is associated with anorexia, lethargy, hyperglycemia, icterus, and sometimes acute death. Chronic pancreatitis is more common in cats and results in intermittent vomiting, anorexia, weight loss, and lethargy. Predisposing causes of chronic pancreatitis in cats include pancreatic flukes, viral infection, hepatic lipidosis, drugs, organophosphate toxicity, and toxoplasmosis.

Clinical signs of acute pancreatitis include sudden severe vomiting, abdominal pain, and lethargy. Depending on the severity of pancreatic inflammation, depression, hypotension, and systemic inflammatory response syndrome (SIRS) may be present. Subacute cases may have minimal clinical signs. Severe pancreatic edema can result in vascular changes and ischemia that perpetuates severe inflammation. Hypovolemic shock and DIC can also decrease pancreatic perfusion. Severe pancreatic edema, autolysis, and ischemia lead to pancreatic necrosis. Duodenal irritation is manifested as both vomiting and diarrhea. Pain may be localized to the right upper abdominal quadrant or may be generalized if peripancreatic saponification occurs. Differential diagnosis of pancreatitis is the same as for any other cause of vomiting.

Complications that occur in patients with severe pancreatitis include dehydration, acid-base and electrolyte abnormalities, hyperlipemia, hypotension, and localized peritonitis. Hepatic necrosis, lipidosis, congestion, and abnormal architecture can develop. Inflammatory mediators (bradykinin, phospholipase A, elastase, myocardial depressant factor, and bacterial endotoxins) stimulate the inflammatory cascade and can lead to SIRS, with severe hypotension, clotting system activation, and DIC. Electrolyte imbalances and hypovolemia secondary to vomiting all can lead to multiple organ dysfunction syndrome (MODS), and ultimately, death. If a patient survives an episode of acute pancreatitis, long-term sequelae can include diabetes mellitus. Monitor patients with recurrent pancreatitis for clinical signs of polyuria, polydipsia, polyphagia, hyperglycemia, and glucosuria.

The diagnosis of pancreatitis is based on the presence of clinical signs (which may be absent in cats), laboratory findings, and ultrasonographic evidence of pancreatic edema and increased peripancreatic echogenicity. Serum biochemistry analyses can sometimes support a diagnosis of pancreatitis; however, serum amylase and lipase are often unreliable indicators of pancreatitis, depending on the chronicity of the process in the individual patient. Both serum amylase and lipase are excreted in the urine. Impaired renal clearance/function can cause artifactual elevations of serum amylase and lipase in the absence of pancreatic inflammation. Furthermore, serum lipase levels can be elevated as a result of gastrointestinal obstruction (e.g., foreign body). Early in the course of the disease, levels can be two to six times normal, but they may decrease to within normal ranges at the time of presentation to the veterinarian. The transient nature of amylase elevation makes this test difficult to interpret, and it is not highly sensitive if a normal value is found. Lipase levels also increase later in the course of the disease. Amylase and lipase should be tested concurrently with the rest of the biochemistry profile.

Other changes often observed are elevations in BUN and creatinine levels secondary to dehydration and prerenal azotemia, hyperglycemia, and hyperlipemia. Hypocalcemia can occur secondary to peripancreatic fat saponification, and its presence warrants a more negative prognosis. A more specific measure is pancreatic lipase immunoreactivity, which becomes elevated in dogs and cats with pancreatitis. This test, combined with ultrasonographic or computed tomography evidence of pancreatitis, is the most sensitive and specific test available for making an accurate diagnosis. However, because the results of this test take time to obtain, animals must be treated in the meantime.

Abdominal effusion or fluid from diagnostic peritoneal lavage can be compared with serum amylase and lipase activity. Abdominal lipase and amylase concentrations in the fluid greater than that in the peripheral blood are characteristic of chemical peritonitis associated with pancreatitis. WBC counts greater than 1000 cells/mm^3, the presence of bacteria, toxic neutrophils, glucose levels less than 50 mg/dL, or lactate levels greater than that of serum are characteristic of septic peritonitis, and immediate exploratory laparotomy is warranted. If a biopsy sample obtained during laparotomy does not demonstrate inflammation, but this does not rule out pancreatitis, because disease can be focal in nature and yet cause severe clinical signs.

Abdominal radiographs may sometimes reveal a loss of abdominal detail or a ground glass appearance in the right upper quadrant. Pancreatic edema and duodenal irritation can displace the gastric axis toward the left, toward the left with dorsomedial displacement of the proximal duodenum (the so-called "backwards 7" or "shepherd's crook" sign). Ultrasonography and CT are more sensitive in making a diagnosis of pancreatitis.

Treatment of pancreatitis is largely supportive in nature and is designed to correct hypovolemia and electrolyte imbalances, prevent or reverse shock, maintain vital organ perfusion, alleviate discomfort and pain, and prevent vomiting (see section on Rule of Twenty). When treating pancreatitis in dogs, all food and water should be restricted. However, food should not be withheld from cats with chronic pancreatitis. Give fresh frozen plasma to replenish alpha-2-macroglobulins. Administer antiemetics such as chlorpromazine (use with caution in a hypovolemic or hypotensive patient), dolasetron, ondansetron, or metoclopramide to prevent or control vomiting. Analgesic drugs can be provided in the form of constant rate infusion (fentanyl, 3-7 µ/kg/hour IV CRI, and lidocaine, 30-50 µ/kg/minute IV CRI), intrapleural injection (lidocaine, 1-2 mg/kg q8h), or intermittent parenteral injections (morphine, 0.25-1 mg/kg SQ, IM; hydromorphone, 0.1 mg/kg IM or SQ). Because the pancreas must be rested, consider using parenteral nutrition.

ACUTE HEPATIC FAILURE

Acute hepatic failure may be associated with toxins, adverse reaction to prescription medication, and bacterial or viral infections. The most frequent clinical signs observed in a patient with acute hepatic failure are anorexia, lethargy, vomiting, icterus, bleeding, and

---

BOX 1-45   CAUSES OF ACUTE HEPATIC FAILURE

ENDOGENOUS HEPATOTOXINS
Bacterial endotoxins

ENVIRONMENTAL TOXINS
Aflatoxin
Carbon tetrachloride
Dimethylnitrosamine
Heavy metals, herbicides
Pesticides
Phosphorus
Pyrrolizidine alkaloids
Selenium

EXOGENOUS DRUGS
Acetaminophen
Arsenicals
Azathioprine
Carprofen
Griseofulvin
Halothane
Ketoconazole

Mebendazole
Methoxyflurane
Phenazopyridine
Phenytoin
Sulfonamides (trimethoprim sulfadiazine, tetracycline)

INFECTIOUS AGENTS
Infectious canine hepatitis
Salmonella spp.
Leptospira spp.
Feline infectious peritonitis virus
Toxoplasma gondii
Bacillus piliformis (Tyzzer's disease)

OTHERS
Pancreatitis
Septicemia
Inflammatory bowel disease
Acute hemolytic anemia

CNS depression or seizures (associated with hepatic encephalopathy). Differential diagnosis and causes of acute hepatic failure are listed in Box 1-45.

Diagnosis of acute hepatic failure is based on clinical signs and biochemical evidence of hepatocellular (AST, ALT) and cholestatic (Alk Phos, T Bili, GGT) enzyme elevations. Ultrasonography may be helpful in distinguishing the architecture of the liver, but unless a mass or abscess is present, cannot provide a specific diagnosis of the cause of the hepatic damage.

Management of the patient with acute hepatic failure includes correction of dehydration and acid-base and electrolyte abnormalities, as shown in the following list:

- Hypoalbuminemia: Plasma or concentrated albumin. Plasma also is an excellent source of clotting factors that can become depleted.
- Clotting abnormalities: Vitamin K_1 (2.5 mg/kg SQ or PO q8-12h) to
- Severe anemia: Fresh or stored blood
- Gastric hemorrhage: Gastroprotectant drugs (omeprazole, ranitidine, famotidine, cimetidine, sucralfate)
- Hypoglycemia: Dextrose supplementation (2.5%-5%)
- Hepatic failure, particularly when hypoglycemia is present: Broad-spectrum antibiotics (ampicillin 22 mg/kg IV q6h; with enrofloxacin, 5 mg/kg IV q24h)
- Hepatic encephalopathy: lactulose or Betadine enemas
- Cerebral edema: Mannitol (0.5-1.0 g/kg IV over 10 to 15 minutes) followed by furosemide (1 mg/kg IV 20 minutes later). Deterioration of clinical signs may signify the development of cerebral edema.

Additional Reading

Applewhite AA, Cornell KK, Selcer BA: Diagnosis and treatment of intussusception in dogs. Comp Cont Educ Pract Vet 24(2):110-126, 2002.

Applewhite AA, Hawthorne JC, Cornell KK: Complications of enteroplication for the prevention of intussusception recurrence in dogs: 35 cases (1989-1999). J Am Vet Med Assoc 219(10): 1415-1418, 2001.

Bertoy RW: Megacolon in the cat. Vet Clin North Am Small Anim Pract 32(4):901-915, 2002.

Coleman M, Robson M: Pancreatic masses following pancreatitis: pancreatic pseudocysts, necrosis and abscesses. Comp Cont Educ Pract Vet 27(2):147-154, 2005.

Ferreri JA, Hardam E, Kimmel SE, et al: Clinical differentiation of acute necrotizing from chronic nonsuppurative pancreatitis in cats: 63 cases (1996-2001). J Am Vet Med Assoc 223(4):469-474, 2003.

Holm JL, Chan DL, Rozanski EA: Acute pancreatitis in dogs. J Vet Emerg Crit Care 13(4): 201-213, 2003.

Junius G, Appeldoorn AM, Schrauwen E: Mesenteric volvulus in the dog: a retrospective study of 12 cases. J Small Anim Pract 45(2):104-107, 2004.

Kemmel SE, Washabau RJ, Drobatz KJ: Incidence and prognostic value of low plasma ionized calcium concentration in cats with pancreatitis: 46 cases (1996-1998). J Am Vet Med Assoc 219(8):1105-1109, 2001.

MacPhail C: Gastrointestinal obstruction. Clin Tech Small Anim Pract 17(4):78-183, 2002.

Mansfield CS, Jones BR: Review of feline pancreatitis. Part 2: Clinical signs, diagnosis and treatment. J Feline Med Surg 3(3):125-132, 2001.

Monnet E: Gastric dilatation-volvulus syndrome in dogs. Vet Clin North Am Small Anim Pract 33(5):987-1105, 2003.

Ruaux CG: Diagnostic approach to acute pancreatitis. Clin Tech Small Anim Pract 18(4): 245-249, 2003.

Ruaux CG: Pathophysiology of organ failure in severe acute pancreatitis in dogs. Comp Cont Educ Pract Vet 22(6):531-542, 2000.

Simpson KW: The emergence of feline pancreatitis. J Vet Intern Med 15(4):327, 2001.

Steiner J: Diagnosis of pancreatitis. Vet Clin North Am Small Anim Pract 33(5):1181-1195, 2003.

Washabau RJ: Gastrointestinal motility disorders and gastrointestinal prokinetic therapy. Vet Clin North Am Small Anim Pract 33(5):1007-1028, 2003.

Watson P, Herrtage M: Chronic pancreatitis in dogs. Vet Rec 152(11):340, 2003.

Watson PT: Exocrine pancreatic insufficiency as an end-stage of pancreatitis in 4 dogs. J Small Anim Pract 44(7):306-312, 2003.

White RN: Surgical management of constipation. J Feline Med Surg 4(3):129-138, 2002.

HYPERTENSION: SYSTEMIC

Systemic hypertension is a recognized syndrome in dogs and cats and occurs most commonly secondary to acute or chronic renal failure, and less commonly as a primary idiopathic disease entity. Risk factors for the development of systemic hypertension in dogs and cats include renal insufficiency, hyperadrenocorticism, hyperthyroidism, pheochromocytoma, diabetes mellitus, polycythemia vera, hyperaldosteronism, hypertensive encephalopathy, acromegaly, intracranial hemorrhage, and CNS trauma.

Often, systemic hypertension is diagnosed when the animal is seen by the veterinarian because of some other clinical sign, such as acute blindness, retinal detachment, hyphema, epistaxis, and CNS signs following intracranial hemorrhage. Diagnosis of systemic hypertension is often difficult in the absence of clinical signs and without performing invasive or noninvasive blood pressure monitoring. Normal blood pressure (BP) measurements in dogs and cats are listed in Table 1-38.

Hypertension is defined as a consistent elevation in systolic BP >200 mm Hg, consistent diastolic BP >110 mm Hg, and consistent mean arterial blood pressure >130 mm Hg. The effects of systemic hypertension include left ventricular hypertrophy, cerebrovascular accident, renal vascular injury, optic nerve edema, hyphema, retinal vascular tortuosity, retinal hemorrhage, retinal detachment, vomiting, neurologic defects, coma, and excessive bleeding from cut surfaces.

TABLE 1-38 Normal Blood Pressure Measurements of Dogs and Cats

Species	Systolic (mm Hg)	Diastolic (mm Hg)	Mean (mm Hg)
Dog	100-160	80-120	90-120
Cat	120-150	70-130	100-150

1

T A B L E   1 - 3 9   Drugs Used to Treat Systemic Hypertension

Drug	Canine dosage	Feline dosage
Angiotensin-converting enzyme inhibitors		
Enalapril	0.5-1.0 mg/kg PO q12-24h	0.25-0.5 mg/kg PO q12-24h
Benazepril	0.25-0.5 mg/kg PO q12-24h	Same as dog
α-Adrenergic blocker		
Prazosin	0.5-2.0 mg PO q12h	Not used
β-Adrenergic blockers		
Propranolol	2.5-10.0 mg PO q8-12h	2.5-5.0 mg PO q8-12h
Atenolol	0.25-1.0 mg/kg PO q12-24h	6.25-12.5 mg PO q12-24h
Calcium channel blockers		
Amlodipine	0.05-0.2 mg/kg PO q24h	0.625-1.25 mg PO q24h
Thiazide diuretics		
Hydrochlorothiazide	20.0-40.0 mg/kg PO q12-24h	
Loop diuretics		
Furosemide	2.0-4.0 mg/kg PO q12-24h	
Phthalazine derivatives		
Hydralazine	0.5-2.0 mg/kg PO q8-12h	2.5 mg PO q12-24h

Patients with systemic hypertension should have a thorough diagnostic work-up to determine the underlying cause. Although uncommon, hypertensive emergencies can occur with pheochromocytoma, acute renal failure, and acute glomerulonephritis. Sodium nitroprusside (1-10 µ/kg/minute IV CRI) or diltiazem (0.3-0.5 mg/kg IV given slowly over 10 minutes, followed by 15 µ/kg/minute) can be used to treat systemic hypertension. With the use of sodium nitroprusside or diltiazem, monitor carefully for hypotension.

Diagnosis is based on consistent elevations in systolic, diastolic, and/or mean arterial BP. Because many of the clinical signs associated with systemic hypertension involve hemorrhage into some closed cavity, other causes of hemorrhage, such as vasculitis, thrombocytopenia, thrombocytopathia, and hepatic or renal failure, should be investigated (see section on coagulation disorders). Diagnostic testing is based on clinical signs and index of suspicion for an underlying disease and may include a complete blood count; urinalysis; urine protein:creatinine ratio; ACTH stimulation test; thoracic and abdominal radiographs; thoracic and abdominal ultrasound; tick serology; brain CT or MRI; and assays of serum electrolytes, aldosterone concentration, T4, endogenous TSH, plasma catecholamine, and growth hormone.

Management of systemic hypertension involves treatment of the primary underlying disorder, whenever possible. Long-term adjunctive management includes sodium restriction in the form of cooked or prescription diets to decrease fluid retention. Obese animals should be placed on dietary restrictions and undergo a weight reduction program. Thiazide and loop diuretics may be used to decrease sodium retention and circulating blood volume. Alpha- and beta-adrenergic blockers may be used, but they are largely ineffective as monotherapeutic agents for treating hypertension. Calcium channel blockers and angiotensin-converting enzyme (ACE) inhibitors are the mainstay of therapy in the treatment of hypertension in dogs and cats (Table 1-39).

Additional Reading

Acierno MJ, Labato MA: Hypertension in dogs and cats. Comp Cont Educ Pract Vet 26(5):336-346, 2004.

Chastain CB, Panciera D, Elliot J, et al: Feline hypertension: clinical findings, and response to antihypertensive treatment in 30 cases. J Am Anim Pract 42(3):122-129, 2002.

Cooke KL, Snyder PS: Diagnosing hypertension in dogs and cats. Vet Med 96(2):145-149, 2001.

DeLaforcade AM, Rozanski EA: Central venous pressure and arterial blood pressure measurements. Vet Clin North Am Small Anim Pract 31(6):1163-1174, 2001.

Littman MP, Fox PR: Systemic hypertension: recognition and treatment. In Fox PR, Sisson D, Moise NS (eds): Textbook of canine and feline cardiology. 2nd Edition. WB Saunders, Philadelphia, 1999.

Selavka CM, Rozanski EA: Invasive blood pressure monitoring. In Wingfield WE (ed): Veterinary emergency medicine secrets. 2nd Edition. Hanley and Belfus, Philadelphia, 2000.

METABOLIC EMERGENCIES

DIABETIC KETOACIDOSIS

Diabetic ketoacidosis (DKA) is a potentially fatal and terminal consequence of unregulated insulin deficiency and possible glucagon excess. In the absence of insulin, unregulated lipolysis results in the beta-hydroxylation of fatty acids by abnormal hepatic metabolism. As a result, ketoacids—namely, acetoacetic acid, beta-hydroxybutyric acid, and acetone— are produced. Early in the course of the disease, patients exhibit clinical signs associated with diabetes mellitus: weight loss, polyuria, polyphagia, and polydipsia. Later, as ketoacids stimulate the chemoreceptor trigger zone, vomiting and dehydration occur, with resulting hypovolemia, hypotension, severe depression, abdominal pain, oliguria, and coma. At the time of presentation, often a strong odor of ketones (acetone) is present on the patient's breath.

Physical examination often reveals dehydration, severe depression or coma, and hypovolemic shock. In extreme cases, the patient exhibits a slow, deep Kussmaul respiratory pattern in an attempt to blow off excess CO_2 to compensate for the metabolic acidosis. A serum biochemistry profile and complete blood count often reveal prerenal azotemia, severe hyperglycemia (blood glucose >400 mg/dL), hyperosmolarity (>330 mOsm/kg), lipemia, hypernatremia (sodium >145 mEq/L), elevated hepatocellular and cholestatic enzyme activities, high anion gap, and metabolic acidosis. Although a whole body potassium deficit is usually present, the serum potassium may appear artifactually elevated in response to metabolic acidosis. With severe metabolic acidosis, potassium moves extracellularly in exchange for a hydrogen ion. Phosphorus too moves intracellularly in response to acidosis, and serum phosphorus is usually decreased. Hypophosphatemia >2 mg/dL can result in intravascular hemolysis. Urinalysis often reveals 4+ glucosuria, ketonuria, and a specific gravity of 1.030 or greater. The urine of all diabetic animals should be cultured to rule out a urinary tract infection or pyelonephritis.

Treatment of a patient with DKA presents a therapeutic challenge. Treatment is aimed at providing adequate insulin to normalize cellular glucose metabolism, correcting acid-base and electrolyte imbalances, rehydration and restoration of perfusion, correcting acidosis, providing carbohydrate sources for utilization during insulin administration, and identifying any precipitating cause of the DKA.

Obtain blood samples for a complete blood count, and serum biochemistry electrolyte profiles. Whenever possible, insert a central venous catheter for fluid infusion and procurement of repeat blood samples. Calculate the patient's dehydration deficit and maintenance fluid requirements and give appropriate fluid and electrolytes over a period of 24 hours. It is advisable to rehydrate patients with severe hyperosmolarity for a minimum of 6 hours before starting insulin administration. Use a balanced electrolyte solution (e.g., Plasmalyte-M, Normosol-R, lactated Ringer's solution) or 0.9% saline solution for maintenance and rehydration. Balanced electrolyte solutions contain small amounts of potassium and bicarbonate precursors that aid in the treatment of metabolic acidosis. Treat animals with severe metabolic acidosis with an HCO_3^- >11 mEq/L or a pH <7.1 with supplemental bicarbonate (0.25–0.5 mEq/kg). Add supplemental dextrose to the patient's fluids as a carbohydrate source during insulin infusion.

Both insulin and carbohydrates are necessary for the proper metabolism of ketone bodies in patients with DKA. The rate and type of fluid and amount of dextrose supplementation will change according to the patient's blood glucose concentration. Serum potassium will drop rapidly as the metabolic acidosis is corrected with fluid and insulin administration. Measure serum potassium every 8 hours, if possible, and supplement accordingly (see section on Fluid Therapy for chart of potassium supplementation). If the patient's potassium requirement exceeds 100 mEq/L, or if the rate of potassium infusion approaches 0.5 mEq/kg/hour in the face of continued hypokalemia, magnesium should be supplemented. Magnesium is required as a cofactor for many enzymatic processes and for normal function of the Na,K-ATPase pump. Hypomagnesemia is a common electrolyte disturbance in many forms of critical illness. Replenishing magnesium (MgCl$_2$, 0.75 mEq/kg/day IV CRI) often helps to correct the refractory hypokalemia observed in patients with DKA. Patients with hypophosphatemia that approaches 2.0 mmol/L should receive potassium phosphate (0.01-0.03 mmol/kg/hour IV CRI). When providing potassium phosphate supplementation, be aware of the additional potassium added to the patient's fluids, so as not to exceed recommended rates of potassium infusion. To determine the amount of potassium chloride (KCl) to add along with potassium phosphate (KPO$_4$), use the following formula:

$$\text{mEq K}^+ \text{ derived from KCl} = \text{Total mEq of K}^+ \text{ to be administered over 24 hours} - \text{mEq}$$

in which K$^+$ is derived from KPO$_4$

Clinical signs of severe hypophosphatemia include muscle weakness, rhabdomyolysis, intravascular hemolysis, and decreased cerebral function that can lead to depression, stupor, seizures, or coma.

Insulin administration

Regular insulin can be administered either IM or as a constant rate infusion in the treatment of patients with DKA. Subcutaneous insulin should not be administered. Because of the severe dehydration present in most patients with DKA, subcutaneous insulin is poorly absorbed and is not effective until hydration has been restored.

In the low-dose intravenous method, place regular insulin (1.1 units/kg for a cat, and 2.2 units/kg for a dog) in 250 mL of 0.9% saline solution. Run 50 mL of this mixture through the intravenous line to allow the insulin to adsorb to the plastic tubing. Administer the patient's insulin fluid rate according to blood glucose levels (Table 1-40). Adjust the patient's total fluid volume according to changes in the insulin fluid rate as necessary. In many cases, multiple bags of fluids are necessary because they must be changed when fluctuations in blood glucose concentrations occur in response to therapy. Infusion of the insulin mixture should be in a separate intravenous catheter. To replenish hydration, use a second intravenous line for the more rapid infusion of non–insulin-containing fluids.

To administer the regular insulin IM, first give 0.22 unit/kg IM and then re-check the patient's blood glucose every hour. Additional injections of regular insulin (0.11 unit/kg

TABLE 1-40 Type of Fluid and Rate of Insulin Infusion, Based on Patient's Blood Glucose Concentration, in the Treatment of Diabetic Ketoacidosis

Blood glucose (mg/dL)	Rate of insulin/0.9% NaCl infusion (mL/hour)	Other fluid type (mL/hour)
>250	10	0.9% NaCl
200-250	7	0.45% NaCl + 2.5% dextrose
150-200	5	0.45% NaCl + 2.5% dextrose
100-150	5	0.45% NaCl + 2.5% dextrose
<100	0	0.45% NaCl + 5% dextrose

IM) should be administered based on the patient's response to subsequent injections. Once the patient's blood glucose falls to 200 to 250 mg/dL, add 2.5% to 5% dextrose to the fluids to maintain the blood glucose concentration at 200 to 300 mg/dL. Continue intramuscular injection of regular insulin (0.1-0.4 unit/kg q4-6h) until the patient is rehydrated, no longer vomiting, and able to tolerate oral fluids and food without vomiting. Even in patients with intramuscular regular insulin therapy, a central venous catheter should be placed for frequent blood sample collection. As the patient begins to respond to therapy, monitor electrolytes, glucose, and acid-base status carefully. Hypokalemia, hypophosphatemia, and hypomagnesemia can occur. When the patient's hydration and acid-base status has normalized and the patient is able to tolerate oral food and water, a longer-acting insulin can be administered as for treatment of a patient with uncomplicated diabetes.

HYPEROSMOLAR NONKETOTIC DIABETES

Extreme hyperosmolarity can result in a coma, if uncorrected. In patients with diabetes mellitus, hyperglycemia and hypernatremia secondary to osmotic diuresis and free water loss can lead to severe hyperosmolarity. In dogs, normal serum osmolality is <300 mOsm/L of serum. Hyperosmolarity is expected when serum osmolality is >340 mOsm/L. If equipment for determining serum osmolarity is not available, osmolarity can be calculated by the following formula:

$$Osm/L = 2(Na + K) + (glucose/18) + (BUN/2.8)$$

Patients with severe dehydration, hyperglycemia, hypernatremia, and azotemia may experience cerebral edema without ketonemia. Treatment is directed solely at rehydrating the patient and slowly reducing blood glucose levels using a hypotonic solution such as 0.45% NaCl + 2.5% dextrose or 5% dextrose in water (D_5W). After the initial rehydration period, administer potassium supplementation conservatively.

HYPOGLYCEMIA

Red blood cells and the brain absolutely depend on the oxidation of glucose for energy. Hypoglycemia can be caused by various systemic abnormalities that can be related to intestinal malabsorption of nutrients, impaired hepatic glycogenolysis or gluconeogenesis, and inadequate peripheral utilization of glucose. Clinical signs of hypoglycemia are extremely variable and can include weakness, tremors, nervousness, polyphagia, ataxia, tachycardia, muscle twitching, incoordination, visual disturbances, and generalized seizures. Clinical signs typically occur when serum glucose levels are <60 mg/dL. The combination of the clinical signs listed previously, documentation of low serum glucose, and alleviation of clinical signs upon glucose administration is known as *Whipple's triad*.

Whenever a patient presents with hypoglycemia, consider the following important factors: the age of onset, the nature of the hypoglycemic episode (transient, persistent, or recurrent), and the pattern based on the patient's history (Box 1-46).

Treatment of hypoglycemia is directed at providing glucose supplementation and determining any underlying cause. Administer supplemental dextrose (25%-50% dextrose, 2-5 mL/kg IV; or 10% dextrose, 20 mL/kg PO) as quickly as possible. Do not attempt oral glucose supplementation in any patient having a seizure or if the airway cannot be protected. Administer intravenous fluids (e.g., Normosol-R, lactated Ringer's solution, 0.9% saline solution) with 2.5%-5% supplemental dextrose until the patient is eating and able to maintain euglycemia without supplementation. In some cases (e.g., insulinoma), eating or administration of supplemental dextrose can promote insulin secretion and exacerbate clinical signs and hypoglycemia. In cases of refractory hypoglycemia secondary to iatrogenic insulin overdose, glucagon (50 mg/kg IV bolus, then 10-40 ng/kg/minute IV CRI) can also be administered along with supplemental dextrose. To make a glucagon infusion of 1000 ng/mL, reconstitute 1 mL (1 mg/mL) of glucagon according to the manufacturer's instructions and add this amount to 1000 mL of 0.9% saline solution.

BOX 1-46 CAUSES OF HYPOGLYCEMIA	
ACCELERATED GLUCOSE REMOVAL Insulin overdose Ethanol poisoning Salicylate toxicity Propranolol Functional islet cell tumor Toxicity Oral hypoglycemic agents Renal glucosuria Hepatoma Endotoxemia **FAILURE OF GLUCOSE SECRETION** Functional hypoglycemia (nonrecognizable lesion) Neonatal hypoglycemia	"Toy breed hypoglycemia" "Hunting breed hypoglycemia" Starvation Hepatic enzyme insufficiencies Hypoadrenocorticism Hepatic insufficiency Malabsorption and starvation Large mesodermal tumors Sepsis Increased extrahepatic glucose substrate utilization Hematoma Hepatic abscess Renal failure Extrahepatic tumors

HYPOCALCEMIA: ECLAMPSIA (PUERPERAL TETANY)

The diagnosis of eclampsia (puerperal tetany) is often made on the basis of history and clinical signs. Clinical signs can become evident when total calcium decreases to <8.0 mg/dL in dogs and <7.0 mg/dL in cats. The disease is often observed in small, excitable dogs, and stress may play a complicating role in the etiology. In most bitches, the disease manifests itself 1 to 3 weeks after parturition. In some cases, however, clinical signs can develop before parturition occurs. Hypophosphatemia may accompany hypocalcemia. Clinical signs of hypocalcemia include muscle tremors or fasciculations, panting, restlessness, aggression, hypersensitivity, disorientation, muscle cramping, hyperthermia, stiff gait, seizures, tachycardia, a prolonged QT interval on ECG, polydipsia, polyuria, and respiratory arrest.

Treatment of eclampsia consists of slow, cautious calcium supplementation (10% calcium gluconate, 0.15 mg/kg IV over 30 minutes). Severe refractory tetanus can be controlled with intravenous diazepam. Supportive care includes intravenous fluid administration and cooling (see section on Hyperthermia and Heat-induced Illness). Instruct the owner to give the patient oral calcium supplements (e.g., 1 to 2 tablets of Tums bid-tid) after discharge from the hospital. Also instruct the owner about how to wean the puppies, allowing the bitch to dry up, in order to prevent recurrence. Recurrence with subsequent pregnancies is common, particularly in patients that receive calcium supplementation during gestation (Table 1-41).

HYPERCALCEMIA

Hypercalcemia can occur from a variety of causes. The GOSH DARN IT mnemonic can be used to remember the various causes of hypercalcemia in small animal patients (Box 1-47).

The gastrointestinal, renal, and nervous systems are most commonly affected, particularly when serum total calcium rises above 16.0 mg/dL. Clinical signs of severe hypercalcemia include muscle weakness, vomiting, seizures, and coma. ECG abnormalities include prolonged PR interval, rapid QT interval, and ventricular fibrillation. The most serious clinical signs are often seen when hypercalcemia is observed in combination with hyperphosphatemia or hypokalemia. Pay special attention to the "calcium × phosphorus product." If this product exceeds 70, dystrophic calcification can occur, leading to renal failure. Renal complications include polyuria, polydipsia, dehydration, and loss of renal tubular concentrating ability. Renal blood flow and the glomerular filtration rate (GFR) are impaired when serum total calcium exceeds 20 mg/dL. The extent, location, and number of renal tubular injuries are the main factors in determining whether renal damage secondary to hypercalcemia is reversible or irreversible.

TABLE 1-41 Treatment of Hypocalcemia

Drug	Preparation	Available calcium	Dosage	Comments	Time for Maximal Effect to Occur	Time for Toxic Effect to Resolve
*Parenteral calcium**						
Calcium gluconate	10% solution	9.3 mg/mL	a. Slow IV to effect (0.5–1.5 mL/kg IV) b. 5–15 mg/kg/hr IV c. 1–2 ml/kg diluted 1:1 with saline SC t.i.d.	Stop if bradycardia or shortened Q-T interval occurs; infusion to maintain normal Ca; may be given SC		
Calcium chloride	10% solution	27.2 mg/mL	5–15 mg/kg/hr IV	Only given IV, as extremely caustic perivascularly		
Oral calcium†						
Calcium carbonate	Many sizes	40% tablet	25–50 mg/kg/day	Most common calcium supplement		
Calcium lactate	325-, 650-mg tablets	13% tablet	25–50 mg/kg/day			
Calcium chloride	Powder	27.2%	25–50 mg/kg/day	May cause gastric irritation		
Calcium gluconate	Many sizes	10%	25–50 mg/kg/day			
Vitamin D						
Vitamin D₂ (ergocalciferol)	Capsules, syrup, parenteral (IM)	–	*Initial:* 4000–6000 units day *Maintenance:* 1000–2000 units/kg once daily to once weekly		5–21 days	1–18 wk
Dihydrotachysterol	Tablets, capsules, oral solution	–	*Initial:* 0.02–0.03 mg/kg/day *Maintenance:* 0.01–0.02 mg/kg q24–48h		1–7 days	1–3 wk
1,25-dihydroxyvitamin D₃ (calcitriol)	Capsules	–	2.5 mg/kg/day		1–4 days	2–24 days

*Do not mix calcium solution with bicarbonate-containing fluids, as precipitation may occur.
†Calculate dose on elemental calcium sontent.
From DiBartola SP: Fluid Therapy in Small Animal Practice, Philadelphia, WB Saunders, 1992, p 169.

BOX 1-47 CAUSES OF HYPERCALCEMIA	
• Granulomatous (fungal disease)	• Renal failure
• Osteogenic	• Neoplasia (lymphoma, multiple myeloma, osteosarcoma)
• Spurious (laboratory error)	
• Hyperparathyroidism	• Idiopathic (cats)
• Vitamin D toxicosis	• Toxins and drugs (overzealous calcium administration; thiazide diuretics)
• Addison's disease (hypoadrenocorticism)	

Emergency therapy of hypercalcemia is warranted when severe renal compromise, cardiac dysfunction, or neurologic abnormalities are present, or if no clinical signs occur but the calcium × phosphorus product exceeds 70. The treatment of choice is correction of the underlying cause of hypercalcemia, whenever possible. In some cases, the results of diagnostic tests take time, and emergency therapy should be initiated immediately, before a definitive cause of the hypercalcemia is found. Emergency management of hypercalcemia consists of reduction of serum calcium levels. Administer intravenous fluids (0.9% saline solution) to expand extracellular fluid volume and promote calciuresis. To promote diuresis, initial intravenous fluid rates should approach two to three times maintenance levels (120-180 mL/kg/day). Potassium supplementation may be required to prevent iatrogenic hypokalemia. Administration of a loop diuretic such as furosemide (2-5 mg/kg IV) will promote calcium excretion. Calcitonin (4 IU/kg IM q12h for cats and 8 IU/kg IM q24h for dogs) can be administered to decrease serum calcium levels. In severe refractory hypercalcemia secondary to cholecalciferol toxicity, more aggressive calcitonin therapy (4-7 IU/kg SQ q6-8h) can be attempted. Side effects of calcitonin treatment include vomiting and diarrhea. Alternatively, bisphosphonates (pamidronate, 1.02-2.0 mg/kg IV) are useful in rapidly reducing serum calcium concentrations.

Glucocorticosteroids reduce calcium release from the bone, decrease intestinal absorption of calcium, and promote renal calcium excretion. Administer glucocorticosteroids only after the underlying cause of hypercalcemia has been determined and appropriate therapy started. Because many forms of neoplasia can result in hypercalcemia as a paraneoplastic syndrome, empiric use of glucocorticosteroids can induce multiple drug resistance, making the tumor refractory to the effects of chemotherapeutic agents.

ACUTE ADRENOCORTICAL INSUFFICIENCY

Hypoadrenocorticism is most commonly observed in young to middle-aged female dogs, but it can occur in animals of any age, gender, and breed. Clinical signs, which are referable to deficiency in glucocorticoid (cortisol) and mineralocorticoid (aldosterone) hormones, may develop slowly over time, leading to a waxing and waning course; acute clinical signs occur when >90% of the adrenal functional reserve has been destroyed. In such cases, complete adrenocortical collapse can result in an addisonian crisis. Lack of aldosterone causes a lack of renal sodium and water retention, and impaired potassium excretion. The most significant clinical signs associated with hypoadrenocorticism are depression, lethargy, weakness, anorexia, shaking, shivering, vomiting, diarrhea, weight loss, abdominal pain, weakness, hypotension, dehydration, and inappropriate bradycardia (Box 1-48).

The diagnosis of hypoadrenocorticism is made based on the patient's clinical signs in combination with electrolyte abnormalities that include hyperkalemia, hyponatremia, and hypochloremia. Serum sodium concentration (115-130 mEq/L) is often greatly reduced, and serum potassium is elevated (>6.0 mEq/L). A sodium:potassium ratio of <27 is characteristic of hypoadrenocorticism, although not exactly pathognomonic. Electrocardiographic changes associated with hyperkalemia include inappropriate bradycardia, absence of p waves, elevated spiked T waves, and widened QRS complexes. Other more variable bloodwork abnormalities include a lack of a stress leukogram, eosinophilia, hypoglycemia, hyperphosphatemia, hypercalcemia, azotemia, and hypocholesterolemia. A definitive diagnosis of hypoadrenocorticism is based on an adrenocorticotropic hormone (ACTH) stimulation test.

BOX 1-48   BREED PREDISPOSITION TO HYPOADRENOCORTICISM

- Bassett Hound
- Bearded Collie
- Great Dane
- Great Pyrenees
- Portuguese Water Dog
- Standard Poodle
- West Highland White Terrier

In patients with hypoadrenocorticism, baseline cortisol levels are usually low, with a lack of appropriate cortisol release after administration of ACTH analogue. Rarely, animals with "atypical" hypoadrenocorticism lose glucocorticoid secreting ability from the zona fasciculata, but retain mineralocorticoid secretory ability from the zona glomerulosa. Atypical addisonian patients have normal serum electrolytes but still have clinical signs of vomiting, diarrhea, weakness, lethargy, inappetence, muscle wasting, and weight loss. The diagnosis is more difficult in such cases because of the presence of normal electrolytes. An ACTH stimulation test should be considered, particularly in predisposed breeds.

Treatment of hypoadrenocorticism includes placement of a large-bore intravenous catheter, infusion of intravenous crystalloid fluids (0.9% saline solution), and replenishment of glucocorticoid and mineralocorticoid hormones. Administer dexamethasone or dexamethasone–sodium phosphate (0.5-1.0 mg/kg IV). Dexamethasone will not interfere with the ACTH stimulation test, unlike other longer-acting steroids (e.g., prednisolone, methylprednisolone sodium succinate, triamcinolone). Depending on the severity of the patient's condition, consider monitoring using the Rule of Twenty. Administer antiemetics and gastroprotectant drugs to treat nausea, vomiting, and hematemesis. Give the patient broad-spectrum antibiotics (ampicillin, 22 mg/kg IV q6h) if hematochezia or hemorrhagic diarrhea is present. If severe gastrointestinal blood loss occurs, whole blood, packed red blood cells, or fresh frozen plasma may be required. Control hypoglycemia with 2.5%-5.0% dextrose. Use sodium bicarbonate, regular insulin with dextrose, or calcium gluconate to correct severe hyperkalemia with atrial standstill (see section on Atrial Standstill).

Chronic therapy for hypoadrenocorticism consists of mineralocorticoid and glucocorticosteroids supplementation for the rest of the animal's life. Mineralocorticoid supplementation can be in the form of desoxycorticosterone pivalate (DOCP) (2.2 mg/kg IM) or fludrocortisone acetate (0.1 mg/2.5-5 kg body weight daily). Fludrocortisone acetate possesses both mineralocorticoid and glucocorticoid activities and can be used as the sole daily treatment of hypoadrenocorticism. (Because fludrocortisone is poorly absorbed in some dogs, it may not completely normalize electrolyte abnormalities in these animals.) DOCP is primarily a mineralocorticoid. Give supplemental glucocorticosteroids in the form of prednis(ol)one (1-0.25 mg/kg/day).

In dogs, iatrogenic hypoadrenocorticism can be caused by abrupt discontinuation of glucocorticosteroid treatment. Long-term glucocorticosteroid supplementation can downregulate the pituitary gland's excretion of endogenous ACTH and the zona fasciculata's ability to excrete cortisol. However, the zona glomerulosa's ability to secrete aldosterone does not appear to be affected. Clinical signs of iatrogenic hypoadrenocorticism include inability to compensate for stress, weakness, lethargy, vomiting, diarrhea, and collapse. Treatment of iatrogenic hypoadrenocorticism is the same as for naturally occurring disease. Following immediate emergency treatment, the patient should be weaned slowly from exogenous glucocorticosteroid supplementation.

THYROTOXICOSIS

Severe hyperthyroidism can manifest as a medical emergency as a result of hypermetabolism. Clinical signs in affected cats with severe thyrotoxicosis include fever, severe tachycardia (heart rate >240 bpm), vomiting, hypertension, congestive heart failure with pulmonary edema, and fulminant collapse. Clinical signs typically are manifested as an end-stage of chronic debilitation associated with hyperthyroidism and are often preceded by polyphagia, weight loss, cardiac murmur, polyuria/polydipsia (PU/PD), vomiting, and diarrhea.

Treatment of thyrotoxicosis includes antagonizing the adrenergic activity by administration of a beta-adrenergic blocker (esmolol, (25-50 μ/kg/minute, or propranolol, 0.02 mg/kg/hour). Administration of glucocorticosteroids (dexamethasone, 1 mg/kg) may inhibit the conversion of thyroxine (T_4) to the active form triiodothyronine (T_3) and decrease peripheral tissue responsiveness to T_3, effectively blocking its effects. Correct hypoglycemia with supplemental dextrose (2.5%). Use care to avoid overhydration in a patient with cardiac failure or insufficiency. Start the patient on methimazole as quickly as possible and consider the use of radioactive iodine therapy.

Additional Reading

Behrend EN: Clinical approach to hypercalcemia. Vet Med 97(10):763-769, 2002.

Chastain CB, et al. Use of Pamidronate to reverse Vitamin D_3–induced toxicosis in dogs. Small Anim Clin Endocrinol 10(2):10, 2000.

Chastain CB, Panciera D, Waters C, et al: Glucagon constant rate infusion: a novel strategy for the management of hyperinsulinemic-hypoglycemic crisis in the dog. Small Anim Clin Endocrinol 10(3):18, 2000.

Connally HE: Critical care monitoring considerations for the diabetic patient. Clin Tech Small Anim Pract 17(2):73-78, 2002.

Drobatz KJ, Casey KK: Eclampsia in dogs: 31 cases (1995-1998). J Am Vet Med Assoc 217(2): 216-219, 2000.

Fincham SC, Drobatz KJ, Gillespie TN, Hess RS: Evaluation of plasma ionized magnesium concentration in 122 dogs with diabetes mellitus: a retrospective study. J Vet Intern Med 18(5):615-617, 2004.

Greco DS: Hypoadrenocorticism in dogs and cats. Vet Med 95(6):468-475, 2000.

Hostutler RA, Chew DJ, Jaeger JQ, et al: Uses and effectiveness of pamidronate disodium for treatment of dogs and cats with hypercalcemia. J Vet Intern Med 19(1):29-33, 2005.

Kerl ME: Diabetic ketoacidosis: pathophysiology and clinical and laboratory presentation. Comp Cont Educ Pract Vet 23(3):220-228, 2001.

Kerl ME. Diabetic ketoacidosis: treatment recommendations. Comp Cont Educ Pract Vet 23(4):330-339, 2001.

Koenig A, Drobatz KJ, Beale AB, King LG: Hyperglycemia, hyperosmolar syndrome in feline diabetics: 17 cases (1995-2001). J Vet Emerg Crit Care 14(1):30-40, 2004.

Lathan P, Tyler J: Canine hypoadrenocorticism: pathogenesis and treatment. Comp Cont Educ Pract Vet 27(2):110-120, 121-133, 2003.

Midkiff AM, Chew DJ, Randolf JF, et al:. Idiopathic hypercalcemia in cats. J Vet Intern Med 14(6):619-626, 2000.

Morrow CK, Volmer PA: Hypercalcemia, hyperphosphatemia, and soft issue mineralization. Comp Cont Educ Pract Vet 24(5):380-388, 2002.

Vasilopulos RJ, Mackin A: Humoral hypercalcemia of malignancy: diagnosis and treatment. Comp Cont Educ Pract Vet 25(2):128-136, 2003.

NEUROLOGIC EMERGENCIES

Four classes of neurologic injuries can seriously jeopardize a patient's life: head injuries, spinal cord and vertebral column injuries, coma, and seizure. The separate entities are discussed in this section.

HEAD INJURIES

Head injuries can be associated with skin and superficial lacerations, concussions, fractures, and hemorrhage (intracranial and extracranial). Fractures include extracranial, linear, and depressed intracranial. Hemorrhage can be extradural, intradural, subdural, subarachnoid, and intracerebral. Immediately perform a baseline physical examination of an animal with head trauma at the time of presentation to assess neurologic status and determine whether progressive deterioration exists (Table 1-42).

During the initial examination, note the patient's ABC's (airway, breathing, and circulation). If necessary, establish an airway. Always supply supplemental oxygen to maintain SpO$_2$ >90%. Place an intravenous catheter and start increments of a shock dose of intravenous fluids (1/4 of 90 mL/kg/hour for dogs: 44 mL/kg/hour for cats). In order

TABLE 1-42 **Localizing Signs in Patients Presenting with Head Trauma**

Clinical sign	Description	Anatomic location
Decerebrate rigidity	Extensor rigidity of all four limbs	Caudal midbrain, pontine, or rostral opisthotonus Cerebellar
Decerebellate	Extensor rigidity of forelimbs, tucked or flexed hind limbs, opisthotonus	Caudal cerebellar
Tetraplegia	Plegia of all four limbs	Pontomedullary or cervical spine
Hemiplegia	Plegia of front and hind limbs on same side, opposite side unaffected	Ipsilateral pontomedullary or cervical spine
Hemiparesis	Paresis of front and hind limbs on same side, opposite side unaffected	Opposite rostral brainstem or cerebrum
Torticollis or head aversion	Neck torsion, turning head and neck to one side	Contralateral midbrain-pontine tegmental

---

BOX 1-49   LEVELS OF CONSCIOUSNESS

Alertness	Alert, responsive, appropriate reaction to external stimuli
Depression	Appears lethargic and has sluggish response to external stimuli
Confusion	May appear confused or aggressive
Delirium	Vocalization, inappropriate response to external stimuli
Semicoma	Unconscious but responds to external noxious stimuli
Coma	Unconscious with no response to noxious stimuli

---

to maintain cerebral perfusion pressure, blood pressure must be normalized. If other concurrent injuries are suspected (e.g., pulmonary contusions), administer synthetic colloid fluids (Dextran-70, 5-10 mL/kg IV, or hetastarch, 5-10 mL/kg IV) to normalize blood pressure. Although the use of colloids is controversial because of their potential to leak into the calvarium, the benefits of reestablishing cerebral perfusion far outweigh the risks of their use. Hypertonic saline (7.5% NaCl, 3-5 mL/kg IV) can also be administered over 10 to 15 minutes to expand intravascular volume. Maintain blood glucose within normal reference ranges whenever possible, because hyperglycemia is a negative prognostic indicator in cases of head trauma. If tremors or seizures cause hyperthermia or increased metabolism, active cooling of the patient is warranted (see sections on Hyperthermia and Heat-Induced Injury). All patients with head trauma should receive care and monitoring based on the Rule of Twenty (see section on Rule of Twenty).

THE EMERGENCY NEUROLOGIC EXAMINATION

Examine the patient's level of consciousness, response to various stimuli, pupil size and reactivity to light, physiologic nystagmus, and cranial nerve deficits. In dogs, damage to the midbrain often produces coma and decerebrate rigidity. Initial consciousness followed by a unconsciousness or stupor usually involves an injury to the brainstem. Brainstem lesions can be caused by compressive skull fractures, extradural or subdural hematomas, or herniation through the foramen magnum from cerebral edema (Box 1-49).

The patient's pupil size and response to light can be used to localize a diagnosis and give a rough prognosis for severity of disease and possibility for return to function. Pupils can be normal in size, mydriatic, or miotic. Whenever a pupil appears miotic, direct ocular injury with uveitis or secondary miosis due to brachial plexus injury should be ruled out. The eyes should always be examined to rule out ocular trauma.

In a patient with head trauma, a change from dilated to constricted to normal pupil size is suggestive of improvement in clinical function. Bilateral mydriatic pupils that are unresponsive to light in an unconscious animal are a grave prognostic sign and usually indicate an irreversible severe midbrain contusion. Bilateral miotic pupils with normal nystagmus and ocular movements are associated with diffuse cerebral or diencephalic lesions. Miotic pupils that become mydriatic indicate a progressive midbrain lesion with a poor prognosis. Unilateral, slowly progressive pupillary abnormalities in the absence of direct ocular injury are characteristic of brainstem compression or herniation caused by progressive brain swelling. Asymmetric pupils are seen in patients with rostral brainstem lesions and can change rapidly. Unresponsive pupils that are seen in the midposition occur with brainstem lesions that extend into the medulla and are a grave sign.

Visual deficits are common with intracranial injury. Lesions that are less severe and limited to the cerebrum produce contralateral menace deficits with normal pupillary light response. Bilateral cerebral edema can cause blindness with a normal response to light if the midbrain is not disturbed. A patient that is severely depressed and recumbent may not respond to menacing gestures, even when visual pathways are intact. Ocular, optic tract, optic nerve, or optic chiasm lesions can interfere with vision and the pupillary light response. Brainstem contusion and cerebral edema may produce blindness and dilated unresponsive pupils due to disturbance of the oculomotor area.

Examine all cranial nerves carefully. Cranial nerve abnormalities can indicate direct contusion or laceration of the neurons in the brainstem or where they exit the skull. Cranial nerves that are initially normal then later lose function indicate a progressively expanding lesion. When specific cranial nerve deficits are present, the prognosis is considered guarded.

Clinical signs such as rolling to one side, torticollis, head tilt, and abnormal nystagmus are usually associated with petrosal bone or cerebellomedullary lesions that produce vestibular neuron dysfunction. Fractures of the petrosal temporal bone often cause hemorrhage and cerebrospinal fluid (CSF) leak from the external ear canal. If the lesion is limited to the membranous labyrinth, the loss of balance will be toward the injured side and the quick phase of the nystagmus will be toward the injured side.

Normal physiologic nystagmus requires that the pathway is between the peripheral vestibular neurons and the pontomedullary vestibular nuclei to the nuclei of the cranial nerves that innervate the extraocular muscles (III, IV, VI). Severe brainstem lesions disrupt this pathway. Disruption of the pathway is manifested as an inability to produce normal physiologic nystagmus by moving the patient's head from side to side. In patients with severe central nervous system depression, this reflex may not be observed.

Next, assess postural changes and motor function abilities. A loss of the normal oculocephalic ("dolls-eye") reflex is an early sign of brainstem hemorrhage and a late sign of brainstem compression and herniation.

Any intracranial injury may be accompanied by a concurrent cervical spinal cord injury. Handle animals with such injuries with extreme care to avoid causing further damage. Whenever there is uncertainty whether a spinal cord lesion exists, strap the patient down to a flat surface and obtain radiographs of the spine. At least two orthogonal views may be required to see fractures; however, do not manipulate the patient until radiography has been completed. Crosstable views, in which the Bucky is turned perpendicular to the patient's spine, with a radiograph plate secured behind the patient, may be required to minimize patient motion. In patients with cerebral lesions, hemiparesis usually resolves within 1 to 3 days.

Evaluation of cranial nerve function at frequent intervals may reveal an initial injury or a progressively expanding lesion in the brain. Signs of vestibular disorientation, marked head tilt, and abnormal nystagmus occur with contusions of the membranous labyrinth and fracture of the petrous temporal bone. Hemorrhage and cerebrospinal fluid otorrhea may be visible from the external ear canal. Rolling movements indicate an injury to the cerebellar-medullary vestibular system.

Respiratory dysfunction and abnormal respiratory patterns are sometimes observed with severe head injury. Lesions of the diencephalon produce Cheyne-Stokes respirations, in which the patient takes progressively larger and larger breaths, pauses, then takes progressively smaller and smaller breaths. Mesencephalic lesions cause hyperventilation and can result in respiratory alkalosis. Medullary lesions result in a choppy, irregular respiratory pattern. Clinical signs of respiratory dysfunction in the absence of primary respiratory damage indicate a guarded prognosis.

After injury, seizures may be associated with intracranial hemorrhage, trauma, or an expanding intracranial mass lesion. Immediately begin medical therapy to control the seizure. Administer diazepam (0.5 mg/kg IV or 0.1-0.5 mg/kg/hour IV CRI) to treat seizures. If diazepam is not effective in combination with other treatments to control intracranial edema, consider giving pentobarbital (3-25 mg/kg IV to effect). Loading doses of phenobarbital (16-20 mg/kg IV divided into 4 or 5 doses, given every 20 to 30 minutes) may be beneficial in preventing further seizures.

Severe refractory seizures or decreased mentation may be associated with cerebral edema and increased intracranial pressure. Mannitol, an osmotic diuretic, is effective at reducing cerebral edema (0.5-1.0 g/kg IV over 10 to 15 minutes). Mannitol also acts as a free radical scavenger that can inhibit the effects of cerebral ischemia-reperfusion injury. Mannitol works synergistically with furosemide (1 mg/kg IV given 20 minutes after the mannitol infusion). Corticosteroids have not been demonstrated to be beneficial in the treatment of head trauma and may induce hyperglycemia. Hyperglycemia has been shown to be a negative prognostic indicator in cases of head trauma. Also, glucocorticoids can suppress immune system function and impair wound healing. Because of the known risks and lack of known benefits of glucocorticosteroids, their use in treatment of head trauma is contraindicated.

The prognosis for any patient with severe head trauma is guarded. Management of head trauma patients may include intense nursing care for a period of weeks to months, depending on the presence and extent of concurrent injuries. If progressive loss of consciousness occurs, surgery for decompression of compressive skull injuries should be considered.

The most common injury associated with head trauma in small animals is a contusion with hemorrhage in the midbrain and pons. Subdural or extradural hemorrhage with space-occupying blood clots is uncommon. Diagnostic tests of head trauma may include skull radiographs, CT, and MRI of the brain. Special studies can help detect edema and hemorrhage in the brain and brainstem, and aid in making an accurate diagnosis and prognosis. A cerebrospinal fluid tap is contraindicated in patients with head trauma because of the risk of causing a rapid decrease in intracranial pressure and brainstem herniation. If a compressive skull fracture is present, the patient should be stabilized for surgery to remove the compression. Surgery to alleviate increased intracranial pressure is rarely performed in veterinary medicine because of the poor prognosis and results. In some cases, when a lesion can be localized to one area, 1- to 2-cm burr holes can be placed through the skull over the affected area of the cerebrum, exposing the underlying brain tissue. Blood clots can be removed through the holes. The bone flap may or may not be replaced, depending on the surgeon's preference and the degree of brain swelling.

Spinal Cord Injuries

Spinal cord injuries may be associated with trauma, disk rupture, fractures, and dislocation of the spinal column. Proceed with caution when moving a patient with suspected spinal cord injury. Avoid flexion, extension, and torsion of the vertebral column. All animals that are unconscious following a traumatic event should be considered to have cervical or thoracolumbar spinal injury until proved otherwise by radiography, CT, or MRI. The animal should be moved onto a flat surface (e.g., board, door, window, picture frame) and taped down to prevent motion and further displacement of vertebrae. Sedation with analgesics or tranquilizers may be necessary to keep the animal immobile and to minimize patient motion. Whenever possible, avoid the use of narcotics in patients with head trauma because of the risk of increasing intracranial pressure. As in other emergencies, the ABCs should be evaluated, and the patient treated for shock, hemorrhage, and respiratory compromise. Once the cardiovascular and respiratory systems have been evaluated and stabilized, a more thorough neurologic examination can be performed.

Thoracolumbar disease: herniated disks and trauma

Protrusion of an intervertebral disk indicates that the disk is bulging into the vertebral canal as a result of dorsal shifting of the nuclear pulposus disk material. Disk extrusion refers to the rupture of the outer disk membrane and extrusion of the nuclear material into the vertebral column. In dogs and cats, there are 36 intervertebral disks that potentially can cause a problem. Chondrodystrophic breeds of dogs are predisposed to endochondral ossification and include the Dachshund, Shih Tzu, French Bulldog, Bassett Hound, Welsh Corgis, American Spaniel, Beagle, Lhasa Apso, and Pekingese.

Initial examination of the patient with suspected intervertebral disk disease includes identifying the neuroanatomic location of the lesion based on clinical signs and neurologic deficits and then establishing a prognosis. The neurologic examination should be carried out without excessive manipulation of the animal. The presence of pain, edema, hemorrhage, or a visible deformity may localize an area of vertebral injury. Once an area of suspected lesion is localized based on physical examination findings, take radiographs to establish a diagnosis and to institute therapy. In most cases, the animal must receive a short-acting anesthestic for proper radiographic technique and to prevent further injury. Lateral and crosstable ventrodorsal (VD) or dorsoventral (DV) radiographs require less manipulation of the animal compared with traditional VD and DV projections. Myelography is often required to delineate the location of the herniated disk material.

Prognosis in spinal cord injury depends on the extent of the injury and the reversibility of the damage. Perception of noxious stimuli, or the presence of "deep pain," by the animal when the stimulus is applied caudal to the level of the lesion is a good sign. To apply a noxious stimulus, apply firm pressure to a toe on one of the rear limbs using a thick hemostat or a pair of pliers. Flexion or withdrawl of the limb is simply a local spinal reflex, and should not be perceived as a positive response to or patient perception of the noxious stimulus. Turning of the head, vocalization, dilation of the pupils, change in respiratory rate or character, or attempts to bite are behaviors that are more consistent with perception of the noxious stimulus. Absence of perception of the noxious stimulus ("loss of deep pain") is a very poor prognosis for return to function.

Focal lesions are usually associated with vertebral fractures and displacement of the vertebral canal. Focal lesions in one or more of the spinal cord segments from T_3 to T_4 can cause complete dysfunction of the injured tissue as a result of concussion, contusion, or laceration. The degree of structural damage cannot be determined from the neurologic signs alone. Transverse focal lesions result in paraplegia, with intact pelvic limb spinal reflexes and analgesia of the limbs and body caudal to the lesion. Clinical signs in patients with spinal injury are summarized in Table 1-43.

Treatment of spinal cord injuries

Carefully evaluate the cardiovascular and respiratory status of patients with spinal injuries. Immediately address specific injuries such as pneumothorax, pulmonary contusions, hypovolemic shock, and open wounds. If there is palpable or radiographic evidence of a vertebral lesion causing compressive injury, surgery is the treatment of choice unless the displacement has compromised most or all of the vertebral canal. Displacements through 50% to 100% of the vertebral canal are associated with a poor prognosis, particularly if deep pain is absent caudal to the lesion. In the absence of a radiographic lesion and in the presence of continued neurologic deficits, an MRI or CT scan or myelography is warranted to localize a potentially correctable lesion. Surgical exploration can be considered: with the objectives of providing spinal cord decompression by hemilaminectomy or laminectomy with removal of disk material or blood clots, realign and stabilize the vertebral column, and perform a meningotomy, if necessary. Place the patient on a backboard or other rigid surface, taped down for transport and sedated, to be transported to a surgical specialist.

TABLE 1-43	**Localizing Signs in Patients with Spinal Trauma/Injuries**
Location of lesion	**Postural and reflex change**
Cranial to C6	Spastic tetraplegia or tetraparesis
	Hyperreflexive all four limbs
	Severe injury can result in death from respiratory failure.
C6-T2	Tetraparesis or tetraplegia
	Depressed thoracic limb spinal reflexes (lower motor neuron)
	Hyperreflexive pelvic limbs (upper motor neuron)
T1-T3	Horner' syndrome (prolapsed nictitans, enophthalmos, and miosis)
T3-L3	Schiff-Sherrington syndrome (extensor rigidity of thoracic limbs, flaccid paralysis with atonia, areflexia, and analgesia of pelvic limbs)

BOX 1-50   CORTICOSTEROID DOSAGE IN ACUTE SPINAL TRAUMA*

Prednisolone sodium succinate or methylprednisolone, 20 to 30 mg/kg IV once, then 10 to 15 mg/kg IV at 3, 6, and 9 hours

*Potentially useful for injuries less than 8 hours old.
Adapted from Shores A: Spinal trauma, Vet Clin North Am Small Anim Pract 22:859, 1992.

The presence of worsening or ascending clinical signs may signify ascending-descending myelomalacia and is characteristic of a very poor prognosis.In acute spinal trauma, the use of glucocorticoids has been the mainstay of therapy; however, controversy exists about whether they actually offer any benefit. Traditional glucocorticosteroid therapy is listed in Box 1-50. More recently, the use of propylene glycol has proved to be beneficial in the treatment of acute traumatic herniated disk. High-dose glucocorticoids should only be used for the first 48 hours after initial injury. Side effects of glucocorticosteroid therapy include gastric and intestinal ulceration. The prophylactic use of gastroprotectant drugs will not prevent gastrointestinal ulcer formation; however, if signs of gastrointestinal ulcer are present, institute gastroprotectant therapy.

Management

Management of the patient with spinal cord injury includes aggressive nursing care and physical therapy. Many patients with spinal cord injury have little to no control over bladder function, which results in chronic dribbling or retention of urine and overdistention of the urinary bladder with overflow incontinence. Urinary bladder retention can lead to urinary tract infection, bladder atony, and overflow incontinence. Manual expression of the bladder several times a day may be enough to keep the bladder empty. Alternatively, place a urinary catheter to maintain patient cleanliness and to keep the bladder decompressed. (see section 5 on Urinary Catheterization).

Paralytic ileus and fecal retention are frequent complications of spinal cord injury. To help prevent constipation, provide highly digestable foods and maintain the patient's hydration with oral and intravenous fluids. Mild enemas or stool softeners can also be used to treat fecal retention. To prevent decubital ulcer formation, turn the patient every 4 to 6 hours, and use clean, dry, soft padded bedding. Apply deep muscle massage and passive range of motion exercises to prevent disuse atrophy of the muscles and dependent edema.

INJURIES TO THE PERIPHERAL NERVOUS SYSTEM

The radial nerve innervates the extensor muscles of the elbow, carpus, and digits. The radial nerve also supplies sensory innervation to the distal craniolateral surface of the forearm and the dorsal surface of the forepaw. Injuries to the radial nerve at the level of the elbow result in an inability to extend the carpus and digits. As a result, the animal walks and bears weight on the dorsal surface of the paw. There is also loss of cutaneous sensation, which leads to paw injury. Injuries to the radial nerve above the elbow (in the shoulder area) results in an inability to extend the elbow and bear weight on the affected limb. It can take weeks before the full extent of the injury and any return to function are manifested. The animal may need to be placed in a carpal flexion sling or have eventual amputation if distal limb injury or self-mutilation occurs.

BRACHIAL PLEXUS

Sciatic nerve

The sciatic nerve primarily innervates the caudal thigh muscles that flex the stifle and extend the hip. The tibial branch of the sciatic nerve innervates the caudal leg muscles that extend the tarsus and flex the digits. The tibial nerve provides the sole cutaneous sensory innervation to the plantar aspect of the paw and digits. The peroneal branch of the sciatic nerve provides the sole sensory cutaneous innervation to the dorsal surface of the paw (Table 1-44). Sciatic nerve injury may occur with pelvic fractures, particularly those that involve the body of the ileum at the greater ischiatic notch, or with sacroiliac luxations that contuse the L6 and L7 spinal nerves that pass ventral to the sacrum to contribute to the sciatic nerve. With sciatic nerve injury, there is decreased stifle flexion and overflexion of the hock (tibial nerve), and the animal walks on the dorsal surface of the paw (peroneal nerve). Clinical signs of tibial or peroneal damage are seen with femur fractures or with inadvertent injection of drugs into the caudal thigh muscles.

Femoral nerve

The femoral nerve innervates the extensor muscles of the stifle. The saphenous branch of the femoral nerve provides the sole cutaneous innervation to an area on the medial distal thigh, the leg, and the paw. The femoral nerve is protected by muscles and is rarely injured in pelvic fractures. Clinical signs of femoral nerve injury are inability to support weight on the pelvic limb, absence of a patellar reflex, and analgesia in the area of cutaneous innervation.

COMA

Coma is complete loss of consciousness, with no response to noxious stimuli. In some animals that present in a coma or stuporous state, the immediate cause will be apparent. In other cases, however, a careful and thorough diagnostic work-up must be performed. A coma scale devised to assist in the clinical evaluation of the comatose patient is shown in Table 1-45. Whenever an animal presents in a comatose state, immediately secure the

TABLE 1-44 **Localizing Signs of Patients with Forelimb Injury/Trauma**

Location of injury	Clinical signs
C6-T2 nerve roots	Radial nerve paralysis
Musculocutaneous nerve	Inability to flex the elbow
Axillary or thoracodorsal	Dropped elbow nerve
Median and ulnar nerves	Loss of cutaneous sensation on the caudal surface of the forearm and palmar and lateral surfaces of the paw; inability to flex the carpus and digits
C8-T1 nerve roots	Radial, median, or ulnar nerve injury
C6-C7 nerve roots	Musculocutaneous, suprascapular, and axillary injury
C7-T3	Horner's syndrome (miosis, enophthalmos, and prolapsed nictitans)

TABLE 1-45 Small Animal Coma Scale (SACS)*

Motor activity	
Normal gait, normal spinal reflexes	6
Hemiparesis, tetraparesis, or decerebrate activity	5
Recumbent, intermittent extensor rigidity	4
Recumbent, constant extensor rigidity	3
Recumbent, constant extensor rigidity with opisthotonus	2
Recumbent, hypotonia of muscles, depressed or absent spinal reflexes	1
Brainstem reflexes	
Normal papillary reflexes and oculocephalic reflexes	6
Slow pupillary light reflexes and normal to reduced oculocephalic reflexes	5
Bilateral unresponsive miosis with normal to reduced oculocephalic reflexes	4
Pinpoint pupils with reduced to absent oculocephalic reflexes	3
Unilateral, unresponsive mydriasis with reduced to absent oculocephalic reflexes	2
Bilateral, unresponsive mydriasis with reduced to absent oculocephalic reflexes	1
Level of consciousness	
Occasional periods of alertness and responsive to environment	6
Depression of delirium, capable of responding to environment but response may be inappropriate	5
Semicomatose, responsive to visual stimuli	4
Semicomatose, responsive to auditory stimuli	3
Semicomatose, responsive only to repeated noxious stimuli	2
Comatose, unresponsive to repeated noxious stimuli	1

*Neurologic function is assessed for each of the three categories and a grade of 1 to 6 is assigned according to the descriptions for each grade. The total score is the sum of the three category scores. This scale is designed to assist the clinician in evaluating the neurologic status of the craniocerebral trauma patient. As a guideline and according to clinical impressions, a consistent total score of 3 to 8 represents a grave prognosis, 9 to 14 a poor to guarded prognosis, and 15 to 18 a good prognosis. (Modified from the Glasgow Coma Scale used in humans.)
From Shores A: Craniocerebral trauma. In Kirk RW, ed: Current Veterinary Therapy X. Small Animal Practice. Philadelphia, WB Saunders, 1989, p 849.

airway by placing an endotracheal tube (see section on Endotracheal Intubation). If necessary, provide respiratory assistance, or at a minimum, supplemental oxygen. Control existing hemorrhage and treat shock, if present.

Take a careful and thorough history from the owner. Make careful note of any seizure, trauma, or toxin exposure, and whether prior episodes of coma have ever occurred. Perform a careful physical examination, taking note of the patient's temperature, pulse, and respiration. An elevated temperature may suggest the presence of systemic infection, such as pneumonia or hepatitis, or a brain lesion with loss of hypothalamic thermoregulatory control. Very high temperatures associated with shock and coma are often observed in animals with heat stroke (see section on Heat Stroke and Heat-Induced Illness). Circulatory collapse or barbiturate overdose can produce coma and hypothermia.

Abnormal respiratory patterns also may be observed in a comatose patient. Hypoventilation may occur with elevated intracranial pressure or barbiturate overdose. Rapid respiratory rate may be associated with pneumonia, metabolic acidosis (DKA, uremia), or brainstem injury.

Examine the skin for any bruises or external trauma. Examine the mucous membranes and make note of color and capillary refill time. Icterus with petechiae or ecchymotic hemorrhage in a comatose patient may be associated with end-stage hepatic failure and hepatic encephalopathy. Smell the patient's breath for the odor of ketones that may signify DKA or end-stage hepatic failure.

Finally, conduct a complete neurologic evaluation. The presence of asymmetric neurologic signs may suggest an intracranial mass lesion (e.g., hemorrhage, neoplasia, injury). Usually, toxicities or metabolic disturbances (e.g., DKA, hepatic encephalopathy) cause symmetric clinical signs of neurologic dysfunction, with cerebral signs predominating. In hepatic encephalopathy, pupils are usually normal in size and responsive to light. In toxicities, the pupils are abnormal in size and may be unresponsive to light.

Obtain a complete blood count, serum biochemistry profile, urinalysis, and specific tests for glucosuria and ketonuria. Findings of a drastically elevated blood glucose with glucosuria, ketonuria, and high specific gravity are characteristic of DKA. Fever and uremic encephalopathy are characterized by severe azotemia with a low urine specific gravity. If barbiturate intoxication is suspected, save urine for later toxin analysis. Evaluate urine sediment for calcium oxalate crystalluria that may indicate ethylene glycol toxicity. Calculate plasma osmolality (see following section) to check for nonketotic hyperosmolar diabetes mellitus. Elevated blood ammonia levels may be associated with hepatic encephalopathy.

Diabetic Coma

In uncontrolled diabetes mellitus, hyperosmolarity can result in clinical signs of disorientation, prostration, and coma. Plasma osmolarity can be calculated from the formula:

$$mOsm/L = 2(Na + K) + (glucose/18) + (BUN/2.8)$$

Clinical signs of hyperosmolarity can occur when the plasma osmolarity exceeds 340 mOsm/L. Treatment of DKA or nonketotic hyperosmolar syndrome is aimed at reducing ketoacid production, stimulating carbohydrate utilization, and impeding peripheral release of fatty acids. The treatment of choice is rehydration and provision of supplemental regular insulin and a carbohydrate source (see section on Diabetic Ketoacidosis). During ketosis, insulin resistance may be present. Slow rehydration with 0.9% saline solution or other balanced crystalloid fluids (e.g., Normosol-R, Plasmalyte-M, lactated Ringer's solution), should occur, with the goal of rehydration over 24 to 48 hours. Too rapid rehydration can result in cerebral edema and exacerbation of clinical signs.

Hepatic Coma

Hepatic encephalopathy (HE) is characterized by an abnormal mental state associated with severe hepatic insufficiency. The most common cause of HE is congenital or acquired

TABLE 1-46

Grade of hepatic encephalopathy	Clinical signs
1	Listlessness, depression, mental dullness
	Personality changes
	Polyuria
2	Ataxia
	Disorientation
	Compulsive pacing or circling, head-pressing
	Apparent blindness
	Personality changes
	Salivation
	Polyuria
3	Stupor
	Severe salivation
	Seizures
4	Coma

portosystemic shunts. Acute hepatic destruction can also be caused by toxins, drugs, or infectious causes. The treatment of HE is considered a medical emergency (Table 1-46). Absorption of ammonia and other nitrogenous substances from the gastrointestinal tract is thought to be one of the complicating factors in HE. Prevent absorption of ammonia and other nitrogenous substances from the gastrointestinal tract by restricting dietary protein to 15% to 20% for dogs, and to 30% to 35% (on a dry matter basis) for cats. Dietary protein should be from a nonanimal plant source (e.g., soybean) whenever possible. Caloric requirements are met with lipids and carbohydrates. Also prescribe cleansing enemas to rid the colon of residual material, and antibiotic therapy to reduce gastrointestinal tract bacteria. Neomycin (15 mg/kg q6h) can be administered as a retention enema. Metronidazole (7.5 mg/kg PO, q8-12h) or amoxicillin-clavulanate (16.25 mg PO q12h) can also be administered. Administer lactulose (2.5-5.0 mL q8h for cats; 2.5-15 mL q8h for dogs) to trap ammonia in the colon to prevent absorption (Table 1-46). Administer lactulose orally to an alert animal, or as a retention enema to a comatose animal. If lactulose is not available, Betadine retention enemas will change colonic pH and prevent ammonia absorption. A side effect of lactulose administration (PO) is soft to diarrheic stool.

EMERGENCY TREATMENT OF SEIZURES

A seizure is a transient disturbance of brain function that is sudden in onset, ceases spontaneously, and has a tendency to recur, depending on the cause. Most seizures are generalized and result in a loss of consciousness and severe involuntary contraction of the skeletal muscles, resulting in tonic-clonic limb activity and opisthotonus. Mastication, salivation, urination, and defecation are common. Partial (petit mal) seizures range from limited limb activity, facial muscle twitching, and episodic behavioral abnormalities to brief loss of consciousness. Similar clinical signs also can occur with syncopal episodes. Conduct a careful cardiac examination in any patient with a history of petit mal seizures. Seizures of any form constitute a medical emergency, particularly when they occur in clusters, or as *status epilepticus*.

Most seizures are of short duration and may have subsided by the time the animal is presented for treatment. Whenever a seizure occurs, however, it is important that the animal does not inadvertently injure itself or a bystander. It is important to evaluate whether the patient has a coexisting disease that can predispose it to seizures, such as hepatic failure, uremia, diabetes mellitus, hypoglycemia, toxin exposure, insulin-secreting tumors, and thiamine deficiency. Many toxins are responsible for clinical signs of tremors or seizures (see section on Poisons and Toxins). Treatment of a primary disease entity can help control seizures, in some cases, provided that the underlying cause is investigated and treated.

Status epilepticus, a state of continuous uncontrolled seizure activity, is a medical emergency. When an animal is in a state of status epilepticus, immediately place a lateral or medial saphenous intravenous catheter and administer diazepam (0.5 mg/kg IV) to help control the seizure. In most cases, the seizure must be controlled before a diagnostic workup is attempted. Whenever possible, however, blood samples should be collected before administration of any anticonvulsant agent because of the risk of incorrect test results. For example, the propylene glycol carrier in diazepam can cause a false-positive ethylene glycol test using an in-house testing kit.

Whenever possible, check blood glucose levels, particularly in young puppies or kittens, to evaluate and treat hypoglycemia as a cause of seizures. If hypoglycemia exists, administer 25% dextrose (1 g/kg IV). If diazepam partially controls the status epilepticus, administer a constant rate infusion (0.1 mg/kg/hour in 5% dextrose in water). Diazepam is sensitive to light, and the bag and infusion line must be covered to prevent degradation of the drug. If diazepam fails to control status epilepticus, give pentobarbital (3-25 mg/kg IV to effect). The animal's airway should be intubated and protected while the patient is kept in the drug-induced coma. Protracted cases of seizures may require mannitol and furosemide therapy to treat cerebral edema.

Administer intravenous fluids (balanced crystalloid at maintenance doses [see section on Intravenous Fluid Therapy]). The patient should be turned every 4 to 6 hours to

1

prevent atelectasis. Insert a urinary catheter for cleanliness, and place the animal on soft dry padded bedding to prevent decubital ulcer formation. Depending on the length of time that the patient is rendered unconscious, apply passive range of motion exercises and deep muscle massage to prevent disuse atrophy of the muscles and dependent or disuse edema. Monitor the patient's oxygenation and ventilation status by arterial blood gas measurement or pulse oximetry and capnometry (see Section 5 on Blood Gas, Pulse Oximetry, and Capnometry). Administer supplemental oxygen to any patient that is hypoxemic secondary to hypoventilation or other causes. Severe refractory seizures can result in the development of neurogenic pulmonary edema. Lubricate the animal's eyes every 4 hours to prevent drying out and corneal abrasions. Depending on the cause of the seizure, administer phenobarbital at a loading dose of 16 to 20 mg/kg IV given in four to five injections, every 20 to 30 minutes; make sure that the patient is rousable in between injections).

Seizures in cats often are associated with structural brain disease. The occurrence of partial focal seizures is unequivocally associated with a focal cerebral lesion and acquired structural brain disease. An initial high frequency of seizures is also a strong indication that structural brain disease is present. Seizure activity in cats may occur as mild generalized seizures or complex partial seizures and may be associated with systemic disorders such as feline infectious peritonitis virus, toxoplasmosis, *Cryptococcus* infection, lymphosarcoma, meningiomas, ischemic encephalopathy, and thiamine deficiency.

Thiamine deficiency in the cat can be a medical emergency characterized by dilated pupils, ataxic gait, cerebellar tremor, abnormal oculocephalic reflex, and seizures. Treatment consists of administration of thiamine (50 mg/day) for three days.

Additional Reading

Barnes HL, Chrisman CL, Mariani CL, Sims M, Alleman AR: Clinical signs, underlying cause, and outcome in cats with seizures: 17 cases (1997-2002). J Am Vet Med Assoc 225(11):1723-1726, 2004.

Gandini G, Cizinauskas S, Lang J, et al: Fibrocartilaginous embolism in 75 dogs: clinical findings and factors influencing the recovery rate. J Small Anim Pract 44(2):76-80, 2003.

Gordon PN, Dunphy ED, Mann FA: A traumatic emergency: handling patients with head injuries. Vet Med 98(9):788-798, 2003.

Johnson J, Murtaugh R: Craniocerebral trauma. In Bonagura J (ed): Kirk's current veterinary therapy XIII. Philadelphia, WB Saunders, 2000.

Knipe MF, Vernau KM, Hornof WJ, LeCouteur RA: Intervertebral disc extrusion in six cats. J Feline Med Surg 3(3):161-168, 2001.

Kraus K: Medical management of acute spinal cord disease. In Bonagura J, editor: Kirk's current veterinary therapy XIII. WB Saunders, Philadelphia, 2000.

Mayhew PD, McLear RC, Ziemer LS, et al: Risk factors for recurrence of clinical signs associated with thoracolumbar intervertebral disk herniation in dogs: 229 cases (1994-2000). J Am Vet Med Assoc 225(8):1231-1236, 2004.

Munana KR, Olby NJ, Sharp NJ, Skeen TM: Intervertebral disk disease in 10 cats. J Am Anim Hosp Assoc 37(4):384-389, 2001.

Olby N, Levine J, Harris T, et al: Long-term functional outcome of dogs with severe injuries of the thoracolumbar spinal cord: 87 cases (1996-2001). J Am Vet Med Assoc 222(6):762-769, 2003.

Platt SR: Feline seizure control. J Am Anim Hosp Assoc 37(6):515-517, 2001.

Platt SR, Haag M: Canine status epilepticus: a retrospective study of 50 cases J Small Anim Pract 43(4):151-153, 2002.

Saito M, Munana KR, Sharp NJ, Olby NJ: Risk factors for development of status epilepticus in dogs with idiopathic epilepsy and effects of status epilepticus on outcome and survival time: 32 cases (1990-1996). J Am Vet Med Assoc 219(5):618-623, 2001.

Sammut V: Skills Laboratory Part I: Performing a neurologic examination. Vet Med 100(2): 118-132, 2005.

Sammut V: Skills Laboratory Part II: Interpreting the results of the neurologic examination. Vet Med 100(2):136-142, 2005.

Somerville ME, Anderson SM, Gill PJ, et al: Accuracy of localization of cervical intervertebral disk extrusion or protrusion using survey radiography in dogs. J Am Anim Hosp Assoc 37(6):563-572, 2001.

Steffen F, Grasmueck S: Propofol for treatment of refractory seizures in dogs and a cat with intracranial disorders. J Small Anim Pract 41(11):496-499, 2000.

Syring RS: Assessment and treatment of central nervous system abnormalities in the emergency patient. Vet Clin North Am Small Anim Pract 35:343-358, 2005.

Syring RS, Otto CM, Drobatz KJ: Hyperglycemia in dogs and cats with head trauma: 122 cases (1997-1999). J Am Vet Med Assoc 218(7):1124-1129, 2001.

OCULAR EMERGENCIES

An ocular emergency is any serious condition that causes or threatens to cause severe pain, deformity, or loss of vision. Treat ocular emergencies immediately, within 1 to several hours after the emergency, whenever possible (Box 1-51, 1-52).

To assess the location and degree of ocular injury, perform a complete ocular examination. In some cases, short-acting sedation or general anesthesia in conjunction with topical local anesthetic may be necessary to perform the examination, because of patient discomfort and blepharospasm. The equipment listed in Box 1-53 may be necessary and may be invaluable in making an accurate diagnosis.

To perform a systematic and thorough ocular examination, first obtain a history from the owner. Has there been any prior incident of ocular disease? Is there any history of trauma or known chemical irritant or exposure? Did the owner attempt any irrigation or medical techniques prior to presentation? When was the problem first noticed? Has it changed at all since the owner noticed the problem?

After a history has been obtained, examine the patient's eyes for discharge, blepharospasm, or photophobia. If any discharge is present, note its color and consistency.

BOX 1-51   OCULAR EMERGENCIES REQUIRING IMMEDIATE THERAPY

- Penetrating injury to the globe
- Proptosis of the globe
- Glaucoma
- Corneal laceration
- Acute corneal abrasion or ulcer
- Acute iritis
- Lid laceration
- Descemetocele
- Orbital cellulitis
- Chemical burns
- Ocular foreign bodies
- Hyphema

BOX 1-52   OCULAR EMERGENCIES THAT CAN CAUSE A SUDDEN LOSS OF VISION

- Hyphema
- Traumatic lid swelling
- Exposure keratitis
- Sudden acquired retinal degeneration
- Retinal hemorrhage
- Retinal detachment
- Intracranial damage
- Vitreous hemorrhage
- Corneal edema
- Acute glaucoma
- Retinal detachment
- Retinal edema
- Traumatic avulsion of the optic nerve
- Proptosis of the globe

BOX 1-53   EQUIPMENT NEEDED TO PERFORM AN OCULAR EXAMINATION

- Loupe
- Direct ophthalmoscope
- Fine-tooth forceps
- Lacrimal probe
- Fluorescein sterile strips
- Proparacaine (0.5%)
- Short-acting mydriatics (tropicamide 1%)
- Monocular indirect ophthalmoscope
- Transilluminator
- Lid retractor
- Sterile saline eye wash in irrigation bottle
- Sterile cotton-tipped swabs
- Schiotz tonometer or Tonopen

Do not attempt to force the eyelids open if the patient is in extreme discomfort. Administer a short-acting sedative and topical local anesthetic such as 0.5% proparacaine. Note the position of the globe within its orbit. If the eye is exophthalmic, strabismus and protrusion of the third eyelid are often visible. Exposure keratitis may be present. In cases of retrobulbar or zygomatic salivary gland inflammation, the patient will resist opening the mouth and exhibit signs of discomfort or pain. Note any swelling, contusions, abrasions, or lacerations of the eyelids. Note whether the lids are able to close completely and cover the cornea. If a laceration of the lid is present, determine the depth of the laceration. Palpate the orbit for fractures, swelling, pain, crepitus, and cellulitis.

Examine the cornea and sclera for penetrating injury or foreign material. The use of lid retractors or small forceps can be very helpful in these cases. If a wound appears to penetrate completely into the globe, look for loss of uveal tissue, lens, or vitreous. Do NOT put any pressure on the globe, because intraocular herniation may result. Examine the conjunctiva for hemorrhage, chemosis, lacerations, and foreign bodies. Examine the superior and inferior conjunctival cul-de-sacs for foreign material. In such cases, placement of a topical anesthetic and use of a moistened cotton swab is invaluable to sweep the conjunctival fornix to pick up foreign bodies. Use a small, fine-tipped forceps to retract the third eyelid away from the globe and examine behind the third eyelid for foreign bodies.

Next, examine the cornea for opacities, ulcers, foreign bodies, abrasions, or lacerations. Place a small amount of fluoroescein stain mixed with sterile water or saline on the dorsal sclera. Close the eye to disperse the stain over the surface of the cornea, then flush gently with sterile saline irrigation. Examine the cornea again for any defects. A linear defect perpendicular to the long axis of the eye should alert the clinician to investigate the conjunctiva for dystechia.

Record the pupil size, shape, and response to light (both direct and consensual). Examine the anterior chamber and note its depth and whether hyphema or aqueous flare are present. Is the lens clear and is it in the normal position? Lens luxation can cause the lens tissue to touch the cornea and cause acute corneal edema. Measure intraocular pressure with a Schiotz tonometer or Tonopen. Finally, dilate the pupil and examine the posterior chamber using a direct or indirect ophthalmoscope to look for intraocular hemorrhage, retinal hemorrhage, retinal detachment, tortuous retinal vessels, optic neuritis, and inflammation.

SPECIFIC CONDITIONS AND TREATMENT

The basic surgical instruments listed in Box 1-54 may be useful in the treatment of ocular lacerations and other ophthalmic injuries:

Injuries of the eyelids

Lid laceration

Bite wounds and automobile trauma commonly cause lacerations and abrasions of the lid margins. The lids can be considered to be two-layer structures, with the anterior composed of the skin and orbicularis muscle and the posterior layer composed of the tarsus and conjunctiva. The openings of the meibomian glands in the lid margin form the approximate line separating the lids into anterior and posterior segments. Splitting the lid into

---

BOX 1-54   BASIC INSTRUMENTS FOR TREATMENT OF OCULAR EMERGENCIES

- Castroviejo or Barraquer lid speculum
- Bishop-Harmon tissue forceps
- Stevens tenotomy scissors
- Castroviejo corneal scissors
- Castroviejo needle holder; standard jaws with lock
- Beaver knife handle and No. 64 blades

- Lacrimal cannula, straight 22 gauge
- Barraquer iris repository
- Foreign body spud
- Enucleation scissors, medium curve
- Suture material: 6-0 silk, 4-0 nylon, 7-0 collagen, 6-0 ophthalmic gut, 7-0 nylon

these two segments facilitates the use of sliding skin flaps to close wound defects, if necessary.

Clean and thoroughly but gently irrigate the wound with sterile saline solution before attempting any lid laceration repair. Use sterile saline solution to irrigate the wound and conjunctiva. A 1% povidone-iodine scrub can be used on the skin, taking care to avoid getting any scrub material in the soft tissues of the eye. Drape the eye with an adhesive ocular drape, if possible, to prevent further wound contamination.

Trim the ragged wound edges, but be very conservative with tissue debridement. Leave as much tissue as possible to insure proper wound contracture with minimal lid deformity. Close a small lid wound with a figure-of-eight or two-layered simple interrupted suture of absorbable suture material or nylon in the skin. The lid margins must be absolutely apposed to prevent postoperative lid notching.

Ecchymosis of the lids

Direct blunt trauma to the eye can cause severe ecchymosis because of the excellent vascular supply of the eyelids. Other associated ocular injuries such as orbital hemorrhage, proptosis, and corneal laceration may also occur. Trauma, allergic reactions, inflammation of the sebaceous glands (hordeolum), thrombocytopenia, and vitamin K antagonist rodenticide intoxication can all cause ecchymoses of the lids.

Treat eyelid ecchymoses initially with cool compresses, followed by warm compresses. Resorption of blood can occur from 3 to 10 days after the initial insult. Ocular allergies respond well to topical application (dexamethasone ophthalmic ointment q6-8h) and systemic administration of glucocorticosteroids, along with cool compresses.

Conjunctival lacerations

In order to fully assess the conjunctiva for abnormalities, it may be necessary to carefully dissect it away from the underlying sclera. When performing this dissection, do not place undue pressure on the globe because of the risk of herniation of the intraocular contents through a scleral wound.

Repair large conjunctival lacerations with 6-0 absorbable sutures, using an interrupted or continuous pattern. Carefully approximate the margins of the conjunctiva to prevent formation of inclusion cysts. When large areas of the conjunctiva have been damaged, advancement flaps may be required to close the defect.

Subconjunctival hemorrhage

Subconjunctival hemorrhage is a common sequela of head trauma, and it may also be observed in various coagulopathies. By itself, it is not a serious problem but may signify severe underlying intraocular damage. A complete ocular examination is indicated. Other causes of subconjunctival hemorrhage include thrombocytopenia, autoimmune hemolytic anemia, hemophilia, leptospirosis, vitamin K antagonist rodenticide intoxication, severe systemic infection or inflammation, and prolonged labor (dystocia). Uncomplicated subconjunctival hemorrhage usually clears on its own within 14 days. If the conjunctiva is exposed because of swelling and hemorrhage, administer a topical protective triple antibiotic ophthalmic ointment every 6 to 8 hours until the conjunctival hemorrhage resolves.

Chemical injuries

Toxic, acid, and alkaline chemical injuries to the eye can sometimes occur. The severity of the injury caused by ocular burns depends on the concentration, type, and pH of the chemical and on the duration of exposure. Weak acids do not penetrate biologic tissue very well. The hydrogen ion precipitates the protein upon contact and therefore provides some protection to the corneal stroma and intraocular contents. Precipitation of corneal proteins produces a ground-glass appearance in the cornea.

Alkaline solutions and very strong acids penetrate tissues rapidly, causing saponification of the plasma membrane, denaturation of collagen, and vascular thrombosis within the conjunctiva, episclera, and anterior uvea.

Severe pain, blepharospasm, and photophobia are produced by exposure of free nerve endings in the corneal epithelium and conjunctiva. Severe alkaline burns cause an increase in intraocular pressure. Intraocular prostaglandins are released, and the intraocular aqueous pH increases, producing changes in the blood–aqueous barrier and secondary uveitis. Uveitis with anterior synechia formation, eventual chronic glaucoma, phthisis, secondary cataract, and corneal perforation can occur.

Healing of the corneal epithelium is usually accomplished by neovascularization and sliding and increased mitosis of the corneal epithelium. Severe stromal burns within the cornea heal by degradation and removal of necrotic debris, followed by replacement of the collagen matrix and corneal epithelial cells. The release of collagenase, endopeptidase, and cathepsins from polymorphonuclear cells serves to cause further corneal breakdown. In severe cases, only PMNs may be present, and fibroblasts may never invade the corneal stroma.

All chemical burns should be washed copiously with any clean aqueous solution available. If any sticky paste or powder is adherent to the conjunctival sac, remove it with moist cotton swabs and irrigation. Begin mydriasis and cycloplegia by topical application of 1% atropine ophthalmic drops or ointment. Start antibiotic therapy with triple antibiotic ophthalmic ointment or Gentocin ointment every 6 to 8 hours. Treat secondary glaucomas with topical carbonic anhydrase inhibitors. To avoid fibrinous adhesions and symblepharon formation, keep the conjunctival cul-de-sacs free of proteinaceous exudate that can form adhesions. Analgesics are required for pain. Oral nonsteroidal antiinflammatory agents such as carprofen, ketoprofen, meloxicam, or aspirin are recommended.

Persistent epithelial erosions may require a conjunctival flap left in place for 3 to 4 weeks or placement of a topical collagen shield (contact lens). Topical antibiotics, mydriatics, and lubricants (Lacrilube or Puralube ointment) should also be used.

Strong acid or alkali burns can result in severe corneal stromal loss. In the past, topical N-acetylcysteine (10% Mucomyst) has been recommended. This treatment is very painful. Other treatments are also available, such as ethylenediaminetetraacetic acid (EDTA) (0.2 M solution) and patient serum to inhibit mammalian collagenase activity. To prepare patient serum, obtain 10 to 12 mL of whole blood from the patient. Spin it down in a serum separator tube after a clot forms and then place the serum in a red-topped tube on the patient's cage. (The contents of the tube are viable for 4 days without refrigeration.) Apply the serum topically to the affected eye every 1 to 2 hours. Avoid using topical steroids because they inhibit fibroblast formation and corneal healing. In severe cases, if conjunctival swelling and chemosis also are present, antiinflammatory doses of oral steroids can be administered short-term. Oral steroids and nonsteroidal antiinflammatory drugs should never be administered to the patient concurrently, because of the risk of gastrointestinal ulcer and perforation.

Corneal abrasions

Corneal abrasions are associated with severe pain, blepharospasm, lacrimation, and photophobia. Animals with such intense pain are often difficult to examine until analgesia has been administered. Topical use of proparacaine (0.5% proparacaine hydrochloride) is usually sufficient to permit relaxation of the eyelids so that the eye can be examined. Using a focal source of illumination and an eye loupe, examine the cornea, inferior and superior conjunctival fornixes, and medial aspect of the nictitans for foreign bodies. Place a sterile drop of saline on a fluorescein-impregnated strip and touch the superior conjunctiva once to allow the stain to spread onto the surface of the eye. Irrigate the eye to remove excess stain and then examine the corneal surface for any areas of stain uptake. If an area of the cornea persistently remains green, there is damage to the corneal epithelium in that area.

Initial treatment consists of application of a topical mydriatic (1 drop of 1% atropine in affected eye q12h) to prevent anterior synechiae and improve cycloplegia. Triple antibiotic ointment is the treatment of choice (a ¼-inch strip in the affected eye q8h) until the ulcer heals. In some cases, nonhealing ulcers (e.g., Boxer ulcer, indolent ulcer) form in which the epithelial growth does not adhere to the underlying cornea. Gently debride the loose edges of the ulcer/erosion with a cotton swab and topical anesthesia. More severe cases in which only minimal healing has occurred after 7 days of treatment require grid keratectomy, in which a 25-gauge needle is used to gently scratch the surface of the abrasion or ulcer in the form of a grid to promote neovascularization. Apply a topical anesthetic before performing the procedure. A collagen contact lens also may be required to promote wound healing. All corneal abrasions should be reevaluated in 48 hours, and then every 4 to 7 days thereafter until they have healed.

Acute infectious keratitis

Acute infectious keratitis secondary to bacterial infection is characterized by mucopurulent ocular discharge, rapidly progressing epithelial and corneal stromal loss, inflammatory cellular infiltrates into the corneal stroma, and secondary uveitis, often with hypopyon formation. Confirmation of infectious keratitis is based on corneal scrapings and a positive Gram stain. Initial treatment for bacterial keratitis consists of systemic antibiotics and topical ciprofloxacin (0.3% eyedrops or ointment).

Penetrating corneal injury

Penetrating injuries through the cornea may result in prolapse of intraocular contents. Frequently, pieces of uveal tissue or fibrin effectively but temporarily seal the defect and permit the anterior chamber to re-form. Avoid manipulation of these wounds until the animal has been anesthetized, as struggling or excitement can promote loss or dislodgement of the temporary seal and cause the intraocular contents to be extruded.

Superficial corneal lacerations need not be sutured and can be treated the same as a superficial corneal ulcer or abrasion. If the laceration penetrates more than 50% the thickness of the cornea, or extends more than 3 to 4 mm, it should be sutured. When placing sutures in the cornea, it is helpful to use magnification. Referral to a veterinary ophthalmologist is advised. If a veterinary ophthalmologist is not available, use 7-0 or 8-0 silk, collagen, or nylon sutures on a micropoint spatula-type needle. Use a simple interrupted suture pattern and leave the sutures in place for a minimum of 3 weeks. Because many corneal lacerations are jagged and corneal edema forms, most of the wound edges cannot be tightly juxtaposed. In such cases, pull a conjunctival flap across the wound to prevent leakage of aqueous fluid. Never suture through the full thickness of the cornea; rather, the suture should pass through the mid-third of the cornea.

Following closure of the corneal wound, the anterior chamber must be re-formed to prevent anterior synechia formation with secondary glaucoma. Taking care to avoid iris injury, use a 25- or 26-gauge needle to insert sterile saline at the limbus. Any defect in the suture line will be apparent because of leakage of the fluid from the site and should be repaired.

Incarceration of uveal tissue in corneal wounds is a difficult surgical problem. Persistent incarceration of uveal tissue can result in development of a chronic wick in the cornea, a shallow anterior chamber, chronic irritation, edema, vascularization of the cornea, and intraocular infection that can lead to panophthalmitis. Referral to a veterinary ophthalmologist is strongly recommended.

Ocular foreign body

The most common foreign bodies associated with ocular injuries in small animals are birdshot, BB pellets, and glass. The site of intraocular penetration of the foreign bodies may be obscured by the eyelids. A foreign body entering the eye may penetrate the cornea and fall into the anterior chamber or become lodged in the iris. Foreign bodies may occasionally penetrate the lens capsule, producing cataracts. Some metallic high-speed foreign bodies may penetrate the cornea, iris, and lens to lodge in the posterior wall of the eye or vitreous chamber.

Direct visualization of a foreign body is the best means of localization. Examination of the eye with an indirect ophthalmoscope or biomicroscope (if available) is invaluable for locating foreign bodies. Indirect visualization of the ocular foreign body can also be achieved through radiographic techniques. Three separate views should be obtained to determine the plane of location of the foreign object. CT or MRI may prove useful, although scatter from the foreign body may make it difficult to directly visualize with these techniques. Ocular ultrasound is perhaps the most useful and refined radiographic technique for locating intraocular foreign bodies.

Before removing any foreign body from the eye, the risk and surgical danger of removing it must be weighed against the risks of leaving it in place. Metallic foreign bodies in the anterior chamber are much easier to remove than nonmagnetic ones. Attempted removal of foreign objects from the vitreous chamber of the eye has consistently produced poor results. For the best chance of recovery, ocular foreign bodies should be removed by a veterinary ophthalmologist whenever possible.

Ocular trauma

Blunt trauma to the globe can result in luxation or subluxation of the lens. The subluxated lens may move anteriorly and make the anterior chamber more shallow. Trembling of the iris (iridodonesis) may be noticed when the lens is subluxated. In complete luxation, the lens may fall totally into the anterior chamber and obstruct aqueous outflow, causing secondary glaucoma. Alternatively, the lens may be lost into the vitreous cavity. Luxation of the lens is almost always associated with rupture of the hyaloid membrane and herniation of the vitreous through the pupillary space.

Emergency surgery for lens luxation is required if the lens is entirely within the anterior chamber or incarcerated within the pupil, causing a secondary pupillary block glaucoma. Acute elevation in intraocular pressure can cause vision loss within 48 hours; thus, lens removal should be accomplished as quickly as possible. Referral to a veterinary ophthalmologist is recommended.

Severe trauma to the globe or a direct blow to the head can result in retinal or vitreous hemorrhage. There may be large areas of subretinal or intraretinal hemorrhage. Subretinal hemorrhage assumes a discrete globular form, and the blood appears reddish-blue in color. The retina is detached at the site of hemorrhage. Superficial retinal hemorrhage may assume a flame-shaped appearance, and preretinal or vitreous hemorrhage assumes a bright-red amorphous appearance, obliterating the underlying retinal architecture. Retinal and vitreous hemorrhage secondary to trauma usually resorbs spontaneously over a 2- to 3-week period. Unfortunately, vitreous hemorrhage, as it organizes, can produce vitreous traction bands that eventually produce retinal detachment.

Expulsive choroid hemorrhage can occur at the time of injury and usually leads to retinal detachment, severe visual impairment, and total loss of vision. Treatment of vitreal and retinal hemorrhage includes rest and correction of factors that may predispose to intraocular hemorrhage. More complicated cases may require vitrectomy performed by a veterinary ophthalmologist.

Hyphema

Hyphema refers to blood in the anterior chamber of the eye. The most common traumatic cause of hyphema is an automobile accident. Hyphema may also present because of penetrating ocular wounds and coagulopathies. Blood within the eye may come from the anterior or posterior uveal tract. Trauma to the eye may result in iridodialysis or a tearing of the iris at its root, permitting excessive bleeding from the iris and ciliary body. Usually, simple hyphema resolves spontaneously in 7 to 10 days and does not cause vision loss. Loss of vision following bleeding into the anterior chamber is associated with secondary ocular injuries such as glaucoma, traumatic iritis, cataract, retinal detachment, endophthalmitis, and corneal scarring.

Treatment of hyphema must be individualized, but there are severe general principles of treatment. First, stop ongoing hemorrhage and prevent further bleeding whenever possible. This may involve correction of the underlying cause, if a coagulopathy is present. Next, aid in the elimination of blood from the anterior chamber, control secondary glaucoma, and treat associated injuries, including traumatic iritis. Finally, detect and treat any late complications of glaucoma.

In most cases of traumatic hyphema, little can be done to arrest or prevent ongoing hemorrhage. It is best to restrict the animal's activity and prohibit exertion. Rebleeding can occur within 5 days, and intraocular pressure must be monitored closely. After 5 to 7 days, the blood in the anterior chamber will change color from a bright red to bluish-black ("eight-ball hemorrhage"). If total hyphema persists and intraocular pressure rises despite therapy, surgical intervention by a veterinary ophthalmologist may be necessary.

The primary route of escape of RBCs from the anterior chamber is via the anterior drainage angle. Iris absorption and phagocytosis play a minor role in the removal of blood from the anterior chamber. Because of the associated traumatic iritis in hyphema, topical administration of a glucocorticoid (1% dexamethasone drops or 1% prednisolone drops) is advised to control anterior chamber inflammation. A cycloplegic agent (1% atropine) should also be used.

The formation of fibrin in the anterior chamber of the eye secondary to hemorrhage can produce adhesions of the iris and secondary glaucoma (see section on Glaucoma Secondary to Hyphema) by blocking the trabecular network. Hyphema secondary to retinal detachment (Collie ectasia syndrome) and end-stage glaucoma are extremely difficult to treat medically and have a poor prognosis.

Proptosis

Proptosis of the globe is common secondary to trauma, particularly in brachycephalic breeds. Proptosis of the globe in dolichocephalic breeds requires a greater degree of initiating contusion than the brachycephalic breeds because the orbits are so much deeper. Therefore, secondary damage to the eye and CNS associated with proptosis of the globe may be greater in the Collie or Greyhound than in the Pug.

When proptosis occurs, carefully evaluate the cardiovascular system for evidence of hypovolemic or hemorrhagic shock. Examine the respiratory and neurologic systems. Be sure to establish an airway and treat shock, if present. Control hemorrhage and stabilize the cardiovascular system before attempting to replace the globe within its orbit or perform enucleation. During the initial management of the cardiovascular and respiratory systems, the eye should be covered with an ophthalmic grade ointment or sponges soaked in sterile saline to prevent the globe from drying out. Proptosis of the globe can be associated with serious intraocular problems including iritis, chorioretinitis, retinal detachment, lens luxation, and avulsion of the optic nerve.

Stain the surface of the eye with fluorescein to look for topical abrasions or ulcers. Carefully examine the sclera, cornea, and conjunctiva for penetrating injuries that may allow aqueous leakage. Evaluate the size, location, and response to light of the pupil. A reactive pupil is better than a mydriatic fixed pupil. Topical administration of a mydriatic (atropine 1%) to prevent persistent miosis and synechia formation is indicated, along with topical and oral antibiotics and oral analgesic therapy.

Reposition the proptosed globe with the patient under general anesthesia. Make a lateral canthotomy incision to widen the palpebral fissure. Lavage the globe with sterile saline irrigation to remove any external debris. Place a copious amount of triple antibiotic ophthalmic ointment on the surface of the eye and then gently press the globe into the orbit using the flat side of a scalpel handle or a moistened sterile surgical sponge. Do not probe the retro-orbital space with a needle or attempt to reduce intraocular pressure by paracentesis. When the globe is replaced in the orbit, close the lateral canthotomy incision with simple interrupted sutures. Place three non-penetrating mattress sutures in the lid margins but do not draw them together. Tighten the lid sutures through small pieces of a red rubber catheter or length of intravenous extension tubing to prevent the sutures from causing lid necrosis. Leave the medial canthus of the eye open in order to allow topical treatment.

Postoperative treatment is directed at preventing further iritis and preventing infection. Administer systemic broad-spectrum antibiotics (Clavamox, 16.25 mg/kg PO bid) and analgesic drugs. Apply topical triple antibiotic ophthalmic ointment (¼ inch in affected eye q6-8h) and atropine (1% in affected eye q12h) to prevent infection, cycloplegia, and anterior synechiae. Antiinflammatory doses of systemic steroids can also be added to the treatment if severe periorbital inflammation is present. Systemic steroids should never be used in conjunction with nonsteroidal antiinflammatory drugs, because of the risk of gastrointestinal ulceration and perforation.

The sutures should remain in place for a minimum of 3 weeks. After this time, remove the sutures and inspect the globe. If proptosis recurs, repeat the treatment.

Following proptosis, strabismus is common secondary to periorbital muscle injury. Even after extensive treatment, vision in the eye may still be lost. Nonvisual eyes can remain in place, but phthisis may develop.

Glaucoma secondary to hyphema

Carbonic anhydrase inhibitors such as acetazolamide and dichlorphenamide decrease aqueous secretion and may effectively reduce intraocular pressure if the trabecular outflow is still functioning at 40% of its capacity. An eye with a poorly functional trabecular outflow system will respond poorly to therapy with carbonic anhydrase inhibitors. Osmotic agents such as mannitol or glycerol may be helpful in controlling glaucoma secondary to hyphema. Reduction in vitreous chamber size can make the anterior chamber deeper and may allow increased aqueous outflow. Evacuation of blood or blood clots from the anterior chamber is not advisable unless the glaucoma cannot be controlled medically or there is no indication after a prolonged period of time that blood is being resorbed.

Tissue plasminogen activator (t-PA) has proved to be useful in may be helpful in lysing blood clots and preventing excessive fibrin formation. The t-PA is reconstituted to make a solution of 250 µ/mL, which is then frozen at −70° C in 0.5-mL aliquots. The thawed, warmed reconstituted t-PA is injected into the anterior chamber.

Blind probing of the anterior chamber of the eye and surgical intervention in an attempt to remove blood clots can cause serious complications such as rebleeding, lens luxation, iris damage, and damage to the corneal epithelium, and therefore is not advised.

Acute glaucoma

Acute glaucoma is a rise in intraocular pressure that is not compatible with normal vision. Glaucoma may present as early acute congestive or noncongestive glaucoma, or as end-stage disease. Cardinal signs of glaucoma are a sudden onset of pain, photophobia, lacrimation, deep episcleral vascular engorgement, edematous insensitive cornea, shallow anterior chamber depth, dilated unresponsive pupil, loss of visual acuity, and buphthalmia. Intraocular pressure usually exceeds 40 mm Hg but may be normal or only slightly increased if glaucoma is secondary to anterior uveitis.

Most forms of clinical glaucoma in dogs are secondary to some other intraocular problem. Primary glaucoma is recognized in some breeds, including the Bassett Hound, Cocker Spaniel, Samoyed, Bouvier des Flandres, and some Terrier breeds either from goniodysgenesis or a predisposition to lens luxation. Other common causes of acute glaucoma are anterior uveitis and intumescent lens secondary to rapid cataract development, particularly in dogs with diabetes mellitus.

Treatment involves investigation of the underlying cause of the sudden rise in intraocular pressure and rapid reduction in intraocular pressure. Permanent visual impairment is often associated with chronically buphthalmic globes or the presence of rippling or striae formation on the cornea. Referral to a veterinary ophthalmologist is recommended.

If the eye is still visual and not buphthalmic, the prognosis is favorable, depending on the cause of the acute glaucoma. Treatment to reduce intraocular pressure consists of improving aqueous outflow, reducing intraocular volume with osmotic agents, and reducing aqueous formation (Table 1-47).

The use of topical mydriatic agents in acute glaucoma is contraindicated because of the risk of making lens luxation or anterior uveitis worse. Referral to a veterinary ophthalmologist for emergency surgery is indicated in cases of iris bombe, intumescent lens, or lens subluxation.

Administer osmotic agents to reduce the size of the vitreous body and the amount of aqueous. Osmotic agents create an osmotic gradient between the intraocular fluids and the

T A B L E 1 - 4 7	Drugs Indicated for the Emergency Management of Acute Glaucoma

Osmotic agents	
Mannitol	1-2 g/kg IV over 20-60 minutes
Glycerol	1.4 g/kg PO; watch for vomiting
Carbonic anhydrase inhibitors	
Dichlorphenamide (Daranide)*	2-10 mg/kg PO q12-24h
Methazolamide (Neptazene)*	5-10 mg/kg PO q8-12h
Dorzolamide (Trusopt)*	1 drop topical q8-12h
β-*Blocker*	
Timolol maleate (Timoptic 0.25 or 0.5%)[†]	1 drop topical q12h
Prostaglandin analogue	
Latanaprost[‡]	1 drop topical q24h

*Vomiting, diarrhea, panting, staggering, and disorientation are side effects.
[†]Do not use in cats with bronchitis (asthma).
[‡]Do not use if uveitis or lens subluxation is present.

vascular bed, thus allowing osmotic removal of fluid independent of the aqueous inflow and outflow systems. If no other treatments are available, oral glycerol (50%, 0.6 mL/kg or 1.4 g/kg) can be used to effectively reduce intraocular pressure. An adverse side effect of oral glycerol treatment is protracted vomiting. Do not use glycerol in a diabetic patient. Mannitol (1-2 g/kg IV over 1 hour) also effectively reduces intraocular pressure but does not cause vomiting.

Carbonic anhydrase inhibitors can be used to reduce intraocular volume by reducing aqueous production. Oral administration of dichlorphenamide, methazolamide, and acetazolamide (2-4 mg/kg) is usually not very effective alone in reducing aqueous volume and intraocular pressure and also can cause metabolic acidosis. Topical carbonic anhydrase inhibitors appear to be more effective (dorzolamide, Trusopt) when used in conjunction with topical beta-blockers (timolol, 0.25% or 0.5% solution q8h). The most effective treatment for acute pressure reduction is use of a topical prostaglandin inhibitor (latanaprost). Usually just one or two drops effectively reduces intraocular pressure in the emergency stages, until the patient can be referred to a veterinary ophthalmologist the following day.

Additional Reading

Abrams KL: Medical and surgical management of the glaucoma patient. Clin Tech Small Anim Pract 16:71-76, 2001.

Blocker T, van der Woerdt A: The feline glaucomas: 82 cases (1995-1999). Vet Ophthalmol 4: 81-85, 2001.

Gelatt KN, Brooks DE: The canine glaucomas. In Gellatt KN (ed): Veterinary ophthalmology. 3rd Edition. Lippincott, Baltimore, 1999.

Gilger BC, Hamilton HL, Wilkie DA, et al: Traumatic ocular protrusion in dogs and cats: 84 cases. J Am Vet Med Assoc 206(8):1186-1189, 1995.

Gionfriddo JR, Powell CC: Traumatic glaucoma in a dog. Vet Med 96(11):830-836, 2001.

Grahn BH, Szentimrey D, Pharr JW, et al: Ocular and orbital porcupine quills in the dog: a review and case series. Can Vet J 36(8):488-493, 1995.

Komaromy AM, Ramsey DT, Brooks DE, et al: Hyphema: pathophysiologic considerations. Comp Cont Educ Pract Vet 21(11):1064-1069, 1999.

Mandell D: Ophthalmic emergencies. Clin Tech Small Anim Pract 15(2):94-100, 2000.

Singh A, Cullen CL, Grahn BH: Alkali burns to the right eye. Can Vet J 45(9):777-778, 2004.

van der Woerdt A: The treatment of acute glaucoma in dogs and cats. J Vet Emerg Crit Care 11(3):199-205, 2001.

ONCOLOGIC EMERGENCIES

Many clinical conditions that are presented as emergencies may be due in part or wholly to the presence of a neoplasm. Paraneoplastic signs are summarized in Table 1-48. Prompt identification of the neoplasia combined with knowledge of treatment, expected response to therapy, and long-term prognosis can aid owners and practitioners in making appropriate treatment decisions.

HEMORRHAGE OR EFFUSION

Hemorrhage or effusion can occur in any body cavity as a result of the presence of benign or malignant tumors. Tumors secrete anticoagulants to allow angiogenesis to grow unchecked. Hemorrhage often occurs as a result of rupture of a neoplasm or invasion of a neoplasm into a major vascular structure. Effusion may be the result of direct fluid production by the mass or may be due to obstruction of lymphatic or venous flow.

TABLE 1-48   Paraneoplastic Syndromes in Dogs and Cats

Paraneoplastic syndrome	Cause/Clinical signs	Tumor type	Treatment
Neutropenia	Immunosuppression, chemotherapy, leukemia and myelophthisis, fever, hypothermia	Lymphoma (stage V), leukemia, multiple myeloma	Granulocyte colony-stimulating factor (G-CSF), antibiotics
Sepsis	Cellular immune dysfunction, indwelling intravenous and urinary catheters, weakness, collapse, fever, vomiting, diarrhea, hypotension, lethargy, melena	Various	G-CSF, intravenous fluids, antibiotics
Thrombocytopenia	Decreased bone marrow production (chemotherapy, hyperestrogenism), increased destruction with microangiopathic disease, disseminated intravascular coagulation (DIC), blood loss from tumor, immune-mediated destruction, petechiae and ecchymosis	Lymphoma, multiple myeloma, hemangiosarcoma, leukemia, gastrointestinal adenocarcinoma, any tumor type	Blood transfusion, treatment of underlying disease
Anemia	Decreased bone marrow production, hemorrhage, microangiopathic disease, DIC, immune-mediated destruction, chemotherapy, weakness, lethargy, tachycardia, tachypnea	Leukemia, lymphoma, hyperestrogenemia, adenocarcinoma, thyroid carcinoma	Blood transfusion, treatment of underlying disease

Continued

TABLE 1-48   Paraneoplastic Syndromes in Dogs and Cats—cont'd

Paraneoplastic syndrome	Cause/Clinical signs	Tumor type	Treatment
Erythrocytosis	Erythropoietin production by tumor or renal hypoxia, lethargy, dementia, vomiting, renal azotemia	Renal carcinoma, lymphoma, primary polycythemia vera	Identification and treatment of underlying cause, hydroxyurea, phlebotomy
DIC	Microangiopathic syndrome	Many	Blood transfusion, heparin, fresh frozen plasma
Hypergammaglobu-linemia	Increased serum viscosity following increased immunoglobulin G production by tumor, ocular hemorrhage and retinal detachment, dementia, seizures, petechiae, bleeding, occult infection	Plasma cell tumor, multiple myeloma	Treatment of underlying cause, melphalan and prednisone
Acute tumor lysis syndrome	Acute tumor cell death after chemotherapy, acute collapse and shock, vomiting, atrial standstill from hyperkalemia, bradycardia, muscle twitching	Lymphoma, leukemia	Crystalloid fluid therapy, treatment of hyperkalemia, monitoring of electrolyte status
Hypercalcemia	Parathyroid-related peptide increased osteoclast activity; vomiting, diarrhea, constipation, polyuria/polydipsia, bradycardia, stupor, hypertension, weakness, seizures	Lymphoma, apocrine gland adenocarcinoma, multiple myeloma, mammary adenocarcinoma, parathyroid adenoma, parathyroid adenocarcinoma	Administration of 0.9% sodium chloride intravenously, prednisolone, bisphosphonates, furosemide, salmon calcitonin
Hypoglycemia	Sepsis, insulin secretion or insulin-like peptide secretion from tumor, catecholamine release, weakness, seizures	Pancreatic beta cell tumor (insulinoma), leiomyosarcoma, leiomyoma, oral melanoma, hepatoma, hepatocellular carcinoma	Surgical removal of tumor, supplemental dextrose in intravenous fluids, parathyroid hormone–related peptide, prednisone, diazoxide, propranolol

Hemorrhagic effusions in the abdominal cavity occur most commonly with neoplastic masses of the spleen or liver. The most common causes are hemangiosarcoma and hepatocellular carcinoma. Clinical signs associated with acute abdominal hemorrhage, regardless of the cause, are related to hypovolemic shock and decreased perfusion and include pale mucous membranes, tachycardia, anemia, lethargy, and acute collapse. Treatment for abdominal hemorrhage includes placement of a large-bore peripheral cephalic catheter and starting one fourth of a shock dose (90 mL/kg/hour for dogs, and 44 mL/kg/hour for cats) of intravenous crystalloid fluids, taking care to carefully monitor perfusion parameters of heart rate, capillary refill time, mucous membrane color, and blood pressure. Administer intravenous colloids such as Dextran-70, Hetastarch, and oxyglobin (5-10 mL/kg IV bolus) to restore intravascular volume and normotension. Treat severe anemia with whole blood or packed RBCs to improve oxygen-carrying capacity and oxygen delivery (see sections on Transfusion Medicine and Treatment of Shock). Confirm the presence of hemoabdomen abdominocentesis (see section on Abdominocentesis). The presence of nonclotting hemorrhagic effusion is consistent with free blood. Packed cell volume of the fluid is usually the same or higher than that of the peripheral blood. An abdominal compression bandage can be placed while further diagnostics are being performed.

In cases of acute hemoabdomen, obtain right lateral, left lateral, and ventrodorsal or dorsoventral thoracic radiographs to help rule out obvious metastasis. Monitor the patient's ECG and correct dysrhythmias as necessary (see section on Cardiac Dysrhythmias). Surgery is indicated once the patient is stabilized. In some cases, hemorrhage is so severe that the patient should be taken immediately to surgery.

When recommending surgery for a hemorrhaging intraabdominal mass, it is important to discuss likely diagnoses and long-term prognosis with the owner. Hemangiosarcoma usually involves the spleen or liver or both. The presence of free abdominal hemorrhage is associated with a malignant tumor in 80% of cases. Even when free abdominal hemorrhage is not present, the tumor is malignant in 50% of cases. Approximately 66% (two thirds) of masses in the spleen are malignant (hemangiosarcoma, lymphoma, mast cell tumor, malignant fibrous histiocytoma, leiomyosarcoma, fibrosarcoma), and approximately one third are benign (hematoma, hemangioma).

Hepatocellular carcinoma usually affects one liver lobe (usually the left), and surgery is the treatment of choice. With complete surgical excision, median survival in dogs is longer than 300 days. If diffuse disease is observed at the time of surgery, the prognosis is poor.

Nonhemorrhagic effusions are associated with mesothelioma, lymphoma, carcinomatosis, or any mass that causes vascular or lymphatic obstruction. Clinical signs of respiratory distress and abdominal distention with nonhemorrhagic effusions are usually slowly progressive in onset and not as severe as those observed with hemorrhage. Treatment is usually aimed at identification of the underlying cause.

Obtain a fluid sample via thoracocentesis or abdominocentesis. To obtain further cells for cytologic evaluation, aspirate fluid from the thoracic or abdominal mass with ultrasound guidance. Cytologic evaluation of the fluid will often elucidate the causative tumor type. An abdominal ultrasound can determine the degree of metastasis. Perform therapeutic abdominocentesis or thoracocentesis if the effusion is causing respiratory difficulty. Rapid re-accumulation of the fluid potentially can cause hypoproteinemia and hypovolemic shock.

Mesothelioma is a rare tumor most commonly observed in urban environments. In humans, mesothelioma has been associated with exposure to asbestos. It is sometimes difficult to differentiate between reactive mesothelial cells and malignant mesothelial cells. Treatment is aimed at controlling the neoplastic effusion. Intracavitary cisplatin has been demonstrated to slow rates of fluid re-accumulation, but is largely a palliative therapy. Lymphoma is another tumor type that can cause thoracic or abdominal effusion. Cytologic evaluation of the fluid usually reveals abundant lymphoblasts. Treatment with multiagent chemotherapy protocols, with or without adjunctive radiation therapy, can prevent tumor remission and stop fluid accumulation.

Carcinomatosis occurs as a result of diffuse seeding of the abdominal cavity with malignant carcinomas and has a poor prognosis. Carcinomatosis may occur de novo or from metastasis of a primary tumor. Treatment consists of fluid removal when respiratory difficulty occurs, with or without intracavitary cisplatin as a palliative measure. Cisplatin should never be used in cats due to fatal acute pulmonary edema.

THORACIC CAVITY

Clinical signs of hemorrhagic thoracic effusion include acute respiratory distress, anemia, hypovolemic or cardiogenic shock, and collapse. Hemorrhagic thoracic effusions are rare in association with neoplastic effusions. A notable exception is intrathoracic hemorrhage in young dogs with osteosarcoma of the rib. Hemorrhage can result when a primary lung tumor erodes through a vessel. Hemangiosarcoma of the lungs or right auricular area can also result in hemorrhagic thoracic effusion. In many cases, hemorrhage may be confined to the pericardial sac with a right auricular mass, causing a globoid cardiac silhouette on thoracic radiographs.

Treatment consists of pericardiocentesis (see section on Pericardial Effusion and Pericardiocentesis) and placement of a pericardial window, or the mass may be removed if it is in the right auricular appendage and resectable. Although surgery can resolve clinical signs of right-sided heart failure, metastatic disease often develops soon afterward.

Nonhemorrhagic thoracic effusion is more common than hemorrhagic thoracic effusion, and is caused most commonly by mesothelioma, lymphoma, carcinomatosis, and thymoma. Clinical signs develop gradually and include respiratory difficulty, cyanosis, and cough. Supplemental oxygen should be administered. In many cases, thoracocentesis can be therapeutic and diagnostic. Obtain thoracic radiographs both before and after thoracocentesis to determine whether a mass effect is present. Following identification of a cause, definitive therapy can be instituted.

Mesotheliomas are rare and are associated with diffuse serosal disease. They are more common in dogs than in cats. Effusions caused by mesotheliomas can affect the pleural or pericardial cavities. Treatment is directed at removing effusion fluid and controlling reaccumulation with use of intracavitary platinum compounds, carboplatin, and cisplatin can be used in dogs. (Cisplatin and carboplatin should never be used in cats.) Chemical or physical pleurodesis may be helpful in controlling reaccumulation of fluid, but it is very painful in small animal patients.

Thoracic effusion secondary to lymphoma often is associated with an anterior mediastinal mass. T-cell lymphoma is the most common type of mediastinal mass observed in dogs. B-cell lymphoma is associated with a decreased response to chemotherapy and shorter survival times. Treatment consists of combination chemotherapy with or without radiation therapy to decrease mass size.

Carcinomatosis is a diffuse disease of the pleural cavity that often is a result of metastasis from a primary pulmonary carcinoma or mammary adenocarcinoma. Treatment is similar to that for mesothelioma and is aimed at controlling the effusion and delaying its recurrence.

Thymomas have been documented in both dogs and cats. Dogs most commonly present with a cough, while cats present with clinical signs of respiratory distress and a restrictive respiratory pattern associated with the presence of pleural effusion. An anterior mediastinal mass is often observed on thoracic radiographs. In some cases, the pleural effusion must be drained via thoracocentesis before a mass is visible. Ultrasound-guided aspiration and cytologic evaluation of the mass reveal a malignant epithelial tumor with small lymphocytes and mast cells. Prognosis is good if the tumor can be completely excised. Treatment consists of surgical removal with or without presurgical radiation therapy to shrink the mass. Paraneoplastic syndromes of myasthenia gravis have been documented in dogs with thymomas. If megaesophagus or aspiration pneumonia is present, the prognosis is more guarded because of the high rate of complications.

NEOPLASIA CAUSING ORGAN SYSTEM OBSTRUCTION

Urinary tract

Obstructive lesions affecting the urinary tract can be extramural (intra-abdominal, pelvic, or retroperitoneal) or intramural (urethral, bladder, or urethral wall). Transitional cell carcinoma is the most common type of bladder tumor observed in dogs. Prostatic adenocarcinoma, or neoplasia of the sublumbar lymph nodes (lymphoma, adenocarcinoma from apocrine gland adenocarcinoma), also can cause urethral obstruction. Treatment is aimed at relieving the obstruction and then attempting to identify the cause of the disease. To alleviate the obstruction, pass a urinary catheter whenever possible. Perform cystocentesis only as a last resort because of the risk of seeding the peritoneal cavity with tumor cells if transitional cell carcinoma is the cause of the obstruction. Institute supportive therapy including intravenous fluids and correction of electrolyte abnormalities.

Plain radiographs may reveal a mass lesion or may not be helpful without double contrast cystography. Abdominal ultrasound is more sensitive in identifying a mass lesion in the urinary bladder. Masses in the pelvic urethra are difficult to visualize with ultrasonography. Double contrast cystourethrography is preferred. Once the patient is stabilized, biopsy or surgery is indicated to identify the cause of the mass and attempt resection. Urine tests for transitional cell carcinoma are available for identification of transitional cell carcinoma in the dog.

Complete surgical excision of transitional cell carcinoma or removal of benign tumors of the urinary bladder yields a favorable prognosis. Poorer prognosis is seen with incomplete excision. Many transitional cell carcinomas are located in the trigone region of the bladder and cannot be completely excised. The nonsteroidal antiinflammatory drug piroxicam is helpful in alleviating clinical signs for a reported 7-month median survival. In some dogs, cisplatin and carboplatin may delay recurrence of transitional cell carcinoma.

Tumors of the prostate gland are always malignant and occur with equal frequency in castrated and uncastrated male dogs. Diagnosis of prostatic tumors is based on ultrasonographic evidence of a mass effect or prostatomegaly and on transrectal or transabdominal aspiration or biopsy. Surgery, chemotherapy, and radiation therapy generally are unrewarding over the long term, although palliative radiation therapy may relieve clinical signs for 2 to 6 months.

Gastrointestinal obstruction

Luminal tumors of the gastrointestinal tract typically cause obstruction, with slowly progressive clinical signs including vomiting, inappetence, and weight loss, or with acute severe protracted vomiting. Extraluminal obstructive lesions usually arise from adhesions, or strangulation may occur, resulting in obstruction. Perforation of the mass through the gastric or intestinal wall can cause peritonitis. Treatment consists of initial stabilization and rehydration, evaluation for evidence of metastasis, and surgical resection of the affected area in cases of adenocarcinoma, leiomyoma, leiomyosarcoma, and obstructive or perforated lymphoma.

Gastric and intestinal adenocarcinoma are the most common gastrointestinal tumors observed in dogs. Affected animals typically have a history of anorexia, weight loss, and vomiting. Obtain an abdominal ultrasound before performing any surgery. Fine needle aspirates of the mass and adjacent lymph nodes are usually diagnostic and can determine whether there is local metastasis. Many tumors are not resectable, and metastasis occurs in approximately 70% of cases. Dogs with smaller tumors that can be resected typically have longer survival times.

Leiomyosarcomas occur in the intestines of dogs, and carry a more favorable prognosis than adenocarcinoma if the mass can be completely resected. With complete resection, the average survival time is longer than 1 year. The paraneoplastic syndrome of hypoglycemia has been observed with this tumor type.

Gastrointestinal lymphoma is the most common tumor of the gastrointestinal tract observed in cats. In comparison, it is relatively rare in dogs. Unless there is complete obstruction or perforation of the gastrointestinal tract, surgical treatment for gastrointestinal lymphoma is not indicated. Rather, multiple chemotherapy drugs are used in combination to achieve remission and resolution of the clinical signs of anorexia, weight loss, and vomiting. Treatment responses unfortunately are poor.

Mast cell tumors of the gastrointestinal tract typically are manifested as gastrointestinal ulceration and hemorrhage in up to 83% of patients. The gastrointestinal hemorrhage that occurs with mast cell tumors results from increased acid secretion as a result of histamine receptor stimulation. Treatment consists of histamine or proton pump inhibition (ranitidine, famotidine, cimetidine, or omeprazole). Bowel perforation is a rare complication.

PARANEOPLASTIC SYNDROMES

Chemotherapy-related toxicities

Many chemotherapy agents exert their effects on rapidly dividing normal and neoplastic cells. Normal tissues that are commonly affected include the bone marrow, gastrointestinal tract, skin and hair follicles, and reproductive organs. Some drugs have unique organ-specific toxicities that must be monitored. Knowledge and recognition of the expected type and onset of complications can alleviate their severity by rapid treatment, when complications occur (see Table 1-48).

Bone marrow toxicity

Neutropenia is the most common bone marrow toxicity observed secondary to chemotherapy in small animal patients (Table 1-49). In most cases, the neutropenia is dose-dependent. The nadir, or lowest neutrophil count, is typically observed 5 to 10 days after chemotherapy treatment. Once the nadir occurs, bone marrow recovery is observed, with an increase in circulating neutrophils within 36 to 72 hours (Table 1-49).

Treatment of myelosuppression is largely supportive to treat or prevent sepsis. Prophylactic antibiotics are recommended in the afebrile patient with a neutrophil count <2000/µL. Acceptable antibiotics include trimethoprim-sulfa and amoxicillin-clavulanate. Granulocyte-colony stimulating factor (G-CSF) (e.g., Neupogen) is a recombinant human product that stimulates the release of neutrophils from the bone marrow, and its use shortens the recovery time following myelosuppressive drug therapy. Disadvantages of G-CSF include antibody production in response to the drug within 4 weeks of use and its high cost. To prevent ongoing neutropenia, subsequent chemotherapy dosages should be decreased by 25%, and the interval in between treatments increased. Whenever possible, overlap of myelosuppressive drugs should be avoided.

Gastrointestinal toxicity

Acute gastrointestinal toxicity can occur within 6 to 12 hours after administration of cisplatin and actinomycin D. In many cases, pretreatment with the antiemetics metoclopramide, butorphanol, chlorpromazine, dolasetron or ondansetron can prevent chemotherapy-induced nausea and vomiting. Vomiting can also occur as a delayed side effect 3 to 5 days after treatment with doxorubicin (Adriamycin), actinomycin D, methotrexate, and Cytoxan. In delayed reactions, vomiting and diarrhea are caused by damage to intestinal crypt cells. Treatment consists of administration of antiemetics, intravenous fluids, and a bland highly digestible diet. Doxorubicin also can cause hemorrhagic colitis within 5 to 7 days of administration. Treatment includes a bland diet, metronidazole, and tylosin tartrate (Tylan Powder).

TABLE 1-49 **Classification Scheme for Myelosuppression Associated with Chemotherapy**

Degree of myelosuppression	Time of nadir	Causative agent
Mild to none	Not observed	Vincristine (low-dose), L-asparaginase, glucocorticosteroids
Moderate	7-10 days	Melphalan, cisplatin, mitoxantrone, actinomycin D
Severe	7-10 days	Doxorubicin, cyclophosphamide, vinblastine

Paralytic ileus can be observed 2 to 5 days after administration of vincristine. This side effect is more common in humans than animals and can be treated with metoclopramide once a gastrointestinal obstruction has been ruled out.

Cardiotoxicity

Doxorubicin (Adriamycin) causes a dose-dependent dilative cardiomyopathy when the cumulative dose reaches 100 to 150 mg/m^2. In many cases, however, clinical signs do not occur until the cumulative dose is 240 mg/m^2. The myocardial lesions are irreversible. Treatment of cardiac dysrhythmias is dependent on the type of dysrhythmia (see section on Treatment of Dysrhythmias). Discontinue doxorubicin and administer diuretics and positive inotropic therapy for dilative cardiomyopathy in order to delay the progression of congestive heart failure (see sections on Treatment of Congestive Heart Failure). If abnormalities are shown on electrocardiography performed before beginning therapy, substitute liposome-encapsulated doxorubicin or mitoxantrone substituted in the chemotherapy protocol. Cardioprotectant drugs such as vitamin E, selenium, and N-acetyl cysteine have shown some promise in the prevention of doxorubicin-induced cardiotoxicity.

Urinary bladder toxicity

Cyclophosphamide can cause a sterile hemorrhagic cystitis. Damage to the urinary bladder mucosa and vessels is caused by the toxic metabolite acrolein. Clinical signs of sterile hemorrhagic cystitis include a history of cyclophosphamide administration, stranguria, hematuria, and pollakiuria. Treatment for sterile hemorrhagic cystitis is discontinuation of the drug, treatment of any underlying urinary tract infection with antibiotic therapy based on susceptibility testing, and intravesicle drug administration. In extremely refractory cases, surgical debridement and cauterization of the bladder mucosa may be necessary.

Prevention of sterile hemorrhagic cystitis includes emptying the bladder frequently and administering the drug in the morning. Concurrent administration of prednisone can induce polyuria and polydipsia. If sterile hemorrhagic cystitis occurs, chlorambucil can be substituted as a chemotherapeutic agent.

Anaphylactic reactions

Anaphylactic reactions have been observed with the administration of L-asparaginase, Adriamycin, etoposide, and paclitaxel. The risk of anaphylaxis increases with repeated administration, although in some animals anaphylaxis will occur on the first exposure to the drug. Treatment consists of administration of epinephrine, diphenhydramine, famotidine, and glucocorticosteroids, as with any other life-threatening allergic reaction (see section on Treatment of Allergic Reactions). To decrease the risk of an adverse reaction, give diphenhydramine (2.2 mg/kg IM) 15 to 30 minutes before drug administration. Slowing the rate of intravenous infusion also can decrease the chance of an anaphylactic reaction.

Species-specific toxicities

Cisplatin can cause a fatal irreversible pulmonary edema in cats, even at low dosages. 5-Fluorouracil (5-FU) can cause a severe neurotoxicity in cats that results in ataxia and seizures. Never use cisplatin or 5-FU in cats.

Additional Reading

Henry CJ: Management of transitional cell carcinoma. Vet Clin North Am Small Anim Pract 33(3):597-613, 2003.

Henry CJ, Tyler JW, McEntee MC, et al: Evaluation of a bladder tumor antigen test as a screening test for transitional cell carcinoma of the lower urinary tract in dogs. Am J Vet Res 64(8):1017-1020, 2003.

Liptak JM, Brutscher SP, Monnet E, et al. Transurethral resection in the management of urethral and prostatic neoplasia in 6 dogs. Vet Surg 33(5):505-516, 2004.

Nyland TG, Wallack ST, Wisner ER: Needle tract implantation following US-guided fine-needle aspiration biopsy of transitional cell carcinoma of the bladder, urethra, and prostate. Vet Radiol Ultrasound 43(1):50- 53, 2002.

Ogilvie GK, Moore AS: Managing the Veterinary Cancer Patient. A Practice Manual. Veterinary Learning Systems, Trenton, NJ, 1997.

Rocha TA, Mauldin GN, Patnaik AK, Bergman PJ: Prognostic factors in dogs with urinary bladder carcinoma. J Vet Intern Med 14(5):486-490, 2000.

Walters JM, Connally HE, Ogilvie GK, et al: EM. Emergency complications associated with chemotherapeutics and cancer. Comp Contin Educ Pract Vet 25(9):676-688, 2003.

POISONS AND TOXINS

Poisoning cases benefit from a rapid, organized approach. Key points in this approach are giving appropriate advice over the telephone, being able to access information sources, and providing appropriate treatment. There are only a few classes of poisons that account for the majority of toxicities reported in dogs and cats.

Every veterinarian should develop a familiarity with the clinical management of rodenticide and insecticide toxicity and be prepared with antidotes on hand. Beyond the most common toxins, the spectrum of possibilities is endless, and the veterinarian must rely on appropriate information resources. It is important to have available a comprehensive source of pharmaceutical and plant identification resources.

Remarkably, considering the myriad of potentially toxic substances to which an animal can be exposed, relatively few specific antidotes are commonly used in veterinary medicine. Because of the lack of specific antidotes, the veterinarian must treat each toxicity with general methods of poison management, applying basic critical care in the treatment of specific clinical signs associated with the poison exposure or toxicity. The adage "Treat the patient, not the poison" often comes into play when the exact toxic substance is unknown, or has no specific antidote.

Advising Clients over the Phone

Before an animal arrives, the staff should be prepared to ask specific questions over the phone, and provide initial advice for clients, particularly if the animal lives some distance from the hospital (Box 1-55.)

Toxicology Resources

It is important to have access to a database of information on toxic substances. Thousands of potentially toxic substances are available on the market today. The American Society for the Prevention of Cruelty to Animals (ASPCA) Animal Poison Control Center provides direct access to veterinary toxicologists 24 hours a day, 365 days a year. For additional information, call the nearest veterinary school or emergency center (Box 1-56). Also, see Section 6 for a table of emergency hotlines.

Human poison control centers

Check your local telephone book for a poison control center listing under Emergency numbers, usually found on the front cover. Although these numbers are for human poisonings, they have access to extensive poison and toxin databases and can potentially provide useful information for veterinarians, particularly regarding antidotal substances suitable for out of the ordinary toxins and human medications. Information on the toxic ingredients in thousands of medications, insecticides, pesticides, and other registered commercial products has been confidentially placed by the government in these poison control centers. As new products are marketed, information regarding toxin ingredients is forwarded to the centers.

Internet

Various e-mail discussion lists can serve as an informative resource for practitioners, but access generally requires an initial subscription and may have the disadvantage of delayed

BOX 1-55   TELEPHONE ADVICE FOR CLIENTS*

1. Questions to ask client:
   Is your animal breathing or does it have respiratory difficulty? What is the color of the gums or tongue?
   Is your animal able to walk?
   Is there any vomiting, diarrhea, trembling, or seizures?
   Does it appear lethargic or hyperactive?
   What is the substance that your animal ingested (was exposed to)?
   Did you witness the ingestion or exposure?
   How much did the animal consume?
   How long ago was the exposure?
   Was the substance swallowed, or is it on the animal's skin or eyes?
   How is the patient acting?
   How long has the animal been acting that way?
   or
   When was the last time you saw your animal act normally?
2. First aid instructions for the client:
   Induce vomiting at home and save the vomitus. Never induce vomiting if the patient is depressed, appears comatose, or is actively seizing. If the animal has ingested a caustic substance (strong alkali or acids) or a petroleum-based product (kerosene or turpentine), NEVER recommend induction of emesis.
   Hydrogen peroxide (3% w/v†)
   5 mL = 1 tsp/10 lb of body weight
   Can repeat once if no vomiting occurs after 10 minutes
3. *Remind the owner* to bring a sample of the toxin and the vomitus in with the patient.
4. Advise the owner to *transport* the patient as rapidly as possible to the nearest veterinary hospital.

*Do not keep the client on the telephone for too long. Lengthy histories can be performed once the animal is at your hospital and you have started to initiate treatment.
†Hair dressing products sometimes have hydrogen peroxide as a 30% w/v; this concentration is not suitable for induction of emesis.

BOX 1-56   TOXICOLOGY DATABASES AND SUPPORTING RESOURCES

ASPCA ANIMAL POISON CONTROL CENTER
1-888-426-4435 or 1-800-548-2423 (inside United States)
1-888-426-4435 (outside United States)
1717 S. Philo Road, Suite #36
Urbana, IL 61802
www.napcc.aspca.org
   A flat fee of $50.00 US will be charged to a major credit card (Mastercard, Visa, Discover, or American Express).
Be ready to provide the following information:
Your name, address, and telephone number
Animal species, age, weight, gender, and number of animals involved
Information concerning exposure (what, how much, how long ago)
Clinical signs and onset of clinical signs after exposure

TEXTBOOKS
There are several excellent veterinary textbooks that provide detailed information on specific toxins:
Gfeller RW, Messonier SP: *Handbook of small animal toxicology and poisoning,* St Louis, 1997, Mosby-Year Book; Veterinary Software Publishing, 1998.
Lorgue G, Lechenet J, Riviere A: *Clinical veterinary toxicology,* Cambridge, Mass, 1996, Blackwell Science.
Plumlee KH: *Clinical veterinary toxicology,* St Louis, 2003, Mosby.

response times. They are useful for ideas on standard and long-term therapy, but not emergency stabilization. An exception to this is the Veterinary Interactive Network (VIN), which posts message board communications. Previous communications from veterinarians who treated a case with the same poison/toxin can be accessed with a subscription.

Manufacturers

Many manufacturers operate an information service about their products. If the product label or name is available, check for a telephone number that may route you to a specialist.

ESSENTIAL STEPS OF EMERGENCY TREATMENT OF TOXICITIES

There are six essential steps in treating toxicities:
1. Performing a physical examination
2. Stabilizing the patient's vital signs
3. Taking a thorough history
4. Preventing continued absorption of the toxin
5. Administering specific antidotes when available
6. Facilitating clearance or metabolism of the absorbed toxin

It is most important to provide symptomatic and supportive care both during and following emergency treatment.

The physical examination

Immediately on presentation, perform a brief but thorough physical examination. Obtain a minimum database as well as serum, urine, or orogastric lavage samples for later toxicologic analyses. It is important at this time to systematically evaluate the patient's physical status, focusing particularly on the toxins most common to a particular geographic location and the organ systems most commonly affected by toxins in veterinary medicine—namely, the neurologic and gastrointestinal tracts. A checklist is useful when performing a complete physical examination (Box 1-57).

Minimum database

The minimium database includes a urine sample, packed cell volume, total protein, serum urea, and serum glucose. The information obtained from these simple cage-side tests is useful for determining dehydration, hemoconcentration, azotemia (renal or prerenal), and hypo- or hyperglycemia. When appropriate, obtain samples for serum biochemistry profiles, serum electrolytes, blood gases, serum osmolality, a complete hemogram, and coagulation profiles. Samples of serum, urine, and any vomitus or orogastric lavage contents should be collected and saved for later toxicologic analyses as required later.

Stabilization of vital signs

Stabilization of vital signs includes four major goals of treatment: maintain respiration, maintain cardiovascular function, control CNS excitation, and control body temperature. In any patient with clinical signs of respiratory distress or respiratory dysfunction, supplemental oxygen should be administered via flow-by, oxygen hood, oxygen cage, nasal, nasopharyngeal, or transtracheal oxygen sources. Ventilatory assistance may be necessary. Irritant or corrosive substances can cause damage to the oropharyngeal mucosa to such an extent that airway obstruction occurs. When necessary, a temporary tracheostomy should be performed. Arterial blood gases, pulse oximetry, and capnometry may be required to monitor oxygenation and ventilation.

At the time of presentation, immediately place an intravenous catheter for administration of intravenous fluids, inotropes, antiarrhythmics, and antidotes, if necessary. The initial fluid of choice is a balanced crystalloid solution such as Normosol-R, Plasmalyte-M, or lactated Ringer's solution. Fluid therapy can later be changed based on the patient's acid-base and electrolyte status. Some toxins can cause severe dysrhythmias and hyper- or hypotension. Monitor blood pressure and perform ECG and correct any abnormalities according to standard therapy (see sections on Hypotension and Cardiac Dysrhythmias).

BOX 1-57   PHYSICAL EXAMINATION CHECKLIST

EYES, EARS, NOSE, AND THROAT
What is the pupil size?
What is the pupil reactivity to light?
Is the ocular examination normal?
What is the sensitivity to light or sound?
Nose: Is it moist, dry, bubbling, or frothy, or caked with dirt?
Throat: Are there any characteristic odors on the breath?
Are there any traces of foreign material on the tongue or in the crevices of the teeth or gums?
Are there petechiae or ecchymosis on the gums or bleeding from the gumline?

CARDIOVASCULAR
What is the mucous membrane color? Is it normal and pink, or dark red (injected), pale, or icteric?
What is the capillary refill time? Is it fast, normal, or slow?
What is the patient's heart rate?
Are there any pulse deficits or dysrhythmias auscultated?
What is the patient's blood pressure?
What is the quality of the femoral pulse? Is it synchronous with the heart rate, or are there dropped pulses? Is the pulse bounding, normal, thready, or not palpable?
What is the patient's electrocardiogram?

RESPIRATORY
What is the patient's respiratory rate?
What is the patient's respiratory character? Is it normal, fast, shallow, or labored?
What do you hear on thoracic auscultation? Do you hear harsh airway sounds or pulmonary crackles?

GASTROINTESTINAL AND HEPATIC
What is the patient's rectal temperature?
Is there excessive salivation?
Is there evidence of vomiting or diarrhea?
Is abdominal palpation painful?
Do the intestinal loops feel normal, or are they fluid-filled or gas-filled?
What is the color and consistency of the feces?

UROGENITAL
Is there a palpable urinary bladder?
Is there urine production?
What is the color of the urine?

MUSCULOSKELETAL AND NEUROLOGIC
What is the patient's gait?
Is the patient weak or recumbent?
Is the patient ataxic?
Does the patient display signs of hypermetria?
Are there muscle fasciculations?
Is there increased extensor tone?
What is the patient's attitude?
Score the animal's level of consciousness on a simple scale:
Alert
Responds to voice
Responds to touch
Responds to pain/noxious stimulus
Unresponsive: unconscious

INTEGUMENT
Are there wet patches that smell of a particular substance?
Is there any evidence of erythema or ulcerations?
Does the muzzle, paws, prepuce, or vulva fluoresce with a black light?

PERIPHERAL LYMPH NODES
Peripheral lymph nodes should be normal in poisonings.

Some toxins cause hemolysis, methemoglobinemia, Heinz body anemia, and coagulopathies. Whole blood, fresh frozen plasma, packed RBCs, or hemoglobin-based oxygen carriers should be available and used if necessary. Treat methemoglobinemia with a combination of ascorbic acid and N-acetylcysteine.

Many toxins affect the CNS, producing clinical signs of excitation and/or seizures. Diazepam is the drug of choice for most but not all seizures and tremors. If an animal has CNS excitation secondary to the ingestion of selective norepinephrine reuptake inhibitors, avoid using diazepam, as it can potentially exacerbate clinical signs. Muscle relaxants such as guaifenesin or methocarbamol may be required to control muscle spasm and tremors associated with some toxicities. Consider animals that are in status epilepticus because of toxin exposure at high risk. Such patients may not require the full dose of anesthetics or sedatives for seizure control. Give phenobarbital (16-20 mg/kg IV) or pentobarbital (3-25 mg/kg IV to effect) for longer-term management of seizures.

Core body temperature can easily increase or decrease secondary to increased muscle activity or coma. Animals may present as hypo- or hyperthermic, depending on the toxin ingested and the stage of toxicity. Manage hypothermia with circulating hot water or hot air blankets, or place bubble wrap or Saran wrap around the animal's peripheral extremities. Manage hyperthermia by placing lukewarm wet towels on the patient until the rectal temperature has decreased to 39.5° C (103° F). (See section on of Hyperthermia and Heat-induced Illness). If sedatives or anesthetics have been used, initial hyperthermia may initially resolve due to hypothalamic loss of thermoregulatory control, cool water bathing should not be performed.

Obtain a thorough history

When the patient is first presented to the veterinarian, have the owner complete a toxicologic history form (Figure 1-56) while the animal is being initially assessed and vital signs are being stabilized. When initial stabilization of vital signs has been accomplished, the veterinarian can discuss the patient's history with the owner. In urgent situations, the veterinarian should obtain a brief history as an initial procedure (Box 1-58).

Knowing when the animal was last seen as normal provides a time frame in which the toxic substance was most likely accessed, allowing differential diagnoses to be ranked in some order of probability by rate of onset. In eliciting a history from the owner about the animal's access to poisons, it is important not to take anything for granted. Many owners do not realize how poisonous some substances can be, such as insecticide products, garbage, cleaning chemicals, and over-the-counter drugs commonly used by humans. Many owners will deny that an animal could have ingested anything that might be toxic, not wanting to believe that the source of the toxin is within their household or property, particularly if recreational drug exposure is suspected. It is useful to phrase questions in a neutral fashion—for example, "Is such-and-such present on the premises?" rather than "Could the dog have eaten such-and-such?" If recreational drug exposure is suspected, another way to question the owners is to ask whether they have had any guests in their house recently that may have had such-and-such (e.g., marijuana, cocaine, methamphetamine). This approach serves to minimize the suggestion of any bias or preconceptions.

When questioning an owner about recent events, it is useful to realize and acknowledge that disruption in the household routine is a distinct factor in the occurrence accidents, including poisonings. Examples of such disruptive events include moving from the house, family member is ill or in the hospital, and renovations or recent construction. While these events are occurring, the safeguards followed by a normally careful owner may be disrupted. Often, doors or gates may be left open, animals may be outside instead of inside (or vice versa), and inexperienced people may be pet-sitters. Once owners are made aware of the importance of assessing such risks, they are often able to provide insight into otherwise baffling circumstances.

Prevent continued absorption of the toxin

Various methods can be used to remove toxins from the gastrointestinal tract, including emesis, orogastric lavage, cathartics, and enemas. Adsorbents, ion exchange resins, or

Toxicologic History Form

1

Date:
Time:

Patient information:
Name of animal:
Age:
Breed:
Gender and Neuter status:
Weight:
Vaccinations last given:
Any current medications (including heartworm prevention and nutriceuticals)

Today's Problem
When did you first notice that something was wrong with your pet?
When was the last time you noticed your pet act normally?
What was the first abnormal sign noticed?
What other conditions have developed and what are they?
How soon did other signs develop?
Have the signs become better or worse since you first saw them?

Information on any suspected poison
What is the name of the product?
Do you have the container with you today?
Is it a liquid concentrate, dilute spray, or solid?
How long ago do you think that your pet was exposed to the poison?
Where do you think it happened?
Do you have any over-the-counter or prescription medications that your animal may have had access to?
Did you give any medications to your animal?
Is there any possibility of recreational drug exposure?

Your pet's recent activity
Did your pet eat this morning or last night?
What is he/she normally fed?
Is there a chance that your pet may have gotten into the garbage?
Have you fed table scraps or anything new recently? If so, what?
Has your pet been off your property in the last 24-48 hours?
Does your pet run loose unattended?
Has your pet had any antiflea/tick medication within the last week?

Your pet's environment
Is your animal kept inside or outside of the house?
Is your pet kept in a fenced-in yard or allowed to run loose unattended?
Does your pet have access to neighboring properties (even for a short time)?
Where has your pet been in the last 24 hours?
Has your pet traveled outside of your immediate geographic location? If so, when?
Has your pet been to rural areas in the last week?

Your household's recent activity
Has there been any gardening work recently?
Does your pet have access to a compost pile?
Any fertilizers or weed killer used in the last week?
Any construction work or renovation recently?
Any mouse or rat poison in your house, yard, or garage?
Any cleaning products used inside or outside the house within the last 48 hours? If so, which?
Have you changed your radiator fluid or does a car leak antifreeze?

Figure 1-56:   Example of a thorough history form when a toxin is suspected.

precipitating or chelating agents may be used. Removal of a toxic substance from the body surface may be necessary, depending on the toxin. The use of both emesis and orogastric lavage is less and less frequent in human medicine because of the risk of aspiration pneumonia and doubts about their efficacy. Currently, management of poisonings in human medicine relies heavily on the use of activated charcoal combined with sorbitol as a cathartic, when appropriate, and supportive critical care. It should be emphasized, however, that the majority of poisonings in humans are due to drug overdoses (illicit or otherwise) (which have a relatively small volume and rapid absorption), for which this treatment is appropriate. Furthermore, adoption of the approach rests on the availability of a hospital intensive care infrastructure, which is not always available in veterinary practice.

Emetics

Induce emesis if the animal's physiology and neurologic status are stable (i.e., does not have respiratory depression or is not actively seizing, obtunded, unable to swallow or protect its airway). Do not administer the same emetic more than twice. If the emetic doesn't work after two doses, give a different emetic or perform orogastric lavage under general anesthesia. *Emetics are strictly contraindicated for toxicity from petroleum-based products and corrosives because of the risk of aspiration pneumonia and further esophageal damage.* Emetics may also be of little value if poisons with antiemetic properties have been ingested, such as benzodiazepines, tricyclic antidepressants, and marijuana (Table 1-50).

Various emetics traditionally have been recommended for use in veterinary medicine. Many have fallen out of favor because of the risk of causing adverse consequences and side effects. Apomorphine (0.04 mg/kg IV or in the conjunctival sac) remains the standard but is less useful in certain situations in which the poison causes CNS excitation or stimulation. It is ineffective in cats. Other emetics include xylazine and hydrogen peroxide. Do NOT use table salt because of the risk of severe oropharyngeal irritation and hypernatremia. Do not use mustard powder or dishwashing liquid detergent because of the risk of severe oropharyngeal, esophageal, and gastric irritation.

Orogastric lavage

Orogastric lavage is described in detail in the section on Emergency Procedures Gastric lavage is contraindicated in treatment of toxicity from petroleum-based compounds and acid/alkali ingestion. The procedure can be messy but is very effective if performed within 1 to 2 hours of ingestion of the poison. To prevent aspiration, the patient should be placed under general anesthesia. Keep the animal's head lowered during the procedure to prevent aspiration of stomach contents into the trachea. It is sometimes helpful to put the animal in both right and left lateral recumbency to allow complete emptying of gastric contents. Repeat the procedure until the fluid runs clear from the stomach. In some cases in which solid material has been ingested, this process can take a long time, so be prepared with a large volume of warm water.

Following successful evacuation and lavage, administer a slurry of activated charcoal through the orogastric tube before removing it. Keep the endotracheal tube cuffed and in place until the animal is semi-conscious, is starting the fight the tube, and is visibly able to swallow and protect its airway.

TABLE 1-50 List of Emetics and Recommended Doses

Name	Mechanism of action	Dose/onset	How supplied	Adverse effects
Apomorphine	Dopaminergic-receptor stimulation in chemoreceptor trigger zone; causes both central nervous system (CNS) depression and stimulation and some respiratory depression	0.02-0.04 mg/kg IV or in conjunctival sac	6.25-mg tablets, can be compounded into sterile capsules for intravenous use	Respiratory and CNS depression Undesirable CNS excitement in metaldehyde toxicosis
Hydrogen peroxide	Gastric irritation	1-2 mL/kg	3% solution PO, can be repeated once every 10 minutes	Protracted vomiting; some formulations have a stabilizing factor that can be converted into acetaminophen; use caution in very small dogs and in cats
Xylazine	Central α2-agonist stimulation	0.5-1.0 mg/kg IM every 10-15 minutes	Solution	Sedation, bradycardia, respiratory depression

---

BOX 1-59 EQUIPMENT NEEDED FOR ENEMA ADMINISTRATION

TUBING
Flexible red rubber catheters
Foley balloon-tipped catheters if a retention enema is required

OBSTETRIC LUBRICANT
Use nonsterile nonspermicidal water-soluble lubricants (K-Y jelly)

FLUID RESERVOIR
Old intravenous fluid bag
Enema bag
60- to 120-mL syringe

FLUID
Warm water, with or without hand or liquid dish soap

Enemas

Enemas are useful to facilitate the action of cathartics and in cases in which the poison is a solid material (e.g., compost, snail bait, garbage) (Box 1-59). It is best to use just lukewarm water. Commercially available phosphate enema solutions can cause severe electrolyte disturbances (hyperphosphatemia, hyponatremia, hypocalcemia, and hypomagnesemia) and acid-base abnormalities (metabolic acidosis); therefore, they are absolutely contraindicated in small animal patients.

The fluid volume required depends on the size of the animal and the state of its lower gastrointestinal tract. As with orogastric lavage, continue the procedure until the water runs clear. If difficulty is encountered emptying the lower gastrointestinal tract, repeat the enema in 1 or 2 hours, rather than be overzealous on the first attempt.

Cathartics

Cathartics are useful for hastening gastrointestinal elimination of toxins, and they are particularly useful for elimination of most solid toxicants (e.g., compost, garbage, snail baits). Cathartics can be used in conjunction with activated charcoal. Do not use magnesium-based cathartics in patients with CNS depression, because hypermagnesemia can worsen this disorder and also cause cardiac rhythm disturbances (Table 1-51).

Activated charcoal (1-4 mL/kg) is the safest and to date the most effective adsorbent for the treatment of ingested toxins. Activated charcoal can be administered after emesis or orogastric lavage or can be administered as the sole treatment. Various preparations are available on the market, including dry powder, compressed tablets, granules, liquid suspensions, and concentrated paste preparations. Commercially available products are relatively inexpensive and should be used whenever possible for ease of administration. Vegetable-origin activated charcoal is the most efficient adsorbent and binds compounds with weak, nonionic bonds. Some preparations are combined with sorbitol to provide simultaneous administration of an adsorbent and a cathartic; this combination has been shown to be most efficacious.

Repeated administration of activated charcoal every 4 to 6 hours has been shown to be beneficial in the management of a toxin that undergoes enterohepatic recirculation. Administration of an oily cathartic or mixing the activated charcoal with food only serves to reduce the absorptive surface of the activated charcoal and therefore is not recommended. In general, substances that are very soluble and are rapidly absorbed are not well adsorbed by activated charcoal, including alkalis, nitrates, mineral acids, ethanol, methanol, ferrous sulfate, ammonia, and cyanide.

Kaolin and bentonite are clays that have been used as adsorbents. Both are usually less effective than activated charcoal. However, they are reported to be better adsorbents than activated charcoal for the herbicide paraquat.

Ion exchange resins

Ion exchange resins can ionically bind certain drugs or toxins. Cholestyramine is one such resin, commonly used in human medicine to bind intestinal bile acids and thereby decrease cholesterol absorption. Its application in toxicology extends to the absorption of

T A B L E 1 - 5 1 List of Cathartics and Recommended Doses	
Product*	**Dose**
Sodium sulfate (Glauber's salts, GoLYTELY)	250-500 mg/kg PO in 10 times volume of water
Sorbitol (70%)	3 mL/kg PO
Mineral oil (paraffin oil)	5-15 mL per dog; 2-6 mL/cat Is not normally absorbed across the intestinal wall; do not use along with dioctyl sodium sulfosuccinate because emulsification can cause accumulation of indigestible oil in the liver; is no longer recommended for organophosphate insecticide and other organic compound ingestions

*Vegetable oil and Epsom salts (magnesium sulfate) are no longer recommended.
Note: Administer all cathartics at least 30 minutes after activated charcoal. Many activated charcoal products have sorbitol or other cathartic with the activated charcoal, so administration of a different cathartic is often unnecessary.

fat-soluble toxins such as organochlorine and certain acidic compounds such as digitalis. Ion exchange resins also have been used to delay or reduce the absorption of phenylbuta- zone, warfarin, chlorothiazide, tetracycline, phenobarbital, and thyroid preparations.

Precipitating, chelating, and diluting agents

Precipitating, chelating, and diluting agents are used primarily in the management of heavy metal intoxications, such as alkaloids or oxalates. They work by binding preferentially to the metal ion and creating a more soluble complex that is amenable to renal excretion. Those chelating agents in common usage are calcium EDTA, deferoxamine, and D-penicil- lamine. Calcium EDTA and deferoxamine should both be on hand in the veterinary hospital because they are necessary to treat zinc and iron toxicity, respectively, both of which have a short window of opportunity for therapeutic intervention. D-Penicillamine has a wide application for a number of metal toxicities but tends to be used for long-term chronic therapy because it can be administered orally. Various agents used for nonspecific dilution of toxins, including Milk of Magnesia and egg whites, although old-fashioned, still have wide application in many cases in which low-grade irritants have been ingested.

Eliminating poison from the skin

Bathing the animal is an important aspect of treatment for topical exposures to toxins such as insecticidal products, petroleum-based products, and aromatic oils. Bathing an animal is not an innocuous procedure. To avoid hypothermia and shock, use warm water at all times. Actively dry the animal to further minimize the risk of hypothermia. When bathing the animal, use rubber gloves and a plastic apron to avoid exposure to noxious agents.

In most cases, a mild dishwashing soap is appropriate. Medicated or antibacterial sham- poos are less appropriate in this situation. For petroleum-based products in particular, Dawn dishwashing liquid that "cuts the grease" works well to remove the oils. If Dawn is not available, mechanics' hand cleaners or coconut oil–based soaps can be used instead. As a general principle, best results are obtained by barely wetting the patient's fur until the detergent is worked well into the fur, keeping the amount of water to a minimum until ready for the rinse. Oil-based paint is best removed by clipping rather than by attempting removal with solvents, because solvents are also toxic.

To remove powder products, brush and vacuum the animal before bathing it to eliminate further toxic exposure. With caustic alkaline or acidic products, the primary treatment is to dilute and flush the skin with warm water; do NOT attempt neutralization. Neutralization can cause an exothermic reaction that causes further damage to the underlying tissues.

Eliminating poison from the eyes

For ocular exposures, irrigate the eyes for a minimum of 20 to 30 minutes with warm (body temperature) tap water or warmed 0.9% sterile saline solution. The use of neutralizing substances is not recommended because of the risk of causing further ocular damage. Following adequate irrigation, treat chemical burns of the eyes with lubricating ointments and possibly a temporary tarsorrhaphy. Atropine may be indicated as a cycloplegic agent. Systemic nonsteroidal antiinflammatory drugs can be used to control patient discomfort.

Daily follow-up examinations are required because epithelial damage may be delayed, especially with alkali burns, and it is difficult to predict the final extent of ocular damage. Topical glucocorticosteroids are contraindicated if the corneal epithelium is not intact. If severe conjunctival swelling is present with a corneal ulcer, parenteral glucocorticosteroids can be administered to help alleviate inflammation, but nonsteroidal antiinflammatory drugs should not be used simultaneously due to the risk of gastrointestinal ulceration or perforation.

Administer antidotes

Whenever possible, administer specific antidotes to negate the effects of the toxin and prevent conversion of the substance to the toxic metabolite. Three categories of agents are used in the management of poisonings.

The first category is specific antidotes. Unfortunately, few specific antidotes are available for use in veterinary medicine. Some "classic" toxins and antidotes are now considered to be rare, such as curare and physostigmine, thallium and Prussian blue, and fluoride and calcium borogluconate. These and a few others have been omitted from the table.

The second, broader category of antidotes includes those drugs used in the symptomatic management of clinical signs, which are part of our routine veterinary stock. Drugs such as atropine, sedatives, steroids, antiarrhythmics, and beta-blockers fall into this category.

The third category comprises nonspecific decontaminants such as activated charcoal, cathartics, and emetics. These were discussed previously.

Facilitate clearance or metabolism of absorbed toxin

Many patients benefit from efforts to enhance clearance or metabolism of the absorbed toxins. Some specific therapies have been developed for this purpose, including 4-methylpyrazole for ethylene glycol toxicity and specific antibodies such as Digibind (digoxin immune Fab [ovine]) for digitalis toxicity. Other strategies are aimed at promoting renal excretion. Renal excretion strategies include diuresis, ion trapping, and peritoneal dialysis or hemodialysis (see section on Peritoneal Dialysis). Diuresis and ion trapping are applicable to a large number of toxins and are discussed here in more detail. Other toxins respond to urine acidification and urine alkalinization.

Enhancing renal excretion of substances is most useful for those organic substances that are present in significant concentrations in the plasma. Substances that are non-ionic and lipid-soluble, such as certain herbicides, are likely to be less affected by attempts to promote rapid renal elimination.

Before starting diuresis or ion trapping, intravenous fluid therapy should be adequate as determined by normal central venous pressure, urine output, and mean arterial blood pressure. If any of these values are less than normal, use other measures to ensure adequate renal perfusion, including but not limited to a constant rate infusion of dopamine.

Simple fluid diuresis can influence the excretion of certain substances. The use of mannitol as an osmotic diuretic may reduce the passive reabsorption of some toxic substances in the proximal renal convoluted tubule by reducing water reabsorption. Dextrose (50%) can be used as an osmotic diuretic. Furosemide can be used to promote diuresis, but again, there is no substitute for intravenous fluid therapy. The use of mannitol, dextrose, and furosemide is contraindicated in hypotensive or hypovolemic patients. Take care to avoid causing dehydration with any diuretic; central venous pressure monitoring is strongly recommended.

Urine acidification and alkalinization

Ion trapping is based on the principle that ionized substances do not cross renal tubular membranes easily, and are not well reabsorbed. If the urinary pH can be changed so that the toxin's chemical equilibrium shifts to its ionized form, then that toxin can be "trapped" in the urine and excreted. Alkaline urine favors the ionization of acidic compounds, and acidic urine favors the ionization of alkaline compounds. Those toxins that are amenable to ion trapping are mostly weak acids and weak bases.

Ammonium chloride can be used to promote urinary acidification. Contraindications to the use of ammonium chloride include a preexisting metabolic acidosis, hepatic or renal insufficiency, and hemolysis or rhabdomyolysis leading to hemoglobinuria or myoglobinuria. Signs of ammonia intoxication include CNS depression and coma. When performing urine acidification, frequently check the serum potassium concentration and urine pH.

Urine alkalinization can be performed with use of sodium bicarbonate. Contraindications to the use of sodium bicarbonate include metabolic alkalosis (particularly with concurrent use of furosemide), hypocalcemia, and hypokalemia. As with urine acidification, monitor the serum potassium concentration and urine pH frequently.

Supportive and Symptomatic Care of the Poisoning Patient

The major steps in management of poisonings discussed here must be accompanied by application of the fundamentals of critical care. Respiratory and cardiovascular support have been discussed previously. Renal and gastrointestinal function and analgesia are particularly important in the management of the poisoning patient.

Maintenance of renal perfusion is a priority in the poisoning patient. Fluid, electrolyte, and acid-base balance must be controlled and be accurate. Poisoning patients are at particularly high risk for renal damage and acute renal failure, whether by primary toxic insult to the renal parenchyma or by acute or prolonged renal hypoperfusion. For this reason, a protocol that aims at preventing oliguria and ensuing renal failure is one of the therapeutic strategies that should be routinely employed. This protocol is described in Box 1-60.

Gastrointestinal protectants

Gastrointestinal protectant drugs may be indicated for the management of those poisons that are gastrointestinal irritants or ulcerogenic. Commonly used gastroprotectant drugs include cimetidine, ranitidine, famotidine, omeprazole, sucralfate, and misoprostol.

Antiemetics

Antiemetics may be used to suppress intractable vomiting. Metoclopramide is commonly used, and it is the drug of choice for centrally mediated nausea. Antiemetics that work by different mechanisms can be used in combination as necessary. Examples are dopamine 2-receptor antagonists such as prochlorperazine, 5-hydroxytryptamine antagonists such as ondansetron and dolasetron, and H-1 receptor antagonists such as diphenhydramine and meclizine.

Analgesics

Analgesics are more appropriate to treat poisonings than once thought. Common effects of poisons including severe gastroenteritis and topical burns or ulcerations may warrant the use of analgesics. Longer-acting analgesics such as morphine, hydromorphone, and buprenorphine are particularly useful.

Nutritional support

Nutritional support may be necessary in the form of enteral or parenteral feeding in patients that have esophageal or gastric damage or that need to be sedated for long periods of time. Endoscopy may be useful in assessing the degree of esophageal and gastric damage, particularly after ingestion of caustic substances.

BOX 1-60   MAINTENANCE OF RENAL PERFUSION

1. Administer crystalloid intravenous fluids at maintenance rates using a balanced electrolyte solution.
2. Perform urinary catheterization and collection to monitor urine output.
3. Monitor serum urea nitrogen and creatinine every 12 hours.
4. Monitor serum electrolytes every 6 to 8 hours.
5. Monitor central venous pressure every 2 to 4 hours.
6. Treat oliguria, defined as a drop in urine output to less than 1 mL/kg/hour.
7. Initiate a fluid challenge with a crystalloid or colloid (5 mL/kg) bolus.
8. Start dopamine at 3 to 5 µg/kg/minute if no response to crystalloid/colloid bolus occurs within 30 minutes.
9a. Consider mannitol (0.5 to 1 g/kg IV) administration if no response to dopamine occurs within 30 minutes.
9b. Consider furosemide (4 to 8 mg/kg IV, or 0.66 to 1 mg/kg/hour IV CRI) if no response to dopamine or mannitol occurs in 30 to 60 minutes.
10. If no response to furosemide, peritoneal dialysis or hemodialysis is indicated immediately, particularly if anuria is present.

1

Treatment of Specific Toxins

Acetaminophen (paracetamol)

Introduction:

Acetaminophen (paracetamol) is the active ingredient in Tylenol and many over-the-counter cold products. Acetaminophen is converted to N-acetyl-P-benzoquinonimine in the liver, a toxic substance that can cause oxidative injury of red blood cells and hepatocytes. Clinical signs of acetaminophen toxicity include respiratory distress from lack of oxygen-carrying capacity, cyanosis, methemoglobinemia (chocolate-brown appearance of the blood and mucous membranes), lethargy, vomiting, and facial and paw swelling (cats). The toxic dose of acetaminophen is >100 mg/kg for dogs, and 50 mg/kg for cats.

Treatment:

Treatment of acetaminophen toxicity includes induction of emesis or orogastric lavage if the substance has been ingested within 30 minutes. Activated charcoal should also be administered. In cases of severe anemia, give supplemental oxygen along with a packed RBC transfusion. Administer intravenous fluids to maintain renal and hepatic perfusion. N-acetylcysteine, vitamin C, and cimetidine are the treatments of choice for methemoglobinemia in patients with acetaminophen toxicity.

Acids/corrosives

Introduction:

Hydrochloric, nitric, and phosphoric acids cause chemical burns through contact with the skin and/or eyes. Localized superficial coagulative necrosis occurs upon contact. Usually, the patient's skin is painful to the touch or the animal may lick or chew at an irritated area that is not visible under the haircoat.

Treatment:

If the chemical is swallowed, do NOT induce emesis or perform orogastric lavage, because of the risk of worsening esophageal irritation. Rinse the patient's skin and eyes with warm water or warm saline for a minimum of ½ hour. Use analgesics and treat corneal ulcers (see section on Corneal Ulcers) as required. Do not attempt chemical neutralization, because of the risk of causing an exothermic reaction and worsening tissue injury.

Aflatoxin

Introduction:

Aflatoxin (*Aspergillus flavus*) is found in moldy feed grains. Clinical signs of toxicity occur after ingestion and include vomiting, diarrhea, and acute hepatitis; abortion may occur in pregnant bitches.

Treatment:

Treatment of suspected aflatoxin ingestion consists of gastric decontamination, administration of activated charcoal, intravenous fluids, and hepatic supportive care (S-Adenosyl Methionine [SAMe], milk thistle).

Alcohols

Introduction:

Drinking (ethanol), rubbing (isopropyl), and methyl (methanol) alcohols can be harmful if ingested (4.1 to 8.0 g/kg PO). All cause disruption of neuronal membrane structure, impaired motor coordination, CNS excitation followed by depression, and stupor that can lead to cardiac and respiratory arrest, depending on the amount ingested. Affected animals may appear excited and then ataxic and lethargic. Contact or inhalant injury can occur, causing dermal irritation and cutaneous hyperemia. Methanol also can cause hepatotoxicity.

Treatment:

Induce and maintain a patent airway and stabilize the patient's cardiovascular and respiratory status. Control CNS excitation with diazepam, if necessary, and control the patient's body temperature (both hypo- and hyperthermia). Induce vomiting if the patient is alert and can protect its airway; otherwise, perform orogastric lavage with the patient under general anesthesia with a cuffed endotracheal tube in place. Alcohols do not bind well with activated charcoal. Treat dermal exposure by bathing the area with warm water.

Alkalis/caustics

Introduction:

If ingested, sodium or potassium hydroxide can cause severe contact dermatitis or irritation of the gastrointestinal tract. Esophageal burns and full-thickness coagulative necrosis can occur.

Treatment:

If an animal ingests a caustic alkali substance, feed the animal four egg whites mixed with 1 quart of warmed water. Perform endoscopy within 24 hours to evaluate the extent of injury and to place a feeding tube, in severe cases. Do NOT induce emesis , and do NOT perform orogastric lavage, because of the risk of worsening esophageal irritation. In cases of contact exposure to the skin or eyes, rinse the exposed area with warm water baths for at least 30 minutes. Administer gastroprotectant, antiemetic, and analgesic drugs as necessary. Avoid neutralization, which can cause a hyperthermic reaction and worsen injury to the skin and gastrointestinal tract.

Amitraz

Introduction:

Amitraz is the active ingredient in ascaricides and anti-tick and anti-mite products such as Mitaban and Taktic. The toxic dose is 10 to20 mg/kg. Amitraz exerts its toxic effects by causing α-adrenergic stimulation, and causes clinical signs similar to those observed with administration of xylazine: bradycardia, CNS depression, ataxia, hypotension, hyperglycemia, hypothermia, cyanotic mucous membranes, polyuria, mydriasis, and emesis. A coma can develop.

Treatment:

Treatment of amitraz intoxication includes cardiovascular support with intravenous crystalloid fluids and induction of emesis in asymptomatic animals. If clinical signs are present, orogastric lavage may be required. Many toxic compounds are impregnated in a collar form. If the patient has ingested a collar and does not vomit it, it should be removed using endoscopy or gastrotomy. Administer activated charcoal to prevent or delay absorption of the toxic compound. Yohimbine or atepamizole, both α-adrenergic antagonists, are the treatment(s) of choice to reverse the clinical signs of toxicity. Avoid the use of atropine, because it can potentially increase the viscosity of respiratory secretions and cause gastrointestinal ileus, thus promoting increased absorption of the toxic compound.

Ammonia, cleaning

Introduction

Ammonium hydroxide, or cleaning ammonia, can be caustic at high concentrations (see Alkalis/Caustics) and cause severe injury to the respiratory system if inhaled. Pulmonary edema or pneumonia can occur, resulting in respiratory distress. Ingestion of ammonia can cause severe irritation to the gastrointestinal tract and cause vomiting and esophageal injury.

Treatment:

If ammonia is ingested, administer a dilute solution of egg white.

Administer gastroprotectant, antiemetic, and analgesic drugs as necessary. If pneumonia or pulmonary edema occurs secondary to aspiration of ammonia into the airways and alveolar spaces, treatment is largely supportive with supplemental oxygen administration, antibiotics, fluid therapy, and mechanical ventilation as necessary. Diuretics may or may not be useful in the treatment of pulmonary edema secondary to ammonia inhalation.

Amphetamine

Introduction

Amphetamines cause CNS excitation due to neurosynaptic stimulation, resulting in hypersensitivity to noise and motion, agitation, tremors, vomiting, diarrhea, and seizures. Clinical signs of amphetamine toxicity include muscle tremors, tachyarrhythmias, mydriasis, ptyalism, and hyperthermia.

Treatment

Amphetamines are rapidly absorbed from the gastrointestinal tract. Treatment includes administration of intravenous fluids to maintain hydration and renal perfusion and correction of hyperthermia. Administer sedative drugs such as chlorpromazine to control agitation and tremors, and diazepam to control seizures. Urinary acidification can promote excretion and prevent reabsorption from the urinary bladder. In severe cases, treat cerebral edema with a combination of mannitol followed by furosemide to control increased intracranial pressure.

Antifreeze: see ethylene glycol

Antihistamines

Introduction

Antihistamines (loratadine, diphenhydramine, doxylamine, clemastine, meclizine, dimenhydrinate, chlorpheniramine, cyclizine, terfenadine, hydroxyzine) are available as over-the-counter and prescription allergy and anti-motion sickness products. Clinical signs of antihistamine toxicity include restlessness, nausea, vomiting, agitation, seizures, hyperthermia, and tachyarrhythmias.

Treatment

Treatment of antihistamine intoxication is largely symptomatic and supportive, as there is no known antidote. If ingestion is recent (within 1 to 2 hours) and the patient is not actively seizing and can protect its airway, induce emesis or perform orogastric lavage, followed by administration of activated charcoal and a cathartic. Monitor the patient's heart rate, rhythm, and blood pressure. Treat cardiac arrhythmias, if present, with appropriate therapies (see section on Cardiac Dysrhythmias). Administer cooling measures and intravenous fluids to treat hyperthermia. A constant rate infusion of guaifenasin can be used to control muscle tremors.

ANTU (α-naphthylthiourea)

Introduction

α-Naphthylthiourea (ANTU) is manufactured as a white or blue-gray powder. The toxic dose in dogs is 10-40 mg/kg, and in cats is 75-100 mg/kg. Younger dogs appear to be more resistant to its toxic effects. ANTU usually causes profound emesis and increased capillary permeability that eventually leads to pulmonary edema.

Treatment

Treatment of ANTU toxicity includes respiratory support. Mechanical ventilation may be required in severe cases of pulmonary edema. If an animal does not vomit, orogastric lavage should be performed. Administer gastrointestinal protectant, antiemetic, and analgesic drugs. Cardiovascular support in the form of intravenous crystalloids should be administered with caution, because of the risk of exacerbating increased capillary permeability and causing pulmonary edema.

Arsenic

Introduction

Inorganic arsenic (arsenic trioxide, sodium arsenite, sodium arsenate) is the active ingredient in many herbicides, defoliants, and insecticides, including ant killers. The toxic dose of sodium arsenate is 100-150 mg/kg; that of sodium arsenite is 1-25 mg/kg. Sodium arsenite is less toxic, although cats are very susceptible. Arsenic compounds interfere with cellular respiration by combining with sulfhydryl enzymes. Clinical signs of toxicity include severe gastroenteritis, muscle weakness, capillary damage, hypotension, renal failure, seizures, and death. In many cases, clinical signs are acute in onset.

Treatment

Treatment of arsenic toxicity involves procuring and maintaining a patent airway. Administer intravenous crystalloid fluids to correct hypotension and hypovolemia, and normalize acid-base and electrolyte balance. If no clinical signs are present and if the compound was ingested within 2 hours, induce emesis. If clinical signs are present, perform orogastric lavage followed by administration of activated charcoal. If dermal exposure has occurred, throughly bathe the animal to prevent further absorption. Dimercaprol (BAL, 3-4 mg/kg IM q8h) can be administered as a chelating agent. *N*-acetylcysteine (Mucomyst) (for cats, 140-240 mg/kg PO IV, then 70 mg/kg PO IV q6h for 3 days; for dogs, 280 mg/kg PO or IV, then 140 mg/kg PO IV q4h for 3 days) has been shown to decrease arsenic toxicity in rats.

Aspirin (acetylsalicylic acid, salicylate)

Introduction

Aspirin causes inhibition of the production of prostaglandins, a high anion gap metabolic acidosis, gastrointestinal ulceration, hypophosphatemia, and decreased platelet aggregation when ingested in high quantities (>50 mg/kg/24 hours in dogs; >25 mg/kg/24 hours in cats). Clinical signs of aspirin toxicity include tachypnea, vomiting, anorexia, lethargy, hematemesis, and melena.

Treatment

Treatment of aspirin toxicity is largely supportive. If the ingestion was recent (within the last hour), induce emesis or perform orogastric lavage followed by administration of activated charcoal. Administer intravenous crystalloid fluids to maintain hydration and correct acid-base abnormalities. Administer synthetic prostaglandin analogues (misoprostol), gastroprotectant drugs, and antiemetics. Alkalinization of the urine can enhance excretion.

Atomoxetine: see Strattera

Baclofen

Introduction

Baclofen is a GABA agonist centrally acting muscle relaxant. Clinical signs of toxicity include vomiting, ataxia, vocalization, disorientation, seizures, hypoventilation, coma, and apnea. Clinical signs can occur at doses as low as 1.3 mg/kg.

Treatment

Treatment of baclofen ingestion includes induction of emesis if the animal is asymptomatic. Otherwise, perform orogastric lavage. Emesis or orogastric lavage should be followed by administration of activated charcoal. Perform intravenous crystalloid fluid diuresis to promote elimination of the toxin, maintain renal perfusion, and normalize body temperature. Supplemental oxygen or mechanical ventilation may be required for hypoventilation or apnea. If seizures occur, avoid the use of diazepam, which is a GABA agonist and can potentially worsen clinical signs. Control seizures with intravenous phenobarbital, pentobarbital, or propofol. Supportive care (eye lubrication, urinary catheter placement for patient cleanliness, passive range of motion exercises, soft heavy bedding to prevent decubitus ulcer formation) is required. Clinical signs usually resolve in several days. Seizures warrant a more guarded prognosis.

β-Adrenergic agonists (asthma inhalers/medications)

Introduction

β-adrenergic agonists, including terbutaline, albuterol (salbutamol), and metaproterenol, are commonly used in inhaled form for the treatment of asthma. Animals commonly are exposed to the compounds after chewing on their owners' inhalers. Clinical signs of β-adrenergic stimulation include tachycardia, muscle tremors, and agitation. Severe hypokalemia can occur.

Treatment

Treatment of β-adrenergic agonist intoxication includes treatment with beta-blockers (propranolol, esmolol, Atenolol), intravenous fluids, and intravenous potassium supplementation. Diazepam or acepromazine may be administered for sedation and muscle relaxation.

Barbecue lighter fluids: see fuels

Barbiturates

Introduction

Barbiturates such as phenobarbital are GABA agonists and induce CNS depression. Clinical signs of barbiturate overdose or toxicity include weakness, lethargy, hypotension, hypoventilation, stupor, coma, and death.

Treatment

Treatment of barbiturate toxicity includes maintenance and support of the cardiovascular and respiratory systems. If clinical signs are absent and the patient can protect its airway, induce emesis followed by repeated doses of activated charcoal. Perform orogastric lavage if emesis is contraindicated. Administer supplemental oxygen if hypoventilation occurs. Some animals may require mechanical ventilation. Administer intravenous fluids to control perfusion and blood pressure. Positive inotropic drugs may be required if dose-dependent decrease in cardiac output and blood pressure occurs. Alkalinization of the urine and peritoneal dialysis can be performed to enhance excretion and elimination. Hemodialysis should be considered in severe cases, if available.

Batteries

Introduction

Automotive and dry cell batteries contain sulfuric acid that can be irritating on contact with the eyes, skin, and gastrointestinal tract. Button batteries, which contain sodium or potassium hydroxide, cause contact irritation if chewed.

Treatment

To treat exposure, rinse the eyes and skin with copious amounts of warm tap water or sterile saline solution for a minimum of 30 minutes. If ingestion occurred, administer gastroprotectant and antiemetic drugs. Induction of emesis and orogastric lavage is absolutely contraindicated because of the risk of aspiration pneumonia and worsening esophageal irritation. No attempt should be made at performing neutralization because of the risk of causing an exothermic reaction and worsening tissue damage. Administer analgesics to control discomfort.

Benzoyl peroxide

Introduction

Benzoyl peroxide is the active ingredient in many over-the-counter acne preparations. Ingestion can result in production of hydrogen peroxide, gastroenteritis, and gastric dilatation. Topical exposure can cause dermal irritation and blistering.

Treatment

If an animal has ingested benzoyl peroxide, do NOT induce emesis, because of the risk of worsening esophageal irritation. Instead, perform orogastric lavage. Administer gastroprotectant and antiemetic medications and closely observe the patient observed for signs of gastric dilatation.

Bismuth subsalicylate (Pepto-Bismol): see aspirin

Bleach, chlorine (sodium hypochlorite)

Introduction

Sodium hypochlorite is available in dilute (3%-6%) or concentrated (50% industrial strength or swimming pool) solutions for a variety of purposes. Sodium hypochlorite can cause severe contact irritation and tissue destruction, depending on the concentration. Affected animals may have a bleached haircoat.

Treatment

Treatment of exposure includes dilution with copious amounts of warm water or saline baths and ocular lavage. Induction of emesis and orogastric lavage is absolutely contraindicated because of the risk of causing further esophageal irritation. To treat ingestion, give the animal milk or large amounts of water, in combination with gastroprotectant and antiemetic drugs, to dilute the contents in the stomach. Administration of sodium bicarbonate or Milk of Magnesia is no longer recommended.

Bleach, nonchlorine

Introduction

Nonchlorine bleaches (sodium peroxide or sodium perborate) have a moderate toxic potential if ingested. Sodium peroxide can cause gastric distention. Sodium perborate can cause severe gastric irritation, with vomiting and diarrhea; renal damage and CNS excitation followed by depression can occur, depending on the amount ingested.

Treatment

To treat dermal or ocular exposure, rinse the skin or eyes with copious amounts of warm tap water or sterile saline for a minimum of 30 minutes; treat ocular injuries as necessary, if corneal burns have occurred. If the bleach has been ingested, DO induce emesis and perform orogastric lavage. Administer Milk of Magnesia (2-3 mL/kg).

Boric acid, borate

Introduction

Boric acid is the active ingredient in many ant and roach killers. The toxic ingredient (in amounts of 1-3 g/kg) can cause clinical signs in dogs by an unknown mechanism. Clinical signs include vomiting (blue-green vomitus), blue-green stools, renal damage, and CNS excitation and depression.

Treatment

Treatment of boric acid or borate ingestion includes gastric decontamination with induction of emesis or orogastric lavage, followed by administration of a cathartic to hasten elimination. Activated charcoal is not useful to treat ingestion of this toxin. Administer intravenous fluid therapy to maintain renal perfusion. Administer gastroprotectant and antiemetic drugs, as necessary.

Botulism

Introduction

Clostridium botulinum endospores can be found in carrion, food, garbage, and the environment. Ingestion of endospores and *C. botulinum* endotoxin rarely can cause generalized neuromuscular blockade of spinal and cranial nerves, resulting in miosis, anisocoria, lower motor neuron weakness, and paralysis. Respiratory paralysis, megaesophagus, and aspiration pneumonia can occur. Clinical signs usually develop within 6 days of ingestion.

Differential diagnosis includes acute polyradiculoneuritis (coonhound paralysis), bromethalin intoxication, and tick paralysis.

Treatment

Treatment of botulism is largely supportive; although an antitoxin exists, it often is of no benefit. Treatment may include administration of intravenous fluids, frequent turning of the patient and passive range-of-motion exercises to prevent disuse muscle atrophy, and supplemental oxygen administration or mechanical ventilation. Administer amoxicillin, ampicillin, or metronidazole. Recovery may be prolonged, up to 3 to 4 weeks in some cases.

Bromethalin

Introduction

Bromethalin is the active ingredient in some brands of mouse and rat poisons. It usually is packaged as 0.01% bromethalin in green or tan pellets, and packaged in 16 – 42.5 g place packs. The toxic dose for dogs is 116.7 g/kg, and for cats 3 g/kg. Bromethalin causes toxicity by uncoupling of oxidative phosphorylation. An acute syndrome of vomiting, tremors, extensor rigidity, and seizures occurs within 24 hours of ingestion of high doses. Delayed clinical signs occur within 3 to 7 days of ingestion of a lower dose and include posterior paresis progressing to ascending paralysis, CNS depression, and coma.

Treatment

Treatment of known bromethalin ingestion includes induction of emesis or orogastric lavage, and repeated doses of activated charcoal every 4 to 6 hours for 3 days, because bromethalin undergoes enterohepatic recirculation. Supportive care includes intravenous fluids, anticonvulsants, muscle relaxants (methocarbamol up to 220 mg/kg/day IV to effect), frequent turning of the patient, and passive range-of-motion exercises. Supplemental oxygen and /or mechanical ventilation may be required in patients with coma and severe hypoventilation. Administer mannitol (0.5-1 g/kg) in conjunction with furosemide (1 mg/kg IV) if cerebral edema is suspected.

Caffeine

Introduction

The majority of caffeine toxicities occur in dogs that ingest coffee beans. Caffeine causes phosphodiesterase inhibition, and can cause cardiac tachyarrhythmias, CNS stimulation (hyperexcitability and seizures), diuresis, gastric ulcers, vomiting, and diarrhea. Muscle tremors and seizures can occur, resulting in severe hyperthermia.

Treatment

Treatment of caffeine toxicity is largely symptomatic and supportive, as there is no known antidote. If clinical signs are not apparent and the patient is able to protect its airway, induce emesis. Alternatively, orogastric lavage can be performed, followed by administration of activated charcoal. Administer diazepam to control seizures. Administer beta-adrenergic blockers (e.g., esmolol, propranolol, atenolol) to control tachyarrhythmias. Give intravenous fluids to maintain hydration and correct hyperthermia. The patient should be walked frequently or have a urinary catheter placed to prevent reabsorption of the toxin from the urinary bladder.

Carbamates

Introduction

Carbamate compounds are found in agricultural and home insecticide products. Examples of carbamates include carbofuran, aldicarb, propoxur, carbaryl, and methiocarb. The toxic dose of each compound varies. Carbamate compounds function by causing acetylcholinesterase inhibition. Toxic amounts cause CNS excitation, muscarinic acetylcholine overload, and SLUD (salivation, lacrimation, urination, and defecation). Miosis, vomiting, and diarrhea result from muscarinic overload. Nicotinic overload produces muscle tremors. Toxicity can result in seizures, coma, and death.

Treatment

Treatment of carbamate intoxication includes maintaining an airway and, if necessary, artificial ventilation. Administer intravenous crystalloid fluids to control the patient's hydration, blood pressure, and temperature. Cooling measures may be warranted. Induce emesis if the substance was ingested within 60 minutes and the animal is asymptomatic. Give repeated doses of activated charcoal if the animal can swallow and protect its airway. Control seizures with diazepam (0.5 mg/kg IV). Bathe the patient thoroughly. Atropine (0.2 mg/kg IV) is useful in controlling some of the muscarinic signs associated with the toxicity. Pralidoxime hydrochloride (2-PAM) is not useful in cases of carbamate intoxication. Control muscle tremors with methocarbamol (up to 220 mg/kg IV) or guaifenesin.

Carbon tetrachloride

Introduction

In humans, ingestion or inhalation of 3-5 mL of carbon tetrachloride can be fatal. Clinical signs of carbon tetrachloride toxicity include vomiting and diarrhea, then progressive respiratory and central nervous system depression. Ventricular dysrhythmias and hepatorenal damage ensue. The prognosis is grave.

Treatment

Treatment of carbon tetrachloride inhalation includes procurement and maintenance of a patent airway with supplemental oxygen, and cardiovascular support. To treat ingestion, administer activated charcoal, and give intravenous fluids to maintain hydration and support renal function.

Chlorinated hydrocarbons

Introduction

Chlorinated hydrocarbons include DDT, methoxychlor, lindane, dieldrin, aldrin, chlordane, chlordecone, perthane, toxaphene, heptachlor, mirex, and endosulfan. The toxic dose of each compound varies. Chlorinated hydrocarbons exert their toxic effects by an unknown mechanism, and can be absorbed through the skin and the gastrointestinal tract. Clinical signs are similar to those observed in organophosphate toxicity: CNS excitation, seizures, SLUD, (salivation, lacrimation, urination, defecation), excessive bronchial secretions, vomiting, diarrhea, muscle tremors, and respiratory paralysis. Secondary toxicity from toxic metabolites can cause renal and hepatic failure. Chronic exposure may cause anorexia, vomiting, weight loss, tremors, seizures, and hepatic failure. The clinical course can be prolonged in small animal patients.

Treatment

Treatment of chlorinated hydrocarbon toxicity is largely supportive in nature, as there is no known antidote. Procure and maintain the patient's airway. Normalize the body temperature to prevent hyperthermia. If the substance was just ingested and the patient is not demonstrating any clinical signs, induce emesis. If the patient is symptomatic, perform orogastric lavage followed by activated charcoal administration. Bathe the patient thoroughly in cases of topical exposure. Administer intravenous crystalloid fluids to maintain hydration. These compounds do not appear to be amenable to fluid diuresis.

Chlorphenoxy herbicides

Introduction:

Chlorphenoxy derivatives are found in 2,4-D, 2,4,5-T, MCPA, MCPP, and Silvex. The LD_{50} of 2,4-D is 100 mg/kg; however, the toxic dose appears to be much lower in small animal patients. Chlorphenoxy derivatives exert their toxic effects by an unknown mechanism, and cause clinical signs of gastroenteritis and muscle rigidity.

Treatment

Treatment of chlorphenoxy derivative toxicity is largely supportive in nature, as there is no known antidote. Secure the patient's airway and administer supplemental oxygen, as necessary. Control CNS excitation with diazepam (0.5 mg/kg IV). Intravenous crystalloid fluid diuresis and urinary alkalinization can promote elimination. Administer gastroprotectant and antiemetic drugs, as needed.

Chocolate

Introduction

The toxic effects of chocolate are related to theobromine. Various types of chocolate have different concentrations of theobromine and thus can cause clinical signs of toxicity with ingestion of varying amounts of chocolate, depending on the type. The toxic dose of theobromine is 100-150 mg/kg in dogs. Milk chocolate contains 44 mg/oz (154 mg/100 g) of chocolate, and has a low toxic potential. Semisweet chocolate contains 150 mg/oz (528 mg/100 g), and baking chocolate contains 390 mg/oz (1365 mg/100 g). Semisweet and baking chocolate, being the most concentrated, have a moderate to severe toxic potential, even in large dogs.

Clinical signs of theobromine intoxication are associated with phosphodiesterase inhibition and include CNS stimulation (tremors, anxiety, seizures), myocardial stimulation (tachycardia and tachyarrhythmias), diuresis, and (at very high doses) gastrointestinal ulceration. With treatment, the condition of most dogs returns to normal within 12 to 24 hours ($t_{1/2}$ = 17.5 hours in dogs). Potential side effects include gastroenteritis and pancreatitis due to the fat content of the chocolate.

Treatment

Treatment of chocolate toxicity includes obtaining and maintaining a protected airway (if necessary), intravenous fluid diuresis, induction of emesis or orogastric lavage followed by administration of repeated doses of activated charcoal, and placement of a urinary catheter to prevent reabsorption of the toxin from the urinary bladder.

Cholecalciferol

Introduction

Cholecalciferol rodenticide ingestion can lead to increased intestinal and renal reabsorption of calcium, causing an increase in serum calcium and dystrophic mineralization of the kidneys and liver at 2-3 mg/kg. Clinical signs include lethargy, anorexia, vomiting, constipation, and renal pain within 2 to 3 days of ingestion. Seizures, muscle twitching, and central nervous system depression may be observed at very high doses. As renal failure progresses, polyuria, polydipsia, vomiting/hematemesis, uremic oral ulcers, and melena may be observed.

Treatment

If the compound was ingested recently (within 2 to 4 hours) induce emesis or perform orogastric lavage, followed by administration of activated charcoal. Check the patient's serum calcium once daily for three days following ingestion. If clinical signs of toxicity or hypercalcemia are present, decrease serum calcium with loop diuretics (furosemide, 2-5 mg/kg PO or IV q12h) and glucocorticosteroids (prednisone or prednisolone, 2-3 mg/kg PO bid) to promote renal calcium excretion. In severe cases, salmon calcitonin (4-6 IU/kg SC q2-12h in dogs) or bisphosphonate compounds may be required. Correct acid-base abnormalities with intravenous crystalloid fluid diuresis and sodium bicarbonate, if necessary. (See section on Hypercalcemia.)

1

Coal, tar-based: see hydrocarbons, aromatic
Coumarins: see vitamin K antagonist rodenticides
Cresol: see hydrocarbons, aromatic
Deicers: see ethylene glycol and alcohols

Denture cleaners
Introduction
Denture cleaners contain sodium perborate as the active compound. Sodium perborate can cause severe direct irritation of the mucous membranes and may also act as a CNS depressant. Clinical signs are similar to those seen if bleach or boric acid compound is ingested, namely vomiting, diarrhea, CNS excitation then depression, and renal failure.

Treatment
Treatment for ingestion of denture cleaner includes gastric decontamination along with induction of emesis or orogastric lavage and administration of a cathartic to hasten elimination. Activated charcoal is not useful for treatment of ingestion of this toxin. Administer intravenous fluid therapy to maintain renal perfusion. Administer gastroprotectant and antiemetic drugs, as necessary.

Deodorants
Introduction
Deodorants are usually composed of aluminum chloride and aluminum chlorohydrate. Both have a moderate potential for toxicity. Ingestion of deodorant compounds can cause oral irritation or necrosis, gastroenteritis, and nephrosis.

Treatment:
Treatment of deodorant ingestion includes orogastric lavage, and administration of antiemetic and gastroprotectant drugs.

Detergents, anionic
Introduction
Anionic detergents include sulfonated or phosphorylated forms of benzene. Dishwashing liquid is an example of an anionic detergent that can be toxic at doses of 1 – 5 g/kg. Anionic detergents cause significant mucosal damage and edema, gastrointestinal irritation, CNS depression, seizures, and possible hemolysis. Ocular exposure can cause corneal ulcers and edema.

Treatment
Treatment of anionic detergent exposure is largely symptomatic, as there is no known antidote. To treat topical toxicity, flush the patient's eyes and skin with warmed tap water or 0.9% saline solution for a minimum of 30 minutes, taking care to avoid hypothermia. To treat ingestion, feed the patient milk and large amounts of water to dilute the toxin. Do NOT induce emesis, because of the risk of worsening esophageal irritation. To dilute the toxin, perform orogastric lavage, followed by administration of activated charcoal. Closely monitor the patient's respiratory status, because oropharyngeal edema can be severe. If necessary, perform endotracheal intubation in cases of airway obstruction. Monitor the patient for signs of intravascular hemolysis. Administer intravenous crystalloid fluids to maintain hydration until the patient is able to tolerate oral fluids.

Detergents, cationic, and disinfectants
Introduction
Cationic detergents and disinfectants include quaternary ammonia compounds, isopropyl alcohol, and isopropanol. Quaternary ammonia compounds have a serious toxic potential

and cause severe irritation and corrosion of the mucous membranes and skin. Some compounds also can cause clinical signs similar to those observed with anticholinesterase compounds, including muscle tremors, seizures, paralysis, and coma. Methemoglobinemia can occur.

Treatment

Treatment of cationic detergent exposure includes careful bathing and ocular rinsing of the patient for a minimum of 30 minutes, taking care to avoid hypotension. Secure the patient's airway and monitor the patient's respiratory status. Administer supplemental oxygen, if necessary. Place an intravenous catheter and administer intravenous crystalloid fluids to maintain hydration. Do NOT induce emesis, because of the risk of causing further esophageal irritation. Give milk or large amounts of water orally, as tolerated by the patient, to dilute the toxin.

Detergents, nonionic

Introduction

Nonionic detergents include alkyl and aryl polyether sulfates, alcohols, and sulfonates; alkyl phenol; polyethylene glycol; and phenol compounds. Phenols are particularly toxic in cats and puppies. Clinical signs of exposure include severe gastroenteritis and topical irritation. Some compounds can be metabolized to glycolic and oxalic acid, causing renal damage similar to that observed with ethylene glycol toxicity.

Treatment

Topical and ocular exposure should be treated with careful bathing or ocular irrigation for at least 30 minutes. Administer activated charcoal to prevent absorption of the compound. As tolerated, give dilute milk or straight tap water orally to dilute the compound. Administer antiemetic and gastroprotectant drugs to control vomiting and decrease gastrointestinal irritation. Administer intravenous crystalloid fluids to maintain hydration and decrease the potential for renal tubular damage. Monitor the patient's acid-base and electrolyte status and correct any abnormalities with appropriate intravenous fluid therapy.

Dichlone

Introduction

Diclone (Phigone) is a dipyridyl compound that is a CNS depressant. The LD_{50} in rats is 25-50 mg/kg. Dichlone reacts with thiol enzymes to cause methemoglobinemia and hepatorenal damage.

Treatment

To treat dichlone ingestion, induce emesis or perform orogastric lavage, followed by administration of activated charcoal and a cathartic. Procure and maintain a patent airway. Perform intravenous fluid diuresis to maintain renal perfusion. *N*-acetylcysteine may be useful in the treatment of methemoglobinemia.

Diethyltoluamide (DEET)

Introduction

Diethyltoluamide (DEET) is the active ingredient in many insect repellants (e.g., Off, Cutters, Hartz Blockade). The mechanism of action of DEET is not fully understood, but it acts as a lipophilic neurotoxin within 5 to 10 minutes of exposure. Cats appear to be particularly sensitive to DEET. A lethal dermal dose is 1.8 g/kg; if ingested, the lethal dose is much less. The toxic dose of dermal exposure in dogs is 7 g/kg. Clinical signs of toxicity include aimless gazing, hypersalivation, chewing motions, and muscle tremors that progress to seizures. Recumbency and death can occur within 30 minutes of exposure at high doses.

Treatment

Treatment of DEET toxicity is largely supportive, as there are no known antidotes. Procure and maintain a patent airway and perform mechanical ventilation, if necessary. Place an intravenous catheter and administer intravenous crystalloid fluids to control hydration and treat hypotension, as necessary. Treat seizures with diazepam (0.5 mg/kg IV) or phenobarbital. Because of the rapid onset of clinical signs, induction of emesis is contraindicated. Perform orogastric lavage if the compound was ingested within the last 2 hours. Administer multiple repeated doses of activated charcoal. Cooling measures should be implemented to control hyperthermia. If dermal exposure has occurred, bathe the patient thoroughly to avoid further exposure and absorption.

Diquat

Introduction

Diquat is a dipyridyl compound that is the active ingredient in some herbicide compounds. The LD_{50} of diquat is 25-50 mg/kg. Like paraquat, diquat induces its toxic effects by causing the production of oxygen-derived free radical species. Clinical signs of diquat intoxication include anorexia, vomiting, diarrhea, and acute renal failure. Massive dehydration and electrolyte imbalances can occur as a result of fluid loss into the gastrointestinal tract.

Treatment

Treatment of diquat intoxication is similar to that for paraquat ingestion. If the animal had ingested diquat within 1 hour of presentation, induce emesis. In clinical cases, orogastric lavage may be required. Both emesis and orogastric lavage should be followed by administration of kaolin or bentonite as an adsorbent, rather than activated charcoal. Place an intravenous catheter and administer crystalloid fluids to restore volume status and maintain renal perfusion. Monitor urine output. If oliguria or anuria occurs, treatment with mannitol, furosemide, and dopamine may be considered.

Ecstasy

Introduction

Ecstasy (3,4-methylenedioxymethylamphetamine; MDMA) is a recreational drug used by humans. Ecstasy causes release of serotonin. Clinical signs of intoxication are related to the serotonin syndrome (excitation, hyperthermia, tremors, and hypertension), and seizures may be observed. A urine drug screening test can be used to detect the presence of MDMA.

Treatment

Treatment of ecstasy intoxication is largely supportive, as there is no known antidote. Administer intravenous fluids to maintain hydration, correct acid-base status, and treat hyperthermia. Serotonin antagonist drugs (cyproheptadine) can be dissolved and administered per rectum to alleviate clinical signs. Intravenous propranolol has additional anti-serotonin effects. Administer diazepam (0.5-2 mg/kg IV) to control seizures. If cerebral edema is suspected, administer mannitol, followed by furosemide.

Ethylene glycol

Introduction

Ethylene glycol is most commonly found in antifreeze solutions but is also in some paints, photography developer solutions, and windshield wiper fluid. Ethylene glycol in itself is only minimally toxic. However, when it is metabolized to glycolate, glyoxal, glyoxylate, and oxalate, the metabolites cause an increased anion gap metabolic acidosis and precipitation of calcium oxalate crystals in the renal tubules, renal failure, and (ultimately) death.

The toxic dose in dogs is 6.6 mL/kg, and in cats is 1.5 mL/kg. The toxin is absorbed quite readily from the gastrointestinal tract and can be detected in the patient's serum within an hour of ingestion. Colorimetric tests that can be performed in most veterinary hospitals can detect larger quantities of ethylene glycol in the patient's serum. In a dog with clinical signs of ethylene glycol intoxication and renal impairment or failure, a negative test for the presence of calcium oxalate crystalluria means that there is no more ethylene glycol in the patient's serum because it has all been metabolized. Cats are very sensitive to the toxic effects of ethylene glycol. In many cases, cat may have ingested a toxic dose, but because the sensitivity of the assay is low, test results will be negative. Lack of treatment can result in death.

There are three phases of ethylene glycol intoxication. In the first 1 to12 hours after ingestion (stage I), the patient may appear lethargic, disoriented, and ataxic. In stage II (12 to 24 hours following ingestion), the patient improves and appears clinically normal. In stage III (24 to 72 hours following ingestion), the patient demonstrates clinical signs of renal failure (polyuria and polydipsia) that progress to uremic renal failure (vomiting, lethargy, oral ulceration). Finally, seizures, coma, and death occur.

Treatment

Begin treatment of known ethylene glycol ingestion immediately. Induce emesis or perform orogastric lavage and adminiser repeated doses of activated charcoal. Place an intravenous catheter and perform crystalloid fluid diuresis with a known antidote. The treatment of choice for dogs is administration of 4-methylpyrrazole (4-MP), which directly inhibits alcohol dehydrogenase, thus preventing the conversion of ethylene glycol to its toxic metabolites. The dose for dogs is 20 mg/kg initially, followed by 15 mg/kg at 12 and 24 hours and 5 mg/kg at 36 hours. 4-MP has been used experimentally at 6.25 times the recommended dose for dogs. In cats, treatment with 4-MP is effective if it is administered within the first 3 hours of ingestion.

Cats will demonstrate signs of sedation and hypothermia with this treatment. If 4-MP is not available, administer ethanol (600 mg/kg IV loading dose, followed by 100 mg/kg/hour), or as a 20% solution (for dogs, 5.5 mL/kg IV q4h for five treatments, then q 6h for five more treatments; for cats, 5 mL/kg q8h for four treatments). Grain alcohol (190 proof) contains approximately 715 mg/mL of ethanol. Antiemetics and gastroprotective agents should be considered. Urinary alkalinization and peritoneal dialysis may enhance the elimination of ethylene glycol and its metabolites.

Fertilizers

Introduction

Many fertilizers are on the market, and may be composed of urea or ammonium salts, phosphates, nitrates, potash, and metal salts. Fertilizers have a moderate toxic potential, depending on the type and amount ingested. Clinical signs of fertilizer ingestion include vomiting, diarrhea, metabolic acidosis, and diuresis. Nitrates or nitrites can cause formation of methemoglobin and chocolate-brown blood. Electrolyte disturbances include hyperkalemia, hyperphosphatemia, hyperammonemia, and hyperosmolality.

Treatment

Treatment of fertilizer ingestion includes cardiovascular support, and administration of milk or a mixture of egg whites and water, followed by induction of emesis or orogastric lavage. Correct electrolyte abnormalities as they occur (see section on Hyperkalemia). Administer antiemetic and gastroprotectant drugs, as necessary. Administer intravenous fluids to control hydration and maintain blood pressure. *N*-acetylcysteine may be useful if methemoglobinemia is present.

Fipronil

Introduction

Fipronil is the active ingredient in Frontline, a flea control product. Fipronil exerts its effects by GABA antagonism and can cause CNS excitation.

Treatment

Treatment of fiprinol toxicity includes treatment of CNS excitation, treatment of hyperthermia by cooling measures, and administration of activated charcoal.

1

Fire extinguisher (liquid)

Introduction

Fire extinguisher fluid contains chlorobromomethane or methyl bromide, both of which have a serious toxic potential. Dermal or ocular irritation can occur. If ingested, the compounds can be converted to methanol, and cause high anion gap metabolic acidosis, CNS excitation and depression, aspiration pneumonitis, and hepatorenal damage.

Treatment

To treat ocular or dermal exposure to fire extinguisher fluids, flush the eyes or skin with warmed tap water or 0.9% saline solution for a minimum of 30 minutes. Do NOT induce emesis or perform orogastric lavage to treat ingestion, because of the risk of causing severe aspiration pneumonitis. Gastroprotectant and antiemetic drugs may be used, if indicated. Administer intravenous fluids to maintain hydration and renal perfusion. Supplemental oxygen or mechanical ventilation may be required in severe cases of aspiration pneumonitis.

Fireplace colors

Introduction

Fireplace colors contain salts of heavy metals—namely, copper rubidium, cesium, lead, arsenic, antimony, barium, selenium, and zinc, all of which have moderate toxic potential, depending on the amount ingested and the size of the patient. Clinical signs are largely associated with gastrointestinal irritation (vomiting, diarrhea, anorexia). Zinc toxicity can cause intravascular hemolysis and hepatorenal damage.

Treatment

To treat ingestion of fireplace colors, administer cathartics and activated charcoal and gastroprotectant and antiemetic drugs. Place an intravenous catheter for intravenous crystalloid fluid administration to maintain hydration and renal perfusion. Specific chelating agents may be useful in hastening elimination of the heavy metals.

Fireworks

Introduction

Fireworks contain oxidizing agents (nitrates and chlorates) and metals (mercury, copper, strontium, barium, and phosphorus). Ingestion of fireworks can cause hemorrhagic gastroenteritis and methemoglobinemia.

Treatment

To treat firework ingestion, induce emesis or perform orogastric lavage and administer activated charcoal. Administer specific chelating drugs if the amount and type of metal are known, and administer gastroprotectant and antiemetic drugs. If methemoglobinemia occurs, administer *N*-acetylcysteine; a blood transfusion may be necessary.

Fuels

Introduction

Fuels such as barbecue lighter fluid, gasoline, kerosene, and oils (mineral, fuel, lubricating) are petroleum distillate products that have a low toxic potential if ingested but can cause severe aspiration pneumonitis if as little as 1 mL is inhaled into the tracheobronchial tree. CNS depression, mucosal damage, hepatorenal insufficiency, seizures, and corneal irritation can occur.

Treatment

If fuels are ingested, administer gastroprotectant and antiemetics drugs. Do NOT induce emesis or perform orogastric lavage, because of the risk of aspiration pneumonia. To treat topical exposure, rinse the skin and eyes copiously with warm tap water or

0.9% saline solution. Administer antiemetic and gastroprotectant drugs, as necessary. Administer intravenous fluids to maintain hydration and treat acid-base and electrolyte abnormalities.

Furniture polish: see fuels

Gasolines: see Fuels

Glue, children's

Introduction

Children's glue contains polyvinyl acetate, which has a very low toxic potential. If inhaled, the compound can cause pneumonitis.

Treatment

Treatment of polyvinyl acetate should be performed as clinical signs of pneumonitis (increased respiratory effort, cough, lethargy, respiratory distress) occur.

Glue, Superglue

Introduction

Superglue contains methyl-2-cyanoacrylate, a compound that can cause severe dermal irritation on contact.

Treatment:

Do NOT induce emesis. Do NOT bathe the animal, and do NOT apply other compounds (acetone, turpentine) in an attempt to remove the glue from the skin. The fur can be shaved, using care to avoid damaging the underlying skin. The affected area should be allowed to exfoliate naturally.

Glyophosate

Introduction

Glyophosate is a herbicide found in Roundup and Kleenup. If applied properly, the product has a very low toxic potential. Clinical signs of toxicity include dermal and gastric irritation, including dermal erythema, anorexia, and vomiting. CNS depression can occur.

Treatment

Treatment includes thorough bathing in cases of dermal exposure, and induction of emesis or orogastric lavage followed by administration of activated charcoal. Administer antiemetic and gastroprotectant drugs as necessary. Administer intravenous crystalloid fluids to prevent dehydration secondary to vomiting.

Grapes and raisins

Introduction

Even small amounts of grapes and raisins can be toxic to dogs. The mechanism of toxicity remains unknown. Clinical signs occur within 24 hours of ingestion of raisins or grapes, and include vomiting, anorexia, lethargy, and diarrhea (often with visible raisins or grapes in the fecal matter). Within 48 hours, dogs demonstrate signs of acute renal failure (polyuria, polydipsia, vomiting) that can progress to anuria.

Treatment

To treat known ingestion of raisins or grapes, induce emesis or perform orogastric lavage, followed by repeated doses of activated charcoal. If clinical signs of vomiting and diarrhea are present, administer intravenous fluids and monitor urine output. Aggressive intravenous fluid therapy, in conjunction with maintenance of renal perfusion, is necessary. In cases of anuric renal failure, dopamine, furosemide, and mannitol can be useful in increasing urine output. Peritoneal or hemodialysis may be necessary in cases of severe oliguric or anuric renal failure. Calcium channel blockers such as amlodipine and diltiazem can be used to treat systemic hypertension. Supportive care includes treatment of hyperkalemia, and administration of gastroprotectant and antiemetic drugs and (if the animal is eating) phosphate binders.

Hashish: see marijuana

Hexachlorophene: see detergents, nonionic

Hydrocarbons, aromatic

Introduction

Aromatic hydrocarbons include phenols, cresols, toluene, and naphthalene. All have a moderate toxic potential if ingested. Toxicities associated with ingestion of aromatic hydrocarbons include CNS depression, hepatorenal damage, muscle tremors, pneumonia, methemoglobinemia, and intravascular hemolysis.

Treatment

If an aromatic hydrocarbon is ingested, do NOT induce emesis, because of the risk of aspiration pneumonia. A dilute milk solution or water can be administered to dilute the compound. Perform orogastric lavage. Carefully monitor the patient's respiratory and cardiovascular status. Administer supplemental oxygen if aspiration pneumonia is present. To treat topical exposure, thoroughly rinse the eyes and skin with copious amounts of warm tap water or 0.9% saline solution.

Ibuprofen: see nonsteroidal antiinflammatory drugs

Imidacloprid

Introduction

Imidacloprid is the compound used in the flea product Advantage. Clinical signs of toxicity are related to nicotinic cholinergic stimulation, causing neuromuscular excitation followed by collapse. The compound may induce respiratory paralysis.

Treatment

To treat imidacloprid toxicity, procure and maintain a patent airway with supplemental oxygen administration. Control CNS excitation with diazepam, phenobarbital, or propofol. Administer enemas to hasten gastrointestinal elimination, and administer activated charcoal. Bathe the animal thoroughly to prevent further dermal absorption. Closely monitor the patient's oxygenation and ventilation status. If severe hypoventilation or respiratory paralysis occurs, initiate mechanical ventilation.

Iron and iron salts

Introduction

Iron and iron salts can cause severe gastroenteritis, myocardial toxicity, and hepatic damage if high enough doses are ingested. Lawn fertilizers are a common source of iron salts.

Treatment:

Treatment of ingestion of iron and iron salts includes cardiovascular support in the form of intravenous fluids and antiarrhythmic drugs, as needed. Induce emesis or perform orogastric lavage for gastric decontamination. A cathartic can be administered to promote elimination from the gastrointestinal tract. Antiemetic and gastroprotectant drugs should be administered to prevent nausea and vomiting. In some cases, radiographs can aid in making a diagnosis of whether the compound was actually ingested. Iron toxicity can be treated with the chelating agent deferoxamine.

Ivermectin

Introduction

Ivermectin is a GABA agonist that is used in commercial heartworm prevention and antihelminthic compounds and can be toxic in predisposed breeds, including Collies, Collie crosses, Old English Sheepdogs, and some Terriers. Clinical signs of ivermectin toxicity include vomiting, ataxia, hypersalivation, agitation, tremors, hyperactivity, hyperthermia, hypoventilation, coma, seizures, signs of circulatory shock, bradycardia, and death. Clinical signs often occur within 2 to 24 hours after ingestion or iatrogenic overdose. Blood ivermectin levels can be measured, but diagnosis is often made based on clinical signs and knowledge of exposure in predisposed breeds. There is no known antidote. The clinical course can be prolonged for weeks to months before recovery occurs.

Treatment

To treat known exposure, induce emesis or perform orogastric lavage if the substance was ingested was within 1 hour of presentation and the patient is not symptomatic. Administer activated charcoal. Control seizures with phenobarbital, pentobarbital, or propofol administered as intermittent boluses or as a constant rate infusion. Diazepam, which potentially can *worsen* central nervous stimulation, is contraindicated. Administer intravenous fluids to maintain perfusion and hydration, and treat hyperthermia. Supportive care may be necessary, including supplemental oxygen (or mechanical ventilation, if necessary), frequent turning of the patient and passive range-of-motion exercises, placement of a urinary catheter to maintain patient cleanliness and monitor urine output, lubrication of the eyes, and parenteral nutrition (see section on Rule of Twenty). Specific antidotes used to treat ivermectin toxicity include physostigmine and picrotoxin. Physostigmine therapy was beneficial in some patients for a short period; picrotoxin caused severe violent seizures and therefore should be avoided.

Kerosene: see fuels

d-Limonene, linalool

Introduction

d-Limonene and linalool are components of citrus oil extracts used in some flea control products. The toxic dose is unknown, but cats appear to be very sensitive to exposure. Clinical signs of toxicity include hypersalivation, muscle tremors, ataxia, and hypothermia.

Treatment

Treatment of d-Limonene and linalool exposure includes treatment of hypothermia, administration of activated charcoal to prevent further absorption, and careful, thorough bathing to prevent further dermal exposure.

Lead

Introduction

Lead is ubiquitous, and is found in some paints, car batteries, fishing equipment/ sinkers, and plumbing materials. Lead can be toxic at doses of 3 mg/kg. If more than than 10-25 mg/kg of lead is ingested, death can occur. Lead causes toxicity by inhibiting sulfur-containing enzymes, leading to increased RBC fragility, and CNS damage. Clinical signs of hyperexcitability, dementia, vocalization, seizures, and lower motor neuron polyneuropathy can occur. Affected animals may appear blind, or vomiting, anorexia, and constipation or diarrhea may occur. If lead toxicity is suspected, blood and urine lead levels can be measured.

Treatment

Treatment of lead toxicity is supportive and is directed at treatment of clinical signs. Control seizures with diazepam or phenobarbital. If cerebral edema is present, administer mannitol (0.5-1.0 g/kg IV), followed by furosemide (1 mg/kg IV 20 minutes after mannitol). Sodium or magnesium sulfate should be administered as a cathartic. Initiate chelation therapy with dimercaprol, penicillamine, or calcium EDTA. If a lead object is identified in the gastrointestinal tract on radiographs, remove the object using endoscopy or exploratory laparotomy.

Loperamide

Introduction

Loperamide is an opioid derivative that is used to treat diarrhea. Clinical signs of loperamide intoxication include constipation, ataxia, nausea, and sedation.

Treatment

Induce emesis or perform orogastric lavage, followed by administration of activated charcoal and a cathartic. Naloxone may be beneficial in the temporary reversal of ataxia and sedation.

Macadamia nuts

Introduction

Ingestion of macadamia nuts can cause clinical signs of vomiting, ataxia, and ascending paralysis in dogs. The toxic principle in macadamia nuts is unknown.

Treatment

There is no known antidote. Treatment consists of supportive care, including administration of intravenous fluids and antiemetics and placement of a urinary catheter for patient cleanliness. Clinical signs resolve in most cases within 72 hours.

Marijuana *(Cannibis sativa)*

Introduction

Marijuana is a hallucinogen that can cause CNS depression, ataxia, mydriasis, increased sensitivity to motion or sound, salivation, and tremors. Along with these findings, a classic clinical sign is the sudden onset of dribbling urine. Urine can be tested with drug test kits for tetrahydrocannabinoid (THC), the toxic compound in marijuana.

Treatment

There is no known antidote for marijuana toxicity; therefore, treatment is largely symptomatic. place an intravenous catheter and administer intravenous fluids to support hydration. Administer atropine if severe bradycardia exists. Induction of emesis can be attempted but because of the antiemetic effects of THC, is usually unsuccessful. Orogastric lavage can be performed, followed by repeated doses of activated charcoal. Clinical signs usually resolve within 12 to 16 hours.

Matches

Introduction

"Strike Anywhere" matches, safety matches, and the striking surface of matchbook covers contain iron phosphorus or potassium chlorate. Both compounds have a low toxic potential but can cause clinical signs of gastroenteritis and methemoglobinemia if large quantities are ingested.

Treatment

Treatment of match and matchbook ingestion includes gastric decontamination with induction of emesis or orogastric lavage and administration of activated charcoal and a cathartic. If methemoglobinemia occurs, administer *N*-acetylcysteine, intravenous fluids, and supplemental oxygen.

Metaldehyde

Introduction

Metaldehyde is the active ingredient in most brands of snail bait. The exact mechanism of toxicity is unknown but may involve inhibition of GABA channels. Clinical signs associated with metaldehyde toxicity include severe muscle tremors, CNS excitation, and

1

hyperthermia, that occurs within 15 – 30 minutes of ingestion. Diarrhea and convulsions can develop. If hyperthermia is severe, renal failure secondary to myoglobinuria and disseminated intravascular coagulation can result. Delayed hepatic failure has been described days after initial recovery. If metaldehyde toxicosis is suspected, analysis of urine, serum, and stomach contents is warranted.

Treatment

To treat metaldehyde toxicity, procure and maintain a patent airway and control CNS excitation and muscle tremors. If an animal has just ingested the metaldehyde and is not symptomatic, induce emesis. If clinical signs are present, perform orogastric lavage. Both emesis and orogastric lavage should be followed by administration of one dose of activated charcoal. Administer intravenous fluids to control hyperthermia, prevent dehydration, and correct acid-base and electrolyte abnormalities. Methocarbamol is the treatment of choice to control muscle tremors. Diazepam can be used to control seizures if they occur.

Methiocarb: see carbamates
Mineral Spirits: see fuels
Mothballs: see naphthalene
Mushrooms
Introduction

Mushroom ingestion most commonly causes activation of the autonomic nervous system, resulting in tremors, agitation, restlessness, hyperexcitability, and seizures. In some cases SLUD (salivation, lacrimation, urination, and defecation) is seen. Some mushrooms (*Amanita* spp.) also can cause hepatocellular toxicity. Clinical signs include vomiting, anorexia, lethargy, and progressive icterus.

Treatment

Treatment of mushroom toxicity is largely supportive. If the mushroom was ingested within the last 2 hours, induce emesis or perform orogastric lavage and then administer activated charcoal. Symptomatic treatment includes intravenous fluids to promote diuresis and treat hyperthermia and skeletal muscle relaxants to control tremors and seizures (methocarbamol, diazepam). If *Amanita* ingestion is suspected, administer hepatoprotectant agents including milk thistle.

Mycotoxins (tremorigenic mycotoxins)
Introduction

Mycotoxins from *Penicillium* spp. are found in moldy foods, cream cheese, and nuts. Clinical signs of intoxication include tremors, agitation, hyperesthesia, and seizures. If tremorigenic mycotoxin toxicity is suspected, a sample of the patient's serum and gastric contents or vomitus can be submitted to the Michigan State University Veterinary Toxicology Laboratory for tremorigen assay.

Treatment

There is no known antidote. Perform orogastric lavage, followed by administration of activated charcoal. Control tremors and seizures with methocarbamol, diazepam, phenobarbital, or pentobarbital. Administer intravenous fluids to control hyperthermia and maintain hydration. In cases in which cerebral edema is suspected secondary to severe refractory seizures, administer intravenous mannitol and furosemide.

Naphthalene
Introduction

Naphthalene is the active ingredient in mothballs and has a high toxic potential. Clinical signs associated with naphthalene toxicity include vomiting, methemoglobinemia, CNS stimulation, seizures, and hepatic toxicity. A complete blood count often reveals Heinz bodies and anemia.

Treatment

DO NOT induce emesis if naphthalene ingestion is suspected. If the ingestion was within 1 hour of presentation, perform orogastric lavage. Control seizures with diazepam or phenobarbital. Administer intravenous fluids to control hyperthermia and maintain hydration. *N*-acetylcysteine can play a role in the treatment of methemoglobinemia. A packed RBC transfusion may be necessary if anemia is severe. Observe the patient for clinical signs associated with hepatitis.

Nicotine

Introduction

Nicotine toxicity occurs in animals as the result of ingestion of cigarettes, nicotine-containing gum, and some insecticides. Nicotine stimulates autonomic ganglia at low doses, and blocks autonomic ganglia and the neuromuscular junction at high doses. Absorption after ingestion is rapid. Clinical signs include hyperexcitability and SLUD (salivation, lacrimation, urination, and defecation). Muscle tremors, respiratory muscle fatigue or hypoventilation, tachyarrhythmias, seizures, coma, and death can occur.

Treatment

If the patient presents within 1 hour of ingestion and has no clinical signs, induce emesis, followed by administration of repeated doses of activated charcoal. In patients with clinical signs of toxicity, perform orogastric lavage. Administer intravenous fluids to maintain hydration and promote diuresis, and treat hyperthermia. Administer atropine to treat cholinergic symptoms. Urinary acidification can promote nicotine excretion.

Nonsteroidal ant-inflammatory drugs

Introduction

Nonsteroidal antiinflammatory drugs (NSAIDs) include ibuprofen, ketoprofen, carprofen, diclofenac, naproxen, celecoxib, valdecoxib, rofecoxib, and deracoxib. NSAIDs cause inhibition of prostaglandin synthesis, leading to gastrointestinal ulceration, renal failure and hepatotoxicity. Ibuprofen toxicity has been associated with seizures in dogs, cats, and ferrets. The toxic dose varies with the specific compound ingested.

Treatment

To treat NSAID toxicity, induce emesis or perform orogastric lavage, followed by administration of multiple repeated doses of activated charcoal. Place an intravenous catheter for crystalloid fluid diuresis to maintain renal perfusion. Administer the synthetic prostaglandin analogue misoprostol to help maintain gastric and renal perfusion. Control seizures, if present, with intravenous diazepam. Administer gastroprotectant and antiemetic drugs to control vomiting and gastrointestinal hemorrhage. Continue intravenous fluid diuresis for a minimum of 48 hours, with frequent monitoring of the patient's BUN and creatinine. When the BUN and creatinine levels are normal or have plateaued for 24 hours, slowly decrease fluid diuresis 25% per day until maintenance levels are restored.

Oils (lubricating, fuel, mineral): see fuels
Onions, garlic, and chives

Introduction

Onions, garlic, and chives contain sulfoxide compounds that can cause oxidative damage of RBCs, leading to Heinz body anemia, methemoglobinemia, and intravascular hemolysis. Clinical signs of toxicity include weakness, lethargy, tachypnea, tachycardia, and pale mucous membranes. Vomiting and diarrhea can occur. Intravascular hemolysis can cause hemoglobinuria and pigment damage of the renal tubular epithelium. Heinz bodies may be observed on cytologic evaluation of the peripheral blood smear.

Treatment

Treatment of onion, chive, and garlic toxicity includes administration of intravenous fluid diuresis, and induction of emesis or orogastric lavage, followed by administration of activated charcoal and a cathartic. In cases of severe anemia, packed RBC transfusion or administration of a hemoglobin-based oxygen carrier should be considered.

Opiates

Introduction

Opiate drugs include heroin, morphine, oxymorphone, fentanyl, meperidine, and codeine. Opiate compounds bind to specific opioid receptors throughout the body and produce clinical signs of miosis or mydriasis (cats), and CNS excitation, followed by ataxia and CNS depression, leading to stupor and coma. Hypoventilation, bradycardia, hypoxia, and cyanosis can occur.

Treatment

To treat known overdose or ingestion of an opiate compound, induce emesis (in asymptomatic animals) or perform orogastric lavage, followed by administration of activated charcoal. Administer intravenous fluids and supplemental oxygen to support the cardiovascular and respiratory systems. Mechanical ventilation may be necessary until hypoventilation resolves. Administer repeated doses of naloxone as a specific antidote to reverse clinical signs of narcosis and hypoventilation. If seizures are present (meperidine toxicity), administer diazepam.

Oral contraceptives
Organophosphates

Introduction

Organophosphate compounds traditionally are used in flea control products and insecticides. Common examples of organophosphates include chlorpyrifos, coumaphos, diazinon, dichlorvos, and malathion. The toxic dose varies, depending on the particular compound and individual animal sensitivity. Organophosphate toxicity causes acetylcholinesterase inhibition, resulting in clinical signs of CNS stimulation, including tremors and seizures. Muscarinic acetylcholine overload causes the classic SLUD signs of salivation, lacrimation, urination, and defecation. Miosis, excessive bronchial secretions, muscle tremors, and respiratory paralysis can occur. An intermediate syndrome of generalized weakness, hypoventilation, and eventual paralysis with ventral cervical ventroflexion that may require mechanical ventilation has been described. If organophosphate toxicity is suspected, whole-blood acetylcholinesterase activity can be measured and will be low.

Treatment

Treatment of toxicity includes careful and thorough bathing in cases of dermal exposure and, if the substance was ingested, gastric decontamination with induction of emesis or orogastric lavage, followed by administration of activated charcoal, and administration of the antidote pralidoxime hydrochloride (2-PAM). Atropine can help control the muscarinic clinical signs. Supportive care in the form of cooling measures, intravenous crystalloid fluids, and supplemental oxygen or mechanical ventilation may be required, depending on the severity of clinical signs.

Paint and varnish removers: see fuels
Paints and varnishes: see fuels
Paintballs

Introduction

Ingestion of large amounts of paintballs can cause neurologic signs, electrolyte abnormalities, and occasionally death. Paintballs are gelatin capsules that contain multiple colors of paint in a sorbitol or glycerol carrier. When large quantities of these osmotically active sugars are ingested, osmotic shifts of fluid cause a sudden onset of neurologic or gastro-intestinal signs, including ataxia, seizures, and osmotic diarrhea caused by massive fluid shifts into the gastrointestinal tract. The loss of water in excess of solute can result in hyper-natremia, a free water deficit, and increased serum osmolality.

Treatment

Following orogastric lavage, treatment of ingestion includes administering warm water enemas to help speed the movement of the paintballs through the gastrointestinal tract. Do NOT administer activated charcoal (usually in a propylene glycol carrier), because the compound's cathartic action will pull more fluid into the gastrointestinal tract. Baseline electrolytes should be obtained and then carefully monitored. If severe hypernatremia develops, administer hypotonic solutions such as 0.45% NaCl + 2.5% dextrose or 5% dextrose in water after calculating the patient's free water deficit. Because of the large volume of fluid loss, intravenous fluid rates may seem excessive but are necessary to normalize acid-base, electrolyte, and hydration status. In most cases, these patients can survive if the problem is recognized promptly and corrected with careful electrolyte moni-toring, aggressive decontamination strategies, and intravenous fluid support.

Paracetamol: see acetaminophen
Paraquat
Introduction

Paraquat, a dipyridyl compound, is the active ingredient in some herbicides. The LD_{50} of paraquat is 25-50 mg/kg. Paraquat initially causes CNS excitation. It also causes produc-tion of oxygen-derived free radical species in the lungs, that can lead to the development of acute respiratory distress syndrome. Initial clinical signs include vomiting, diarrhea, and seizures. Within 2 to 3 days, clinical signs associated with severe respiratory distress and acute respiratory distress syndrome (ARDS) can develop, leading to death. Chronic effects include pulmonary fibrosis, if the patient survives the initial toxicity period. The prognosis for paraquat toxicity is generally unfavorable.

Treatment

To treat Paraquat ingestion, remove the toxin from the gastrointestinal tract as rapidly as possible after ingestion. There are no known antidotes. If the compound was ingested within the past hour and the animal is able to protect its airway, induce emesis. Otherwise, perform orogastric lavage. Activated charcoal is not as effective as clay or bentonite adsor-bents for removing this particular toxin. Early in the course of paraquat toxicity, oxygen therapy is contraindicated because of the risk of producing oxygen-derived free radical species. Later, oxygen therapy, including mechanical ventilation, is necessary if ARDS develops. Experimentally, free radical scavengers (*N*-acetyl cysteine, vitamin C, vitamin E, sAME) have been shown to be useful in preventing damage caused by oxygen-derived free radical species. Hemoperfusion may be useful in eliminating the toxin, if it is performed early in the course of toxicity.

Paraffin wax: see fuels
Pennies: see zinc and zinc oxide
Pennyroyal oil
Introduction

Pennyroyal oil is an herbal flea control compound that contains menthofuran as its toxic compound. Menthofuran is hepatotoxic and may cause gastrointestinal hemorrhage and coagulopathies.

Treatment

To treat toxicity, administer a cathartic and activated charcoal and antiemetic and gastro-protectant drugs, and thoroughly bathe the animal to prevent further dermal exposure.

Petroleum distillates: see fuels

Phenobarbital: see barbiturates

Phenylcyclidine (angel dust)

Introduction

Phenylcyclidine (Angel Dust) is an illicit recreational drug that causes both CNS depression and excitation, decreased cardiac output, and hypotension.

Treatment

To treat phenylcyclidine toxicity, place an intravenous catheter, and administer intravenous fluids and antiarrhythmic drugs to maintain organ perfusion. Administer supplemental oxygen, and administer diazepam to control seizures. Urine alkalinization can help eliminate the compound.

Phenylephrine

Introduction

Phenylephrine is an α-adrenergic agonist in many over-the-counter decongestant preparations. Clinical signs of intoxication include mydriasis, tachypnea, agitation, hyperactivity, and abnormal flybiting and staring behavior. Tachycardia, bradycardia, hypertension, hyperthermia, and seizures can occur.

Treatment:

To treat phenylephrine toxicity, place an intravenous catheter and give intravenous fluids to maintain hydration, promote diuresis, and treat hyperthermia. Administer prazosin or sodium nitroprusside to treat hypertension, antiarrhythmic drugs as necessary, and diazepam to control seizures.

Phenylpropanolamine

Introduction

Phenylpropanolamine has both α- and β-adrenergic agonist effects, and is used primarily in the treatment of urinary incontinence in dogs. The drug was taken off of the market for use in humans because of the risk of stroke. Clinical signs of phenylpropanolamine intoxication include hyperactivity, hyperthermia, mydriasis, tachyarrhythmias or bradycardia, hypertension, agitation, and seizures.

Treatment

To treat toxicity, administer prazosin or nitroprusside to control hypertension, a beta-blocker (esmolol, propranolol, atenolol) to control tachyarrhythmias, diazepam to control seizures, and intravenous fluids to maintain hydration and promote diuresis. Urine acidification may aid in facilitating excretion. If bradycardia occurs, do NOT use atropine.

Pseudoephedrine

Introduction

Pseudoephedrine is an α- and β-adrenergic agonist that is a component of many over-the-counter decongestants and is used in the manufacture of crystal methamphetamine. Clinical signs of toxicity include severe restlessness, tremors, mydriasis, agitation, hyperthermia, tachyarrhythmias or bradycardia, hypertension, and seizures.

Treatment

To treat toxicity, administer activated charcoal, intravenous fluids to promote diuresis and treat hyperthermia, chlorpromazine to combat α-adrenergic effects, a beta-blocker (propranolol, esmolol, atenolol) to treat β-adrenergic effects, and cyproheptadine (per rectum) to combat serotoninergic effects.

Photographic developer solutions: see detergents, nonionic

Pine oil disinfectants: see detergents, nonionic, and alcohols

Piperazine

Introduction

Piperazine is a GABA agonist, and causes cervical and truncal ataxia, tremors, seizures, coma, and death.

Treatment

If ingestion was recent and if no clinical signs of toxicity are present, induce emesis or perform orogastric lavage, followed by administration of a cathartic and activated charcoal. There is no known antidote. Treatment includes supportive care in the form of intravenous fluids and administration of phenobarbital or methocarbamol to control seizures and tremors. Diazepam, a GABA agonist, is contraindicated, because it can potentially worsen clinical signs. Urine acidification may hasten elimination. Clinical signs can last from 3 to 5 days.

Pyrethrin and pyrethroids

Introduction

Pyrethrin and pyrethroid compounds are extracted from chrysanthemums, and include allethrin, decamethrin, tralomethrin, fenpropanthrin, pallethrin, sumethrin, permethrin, tetramethrin, cyfluthrin, and resemethrin. The oral toxicity is fairly low; however, the compounds can be significantly harmful if inhaled or applied to the skin. Pyrethrin and pyrethroid compounds cause depolarization and blockade of nerve membrane potentials, causing clinical signs of tremors, seizures, respiratory distress, and paralysis. Contact dermatitis can occur. To distinguish between pyrethrin/pyrethroid toxicity and organophosphate toxicity, acetylcholinesterase levels should be obtained; they will be normal if pyrethrins are the cause of the animal's clinical signs.

Treatment

Treatment of toxicity is supportive, as there is no known antidote. Carefully bathe the animal in lukewarm water to prevent further oral and dermal exposure. Both hyperthermia and hypothermia can worsen clinical signs. Administer activated charcoal to decrease enterohepatic recirculation. Atropine may control clinical signs of excessive salivation. To control muscle tremors, administer methocarbamol to effect. Administer diazepam or phenobarbital to control seizures, as necessary.

Radiator fluids: see ethylene glycol

Raisins: see grapes and raisins

Rotenone

Introduction

Rotenone is used as a common garden and delousing insecticide. Fish and birds are very susceptible to rotenone toxicity. Rotenone inhibits mitochondrial electron transport. Clinical signs of tissue irritation and hypoglycemia can occur after topical or oral exposure. If the compound is inhaled, CNS depression and seizures can occur.

Treatment

To treat toxicity, perform orogastric lavage, followed by administration of a cathartic and activated charcoal. Bathe the animal carefully to prevent further dermal exposure and further ingestion. Administer diazepam or phenobarbital to control seizures. The prognosis generally is guarded.

Rubbing alcohol: see alcohols

Rust removers: see acids/corrosives

Salicylates: see aspirin

Salt, thawing

Introduction

Salt used for thawing ice commonly contains calcium chloride, a compound that has a moderate toxic potential. Calcium chloride produces strong local irritation and can cause gastroenteritis and gastrointestinal ulcers if ingested.

Treatment

Treatment of ingestion includes dilution with milk, water, or egg whites. Perform orogastric lavage, followed by administration of activated charcoal. Administer intravenous crystalloid fluids to maintain hydration. Administer antiemetic and gastroprotectant drugs to treat gastroenteritis and vomiting.

Shampoos, nonmedicated: see detergents, nonionic

Shampoos, selenium sulfide

Introduction

Selenium sulfide shampoos (e.g., Selsun Blue) have a low toxic potential, and primarily cause gastroenteritis.

Treatment

Treatment of ingestion includes dilution with water, milk, or egg whites and administration of activated charcoal. Carefully and thoroughly rinse the skin and eyes to prevent further exposure. Administer antiemetic and gastroprotectant drugs in cases of severe gastroenteritis.

Shampoos, zinc-based (anti-dandruff)

Introduction

Zinc-based (zinc pyridinethione) anti-dandruff shampoos have a serious toxic potential if ingested or if ocular exposure occurs. Gastrointestinal irritation, retinal detachment, progressive blindness, and exudative chorioretinitis can occur.

Treatment

Treatment of ingestion includes gastric decontamination. Induce emesis or perform orogastric lavage, followed by administration of a cathartic and activated charcoal.

To treat ocular exposure, thoroughly rinse the patient's eyes for a minimum of 30 minutes. Carefully monitor the animal for clinical signs of blindness. Implement intravenous fluid to maintain hydration and renal perfusion in cases of severe gastroenteritis.

Shoe polish: see aromatic hydrocarbons

Silver polish

Introduction

Silver polish contains the alkali substance sodium carbonate and cyanide salts, and has a serious toxic potential. Ingestion results in rapid onset of vomiting and possibly cyanide toxicity.

Treatment

To treat ingestion, monitor and maintain the patient's respiration and cardiovascular status and administer intravenous crystalloid fluids. Induce emesis, followed by administration of activated charcoal. Administer sodium nitrite or sodium thiosulfate IV for cyanide toxicity.

Soaps (bath, bar soap)

Introduction

Bath soap (bar soap) usually has low toxic potential and causes mild gastroenteritis with vomiting if ingested.

Treatment

To treat ingestion, include dilution with water, administration of intravenous fluids to maintain hydration, and administration of antiemetic and gastroprotectant drugs to treat gastroenteritis.

Sodium fluoroacetate (1080, 1081)

Introduction

Sodium fluoroacetate is a colorless, odorless, tasteless compound that causes uncoupling of oxidative phosphorylation. The toxic dose in dogs and cats is 0.05-1.0 mg/kg. Clinical signs of toxicity include CNS excitation, seizures, and coma secondary to cerebral edema. The prognosis is guarded.

Treatment

To treat toxicity, procure and maintain a patent airway, monitor and stabilize the cardiovascular status, and control hyperthermia. Perform orogastric lavage, followed by administration of activated charcoal. If clinical signs are not present at the time of presentation, induce emesis. Administer intravenous fluids and supplemental oxygen, as necessary.

Strattera (selective norepinephrine reuptake inhibitor)

Introduction

Strattera (atomoxetine hydrochloride) is a selective norepinephrine reuptake inhibitor used in the treatment of attention deficit hyperactivity disorder (ADHD) in humans. Peak serum concentrations occur in dogs within 3 to 4 hours of ingestion, with a peak half-life at 4 to 5 hours following ingestion. Clinical signs of toxicity include cardiac tachyarrhythmias, hypertension, disorientation, agitation, trembling, tremors, and hyperthermia.

Treatment

Treatment of intoxication is largely symptomatic and supportive in nature. First, induce emesis if the patient is conscious and has an intact gag reflex. Orogastric lavage can also be performed. Administer one dose of activated charcoal to prevent further absorption of the compound from the gastrointestinal tract. Identify cardiac dysrhythmias and treat accordingly. Control hypertension with sodium nitroprusside or diltiazem as a constant rate infusion. Administer acepromazine or chlorpromazine to control agitation. DO NOT use diazepam, because it can potentially worsen clinical signs. Administer intravenous fluids to maintain hydration and promote diuresis.

Strychnine

Introduction

Strychnine is the active ingredient in pesticides used to control rodents and other vermin. The toxic dose in dogs is 0.75 mg/kg, and in cats is 2 mg/kg. Strychnine antagonizes spinal inhibitory neurotransmitters and causes severe muscle tremors, muscle rigidity, and seizures. Clinical signs are stimulated or exacerbated by noise, touch, light, and sound. Mydriasis, hyperthermia, and respiratory paralysis can occur. If strychnine toxicity is suspected, gastric contents should be collected and saved for analysis.

Treatment

If the animal is asymptomatic at the time of presentation, induce emesis. If clinical signs are present, perform orogastric lavage. Both emesis and orogastric lavage should be followed by the administration of activated charcoal. Administer intravenous crystalloid fluids to support the cardiovascular system, aid in cooling measures, and improve renal diuresis. Treat CNS stimulation with methocarbamol, diazepam, or phenobarbital. The animal should have cotton packed in its ears to prevent noise stimulation, and should be placed in a quiet, dark room.

Styptic pencil

Introduction

Styptic pencils contain potassium alum sulfate, a compound with a low toxic potential. Ingestion of styptic pencils is corrosive due to the release of sulfuric acid during hydrolysis of the salt.

Treatment

Treatment of ingestion includes dilution with Milk of Magnesia or water, administration of antiemetic and gastroprotectant drugs, and administration of intravenous crystalloid fluids to maintain hydration. Do NOT induce emesis, because of the risk of causing further esophageal irritation.

Sunscreen: see zinc and zinc oxide
Suntan lotion: see shampoos, zinc-based, and alcohols
Tar: see fuels
Tea tree oil (melaleuca oil)

Introduction

Tea tree (melaleuca) oil is an herbal-origin flea-control product. The toxic principles in tea tree oil are monoterpenes, which produce clinical signs of neuromuscular weakness, and ataxia.

Treatment

Treatment of tea tree oil toxicity includes administration of cathartics and activated charcoal to prevent further absorption. Carefully bathe the animal to prevent further dermal exposure.

Tetanus

Introduction

Tetanus spores from *Clostridium tetani* organisms are ubiquitous in the soil and feces, particularly in barnyards. Cases have been reported in dogs after tooth eruption and after abdominal surgeries performed with cold sterilization packs. Anaerobic wound infections can contain tetanus spores. The neurotoxin from *C. tetani* inhibits spinal inhibitory neurons, causing motor neuron excitation. Extensor muscle rigidity ("sawhorse stance"), erect ears, and risus sardonicus (a sardonic grin) are characteristic features of tetanus.

Treatment:

Administer tetanus antitoxin if toxin has not already been bound in the CNS. To eliminate the source of the toxin (e.g., abscess), open and debride all wounds. Intravenous administration of ampicillin or penicillin G is the treatment of choice for tetanus. Supportive care in the form of skeletal muscle relaxants, intravenous fluids and parenteral nutrition, and nursing care to prevent decubitus ulcer formation is required. In extreme cases, mechanical ventilation may be necessary.

Toilet bowl cleaners: see acids/corrosives
Triazenes

Introduction

Triazene compounds include atrazine, prometone, and monuron (Telvar). The toxic mechanism of triazene compounds is unknown. Clinical signs of toxicity include salivation, ataxia, hyporeflexia, contact dermatitis, hepatorenal damage, muscle spasms, respiratory difficulty, and death.

Treatment

Treatment of triazene exposure includes cardiovascular and renal support in the form of intravenous crystalloid fluids, inotropic drugs, and antiarrhythmic agents, as necessary. If the exposure is recent, induce emesis. Perform orogastric lavage in animals that cannot protect the airway. Emesis and orogastric lavage should be followed by the administration of activated charcoal and a cathartic. Carefully bathe the patient to prevent further dermal absorption.

Tricyclic antidepressants

Introduction

A variety of tricyclic antidepressants are available for use in both humans and animals, including amitriptyline, amoxapine, desipramine, doxepine, fluoxetine (Prozac), fluvoxamine (Luvox), imipramine, nortriptyline, paroxetine (Paxil), protriptyline, sertraline (Zoloft), and trimipramine. Selective serotonin reuptake inhibitors (SSRIs) are rapidly absorbed from the digestive tract, with peak serum concentrations occurring 2 to 8 hours after ingestion. The elimination half-life for each drug differs in dogs, but typically last 16 to 24 hours. SSRIs inhibit the reuptake of serotonin, causing serotonin to accumulate in the brain. This can cause "serotonin syndrome," characterized by trembling, seizures, hyperthermia, ptyalism or hypersalivation, cramping or abdominal pain, vomiting, and diarrhea. Other clinical signs of SSRI intoxication include depression, tremors, bradycardia, tachyarrhythmias, and anorexia. Any animal that has ingested an SSRI should be promptly treated and carefully observed for at least 72 hours for side effects.

Treatment

The treatment of suspected SSRI intoxication involves gastric decontamination if the patient is not depressed and has an intact gag reflex. Perform orogastric lavage and administer activated charcoal to prevent further toxin absorption and hasten elimination from the gastrointestinal tract. Treat other clinical signs symptomatically. Administer intravenous diazepam to control seizures. Treat tachyarrhythmias according to type. Administer methocarbamol to control muscle tremors. Cyproheptadine (1 mg/kg), a serotonin antagonist, can be dissolved in water and administered per rectum.

Turpentine: See Fuels

Vitamin K antagonist rodenticides

Introduction

Vitamin K antagonist rodenticides, which are commonly found in pelleted or block form, inhibit the activation of the vitamin K–dependent coagulation factors II, VII, IX, and X. Clinical signs of hemorrhage occur within 2 to 7 days of exposure. Hemorrhage can occur anywhere in the body, and can be manifested as petechiation of the skin or mucous membranes, hemorrhagic sclera, epistaxis, pulmonary parenchymal or pleural hemorrhage, gastrointestinal hemorrhage, pericardial hemorrhage, hematuria, retroperitoneal hemorrhage, hemarthrosis, and central nervous system hemorrhage. Clinical signs include respiratory distress, cough, bleeding from the gums or into the eyes, ataxia, paresis, paralysis, seizures, hematuria, joint swelling, lameness, lethargy, weakness, inappetence, and collapse.

Diagnosis is made based on clinical signs and a prolonged activated clotting time, or prothrombin time. The PIVKA (proteins induced by vitamin K antagonism) test may be helpful but usually cannot be performed in-house. Slight thrombocytopenia may be present secondary to hemorrhage; however, blood levels usually do not reach the critical level of <50,000 platelets/μL to cause clinical signs of hemorrhage. In some cases, severe stress-induced hyperglycemia and glucosuria may be present but resolves within 24 hours.

Treatment

If the rodenticide was ingested within the last 2 hours, induce emesis. Alternatively, orogastric lavage can be performed in an uncooperative patient. Both emesis and orogastric lavage should be followed by administration of activated charcoal. The stomach contents can be submitted for analysis. Following successful treatment, administer oral vitamin K for 30 days after the exposure; or a check prothrombin time 2 days after gastric decontamination. If the prothrombin time is prolonged, administer fresh frozen plasma and Vitamin K.

If the prothrombin time is normal, gastric decontamination was successful, and no further treatment is necessary.

If an animal presents with clinical signs of intoxication, administer activated clotting factors in the form of fresh frozen plasma (20 mL/kg), and vitamin K_1 (5 mg/kg SQ in multiple sites with a 24-gauge needle). Packed RBCs or fresh whole blood may be required if the patient is also anemic. Supportive care in the form of supplemental oxygen may be necessary in cases of pulmonary or pleural hemorrhage. Following initial therapy and discharge, the patient should receive vitamin K_1 (2.5 mg/kg PO q8-2h for 30 days), and prothrombin time should be checked 2 days after the last vitamin K capsule is administered. In some cases, depending on the type of anticoagulant ingested, an additional 2 weeks of vitamin K1 therapy may be required.

Window cleaner: see ethylene glycol

Xylitol

Introduction

Xylitol is a sugar alcohol that, when ingested by humans, does not cause a significant increase in blood glucose, and therefore does not stimulate insulin release from the human pancreas. In dogs, however, xylitol causes a massive rapid and dose-dependent release of insulin from pancreatic beta-cells. Following insulin release, clinically significant hypoglycemia can develop, followed by signs of vomiting, weakness, ataxia, mental depression, hypokalemia, hypoglycemic seizures, and coma. Clinical signs associated with xylitol ingestion can be seen within 30 minutes of ingestion and can last for more than 12 hours, even with aggressive treatment.

Treatment

Known xylitol ingestion should be treated as for other toxin ingestion. If no neurologic abnormalities exist at the time the patient is seen, induce emesis, followed by administration of activated charcoal. It remains unknown at this time whether activated charcoal actually delays or prevents the absorption of xylitol from the canine gastrointestinal tract. If clinical signs have already developed, perform orogastric lavage and gastric decontamination. Blood glucose concentrations should be analyzed and maintained with supplemental dextrose as a constant rate infusion (2.5%-5%) until normoglycemia can be maintained with multiple frequent small meals. Hypokalemia may develop because it is driven intracellularly by the actions of insulin. Treat hypokalemia with supplemental potassium chloride by infusion, not to exceed 0.5 mEq/kg/hour.

Zephiran: see detergents, cationic

Zinc and zinc oxide

Introduction

Pennies minted in the U.S. after 1982 contain large amounts of zinc rather than copper. Other sources of zinc include zinc oxide ointment and hardware such as that found in metal bird cages. Zinc toxicity causes intravascular hemolysis, anemia, gastroenteritis, and renal failure.

Treatment

If zinc toxicity is suspected, take an abdominal radiograph to document the presence of the metal in the stomach or intestines. (If zinc-containing ointment was ingested, this will not be visible on radiographs.) Induce emesis or perform orogastric lavage, depending on the size of the object ingested. Often, small objects such as pennies can be retrieved using endoscopy or surgical gastrotomy/enterotomy. Always take an additional radiograph after the removal procedure to ensure that all objects have been successfully removed. Administer intravenous fluids to maintain renal perfusion and promote fluid diuresis. Administer gastroprotectant and antiemetic drugs. Chelation therapy with succimer, calcium EDTA, dimercaprol, or penicillamine may be necessary. Do NOT administer calcium EDTA if the patient is dehydrated, because renal failure can result. Severe anemia should be treated with packed RBCs or hemoglobin-based oxygen carriers.

Additional Reading

Cope RB:. Four new small animal toxicoses. Aust Vet Pract 34(3):121-123, 2004.

Donaldson CW: Paintball toxicosis in dogs. Vet Med 98(12):995-998, 2003.

Dunayer ER: Hypoglycemia following canine ingestion of xylitol-containing gum. Vet Hum Toxicol 46(2):87-88, 2004.

Gfeller RW, Messonnier SP: Handbook of small animal toxicology and poisonings, ed 2, St. Louis, 2004, Mosby.

Hansen SR: Macadamia nut toxicosis in dogs. Vet Med 97(4):274-276, 2002.

Hopper K, Aldrich J, Haskins S: The recognition and treatment of the intermediate syndrome of organophosphate poisoning in a dog. J Vet Emerg Crit Care 12(2):99-103, 2002.

Mazzaferro EM, Eubig PA, Hackett TB et al: Acute renal failure in four dogs after raisin or grape ingestion (1999-2002). J Vet Emerg Crit Care 14(3):203-212, 2004.

Plum Lee KH: Clinical veterinary toxicology. Mosby, St. Louis, 2004.

Roder JD: Veterinary toxicology. Butterworth-Heinemann, Woburn, Mass, 2001.

RESPIRATORY EMERGENCIES

Respiratory emergencies consist of any problem that impairs delivery of oxygen to the level of the alveoli or diffusion of oxygen across the alveolar capillary membrane into the pulmonary capillary network. Decreased respiratory rate or tidal volume can result in hypoxia and buildup of carbon dioxide, or hypercarbia, leading to respiratory acidosis. Conditions most frequently encountered result in airflow obstruction, prevention of normal lung expansion, interference with pulmonary gas exchange (ventilation-perfusion mismatch), and alterations of pulmonary circulation. Evaluation of the patient with respiratory distress is often challenging, because the most minimal stress can cause rapid deterioration, or even death in critical cases. Careful observation of the patient from a distance often allows the clinician to determine the severity of respiratory distress and localize the lesion based on the patient's respiratory pattern and effort.

Animals in respiratory distress often have a rapid respiratory rate (>30 breaths per minute). As respiratory distress progresses, the patient may appear anxious and start open-mouth breathing. The animal often develops an orthopneic posture, characterized by neck extension, open-mouthed breathing, and elbows abducted or pulled away from the body. Cyanosis of the mucous membranes often indicates extreme decompensation. Clinical signs of respiratory distress can develop acutely, or from decompensation of a more chronic problem that was preceded by a cough, noisy respirations, or exercise intolerance.

Localization of the cause of respiratory distress is essential to successful case management. In any patient with clinical signs of respiratory distress, the differential diagnosis should include primary pulmonary parenchymal disease, airway disease, thoracic cage disorders, congestive heart failure, dyshemoglobinemias (carbon monoxide, methemoglobin), and anemia. Careful observation of the patient's respiratory pattern can aid in making a diagnosis of upper airway disease/obstruction, primary pulmonary parenchymal disease, pleural space disease, and abnormalities of the thoracic cage. It is often helpful to rest a hand on the patient and breathe along with the patient's effort, to confirm the periods of inhalation and exhalation.

The pharynx, larynx, and extrathoracic trachea comprise the upper airway. Obstructive lesions are associated with a marked inspiratory wheeze or stridor and slow deep inspiratory effort. Auscultation of the larynx and trachea may reveal more subtle obstructions of normal air flow. Stridor can usually be auscultated without the use of a stethoscope. Lung sounds are usually normal. The neck should be carefully palpated for a mass lesion, tracheal collapse, and subcutaneous emphysema. Subcutaneous emphysema suggests tracheal damage or collapse secondary to severe trauma. In some cases, there is a history of voice, or bark, change secondary to laryngeal dysfunction. Differential diagnosis is usually based on the patient's signalment, history, and index of suspicion of a particular disease process. Differential diagnoses of upper airway obstruction are listed in Box 1-61.

1

BOX 1-61   DIFFERENTIAL DIAGNOSES OF UPPER AIRWAY OBSTRUCTION

- Abscess
- Brachycephalic airway syndrome
- Granuloma
- Laryngeal collapse
- Laryngeal paralysis
- Nasopharyngeal polyp
- Neoplasia
- Obstructive laryngitis
- Pharyngeal foreign body
- Tracheal collapse
- Tracheal foreign body
- Traumatic fracture of larynx or tracheal cartilage

Diseases of the pleural space often are associated with a restrictive respiratory pattern. Inspiratory efforts are short, rapid, and shallow, and there is often a marked abdominal push. The pattern has been referred to as a choppy "dysynchronous" respiratory pattern. Depending on the disease present, lung sounds may be muffled ventrally and enhanced dorsally. Percussion of the thorax reveals decreased resonance if fluid is present. Increased resonance is present with pneumothorax. Decreased compressibility of the anterior thorax may be present with an anterior mediastinal mass lesion, particularly in cats and ferrets. A pneumothorax or diaphragmatic hernia is commonly associated with evidence of trauma, with or without rib fractures. Respiratory distress due to hemothorax may be exacerbated by anemia. Differential diagnoses for patients with evidence of pleural cavity disease include pneumothorax, diaphragmatic hernia, neoplasia, and various types of pleural effusion.

Primary pulmonary parenchymal disease can involve the intrathoracic airways, alveoli, interstitial space, and pulmonary vasculature. A rapid, shallow, restrictive respiratory pattern may be observed with a marked push on exhalation, particularly with obstructive airway disease such as chronic bronchitis (asthma) in cats. Crackles or wheezes are heard on thoracic auscultation. Differential diagnoses for pulmonary parenchymal disease include cardiogenic and noncardiogenic pulmonary edema, pneumonia, feline bronchitis (asthma), pulmonary contusion, aspiration pneumonitis, pulmonary thromboembolism, neoplasia, infection (bacterial, fungal, protozoal, viral), and/or chronic bronchitis.

Other abnormal respiratory patterns may be evident, and warrant further consideration. Tachypnea present in the absence of other signs of respiratory distress can be a normal response to nonrespiratory problems, including pain, hyperthermia, and stress. A restrictive respiratory pattern with minimal thoracic excursions can be associated with diseases of neuromuscular function, including ascending polyradiculoneuritis, botulism, and tick paralysis. If adequate ventilation cannot be maintained by the patient, mechanical ventilation may be indicated. Kussmaul respiration manifests as very slow, very deep respirations when a metabolic acidosis is present. This type of respiratory pattern typically is observed in patients with severe diabetic ketoacidosis and renal failure in a compensatory attempt to blow off carbon dioxide. Cheyne-Stokes respiration is usually observed with a defect in the central respiratory control center. The classic pattern of Cheyne-Stokes respiration is normal or hyperventilation followed by a period of apnea or hypoventilation. In cases of lower cervical cord damage or damage to the central respiratory control center in the CNS, the diaphragm alone may assume most of the ventilatory movement. With diaphragmatic fatigue, severe hypoventilation and resultant hypoxemia may require mechanical ventilation.

IMMEDIATE MANAGEMENT

Immediate management of any patient in respiratory distress is to minimize stress at all costs. Relatively benign procedures such as radiography or intravenous catheter placement can be fatal in patients with severe respiratory compromise. Stabilization should always precede further diagnostic evaluation. In some cases, sedation may be required before performing any diagnostics, to prevent further stress. All patients should receive some form of supplemental oxygen, either by mask, cage, or flow-by techniques. In cases in which a severe pneumothorax or pleural effusion is suspected, perform therapeutic and diagnostic thoracocentesis bilaterally to allow lung re-expansion and alleviate respiratory distress, whenever possible. If thoracocentesis alone is not effective at maintaining lung re-expansion, place a thoracostomy tube (particularly in cases of tension pneumothorax). If hypovolemic/ hemorrhagic shock is present, initiate treatment while stabilizing the respiratory system (see section on Shock).

If an animal is suspected of having an upper airway obstruction, reestablish airflow. In cases of laryngeal paralysis, tracheal collapse, and brachycephalic airway syndrome, sedation is often very useful in alleviating the distress of airway obstruction. In cases of laryngeal collapse, however, sedation may make the condition worse. If laryngeal edema is severe, administer a dose of short-acting glucocorticosteroids (dexamethasone sodium phosphate) to decrease laryngeal inflammation and edema. If a foreign body is lodged in the pharynx, perform the Heimlich maneuver by thrusting bluntly several times on the patient's sternum. Objects such as balls or bones may be small enough to enter the larynx but too large to be expelled, and will require rapid-acting general anesthesia to facilitate dislodgement and removal. If the obstruction cannot be removed, bypassing the obstruction with an endotracheal tube or temporary tracheostomy should be considered.

In an emergency, a temporary transtracheal oxygen catheter can quickly be placed in the following manner. Connect a 20- or 22-gauge needle to a length of intravenous extension tubing and a 3-mL syringe. Place the male connector of the syringe into the female portion of the extension tubing. Cut off the syringe plunger and connect the resulting blunt end to a length of flexible tubing attached to a humidified oxygen source. Run the oxygen at 10 L/minute to provide adequate oxygenation until a tracheostomy can be performed. (See sections on Oxygen Supplementation and Tracheostomy).

Once the animal's condition has been stabilized, specific diagnostic tests, including arterial blood gas analyses, thoracic radiographs, and/or transtracheal wash, can be performed, depending on the patient's condition and needs. Specific therapies for management of upper airway obstruction, pleural space disease, and pulmonary disease are discussed next.

Management of upper airway obstruction

Upper airway obstruction can occur as a result of intraluminal or extraluminal mass lesions or foreign bodies in the oropharynx (abscess, neoplasia), laryngeal paralysis, trauma, and anatomic abnormalities. Clinical signs of an upper airway obstruction are associated with an animal's extreme efforts to inhale air past the obstruction. Marked negative pressure occurs in the extrathoracic airways and can cause worsening of clinical signs. Mucosal edema and inflammation further worsen the obstruction.

Therapy for upper airway obstruction is aimed at breaking the cycle of anxiety and respiratory distress. Administer the anxiolytic tranquilizer acepromazine (0.02-0.05 mg/kg IV, IM, SQ) to decrease patient anxiety. Many animals develop hyperthermia from increased respiratory effort and extreme anxiety. Implement cooling measures in the form of cool intravenous fluids and wet towels soaked in tepid water placed over the animal (see section on Hyperthermia). Administer supplemental oxygen in a manner that is least stressful for the animal. Short-acting glucocorticosteroids can also be administered (dexamethasone sodium phosphate, 0.25 mg/kg IV, SQ, IM) to decrease edema and inflammation.

If the airway obstruction is severe and there is no response to initial measures to alleviate anxiety and decrease inflammation, establish control of ventilation by placement of an endotracheal tube (see section on Endotracheal Intubation), tracheal oxygen catheter, or temporary tracheostomy. To obtain airway control, administer a rapid-acting anesthetic (propofol, 4-7 mg/kg IV to effect), and intubate with a temporary tracheostomy. An intratracheal oxygen catheter can be placed with sedation and/or a local anesthetic (see technique for transtracheal wash).

LARYNGEAL PARALYSIS

Laryngeal paralysis is a congenital or acquired condition that occurs primarily in large-breed dogs secondary to denervation of the arytenoid cartilages by the recurrent laryngeal nerve. Congenital laryngeal paralysis occurs in the Bouvier des Flandres, Siberian Husky, and Bull Terrier. Acquired laryngeal paralysis occurs in Labrador Retrievers, Saint Bernards, and Irish Setters. Acquired laryngeal paralysis can be idiopathic, acquired secondary to trauma to the recurrent laryngeal nerve, or can be a component of systemic neuromuscular disease. Although rare, this condition also occurs in cats.

With dysfunction of the recurrent laryngeal nerve, the intrinsic laryngeal muscles atrophy and degenerate. As a result, the vocal folds and arytenoid cartilage move in a paramedian position within the airway and fail to abduct during inhalation, causing airway obstruction. Laryngeal paralysis can be partial or complete, unilateral or bilateral. In many cases, a change in bark is noted prior to the development of clinical signs of respiratory distress or exercise intolerance. When a patient presents with severe inspiratory stridor (with or without hyperthermia) initiate stabilization with anxiolytic tranquilizers, supplemental oxygen, and cooling measures. Once the patient's condition has been stabilized, definitive measures to accurately document and assess the patient's airway should be considered. Place the patient under very heavy sedation with short-acting barbiturates or propofol (4-7 mg/kg IV) and observe the arytenoid cartilages closely in all phases of respiration. Administer just enough drug to allow careful examination without getting bitten. If the arytenoid cartilages do not abduct during inhalation, administer Dopram (doxapram hydrochloride, 1-5 mg/kg IV) to stimulate respiration.

Absent or paradoxical laryngeal motion (closed during inspiration and open during exhalation) is characteristic of laryngeal paralysis. Correction of the defect involves documentation and treatment of any underlying disorder and surgical repair of the area to open the airway. Partial laryngectomy, arytenoid lateralization ("tie-back" surgery), or removal of the vocal folds has been used with some success. Aspiration pneumonitis is common following these procedures.

Brachycephalic Airway Syndrome and Laryngeal Collapse

Brachycephalic airway syndrome is associated with a series of anatomic abnormalities that collectively increase resistance to airflow. Affected animals typically have stenotic nares, an elongated soft palate, and a hypoplastic trachea. Components of the syndrome can occur alone or in combination. In severe cases, laryngeal saccular edema and eversion, and eventual pharyngeal collapse, can occur secondary to the severe increase in intrathoracic airway pressure required to overcome the resistance of the upper airways. Specific airway anomalies can be identified with general anesthesia and laryngoscopy.

Severe respiratory distress should be treated as discussed previously. Treatment requires surgical correction of the anatomic abnormalities. In animals with laryngeal collapse, surgical correction may not be possible, and a permanent tracheostomy may be required. Because an elongated soft palate and stenotic nares can be identified before the onset of clinical signs, surgical correction to improve airflow when the animal is young may decrease the negative intra-thoracic pressure necessary to move air past these obstructions. The chronic consequences of everted laryngeal saccules and laryngeal collapse potentially can be prevented.

Tracheal Collapse

Tracheal collapse is common in middle-aged and older toy and small-breed dogs. The owner typically reports a chronic cough that is readily induced by excitement or palpation of the trachea. The cough often sounds like a "goose honk." Diagnostic confirmation is obtained by lateral radiography or fluoroscopy of the cervical and thoracic trachea during all phases of respiration. Acute decompensation is uncommon but does occur, particularly with excitement, exercise, and increased environmental temperatures or ambient humidity.

Therapy of the patient with acute respiratory distress secondary to tracheal collapse includes sedation, administration of supplemental oxygen, and provision of cooling measures to treat hyperthermia. Cough suppressants (hydrocodone bitartrate–homatropine methylbromide, 0.25 mg/kg PO q8-12h, or butorphanol, 0.5 mg/kg PO q6-12h) are useful. Tracheal collapse is a dynamic process that usually involves both the upper and lower airways. Because of this, bypassing the obstruction is often difficult. Tracheal stents have been used with limited success in combination with treatment of chronic lower airway disease.

TRAUMA

Crush or bite injuries to the neck can result in fractures or avulsion of the laryngeal or tracheal cartilages. Bypassing the obstructed area may be necessary until the patient is stable and can undergo surgical correction of the injury. If there is avulsion of the cranial trachea, it may be difficult to intubate the patient. A long, rigid urinary catheter can be inserted past the area of avulsion into the distal segment, and an endotracheal tube passed over the rigid catheter, to establish a secure airway. Neck injury can also result in damage to the recurrent laryngeal nerve and laryngeal paralysis.

FOREIGN BODIES

Foreign bodies can lodge in the nasal cavity, pharynx, larynx, and distal trachea. Signs of foreign bodies in the nares include acute sneezing and pawing at or rubbing the muzzle on the ground. If the object is not removed, sneezing continues and a chronic nasal discharge develops. Respiratory distress is uncommon, but the foreign body is severely irritating. Pharyngeal and tracheal foreign bodies can cause severe obstruction to airflow and respiratory distress. Diagnosis of a foreign body is based on the patient history, physical examination findings, and thoracic or cervical radiographs. Smaller foreign bodies lodged in the distal airways may not be apparent radiographically but can cause pulmonary atelectasis.

Foreign bodies of the nose or pharynx can often be removed with an alligator forceps with the patient under anesthesia. If removal is not possible with a forceps, flushing the nasal cavity from cranial to caudal (pack the back of the mouth with gauze to prevent aspiration) can sometimes dislodge the foreign material into the gauze packing. Rhinoscopy may be necessary. If an endoscope is not available, an otoscope can be used.

Foreign objects lodged in the trachea can be small and function like a ball valve during inhalation and exhalation, causing episodic hypoxia and collapse. When attempting to remove these objects, suspend the patient with its head down. Remove the object with an alligator forceps, using a laryngoscope to aid in visualization. Foreign bodies lodged in the trachea or bronchi require removal with endoscopic assistance.

INTRALUMINAL MASSES

Nasopharyngeal polyps (in cats, tumors, obstructive laryngitis, granulomas, abscesses, and cysts) can cause upper airway obstruction. Clinical signs are usually gradual in onset. The lesions can be identified through careful laryngoscopic examination performed with the patient under general anesthesia. The nasopharynx above the soft palpate should always be included in the examination. Pedunculated masses and cysts are excised at the time of evaluation. Biopsy of diffusely infiltrative masses is indicated for histologic examination and prognosis. It is impossible to distinguish obstructive laryngitis from neoplasia based on gross appearance alone. Whenever possible, material should be collected from abscesses and granulomas for cytologic evaluation and bacterial culture.

EXTRALUMINAL MASSES

Extraluminal masses impinge on and slowly compress the upper airways, resulting in slow progression of clinical signs. Masses are usually identified by palpation of the neck. Enlarged mandibular lymph nodes, thyroid tumors, and other neoplasms may be present. Diagnosis is usually based on a combination of radiography and ultrasonography. CT and/or MRI are helpful in identifying the full extent and invasiveness of the lesion. Definitive diagnosis is made with a fine-needle aspirate or biopsy. Many thyroid tumors bleed excessively.

PLEURAL CAVITY DISEASE

The inside of each side of the hemithorax is covered in parietal pleura. The lung lobes are covered in visceral pleura. The two surfaces are in close contact with each other, and are contiguous at the hilum under normal circumstances. Pneumothorax refers to free air within the pleural space, accumulating in between the parietal and visceral pleura. The term *pleural effusion* refers to fluid accumulation in that area but does not reflect the amount or type of fluid present. The mediastinal reflections of the pleura typically are thin in dogs and cats, and usually, but not always, connect. Bilateral involvement of pneumothorax or pleural effusion is common. Both pneumothorax and pleural effusion compromise the lungs' ability to expand and result in hypoxia and respiratory distress.

Pneumothorax

Pneumothorax can be classified as open versus closed, simple versus complicated, and tension. An open pneumothorax communicates with the external environment through a rent in the thoracic wall. A closed pneumothorax results from tears in the visceral pleura but does not communicate with the outside. A tension pneumothorax occurs as a result of a tear in the lung or chest wall that creates a flap valve, such that air is allowed to leave the lung and accumulate in the pleural space during inhalation, and closes to seal off exit of air from the pleural space during exhalation. Tension pneumothorax can cause rapid decline in cardiopulmonary status and death if not recognized and treated immediately. A simple pneumothorax is one that can be controlled with a simple thoracocentesis. Complicated pneumothorax involves repeated accumulation of air, requiring placement of a thoracic drainage catheter.

In many cases, pneumothorax develops as a result of trauma. Spontaneous pneumothorax occurs with rupture of cavitary lesions of the lung that may be congenital or acquired as a result of prior trauma, heartworm disease, airway disease (emphysema), paragonimiasis, neoplasia, or lung abscess. Pneumothorax also rarely occurs as a result of esophageal tears or esophageal foreign bodies.

Rapid circulatory and respiratory compromise following traumatic pneumothorax can develop as a result of open or tension pneumothorax, rib fractures, airway obstruction, pulmonary contusions, hemothorax, cardiac dysrhythmias, cardiac tamponade, and hypovolemic shock. Any patient that is rapidly decompensating after a traumatic episode must be quickly assessed, and emergency therapy initiated (see section on Immediate Management of Trauma, a CRASH plan).

Diagnosis of pneumothorax is usually made based on a history of trauma, a rapid, shallow, restrictive respiratory pattern, and muffled heart and lung sounds on thoracic auscultation. The clinical signs and history alone should prompt the clinician to perform a bilateral diagnostic and therapeutic thoracocentesis before taking thoracic radiographs (see section on Thoracocentesis). The stress of handling the patient for radiography can be deadly in severe cases of pneumothorax. Although the mediastinum on both sides of the thorax connects, it is necessary to perform thoracocentesis on both sides to ensure maximal removal of free air in the pleural space and allow maximal lung expansion. If negative pressure cannot be obtained, or if the patient rapidly reaccumulates air, place a thoracostomy tube connected to continuous suction. (See section on Thoracostomy Tube Placement).

Management of open sucking chest wounds in pneumothorax

Treat all penetrating wounds to the thorax as open sucking chest wounds unless proved otherwise. To "close" an open sucking chest wound, clip the fur around the wound as quickly as possible, and place sterile lubricant jelly or antimicrobial ointment circumferentially around the wound. Cut a sterile glove to provide a covering. Place the covering over the wound, making sure to cover all of the sterile lubricant, thus creating a seal to close the wound temporarily from the external environment. Evaluate the patient's thorax via thoracocentesis while placing a thoracostomy tube. Once the patient is stable, the open chest wound can be surgically explored, lavaged, and definitively corrected. All animals with open chest wounds should receive antibiotics (first-generation cephalosporin) to prevent infection. Following stabilization, radiographs can be taken and evaluated. Pneumothorax is confirmed by evidence of elevation of the cardiac silhouette above the sternum, increased density of the pulmonary parenchymal tissue, free air in between the parietal and visceral pleura (making the outline of the lungs visible), and absence of pulmonary vascular structures in the periphery. Parenchymal lesions within the lungs are best identified after as much air as possible has been removed from the thorax. Obtain left and right lateral and ventrodorsal or dorsoventral views. A standing lateral view may reveal air- or fluid-filled cavitary masses. If underlying pulmonary disease is suspected as a cause of spontaneous pneumothorax, a transtracheal wash, fecal flotation, and heartworm test may be indicated.

Treatment of pneumothorax

Treatment of pneumothorax includes immediate bilateral thoracocentesis, covering of any open chest wounds, administration of supplemental oxygen, and placement of a thoracostomy tube if negative pressure cannot be obtained or if air rapidly reaccumulates. Serial radiography, CT, or MRI should be performed in dogs with spontaneous pneumothorax, because the condition can be associated with generalized pulmonary parenchymal disease. Strict cage rest is required until air stops accumulating and the thoracostomy tube can be removed. The patient's chest tube should be aspirated every 4 hours after discontinuing continuous suction. If no air reaccumulates after 24 hours, the chest tube can be removed. Exercise restriction is indicated for a minimum of 1 week. If bullae or mass lesions are present, exploratory thoracotomy should be considered as a diagnostic and potentially therapeutic option for long-term management in prevention of recurrence.

Pleural effusion

Pleural fluid cytologic analysis is indicated for all patients with pleural effusion before administration of antibiotics. The general term *pleural effusion* means a collection of fluid in the space between the parietal and visceral pleura but does not indicate what kind or how much fluid is present. Clinical signs associated with pleural effusion depend on how much fluid is present, and how rapidly the fluid has accumulated. Clinical signs associated with pleural effusion include respiratory distress, reluctance to lie down, labored breathing with an abdominal component on exhalation, cough, and lethargy. Auscultation of the thorax may reveal muffled heart and lung sounds ventrally and increased lung sounds dorsally, although pockets of fluid may be present, depending on the chronicity of the effusion. Percussion of the thorax may reveal decreased resonance.

In stable patients, the presence of pleural effusion can be confirmed radiographically. Radiographic confirmation of the pleural effusion should include right and left lateral and dorsoventral or ventrodorsal views. A handling or standing lateral view should be obtained if an anterior mediastinal mass is suspected. The standing lateral view will allow the fluid to collect in the costophrenic recess.

In patients with respiratory distress, muffled heart and lung sounds, and suspicion of pleural effusion, thoracocentesis should be performed immediately. Thoracocentesis can be both therapeutic and diagnostic. Radiography is contraindicated because the procedure can cause undue stress and exacerbation of clinical signs in an unstable patient. Pleural effusion can cause severe respiratory distress, and can be the result of a number of factors that must be considered when implementing an appropriate treatment plan. Pathology of the pleura is almost always a secondary process except for primary bacterial pleuritis and pleural mesotheliomas. Causes of pleural effusion in the cat and dog include pyothorax, feline infectious peritonitis, congestive heart failure, chylothorax, heartworm disease, hemothorax, hypoalbuminemia, lung lobe torsions, neoplasia, diaphragmatic hernia, and pancreatitis (Box 1-62). In stable animals, diagnosis of pleural effusion can be made based

---

BOX 1-62   PHYSIOLOGIC PROCESSES ASSOCIATED WITH PLEURAL EFFUSION

- Imbalance of transpleural or hydrostatic or protein osmotic forces
- Change in membrane permeability
- Decrease in rate of fluid reabsorption
- Combination of foregoing mechanisms

on thoracic radiography or ultrasound. Thoracic radiographs can show whether the pleural effusion is unilateral or bilateral. Effusions in dogs and cats are usually bilateral. The lung parenchyma and the cardiac silhouette cannot be fully evaluated until most of the fluid has been evacuated from the pleural cavity. Following thoracocentesis, radiography should be performed with left and right lateral and ventrodorsal or dorsoventral views. In cases of suspected heart failure, echocardiography also is necessary.

Pleural fluid cytologic analysis is indicated for all patients with pleural effusion. Collect specimens before administering antibiotics, whenever possible, because treatment with antibiotics can make a septic condition (pyothorax) appear nonseptic. The remainder of the diagnostic workup and treatment is based on the type of fluid present (Table 1-52). The fluid may be a transudate, nonseptic exudate, septic exudate, chylous, hemorrhagic, or neoplastic. Ultrasonographic evaluation of the thorax can be helpful in identifying intrathoracic masses, diaphragmatic hernias, lung lobe torsions, and cardiac abnormalities. Unlike radiography, ultrasonography is facilitated by the presence of fluid in the pleural space.

Pyothorax

Pyothorax refers to a septic effusion of the pleural cavity. The infection is generally the result of a combination of aerobic and anaerobic bacteria. Rarely, fungal organisms are present. The source of the underlying organisms is rarely identified, particularly in cats, but can be caused by penetrating wounds through the chest wall, esophagus, migrating foreign bodies (especially grass awns), or primary lung infections. The most common organisms associated with pyothorax in the cat are *Pasteurella*, *Bacteroides*, and *Fusobacterium*. Fever is often present in addition to clinical signs of pleural effusion. Septic shock is ununcommon.

Diagnosis of pyothorax is made based on cytologic analysis and the demonstration of intracellular and extracellular bacteria, toxin neutrophils and macrophages, and sometimes the presence of sulfur granules. Gram stains of the fluid can assist in the initial identification of some organisms. Bacterial cultures are indicated for bacteria identification and antibiotic susceptibility testing. Administration of antibiotics before cytologic evaluation can cause a septic effusion to appear nonseptic.

Emergency treatment for pyothorax involves placement of an intravenous catheter, intravenous fluids to treat hypovolemic shock, and broad-spectrum antibiotics (ampicillin, 22 mg/kg IV q6h, and enrofloxacin, 10 mg/kg IV q24h). Chloramphenicol also is an appropriate antibiotic to use for penetration into pockets of fluid. Administration of a beta-lactam antibiotic (ampicillin or amoxicillin) with a beta-lactamase inhibitor (amoxicillin clavulanate or ampicillin sulbactam) is helpful in achieving better coverage of *Bacteroides* spp.

Treatment of pyothorax differs in the cat and dog. In the cat, placement of one or two thoracic drainage catheters is recommended to allow continuous drainage of the intrathoracic abscess. Inadequate drainage can result in treatment failure. Fluid should be evaluated and the pleural cavity lavaged with 10 mL/kg of warmed 0.9% saline or lactated Ringer's solution every 8 hours. Approximately 75% of the infused volume should be recovered after each lavage.

In dogs, or in cats with refractory pyothorax, perform an exploratory thoracotomy to remove any nidus of infection. Rarely a foreign body is visible that can be removed at the time of surgery, but this finding is rare. Antibiotics are indicated for a minimum of 6 to 8 weeks after removal of the thoracostomy tube. Early diagnosis and aggressive treatment result in a good prognosis in the majority of patients with pyothorax. In cats, clinical signs of ptyalism and hypothermia at the time of presentation worsen the prognosis.

Chylothorax

Chylothorax refers to the abnormal accumulation of chyle (lymphatic fluid) in the pleural cavity. The cisterna chili is the dilated collection pool of lymphatic ducts in the abdomen that accumulate chyle prior to entry into the thoracic duct located within the thoracic cavity.

TABLE 1-52 Analysis of Pleural Effusions

	Transudates	Exudates				
		Modified transudates	Nonseptic exudates	Septic exudates	Chylous effusions	Hemorrhagic effusions
Color	Pale yellow	Yellow-pink	Yellow-pink	Yellow	White-pink	Red
Transparency	Clear	Clear to cloudy	Cloudy	Cloudy to flocculent	Opaque	Opaque
Protein (g/dL)	<2.5	<3.5	>3.0	>3.0	>2.5	>3.0
RBCs	Absent to rare	Variable	Variable	Variable	Variable	Acute: high number Chronic: moderate number
Nucleated cells/mL	<500	<5000	>5000	>5000	400-10,000	>1000
Neutrophils	Rare	Variable number Nondegenerative	Moderate Nondegenerative	Moderate to high number Nondegenerative to degenerative	Acute: low number Chronic: moderate number Nondegenerative	Variable number Nondegenerative
Lymphocytes	Rare	Variable	Variable	Variable	Acute: high number Chronic: low number	Variable
Macrophages	Occasional	Variable	Increased number Contain ingested debrides	Increased number	Present	Chronic: moderate number Contain ingested RBCs
Mesothelial cells	Occasional	Occasional	Rare	Rare	Occasional	Chronic: present
Fibrin	Absent	Absent	Present	Present	Chronic: present	Variable

Continued

1

TABLE 1-52 Analysis of Pleural Effusions—cont'd

	Transudates		Exudates				
	Transudates	Modified transudates	Nonseptic exudates	Septic exudates	Chylous effusions	Hemorrhagic effusions
Bacteria	Absent	Absent	Absent	Present intra-and extracellularly	Absent	Absent
Lipid	Absent	Absent	Absent	Absent	High triglycerides relative to low serum cholesterol; positive to lipotrophic stains	Absent
Etiology	Right heart failure Hypoproteinemia	Chronic transudates Diaphragmatic hernia Neoplasia Right heart failure Pericardial disease	Neoplasia Feline infectious peritonitis Chronic diaphragmatic hernia Lung torsions Pyothorax	Foreign body Penetrating wound Idiopathic pyothorax	Idiopathic Congenital Lymphangiectasia Trauma Neoplasia Cardiac disease Pericardial disease Dirofilariasis	Trauma Neoplasia Bleeding disorders Lung torsions

The thoracic duct enters the thorax at the aortic hiatus. Numerous tributaries or collateral ducts exist. The functions of the lymphatic vessels collectively serve to deliver triglycerides and fat-soluble vitamins into the peripheral vascular circulation. Damage of the thoracic duct or lymphatic system or obstruction to lymphatic flow can result in the development of chylous effusion in the pleural or peritoneal space.

It is difficult to identify chylous effusions based on their milky appearance alone. To identify a chylous effusion versus a pseudochylous effusion, the triglyceride and cholesterol levels of the fluid must be compared with those of peripheral blood. Chylous effusions have a higher triglyceride and lower cholesterol levels than peripheral blood. Pseudochylous effusions have a higher cholesterol and lower triglyceride levels than peripheral blood.

Disease processes that can result in chylous effusions are listed in the Box 1-63. Clinical signs associated with chylous effusion are typical of any pleural effusion and of the disease process that caused the effusion. Weight loss may be evident, depending on the chronicity of the process.

The diagnosis is made based on thoracocentesis, cytology, and biochemical evaluation of the fluid (i.e., triglyceride and cholesterol levels). The fluid often appears milky or blood-tinged but can be clear if the patient has significant anorexia. Typical cytologic characteristics are listed in Table 1-52. Lymphangiography can be used to confirm trauma to the thoracic duct, but this is usually not necessary unless surgical ligation is going to be attempted. The diagnostic evaluation must also attempt to identify an underlying cause.

Therapy for chylothorax is difficult and primarily involves documentation and treatment of the underlying cause. If an underlying cause is not found, treatment is largely supportive and consists of intermittent thoracocentesis to drain the fluid as it accumulates and causes respiratory dysfunction, nutritional support, and maintenance of fluid balance. A variety of surgical techniques, including ligation of the thoracic duct, pleural-peritoneal shunts, and pleurodesis, have been attempted but have had limited success. Most recently, the combination of thoracic duct ligation with subtotal pericardectomy has been shown to improve surgical success rates in the treatment of chylothorax. Rutin, a bioflavinoid, has been used with limited success in the treatment of idiopathic chylothorax in cats. Prognosis in many cases of chylothorax is guarded.

Hemothorax

Extensive hemorrhage into the pleural cavity can cause fulminant respiratory distress due to sudden hypovolemia and anemia and interference with lung expansion. Hemothorax typically is associated with trauma, systemic coagulopathy, lung lobe torsions, and erosive lesions within the thorax (usually neoplasia). Diagnosis of hemothorax involves obtaining a fluid sample via thoracocentesis. Hemorrhagic effusion must be differentiated from systemic blood inadvertently collected during the thoracocentesis procedure. Unless the hemorrhage is peracute, fluid in cases of hemothorax is rapidly defibrinated and will not clot, has a packed cell volume less than that of venous blood, contains RBCs and macrophages. Hemorrhagic effusions also usually contain a disproportionately higher number of white blood cells compared with peripheral blood.

Hemothorax commonly is the sole clinical sign observed in animals with vitamin K antagonist rodenticide intoxication and systemic coagulopathy. Whenever an animal presents

---

BOX 1-63   CAUSES OF CHYLOUS EFFUSION

- Cardiac disease
- Diaphragmatic hernia
- Heartworm disease
- Idiopathic
- Immune-mediated lymphadenitis
- Lung lobe torsion
- Pericardial disease
- Thoracic duct rupture
- Thoracic lymphangiectasia
- Thoracic neoplasia
- Trauma
- Venous thrombi

1

with signs of a hemorrhagic pleural effusion, perform coagulation testing immediately to determine whether a coagulopathy exists. The prothrombin time test is fast and can be performed as a cage-side test (see section on Coagulopathy).

Therapy for hemorrhagic pleural effusions should address the blood and fluid loss. Administer intravenous crystalloid fluids and RBC products (see section on Transfusion Therapy). When necessary, administer coagulation factors in the form of fresh whole blood or fresh frozen plasma, along with Vitamin K_1 (5 mg/kg SQ in multiple sites with a 25-gauge needle). If severe respiratory distress is present, evacuate the blood within the pleural space via thoracocentesis until clinical signs of respiratory distress resolve. Fluid that remains aids in the recovery of the patient, because RBCs and proteins eventually will be reabsorbed. Autotransfusion can be performed to salvage blood and reinfuse it into the anemic patient. In cases of neoplastic or traumatic uncontrollable hemorrhagic effusions, surgical exploration of the thorax is warranted.

DIAPHRAGMATIC HERNIA

Diaphragmatic hernia, or a rent in the diaphragm, can result in the protrusion of abdominal organs into the thoracic cavity and impair pulmonary expansion. Organs that are commonly herniated into the thorax include the liver, stomach, and small intestines. Diaphragmatic hernia usually is secondary to trauma but can occur as a congenital anomaly. In cases of trauma, rib fractures, pulmonary contusions, traumatic myocarditis, hemothorax, and shock are also often present concurrently with diaphragmatic hernia. Respiratory distress can be caused by any one or a combination of the above lesions. Animals with prior or chronic diaphragmatic hernias may have minimal clinical signs despite the presence of abdominal organs within the thorax. Clinical signs of acute or severe diaphragmatic hernia include respiratory distress, cyanosis, and shock.

A diagnosis of diaphragmatic hernia is made based on the patient's history (traumatic event), clinical signs, and radiographs. In some cases, ultrasonography or contrast peritoneography is necessary to confirm the diagnosis. Contrast radiographs may show the presence of the stomach or intestines within the thorax following oral administration of barium. Never administer barium directly into the peritoneal cavity or in cases of suspected gastrointestinal rupture.

Treatment of a patient with a diaphragmatic hernia includes cardiovascular and respiratory system stabilization before attempting surgical repair of the diaphragm. If the stomach is within the thorax, or if the patient's respiratory distress cannot be alleviated with medical management alone, immediate surgery is necessary. If the respiratory distress is minimal and the stomach is not located within the thorax, surgery can be postponed until the patient is a more stable anesthetic candidate. At the time of surgery, the abdominal organs are replaced into the abdominal cavity, and the rent in the diaphragm is closed. Air must be evacuated from the thorax following closure of the diaphragm. If chronic diaphragmatic hernia is repaired, the complication of reexpansion pulmonary edema can occur.

CARDIAC CHANGES ASSOCIATED WITH THORACIC TRAUMA

Cardiac injury is a common complication secondary to blunt thoracic trauma. In most cases, cardiac injury is manifested as arrhythmias, including multiple premature ventricular contractions, ventricular tachycardia, ST segment depression or elevation secondary to myocardial hypoxemia, and atrial fibrillation (See section on Cardiac Emergencies). Myocardial infarction and cardiac failure can occur. Careful and repeated assessments of the patient's blood pressure and ECG tracing should be a part of any diagnostic work-up for a patient that has sustained blunt thoracic trauma.

RIB FRACTURES AND FLAIL CHEST

Rib fractures are associated with localized pain and painful respiratory movements. Radiographs are helpful to confirm the diagnosis. Careful palpation may reveal crepitus and instability of the fractured ribs. Common problems associated with rib fractures include pulmonary contusions, pericardial laceration, traumatic myocarditis, diaphragmatic hernia, and splenic laceration or rupture.

A flail segment results from rib fractures of more than three adjacent ribs that produce a "floating segment" of the chest wall. The flail segment moves paradoxically with respiration—that is, it moves inward during inhalation and outward during exhalation. Respiratory distress is associated with the pain caused by the fractures and the presence of traumatic underlying pulmonary pathology.

Therapy for rib fractures and flail chest includes administration of supplemental oxygen, treatment of pneumothorax or diaphragmatic hernia, and administration of systemic and local anesthesia to alleviate the discomfort associated with the fractures. Although controversial, positioning the patient with the flail segment up may reduce pain and improve ventilation. Avoid the use of chest wraps, which do nothing to stabilize the flail segment and can further impair respiratory excursions. Following administration of a systemic analgesic, administer a local anesthetic at the dorsocaudal and ventrocaudal segment of each fractured rib, and in one rib in front of and behind the flail segment. Often, pulmonary function will improve once the pain associated with rib fractures has been adequately treated. In rare cases in which the flail segment involves five or more ribs, surgical stabilization may be necessary. Single rib fractures or smaller flail segments are allowed to heal on their own.

PULMONARY DISEASES

FELINE BRONCHITIS (FELINE LOWER AIRWAY DISEASE, ASTHMA)

Feline bronchitis has a variety of names (bronchial asthma, asthma, acute bronchitis, allergic bronchitis, chronic asthmatic bronchitis, feline lower airway disease) and refers to the acute onset of respiratory distress secondary to narrowing of the bronchi. Cats may present with an acute onset of severe restrictive respiratory pattern associated with lower airway obstruction. Acute bronchitis in cats typically has an inflammatory component in the lower airways, resulting in acute bronchoconstriction, excessive mucus production, and inflammatory exudates. In cats with chronic bronchitis, there may be damage of the bronchial epithelium and fibrosis of the airways. These patients often have a history if intermittent exacerbation of clinical signs, intermittent cough, and periods of normality throughout the year. Because there appears to be an allergic or inflammatory component in feline bronchitis, clinical signs can be acutely exacerbated by stress and the presence of aerosolized particles such as perfume, smoke, and carpet powders. Causes of feline bronchitis include heartworm disease, parasitic infestation (lungworms), and (rarely) bacterial infection.

Immediate action

On presentation, the patient should be placed in an oxygen cage and allowed to rest while being observed from a distance. Postpone performing stressful diagnostic procedures until the patient's respiratory status has been stabilized. After careful thoracic auscultation, administer a short-acting bronchodilator (terbutaline, 0.01 mg/kg SQ or IM) along with a glucocorticosteroid (dexamethasone sodium phosphate 1 mg/kg IM, SQ, IV) to alleviate immediate bronchospasm and airway inflammation.

Diagnosis

Clinical signs of feline bronchitis are characterized by a short, rapid respiratory pattern with prolonged expiration with an abdominal push. Wheezes may be heard on thoracic auscultation. In some cases, no abnormalities are found on auscultation, but become acutely worse when the patient is stimulated to cough by tracheal palpation. Radiographs may reveal a hyperinflated lung field with bronchial markings and caudal displacement of the diaphragm. In some cases, consolidation of the right middle lung lobe is present. A complete blood count and serum biochemistry profile can be performed, but results usually are unrewarding. In endemic areas, a heartworm test is warranted. Fecal examination by flotation and the Baermann technique is helpful in ruling out lungworms and other parasites. Bronchoalveolar lavage or transtracheal wash is useful for cytologic and bacterial examination.

Management

Long-term management of feline bronchitis includes isolation from environmental exposure to potential allergens (litter dust, perfumes, smoke, incense, carpet powders) and treatment of bronchoconstriction and inflammation with a combination of oral and inhaled glucocorticosteroids and bronchodilators (Table 1-53). Antibiotic therapy is contraindicated unless a pure culture of a pathogen is documented. Oral therapy with steroids and bronchodilators should be used for a minimum of 4 weeks after an acute exacerbation and then gradually decreased to the lowest dose possible to alleviate clinical signs. Metered dose inhalers are now available (aerokat.com) for administration of inhaled bronchodilators and steroids. Fluticasone (Flovent, 100 mcg/puff) can be administered initially every 12 hours for 1 week and then decreased to once daily, in most cases. Inhaled glucocorticosteroids are not absorbed systemically, and therefore patients do not develop the adverse side effects sometimes documented with oral glucocorticosteroid administration. Because it takes time for glucocorticosteroids to reach peak effects in the lungs, administration of inhaled glucocorticosteroids should overlap with oral prednisolone administration for 5 to 7 days.

PULMONARY CONTUSIONS

Pulmonary contusions are a common sequela of blunt traumatic injury. A contusion basically is a bruise characterized by edema, hemorrhage, and vascular injury. Contusions may be present at the time of presentation or can develop over the first 24 hours after injury. A diagnosis of pulmonary contusion can be made based on auscultation of pulmonary crackles, presence of respiratory distress, and the presence of patchy interstitial to alveolar infiltrates on thoracic radiographs. Radiographic signs can lag behind the development of clinical signs of respiratory distress and hypoxemia by 24 hours.

TABLE 1-53   Drugs to Use in the Immediate and Long-Term Management of Feline Bronchitis

Drug	Emergency treatment	Long-term management
Bronchodilators		
Aminophylline	4 mg/kg IM (emergency)	5 mg/kg PO q8-12h
Terbutaline	0.01 mg/kg SQ	0.625 mg/cat PO q12h
Theophylline		50-100 mg/cat PO q24h
Albuterol MDI*	90 μg	90 μg as needed up to q6h
Glucocorticosteroids		
Dexamethasone sodium phosphate	1 mg/kg IV, IM, SQ	
Dexamethasone		0.25 mg/kg PO q8-12h, then taper to q24h for 1-2 months
Prednisolone		1 mg/kg PO q12h, then taper
Prednisolone sodium succinate	50-100 mg/cat IV	0.1-0.625 mg/kg PO q12h
Triamcinolone	0.11 mg/kg SQ, repeat	0.11 mg/kg PO q12-24h, then taper in 10-14 days
Fluticasone MDI	110 μg/puff	110 μg MDI q12h
Beclomethasone	220 μg/puff	220 μg MDI q6-8h

*MDI, Metered dose inhaler.

Treatment of pulmonary contusions is supportive. Administer supplemental oxygen in a manner that is least stressful for the animal. Arterial blood gas analysis or pulse oximetry can determine the degree of hypoxemia and monitor the response to therapy. Intravenous fluids should be administered with caution to avoid exacerbating pulmonary hemorrhage or fluid accumulation in the alveoli. Treat other conditions associated with the traumatic event. Possible complications of pulmonary contusions are rare but include bacterial infection, abscessation, lung lobe consolidation, and the development of cavitary lesions. The routine use of antibiotics or steroids in cases of pulmonary contusions is contraindicated unless external wounds are present. Empiric antibiotic use without evidence of external injury or known infection can potentially increase the risk of a resistant bacterial infection. Steroids have been shown to decrease pulmonary alveolar macrophage function and impair wound healing and are contraindicated.

Aspiration Pneumonia

Aspiration pneumonia can occur in animals as a result of abnormal laryngeal or pharyngeal protective mechanisms or can be secondary to vomiting during states of altered mentation, including anesthesia, recovery from anesthesia, and sleep. Megaesophagus, systemic polyneuropathy, myasthenia gravis, and localized oropharyngeal defects such as cleft palate can increase the risk of developing aspiration pneumonitis. Iatrogenic causes of aspiration pneumonia include improper placement of nasogastric feeding tubes, overly aggressive force-feeding, and oral administration of drugs. Aspiration of contents into the airways can cause mechanical airway obstruction, bronchoconstriction, chemical damage to the alveoli, and infection. Severe inflammation and airway edema are common. Pulmonary hemorrhage and necrosis can occur.

Diagnosis of aspiration pneumonia is based on clinical signs of pulmonary parenchymal disease, a history consistent with vomiting or other predisposing causes, and thoracic radiographs demonstrating a bronchointerstitial to alveolar pulmonary infiltrate. The most common site is the right middle lung lobe, although the pneumonia can occur anywhere, depending on the position of the patient at the time of aspiration. A transtracheal wash or bronchoalveolar lavage is useful for bacterial culture and susceptibility testing.

Treatment of aspiration pneumonia includes antibiotic therapy for the infection, administration of supplemental oxygen, and loosening the debris in the airways. Administer intravenous fluids to maintain hydration. Nebulization with sterile saline and chest physiotherapy (coupage) should be performed at least every 8 hours. Antibiotics to consider in the treatment of aspiration pneumonia include ampicillin/enrofloxacin, amoxicillin-clavulanate, ampicillin-sulbactam, trimethoprim sulfa, and chloramphenicol. The use of glucocorticosteroids is absolutely contraindicated. Continue antibiotic therapy for a minimum of 2 weeks after the resolution of radiographic signs of pneumonia.

Pulmonary Edema

Pulmonary edema arises from the accumulation of fluid in the pulmonary interstitial alveolar spaces, and airways. Ventilation-perfusion abnormalities result in hypoxia. Pulmonary edema can be caused by increased pulmonary vasculature hydrostatic pressure, decreased pulmonary oncotic pressure, obstruction of lymphatic drainage, or increased capillary permeability. Multiple factors can occur simultaneously. The most common cause of edema is increased pulmonary hydrostatic pressure resulting from left-sided congestive heart failure. Decreased plasma oncotic pressure with albumin <1.5 g/dL can also result in accumulation of fluid in the pulmonary parenchyma. Overzealous intravenous crystalloid fluid administration can result in dilution of serum oncotic pressure and vascular overload. Obstruction of lymphatic drainage is usually caused by neoplasia. Other causes of pulmonary edema include pulmonary thromboembolic disease, severe upper airway obstruction (noncardiogenic pulmonary edema), seizures, and head trauma.

Increased capillary permeability is associated with a variety of diseases that cause severe inflammation (systemic inflammatory response syndrome). The resultant pulmonary edema contains a high amount of protein and is known as acute respiratory distress syndrome (ARDS). ARDS can be associated with pulmonary or extrapulmonary causes, including direct lung injury from trauma, aspiration pneumonia, sepsis, pancreatitis, smoke inhalation, oxygen toxicity, electrocution, and immune-mediated hemolytic anemia with disseminated intravascular coagulation.

Diagnosis of pulmonary edema is made based on clinical signs of respiratory distress and the presence of crackles on thoracic auscultation. In severe cases, cyanosis and fulminant blood-tinged frothy edema fluid may be present in the mouth and nostrils. Immediate management includes administration of furosemide (4-8 mg/kg IV, IM) and supplemental oxygen. Sedation with low-dose morphine sulfate (0.025-0.1 mg/kg IV) is helpful in dilating the splanchnic capacitance vasculature and relieving anxiety for the patient. If fluid overload is suspected secondary to intravenous fluid administration, fluids should be discontinued. Severely hypoalbuminemic patients should receive concentrated human albumin (2 mL/kg of a 25% solution) or fresh frozen plasma. Furosemide as a constant rate infusion (0.66-0.1 mg/kg/hour) also can dilate the pulmonary vasculature and decrease fluid accumulation in cases of ARDS. Following initial stabilization of the patient, thoracic radiographs and an echocardiogram should be assessed to determine cardiac side, pulmonary vascular size, and cardiac contractility. Further diagnostic testing may be required to determine other underlying causes of pulmonary edema.

Heart failure is managed with vasodilators, diuretics, oxygen, and sometimes positive inotropes. Treatment ultimately consists of administration of supplemental oxygen, minimal stress and patient handling, and judicious use of diuretics. In cases of cardiogenic pulmonary edema, administer furosemide (4-8 mg/kg IV, IM) every 30 to 60 minutes until the patient loses 7% of its body weight. Positive inotropic and antiarrhythmic therapy may be necessary to improve cardiac contractility and control dysrhythmias. The clinician should determine whether the cause of the pulmonary edema is secondary to congestive heart failure with pulmonary vascular overload, volume overload, hypoalbuminemia, or increased permeability (ARDS). Pulmonary edema secondary to ARDS typically is refractory to supplemental oxygen and diuretic therapy. In many cases, mechanical ventilation should be considered.

PULMONARY THROMBOEMBOLISM

A diagnosis of pulmonary thromboembolism (PTE) is difficult to make and is based on clinical signs of respiratory distress consistent with PTE, lack of other causes of hypoxemia, a high index of suspicion in susceptible animals, the presence of a condition associated with PTE, and radiographic findings. Virchow's triad consists of vascular endothelial injury, sluggish blood flow with increased vascular stasis, and a hypercoagulable state as predisposing factors for thromboembolic disease. Clinical conditions that predispose an animal to PTE include hyperadrenocorticism, disseminated intravascular coagulation (DIC), catheterization of blood vessels, bacterial endocarditis, protein-losing nephropathy or enteropathy, hyperviscosity syndromes, heat-induced illness, pancreatitis, diabetes mellitus, inflammatory bowel disease, and immune-mediated hemolytic anemia. Definitive diagnosis requires angiography or a lung perfusion scan.

Clinical signs associated with PTE include an acute onset of tachypnea, tachycardia, orthopnea, and cyanosis. If the embolism is large, the patient may respond poorly to supplemental oxygen administration. Pulmonary hypertension can cause a split second heart sound on cardiac auscultation. In some cases, a normal thoracic radiograph is present in the face of severe respiratory distress. This is a classic finding in cases of PTE. Potential radiographic abnormalities include dilated, tortuous, or blunted pulmonary arteries; wedge-shaped opacities in the lungs distal to an obstructed artery; and interstitial to alveolar infiltrates. The right heart may be enlarged.

Echocardiography can show right heart enlargement, tricuspid regurgitation, pulmonary hypertension, and evidence of underlying cardiac disease, possibly with clots in the atria. Measurement of antithrombin (AT) and D-dimer levels can be useful in the identification of hypercoagulable states, including DIC. Treatment of any patient with AT deficiency or DIC includes replenishment of AT and clotting factors in the form of fresh frozen plasma.

Treatment of PTE includes therapy for cardiovascular shock, oxygen supplementation, and thrombolytic therapy (see section on Thromboembolic Therapy). For short-term treatment, administer heparin (heparin sodium, 200-300 units/kg SQ once, followed by 100 units/kg q8h of unfractionated heparin; or fractionated heparin). Thrombolytic therapy may include tissue plasminogen activator, streptokinase, or urokinase. Long-term therapy with low molecular weight heparin or warfarin may be required to prevent further thromboembolic events. Ideally, management should include treatment and elimination of the underlying disease.

SMOKE INHALATION

Smoke inhalation commonly occurs when an animal is trapped in a burning building. The most severe respiratory complications of smoke inhalation are seen in animals that are close enough to the flames to also sustain burn injuries (see section on Burn Injury). At the scene, many animals are unconscious from the effects of hypoxia, hypercapnia, carbon monoxide intoxication, and hydrogen cyanide gases that accumulate in a fire. Carbon monoxide produces hypoxia by avidly binding to and displacing oxygen binding to hemoglobin, resulting in severe impairment of oxygen-carrying capacity. The percentage of carboxyhemoglobin in peripheral blood depends on the amount or carbon monoxide in inhaled gases and the length of time of exposure. Clinical signs of carbon monoxide intoxication include cyanosis, nausea, vomiting, collapse, respiratory failure, loss of consciousness, and death.

Smoke inhalation of superheated particles also causes damage to the upper airways and respiratory tree. The larynx can become severely edematous and obstruct inspiration. Emergency endotracheal intubation, tracheal oxygen, or tracheostomy tube may be required in the initial resuscitation of the patient, depending on the extent of airway edema. Inhalation of noxious gases and particles can cause damage to the terminal respiratory bronchioles. Specific noxious gases that can cause alveolar damage include combustible particles from plastic, rubber, and other synthetic products. Pulmonary edema, bacterial infection, and ARDS can result.

In any case of smoke inhalation, the first and foremost treatment is to get the animal away from the source of the flames and smoke and administer supplemental oxygen at the scene. At the time of presentation, carefully examine the animal's eyes, mouth, and oropharynx Suction soot and debris from the mouth and upper airways. Evaluate the patient's respiratory rate, rhythm, and pulmonary sounds. Arterial blood gases should be analyzed with co-oximetry to evaluate the PaO_2 and carboxyhemoglobin concentrations. Evaluation of SaO_2 by pulse oximetry is not accurate in cases of smoke inhalation, as the PaO_2 may appear normal, even when large quantities of carboxyhemoglobin are present. Radiographs are helpful in determining the extent of pulmonary involvement, although radiographic signs may lag behind the appearance of clinical respiratory abnormalities by 16 to 24 hours. Bronchoscopy and bronchoalveolar lavage provide a more thorough and accurate evaluation of the respiratory tree; however, these procedures should be performed only in patients whose cardiovascular and respiratory status is stable.

Management of the patient with smoke inhalation includes maintaining a patent airway, administration of supplemental oxygen, correction of hypoxemia and acid-base abnormalities, preventing infection, and treating thermal burns (See section on Burn Injury). If severe laryngeal edema is present, a temporary tracheostomy may be necessary to allow adequate oxygenation and ventilation. Glucocorticosteroids should NOT be empirically used in the treatment of smoke inhalation, because of the risk of decreasing pulmonary alveolar macrophage function and increasing the potential for infection. In cases of severe laryngeal edema, however, glucocorticosteroids may be necessary to decrease edema and inflammation. The use of empiric antibiotics is contraindicated unless clinical signs of deterioration and bacterial pneumonia develop.

EPISTAXIS

Epistaxis can be caused by facial trauma, a foreign body, bacterial or fungal rhinitis, neoplasia, coagulopathies, and systemic hypertension. Acute, severe bilateral hemorrhage without exudate is suggestive of a systemic disorder. A history of chronic nasal discharge usually accompanies nasal disease. Acute unilateral epistaxis can occur with nasal or systemic disease.

In most cases, cage rest is sufficient to temporarily diminish blood loss. Sedation (acepromazine, 0.02-0.05 mg/kg IV, IM, SQ) may be helpful in alleviating anxiety and decreasing blood pressure. The hypotensive effects of acepromazine are potentially harmful if severe blood loss has occurred. If evidence of hypovolemia is present (see section on Hypovolemic Shock), intravenous fluid resuscitation should be administered.

Rapid assessment of clotting ability, with a platelet count estimate and clotting profile (ACT or APTT and PT), should be performed. If epistaxis secondary to Vitamin K antagonist rodenticide intoxication is suspected, administer vitamin K_1 and fresh frozen plasma or fresh whole blood.

Persistent hemorrhage from a nasal disorder can be treated with dilute epinephrine (1:100,000) into the nasal cavity with the nose pointed toward the ceiling to promote vasoconstriction. If this fails, the animal can be anesthetized, and the nasal cavity packed with gauze, and the caudal oropharynx and external nares covered with umbilical tape to control hemorrhage. A rhinoscopy should be performed to determine the cause of ongoing hemorrhage. Continued excessive hemorrhage can be controlled with ligation of the carotid artery on the side of the hemorrhage, or with percutaneous arterial embolization.

Additional Reading

Buerge HCD: Pleural effusion in cats. Vet Med 97(11):812-818, 2002.

Campbell VL, King LG: Pulmonary function, ventilator management, and outcome of dogs with thoracic trauma and pulmonary contusions: 10 cases (1994-1998). J Am Vet Med Assoc 217(10):1505-1509, 2000.

Carpenter DH, Macintire DK, Tyler JW: Acute lung injury and acute respiratory distress syndrome. Comp Cont Educ Pract Vet 23(8):712-725, 2001.

Drobatz KJ, Walker LM, Hendricks JC: Smoke exposure in cats: 22 cases (1986-1997). J Am Vet Med Assoc 215(9):1312-1316, 1999.

Drobatz KJ, Walker LM, Hendricks JC: Smoke exposure in dogs: 27 cases (1988-1997) J Am Vet Med Assoc 215(9):1306-1311, 1999.

Fossum TW, Mertens MM, Miller MW, et al: Thoracic duct ligation and pericardectomy for treatment of idiopathic chylothorax. J Vet Intern Med 18(3):307-310, 2004.

Gellasch KL, De Costa Gomez T, McAnulty JF, Bjorling DE, et al. Use of intraluminal nitinol stents in the treatment of tracheal collapse in a dog. J Am Vet Med Assoc 221(12):1719-1723, 2002.

Gieger T, Northrup N: Clinical approach to epistaxis. Comp Cont Educ Pract Vet 26(1):30-43, 2004.

Hughes D: Pulmonary edema. In Wingfield WE, Raffe MR (eds): The Veterinary ICU Book. Teton NewMedia, Jackson, Wyo, 2001.

Hyun C: Radiographic diagnosis of diaphragmatic hernia: review of 60 cases in dogs and cats. J Vet Sci 5(2):157-162, 2004.

Johnson L: Tracheal collapse: diagnosis and medical and surgical management. Vet Clin North Am Small Anim Pract 30(6):1253-1266, 2000.

King LG, Waddell LS: Acute respiratory distress syndrome. In Wingfield WE, Raffe MR (eds): The Veterinary ICU Book. Teton NewMedia, Jackson, Wyo, 2001.

Koch DA, Arnold S, Hubler M, Montavon PM: Brachycephalic syndrome in dogs. Comp Cont Educ Pract Vet 25(1):48-55, 2003.

MacPhail CM, Monnet E: Outcome and postoperative complications in dogs undergoing surgical treatment of laryngeal paralysis: 140 cases (1985-1998). J Am Vet Med Assoc 218(12):1949-1956, 2001.

Mariani CL: Full recovery following delayed neurologic signs after smoke inhalation in a dog. J Vet Emerg Crit Care 13(4):235-239, 2003.

Mazzaferro EM: Aspiration pneumonitis. In Wingfield WE, Raffe MR (eds): The Veterinary ICU Book. Teton NewMedia, Jackson, Wyo, 2001.

Mazzaferro EM: Respiratory Injury. In Wingfield WE, Raffe MR (eds): The Veterinary ICU Book. Teton NewMedia, Jackson, Wyo, 2001.

McKiernan BC, Miller C: Allergic airway disease. In Wingfield WE, Raffe MR (eds): The Veterinary ICU Book. Teton NewMedia, Jackson, Wyo, 2001.

Mellanby RJ, Villiers E, Herrtage ME: Canine pleural and mediastinal effusion, a retrospective study of 81 cases. J Small Anim Pract 43(10):447-451, 2002.

Mueller ER: Suggested strategies for ventilatory management in veterinary patients with acute respiratory distress syndrome. J Vet Emerg Crit Care 11(3):191-197, 2001.

Reiss AJ, McKiernan BC: Laryngeal and tracheal disorders. In Wingfield WE, Raffe MR, editors: The veterinary ICU book, Jackson,Wyo, 2001, Teton NewMedia,.

Reiss AJ, McKiernan BC. Pneumonia. In Wingfield WE, Raffe MR (eds): The Veterinary ICU Book. Teton NewMedia, Jackson, Wyo, 2001.

Rooney MB, Monnet E: Medical and surgical treatment of pyothorax in dogs: 26 cases (1991-2001). J Am Vet Med Assoc 221(1):86-92, 2002.

Schmidt CW, Tobias KM, McCrackin Stevenson MA: Traumatic diaphragmatic hernia in cats: 34 cases (1991-2000). J Am Vet Med Assoc 229(9):1237-1240, 2003.

Scott JA, Macintire DK: Canine Pyothorax: Clinical presentation, diagnosis, and treatment. Comp Cont Educ Pract Vet 25(3):180-194, 2003.

Scott JA, Macintire DK: Canine pyothorax: pleural anatomy and pathophysiology. Comp Cont Educ Pract Vet 25(3):172-179, 2003.

Smeak DD, Birchard SJ, McLoughlin MA, et al: Treatment of chronic pleural effusion with pleuroperitoneal shunt in dogs: 14 cases (1985-1999). J Am Vet Med Assoc 219(11): 1590-1597, 2001.

Tobias KM, Jackson AM, Harvey RC: Effects of doxapram hydrochloride on laryngeal function of normal dogs and dogs with naturally occurring laryngeal paralysis. Vet Anaesth Analg 31(4):258-263, 2004.

Vassilev E, McMichael M: An overview of positive pressure ventilation. J Vet Emerg Crit Care 14(1):15-21, 2004.

Waddell LS, Brady CA, Drobatz KJ: Risk factors, prognostic indicators, and outcome of pyothorax in cats: 80 cases (1986-1999). J Am Vet Med Assoc 221(6):819-824, 2002.

Weiss C, Nicholson ME, Rollings C, et al: Use of percutaneous arterial embolization for the treatment of intractable epistaxis in 3 dogs. J Am Vet Med Assoc 224(8):1307-1311, 2004.

SUPERFICIAL SOFT TISSUE INJURIES

Wounds have been classified in several ways according their degree of tissue integrity, etiologic force, degree of contamination and duration, and degree of contamination and infection (Table 1-54). There are also unique causes of wounds such as burns, psychogenic dermatoses, frostbite, decubital ulcers, and snake bite.

The animal should be transported to the nearest veterinary facility for definitive care. The wound should be covered or packed with dry gauze or clean linen to protect the wound, and to prevent further hemorrhage and contamination. If an open fracture is present, the limb should be splinted without placing the exposed bone back into the wound. Replacing the exposed bone fragment back through the skin wound can cause further damage to underlying soft tissue structures and increase the degree of contamination of deeper tissues. If a spinal fracture is suspected, the patient should be transported on a stable flat surface to prevent further spinal mobilization and neurologic injury.

At the time of presentation, first refer to the ABCs of trauma, taking care to evaluate and stabilize the patient's cardiovascular and respiratory status. After a complete physical examination and history, ancillary diagnostic techniques can be performed if the patient is hemodynamically stable (see section on Triage, Assessment, and Treatment of Emergencies).

WOUND MANAGEMENT

Initially, every patient with superficial wound should receive some degree of analgesia and an injection of a first-generation cephalosporin, preferably within 3 hours of the injury. Evaluate the wound after the patient's cardiovascular and respiratory status have been stabilized. Always cover an open wound before taking an animal to the hospital to prevent a nosocomial infection. Evaluate limb wounds for neural, vascular, and orthopedic abnormalities. Carefully examine the structures deep to the superficial wounds.

When there has been a delay in assessment of the wound, obtain samples for culture and antimicrobial susceptibility testing. If the wound is older and obviously infected, a Gram stain can help guide appropriate antimicrobial therapy pending results of culture

1

TABLE 1-54   Classification of Soft Tissue Wounds

Classification	Characteristics
Tissue integrity	
Open	Lacerations or skin loss
Closed	Crushing injuries and contusions
Etiologic force	
Abrasion	Loss of epidermis and portions of dermis, usually caused by shearing between two compressive surfaces
Avulsion	Tearing of tissue from its attachment because of forces similar to those causing abrasion but of a greater magnitude
Incision	Wound created by a sharp object; wound edges are smooth and there is minimal trauma in the surrounding tissues
Laceration	Irregular wound caused by tearing of tissue with variable damage to the superficial and underlying tissue
Puncture	Penetrating wound caused by a missile or sharp object; superficial damage may be minimal; damage to deeper structures may be considerable; contamination by fur and bacteria with subsequent infection is common
Degree of contamination and duration	
Class I	0-6 hours with minimal contamination
Class II	6-12 hours with significant contamination
Class III	>12 hours with gross contamination
Degree of contamination or infection	
Clean wound	Surgically created under aseptic conditions; no invasion of the respiratory, gastrointestinal, or genitourinary tracts, or of the oropharyngeal cavity
Clean contaminated wound	Minimal contamination, and contamination can be removed effectively; includes operative wounds involving the respiratory, gastrointestinal, and genitourinary tracts
Contaminated wound	Open traumatic wound with heavy contamination and possibly foreign debris; includes operative wounds with major breaks in aseptic technique and incisions in areas of acute nonpurulent inflammation adjacent to inflamed or contaminated skin
Dirty/infected wound	Old traumatic wound and wounds with clinical signs of infection or perforated viscera

Modified from Swaim SF, Henderson RA: *Small animal wound management*, ed 2, Media, Pa, 1997, Williams & Wilkins.

and susceptibility testing. Place a support bandage saturated with a water-soluble antibiotic ointment or nonirritating antimicrobial solution (e.g., 0.05% chlorhexidine, if bone or joint tissue is not exposed) around the wound. In addition to a first-generation cephalosporin, other appropriate antibiotic choices include amoxicillin-clavulanate, trimethoprim-sulfadiazine, amoxicillin, and ampicillin. If gram-negative flora are present, administer enrofloxacin. Administer the antibiotics of choice for a minimum of 7 days unless a change of antibiotic therapy is indicated.

At the time of wound cleansing or definitive wound repair, the patient should be placed under general anesthesia with endotracheal intubation, unless the procedure will be brief (i.e., less than 10 minutes). In such cases, a short-acting anesthetic combination

1

(analgesia + propofol, analgesia + ketamine/diazepam) can be administered to effect. Heavy sedation with infiltration of a local anesthetic may also be appropriate for very small wounds, depending on the location of the wound and temperament of the patient. Protect the wound by packing it with sterile gauze sponges soaked in sterile saline, or with water-soluble lubricating gel such as K-Y jelly.

Clip the fur surrounding the wound, moving from the inner edge of the wound outward, to help prevent wound contamination with fur or other debris. Scrub the wound and surrounding skin with an antimicrobial soap and solution such as dilute chlorhexidine until the area is free of all gross debris. Gross debris within the wound itself can be flushed using a 30-mL syringe filled with sterile saline or lactated Ringer's solution and an 18-gauge needle. Pressure-lavage systems are also available for use, if desired. Grossly contaminated wounds can be rinsed first with warm tap water to eliminate gross contamination, and then prepared as just described.

Debride the wound, removing skin and other soft tissue that is not obviously viable. Obviously viable and questionable tissue should remain, and the wound left open for frequent reassessment on a daily basis. Remove any dark or white segments of skin. Questionable skin edges may or not regain viability and should be left in place for 48 hours, so the wound can fully reveal itself. Excise grossly contaminated areas of fat and underlying fascia. Blood vessels that are actively bleeding should be ligated to control hemorrhage, if collateral circulation is present.

If nerve bundles are ligated cleanly in a clean wound, the nerve edges should be reapposed and anastomosed. If gross contamination is present, however, definitive neurologic repair should be delayed until healthy tissue is present. Excise contaminated muscle until healthy bleeding tissue is present. Anastamoe tendon lacerations if the wound is clean and not grossly contaminated. If gross contamination is present, the tendon can be temporarily anastomosed and a splint placed on the limb until definitive repair of healthy tissue is possible.

Thoroughly lavage open wounds to a joint with sterile saline or lactated Ringer's solution. Infusion of chlorhexidine or povidone-iodine solution into the joint can cause a decrease in cartilage repair and is contraindicated. Smooth sharp edges and remove any obvious fragments. Whenever possible, the joint capsule and ligaments should be partially or completely closed. After removing bullets and metal fragments, the subcutaneous tissue and skin should be left open to heal by second intention, or should be partially closed with a drain. The joint should then be immobilized.

Injuries and exposed bone should be carefully lavaged, taking care to remove any gross debris without pushing the debris further into the bone and wound. The bone should be covered with a moist dressing and stabilized until definitive fracture repair can be made. This type of injury typically is seen with shearing injuries of the distal extremities caused by interaction with slow-moving vehicles. Perform wet-to-dry or enzymatic debridement until a healthy granulation bed is present.

If large areas of contamination are present (e.g., necrotizing fasciitis), en bloc debridement may be necessary. En bloc debridement consists of complete excision of badly infected wounds without entering the wound cavity, to prevent systemic infection. This technique should be used only if there is sufficient skin and soft tissue to allow later closure and it can be performed without damaging any major nerves, tendons, or blood vessels.

OPEN WOUNDS

Open wounds often are managed by second intention healing, delayed primary closure, or secondary closure. See section on Wound Management and Bandaging for a more complete discussion on the use of various bandaging materials in the treatment of open wounds.

CLOSED WOUNDS

If an animal is presented very shortly after a wound has occurred and there is minimal contamination and trauma, the wound can be closed after induction of anesthesia and careful preparation of the wound and surrounding tissues. Close any dead space under the skin with absorbable suture material in an interrupted suture pattern. Avoid incising major blood vessels or nerves. Close the subcutaneous tissues with absorbable suture material in an interrupted or continuous suture pattern. Take care that there is not too much tension on the wound, or else surgical dehiscence will occur with patient movement. Close the skin with nonabsorbable suture or surgical staples (2-0 to 4-0).

If there is any doubt at the time of repair about tissue status or inability to close all dead space, place a passive drain (Penrose drain) so that the proximal end of the drain is anchored in the proximal aspect of the wound with a suture(s). Leave the ends long so that the suture can be accurately identified at the time of drain removal. Pass the suture through the skin, through the drain, and out the other side of the skin. Place the rest of the drain into the wound and then secure it at the most ventral portion of the wound or exit hole in the most dependent area of the body, to allow drainage and prevent seroma formation. Close the subcutaneous tissue over the drain before skin closure. During wound closure, be sure to not incorporate the subcutaneous or skin sutures into the drain, or it will not be possible to remove the drain without reopening the wound. Bandage the area to prevent contamination. The drain can be removed once drainage is minimal (usually 3 to 5 days).

Active drains can be constructed or purchased; their use is indicated in wounds that are free of material that can plug the drain. To construct a small suction drain, remove the female portion or catheter hub at the end of a butterfly catheter. Fenestrate the tubing so that there are multiple side holes, taking care to avoid making the holes larger than 50% of the circumference of the tubing. Place the tubing into the wound via a small stab incision distal to the wound. Use a purse-string suture around the tubing to facilitate a tight seal and prevent the tubing from exiting the wound. Following wound closure, insert the butterfly needle into a 5- to 10-mL evacuated blood collection tube to allow fluid to drain into the tube. Incorporate the tube into the bandage, and replace it when it becomes full.

Alternatively, the butterfly portion of the system can be removed and the tube fenestrated as described previously. Place the tube into the wound and suture it in place to create a tight seal. Secure the catheter hub to a syringe in which the plunger has been drawn back slightly to create suction. Insert a metal pin or 16- to 18-gauge needle through the plunger at the top of the barrel to hold it at the desired level. Incorporate the suction apparatus into the bandage and replace it when it becomes full.

DELAYED PRIMARY CLOSURE

Delayed primary closure should be considered when there is heavy contamination, purulent exudate, residual necrotic debris, skin tension, edema and erythema, and lymphangitis. Delayed primary closure usually is made 3 to 5 days after the initial wound infliction and open wound management has been performed. Once healthy tissue is observed, the skin edges should be debrided and the wound closed as with primary closure.

SECONDARY WOUND CLOSURE

Secondary wound closure should be considered when infection and tissue trauma necessitate open wound management for more than 5 days. Secondary wound closure is performed after the development of a healthy granulation bed. This technique also is useful when a wound has dehisced and has formed granulation tissue.

If the wound edges can be manipulated into apposition and if epithelialization has not begun, the wound can be cleansed and the wound edges apposed and sutured. This is known as early secondary closure.

Late secondary closure should be performed whenever there is a considerable amount of granulation tissue, the edges of the wound cannot be manipulated into position, and epithelialization has already started. In such cases, the wound should be cleaned, and the skin edges debrided to remove the epithelium. The remaining wound edges are then sutured over the granulation tissue (Table 1-55).

1

TABLE 1-55   Complicating Factors Involving the Management of Superficial Soft Tissue Wounds

Circumstance	Potential problem(s)
Improper handling of animal during transport	Further tissue and neurologic damage may occur (e.g., improper limb or spine immobilization).
Inadequate assessment of animal's general condition or wounded tissues	Animal's condition may worsen or animal may succumb; tissue injuries may be overlooked.
Inadequate wound protection during assessment, resuscitation, or stabilization procedures	Further wound contamination may occur at veterinary facility.
Inadequate wound protection while preparing the surrounding area	Further wound contamination with fur and debris may occur.
Insufficient wound lavage	Wound infection may occur.
Hydrogen peroxide wound lavage	Lavage offers little bactericidal activity and contributes to irritation of tissues and delayed healing.
Povidone-iodine wound lavage	Lavage has short residual activity and absorption with large wound.
Overly aggressive initial layered debridement	Debridement may result in the removal of viable tissue.
En bloc debridement	Debridement results in removal of large amounts of tissue and a large defect for closure.
Use of drains	Potential exists for bacteria to ascend along the drain, for drain removal by the animal or breakage of the drain, and for possible tissue emphysema with air being sucked under the skin with patient movement.
Tube-type drains	Drains may cause postoperative discomfort; fenestrations may become occluded to stop intraluminal drainage.
Deeply placed sutures in the presence of a drain	Drain may be incorporated into the repair and prevent drain removal.
Active drains	High negative pressure may cause tissue injury; highly productive wounds may necessitate changing the evacuated blood tubes several times a day with constructed drains.

Additional Reading

Swaim SF, Henderson RA: small animal wound management. 2nd Edition. Williams and Wilkins, Media, Pa, 1997,

SHOCK

Shock is defined as a state of inadequate circulating volume and inability to meet cellular oxygen demands. There are three types of shock: hypovolemic, cardiogenic, and septic. Early recognition of the type of shock present is crucial in the successful clinical management of shock syndrome. Tissue oxygen delivery is based on cardiac output and arterial oxygen concentration. Knowledge of the components of normal oxygen delivery is essential to the treatment of shock in the critical patient.

$$\text{Oxygen delivery (DO}_2) = \text{cardiac output (Q)} \times \text{arterial oxygen content (CaO}_2)$$

where Q = heart rate × stroke volume. Stroke volume is affected by preload, afterload, and cardiac contractility.

$$CaO_2 = (1.34 \times [Hb] \times SaO_2) + (0.003 \times PaO_2)$$

where Hb = hemoglobin concentration, SaO_2 = oxygen saturation, and PaO_2 = arterial partial pressure of oxygen in mm Hg.

Thus, factors that can adversely affect oxygen delivery include inadequate preload or loss of circulating volume, severe peripheral vasoconstriction and increased afterload, depressed cardiac contractility, tachycardia and decreased diastolic filling, cardiac dysrhythmias, inadequate circulating hemoglobin, and inadequate oxygen saturation of hemoglobin. During septic shock, enzymatic dysfunction and decreased cellular uptake and utilization of oxygen also contribute to anaerobic glycolysis.

An inadequate circulating volume may develop secondary to maldistribution of available blood volume (traumatic, septic, and cardiogenic origin) or as a result of absolute hypovolemia (whole blood or loss of extracellular fluid). Normally, the animal compensates by (1) splenic and vascular constriction to translocated blood from venous capacitance vessels to central arterial circulation, (2) arteriolar constriction to help maintain diastolic blood pressure and tissue perfusion, and (3) an increase in heart rate to help maintain cardiac output. Arteriolar vasoconstrictions support perfusion to the brain and heart at the expense of other visceral organs. If vasoconstriction is severe enough to interfere with delivery of adequate tissue oxygen for a sufficient period of time, the animal may die.

Hypovolemic Shock

Hypovolemic shock can result from acute hemorrhage or from severe fluid loss from vomiting, diarrhea, or third spacing of fluids. Early in shock, baroreceptors in the carotid body and aortic arch sense a decrease in wall stretch from a decrease in circulating fluid volume. Tonic inhibition of sympathetic tone via vagal stimulation is diminished, and heart rate and contractility increase and peripheral vessels constrict to compensate for the decrease in cardiac output. The compensatory mechanisms protect and support blood supply to the brain and heart at the expense of peripheral organ perfusion. This is called *early compensatory shock.*

Early compensatory shock is characterized by tachycardia, normal to fast capillary refill time, tachypnea, and normothermia. As shock progresses, the body loses its ability to compensate for ongoing fluid losses. Early decompensatory shock is characterized by tachycardia, tachypnea, delayed capillary refill time, normotension to hypotension, and a fall in body temperature. End-stage decompensatory shock is characterized by bradycardia, markedly prolonged capillary refill time, hypothermia, and hypotension. Aggressive treatment is necessary for any hope of a favorable outcome.

Septic Shock

Septic shock should be considered in any patient with a known infection, recent instrumentation that could potentially introduce infection (indwelling intravenous or urinary catheter, surgery or penetrating injury), disorders or medical therapy that can compromise immune function (diabetes mellitus, immunodeficiency virus, parvovirus or feline panleukopenia virus infection, stress, malnutrition, glucocorticoids, chemotherapy). The presence of bacteria, viruses or rickettsiae, protozoa, or fungal organisms in the blood constitutes septicemia. Septic shock is characterized by the presence of sepsis and refractory hypotension that is unresponsive to standard aggressive fluid therapy and inotropic or pressor support. Septic shock and other causes of inflammation can lead to systemic inflammatory response syndrome (SIRS). In animals, the presence of two or more of the criteria in Table 1-56 in the presence of suspected inflammation or sepsis constitutes SIRS (Table 1-56).

TABLE 1-56 **Summary of Systemic Inflammatory Response Syndrome Criteria**

Criteria	Dogs	Cats
Temperature	<100° F or >103.5° F	<100° F or >103.5° F
Heart rate	>120 beats/minute in dogs	<140 or >250 beats/minute in cats
Respiratory rate	>20 breaths/minute or Pa_{CO_2} <32 mm Hg	>40 breaths/minute or Pa_{CO_2} <32 mm Hg
White blood cell count	>18,000 cells/μL or <4000 cells/μL or >10% bands	19,000 cells/μL or <5000 cells/mL or >10% bands

Clinical signs associated with sepsis may be vague and nonspecific, including weakness, lethargy, vomiting, and diarrhea. Cough and pulmonary crackles may be associated with pneumonia. Decreased lung sounds may be associated with pyothorax. Abdominal pain and fluid may be associated with septic peritonitis. Vaginal discharge may or may not be present in patients with pyometra. Diagnostic tests should include a white blood cell count, serum biochemical profile, coagulation tests, thoracic and abdominal radiographs, and urinalysis.

The white blood cell count in a septic patient that is appropriately responding to the infection will be elevated with a left-shifted neutrophilia and leukocytosis. A degenerative left shift, in which leukopenia with elevated band neutrophils suggests an overwhelming infection. Biochemical analyses may demonstrate hypoglycemia and nonspecific hepatocellular and cholestatic enzyme elevations. In the most severe cases, metabolic (lactic) acidosis, coagulopathies, and end-organ failure, including anuria and ARDS, may be present.

CARDIOGENIC SHOCK

Cardiogenic shock occurs as a result of cardiac output inadequate to meet cellular oxygen demands. Cardiogenic shock is associated with primary cardiomyopathies, cardiac dysrhythmias, pericardial fluid, and pericardial fibrosis. Abnormalities seen on physical examination often are similar to those seen in other categories of shock, but they can also include cardiac murmurs, dysrhythmias, pulmonary rales, bloody frothy pulmonary edema fluid from the nares or mouth, orthopnea, and cyanosis. It is important to distinguish the primary cause of shock before implementing treatment (Table 1-57), whenever possible, because treatment for a suspected ruptured hemangiosarcoma differs markedly from the treatment for end-stage dilatative cardiomyopathy. The patient's clinical signs may be similar and include a peritoneal fluid wave, but the treatment for hypovolemia can dramatically worsen the congestive heart failure secondary to dilatative cardiomyopathy.

When a patient presents with some form of shock, immediate vascular access is of paramount importance. Place a large-bore peripheral or central venous catheter for the infusion of crystalloid or colloid fluids, blood component therapy, and drugs. Monitor the patient's cardiopulmonary status (by ECG), blood pressure, oxygen saturation (as determined by pulse oximetry or arterial blood gas analyses), hematocrit, BUN, and glucose. Ancillary diagnostics, including thoracic and abdominal radiography, urinalysis, serum biochemistry profile, coagulation tests, complete blood count, abdominal ultrasound, and echocardiography, should be performed as determined by the individual patient's needs and the type of shock.

MANAGEMENT OF THE SHOCK PATIENT

THE RULE OF TWENTY

The following list, called the "Rule of Twenty," is a guideline for case management of the shock patient. Consideration of each aspect of the Rule of Twenty on a daily basis ensures

TABLE 1-57   Clinical Signs of Shock Syndrome

Parameter	Traumatic/ Hypovolemic	Septic	Cardiogenic
Heart rate	Increased	Increased	Increased
Pulse character	Weak	Strong early, weak late	Weak
Mucous membrane color	Pale	Injected early, pale late	Pale
Capillary refill time	Prolonged	Rapid early, prolonged late	Prolonged
Respiratory rate	Increased	Increased	Increased
Core temperature	Low/normal	Elevated early, low late	Low/normal
Peripheral temperature	Low	Low/elevated	Low
Urine output	Low	Low	Low
Blood pressure	Normal to high early, low late	Low	Low

that major organ systems are not overlooked. The list also provides a means to integrate and relate changes in different organ systems functions with one another.*

1. Fluid balance

The treatment of hypovolemic and septic shock requires the placement of large-bore intravenous catheters in peripheral and central veins. If vascular access cannot be obtained percutaneously or by cutdown methods, intraosseous catheterization should be considered. Once vascular access is achieved, rapidly administer large volumes of crystalloid or colloid fluids. As a rule of thumb, administer ¼ of a calculated shock dose of fluids—that is, ¼ × (90 mL/kg/hour) in dogs and ¼ × (44 mL/kg/hour) in cats) of a balanced crystalloid fluid (Normosol-R, Plasmalyte-M, lactated Ringer's solution, or 0.9% sterile saline). Reassess the patient's perfusion parameters (heart rate, capillary refill time, blood pressure, urine output) on a continual basis to direct further fluid therapy. Synthetic colloid fluids (hetastarch, dextran 70, or Oxyglobin) can also be administered in the initial resuscitation from shock. A guideline is to administer 5 to 10 mL/kg of hetastarch or dextran as a bolus over 10 to 15 minutes and then reassess perfusion parameters. Hypertonic saline (0.7% NaCl, 4 mL/kg) can be used in cases of hemorrhagic shock to temporarily restore intravascular fluid volume by drawing fluid from the interstitial space. because this type of fluid resuscitation is short-lived, hypertonic saline should always be used with another crystalloid or colloid fluid, and it should not be used in patients with interstitial dehydration. If hemorrhagic shock is present, the goal should be to return a patient's blood pressure to normal (not supraphysiologic) levels (i.e., systolic pressure 90-100 mm Hg, diastolic pressure >40 mm Hg, and mean arterial pressure ≥60 mm Hg) to avoid iatrogenically causing clots to fall off and hemorrhage to re-start.

In critically ill patients, fluid loss can be measured in the form of urine, vomit, diarrhea, body cavity effusions, and wound exudates. Additionally, insensible losses (those that cannot be readily measured from sweat, panting, and cellular metabolism) constitute 20 mL/kg/day. Measurement of fluid "ins and outs" in conjunction with the patient's central venous pressure, hematocrit, albumin, and colloid oncotic pressure can help guide fluid therapy (see also section on Fluid Therapy).

---

*From Purvis D, Kirby R. Systemic inflammatory response syndrome: septic shock. *Vet Clin North Amer Small Anim Pract* 24(6):1225-1247, 1994.
Kirby R: Septic shock. In Bonagura JD, editor: Kirk's current veterinary therapy XII. Philadelphia, 1995, WB Saunders.

T A B L E 1 - 5 8 Sympathomimetic Drugs Used to Treat Cardiogenic Shock

Drug	Receptor activity	Dosage (IV)
Dopamine	DA_1, DA_2, α^{+++}, β^{+++}	5-25 µg/kg/minute (blood pressure support)* 1-5 µg/kg/minute (renal afferent diuresis)
Dobutamine	α^+, β^{+++}	3-20 µg/kg/minute* (blood pressure support, positive inotrope)
Norepinephrine	α^{+++}, β^+	0.05-0.3 mg/kg/minute; 0.01-0.02 mg/kg
Phenylephrine	α^{+++}, β^0	0.05-0.2 mg/kg
Epinephrine	α^{+++}, β^{+++}	0.02-0.5 mg/kg, 0.05-0.2 mg/kg/minute

+++, Strong receptor activity; *0*, no receptor activity; +, weak receptor activity.
*Monitor for tachyarrhythmias at higher doses.

2. Blood pressure

Maintenance of normotension is necessary for adequate oxygen delivery to meet cellular energy demands. Blood pressure can be measured using direct arterial catheterization, or through indirect means such as Doppler plesthymography or oscillometric methods. The systolic pressure should remain at or greater than 90-100 mm Hg at all times. The diastolic pressure is very important, too, as it constitutes two thirds of the mean arterial pressure; it must be greater than 40 mm Hg for coronary artery perfusion. The mean arterial pressure should be greater than 60 mm Hg for adequate tissue perfusion.

If fluid resuscitation and pain management are not adequate in restoring blood pressure to normal, vasoactive drugs including positive inotropes and pressors should be considered (Table 1-58).

In cases of cardiogenic shock, vasodilator drugs (Table 1-59) can be used to decrease vascular resistance and afterload. Low-dose morphine (0.05 mg/kg, IV, IM) dilates splanchnic vessels and helps reduce pulmonary edema. Furosemide (1 mg/kg/hour) also can dilate pulmonary vasculature and potentially reduce edema fluid formation in cases of ARDS.

3. Heart rate, rhythm, contractility, and pulse quality

Cardiac output is a function of both heart rate and stroke volume. Stroke volume or (the amount of blood that the ventricle pumps in 1 minute) is affected by preload, afterload, and contractility. During hypovolemic shock, there is a fall in cardiac preload due to a decrease in circulating blood volume. During septic and cardiogenic shock, there is a decrease in contractility secondary to inherent defects of the myocardium or due to the negative inotropic effects of inflammatory cytokines such as TNF-alpha, myocardial depressant factor, IL-1, and IL-10 released during sepsis and systemic inflammation. Afterload also may be increased because of the compensatory mechanisms and neuro-humoral activation of the renin-angiotensin-aldosterone axis in hypovolemic or cardiogenic shock. As heart rate increases to compensate for a decline in cardiac output, myocardial oxygen demand increases and diastolic filling time becomes shorter. Because the coronary arteries are perfused during diastole, coronary perfusion can be impaired, and myocardial lactic acidosis can develop, causing a further decline in contractility. In addition to lactic acidosis, acid-base and electrolyte abnormalities, inflammatory cytokines, direct bruising of the myocardium from trauma, and areas of ischemia can further predispose the patient to ventricular or atrial dysrhythmias.

Cardiac dysrhythmias should be controlled whenever possible. Treatment of bradycardia should be directed at treating the underlying cause. Administer anticholinergic drugs such as atropine (0.04 mg/kg IM) or glycopyrrolate (0.02 mg/kg IM) as necessary. In cases of third-degree or complete atrioventricular (AV) block, administer a pure beta-agonist such as isoproterenol (0.04-0.08 µg/kg/minute IV CRI, or 0.4 mg in 250 mL of 5% dextrose in water IV slowly). Perform passive rewarming if the patient is hypothermic.

TABLE 1-59 Drugs and Doses Used to Induce Vasodilatation

Drug	Mechanism of action	Dose and method of administration (onset, peak, duration)	Potential adverse effects
Captopril	Angiotensin-converting enzyme inhibitor	0.5-2 mg/kg PO tid	Azotemia
Enalapril	Angiotensin-II-converting enzyme inhibitor	0.25-0.5 mg/kg/PO q12-24h	Azotemia
Hydralazine	Direct arteriolar smooth muscle relaxant; little effect on venous capacitance vessels	0.2-0.5 mg/kg (10-20 minutes; 10-80 minutes, 2-8 hour)	Blood dyscrasias, neuritis with prolonged use
Lisinopril	Angiotensin-II-converting enzyme inhibitor		
Morphine	Splanchnic capacitance vessel dilatation	0.025-0.05 mg/kg IV, IM, SQ	Vomiting
Nitroglycerine paste	Venous and some arteriolar dilatation	¼ to ¾ inch topically on skin every 8 hours	Tolerance after 48 hours
Prazosin	α-Receptor blockade; arteriolar and venous dilatation	1-3 mg/kg PO bid	Anorexia, vomiting, diarrhea
Sodium nitroprusside	Direct arteriolar and venular dilatation	0.5-10 µg/kg/minute CRI; dilute in 5% dextrose in water Intravenous line with continuous blood pressure monitoring (immediately; 1 minute; 2 minutes)	Hypotension, tolerance, cyanide toxicity at higher doses, avoid in hepatic or renal failure; thiocyanate accumulation (disorientation); is light sensitive and must be covered in foil and not kept for longer than 4 hours

Correct any underlying electrolyte abnormalities such as hyperkalemia and hypo- and hypermagnesemia.

Treat ventricular dysrhythmias such as multifocal premature ventricular contractions (PVCs), sustained ventricular tachycardia >160 beats per minute, and R on T phenomenon (the T wave of the preceding beat occurs superimposed on the QRS complex of the next beat, and there is no return to isoelectric shelf), or if runs of ventricular tachycardia cause a drop in blood pressure. Intravenous lidocaine and procainamide are the first drugs of choice for ventricular dysrhythmias. Supraventricular tachycardia can impair cardiac output by impairing diastolic filling time. Control supraventricular dysrhythmias with calcium channel blockers, beta-adrenergic blockers, or quinidine (Table 1-60).

1

TABLE 1-60 Antiarrhythmic Drugs of Choice Used for the Treatment of Ventricular and Supraventricular Tachycardias

Drug	Mechanism of action	Dose
Lidocaine	Fast sodium channel inhibition	1-4 mg/kg IV slowly, then 50-100 µg/kg/minute (dog); 0.25-1.0 mg/kg IV (cat)*
Procainamide	Fast sodium channel inhibition	1-8 mg/kg IV,[†] then 20-40 µg/kg/minute; 6-20 mg/kg PO tid
Tocainide	Fast sodium channel inhibition	5-20 mg/kg PO Q8h[‡] (dog)
Quinidine	Fast sodium channel inhibition	6-10 mg/kg PO qid
Propranolol	β-Adrenergic blocker	0.02-0.06 mg/kg IV; 0.02-1.0 mg/kg PO
Esmolol	β-Adrenergic blocker	0.5 mg/kg IV, then 50-200 µg/kg/minute IV CRI
Verapamil	Slow calcium channel blocker	0.01-1 mg/kg IV; 5-10 mg/kg PO q8h
Diltiazem	Calcium channel blocker	0.25 mg/kg IV, 0.5-1.5 mg/kg PO q8h (dogs) 1.75-2.5 mg/kg PO q8h
Pimobendan	Phosphodiesterase inhibition Positive inotrope	0.1-0.3 mg/kg PO q12h

*Use caution with lidocaine in cats because of neurotoxicity and seizures.
† Monitor for hypotension.
‡Is not to be used for more than 2 weeks due to idiosyncratic blindness.

4. Albumin

Albumin can decrease as a result of loss from the gastrointestinal tract, urinary system, and wound exudates, or into body cavity effusions. Albumin synthesis can decrease during various forms of shock due to a preferential increase in hepatic acute phase protein synthesis. Serum albumin contributes 80% of the colloid oncotic pressure of blood, in addition to its important roles as a free radical scavenger at sites of inflammation and as a drug and hormone carrier. Albumin levels <2.0 g/dL have been associated with an increase in morbidity and mortality in human and veterinary patients. Administer fresh frozen plasma (20 mL/kg) or concentrated human albumin (2 mL/kg of 25% solution) to maintain serum albumin ≥2.0 g/dL. Additional oncotic support can be in the form of synthetic colloids, as indicated.

5. Oncotic pressure

Colloid oncotic pressure within the intravascular and interstitial spaces contributes to fluid flux. Oncotic pressure can be measured with a colloid osmometer. Normal oncotic pressure is 15 mm Hg. In cases of sepsis and SIRS, increased vascular permeability increases the tendency for leakage of fluids into the interstitial spaces. Colloids that can be administered until the source of albumin loss resolves include the synthetic colloids hetastarch and dextran 70 (20-30 mL/kg/day), synthetic hemoglobin-based oxygen carriers (oxyglobin, 3-7 mL/kg/day), concentrated human albumin (25% albumin, 2 mL/kg), and plasma (20 mL/kg).

6. Oxygenation and ventilation

Oxygenation and ventilation can be evaluated by arterial blood gas analysis or by the noninvasive means of pulse oximetry and capnometry (see sections on Pulse Oximetry and Capnometry). Oxygen delivery can be impaired in cases of hypovolemic shock because of hemorrhage and anemia, and thus a decrease in functional capacity to carry oxygen, and in cases of cardiogenic shock as a result of impaired ability to saturate hemoglobin due to pulmonary edema in the lungs, or decrease in cardiac output. In septic shock, decreases in cardiac output due to inflammatory cytokines and a decrease in cellular oxygen extraction can lead to lactic acidosis. Increased cellular metabolism and decreases in respiratory function can lead to respiratory acidosis as CO_2 increases.

Administer supplemental oxygen as flow-by, nasal or nasopharyngeal catheter, oxygen hood, or oxygen cage. Supplemental oxygen should be humidified, and delivered at 50-100 mL/kg/minute. If oxygenation and ventilation are so impaired that the PaO_2 remains <60 mm Hg with the patient on supplemental oxygen, a $PaCO_2$ >60 mm Hg, or severe respiratory fatigue, develops, and mechanical ventilation should be considered.

7. Glucose

Glucose is a necessary fuel source for red blood cells and neuronal tissues, and serum glucose should be maintained within normal reference ranges. Glucose supplementation can be administered as 2.5-5% solutions in crystalloid fluids, or in parenteral and enteral nutrition products.

8. Acid-base and electrolyte and lactate status

Arterial and venous pH can be measured by performing blood gas analyses. Decrease in tissue perfusion, impaired oxygen delivery, and decreased oxygen extraction in the various forms of shock can lead to anaerobic metabolism and metabolic acidosis. In most cases, improving tissue perfusion and oxygen delivery with crystalloid and colloid fluids, supplemental oxygen, and inotropic drugs will help normalize metabolic acidosis. Serial measurements of serum lactate (normal, <2.5 mmol/L) can be used as a guide to evaluate the tissue response to fluid resuscitative efforts.

Serum electrolytes often become severely deranged in shock states. Serum potassium, magnesium, sodium, chloride, and total and ionized calcium should be maintained within normal reference ranges.

If metabolic acidosis is severe, sodium bicarbonate can be administered by calculating the formula

$$\text{Base deficit} \times 0.3 \times \text{body weight in kg} = \text{mEq bicarbonate to administer}$$

Because iatrogenic metabolic alkalosis can occur, a conservative approach is to administer ¼ of the calculated dose and then recheck the patient's pH and bicarbonate levels. If the base excess is unknown, sodium bicarbonate can be administered in incremental doses of 1 mEq/kg until the pH is above 7.2. Complications associated with bicarbonate therapy include iatrogenic hypocalcemia, metabolic alkalosis, paradoxical cerebrospinal fluid acidosis, hypotension, restlessness, and death.

9. Coagulation

Massive trauma, neoplasia, sepsis, and systemic inflammation can all lead to coagulation abnormalities, including disseminated intravascular coagulation (DIC). Cage-side coagulation monitors are available for daily measurement of prothrombin time (PT), activated partial thromboplastin time (APTT), and platelet counts. Fibrin degradation products (fibrin split products) become elevated in DIC, trauma, hepatic disease, and surgery. Coagulation proteins (clotting factors) and antithrombin often are lost with other proteins in hypoproteinemia or are consumed when microclots are formed and then dissolved. Antithrombin levels can be measured by commercial laboratories. Antithrombin and clotting factors can be replenished in the form of fresh frozen plasma transfusions. A more sensitive and specific test for DIC is the detection of D-dimers, which can be measured by commercial laboratories.

Treatment for DIC involves treatment and resolution of the underlying disease and administration of antithrombin and clotting factors in the form of fresh frozen plasma (20 mL/kg) and heparin (unfractionated, 50-100 units/kg SQ tid; fractionated [Lovenox], 1 mg/kg SQ bid).

10. Mentation

Monitor the patient for changes in mental status, including stupor, coma, decreased ability to swallow and protect the airway, and seizures. Elevation of the patient's head can help to protect the airway and decrease the risk of increased intracranial pressure. Serum glucose should be maintained within normal levels to prevent hypoglycemia-induced seizures.

11. Red blood cell and hemoglobin concentration

One of the major components of oxygen delivery is the binding to hemoglobin. Packed cell volume must be kept above 20-30% for adequate cellular oxygen delivery. Acid-base status can adversely affect oxygen offloading at the tissue level if metabolic or respiratory alkalosis is present. Oxygen-carrying capacity and hemoglobin levels can be increased with administration of RBC component therapy or with hemoglobin-based oxygen carriers.

12. Renal function

Monitoring of renal function includes daily measurement of BUN, creatinine, and urine output. Normal urine output in a hydrated euvolemic patient is 1-2 mL/kg/hour. Fluid ins and outs should be measured in cases of suspected oliguria or anuria. In patients with oliguria or anuria, furosemide can be administered as a bolus (4-8 mg/kg) or by constant rate infusion (CRI)(0.66-1 mg/kg/hour). Mannitol should also be administered (0.5-1 g/kg over 10 to 15 minutes). Dopamine (1-5 µg/kg/minute CRI) can be administered to dilate renal afferent vessels and improve urine output.

13. White blood cell count, immune function, antibiotic dose and selection

The patient's white blood cell count may be elevated, normal, or decreased, depending on the type of shock. The decision to administer antibiotics should be made on a daily basis. Superficial or deep *Staphylococcus* or *Streptococcus* infection usually can be treated with a first-generation cephalosporin (cefazolin, 22 mg/kg IV tid). If a known source of infection is present, administer a broad-spectrum antibiotic (cefoxitin, 22 mg/kg IV tid; ampicillin, 22 mg/kg qid, or enrofloxacin, 5-10 mg/kg once daily) pending results of culture and susceptibility testing. If broader anaerobic coverage is required, metronidazole (10 mg/kg IV tid) should be considered. Gentamicin (3-5 mg/kg IV once daily) is a good choice for gram-negative sepsis, provided that the patient is well hydrated and has normal renal function. Ideally, patients receiving any aminoglycoside antibiotic should have a daily urinalysis to check for renal tubular casts that signify renal damage.

14. Gastrointestinal motility and integrity

In dogs, the gut is the shock organ. Impaired gastrointestinal motility and vomiting should aggressively be treated with antiemetics and promotility drugs (dolasetron, 0.6 mg/kg IV once daily, and metoclopramide, 1-2 mg/kg/day IV CRI). Metoclopramide is contraindicated in cases of suspected gastrointestinal obstruction. Histamine-receptor blockers such as famotidine (0.5 mg/kg bid IV) and ranitidine (0.5 to 2 mg/kg IV bid, tid) or proton-pump inhibitors (omeprazole, 0.5-1 mg/kg PO once daily) can be administered for esophagitis. Administer sucralfate (0.25-1 g PO tid) to treat gastric ulceration. If the gastrointestinal barrier function is diminished due to poor perfusion, infection, or inflammation, administer broad-spectrum antibiotics such as ampicillin (22 mg/kg IV qid) to prevent gastrointestinal bacterial translocation.

15. Drug doses and metabolism

The course of drug therapy should be reviewd daily and the patient should be monitored for potential drug interactions. For example, metoclopramide and dopamine, working at the same receptor, can effectively negate the effects of each other. Cimetidine, a cytochrome P450 enzyme inhibitor, can decrease the metabolism of some drugs. Drugs that are avidly protein-bound may have an increase in unbound fraction with concurrent hypoalbuminemia or when hypoalbuminemia is present. Decreased renal function may impair the renal clearance of some drugs, requiring increased dosing interval or decreased dose.

16. Nutrition

Nutrition is of utmost importance in any critically ill patient. Patients with septic shock may become hypermetabolic and require supraphysiologic nutrient caloric requirements, while others may actually become hypometabolic. Enteral nutrition is preferred, whenever possible, because enterocytes undergo atrophy without luminal nutrient stimulation. A variety of enteral feeding tubes can be placed, depending on what portion of the gut is functional, to provide enteral nutrition in an inappetent patient. Loss of gastrointestinal mucosal barrier function may predispose the patients to the development of bacterial translocation and may contribute to sepsis. If enteral nutrition is impossible because of protracted vomiting or gastrointestinal resection, glucose, lipid, and amino acid products are available that can be administered parenterally to meet nutrient needs until the gastrointestinal tract is functioning and the patient can be transitioned to enteral nutrition.

17. Analgesia and pain control

Assessment of pain in animals in shock can be challenging. Pain can result in the release of catecholamines and glucocounterregulatory hormones that can impair nutrient assimilation and lead to negative nitrogen balance, impaired wound healing, and immunocompromise. In any animal determined to be in pain, analgesic drugs should be administered to control pain and discomfort at all times. Opioids are cardiovascularly friendly, and their effects can easily be reversed with naloxone if adverse effects such as hypotension and hypoventilation occur.

18. Nursing care and patient mobilization

If the patient is nonambulatory, rotate the animal from side to side every 4 to 6 hours to prevent lung atelectasis. Passive range-of-motion exercises and deep muscle massage should be performed to increase tissue perfusion, decrease dependent edema, and prevent disuse atrophy. Animals should be kept completely dry on soft, padded bedding to prevent the development of decubital ulcers.

19. Wound care/bandage care

All bandages, wound sites, and catheter sites should be checked daily for the presence of swelling, erythema, and pain. Soiled bandages should be changed to prevent strike-through and contamination of the underlying catheter or wound.

20. TLC (tender loving care)

Hospitalization can be a stressful experience for patient and client alike. Allowing brief visits and walks outside in the fresh air can improve a patient's temperament and decrease stress. The preemptive use of analgesic drugs on a regular schedule (not PRN) should be used to prevent pain *before* it occurs. Pain decreases the patient's ability to sleep. Lack of sleep can promote further stress and impaired wound healing.

OTHER CONSIDERATIONS AND CONTROVERSIES IN SHOCK THERAPY

Glucocorticosteroids and antiprostaglandins

The use of glucocorticosteroids and antiprostaglandins in shock therapy remains a topic of wide controversy. Although the use of these agents potentially may stabilize membranes, decrease the absorption of endotoxin, and decrease prostaglandin release, the routine use of glucocorticosteroids and antiprostaglandins can decrease renal perfusion and gastrointestinal blood flow, promoting gastrointestinal ulceration and impaired renal function. The administration of supraphysiologic levels of glucocorticosteroids in patients in any type of shock can increase sodium and water retention, depress cellular immune function, and impair wound healing. In clinical studies of small animal patients, the routine use of glucocorticosteroids and antiprostaglandins has not demonstrated definite improved survival. The risks of therapy do outweigh the anecdotal reported benefits, and therefore the empiric use of glucocorticosteroids and antiprostaglandins in any shock patient is absolutely contraindicated. The administration of glucocorticosteroids to patients with cardiac disease has been shown to promote sodium and water retention and can actually predispose to the development of congestive heart failure.

Additional Reading

Brady CA, Otto CM: Systemic inflammatory response syndrome, sepsis, and multiple organ dysfunction. Vet Clin North Am Small Anim Pract 31(6):1147-1162, 2000.

Buston R: Treatment of congestive heart failure. J Small Anim Pract 44(11):516, 2003.

Chan DL, Rozanski EA, Freeman LM, Rush JE: Colloid osmotic pressure in health and disease. Compend Contin Educ Pract Vet 23(10):896-904, 2001.

Cote E: Cardiogenic shock and cardiac arrest. Vet Clin North Am Small Anim Pract 31(6): 1129-1145, 2001.

DeLaforcade AM, Freeman LM, Shaw SP, Brooks MB, et al: Hemostatic changes in dogs with naturally occurring sepsis. J Vet Intern Med 17(5):674-679, 2003.

Johnson V, Gaynor A, Chan DL, et al: Multiple organ dysfunction syndrome in humans and dogs. J Vet Emerg Crit Care 14(3):158-166, 2004.

Lagutchik MS, Ogilvie GK, Hackett TB, et al: Increased lactate concentrations in ill and injured dogs. J Vet Emerg Crit Care 8(2):117-127, 1998.

Mazzaferro EM, Rudloff E, Kirby R: The role of albumin in health and disease. J Vet Emerg Crit Care 12(2):113-124, 2002.

Moore KE, Murtaugh RJ: Pathophysiologic characteristics of hypovolemic shock. Vet Clin North Am Small Anim Pract 31(6):1115-1128, 2001.

Okano S, Yoshida M, Fukuahima U, et al: Usefulness of systemic inflammatory response syndrome criteria as an index for prognosis judgement. Vet Rec 150(8):245-246, 2002.

Otto CM: Sepsis. In Wingfield WE, Raffe M (eds): The Veterinary ICU Book. Teton New Media, Jackson,Wyo, 2001.

Rossmeisl JH: Current principles and application of D-dimer analysis in small animal practice. Vet Med 98(3):224-234, 2003.

Rozanski E, Rondeau M: Choosing fluids in traumatic hypovolemic shock: the role of crystalloids, colloids and hypertonic saline. J Am Anim Hosp Assoc 38(6):499-501, 2002.

Rudloff E, Kirby R: Colloid and crystalloid resuscitation. Vet Clin North Am Small Anim Pract 31(6):1207-1229, 2001.

THROMBOEMBOLISM: SYSTEMIC

Systemic thromboembolism is most commonly recognized in cats with cardiomyopathies (hypertrophic, restrictive, unclassified, and dilatative) but can also occur in dogs with hyperadrenocorticism, disseminated intravascular coagulation (DIC), systemic inflammatory response syndrome (SIRS), protein-losing enteropathy and nephropathy, and tumors affecting the aorta and vena cava. Thrombosis occurs through a complex series of mechanisms when the components of Virchow's triad (hypercoaguable state, sluggish blood flow, and vascular endothelial injury or damage) are present. In cats, blood flow through a severely stretched left atrium is a predisposing factor to the development of clots and thromboembolism.

The most common site of embolism is the aortic bifurcation, or "saddle thrombus." Other, less common locations of thromboembolism include the forelimbs, kidneys, gastrointestinal tract, and cerebrum. Diagnosis usually is made based on clinical signs of cool extremities, the presence of a cardiac murmur or gallop rhythm, auscultation of pulmonary crackles resulting from pulmonary edema, acute pain or paralysis of one or more peripheral extremities, respiratory distress, and pain and lack of a palpable pulse in affected limbs. The affected nailbeds and paw pads are cyanotic, and nails do not bleed when cut with a nail clipper.

Client education is one of the most important aspects of emergency management of the patient with thromboembolic disease. Concurrent congestive heart failure (CHF) occurs in 40% to 60% of cats with arterial thromboembolism. More than 70% of cats are euthanized during the initial thromboembolic event because of the poor long-term prognosis and the high risk of recurrence within days to months after the initial event, even with aggressive therapy. Although the long-term prognosis varies from 2 months to 2 years after initial diagnosis and treatment, in the majority of cats thromboembolic disease recurs within 9 months. Rectal temperature hypothermia and bradycardia on presentation are negative prognostic indicators.

Immediate treatment of a patient with CHF and thromboembolic disease involves management of the CHF with furosemide, oxygen, and vasodilators (nitroglycerine paste, morphine, nitroprusside). Additional management includes analgesia (butorphanol, 0.1-0.4 mg/kg IV, IM) and prevention of further clot formation. Aspirin (10 mg/kg PO q48h) is beneficial bcause of its antiplatelet effects. Heparin works in conjunction with antithrombin to prevent further clot formation (100-200 units/kg IV, followed by 250-300 units/kg SQ q8h in cats, and 100-200 units/kg SQ q8h in dogs). Acepromazine can cause peripheral vasodilation and decreased afterload but also can promote hypotension in a patient with concurrent CHF. Acepromazine (0.01-00.02 mg/kg SQ) should be used with extreme caution, if at all.

Thrombolytic therapy can also be attempted, but in most cases is not without risk, and may be cost-prohibitive for many clients. Streptokinase (90,000 units IV over 30 minutes and then 45,000 units/hour IV CRI for 3 hours) was administered with some success in cats; however, many died of hyperkalemia or other complications during the infusion. Tissue plasminogen activator (0.25-1 mg /kg/hour IV CRI, up to 10 mg/kg total dose, to effect) has been used with some success but is cost-prohibitive for most clients. Side effects of thrombolytic therapy include hyperkalemia with reperfusion and hemorrhage.

In cats, the primary cause of arterial thromboembolism is cardiomyopathy. Once an animal is determined to be stable enough for diagnostic procedures, lateral and DV thoracic radiographs and an echocardiogram should be performed. Ultrasound of the distal aorta and renal arteries should also be performed to determine the location of the clot and help establish the prognosis.

Other diagnostic procedures to evaluate the presence and cause of thromboembolism include a complete blood count, serum biochemistry profile, urinalysis (to rule out protein-losing nephropathy), urine protein:creatinine ratio, antithrombin levels, ACTH stimulation test (to rule out hyperadrenocorticism), heartworm antigen test (in dogs), thyroid profile (to rule out hyperthyroidism in cats, and hypothyroidism in dogs), thoracic radiographs, arterial blood gas analyses, coagulation tests, and Coombs' test. Selective and nonselective angiography can also be performed to determine the exact location of the thrombus.

Long-term management of thromboembolism involves management of the underlying disease process and preventing further clot formation. Begin therapy with heparin until the APTT becomes prolonged 1.5 times; then administer warfarin (0.06-0.09 mg/kg/day). Monitoring therapy based on prothrombin time and the international normalized ratio (INR, 2.0-4.0) is recommended. Low-dose aspirin (5-10 mg/kg q48h) also has been recommended. Physical therapy with warm water bathing, deep muscle massage, and passive range-of-motion exercises should be performed until the patient regains motor function. Future therapy may involve the use of platelet receptor antagonists to prevent platelet activation and adhesion.

Additional Reading

Good LI, Manning AM: Thromboembolic disease: predispositions and management. Comp Contin Educ Pract Vet 25(9):660-674, 2003.

Marks SL: Systemic arterial thromboembolism. In Wingfield WE (ed): Veterinary Emergency Medicine Secrets. Hanley and Belfus, Philadelphia, 2001.

Moore KE, Morris N, Dhupa N, et al: Retrospective study of streptokinase administration in 46 cats with arterial thromboembolism. J Vet Emerg Crit Care 10(4):245-257, 2000.

Schoeman JP: Feline distal aortic thromboembolism: a review of 44 cases (1990-1998). J Feline Med Surg 1:221-231, 1999.

Smith SA, Tobias AH: Feline arterial thromboembolism: an update. Vet Clin North Am Small Anim Pract 34(5):1245-1271, 2004.

Smith SA, Tobias AH, Jacob KA, et al: Arterial thromboembolism in cats: acute crises in 127 cases (1992-2001) and long-term management with low-dose aspirin in 24 cases. J Vet Intern Med 17(1):73-83, 2003.

1

URINARY TRACT EMERGENCIES

AZOTEMIA

Azotemia occurs when 75% or more of the nephrons are nonfunctional. The magnitude of the azotemia alone cannot be used to determine whether the azotemia is prerenal, renal, or postrenal in origin, or whether the disease process is acute or chronic, reversible or irreversible, progressive or nonprogressive. Before beginning treatment for azotemia, the location or cause of the azotemia must be identified. Take a thorough history and then perform a physical examination. Obtain blood and urine samples before initiating fluid therapy, for accurate assessment of the location of the azotemia.

For example, an azotemic animal with a history of vomiting and diarrhea that appears clinically dehydrated on physical examination, normally should have a concentrated urine specific gravity (>1.045) reflecting the attempt to conserve fluid. If this level is found, the azotemia is much less likely to be renal in origin, and the azotemia will likely resolve after rehydration.

If, however, the urine specific gravity is isosthenuric or hyposthenuric (1.007-1.015) in the presence of azotemia and dehydration, primary intrinsic renal insufficiency is likely present. If the azotemia resolves with fluid therapy, the patient has prerenal and primary renal disease. If the azotemia does not resolve after rehydration, the patient has prerenal and primary renal failure. Dogs with hypoadrenocorticism can have both prerenal and primary renal disease secondary to the lack of mineralocorticoid (aldosterone) influence on the renal collecting duct and renal interstitial medullary gradient. Medullary washout can occur, causing isosthenuric urine in the presence of dehydration from vomiting and diarrhea. The patient often has azotemia due to fluid loss (dehydration and urinary loss) and gastric or intestinal hemorrhage (elevated BUN). The prerenal component will resolve with treatment with glucocorticoids and crystalloid fluids, but the renal component may take several weeks to resolve, until the medullary concentration gradient is reestablished with the treatment and influence of mineralocorticoids. Drugs such as corticosteroids and diuretics can influence renal tubular uptake and excretion of fluid, and cause a prerenal azotemia and isosthenuric urine in the absence of primary renal disease.

Treatment of azotemia includes calculation of the patient's dehydration estimate and maintenance fluid volumes, and administering that volume over the course of 24 hours. Identify and treat underlying causes of prerenal azotemia (shock, vomiting, diarrhea). Monitor urine output closely. Once a patient is euvolemic, oliguria is defined as urine output <1-2 mL/kg/hour. Urine output should return to normal in patients with prerenal azotemia as rehydration occurs. If a patient remains oliguric after rehydration, consider the possibility of oliguric acute intrinsic renal failure, and administer additional fluid therapy based on the patient's urine output, body weight, central venous pressure, and response to other medical therapies.

PRERENAL AZOTEMIA

Prerenal azotemia is caused by conditions that decrease renal perfusion, including hypovolemic shock, severe dehydration, hypoadrenocorticism, congestive heart failure, cardiac tamponade, cardiac dysrhythmias, and hypotension. Once renal perfusion is restored, the kidneys can resume normal function. Glomerular filtration rate decreases when the mean arterial blood pressure falls to less than 80 mm Hg in a patient with normal renal autoregulation. Renal autoregulation can be impaired in some diseases. Passive reabsorption of urea from the renal tubules can occur during states of low tubular flow (dehydration, hypotension) even if glomerular filtration is not decreased. If renal hypoperfusion is not quickly restored, the condition can progress from prerenal disease to acute intrinsic renal failure. Prerenal and renal azotemia can coexist in animals with primary renal disease, as a result of vomiting and ongoing polyuria in the absence of any oral fluid intake. The treatment of prerenal azotemia consists of rehydration, antiemetic therapy, and treatment of the underlying cause of vomiting, diarrhea, or third spacing of fluids.

1

ACUTE INTRINSIC RENAL FAILURE

Acute intrinsic renal failure is characterized by an abrupt decline in renal function to the extent that azotemia and an inability to regulate solute and fluid balance. Patients with acute intrinsic renal failure may be oliguric or polyuric, depending on the cause and state of renal failure. In small animals, the most common causes of acute intrinsic renal failure are renal ischemia and toxins.

There are three phases of acute intrinsic renal failure: induction, maintenance, and recovery. During the induction phase, some insult (ischemia or toxin) to the kidneys occurs, leading to a defective concentrating mechanism, decreased renal clearance of nitrogenous waste (azotemia), and polyuria or oliguria. If treatment is initiated during the induction phase, progression to the maintenance phase potentially can be stopped. As the induction phase progresses, there is worsening of the urine-concentrating ability and azotemia. Renal tubular epithelial cells and renal tubular casts can be seen on examination of the urine sediment. Glucosuria may be present.

The maintenance phase of acute intrinsic renal failure occurs after a critical amount of irreversible nephron injury. Correction of the azotemia and removal of the cause of the problem do not result in return to normal function. In patients with oliguria, the extent of nephron damage is greater than that observed in patients with polyuria. The maintenance phase may last for several weeks to months. Recovery of renal function may or may not occur, depending on the extent of injury. The most serious complications (overhydration and hyperkalemia) are observed in patients with oliguria.

The recovery phase occurs with sufficient healing of damaged nephrons. Azotemia may resolve, but concentrating defects may remain. If the patient was oliguric in the maintenance phase, a marked diuresis develops during the recovery phase that may be accompanied by fluid and electrolyte losses. This phase may last for weeks to months.

Treatment of acute intrinsic renal failure consists of determining the cause and ruling out obstruction or uroabdomen whenever possible. A careful history can sometimes determine whether there has been exposure to nephrotoxic drugs, chemicals, or food items. If ingestion or exposure to a toxic drug, chemical, or food occurred recently (within 2 to 4 hours), induce emesis with apomorphine (0.04 mg/kg IV). Next, administer activated charcoal either orally or via stomach tube, to prevent further absorption of the toxin. Obtain blood and urine samples for toxicologic analysis (e.g., ethylene glycol) and to determine whether azotemia or abnormalities in the urine sediment exist. (See section on Ethylene Glycol, Grapes and Raisins, and Nonsteroidal Antiinflammatory Drugs). Obtain a complete blood count, biochemical profile, and urinalysis to determine the presence of signs of chronic renal failure, including polyuria, polydipsia, and nonregenerative anemia. Radiographs and abdominal ultrasound can help in determining the chronicity of renal failure. Normal renal size is 2.5-3.5 times the length of L2 in dogs and 2.4-3.0 times the length of L2 in cats. Monitor the patient's body weight at least twice a day to avoid overhydration.

Also monitor urine output; normal output is 1-2 mL/kg/hour. In cases of polyuric renal failure, massive fluid and electrolyte losses can occur. Place a urinary catheter for patient cleanliness and to facilitate urine quantitation. Measure fluid ins and outs (see section on Fluid Therapy). After the patient has been rehydrated, the amount of fluids administered should equal maintenance and insensible needs plus the volume of urine produced each day. If a urinary catheter cannot be placed or maintained, serial body weight measurements and central venous pressure should be used to monitor the patient's fluid balance and prevent overhydration.

If the patient is oliguric (urine output <1-2 mL/kg/hour), pharmacologic intervention is necessary to increase urine output. First, administer furosemide (2-4 mg/kg or 0.66 mg/kg/hour IV CRI). Repeat bolus doses of furosemide if there is no response to initial treatment. If necessary, administer low-dose dopamine (3-5 µg/kg/minute IV CRI) to increase renal afferent dilatation and renal perfusion. Dopamine and furosemide may be synergistic if administered together. If dopamine and furosemide therapy is ineffective, administer mannitol (0.25-0.5 g/kg IV) *once only*. If polyuria is present, management is simplified because of the decreased risk of overhydration. If oliguria cannot be reversed, monitor the central venous pessure, body weight, and respiratory rate and effort, auscultate for crackles, and examine the patient carefully for signs of chemosis and the presence of serous nasal discharge.

Correct hyperkalemia with sodium bicarbonate (0.25-1.0 mEq/kg IV) or with insulin (0.25 units/kg) plus dextrose (1 g/unit of insulin IV, followed by 2.5% dextrose IV CRI). Treat severe metabolic acidosis (pH <7.2 or HCO_3^- <12 mEq/L) with sodium bicarbonate. If anuria develops or oliguria is irreversible despite this therapy, begin peritoneal dialysis. Obtain a renal biopsy to establish a diagnosis and prognosis (See section on Renal Biopsy). Administer gastroprotectant drugs and antiemetics to control nausea and vomiting. If possible, avoid the use of nephrotoxic drugs and general anesthesia. Initiate nutritional support in the form of an enteral feeding tube or parenteral nutrition as early as possible.

Once the patient enters the recovery phase, diuresis may occur that can lead to dehydration and electrolyte imbalances (hyponatremia, hypokalemia). Dehydration and electrolyte imbalances can be treated with parenteral fluid and electrolyte supplementation.

POSTRENAL AZOTEMIA

Postrenal azotemia is primarily caused by urethral obstruction or leakage from the urinary tract into the abdomen (uroabdomen). Complete urinary tract obstruction and uroabdomen are both ultimately fatal within 3 to 5 days if left untreated. In dogs, the most common causes of urethral obstruction are urinary (urethral) calculi or tumors of the urinary bladder or urethra. In male cats, feline urologic syndrome (FUS) is the most common cause of urethral obstruction, although there has been an increased incidence of urethral calculi observed in recent years. A ruptured urinary bladder is the most common cause of uroabdomen and is usually secondary to blunt trauma.

URINARY TRACT OBSTRUCTION

Clinical signs of urinary tract obstruction include dysuria, hematuria, inability to urinate or initiate an adequate stream of urine, and a distended painful urinary bladder. Late in the course of obstructive disease, clinical signs referable to uremia and azotemia (vomiting, oral ulcers, hematemesis, dehydration, lethargy, and anorexia) occur.

The initial goal of treatment of urinary tract obstruction is to relieve the obstruction. In male dogs, a lubricated catheter can be inserted past the area of obstruction with the animal under heavy sedation or general anesthesia (see section on Urohydropulsion). Depending on the chronicity of the obstruction, serum electrolytes should be measured;an ECG should be obtained before administering any anesthetic drugs, because of the cardiotoxic effects of hyperkalemia (see section on Atrial Standstill). Correct fluid, electrolyte, and acid-base abnormalities. If a urinary catheter cannot be placed, perform cystocentesis only as a last resort, because of the risk of urinary bladder rupture.

Definitive treatment includes identification and treatment of the underlying cause (tumor versus urinary calculi). In most cases, surgical intervention is necessary. If an unresectable tumor is present, a low-profile permanent cystostomy tube can be placed, if the owner desires. Administration of piroxicam (Feldene, 0.3 mg/kg PO q24-48h) with or without chemotherapy may shrink the tumor mass and delay the progression of clinical signs.

FELINE LOWER URINARY TRACT DISEASE

A complete discussion of this disorder is beyond the scope of this text (See Additional Reading for other sources of information). Feline lower urinary tract disease can cause urethral obstruction, particularly in male cats. Clinical signs include stranguria, dribbling of small amounts of urine, lethargy, inappetence, and vomiting. Often, owners call with the primary complaint of constipation, because the cat is making frequent trips to the litterbox and straining. Cases with a duration of obstruction <36 hours are considered uncomplicated; those with a duration >36 hours are complicated.

Treatment of urethral obstruction includes stabilizing and normalizing the patient's electrolyte status, induction of sedation or general anesthesia, and relieving the obstruction.

Obtain blood samples for analysis of electrolyte abnormalities. Treat hyperkalemia ($K^+ > 6.0$ mEq/L) with sodium bicarbonate (0.25-1.0 mEq/kg IV), regular insulin (0.25 unit/kg IV) plus dextrose (1 g//unit of insulin IV), followed by 2.5% dextrose IV CRI to prevent hypoglycemia; or calcium gluconate (0.2 mL/kg 10% IV slowly). Administer non–potassium-containing intravenous fluids in 0.9% saline solution. Obtain an ECG to detect atrial standstill (see section on Atrial Standstill).

In some cases, a urethral plug is visible at the tip of the penis. The urethral plug can sometimes be manually extracted or massaged from the penis, and the obstruction temporarily relieved. In such cases, it is still necessary to pass a urethral catheter to flush sediment from the urethra and urinary bladder. Unless a patient is obtunded, administer an anesthetic such as ketamine, atropine, or propofol (4-7 mg/kg IV) with diazepam IV for patient comfort and muscle relaxation.

Once the patient is under anesthesia or heavily sedated, urinary catheterization should be performed. In some cases, it will be difficult to advance the catheter. Lubricate a closed-ended Tomcat catheter and pass the tip into the distal urethra. Fill a 12-mL syringe with sterile saline and sterile lubricant and connect the syringe to the hub of the catheter. Pulse the fluid into the catheter as you gently move the catheter tip back and forth against the urethral obstruction. When the catheter has been passed into the urinary bladder, obtain a urine sample for urinalysis. Drain the bladder and flush with sterile saline solution until the urine efflux appears clear. Remove the Tomcat catheter and insert a 3-5 Fr red rubber tube or Argyle infant feeding catheter into the urethra for urine collection and quantitation. Secure the urinary catheter to prepuce with a butterfly strip of 1-inch adhesive tape secured around the catheter and then sutured to either side of the prepuce. The catheter should be connected to a closed urinary collection system for cleanliness and to reduce the risk of ascending bacterial infection. An Elizabethan collar should be placed at all times to prevent the patient from damaging or removing the catheter.

When the urethral obstruction has been relieved and the catheter placed, continue intravenous fluid diuresis to alleviate postrenal azotemia. Monitor the urine for bacteria and other sediment. In some cases, postobstructive diuresis can be severe. Carefully monitor fluid ins and outs, along with body weight, to maintain adequate hydration and perfusion. Remove the urinary catheter can be removed after 24 to 48 hours. Palpate the bladder frequently to make sure that the patient is voiding normally and to detect the recurrence of obstruction.

In patients with severe penile or urethral trauma or edema, administer a short-acting steroid (dexamethasone sodium phosphate, 0.25 mg/kg IV, IM, SQ). At the time of initial diagnosis and again at the time of discharge, the clients need to be instructed about the long-term management of feline lower urinary tract disease at home, and informed of the risks and consequences of recurrence.

UROABDOMEN

Uroabdomen can occur from trauma or leakage from the kidneys, ureter, or urinary bladder. Clinical signs of uroabdomen (azotemia, uremia, hyperkalemia) can also occur secondary to third spacing of urine and leakage into muscular tissue from a ruptured urethra. In most cases, urinary bladder trauma and rupture are secondary to blunt trauma. Abdominocentesis should be performed in any animal with suspected blunt abdominal trauma, and any fluid obtained should be analyzed for creatinine or potassium and compared with the patient's serum levels. An abdominal effusion that has a low packed cell volume and a potassium or creatinine level greater than that of the patient's serum is consistent with the diagnosis of uroabdomen.

Uroabdomen is not a surgical emergency. However, medical management consists of placement of a temporary abdominal drainage catheter into the abdomen, to facilitate removal of urine from the peritoneal cavity. To place the catheter, position the patient in dorsal or lateral recumbency, shave the ventral abdomen, as for any exploratory laparotomy. Aseptically scrub the clipped area, and instill a local anesthestic (lidocaine, 1-2 mg/kg) caudal and to the right of the umbilicus, through the skin, subcutaneous tissues, and rectus

1

abdominis muscles, inserting the lidocaine as you pull the needle out, thus creating an anesthetized tunnel. Aseptically scrub the area again and drape with sterile field towels; then make a small stab incision through the skin. Bluntly dissect through the subcutaneous tissue to the level of the external rectus abdominis. Pick up the muscle with a thumb forceps, and make a small stab incision into the abdominal cavity. Cut multiple holes in the side of a 14-16 Fr red rubber tube or thoracic drainage catheter, using care not to make the cut wider than 50% of the circumference of the tube. Insert the catheter into the abdominal cavity in a dorsal caudal direction. Make sure that all incisions within the abdomen. Secure the tube by placing a pursestring suture around the tube entrance site in the abdominal musculature with absorbable suture material. Close the dead space in the subcutaneous tissues with absorbable suture. Close the skin around the tube with another purse-string suture secured using a finger-trap technique. Connect the tube to a closed urinary collection system and bandage the catheter to the abdomen. The tube can remain in place until the patient's cardiorespiratory status is stabilized enough to allow anesthesia and definitive repair of the urinary tract defect.

Additional Reading

Forrester SD, McMillan NS, Ward DL: Retrospective evaluation of acute renal failure in dogs. J Vet Intern Med 16:354, 2002.

Gannon KM, Moses L: Uroabdomen in dogs and cats. Comp Cont Educ Pract Vet 248: 604-612, 2002.

Geor RJ: Drug-induced nephrotoxicity: recognition and prevention. Comp Cont Educ Pract Vet 22(9):876-888, 2000.

Labato MA: Peritoneal dialysis in emergency and critical care. Clin Tech Small Anim Pract. 15:126-135. 2000

Langston CE: Acute renal failure caused by lily ingestion in six cats. J Am Vet Med Assoc 220(1):49-52, 2002.

Lees GE: Early diagnosis of renal disease and renal failure. Vet Clin North Amer Sm Anim 34:867-885, 2004.

Mazzaferro EM, Eubig PE, Hackett TB, et al: Acute renal failure in four dogs after raisin or grape ingestion (1999-2002). J Vet Emerg Crit Care 14(3):203-212, 2004.

Osborne CA, Kruger JM, Lulich JP, et al: Disorders of the feline lower urinary tract. In Osborne CA, Finco DR, editors: Canine and feline nephrology and urology, Baltimore, 1995,Williams and Wilkins.

Rieser TM: Urinary tract emergencies. Vet Clin North Am Small Anim Pract 35:359-373, 2005.

Salinardi BJ, Marks SL, Davidson JR, Senior DF: The use of a low-profile cystostomy tube to relieve urethral obstruction in a dog. J Am Anim Hosp Assoc 39(4):403-405, 2003.

Stokes JE, Forrester SD: New and unusual cases of acute renal failure in dogs and cats. Vet Clin North Am Small Anim Pract 34:909-922, 2004.

Vaden SL: Renal biopsy: methods and interpretation. Vet Clin North Am Small Anim Pract 34:887-908, 2004.

Westropp JL, Buffington CAT: Feline idiopathic cystitis: current understanding of pathophysiology and management. Vet Clin North Am Small Anim Pract 34:1043-1055, 2004.

Patient Evaluation and Organ System Examination

Patient Evaluation, *293*
    The "BEETTS" Test: Owner Assessment of Pet Health, *293*
The Medical Record, *301*
    Medical Record Content, *302*
The Organ System Examination, *304*
    The Alimentary Tract, *304*
    Cardiopulmonary Examination, *315*
    Integument (Skin, Hair Coat, and Toenails), *332*
    Ophthalmic (Ocular) Examination, *341*
    Otic (Ear) Examination, *347*
    Lymph Nodes and Thyroid Examination, *350*
    Musculoskeletal (Orthopedic) Examination, *351*
    Nervous System Examination, *356*
    Reproductive Tract Examination: Male, *373*
    Reproductive Tract Examination: Female, *374*
    Respiratory Tract Examination: Upper, *376*
    Respiratory Tract Examination: Lower, *377*
    Normal Breeding Behavior and Physiology, *382*
    Urinary Tract Examination, *384*

PATIENT EVALUATION

THE "BEETTS" TEST: OWNER ASSESSMENT OF PET HEALTH

Most pet owners, particularly first-time owners, have little or no understanding of animal anatomy or physiology. It's not surprising, therefore, that the majority of pet owners are not well prepared to even *recognize* early signs of illness in a pet dog or cat. Therefore, many common medical disorders either are not recognized by owners at all (e.g., accumulation of dental tartar and gingival erosion) or are delayed until the pet has advanced illness (e.g., increased water consumption associated with renal failure).

    Ironically, few veterinary practices take time to teach owners how to recognize potentially significant health problems in a pet dog or cat. Simply educating owners about how to perform a routine, simple examination on their own pet not only encourages early awareness of potential health problems but also supports earlier intervention by a veterinarian.

A simple-to-remember, owner-prescribed examination is the "BEETTS" (pronounced: BEETS) test. This acronym represents a means for willing owners to assess significant changes in a pet's activity or physical appearance that will alert them to common minor problems as well as more serious health problems, thereby avoiding the consequences of delayed diagnosis and treatment.

Note: The majority of pet owners are not well prepared to even **recognize** early signs of illness in a pet dog or cat. Ironically, few veterinary practices take time to teach owners how to recognize potentially significant health problems.

B for Behavior

Know your pet!
Owners should be taught that subtle changes in behavior may be the first sign of underlying illness. Several such behavior changes—such as reduced or no appetite and associated weight loss, increased demand for water, frequent need to urinate or defecate, unexplained aggression, reluctance to play, difficulty standing, or persistent licking of skin (particularly in one location)— justify a physical examination and laboratory profile.

E for Eyes

Asymmetry of the eyes and eyelids (denoting pain or injury) is as important as discoloration of the eye (cataracts, intraocular hemorrhage) or the accumulation of mucous. Some owners allow hair to completely cover a pet's eyes, suggesting the need to encourage even a cursory look at the eyes.

E for Ears

Owners are advised about signs that might indicate an ear infection (e.g., head tilt or scratching, pain on manipulating the ears, ear abrasions, malodor) and are told to at least look at the inside on the pinnae for evidence of discharge or accumulation of excess hair. Owners are told to avoid inserting any instrument or medication into a pet's ears unless specifically instructed to do so.

T for Teeth (and Gingiva)

The relationship between halitosis and serious dental/gingival disease is important and can easily be missed if the teeth are not examined on a regular basis. Owners are encouraged to lift the lip and visually examine the teeth for evidence of damaged or discolored teeth. While most pet owners are comfortable opening their dog's mouth, it is not necessary to do so during a home dental examination. It is sufficient for the owner to assess the appearance of the labial surfaces of the teeth and gingiva once or twice annually.

T for Toes (and Toenails)

Most owners are not aware of when or how to examine a pet's toenails. While cats nails shed periodically and usually do not require clipping, the toenails of sedentary dogs living predominantly indoors deserve attention as often as monthly. Owners are instructed to listen to their dog walk across a noncarpeted surface. If the owner can hear toenails clicking against the floor as the pet walks, clipping is indicated. While some owners are interested in clipping their pet's toenail and will accept instructions, most are not willing to accept this potentially challenging procedure.

S for Skin (and Hair Coat)

Variability in hair coat type, length, and density makes examining the skin one of the home examinations that pet owners least often accomplish. However, examining the skin is one of the most important home examinations. The skin is the largest organ of the body, and serious disorders may develop many weeks or months before they become evident by observing the dog. This is particularly true in long-haired pets. In addition to routine brushing, which benefits *all* dogs and cats, and the occasional bath, owners are instructed to thoroughly touch their pet's skin and hair coat in a systematic manner. One technique owners find appealing begins with the owner standing behind the pet. Starting at the pet's head with one hand around each ear, the owner uses his or her fingers to "crawl" from the head to the tail while gently massaging the pet and touching the entire surface of the skin over the thorax and abdomen. Then, gently grasping one leg at a time with one hand, the owner massages each limb from the point closest to the body to the toes. Quite likely, the pet will enjoy this as much as the owner!

CLINICIAN ASSESSMENT: THE "PROBLEM LIST"

A correct diagnosis is based on the clinician's ability to assess and define constituent problems affecting the patient. Sounds simple enough. However, unless the term "problem" is defined, actually doing a thorough diagnostic assessment of the patient is simply not possible. When pursuing a diagnosis, the astute clinician works from a clear definition of a "problem":

1. The **clinical history**: Any abnormality described by the owner (whether or not the owner's interpretation is correct) is a problem.
2. The **physical examination**: Any abnormality discovered during the physical examination is a problem.
3. Any **imaging** (radiographic/ultrasound) or **laboratory** abnormalities are considered to be problems.

The **problem list**, once acquired, becomes the foundation on which a diagnosis is built. Problems that are obviously related are grouped and may either confirm the diagnosis or determine which additional diagnostic studies need to be performed to elucidate the diagnosis.

THE CLINICAL HISTORY

The **clinical history** is a fundamental component of the patient's problem list and frequently is the single most revealing part of the diagnostic assessment of a given patient. It requires unique skills and experience to elicit an unbiased, pertinent clinical history about a pet's illness. Some owners are astute observers and can readily communicate important information, whereas others either may not be aware of certain abnormalities or may purposely withhold information. The clinical history is centered around, but not limited to, the chief complaint. The **chief complaint** is the reason the patient is being presented. What should be recorded is a sign (vomiting), not a diagnosis (enteritis), because what the owner interprets as a sign (vomiting, for example) may actually be expectoration associated with tracheitis. Note the duration or frequency the sign. Determine whether the duration/frequency has increased, decreased, or remained unchanged since onset. It is important to determine whether or not the pet's overall condition since the onset of illness has improved, worsened, or remained the same.

When obtaining the history, ask neutral questions—ones that will not prejudice the owner's answers—such as "Tell me about your dog's water consumption." Direct or leading questions can be asked, provided that one realizes that such questions may introduce bias. Comments such as "Anything else?" "How do you mean?" or "Tell me about that" are helpful in inducing the owner to elaborate. Given the widespread usage of health care medications in pets (e.g., heartworm, flea, tick preventative), a complete list of drugs/medications is a critical part of the clinical history. If the same sequence of history taking and physical examination is followed each time, the procedure gradually requires less time and important facts are less likely to be omitted.

The clinical history is not inherently distinct from the physical examination. It is not uncommon for the client to be completely unaware that a physical abnormality is present until it is pointed out. When examining the patient, any unusual or unexpected physical findings justify additional inquiry as to causal relationships with the pet's environment, diet, exposure to other animals, and so forth. For example, discovering severe abrasions on the footpads of both rear feet should prompt additional inquiry into possible causes.

> **Note:** Failing to obtain a thorough clinical history is the first step in a missed diagnosis!

The Physical Examination

The **physical examination** is the means whereby the clinician evaluates the health status of the patient through a methodical, "hands-on" organ system evaluation. It is a critical step in problem definition and objective diagnostic assessment of the patient. The physical examination is predicated on the clinician's ability to distinguish normal from abnormal.

The extent of examination carried out on the individual patient varies. The "well patient" physical examination is characteristically employed when evaluating healthy animals presented for routine health care (i.e., there is *no* chief complaint). The basic elements to be included in the well patient examination are explained next.

Vital signs

Temperature, pulse, respiration, and weight are the most fundamental health parameters evaluated when examining the patient. Capillary refill time (CRT) is commonly recorded (normal: ≤ 2 seconds) but is a relatively poor test of peripheral vascular perfusion. Blood pressure (see Section 4) is more sensitive, but requires some operator experience to obtain reliable reading and multiple measurements in the individual patient to obtain a reasonable value. While not strictly a "vital" sign, all patients should be weighed at *every* visit.

Behavior and mentation

Observing the patient's behavior, activity, and alertness in the examination room can be particularly helpful in assessing patients with significant neurologic (brain) disease. Even animals that are nervous or scared in the hospital can be assessed and should manifest reasonable awareness of their surroundings. Dogs and cats that are particularly aggressive need to be handled with extreme care, yet evaluated for possible organic brain or neurologic disease.

Conformation and body condition score

Several methods exist for documenting conformation and body condition in dogs and cats. One commonly applied scale entails use of a 5-point grading system. Making appropriate entries in the medical record allows the clinician to assess, over time, changes in conformation other that just weight. Parameters for the 5-point grading scale are listed as follows:

Grade 1/5 emaciated

Ribs, backbone, and pelvic bones easily seen, even from a distance
No body fat
Obvious loss of muscle mass
   See Figure 2-1.

Grade 2/5: underweight

- Ribs can be seen and easily felt
- Pelvic bones are prominent
- Obvious waist and abdominal tuck

Grade 3/5: ideal body score

- Ribs can be felt
- Waist obvious when viewed from above
- Abdominal tuck evident

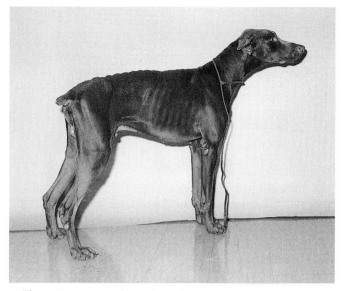

Figure 2-1: Dog with a body condition score (BCS) of 1 out of 5.

Grade 4/5: overweight
- Ribs hard to feel, covered by fat
- Noticeable fat deposits over back and base of tail
- Waist and abdominal tuck barely discernible

Grade 5/5: obese
- Ribs cannot be felt under heavy fat covering
- Massive fat deposits over back and base of tail
- No waist or abdominal tuck
  See Figure 2-2.

The 9-point body condition score (BCS)

An alternative 9-point body condition score for cats and dogs has also been described. In this scoring format, a BCS of 4 to 5 represents the ideal weight and conformation. A BCS of less than 4 represents underfed, underweight dogs and cats, while a BCS of 6 to 7 and higher represents overfed, overweight animals.

General appearance

Note body condition and conformation, state of nutrition, apparent age (compared to that reported), degree of grooming care, type of disposition, mental alertness, gross deformities, and striking findings (e.g., dyspnea, weakness, and lethargy).

Skin

Inspect and palpate. Note the color, texture, degree of moisture or oil present; amount, texture and distribution of hair, symmetry of hair coat, ease of epilation; presence of parasites; and types and distribution of primary and secondary skin lesions. Palpate all superficial nodes and the spleen. Note enlargement, consistency, mobility, and pain.

Eyes

Evaluate the symmetry of the eyes and eyelids. Examine the conjunctiva and sclera for injection, exudation, and petechiae. Assess the clarity of the cornea and adequacy of

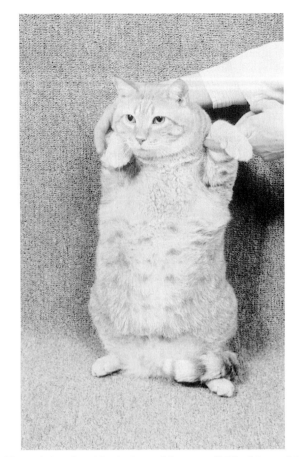

Figure 2-2:   Cat with a body condition score (BCS) of 5 out of 5.

tear production. Elicit the pupillary reflex. Perform an ophthalmoscopic examination (cornea, iris, lens, and retina).

Ears

Look for discharge and perform an otoscopic examination for exudates or parasites. Note the appearance of the tympanic membranes if practical.

Nares/nasal cavity

Look for symmetry, evidence of discharge, erosions of the nasal planum, and patency of nostrils.

Oral cavity

Note any evidence of halitosis (usually not hard to find!); assess the gingiva and tongue for evidence of injury, infection, ulceration, or bleeding; assess the teeth for symmetry, fractures, abnormal accumulations of plaque/calculus, and tooth loss; note any discharges or excess saliva; and observe the color and appearance of mucous membranes, the pharynx, and the tonsils.

Neck and back

Assess the extent of rigidity or range of motion, deformities, and pain (usually characterized by altered posture, such as neck "guarding.")

Respiratory

Evaluate larynx (externally), cervical trachea, and thorax for conformation, abnormal sounds, and respiratory effort. Auscultate the thorax systematically from the dorsal to the ventral aspects and compare left side to right side. Remember, the most clinically important lung sounds are lung sounds that are difficult to hear.

Heart

Auscultate the heart, noting the intensity of apex beat and the presence of thrills. Evaluate rate, rhythm, quality of sounds, bruit (pronounced: "brew-y," which is any abnormal sound, including murmurs), or rubs. Record the heart rate and assess the femoral pulse rate for evidence of pulse deficits. Auscultate the heart from the left and right sides of the thorax.

Abdomen

Assess abdominal symmetry. Auscultate the abdomen for evidence of excessive bowel sounds. Palpate the abdomen, preferably with the patient positioned in right lateral recumbency (Figure 2-3). Evaluate for the presence of masses, peritoneal fluid, rigidity, or unusual pain.

Genitalia, male

Palpate and inspect the scrotum, testes (if present), and penis; inspect the prepuce for abnormal discharges. In older adult males, digital examination of the prostate (per rectum) for symmetry and sensitivity is indicated. (Prostate examination is not routinely performed on healthy young dogs and small breeds).

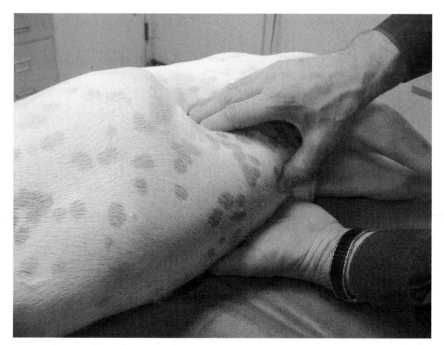

Figure 2-3: Recommended position and technique for abdominal palpitation.

2

TABLE 2-1   Components of the Minimum Laboratory Database (MDB) for Dogs and Cats

	Canine	Feline
Hematology	Complete blood count (CBC) includes the following: - Total RBC count - Hematocrit or packed cell volume - Hemoglobin - Total WBC count - Differential cell count - Total solids - Estimation of platelet numbers - Reticulocyte count *if patient's hematocrit is low (e.g., < 30%)* NOTE: Some laboratories will also provide values for the red blood cell indices: MCV, MCH, and MCHC.	Complete blood count (CBC) includes the following: - Total RBC count - Hematocrit or packed cell volume - Hemoglobin - Total WBC count - Differential cell count - Total solids - Estimation of platelet numbers - *Aggregate* reticulocyte count *if patient's hematocrit is low (e.g., < 30%)* NOTE: Some laboratories will also provide values for the red blood cell indices: MCV, MCH, and MCHC.
Biochemistry	Individual analytes included on biochemistry panels will vary among laboratories. (See Section 5 for a comprehensive review of the various analytes that are likely to be included.)	Individual analytes included on biochemistry panels will vary among laboratories. (See Section 5 for a comprehensive review of the various analytes that are likely to be included.)
Urinalysis	Includes the following: - Specific gravity, color, and appearance - Biochemistry usually includes protein, glucose, ketones, blood (hemoglobin), and urobilinogen - Microscopic includes a description of cell types and number as well as presence of crystals, casts, bacteria, fat	Includes the following: - Specific gravity, color, and appearance - Biochemistry usually includes protein, glucose, ketones, blood (hemoglobin), and urobilinogen - Microscopic includes a description of cell types and number as well as presence of crystals, casts, bacteria, fat, etc.
Parasites	- Fecal flotation for intestinal parasites - Heartworm antigen test	- Fecal flotation for intestinal parasites
Other		Feline leukemia (antigen) test and feline immunodeficiency (antibody) test

Genitalia, female

Assess the mammary glands for symmetry; palpate each gland/nipple for evidence of lactation and tumor; evaluate the perineum for symmetry, ulceration, presence of urine contamination (incontinence), and infection; the vulva should be symmetric, free of discharge, and not painful to the touch.

Anal sacs and anus

Assess the perineum and perianal skin for symmetry, ulceration, and pain. There is no indication to express fluid from the anal sacs in a normal dog or cat. In the healthy dog and cat, a digital rectal examination is not routinely done.

Extremities

Watch the animal walk to assess gait, symmetry, and evidence of lameness. Examine and palpate the legs and joints. Note the presence of pain, heat, swelling, deformities, or limitations to range of motion.

Nervous system

Watch the animal walk. Evaluate hearing and sight. If practical, place in lateral recumbency and observe standing/posture. Palpate muscles and compare tonus and balance with opposite numbers. Evaluate response to tendon reflexes and sensory responses.

2

Note: A more comprehensive organ system examination is indicated when (1) a "well patient" examination reveals an abnormality or evidence of an underlying problem or (2) the owner presents the patient for evaluation of one or more concerning problems, (i.e., the CHIEF COMPLAINT).

THE LABORATORY DATABASE

Clinical evaluation of the sick patient entails obtaining a laboratory profile to assess and characterize biochemical and hematologic abnormalities. Laboratory test abnormalities are a critical component of the diagnostic evaluation and are necessarily included, individually, on the patient's problem list. In companion animal practice, performing a laboratory profile meets the standard of care accepted in veterinary medicine. While the specific test methods used and analytes assayed will vary from practice to practice, the laboratory database on any ill dog or cat should include most or all of the tests listed in Table 2-1.

The availability of numerous supplemental laboratory tests (see Section 5) dictates careful assessment of the initial laboratory database described. The decision to perform additional or specialized laboratory tests is based on the clinician's interpretation of initial test results and physical examination findings.

IMAGING AND SPECIAL DIAGNOSTICS

The results of any abnormal findings observed with conventional radiography, ultrasound examination, echocardiography, or as a result of performing special diagnostic procedures are defined and included individually on the patient's problem list. Routine, special, and invasive diagnostic procedures are described in Section 4.

THE MEDICAL RECORD

Documenting health care delivery and administration of medical procedures is said to date as far back as ancient Egypt when early physicians recognized a need to record (on papyrus) details of surgery and prescriptions. Since that time, those involved in healing or treatment have acknowledged the importance of documenting health care and communicating details of successful procedures or potions either by written methods or through an oral tradition.

In 1969, Dr. Lawrence Weed introduced the problem oriented medical record (POMR) into human medicine. This defined format for clinical recording consists of a **problem list**, **a database** (i.e., results of the history, physical examination, and laboratory findings), and then, written out separately for each problem, **a plan** (diagnostic, therapeutic, and educational), and a daily **SOAP** (subjective, objective, assessment, and plan) entered into the medical record as a progress note. The "Master" problem list was kept at the front of the medical record and served as an index for the reader so that each problem could be followed through until it was resolved. This system widely influenced note keeping by recognizing four distinct phases of the clinical decision-making process: collecting data, formulating problems (not necessarily diagnoses), devising a management plan, then reviewing the situation and revising the plan if necessary.

> **Note:**   There is broad agreement today that the primary purpose of the medical record is to benefit the patient by documenting the standard of care provided at the time of need **and** to support the provision of health care by the same or another clinician in the future.

2

In human medicine, however, the POMR was not widely adopted exactly as Weed proposed because it proved to be too time consuming. In veterinary medicine, a modified version of Weed's POMR is commonly taught in veterinary schools and is widely used in clinical practice. Unfortunately, despite the availability of published guidelines, there are no generally ascribed to standards for either making medical record entries or for maintaining individual patient records in veterinary medicine. This fact becomes most apparent when veterinary medical records are subpoenaed and become the subject of legal scrutiny.

There is broad agreement today that the **primary purpose** of the medical record is to benefit the patient by documenting the standard of care provided at the time of need *and* to support the provision of health care by the same or another clinician in the future. The **secondary purpose** of the record is to provide a medicolegal record of the care provided should there be any reason to investigate the competence of the clinicians providing care. Hence the secondary purpose of the medical record is to demonstrate the competence of the clinicians. The medical record must be respected as a legitimate, legal document and must not jeopardize the primary and secondary purposes.

Thus, a health care record can operate in the interests of a number of people and has a potentially wide audience. It is a key element in individual care, acute and preventative care, supporting and authorizing clinical care, and decision support. It provides the basis for liability in case of negligence and is a source of health care statistics.

MEDICAL RECORD CONTENT

Legal standards outlining the content of veterinary medical records have not been established in the United States. However, the clinician and technical support staff should consider the following information as reasonable content to include in the patient's medical record:

IN-PATIENT MEDICAL RECORD

1. Patient identification data, including patient's name, date of birth, breed, gender, current owner's address, and medical record identifier/number
2. Admission and discharge date (and time)
3. Existing diagnosis(es) and date
4. Medical history, to include the following:
   - Chief complaint (reason for presentation)
   - Details of present illness and current medications
   - Relevant past, social, and family histories
   - Summary of relevant past examinations
5. Statement on the conclusions or impressions drawn from the admission history and physical examination
6. Statement on the course of action planned for this episode of care and its periodic review, as appropriate
7. Diagnostic tests ordered/recommended and therapeutic orders
8. Evidence of appropriate informed consent, as appropriate

9. Clinical observations and progress notes, including the results of therapy and the patient's response to treatment
10. Information on every medication ordered or prescribed and administered, to include dosage and any adverse drug reaction
11. Reports of all operative and other invasive procedures performed
12. Reports of any diagnostic and therapeutic procedures and test results
13. Final diagnosis(es)
14. Recommended: Conclusions at termination of hospitalization to include a discharge summary, condition at discharge, disposition of care, and provisions for follow-up care
15. If applicable, cause of death and necropsy results

Out-Patient Medical Record

1. Patient identification data, including patient's name, date of birth, breed, gender, current owner's address, and medical record identifier/number
2. Admission and discharge date and time
3. Relevant history of the illness or injury and physical findings
4. Diagnostic and therapeutic orders
5. Clinical observations, including results of treatment
6. Evidence of appropriate informed consent, as appropriate
7. Report of procedures, tests, and results
8. Diagnostic impressions
9. Patient disposition and pertinent instructions given to owner for follow-up care
10. Immunization record

Note: In human medicine, a list of significant medical diagnoses and conditions, known operative and invasive procedures, known adverse and allergic drug reactions, and medications known to be prescribed for or used by the patient must be started not later than the third outpatient visit.

Emergency Patient Medical Record

1. Patient identification data, including patient's name, date of birth, breed, gender, current owner's address, and medical record identifier/number
2. Admission and discharge date and time
3. Emergency care provided to the patient by the owner or other veterinarian before arrival, if any
4. History of disease or injury
5. Physical findings
6. Results of diagnostic tests, if applicable
7. Diagnosis(es)
8. Record of treatment
9. Conclusions at the termination of treatment are documented, to include the following:
   • Final disposition
   • Condition at discharge
   • Instructions for follow-up care
10. Notation when owner refused medical care
11. Patient transfer information provided to other facilities (e.g., an after-hours emergency practice), when applicable, to include the following:
    • Reason for transfer
    • Stability of patient
    • Acceptance by the receiving organization and location (address)
    • Responsibility during transfer
    • Documentation that relevant patient information accompanied the patient

THE ORGAN SYSTEM EXAMINATION

Note: In a given patient, presented for a defined (or "chief") complaint, it is appropriate to pursue a more comprehensive examination of the organ system(s) believed to be involved. The sections that follow address indications, options, and techniques for performing such examinations on the individual patient. The organ system examinations outlined here are merely intended to serve as a guide for evaluating the ill patient. The challenge for the clinician is not limited to the examination technique but entails determining *which* organ systems should become the subject of a more comprehensive examination. Referral of the patient to a specialty practice or teaching hospital is indicated when results of the organ system examination are not diagnostic.

2

THE ALIMENTARY TRACT

THE DENTAL EXAMINATION

Before examining specific areas of the alimentary system, carefully observe the general physical status of the animal, particularly noting any evidence of emaciation, abdominal enlargement or asymmetry, the position of the animal at rest, and body carriage while moving (tucked up abdomen, stiffness, etc.).

In most animals, a routine examination of the mouth can be done without anesthesia or tranquilization. Gently retract the lips, and examine the teeth and gingiva. When examining the teeth and gingiva of a cat or a puppy, using a cotton-tipped applicator to lift the lips and even open the mouth is particularly effective.

Normal dentition: canine

Formula for deciduous teeth: 2 (Di3/3 Dc1/1 Dm3/3) = 28 (total)

Formula for permanent teeth: 2 (I3/3 C1/1 P4/4 M2/3) = 42 (total)

Canine eruption dates (shown in Table 2-2)
In dogs, deciduous teeth should be in place by 7 to 8 weeks. Permanent teeth begin to replace the deciduous teeth by about 4 months of age. All permanent teeth should be in place at about 7 months. In some breeds, all the permanent teeth may not erupted until about 1 year of age.

T A B L E 2 - 2 Eruption Dates of Deciduous and Permanent Teeth—Canine

Teeth	Age at eruption	
	Deciduous (wk)	Permanent (mo)
Incisor 1	4–5	4–5
Incisor 2	4–5	4–5
Incisor 3	5–6	4–5
Canine	3–4	5–6
Premolar 1	–	4–5
Premolar 2	–	5–6
Premolar 3	–	5–6
Premolar 4	–	5–6
Molar 1	4–6	4–5
Molar 2	4–6	5–6
Molar 3	6–8	6–7

Normal dentition: feline

> Formula for deciduous teeth: 2 (Di3/3 Dc1/1 Dm3/2) = 26 (total)

> Formula for permanent teeth: 2 (I3/3 C1/1 PM3/2 M1/1) = 30 (total)

Feline eruption dates (shown in Table 2-3)

Examine individual teeth for caries, faulty enamel, exposure of roots, deposition of calculus and plaque, and periodontitis, as well as loose, crooked, or sharp-edged (fractured) teeth. Determine the apposition of the maxilla and mandible for prognathism (undershot jaw) or brachygnathism (overshot jaw). Several systemic abnormalities, including infectious disease, renal failure, hypoadrenocorticism, diabetes mellitus, and hypoparathyroidism, can produce oral pathology.

Dental terminology and anatomy (see Figure 2-4)

Crown. Portion above the gum line and covered by enamel.

Neck. Construction of the tooth located at the gum line where the enamel ends and the dentin covered by cementum begins.

Root. Portion below the gum line and covered by cementum.

Furcation. Visible space between roots of a multirooted tooth representing advanced dental disease.

Apex. Most terminal portion of the root.

Apical delta. Numerous small openings found at the apex allowing the nerves and vessels of the tooth to enter.

Enamel. Outer covering of the crown; very shiny, hard substance. It is the hardest substance in the body and is made up of less than 5% of organic material.

Dentin. Dense, bonelike material underlying the enamel and making up the substance of the tooth. It can be sensitive to heat and cold and is made up of 26% to 28% of organic material. It continues to be formed in the healthy tooth by odontoblasts, cells that line the pulp chamber.

Cementum. Layer of bony tissue that covers the root of the tooth and is attached to the alveolar bone by the periodontal ligament fibers.

Pulp. The soft tissues of the tooth: the nerves, which contain sensory fibers only, and the vessels coming in through the apical delta extending through the length of the tooth in the root canals.

TABLE 2-3 Eruption Dates of Deciduous and Permanent Teeth—Feline

Teeth	Age at eruption	
	Deciduous (wk)	Permanent (mo)
Incisor 1	2–3	3½–4
Incisor 2	2–4	3½–4
Incisor 3	3–4	4–4½
Canine	–	5
Premolar 1	–	–
Premolar 2	–	4½–5*
Premolar 3	–	5–6
Premolar 4	–	5–6
Molar 1	–	4–5
Molar 2	4–5*	–
Molar 3	4–6	–

*Upper only

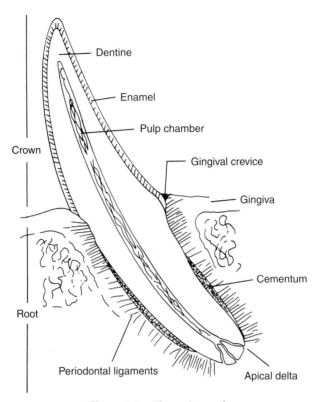

Figure 2-4:   The canine tooth.

Periodontal ligaments. Network of fibrous connective tissue that attaches the tooth to
    the alveolar bone and to other teeth and the gingiva to the alveolus.
Gingiva. Oral mucous membranes (or "gums").

Surfaces of the tooth
Buccal (vestibular). The surface toward the cheek (molars).
Labial (vestibular). The surface toward the lips (incisors, canines, premolars).
Lingual. The surface toward the tongue, lower jaw.
Palatal. The surface toward the tongue, upper jaw.
Occlusal. The surfaces that face the antagonist in the opposite jaw. There are no true
    occlusal surfaces in carnivores such as cats.
Contact. The surface that faces adjacent teeth.
Mesial. The surface closest to the midline.
Distal. The surface most distant from the midline.

The dental record
Like all medical disciplines, dentistry has its special forms. Diagnostic and therapeutic
procedures should be carefully recorded. Figures 2-5 and 2-6 are examples of dental record
forms.

Occlusion and dentition
The major malocclusion defects that are inherited are brachygnathism and prognathism.
In brachygnathism, the upper jaw is longer than the lower (overshot). In prognathism, the

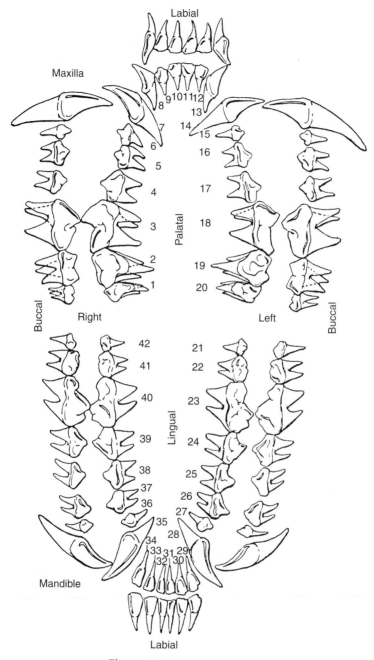

Figure 2-5:   Canine dental chart.
(Courtesy of North Carolina State University, Veterinary Teaching Hospital, Raleigh.)

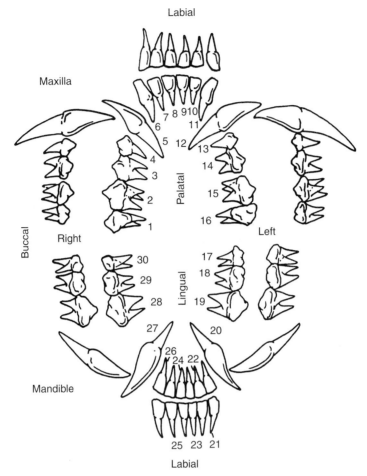

Figure 2-6: Feline dental chart.
(Courtesy of North Carolina State University, Veterinary Teaching Hospital, Raleigh.)

mandible is longer than the maxilla (undershot). This condition is the standard for brachycephalic breeds, including boxers, bulldogs, and Pekingese, but it is not anatomically normal. Any occlusion other than the normal "scissors" occlusion predisposes the patient to dental disease. There can be crowding or rotation of teeth (early onset of periodontal disease) in the short jaw and trauma to the soft tissues or teeth in the long and short jaw (abnormal attrition).

Supernumerary teeth occur occasionally in the maxilla and mandible and should be extracted if they are causing problems. Oligodontia (too few teeth) can be diagnosed in large or small breeds. Radiographs should be taken to confirm tooth absence. Enamel hypoplasia (Figure 2-7) may occur during the ameloblastic phase (2 to 5 months of age). Those are commonly called "distemper teeth" and are usually rough and dark-staining. Tetracyclines or tetracycline derivatives should be avoided in pregnant patients and patients less than 5 months old. Yellow staining of deciduous or permanent teeth can result following 10 or more days of consecutive treatment.

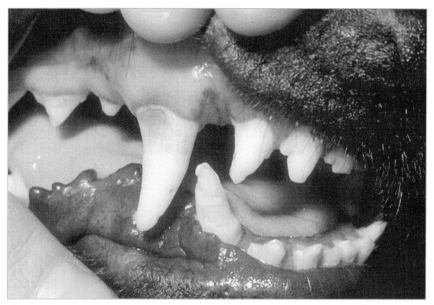

Figure 2-7:   Enamel hypoplasia in a dog that recovered from canine distemper infection as a puppy.

Dental/periodontal abscess

Abscessed teeth are often associated with advanced periodontal disease. A periodontal probe is inserted into the gingival sulcus to locate periodontal pockets (Figure 2-8), where tissue and bone have been lost. Loose teeth can sometimes be salvaged using techniques such as root planing and subgingival curettage. If only one root of a multirooted tooth is involved, a dental bar in a high- or low-speed dental handpiece can be used to section the tooth. The affected root is removed and a pulpotomy performed on the remaining tooth. This is an especially useful procedure for small, old dogs with one root of the lower first molar involved and the other root healthy.

Dental fractures

Fractured teeth with an exposed pulp chamber often form periapical abscesses. An infraorbital abscess indicates a problem with the upper fourth premolar. This problem will not resolve permanently unless endodontic therapy or extraction is performed. A fractured lower first molar may drain into the oral cavity or through the ventral aspect of the mandible. A fractured upper canine tooth may drain into the nasal cavity or through a fistulous tract at the level of the upper first or second premolar. An inapparent (the tooth is in place) oronasal fistula may also be present (this is seen often in old, small-breed dogs secondary to periodontal disease). A fractured lower canine tooth may drain internally or externally. Endodontic therapy and crown restoration have returned many patients to dental health.

ORAL CAVITY EXAMINATION

The normal oral mucosa is pink, partially pigmented, or completely pigmented, depending on the breed. The oral cavity should be moist, and evidence of excessive salivation and malodorous breath should be lacking. Examine the gingiva for color; petechiae or gross hemorrhage; hypertrophy or recession of the gingiva; any discharge around the base of the teeth; or any inflammation, swelling, or growth. Examine the hard palate for the presence of foreign bodies. Dogs and cats presenting with a history of sneezing and nasal discharge

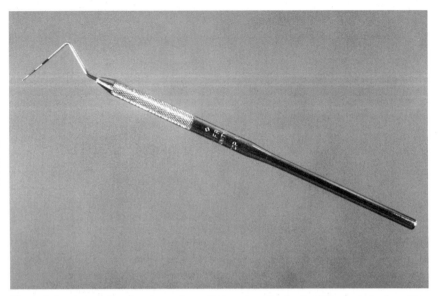

Figure 2-8:   A periodontal probe can be used to measure the depth of the gingival sulcus. Note the probe is marked in 3 mm increments. Normal depth ranges from 1 to 3 mm.

must be examined for evidence of an oronasal fistula (dental probe of the medial aspect of the upper canine teeth) or cleft palate. Inflammation of the mucous membranes of the mouth, stomatitis, can be associated with a variety of primary infectious agents, as well as being secondary to systemic (metabolic) diseases (e.g., chronic renal failure). Stomatitis may be associated with foreign bodies; metabolic disorders (e.g., uremia, diabetes mellitus); heavy metal poisoning (such as thallium); viral infections (especially those of the respiratory system in the cat); mycotic infections associated with *Candida albicans (Monilia)*; and chemical, thermal, or electrical burns.

Technique for examining the oral cavity varies among clinicians. However, the technique used to examine a dog may not work equally as well in a cat. Use of disposable examination gloves is recommended whenever examining the oral mucosa, the tongue, or related tissues. Cooperative dogs will allow the clinician to open the mouth briefly and examine at least the dorsal surface of the tongue, the hard palate, teeth (albeit to a limited extent), and tonsils. One single-handed, yet professional-appearing, method of performing this exam is to place the thumb of one hand in direct contact with the hard palate while gently placing the fingers of the same hand across the nose. Most dogs will open the mouth, allowing at least a limited examination. To facilitate visualizing critical structures, the fingers of the opposite hand are used to *gently* depress the tongue and position the head as needed (Figure 2-9).

Examination of the gingiva and the buccal surface of the teeth in cats is safely accomplished using a cotton-tipped applicator (Figure 2-10). This technique is not only a more professional approach to examining the mouth, especially in the presence of the client, but is better tolerated by many cats than the use of one's fingers. The technique used to actually open the mouth of cats, and small dogs, entails gently touching the hard palate with a cotton-tipped applicator rather than a finger. The stem of the applicator may then be positioned behind the lower canine teeth to facilitate opening the mouth and visualizing the oral cavity.

Note: It is NOT possible to adequately examine any structure caudal to the oral cavity without administering an anesthetic.

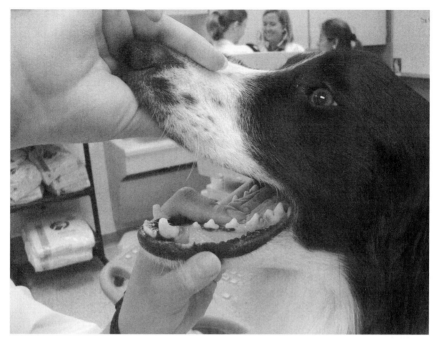

Figure 2-9: Use of only the thumb of one hand to entice a cooperative dog to open its mouth. Use of the opposite hand to facilitate examination of the teeth and oral cavity in the same cooperative dog.

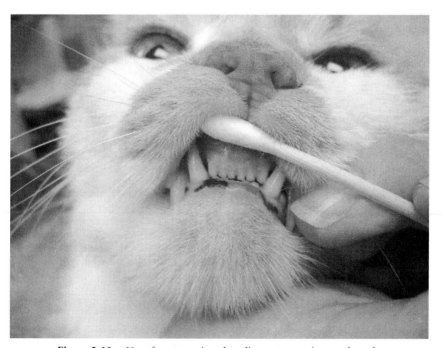

Figure 2-10: Use of a cotton-tipped applicator to examine a cat's teeth.

2

Periodontal disease

Periodontal disease is the most common oral disease in dogs and cats. Eighty-five percent to 95% of dogs and cats over 6 years of age have periodontal disease that is completely preventable. Periodontal disease is progressive and has two phases: gingivitis (reversible) and periodontitis (irreversible, but usually controllable). It is caused by the accumulation of plaque on teeth. Plaque is a soft, sticky, bacteria-ladened film of saliva and debris. The bacteria and bacterial byproducts cause soft tissue inflammation. Plaque mineralizes to form calculus, which then migrates into the gingival sulcus, causing further inflammation, periodontal ligament loss, bone loss, and, eventually, tooth loss. The overall health of the patient with periodontal disease can be expected to decline until such time the destructive process is stopped.

The tongue

Examine the tongue for the presence of any abnormal discoloration, membrane or pseudomembrane, foreign bodies, inflammation, ulcers, growth, or hyperplasia. Note whether the tongue protrudes normally and whether both halves are bilaterally symmetric. The underside of the tongue should be examined for ulcers, foreign bodies such as string wrapped around the base of the tongue (in cats), hyperplasia (indicating a gum chewer syndrome), and swelling of the lingual frenulum.

Palate, pharynx, and buccal mucosa

The ability of the animal to swallow effectively should be tested by stimulating the pharyngeal area. Dysphagia (see Section 3) refers to difficulty in swallowing and can be associated with localized diseases of the oropharynx or central nervous system (CNS) diseases. Thorough examination of the soft palate, oropharynx, and buccal mucosa requires administration of an anesthetic. Use of a focal light source, a tongue depressor or laryngoscope, and a spay hook (for limited examination of the nasopharynx) is important. Samples may be cultured or tissue biopsy may be obtained as needed.

Retropharyngeal tumors or abscesses may produce a ventral displacement of the pharynx and larynx. Careful digital exploration of the retropharyngeal tissues may reveal a palpable mass that otherwise is not visible. Fractures involving one or more bones of the hyoid apparatus may cause dysphagia. Persistent stertor (snorting) in dogs is characteristically associated with foreign matter, occasionally tumors, trapped above the soft palate in the nasopharynx. In dogs, melanoma, squamous cell carcinoma, and fibrosarcoma are the most common oral and pharyngeal neoplasms. In cats, squamous cell carcinoma and fibrosarcoma are the most common tumors involving the oral cavity.

Tonsils

Inspect the oral mucous membranes for changes in color, hemorrhage, inflammation, abrasions, ulceration, abnormal discharges, membranes or pseudomembranes, and abnormal growths. The tonsils should be examined for symmetry, size, color, and consistency; the surrounding tissues should be examined. Conclusive diagnosis of the cause of tonsillar enlargement may depend on the results of a biopsy. Examine the uvula and note its length. Foreign bodies may lodge at the opening of the posterior nares. Only the caudal aspect of the nasopharynx can be examined without use of an endoscope (pharyngoscopy). Pharyngoscopy is required to adequately visualize and biopsy the posterior nares (choanae). Examine the hard and soft palate for the presence of tumors or foreign bodies. Fractures of the hard palate are frequently seen in cats that fall from high elevations.

Note: Halitosis   One of the **most** common complaints registered by owners about a pet dog, halitosis may be caused by the accumulation of bacteria on teeth (plaque), ulcerations (including tumors) of the lip folds, tongue, or the mucous membranes (buccal mucosa), and tonsillitis. Uremia produces an ammonia-like odor (that not everyone equally perceives); diabetic ketosis may cause the smell of acetone; suppurative lung disease may cause a putrid odor to the breath. Interestingly, many owners delay having a pet's bad breath examined believing that halitosis is nothing more than "dog breath."

Examination of the Cervical Esophagus

Examination of the esophagus entails observation and palpation. Observation of swallowing can be simply evaluated by offering a small dose of water administered orally. Animals that manifest painful, frequent, or spontaneous attempts to swallow have dysphagia (see Section 3) and should be subjected to a more comprehensive examination. Careful palpation of the neck for evidence of obstructive lesions is an important part of the exam. However, lesions inside the esophagus must be evaluated with the use of radiography or gastroscopy. The signs of esophageal disease include regurgitation; spontaneous, frequent or painful swallowing; and weight loss. Dogs with regurgitation associated with an esophageal lesion frequently have aspiration pneumonia and pharyngitis.

Abdominal Palpation

Initial examination of the abdomen involves observing abdominal conformation while the patient is standing on the examination table or walking. Unusual abdominal enlargement as well as a particularly small or tensed abdomen should be noted. Determine whether the abdominal wall moves normally during respiration. Abnormal movement may reflect pain from peritonitis. Animals manifesting abdominal pain typically stand with the hindlegs drawn forward well under the body and the back appearing arched. The patient may walk with a shorter than normal stride. When in severe abdominal pain, some animals will assume a "praying position" (lie down with front legs extended, stand up on hindlegs). Look for soft tissue edema, as well as abnormal distention of the abdominal wall.

Following visual inspection, palpate the abdomen. The most effective technique for abdominal palpation entails placing the patient in right (side down) lateral recumbency. This position places the spleen, located in the left upper portion of the abdomen, in a superficial position, accessible to examination. Right-handed individuals should place their left hand beneath the patient's abdomen, palm up. Using the fingertips of the left hand, gently depress the right abdominal wall to assess when the abdominal musculature relaxes.

> **Note:** Dogs that are standing during abdominal palpation cannot completely relax abdominal muscles, making careful assessments of internal anatomy difficult.

While keeping the right hand positioned approximately over the left hand, the examination proceeds using the fingertips, *not* the metacarpals or palms, to discern the location, size, and consistency of abdominal organs. For consistency, the examination proceeds in a clockwise manner starting at the lower left position of the lateral abdomen (i.e., at the level of the xyphoid cartilage) to assess the ventral-most aspect of the liver. The exam continues dorsally along and beneath the costal arch assessing liver and, if palpable, the spleen. The stomach of the dog and cat cannot normally be palpated. Large tumors of the gastric wall and gastric torsion may cause the stomach to be displaced and palpable.

At the junction of the costal arch and the lumbar veterebrae, the examiner should attempt to palpate the caudal pole of the left kidney. In some dogs and virtually all cats, the entire kidney can be palpated. Palpation parallel to and below the lumbar vertebrae allows palpation of the colon. Opposing the fingers of the left and right hands between the lumbar vertebra and the colon allows the clinician to feel the tube-shaped colon positioned beneath and parallel to the lumbar vertebrae. Even an empty colon can be palpated in most patients.

Palpation continues as the clinician positions the hands at the level of the caudal abdomen. With the hands opposed above and below the urinary bladder, the clinician should attempt to assess the size, location, and consistency of the bladder. The prostate gland of male dogs cannot normally be palpated from this position. However, in some dogs, prostatic enlargement may be so extreme that the examiner can feel the ventral prostate gland. Following examination of the caudal abdomen, attention turns to the center of the abdomen. Objectively, the location and consistency of the small bowel mass and occasionally the spleen can be palpated.

Palpation of a normal abdomen typically takes 20 to 30 seconds. Most dogs, although fewer cats, tolerate this technique. Abdominal palpation in uncooperative cats can usually

ABDOMINAL PALPATION	
WHAT CAN NORMALLY BE PALPATED	**WHAT CANNOT CONSISTENTLY BE PALPATED**
Ventral aspect of the liver	Cranial aspect of the liver
Caudal pole of the LEFT kidney	Gall bladder
LEFT kidney	Stomach
RIGHT kidney (cat, occasionally dog)	RIGHT kidney (dog)
Colon	Cecum
Urinary bladder	Intraabdominal lymph nodes
Small bowel mass	Prostate gland (see Rectal Examination)
Uterine horns (occasionally dog)	Adrenal glands
Spleen	Posterior vena cava and abdominal aorta

be achieved with the patient standing on the examination table. Obesity is perhaps the most significant factor to compromise abdominal palpation. Pregnancy, depending on the stage, can also make it very difficult to distinguish discrete anatomic structures.

> **Note:** Abdominal palpation is a clinical technique that does improve with experience. It is this experience that allows the skilled clinician to distinguish normal internal anatomy from abnormal.

Abdominal percussion

Following palpation, percuss the abdomen. The normal abdomen yields a tympanitic note throughout except over a solid organ such as the liver, spleen, or a full bladder. Increased accumulations of air in the stomach or abdomen may result in a greater area of tympanitic sounds.

Free fluid in the peritoneum (ascites) may shift as the patient is moved. When ascites is suspected, place one hand on one side of the abdomen over the lumbar area and, with the other hand, "flick" or tap the opposite abdominal wall. A distinct impact is felt from one hand to the other if fluid under tension is present.

Abdominal auscultation

Carry out auscultation in a quiet room. Normal bowel sounds occur at frequent and regular intervals as liquid ingesta mixes with air during peristalsis. The absence of bowel sounds is abnormal and justifies further evaluation (e.g., abdominal radiography). Increased and decreased bowel sounds are subjective assessments and may only be variations of normal. Borborygmus, an audible rumbling noise emanating from the abdomen as air passes through the intestines, is sufficiently loud in dogs that the owner can actually hear the noise without use of a stethoscope.

Ballottement

The ability to palpate an organ floating in a fluid-filled cavity (e.g., a uterus or tumor in a fluid-filled abdomen) refers to ballottement. In patients having significant ascites, it may be possible to identify abnormal structures by ballottement. However, definitive assessment requires additional examination techniques (e.g., abdominal ultrasound or surgical exploration).

EXAMINATION OF THE RECTUM, ANUS, AND ANAL SACS

The rectum is the caudal 5 to 6 cm of the colon that communicates with the anus. Its diameter varies with the breed and size of the animal. Innervation to the anorectal area is supplied by the pudenal nerve (formed by S1, S2, and S3), which also provides motor nerves to the external anal sphincter and to the skin of the anus and perianal region. The rectum and internal anal sphincter are supplied by nerves from the pelvic plexus.

Tenesmus and dyschezia are the primary signs in anorectal diseases. Carefully examine the external anal area and perineum for evidence of inflammation, swelling, neoplasms, and crypts at the mucocutaneous junction.

Conclude the examination of the intestinal tract by performing a rectal examination. Digital examination (a disposable examination glove is highly recommended) will reveal the color and consistency of the stool in the rectum, any narrowing of the rectum, the possibility of a fractured pelvis, the assymetry of the pelvic canal, impaction or tumors of the anal glands, and the presence of rectal polyps or tumors. In medium- to large-breed male dogs, the rectal exam is an opportunity to assess the size of the prostate gland. Following digital examination of the rectum, direct visualization of the rectal canal can be accomplished by use of a proctoscope or an anoscope. This procedure, however, may require sedation or anesthesia.

A careful examination of the alimentary tract and abdomen may indicate that further diagnostic work is needed. Passage of a stomach tube, esophagoscopy, radiography, ultrasonography, test meals, proctoscopy, or clinicopathologic tests may be required. Do not hesitate to perform tests that may help in arriving at a definitive diagnosis.

CARDIOPULMONARY EXAMINATION

When initial physical examination findings suggest that further evaluation of the heart and lungs is warranted, the examination should encompass assessment of patient's behavior, at rest and during exertion, character of respirations, assessment of pulse character, presence (or absence) of peripheral edema or ascites, careful cardiac auscultation, thoracic radiography, electrocardiography, and, when indicated, echocardiography. Familiarity with normal and conformational variations between breeds and species will allow the veterinarian to distinguish between normal and abnormal findings.

CLINICAL HISTORY

Assessment of the patient suspected of having cardiovascular disease entails obtaining additional historical information from the client. The following questions are representative:

1. *Is there intolerance to exercise?* Most patients with significant cardiac disorders have exercise intolerance at some level of exertion, be it walking, running, prolonged play, or prolonged physical effort.
2. *Is either coughing or dyspnea present?* If so, under what circumstances? The most frequent presenting complaint associated with heart disease is a cough, which may be aggravated by exercise or excitement.
3. *When was the onset and what is the duration of signs?* In most instances, cardiac disease begins somewhat insidiously, with a slow progression over a period of several months to years.
4. *Are the problems progressively worsening?* Cardiac disease, although usually progressive, may be characterized by short periods of clinical stability or even improvement without therapy.
5. *Is weakness or syncope present?* Weakness usually implies a significant decrease in cardiac function that results in tissue hypoxia. Syncope may signify the presence of an arrhythmia.
6. *Are medications currently being administered?* If so, for how long? At what levels? Have they been effective? The knowledge of a prior response or lack of response to therapy is invaluable in formulating an effective therapeutic plan for the cardiac patient.
7. *What is the patient's current diet and feeding regimen?* Sodium and caloric restrictions are frequently part of the management plan for canine and feline cardiac patients.
8. *What is the medical history of the parents and siblings of the patient?* A positive genetic history of cardiac disease in previous generations or littermates is a common finding when such information is available.

9. *Do other problems exist?* Cardinal signs of illness should be investigated in the cardiac patient as in any other patient. These signs include anorexia, polydipsia, polyuria, vomiting, diarrhea, and previous illness. It is well known that cardiac disease may affect the kidney and the liver; thus, dysfunctions of these organs must always be investigated in the medical evaluation of the cardiac patient.

PATIENT ASSESSMENT

Dogs and cats with cardiovascular disease may present as healthy appearing animals. Even the owner may not be aware of subtle signs suggestive of heart disease. However, animals with cardiovascular disease can manifest a wide range of clinical signs, most of which are not directly referable to the heart (e.g., cough, weakness, tachypnea, or weight loss). All patients undergoing evaluation for cardiovascular disease should be observed for general appearance, attitude, and body condition, as well as respiratory rate and character.

Body condition

Note if the patient is overweight or underweight. Animals with advanced heart disease can be very thin (cardiac cachexia). Also note if abdominal distention is present. Abdominal effusion (ascites), hepato- and splenomegaly may be present in animals with right heart failure.

Respiratory character

Observe the animal for both respiratory rate and breathing effort while at rest. The normal respiratory rate for a dog at rest ranges from approximately 12 to 30 breaths per minute. Normal respiratory rate in cats ranges from approximately 20 to 30 breaths per minute.

An increase in respiratory rate and effort in a dog or cat at rest suggests dyspnea. A normal animal should not use its abdominal muscles for breathing. A dyspneic animal may breathe with its mouth open and may recruit its abdominal muscles to aid in respiration. It may also have an anxious facial expression with eyes bulging, nostrils flaring, and head and neck extended. There are several types of dyspnea, depending on which phase of respiration is most prolonged. Inspiratory dyspnea is characterized by a longer than normal inspiratory phase, usually accompanied by stridor (noisy breathing). Inspiratory dyspnea suggests upper airway obstruction, such as laryngeal paralysis or brachycephalic syndrome. Expiratory dyspnea is characterized by forced, abdominal respirations during the expiratory phase. This type of breathing pattern suggests asthma or chronic obstructive pulmonary disease. Dyspnea throughout inspiration and expiration is typical of pulmonary diseases and pulmonary edema. The terminology used to describe normal and abnormal lung sounds is described in Table 2-4.

Body posture and gait

Cats with cardiomyopathy may present with systemic arterial thromboembolization (saddle thrombus), resulting in acute onset and painful paraparesis (weakness in the hindlegs). Animals with saddle thrombus will also have an absent or diminished femoral pulse and have cool, pale, or cyanotic footpads.

The neck

Palpate the trachea in an animal that presents with cough to assess its sensitivity. Animals with collapsing trachea and tracheobronchitis (kennel cough) will usually have a cough induced by tracheal palpation. Beware, as even a normal animal will cough with excessive tracheal palpation. Palpate the neck for a thyroid nodule in cats over 6 years of age, especially if the cat has a heart murmur or tachycardia.

The jugular vein

Assess the jugular vein for distention and pulsation. *Jugular venous distention* suggests increased central venous pressure (CVP) and is a sign of right heart failure. Jugular venous distention may occur with conditions causing tricuspid regurgitation or impaired filling of the right heart such as pericardial effusion, constrictive pericarditis, or a mass lesion in the right heart or cranial thorax. All animals with ascites should have the jugular vein carefully

TABLE 2-4   **Classification and Characterization of Normal and Abnormal (Adventitial) Breath Sounds Audible during Thoracic Auscultation**

Normal breath sounds	Description
Bronchial sounds	Low-pitched sounds made as air passes in and out of large airways and the trachea. Loudest over the trachea and larynx. Least audible over the caudal thorax.
Bronchovesicular sounds (also referred to as "vesicular sounds")	Soft, low-pitched sounds characterized as a rustling sound. Most audible over the peripheral lung fields during inspiration.

Abnormal breath sounds	Description
Crackles (also called "rales")	Discontinuous, clicking or popping sounds that originate in the airways. Most audible during inspiration but may be heard on expiration. Also described as "coarse crackles" (moist rales) and "fine crackles" (dry rales). Clinically significant since they are associated with presence of increased quantities of secretions in the lumen of bronchi and lower airways; may also heard in patients with airway collapse.
Wheezes (also called "ronchi")	Continuous sounds described as a musical or whistling noise heard during either inspiration or expiration. Also described as sibilant wheezes (high pitched) and sonorous wheezes (low pitched). May be most audible at end expiration or early inspiration. Associated with restriction of airflow through the glottis, trachea, or lower airways. Careful auscultation of the larynx, trachea, and lung fields is critical to determine the point of maximum intensity and thereby localize the source of the airway restriction.
Friction rub (pleural)	Combination of both continuous and discontinuous sounds caused by movement of inflamed visceral pleura over inflamed parietal pleura.
"Silent lung"	The absence of breath sounds (in a patient that is obviously breathing) is as important as the presence of abnormally loud breath sounds. This term is used to describe profoundly decreased, or totally inaudible, breath sounds. Clinical significance is that this is associated with significant, life-threatening airway obstruction, pneumothorax, accumulation of a large volume of fluid in the pleural space, and space-occupying lesions (e.g., diaphragmatic hernia, neoplasia). Extreme obesity and low tidal volume (especially in cats) may also be interpreted as "silent lung."

2

DESCRIPTIVE TERMINOLOGY FOR ABNORMAL RESPIRATION

Dyspnea: difficult or labored breathing, usually associated with an increased respiratory rate at rest.
Tachypnea: abnormal increase in the rate of respiration.
Hyperpnea: abnormal increase in both rate and depth of respiration.
Orthopnea: inability to breathe unless in a sitting or standing position, often with elbows abducted; positional breathing at rest.

evaluated and a hepatojugular reflex performed. A positive *hepatojugular reflex* suggests right heart failure and occurs when the jugular vein becomes distended with upward compression of the cranial abdomen. Also observe for jugular venous pulsation. A *jugular pulse* traveling more that one-third the way up the neck is abnormal and is generally associated with tricuspid valve insufficiency (i.e., congenital tricuspid valve dysplasia, or tricuspid valve insufficiency caused by chronic degeneration, pulmonary stenosis, heartworm disease, and pulmonary hypertension). An arrhythmia causing atrioventricular (AV) dissociation, such as a ventricular premature complex and second- or third-degree AV block, may also cause a jugular pulse. The atria contract against a closed AV valve causing the pulsation. In thin animals, beware of the carotid pulse beneath the jugular vein, which may be confused with a jugular pulse.

The thorax

With the patient standing, palpate the thorax for any trauma or deformities. One may also assess the compressibility of the chest in a cat. *Compressibility* is variable even in a normal cat, but this physical examination maneuver may be helpful in cats with space-occupying lesions such as pleural effusion, which will cause decreased compressibility. Cats with cranial mediastinal masses will have reduced compressibility in the cranial thorax.

Palpate the precordium

Palpate the precordium (area of chest wall next to the heart) for the *apex beat*. The palm of the hand, ventral surface of the proximal metacarpals, as well as the fingertips should be used for optimal appreciation of the precordium. The apex beat is the point of maximum intensity of the heartbeat. The normal location is at the left fifth intercostal space around the costochondral junction. *Displacement of the normal apex beat may result from right heart enlargement or a thoracic mass.* The intensity of the apex beat may be decreased or increased. An increased apex beat may occur in thin animals, hyperdynamic states (anemia, hyperthyroidism), mitral valve regurgitation (or other volume-overloaded state with maintained myocardial contractility), and hypertrophic cardiomyopathy. Decreased intensity of the apex beat may occur in dilated cardiomyopathy and pleural or pericardial effusion.

Precordial thrill

Precordial thrill is the vibration felt on the surface of the chest caused by a murmur. The location of the thrill is always the point of maximum intensity of the murmur.

Thoracic percussion

This may be helpful in animals with restrictive breathing patterns and quiet breath sounds. This technique may not be helpful in obese animals. First, the flat part of a fingertip is placed in the intercostal space. Then the fingertip (usually the middle finger) of the other hand briskly strikes the finger on the intercostal space producing a resonating sound. Percussion of the chest should be done systematically from dorsal to ventral, evaluating the entire chest. The sound produced by percussion may be increased or hyperresonant in pneumothorax or asthma. The resonance may be decreased with pleural effusion, consolidated lung (lung filled with fluid or exudate), or a thoracic mass.

The abdomen

Palpate for ascites and hepatic or splenic enlargement, which may accompany right heart failure in the dog. Ascites is an uncommon sign of right heart failure in the cat. *Ballottement* is a palpation technique used to help determine if abdominal distention is caused by fluid. One taps the abdomen (once or twice) with the fingertips to evaluate a fluid wave or rebound of an abdominal organ floating in fluid.

Mucous membranes

The color of the mucous membranes is usually assessed in the mouth, but some animals have pigmented gums, and the vulva, penis, or conjunctiva should be examined. The normal mucous membrane color is pink. Alterations in color may suggest various conditions pertinent to the cardiopulmonary systems such as the following:

Cyanosis (blue discoloration) suggests hypoxia as a result of a congenital right-to-left shunting defect (tetralogy of Fallot) or as a result of respiratory disease (upper airway obstruction or pulmonary disease). If cyanosis is suspected in the oral mucous membrane, the caudal mucous membrane should also be observed for differential cyanosis. Animals with a reverse (right-to-left) patent ductus arteriosus (PDA) will have more cyanosis in the caudal mucous membrane (penis or vulva) than in the oral mucous membrane (differential or caudal cyanosis).

A pale mucous membrane (light pink or white discoloration) suggests anemia or poor perfusion, usually associated with low cardiac output. Hyperemia of the mucous membrane (bright red) suggests peripheral vasodilation as seen in septic shock or exercise.

Capillary refill time (CRT)

Using the gingival mucosa (nonpigmented tissue is required) above the maxillary canine tooth, gently press a finger against the tissue causing it to blanch. The CRT is the time required for blood to reperfuse the mucosal capillaries and the tissue to return to a pink color. Reperfusion of gingiva should be apparent within 2 seconds. Prolonged CRT may indicate poor peripheral perfusion or low cardiac output.

Note: A normal CRT may be observed in animals up to 3 hours following death.

The arterial pulse

Assessment of the pulse, usually the femoral pulse, is a basic and important part of the cardiovascular physical examination. The normal pulse should feel full, with a rapid rise and fall. The arterial pulse is pressure defined as the difference between systolic and diastolic blood pressures (e.g., in a normal dog: 120 mm Hg – 80 mm Hg = 40 mm Hg pulse pressure). Femoral pulses may be difficult to assess in normal cats and obese dogs and cats. Evaluate the pulse quality as well as the rate.

CARDIAC AUSCULTATION

The stethoscope

The main components of the stethoscope are the bell, diaphragm, tubing, and earpieces. The bell transmits both low-frequency and high-frequency sounds. The diaphragm attenuates low-frequency sounds and selectively transmits the high-frequency sounds. The diaphragm also transmits louder sounds than the bell by virtue of its size. The tubing should not be too long because sounds attenuate in the longer tubing. The earpieces should fit comfortably without entering the ear canals. A properly fitted stethoscope is the first step to successful auscultation. In addition to a good stethoscope, a *quiet room and properly restrained patient* are essential. Whenever possible, perform auscultation with the animal in a standing position. Control respirations if necessary by holding the mouth closed or occluding a nostril transiently. Sometimes, if the animal is overly excited, auscultate again after the animal relaxes. Purring in cats may interfere with auscultation, and running tap

---

ABNORMAL PULSES

Pulse deficits: For every heartbeat, there should be a pulse. A PULSE DEFICIT occurs when there is a heartbeat without a corresponding pulse—typically occurs with arrhythmias such as ventricular premature complexes or atrial fibrillation.

Hyperkinetic pulse: (SYN: bounding, BB-shot or water-hammer pulse) an unusually strong pulse, which rises quickly and decays quickly. Associated conditions include PDA and aortic insufficiency or hyperdynamic conditions such as anemia, fever, and hyperthyroidism.

water or the smell of alcohol may stop the purring. Care should be taken not to confuse respiratory sounds, shivering, or rubbing of the hair for heart sounds.

Proper use of the bell and diaphragm is also important for accurate auscultation. Most of the auscultation should be performed with the diaphragm firmly placed on the chest. The bell is used to hear low-frequency sounds such as gallop sounds or low-frequency murmurs. The bell should be used with light pressure; too much pressure on the bell tightens the skin and creates a diaphragm. Auscultation with the bell should be used in animals with an extra heart sound (auscultated with the diaphragm), all cats (to screen for gallop sounds), and dogs suspected of cardiomyopathy or with congestive heart failure. Develop a *systemic approach to auscultation*. Determine heart rate and rhythm and correlate it with the femoral pulse. *Auscultate over all valve areas* for any abnormal heart sounds.

Normal heart rate and rhythm

Certainly heart rate can vary in a normal animal depending on the state of excitement and fitness. Sometimes true resting heart rates can only be determined in the home environment by the owner. In general, the heart rate increases (tachycardia) with excitement, pain, shock, hyperdynamic states (anemia, fever, hyperthyroidism), and congestive heart failure of various causes. Slow heart rates (bradycardia) may be noted in athletic animals, hypothyroidism, increases in vagal tone, or a conduction abnormality of the heart (sick sinus syndrome, advanced AV block).

Heart rhythm is typically regular in cats and dogs. However, *many normal dogs (especially brachycephalic breeds) have respiratory sinus arrhythmia*. In respiratory sinus arrhythmia, the heart rate increases with inspiration and decreases with expiration.

Normal heart sounds

There are four principal anatomic areas for cardiac auscultation (Figure 2-11):
1. *Mitral valve (left AV valve).* The left fifth intercostal space around the costochondral junction—in the normal animal, the area of the apex beat. Usually in the standing animal, the area opposite to the point of the elbow. First heart sounds are heard better at the mitral valve.
2. *Aortic valve.* The left fourth intercostal space dorsal to the mitral valve (usually the level of the point of the shoulder). The second heart sound is heard better at the aortic and pulmonary valves.
3. *Pulmonary valve.* The left third intercostal space at the sternal border (usually at the axilla).
4. *Tricuspid valve (right AV valve).* The right third to fourth intercostal space at the costochondral junction.

The intensity of normal heart sounds may be increased with conditions such as a thin body, young age, and hyperdynamic states (anemia, fever, hyperthyroidism). The intensity may also be decreased with obesity or in a heavily muscled animal, in addition to pathologic conditions such as pericardial effusion or pleural effusion.

The **first heart sound (S_1)** is associated with closure of the atrial-ventricular (AV) valves causing a phonetic sound "**lubb.**" S_1 is typically loudest over the mitral and tricuspid valve areas. The pulse occurs just after S_1.

The **second heart sound (S_2)** is associated with closure of the semilunar valves (**pulmonary and aortic valves**) causing a phonetic sound "**dupp.**" S_2 is typically heard the loudest over the pulmonary and aortic valves.

NORMAL HEART RATE (DOG)
Large dogs: 60 to 100 bpm **Medium-size dogs:** 80 to 120 bpm **Small dogs:** 90 to 140 bpm

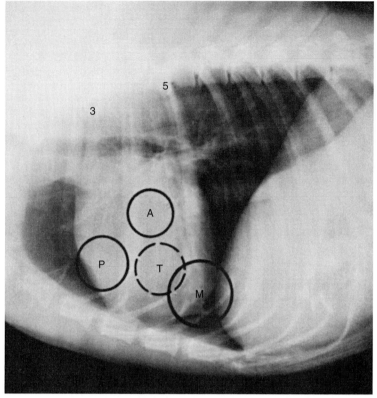

Figure 2-11: Left lateral radiograph of the canine thorax. Circles identify the valve areas: M, mitral valve area; P, pulmonic valve area; A, aortic valve area; T, tricuspid valve area. Because the tricuspid valve area is located on the right side of the thorax, it is indicated by a broken circle. The numbers represent the third and fifth ribs.
(From Ettinger SJ, Suter PF: Canine cardiology. Philadelphia, 1970, WB Saunders.)

Transient heart sounds

Split S_1. Asynchronous closure of the AV valves. May be a normal variant in a large-breed dog. Other causes include a ventricular premature complex or bundle-branch block.

Split S_2. Asynchronous closure of the pulmonic and aortic valves. Associated conditions include heartworm disease or other causes of pulmonary hypertension, pulmonic stenosis, aortic stenosis, and atrial septal defects.

Midsystolic click. A high-frequency sound in the middle of systole usually associated with early mitral valve disease. May precede a murmur in some animals.

S_3 gallop. A low-frequency, diastolic sound associated with rapid ventricular filling. Abnormal in the small animal patient and represents ventricular stiffness. A common associated condition is dilated cardiomyopathy.

S_4 gallop. A low-frequency, diastolic sound associated with atrial contraction. Abnormal in the small animal and represents ventricular stiffness. A common associated condition is hypertrophic cardiomyopathy.

Heart Murmurs

A heart murmur is produced by an interruption of laminar blood flow through the heart or great vessels (i.e., turbulent blood flow). The majority of heart murmurs are caused by a lesion at a level of the heart valves, causing turbulence. However, some murmurs may be physiologic such as murmurs associated with severe anemia or shock. Murmurs can be classified in several ways: timing in the cardiac cycle, intensity, location, point of maximum intensity (PMI), quality (subjective), phonographic configuration, and frequency.

Timing

Systolic murmur occurs during systole (with pulse). These murmurs are heard between S_1 and S_2. Most murmurs are systolic and associated conditions include mitral and tricuspid valve insufficiency, aortic or pulmonary stenosis, and ventricular septal defect (VSD).

Diastolic murmur occurs during diastole (after the pulse), after S_2. Diastolic murmurs are rare and occur most commonly with aortic insufficiency.

Continuous murmur occurs throughout systole and diastole. PDA is the most common cause of a continuous murmur.

One could further classify the timing of the murmur by commenting on the duration and position in the cardiac cycle such as holosystolic (entire systole), versus early-, mid-, or late-systolic murmurs.

Intensity

Intensity is a subjective determination of the loudness of the murmur. In most cases, murmur intensity does not correlate with the severity of heart disease. Murmurs are usually graded on a scale of I to VI:

Grade I. Very faint murmur requiring concentration and a quiet room to be heard

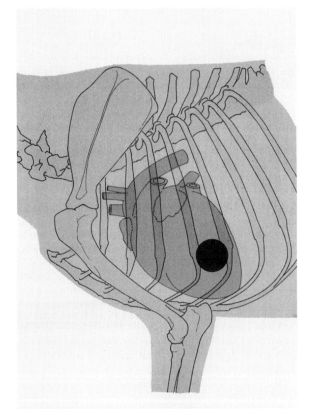

Figure 2-12:   Point of maximum intensity for murmurs associated with the mitral valve (left thorax).

Grade II. Soft murmur that is consistently auscultated over only one valve area

Grade III. Moderate-intensity murmur, readily auscultable, usually radiating to another valve area

Grade IV. Loud murmur without a precordial thrill, usually radiating to both sides of the chest

Grade V. Loud murmur with a precordial thrill

Grade VI. Loud murmur with a precordial thrill and still audible with the stethoscope off the chest wall

Location

Note the valve area where the murmur is loudest (point of maximal intensity or PMI). Also note where the murmur radiates. In some cases of severe subaortic stenosis, the murmur can radiate up the carotid arteries. Figures 2-12 through 2-15 illustrate the location of the PMI for each of the heart valves.

2

> **Note:** Closure of three of the four heart valves is heard best over the left thorax (pulmonary, aortic, and mitral), while the PMI for the tricuspid valve is on the right thorax.

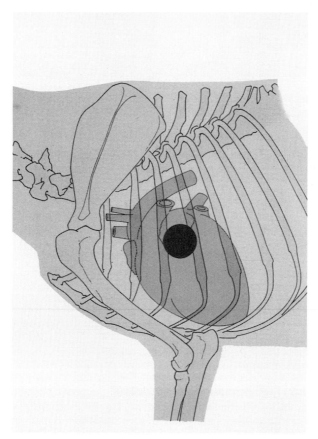

Figure 2-13: Point of maximum intensity for murmurs associated with the aortic valve (left thorax).

2

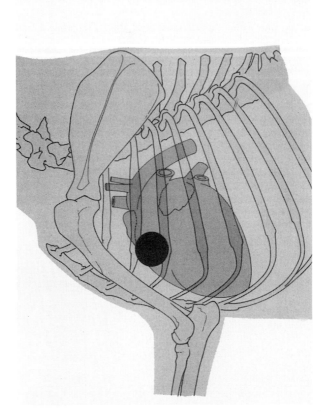

Figure 2-14:   Point of maximum intensity for murmurs associated with the pulmonic valve (left thorax).

Quality

Regurgitant-quality (**plateau**-shaped) murmur is the most common and is associated with AV valve insufficiency.

Ejection-quality (**crescendo-decrescendo** or **diamond**-shaped) murmur is associated with aortic and pulmonary stenosis.

Machinery-quality murmur is a continuous murmur most commonly associated with PDA.

Decrescendo murmur is most commonly associated with VSD or AV valve insufficiency.

Frequency

Low frequency. 30 to 80 cps, low rumbling sound (usually aortic insufficiency, PDA)
High frequency. 120 cps (aortic or pulmonary stenosis)
Mixed frequency. 80 to 120 cps (usually AV valve insufficiency)

Common types of heart murmur (see also Table 2-5)

Mitral valve insufficiency (regurgitation). Early systolic to holosystolic regurgitant (plateau) or occasionally decrescendo murmur with PMI over the left apex (mitral valve area). This is the most commonly heard murmur and is usually associated with chronic degenerative mitral valve disease in the older small-breed dog.

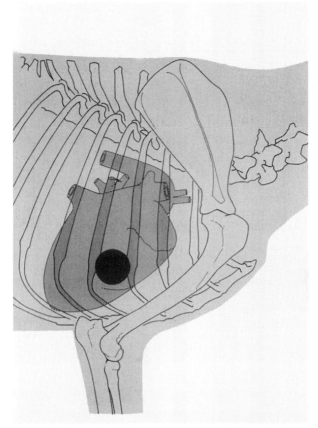

Figure 2-15: Point of maximum intensity for murmurs associated with the tricuspid valve (right thorax).

Tricuspid valve insufficiency (regurgitation). Systolic regurgitant murmur heard loudest in the tricuspid valve area (right apex).

Patent ductus arteriosus. Usually a loud continuous machinery murmur with PMI at the left heart base (pulmonary and aortic valve areas). PDA is the most common congenital defect in the dog.

Pulmonary stenosis. Usually a loud, high-frequency, harsh holosystolic crescendo-decrescendo ejection murmur with a PMI at the left heart base (pulmonary valve area). The murmur usually peaks in midsystole and radiates well caudally and to the right.

Subaortic stenosis. Usually a loud, harsh mixed or high-frequency holosystolic crescendo-decrescendo ejection murmur with a PMI at the left heart base. Sometime the PMI is the right heart base. The murmur radiates well to the right side and up the thoracic inlet and up the carotids. It is sometimes associated with aortic insufficiency.

Ventricular septal defect. Usually a holosystolic murmur with PMI at the right side near the sternum. VSD is the one of the most common congenital defects in the cat.

RADIOGRAPHY OF THE HEART

In the absence of echocardigraphy, survey lateral and ventrodorsal radiographs are critical in assessing patients suspected of having cardiac disease. Figure 2-16 and Figure 2-17 depict the critical anatomic features of the canine heart as seen in properly positioned and

TABLE 2-5 Characterization of Heart Murmurs Heard During Cardiac Auscultation

	Mitral insufficiency	Patent Ductus arteriosus	Aortic stenosis	Pulmonic stenosis	Ventricular septal defect	Anemic murmur	Physiologic (functional) murmur
Timing Duration	Systolic Holosystolic	Continuous Holosystolic, holodiastolic	Systolic Midsystolic (crescendo-decrescendo or diamond-shaped murmur)	Systolic Midsystolic (crescendo-decrescendo or diamond-shaped murmur)	Systolic Holosystolic	Systolic Early systolic	Systolic Early systolic
Pitch	Early–high frequency Later–mixed frequency	Mixed frequency with low frequency components	Harsh mixed frequency, with some high-frequency components	High frequency	Mixed frequency	High frequency	High frequency
Intensity	Usually moderate to loud	Usually loud	Usually loud	Usually loud	Usually loud	Usually very soft; may wax and wane	Very soft; may wax and wane; usually disappears by 8 wk of age
Valve area	Mitral valve area	Anterior on chest in area of pulmonary and aortic valve areas; may have PMI on ventral sternum cranial to left foreleg	Aortic valve area	Pulmonic area on left	Mitral area on left; anterior midthorax on right	Mitral area Aortic area	Mitral area Aortic area
Radiation	Rightward, cranioventral, or dorsal	Craniodorsal	Cranial and rightward; thoracic inlet	Tends not to radiate beyond thoracic inlet; radiates to right	Heard on both sides of chest, but PMI is on right side	None	None

PMI, point of maximal intensity.

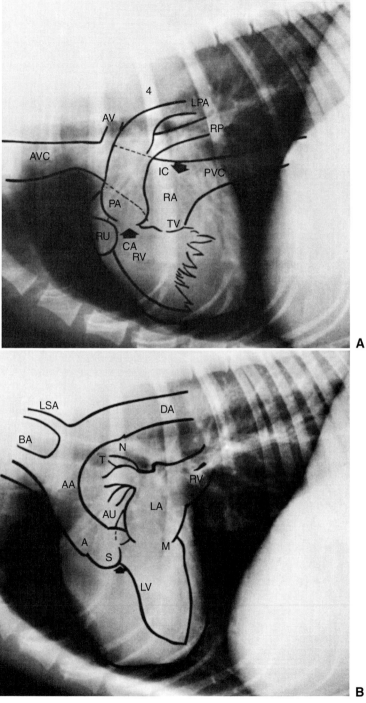

Figure 2-16: **A,** Radiographic anatomy of the RIGHT heart, LATERAL VIEW. **B,** Radiographic anatomy of the LEFT heart, LATERAL VIEW. (From Ettinger SJ, Suter PF: *Canine cardiology,* Philadelphia, 1970, WB Saunders.)

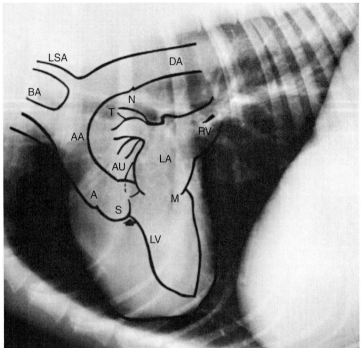

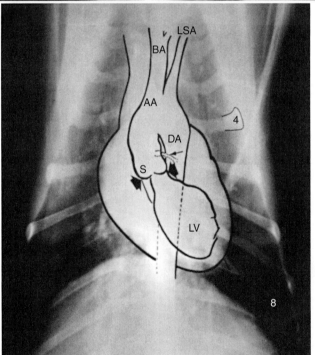

Figure 2-17: **A,** Radiographic anatomy of the RIGHT VENTRICLE and pulmonary artery, DORSOVENTRAL VIEW. **B,** Radiographic anatomy of the LEFT VENTRICLE and Aorta-DORSOVENTRAL VIEW.

(From Ettinger SJ, Suter PF: *Canine cardiology*, Philadelphia, WB Saunders, 1970.)

exposed radiographs. In addition, knowledge of the position and size of major vessels becomes critical in the assessment of patients with heart disease. Changes in lung vasculature may be evident on radiographs. With pulmonary congestion, the pulmonary veins are engorged with blood. With pulmonary overcirculation, the pulmonary arteries and veins are engorged. On lateral radiographic films, the veins appear indistinct and tortuous and are seen emanating from the area of the left atrium. On the other hand, the pulmonary arteries appear straight and branching, like a tree. On the dorsoventral view, veins are medial and arteries are lateral to each bronchus. Decompensated mitral insufficiency causes pulmonary venous congestion; heartworm disease, chronic lung disease, and congenital left-to-right shunt pulmonary artery enlargement.

The mediastinum is a compartment of the thorax between the medial aspects of the two pleural sacs. The mediastinal pleural layers are thin, and disease processes such as pneumothorax and pleural effusion seldom remain unilateral. Signs related to abnormalities in the mediastinal area may be dysphagia, regurgitation, coughing and dyspnea, syncope, head and neck edema, thoracic pain, abdominal breathing, Horner's syndrome, and emphysema.

2

Survey radiographs of the heart

1. The normal canine heart is on a 45-degree angle with the sternum.
2. The heart extends from T1 to T8.
3. Breed variation can greatly affect the appearance of the cardiac silhouette, as can the respiratory and cardiac cycle.
4. Thoracic radiographs should be taken at the height of inspiration.
5. The heart of the cat assumes a more elongated and elliptic position than that of the dog; the feline heart occupies 2 to 2½ intercostal spaces, and the caudal border is separated from the diaphragm by one or two intercostal spaces.
6. In ventrodorsal (VD) and dorsoventral (DV) positions, the canine heart has a curved right border and a straight left border with the long axis oriented at a 30-degree angle to the spine and to the left of the midline.
7. The feline heart is more oval in appearance in the VD position; in the DV view, the cardiac apex is just to the left of the midline; the ratio of the longitudinal axis to the transverse axis is 1.4:1.

Radiograph evaluation of the cardiovascular system and lungs is important in the differential diagnosis of cardiovascular disease. It is especially important to evaluate (1) enlargement of cardiac chambers; (2) dilation of great vessels; (3) increased or decreased pulmonary circulation; (4) venous congestion, pulmonary edema, and pleural effusion; and (5) mediastinal space.

When viewing thoracic radiographs to determine whether there is evidence of cardiovascular disease concomitant with clinical findings, ask the following questions:

1. Is the cardiac silhouette larger or smaller than normal?
2. Is the cardiac apex pointing to the right or left?
3. Are cardiac chamber shapes normal or abnormal?
4. Are there changes in size, shape, or position of cardiac or intrathoracic vessels or of trachea and bronchi?
5. Is there evidence of pleural fluid accumulation?
6. Is there evidence of pulmonary edema?
7. Is there evidence of intrathoracic disease other than cardiovascular in origin?
8. Is the mediastinum normal or abnormal?

When interpreting changes in cardiac size and shape, note the consistency of the radiographic technique. Short radiographic exposure times of 1/60 or 1/120 second with radiographs taken at full inspiration give the best results.

Enlargement of right atrium

Right atrial enlargement is usually associated with right ventricular enlargement.

1. Bulging cranial heart border on lateral view.
2. Bulging at the 9- to 11-o'clock position on VD (DV) view.

Right ventricle

1. Cranial border of heart is more rounded with increased sternal contact (>3 sternebrae), and the heart may be elevated dorsally on lateral view.
2. Overall width of heart is increased.
3. Elevation of trachea, cranial to tracheal bifurcation.
4. VD (DV) view: heart rounded from 6- to 11-o'clock position.
5. Distance between right heart border and thoracic wall is decreased.

Left atrium

1. Bulging caudal dorsal heart border on lateral view.
2. Loss of caudal waist on lateral view.
3. Elevation of trachea, compression of main stem bronchi.
4. Bulging at 2- to 3-o'clock position on VD (DV) view.
5. Increased size of pulmonary veins.

Left ventricle

1. Elongation of cardiac silhouette on either lateral or VD (DV) view.
2. Elevation of trachea.
3. Rounded caudal border of the heart.
4. Distance between left heart border and thoracic wall is decreased on VD (DV) view.

Biventricular enlargement

1. Heart appears rounded on both views.
2. Increased sternal contact on lateral view, with elongation and widening of the heart shadow.
3. May mimic pericardial effusion if uniform and severe.

Decrease in size of cardiac silhouette

1. Heart elevated off the sternum.
2. Increase in ratio of longitudinal axis to transverse axis to more than 1.4:1.
3. Shifting of heart away from midline.
4. Small caudal vena cava.
5. Seen in Addison's disease, hypothyroidism, shock, and pneumothorax.

Differential diagnoses based on survey radiographs (Table 2-6)

A severe degree of cardiomegaly with evidence of right heart failure suggests advanced mitral and tricuspid valvular fibrosis, dilated cardiomyopathy, or pericardial effusion. Nonselective angiocardiography can be helpful in distinguishing between cardiomyopathy, congenital cardiac abnormalities, and pericardial effusion.

Radiographic appearance of the lungs in left-sided heart failure

1. Pulmonary congestion. Engorgement and distention of pulmonary veins, especially at the junction of the veins with the left atrium. Pulmonary radiodensity is unchanged.
2. *Pulmonary interstitial lung edema phase.* Pulmonary radiodensity is increased, and lungs appear hazy. Accumulated fluid in perivascular spaces makes the vascular markings appear hazy.
3. *Alveolar edema.* Fluid enters the alveoli and peripheral bronchioles, creating alveolar radiodensity and air bronchograms. Alveolar radiodensity is most severe in the perihilar area.

   The lung fields should also be carefully reviewed for evidence of vascular changes compatible with heartworm disease or pulmonary embolism.

Disease processes that alter mediastinal position

1. Unilateral pleural or pulmonary masses.
2. Unilateral pneumothorax or pleural effusion.

TABLE 2-6   **Differential Diagnoses for Patients with Cardiomegaly**

Left-sided cardiomegaly	Right-sided cardiomegaly	Generalized cardiomegaly
Dilation	*Dilation*	Chronic valvular disease
Mitral regurgitation	Tricuspid regurgitation	Dilated cardiomyopathy
R-to-L shunting (PDA)[a]	Atrial septal defect	Congenital shunts:
Aortic insufficiency	Dilated cardiomyopathy	PDA
Dilated cardiomyopathy		VSD[b]
Feline hyperthyroidism		Chronic anemia
		Pericardial effusion
Hypertrophy	*Hypertrophy*	
Aortic stenosis	Pulmonic stenosis	
Hypertension	Tetralogy of fallot	
Hypertrophic	Cor pulmonale	
cardiomyopathy	Heartworm disease	
(myocardial infarction)	- pulmonary hypertension	
	Feline hypertrophic	
	cardiomyopathy	
	Feline restrictive	
	cardiomyopathy	

[a]PDA = patent ductus arteriosus. (NOTE: In patients with R-to-L shunting PDA, the characteristic "machinery murmur" becomes systolic.)
[b]VSD = ventricular septal defect.
See also Herrtage ME: Cardiovascular disorders. In Schaer M, editor: *Clinical medicine of the dog and cat.* Iowa State Press, Ames, 2003. pp. 121-162, and Belanger MC: Echocardiography. In Ettinger SJ, Feldman EC, editors: *Textbook of veterinary internal medicine,* ed 6, St. Louis, 2005, Elsevier-Saunders, pp. 311-326.

ANCILLARY RADIOGRAPHIC SIGNS ASSOCIATED WITH HEART DISEASE

- Ascites
- Liver enlargement
- Increased size of portal venous circulation
- Decreased pulmonary circulation

---

3. Lung lobe collapse, agenesis, hypoplasia, or resection.
4. Pleural adhesions.
5. Hypostatic congestion of a lung.

Diseases that result in mediastinal widening

1. Accumulation of mediastinal fat or fluid.
2. Inflammation secondary to tracheal or esophageal puncture.
3. Hemorrhage.
4. Tumor formation (lymphosarcoma, thymoma).
5. Heart base tumors.
6. Enlargement of tracheobronchial lymph nodes.

The intrathoracic trachea is about three times the width of the proximal third rib but increases in diameter on inspiration and decreases on expiration. Normal trachea enters the thoracic inlet in the dorsal third of the inlet. The intrathoracic trachea may collapse on expiration, which may extend to the carina and main stem bronchi.

Congenital tracheal hypoplasia is seen in the English bulldog. Tracheal compression or left main stem bronchus compression may be associated with enlargements of tracheobronchial lymph nodes or of the left atrium.

Advanced diagnostic tests

Section 4 of this text describes in detail the basic requirements for performing advanced cardiac examination, including electrocardiography and echocardiography.

Additional Reading

Fox PR, Sisson D: *Canine and feline cardiology,* ed 2, Philadelphia, 1999, WB Saunders.

Herrtage ME: Cardiovascular disorders. In Schaer M, editor: *Clinical medicine of the dog and cat,* Ames, 2003, Iowa State Press (Blackwell), pp. 121-162.

Tilley LP, Goodwin J-K: *Manual of canine and feline cardiology,* ed 3, Philadelphia, 2002, WB Saunders.

INTEGUMENT (SKIN, HAIR COAT, AND TOENAILS)

CLINICAL HISTORY

The owner's chief complaint is often the major sign used in compiling a differential diagnosis for animals with skin disease. It is important that the questions presented to the client do not suggest answers. The clinician should obtain a complete medical history. Some dermatologists prefer to examine the skin quickly at first, so that they can emphasize pertinent questions in taking the history and omit inappropriate items. However, it is vital to use a systematic, detailed method of examination and history taking so that important information is not overlooked.

Some dermatologic disorders are age related, so age is important in the dermatology history. For example, demodicosis usually begins in young dogs before sexual maturity. Allergies tend to appear in more mature individuals, probably because repeated exposure to the antigen must occur before clinical signs develop. Hormonal disorders tend to occur in animals between 6 and 10 years of age, and most neoplasms develop in mature to older patients.

The sex of the patient obviously limits the incidence of certain problems, but it is especially important in sex hormone imbalances. Perianal adenomas are seen almost exclusively in male dogs. One should determine whether the patient is sexually intact and, if so, whether the skin problem bears any relationship to the estrous cycle.

Breed predilection determines the incidence of some skin disorders. For example, seborrhea is common in cocker spaniels; acanthosis nigricans usually occurs in Dachshunds; adult-onset hyposomatotropism occurs in Pomeranians, Keeshonds, and Chow Chows; dermatomyositis is found in Shetland Sheepdogs and Collies; zinc-responsive dermatosis occurs in Siberian Huskies and Alaskan Malamutes; and many of the wire-coated terrier breeds (Scotties, Cairns, Sealyhams, West Highland Whites, Irish Terriers, and Welsh Terriers) seem to be particularly predisposed to allergic skin disease.

Next, the following information should be obtained from the owner's history sheet: date of onset, original locations of the lesions, description of the initial lesions, tendency to progression or regressions, factors affecting the course and duration, and previous treatment (home, proprietary, or pet shop remedies used, as well as prescribed therapies).

EXAMINATION

Recording historical facts, physical findings, and laboratory data in a systematic way is particularly important for patients with skin disease. Many dermatoses are chronic, and skin lesions are slow to change. For this reason, outline sketches of the patient enable the clinician to draw in the location and extent of lesions. One sketch is worth many words, and comparison of sketches made at different intervals graphically portrays changes in the lesions over time.

Figure 2-18 illustrates a conventional record form for noting physical and laboratory findings for dermatology cases. The special form enables one to circle pertinent descriptive terms, saves time, and ensures that no important information is omitted. This form details only dermatologic data and should be used as a supplement to the general history and physical examination record. A special dermatologic history form, completed by the client, is also useful for patients with documented allergy or other chronic skin disease (Figure 2-19).

2

DERMATOLOGY EXAMINATION

DISTRIBUTION OF LESIONS

Weight ———

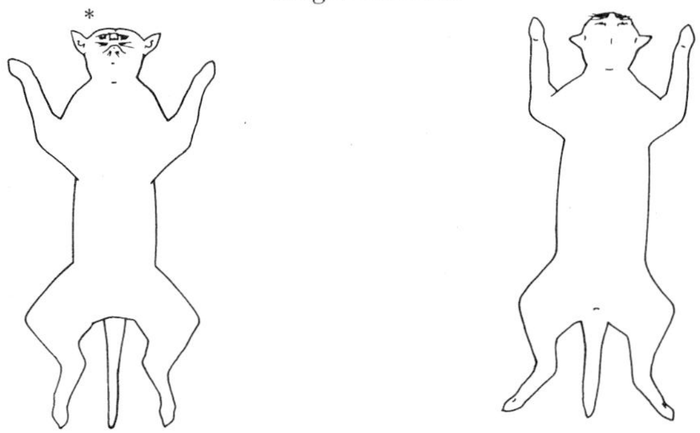

Ventral

Dorsal

PRIMARY LESIONS (Check)

Macule	———	Patch	———	Purpura	———	Wheal	———
Papule	———	Nodule	———	Plaque	———	Tumor	———
Pustule	———	Vesicle	———	Bullae	———	Cyst	———
Abscess	———				

SECONDARY LESIONS (Check)

Scale ——— Crust ——— Alopecia ——— Erythema ———
Erosion ——— Ulcer ——— Fissure ——— Scar ———
Excoriation ——— Collarettes ——— Nikolsky ———
Hyperpigmentation ——— Hypopigmentation ——— Callus ———
Hyperkeratosis ——— Lichenification ——— Comedone ———
Sinus ——— Hyperhidrosis ——— Necrosis ———

SKIN CHANGES (Check)

Normal ——— Thick ——— Thin ——— Fragile ———
Hypotonic ——— Hyperextensible ——— Increased Laxity ———

OTHER FINDINGS

Pinal-Pedal Reflex ———
Lymph Nodes ———

Figure 2-18: Example: Physical examination form appropriate for use in patients presented for complex or chronic dermatologic problems.

Continued

HAIRCOAT CHANGES (Check)

Alopecia ___	Hypotrichosis ___	Hypertrichosis ___
Dry Coat ___	Brittle Coat ___	Oily Coat ___
Easy Epilation ___	1°Hairs ___ 2°Hairs ___	Both ___
Hair Casts ___	Color Associated Hair Loss ___	

CONFIGURATION OF LESIONS (Check)

Linear ___	Follicular ___	Grouped ___
Annular ___	Other ___	

PRURITUS (Check)

Seasonal ___	Nonseasonal ___	Lesional ___
Face ___	Ears ___	Feet/Legs ___ Rump ___
Axillae ___	Abdomen ___	Other ___

CUTANEOUS PAIN (Check)

Absent ___	Mild ___	Moderate ___	Severe ___

PARASITES (Check)

Fleas ___	Flea Dirt ___	Lice ___ Ticks ___
Ear Mites ___	Other ___	

*Can have either dog or cat outline here

Ears L ___
R ___

Oral ___
Anogenital ___
Footpads ___
Nails ___
Other ___

LABORATORY

Scrape ___
Scotch Tape ___
Fungal Cult ___
Wood's Light ___
Hair Exam ___
ID Hist ___ Flea 15 ___ Flea 24 ___
Cytology ___
1. ___
2. ___
3. ___
4. ___

DIAGNOSIS/DIFFERENTIAL

___
___
___
___

Figure 2-18, contd.

2

When was the problem first noted? ———— Day ———— Month ———— Year

Where on the body did the problem begin? ————

Is the problem: ———— Year Round ———— Seasonal ———— Unknown

If seasonal, in which season(s) is it worse? ———— Spring ———— Summer ———— Fall ———— Winter

If nonseasonal, is it worse in any season? ————

Does the animal itch (scratch, chew, lick, rub)? ———— Yes ———— No

Is the itching: ———— Mild ———— Moderate ———— Severe ———— Constant ———— Periodic

Where does the animal itch? Check those areas which are itchy.

Face: ————	Abdomen: ————	Lower Back: ————
Ears: ————	Front Feet/Legs: ————	All Over: ————
Arm Pits: ————	Back Feet/Legs: ————	

What medications have been used?

Drug   *How Much*   *How Often*   *Did It Help?*

———— ———— ———— ————

———— ———— ———— ————

———— ———— ———— ————

Do parents, littermates, other animals in the house or other animals in the area have a similar problem? ———— Yes ———— No

On the reverse side, please provide any information which you feel is important.

Figure 2–19: Example: Dermatology history form for owners to complete on patients with complex or chronic dermatologic problems.

Continued

DERMATOLOGY HISTORY

Chief Complaint:

_____   Itching   _____   Sores

_____   Hair loss   _____   Ear Disease

_____ Other _____

Aside from the skin problem is the animal healthy?

_____ Yes _____ No

(Please Specify) _____

_____

_____

_____

_____

_____

Figure 2-19, contd.

The examination should be performed with good lighting. Normal daylight without glare is best, but any artificial light of adequate candlepower is sufficient if it produces bright, uniform lighting. The lamp should be adjustable to illuminate all body areas. A combination loupe and light magnifies and illuminates the field. Before evaluating individual lesions, the entire animal should be observed from a distance for a general impression of abnormalities and to observe distribution patterns. Does the animal appear to be in good health? Is it fat or thin, unkempt or well groomed? Is the problem generalized or localized? What is the distribution of the lesions? Are they bilaterally symmetric or unilaterally irregular?

Palpation of the skin is important. What is the texture of the hair? Is it coarse or fine, dry or oily, and does it epilate easily? A change in the amount of hair present is often a dramatic finding. Alopecia is a complete lack of hair in areas where hair is normally present. Hypotrichosis implies a partial alopecia that may be developmental, hormonal, neoplastic, inflammatory, or idiopathic. Hypertrichosis is excess hair and, although very rare in animals, is usually hormonal or developmental in nature.

The texture, elasticity, and thickness of the skin should be determined and impressions of heat or coolness recorded. It is important to examine every inch of skin and mucous membranes. It is easier to find important skin lesions in some breeds than in others, depending on the thickness of the coat. The density of an individual's coat varies in different body areas. Lesions can be discerned more easily in sparsely haired regions. However, the clinician must part or clip the hair in many areas to observe and palpate lesions that are partially covered. It is useful to clip hair over an area of abnormal skin with a surgical clipper blade to expose the area for identification of lesions. The clipped area is then cleansed with alcohol. Lesions previously hidden by hair and debris can now be clearly seen and interpreted. It is as if a window appears giving a new view of the skin disease. When abnormalities are discovered, it is important to establish their general distribution as well as their configuration within an area. Are they single, multiple, discrete, diffuse, grouped, or confluent? With sharp observation, linear or annular configuration of the lesions may be noted.

Assessment of individual lesions

The evolution of lesions should be determined from the history or by finding different stages of lesions on the same patient (Table 2-7). Papules often develop into vesicles and pustules, which may rupture to leave erosions or ulcers with epidermal collarettes and finally crusts. An understanding of these processes helps in the diagnostic process. As lesions

---

TABLE 2-7 Classification of Skin Lesions

Primary lesions (lesions of first diagnostic importance)

Macule–patch	Pustule	Tumor–neoplasm	
Papule–plaque	Nodule	Vesicle–bulla	Wheal

Secondary lesions (evolutionary or complicating lesion of secondary diagnostic importance)

Scale–epidermal collarette	Comedo	Pigmentary abnormalities
Crust	Fissure	(hyperpigmentation or
Scar	Excoriation	hypopigmentation)
Erosion–ulcer	Lichenification	Hyperkeratosis–callus

From Muller GH, Kirk RW, Scott DW: *Small animal dermatology,* ed 4. Philadelphia, WB Saunders, 1989, p 104.

---

develop in special patterns, they also involute in characteristic ways. Acute lesions often appear suddenly and disappear quickly and completely. Chronic lesions may leave diagnostically important pigmentation or scars that persist for months or become permanent (i.e., chronic generalized demodicosis and juvenile cellulitis, respectively).

Morphology of skin lesions is the essential feature of dermatologic diagnosis and sometimes is the *only* guide if laboratory procedures yield no useful information. *Most skin diseases are characterized by a single type of lesion.*

The clinician must learn to recognize primary and secondary lesions. A **primary skin lesion** is one that develops spontaneously as a direct reflection of underlying disease. A **secondary skin lesion** evolves from primary lesions or are artifacts induced by the patient or by external factors such as trauma or medications (Table 2-8). Careful inspection of the diseased skin will frequently reveal a primary lesion suggestive of a specific dermatosis. In many cases, however, the significant lesion must be differentiated from the mass of secondary debris. The ability to discover a characteristic lesion and understand its significance is the first step toward mastering dermatologic diagnosis. Variations are common, since early as well as advanced stages exist in most skin diseases. In addition, the appearance of skin lesions may change with medication, self-inflicted trauma, and secondary infection.

The following basic tests are indicated in assessing the severity and extent of dermatologic lesions in dogs and cats:

Several simple techniques for initial examination of skin lesions should be considered:

1. **Diascopy.** This technique entails pressing a clear piece of plastic or glass (a clean microscope slide) over an erythematous lesion. If the lesion blanches on pressure, the erythema is due to vascular engorgement. If the lesion does not blanch, there is hemorrhage into the skin (petechiae or ecchymoses).

2. **Nikolsky's sign.** This sign is elicited by applying pressure on a vesicle or pustule or at the edge of an ulcer or erosion or even on normal skin. The result is positive when the outer layer of the skin is easily rubbed off or pushed away. This indicates poor cellular cohesion, as found in the pemphigus complex, pemphigoid, and toxic epidermal necrolysis.

3. **Skin scrapings.** This procedure can be performed (gently) with a No. 10 surgical blade, mineral oil (as a vehicle to suspend material in), and a glass slide. Assessment centers on identification of ectoparasites, using a microscope.

4. **Wood's lamp.** This ultraviolet light source with a cobalt or nickel filter is used to *screen* patients for the presence of dermatophytes. Some experience is required in making accurate interpretations as keratinized skin, and debris in the hair may appear to fluoresce. The Wood's lamp test is not positive in all dermatophytoses. In fact, it's estimated that less than half of the patients with fungal skin disease will have a positive Wood's lamp test. A negative Wood's lamp test does NOT rule out dermatophytosis as the diagnosis.

TABLE 2-8   Systemic Diseases With Cutaneous Lesions

Disease	Skin lesions or signs
Atopy	Pruritus
Castration-responsive dermatosis	Alopecia
Cold agglutinin diseases	Erytherma, purpura, necrosis, ulceration
Diabetes mellitus	Atrophy, ulceration, pyoderma, seborrhea
Dirofilariasis	Erythema, alopecia, pruritus, nodules
Erythema multiforme	Macules, papules, vesicles, wheals
Feline leukemia virus infection	Pyoderma, seborrhea, poor healing, cutaneous horns on footpads
Hepatocutaneous syndrome	Mucocutaneous crusts and ulcers, footpad hyperkeratosis and ulcers
Hyperadrenocorticism	Alopecia, hyperpigmentation, calcinosis cutis, pyoderma, seborrhea, phlebectasias, thin and hypotonic skin
Hypothyroidism	Alopecia, hypothermia, seborrhea, pyoderma, hyperpigmentation, myxedema, galactorrhea
Leishmaniasis	Erythema, nodules, ulceration, exfoliative dermatitis
Male feminizing syndrome	Alopecia, seborrhea, hyperpigmentation, gynecomastia, galactorrhea
Mycoses, deep	Nodules, ulceration, fistulas
Mycosis fungoides	Erythroderma, plaques, nodules, ulceration
Ovarian inbalances	Alopecia, hyperpigmentation, seborrhea
Pemphigus	Purulent exudate, crusting, vesiculation, ulceration/erosion
Pituitary dwarfism	Alopecia, cutaneous degeneration, hyperpigmentation
Sertoli cell tumor	Alopecia, gynecomastia, hyperpigmentation
Systemic lupus erythematosus	Pyoderma, seborrhea, ulceration, pruritus, erythema
Thallium toxicosis	Alopecia, erytherma, ulceration
Toxic epidermal necrolysis	Ulceration, blisters, pain
Tuberculosis	Nodules, ulceration, fistulas

From Muller GH, Kirk RW, Scott DW: *Small animal dermatology,* ed 4. Philadelphia, WB Saunders, 1989, p 100.

5. **Culture.** Submission of samples for bacterial or fungal cultures may be indicated in patients with particularly complex, chronic lesions that do not respond to empiric therapy. Hair samples from patients suspected of having a dermatophyte infection can be inoculated onto dermatophyte test medium (DTM). In addition, direct cytologic examination of skin scrapings and pustules may be helpful in assessing the underlying cause.

6. **Acetate tape.** Applying acetate (clear) adhesive tape to the hair coat may actually capture diagnostic organisms (e.g., *Chyletiella* spp. mites ["walking dandruff"]). In addition, the acetate tape may be stained with lactophenol cotton blue or Diff-Quick for further cytologic evaluation.

7. **Skin biopsy.** Using 4-mm, 6-mm, or 8-mm punch biopsy instruments, full-thickness skin biopsies, obtained from the *appropriate locations,* can be particularly useful in establishing a diagnosis. Location of the biopsy is critical in obtaining diagnostic tissue. Generally, multiple lesions should be biopsied. *Surgical preparation of the skin is NOT recommended,* as this will alter the histologic appearance of the sample and may compromise the ability to establish a diagnosis.

8. **Allergen-specific IgE serology.** Serum is submitted to a diagnostic laboratory for in vitro testing of atopic dermatitis.

Note: IgE serology is not indicated for patients with suspected food allergy. Although the quality of serologic assays for allergic skin disease has improved, some concerns are expressed by dermatologists over the predictive value of these tests.

9. **Intradermal skin testing.** This testing platform is valuable in diagnosing and managing allergic skin disease *but* must be performed and interpreted by a dermatologist or an individual with considerable experience with intradermal skin testing.

Cutaneous manifestations of systemic disease

Cutaneous changes that accompany internal disease may result from simultaneous involvement of skin and internal organs with identical pathologic mechanisms (multicentric disease), direct extension of an internal disease process to the skin, immunologic manifestations of a deficient or hyperactive immune system, hormonal deficiency or excess, or metabolic derangements. These cutaneous changes may be obvious or subtle, mild or extensive, or incidental or specific. When the cutaneous change has a high correlation to a specific internal disease process, the lesions are referred to as a marker of internal disease (Table 2-9). Clinicians must examine the patient with dermatologic disease while considering internal pathologic factors.

2

TABLE 2-9   Systemic Diseases Having a Primary Dermatologic Presentation

Category	Representative diseases	Manifestions
Fungal	> Deep mycoses -Blastomycosis -Histoplasmosis -Crytococcosis -Coccidioidomycosis > *Pithium insidiosum* > *Lagenidium* spp.	Nodules Draining tracts Suppurative ulceration (can be aggressive in patients with *Pithium isidiosum* infection) Plaques
Viral	> Canine distemper virus > Feline herpesvirus-1 and calicivirus > Feline leukemia virus and feline immunodeficiency virus	> Hyperkeratosis (foot pads and nasal planum) > Oral and cutaneous ulceration, keratitis > Gingivitis, stomatitis, pyoderma, recurrent abscesses, demodectic mange, dermatophytosis
Bacterial	> Tick-borne infections - Rocky Mountain spotted fever group - *Ehrlichia* spp. > Leptospirosis	> Petechiae, ecchymoses, edema > Icterus, petechiae
Parasitic	> Leishmaniasis (protozoa) > Demodicosis (mite)	> Exfoliative dermatitis on the head, neck, and extremities; periocular alopecia, ulcerative dermatitis > Focal, regional, or generalized alopecia, erythema, superficial or deep pyoderma (secondary bacterial dermatitis)

Continued

TABLE 2-9 Systemic Diseases Having a Primary Dermatologic Presentation—cont'd

Category	Representative diseases	Manifestions
Immune mediated	> Pemphigus and the bullous dermatoses.	> Cutaneous ulcerations and secondary pyoderma
	> Erythema multiforme	> Erythematous macule and papules (often associated with neoplasia)
	> Systemic lupus erythematosus (SLE)	> Highly variable; includes seborrhea, alopecia, regionally erythema, nasal dermatitis, etc.
	> Ischemic vasculitis	> Ulcerative skin lesions (hypersensitivity reaction) to drugs, vaccines, insect bites
	> Hemolytic uremic syndrome	> Described in Greyhounds as cutaneous ulceration in patients with renal failure (associated with *E. coli* toxin in consumed raw beef)
	> Dermatomyositis	> Pustules, vesicles, papules that progress to alopecia/crusting on the tips of the ears, face, and carpus and tarsus; seen in collies and Shetland sheepdogs primarily
Neoplasia	> Feline vaccine-associated sarcoma (VAS)	> Aggressive fibrosarcoma associated primarily with adjuvanted FeLV and Rabies vaccines in cats; may occur months to years following inoculation
	> Multiple primary skin tumors	> Mast cell tumor, lymphoma, squamous cell carcinoma, etc.; melanoma in skin of dogs is reported but is typically benign, despite histological appearance of cells
	> Nodular dermatofibrosis	> Subcutaneous nodules (coalescing) with associated alopecia and hyperpigmentation; seen most often in German shepherds, Boxers, and golden retrievers, but seen occasionally in other breeds; may be associated with renal disease
	> Testicular neoplasia	> Male feminization syndrome
	> Pheochromocytoma	> Intermittent flushing, especially of the pinnae; other systemic signs are associated with this tumor
	> Paraneoplastic syndromes	> Various focal and regional changes in skin are reported, including fissures, nodular skin disease, pemphigus vulgaris, necrotizing panniculitis, and exfoliative dermatitis in cats (thymoma)
Endocrine	> Hypothyroidism, canine	> Dry hair coat, symmetric, nonpruritic (usually) truncal alopecia, hyperpigmentation, seborrheic skin disease
	> Hyperthyroidism, feline	> Poor hair coat, matting, excessive shedding, increased nail growth
	> Hyperadrenocorticism (canine Cushings syndrome)	> Symmetric, truncal alopecia, comedones, thinning of the skin, failure of hair regrowth after clipping; calcinosis cutis (~5% of cases)
	> Diabetes mellitus	> Otitis externa, pyoderma, demodectic mange, thin skin, pyoderma, seborrheic skin disease, and in cats, xanthoma formation
Nutritional	> Vitamin E deficiency in cats	> Pansteatitis

Systemic disease should be suspected in patients with dermatologic disorders when the following conditions are observed:

1. Dermatologic disease concurrent with systemic illness, such as fever, depression, or clinical signs consistent with a particular organ system (e.g., diarrhea, lameness).
2. Bizarre or atypical dermatoses.
3. Chronic recurring dermatoses, including pyoderma, scaling, and so forth.
4. Dermatoses in unexpected patients (e.g., age, breed, sex).
5. Dermatologic signs following illness or drug administration.

Distribution patterns of skin lesions

A dramatic change becomes apparent when a skin disorder affects an animal whose body is covered with a dense hair coat. Even the most casual observer is aware of the loss or hair in certain areas. The alopecic pattern, which is often sharply demarcated, assumes a new meaning when it is accurately interpreted. When alopecia and other hair changes are evaluated according to their distribution pattern over the entire body, significant diagnostic clues appear. Comparatively speaking, only on the human scalp is alopecia as striking and meaningful.

In animals, the primary or secondary skin lesions are often hidden under the hair coat; in fact, it requires painstaking observation to see them. In short-coated animals, if you stand behind the animal and use both hands to roll the skin into a horizontal fold, it is possible to see between the erected hair shafts to the skin surface. By rolling the fold backward, you can see progressively new areas of skin surface and get an impression of the distribution of lesions. Only when the animal is clipped can one see the distribution pattern of such lesions with ease and accuracy. Consequently, in animals there are two distinctly different patterns that aid in diagnosis: (1) the changes in external hair coat and (2) the definition and distribution of primary and secondary skin lesions. These two factors do not necessarily have a reciprocal relationship. In addition, it is important to recognize whether the lesions present a symmetric distribution on either side of the midline or an asymmetric distribution.

Stages of skin disease

As a skin disease progresses from its earliest appearance to its final fully developed state, the pattern necessarily changes. A small patch or alopecia can enlarge into almost total hair loss in some cases. Obviously, if all intermediate stages of such a disease were drawn diagrammatically, the result would be more confusing than helpful. Therefore, it is necessary to select for each skin disorder the single distribution pattern that is of greatest diagnostic value. Different stages of each disease exist, and the total impact of the diagram should be interpreted with that fact always in mind. In addition, note that the distribution pattern represents alopecia or changes of the skin surface or both.

Additional Reading

Ihrke PJ: Pruritus. In Ettinger SJ, Feldman EC, editors: *Textbook of veterinary internal medicine,* ed 6, St. Louis, 2005, Elsevier, pp. 38-43.

Lewis DT: Dermatologic disorders. In Schaer M, editor: *Clinical medicine of the dog and cat,* Ames, 2003, Iowa State Press (Blackwell), pp. 9-43.

Scott DW, Miller WH, Griffin CE: *Muller and Kirk's small animal dermatology,* ed 6, Philadelphia, 2001, WB Saunders.

OPHTHALMIC (OCULAR) EXAMINATION

THE GLOBE AND ADNEXA

A general inspection of the globe and external ocular structures should be conducted before any detailed examination of the eye is undertaken. Inspect the globe in normal daylight or room light and observe the relationship of the globe to the orbit and the eyelids. Note whether the eyes are in the same visual axis or whether atropia is present. Observe any undue prominence of either or both eyes. Note the presence of any other facial lesions (e.g., facial paralysis) that may affect the symmetry of the orbit. Inspect the external ocular structures (lids, conjunctiva, cornea, sclera, and lacrimal apparatus). Note the position of the eyelids; the size of the palpebral aperture; the position of the nictitating membrane; and the presence of nystagmus (involuntary, rapid oscillations of the eyes), anisocoria (unequal pupils), blepharospasm (tonic spasm of the eyelids), lagophthalmos (drooping of the eyelid), or ocular discharges.

The tonic eye reflexes

Tonic eye reflexes are used to assess extraocular muscle function and localization of lesions in the CNS. Cranial nerves III (oculomotor), IV (trochlear), and VI (abducent) innervate the extraocular striated muscles and are examined together. Cranial nerve IV innervates the obliquus dorsalis; cranial nerve VI innervates the rectus lateralis and part of the retractor bulbi; and cranial nerve III innervates the rectus medialis and rectus ventralis, obliquus ventralis, and levator palpebrae superioris. Pupillary dilation is controlled by preganglionic neurons in the first three thoracic spinal cord segments, the cranial thoracic and cervical sympathetic trunks, and by postganglionic neurons in the cranial thoracic and cervical trunks, and in the cranial cervical and sympathetic nerves that course through the middle ear to reach the orbit and the dilator pupillae muscle. Parasympathetic fibers in cranial nerve III innervate the sphincter pupillae muscle. The integrity of cranial nerve III may be evaluated by examining (1) the size and symmetry of the pupils; (2) the reaction of the pupil to light; (3) the presence or absence of ptosis (drooping of the upper eyelid) because of paralysis of the levator palpebrae superioris muscle; and (4) the medial deviation of the eye, which occurs in oculomotor nerve palsy (different from humans). In oculomotor nerve palsy with a normal pupillary response, if all the extraocular muscles innervated by cranial nerve III are affected, an intracranial lesion should be suspected. If individual extraocular muscles are involved, a peripheral nerve lesion may exist. If an oculomotor nerve palsy exists in association with a dilated pupil, an intraorbital or intracranial lesion should be suspected.

Paralysis of the trochlear nerve produces a transient strabismus and results in a slight upward deviation of the eye (rarely seen). The affected animal may compensate for this by developing a head tilt. Paralysis of the abducent nerve results in a medial deviation of the affected eye with inability to gaze laterally.

It is important to examine tonic neck and eye reflexes when evaluating the extraocular muscles. When the nose is elevated, the forelimbs extend and the hindlimbs flex. As the nose is elevated, the eye should remain focused within the center of the palpebral fissure. Deviating the head to the left (or right) results in increased extensor tonus on the right (or left) side of the neck. Nystagmus is an abnormal, involuntary rapid movement of the eye that denotes a disorder (stimulation) at some level of the vestibular tract; movement may be horizontal, vertical, rotory, or mixed. In a normal animal, nystagmus can be observed during lateral deviation of the head (with the quick phase toward the side of the deviation). Normal tonic eye reflexes signify a healthy brain stem and peripheral vestibular system and motor efferent pathways to the eyes. Tonic eye reflexes are not dependent on vision.

Pupillary light reflexes (PLR)

Cranial nerve II (optic) has its origin in the retina at the optic disk. About 66% of the optic nerve fibers in the cat and about 75% in the dog decussate (cross over) at the optic chiasm. The optic nerve has two components: one is composed of the fibers that pass to the pupillary centers within the brain stem; the other is composed of fibers that synapse in the thalamus and project impulses to the visual cortex of the brain. The normal pupillary response requires that nerves II and III be intact. The normal DIRECT pupillary light reflex entails centering a beam of focused light into one eye and observing pupillary constriction (miosis). Recovery should be immediate following removal of the light. The normal consensual pupillary light reflex entails directing a beam of focused light into one eye then noting pupillary constriction in the opposite eye.

External appearance of the eye

Note the color of the sclera, and look for nodules, hemorrhages, lacerations, cysts, and tumors. Normal sclera is white to blue-white. The sclera may appear blue when it is abnormally thinned and the uveal tract shows through. Look for staphylomas and for any injection of the scleral vessels and accompanying edema. Episcleritis can produce local scleral inflammation, whereas deep-seated ocular diseases such a glaucoma and uveitis produce generalized scleral vessel injection.

The cornea should be smooth, moist, free of blood vessels, and transparent. Note any ulceration or opacity of the cornea. Slight opacities are termed nebulae; dense ones are called leukomas. In puppies, the cornea tends to be hazy, which restricts ophthalmoscopic examination until the animals are 4 to 6 weeks of age. Diseases of the cornea, such as corneal inflammation, pigmentation, degeneration, trauma, and neoplasia, frequently may alter its transparency. Test the corneal sensitivity by touching the cornea with a wisp of dry cotton.

Topically applied ophthalmic fluorescein stains are routinely used to diagnose lesions of the cornea. Any break in the epithelial barrier permits rapid penetration of fluorescein into the stroma as a deep green color outlining the lesion. It cases of deep corneal ulcers, fluorescein may actually penetrate into the anterior chamber. When the epithelial surface has regenerated, the green color no longer appears. Rose bengal dye stains cells and their nuclei. The dye selectively stains devitalized corneal and conjunctival epithelium a readily visible red. The main use of this dye has been in the identification of corneal and conjunctival lesions caused by keratitis sicca.

If an ulcer is present, note whether the borders are regular or irregular and whether the ulcer is superficial or deep. With ulcers that are progressive and deep, the prognosis is guarded. It is advisable to culture deep ulcers and to take scrapings of their borders. The scrapings should be stained with Giemsa, and the type of cells should be determined. If the ulcer appears to be deep, look for evidence of anterior synechiae, prolapsed iris, iridocyclitis, cataract, extrusion of the lens, fistula, or hemorrhage.

Note the presence of blood vessels in the cornea. The depth at which vascularization is taking place is usually directly related to the cause of the vascularization. Superficial vascularization is commonly associated with superficial keratitis, superficial ulcers, or pannus. Deep vascularization usually indicates a deep corneal stromal lesion, uveitis, or glaucoma.

Look for deposits on the posterior surface of the cornea (keratic precipitates). These precipitates vary in size and shape, but they are usually indicative of a disease of infectious disease (e.g., feline infectious peritonitis virus) (Figure 2-20).

ASSESSMENT OF VISION

Objective signs and reflexes must be used to assess vision in dogs and cats. A vision test often used to assess vision is the "menace reaction." This test involves passing the hand or an object in front of the animal's eyes and noticing the presence or absence of a blink reflex. However, movement of air across the cornea may prompt a blink reflex in a blind animal. Preferably, a cotton ball can be tossed repeatedly in front of an animal to assess its ability to visually track movement. In some cases, it may be important to assess vision in each eye independently. A temporary blindfold can be made with adhesive or masking tape sufficient to cover one eye. Tracking is assessed using a cotton ball. The test is repeated with the opposite eye covered. An obstacle course can also be valuable in assessing visual function. Styrofoam cylinders mounted on a platform can be used to create the course. The light intensity in the examining room can be varied, and alternate patching of the eyes can be helpful for detecting lesions.

Note: Blind dogs and cats do memorize obstacles within their environment and at home, commonly giving the owner the impression that vision is normal.

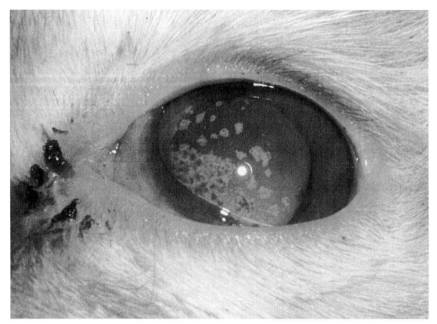

Figure 2-20:   Keratic precipitates in a cat infected with the feline infectious peritonitis (FIP) virus.

EXAMINATION OF THE ORBIT

Observe the orbit for size. Look for swelling, depression, fistulas, or laceration of the orbital margin. If the orbit is enlarged, note whether the swelling is hard or soft, painful or nonpainful. Retrobulbar abscesses produce exophthalmos (protrusion of the globe) accompanied by pain, immobility of the eye, chemosis (swelling of the conjunctiva), edema of the eyelids, and pain on opening of the mouth. Orbital tumors may not be painful. Orbital retrobulbar hemorrhage or orbital fracture may occur following severe head trauma from automobile accidents. Enophthalmos, abnormal retraction of the eye, may result from shrinkage of orbital contents (as in pthisis bulbi following ocular injury), from paralysis of the sympathetic nerve in Horner's syndrome, or from loss of retrobulbar fat in emaciation and dehydration.

EXAMINATION OF THE EYELIDS

Note any inflammation along the margins of the eyelids and any inability to close the lids (lagophthalmos). The eyelids should touch the globe, thus preventing accumulation of tears and debris. The cilia or eyelashes on the dog's upper eyelids are arranged in three irregular rows. The lower eyelids of dogs and both eyelids of cats are devoid of cilia (eyelashes). When examining the lids for the presence of entropion (inversion of the eyelid margin) or ectropion (eversion of the eyelid margin), do not manipulate the head since this may distort the normal lid-globe relationship. The lids of dogs and cats have a very poorly developed tarsal plate, which makes manipulation relatively easy. Observe the edges of the lids for signs of entropion, ectropion, trichiasis (aberrant eyelashes directed at the cornea), or distichiasis (a double row of eyelashes some of which are directed at the cornea). Observe the eyelids for symblepharon (adhesion between the conjunctiva of the eyelid and the globe) or for swelling, edema, redness, or localized inflammation, which may indicate an internal or external hordeolum (sty, or inflammation of the sebaceous glands of the eyelid). Examine the lid margins for indication of any growths. The most common or benign, epithelial growth observed on the lids of older dogs is the papilloma. The most common benign, adnexal-derived growth observed in older dogs is the sebaceous gland adenoma.

EXAMINATION OF THE CONJUNCTIVA

Note whether the conjunctiva is pale, injected (hyperemic), pigmented, hemorrhagic, or jaundiced. The inferior or ventral conjunctiva normally is more hyperemic than the upper conjunctiva. Pigmentation is occasionally present in normal dogs and cats, especially on the superior bulbar conjunctiva. Usually, a few follicles are visible on the conjunctival surface, especially that of the third eyelid in normal animals. Note whether the conjunctiva is relatively smooth and dry, excessively moist, or abnormally congested. Note any lacerations or erosions of the conjunctiva. Lacerations or erosions may be demonstrated using fluorescein. After initial inspection of the conjunctiva, additional tests may be required, such as the Schirmer tear test, culture, cytologic examination, or the use of stains.

Conjunctivitis (also called "red eye") is a common, yet complex, presenting sign that can involve one or both eyes. It is critical, when assessing a dog or cat that presents with a "red eye," to determine whether the underlying problem is caused by congestion of superficial vessels of the eye or a problem deeper within the eye. The differential diagnoses for "red eye" are listed in Table 2-10.

Nictitating membrane (also called "third eyelid")

The palpebral (outer) and bulbar (inner) surfaces of the nictitating membrane should be inspected. The anterior surface of the membrane is normally smooth, and the leading edge is frequently pigmented. The bulbar surface can be examined by placing two to three drops of topical anesthetic (proparacaine hydrochloride) onto the eye. Using a cotton-tipped

TABLE 2-10 Differential Diagnosis Distinguishing between Conjunctivitis, Iritis, and Glaucoma

	Acute conjunctivitis	Acute iritis	Acute glaucoma
Onset	Gradual	Acute	Acute
Pain	None to mild irritation	Fairly severe	Fairly severe
Discharge	Mucopurulent or purulent	Tearing	None
Vision	Unaffected	Slightly reduced	May be markedly reduced
Conjunctiva	Superficial congestion	Deep circumcorneal and ciliary congestion	Deep conjuctival, episcleral, and ciliary congestion
Cornea	Clear	Keratic precipitates may be present	Steamy and insensitive
Iris	Unaffected	Muddy and congested; posterior synechiae may be present	Congested and displaced forward
Pupil	Normal	Contracted	Dilated
Anterior chamber	Unaffected	May contain cells, opacities, and exudates	Shallow
Tenderness	Absent	Present over ciliary body	Usually absent
Intraocular pressure	Unaffected	Lower than normal	Increased
Constitutional signs	Absent	Slight	Slight to moderate

applicator or small, atraumatic thumb forceps, the third eyelid can be everted and the area of the glans nictitans can be examined. The bulbar surface normally contains a few small follicles. The following abnormalities are frequently associated with the third eyelid: laceration, eversion of the cartilage, protrusion, inflammation and hypertrophy of the glans nictitans (also called "cherry eye"), foreign bodies, and neoplasia.

Examination of the Lacrimal System

Excessive tearing (epiphora) and decrease of tear secretion (sicca) are important disorders that can be easily assessed by measuring tear production with the Schirmer Tear Test strips. Basic tear secretion comes mainly from the tarsal and conjunctival glands and the accessory tarsal glands. Reflex tear production comes from the main lacrimal gland and accessory lacrimal glands. The Schirmer Tear Test is performed by placing a single tear strip over the lower eyelid and holding in place 1 minute. In normal dogs, wetting of Schirmer test papers ranges from 10 to 25 mm in 1 minute. Both eyes should be tested.

Note any swelling, redness, or pain in the area of the lacrimal puncta and the lacrimal sac. Excessive tearing may be real, apparent, or physiologic. When excessive tearing exists, it must be determined whether the tearing is real (i.e., due to increased lacrimal secretion from chronic ocular irritation, as in distichiasis or trichiasis), is apparent (i.e., due to partial or complete obstruction of the excretory duct system), or is physiologic (i.e., due to transient stimulation, such as corneal drying resulting from the dog holding its head out the window of the car during the trip to the hospital).

Fluorescein dye can be used to assess patency of the nasolacrimal duct. To perform this exam, place a drop of fluorescein dye from a sterile fluorescein strip into the eye and add one to two drops of a sterile eyewash. After 2 to 5 minutes, examine the external nares with the aid of a cobalt blue filter or Wood's light for the presence or absence of fluorescence. If dye is present, the lacrimal excretory system is patent and functioning. If epiphora exists but the primary dye test indicates that the lacrimal excretory system is patent, hypersecretion of tear fluid may be implicated as the cause of the epiphora.

Irrigation of the nasolacrimal system is indicated if the primary dye test is negative. In the dog, the nasolacrimal puncta are located 1 to 3 mm from the medial canthus on the mucocutaneous border of the upper and lower lids. In the dog, a 20- to 22-gauge (in the cat, a 23-gauge) nasolacrimal cannula should be used, often under topical anesthesia. A 3-mL syringe is filled with 1 to 2 mL of sterile saline. The lacrimal cannula is attached and passed into the lacrimal puncta of the upper lid; the technique is repeated on the lower lid (see Section 4 for a description of how to flush the nasolacrimal ducts).

Several points should be made about evaluating the nasolacrimal system. Brachycephalic breeds of dogs and cats may occasionally have a negative primary dye test, although no blockage in the nasolacrimal system exists. In flushing the nasolacrimal system of some animals, fluid may not appear at the nose; however, the animal may gag and exhibit swallowing movements, indicating that the fluid has entered the mouth and the system is patent.

Examination of the Anterior Chamber

Examine the anterior chamber, and observe its depth; note changes in the transparency of the ocular media, such as hypopyon, hyphema, fibrin, or foreign bodies. Look for anterior synechiae, and make sure the lens is in the normal position. The anterior drainage angle cannot be visualized readily in the dog without the use of a gonioscopic contact lens (discussed later). Large tumors and some anterior synechiae can be visualized with a loupe and a focal light source.

NORMAL TEAR SECRETION
Dogs: 10 to 25 mm in 1 minute **Cats:** > 10 mm in 1 minute

EXAMINATION OF THE IRIS

The color of the iris in each eye may vary. Observe the shape and size of the iris. An iris that is thickened and muddy in color indicates an infiltration of the uveal tract. Look for evidence of atrophy, tears, synechiae, persistent pupillary membranes, iridodonesis, iridodialysis, nodules, tumors, cysts, or colobomas. Examine the pupillary border of the iris for signs of atrophy or posterior synechiae to the anterior lens capsule. Complete posterior synechia results in iris bombé and secondary glaucoma.

Examine the pupil of each eye by diffuse and focal illumination. Note the size, shape, and symmetry of the pupils and perform both direct and consensual pupillary light reflex. Note any inequalities between the two pupils. Note whether the pupil of one eye is equal in size to the pupil of the other and whether the size remains equal with changes in the degree of illumination. Inequality of pupil size (anisocoria) may be caused by physiologic or pathologic factors.

2

> **Note:**   Sympathetic stimulation DILATES the pupil.
> Parasympathetic stimulation CONSTRICTS the pupil.

EXAMINATION OF THE LENS

The pupil must be dilated to properly examine the lens. The lens may be examined with a focal source of illumination, an ophthalmoscope or a slit lamp. Examine the lens for the presence of pigment, adhesions, opacities (cataract), the position of the lens (subluxation or luxation), or absence of the lens (aphakia). Normal refractive changes in the lens occur with aging and can be observed in dogs over 7 years and in cats over 8 years of age. This condition is called *nuclear sclerosis* and appears as a cloudy, white, or light-blue pupil often interpreted by owners as cataracts. Animals with nuclear sclerosis have functional vision. True opacities, however, of the lens, called *cataracts,* may impair vision and, if complete, can cause blindness.

EXAMINATION OF THE RETINA

The fundus is the portion of the inner eye that includes the optic disk or papilla, retinal vessels, tapetum lucidum, and tapetum nigrum. Complete visualization of the fundus requires the iris be dilated (using a 1% tropicamide topical ophthalmic solution). Dilation requires 15 to 20 minutes following instillation of the drug. Examine each fundus in a dark room. To examine the right fundus, hold the ophthalmoscope in the right hand and view the fundus with the right eye. Starting with the ophthalmoscope at 0 diopter setting, hold the ophthalmoscope about 20 inches from the patient's eye. Observe the pupil and the tapetal reflex. Bring the ophthalmoscope to within 1 inch of the patient's eye, and place the setting on 1 to 3 diopters (red numbers 1 to 3 on the rotating scale) to view the optic disk and retina. If the disk is not seen immediately, follow the retinal vessels back to the disk. Inserting more positive diopters (black numbers) into the ophthalmoscope focuses the instrument on more anterior structures within the eye.

OTIC (EAR) EXAMINATION

Among the most important aspects of the ear examination is careful observation of the patient at rest. Physical evidence of a painful ear (e.g., loss of hair around the ear, scratching or rubbing, frequent head-shaking, or head tilt) may facilitate localizing which ear, and which part of the ear, is affected. Externally compare one ear with the other. Observe the skin for signs of inflammation (swelling, redness, or desquamation of the epithelium). Movement and handling of the normal pinna should not produce pain. Look for discharges or blood emanating from the external ear canal.

An otoscope is required to examine the auditory canal. Use a clean or sterile otoscope speculum. Do not examine a noninfected ear with the speculum used in an infected ear. When feasible, always examine the noninfected or normal ear first. To examine the ear,

2

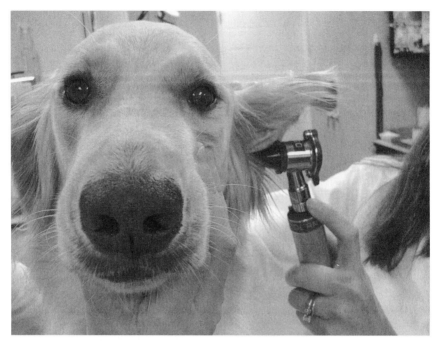

Figure 2-21: Position of the otoscope during examination of the external ear canal. Once the speculum is properly positioned in the ear canal, the pinna must gently be pulled downward and away from the head to facilitate visualization of the entire ear canal and tympanic membrane.

hold the otoscope with one hand and the pinna between the thumb and first two fingers of the other hand (Figure 2-21). Gently insert the speculum without using force while observing the external ear canal through the speculum. Slowly and carefully draw the ear laterally and turn the tip of the instrument medially to straighten the external canal. Otoscopes are provided with speculae of varying diameters.

Note: The largest diameter speculum may *not* necessarily provide the best visualization.

The tympanic membrane (eardrum) is a thin gray membrane through which a white curved bone (the malleus) and blood vessels can be observed along the dorsal margin (Figure 2-22). Every effort should be made to visualize the eardrum. However, considering that a dog's external ear canal is far more tortuous and much longer than a human external ear canal, deep examination of the ear canal in either a dog or cat is an uncomfortable procedure and may not be practical without sedation or general anesthesia. The tympanic membrane consists of a small upper portion, the pars flaccida, and a large lower part, the pars tensa. The membrane separates the horizontal portion of the external auditory canal from the middle ear. The posterior portion of the pars tensa is the part that is usually visualized to the greatest extent with the otoscope. The tense part of the tympanic membrane appears darker because the tympanic bulla of the middle ear can be seen through the eardrum. The eardrum can usually be seen in normal dogs younger than 1 year of age. It may be difficult to visualize the eardrum in older dogs, because the meatus is narrowed, the tense part of the eardrum is obscured by the flaccid part, the lining of the meatus obscures the eardrum, or the eardrum is ruptured, a common occurrence in dogs with chronic otitis externa.

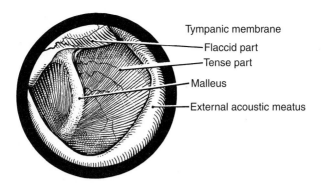

Tympanic membrane
Flaccid part
Tense part
Malleus
External acoustic meatus

2

Figure 2-22: The normal tympanic membrane ("eardrum") of a dog. (From Habel RE, deLahunta A: *Applied veterinary anatomy.* Philadelphia, 1986, WB Saunders.)

Any abnormal changes in the tympanic membrane, such as swelling, redness, loss of translucency, or absence of the membrane, should be recorded. Any concern that the tympanic membrane may have been penetrated or a thorough examination of the external ear canal is indicated justifies the use of general anesthesia.

CLEANING THE EAR CANAL

Otitis externa is associated with the accumulation of cerumen, exudate, bacteria, and tissue debris in the lumen and skin of the external ear canal. In many breeds, but especially Poodles, Bedlington Terriers, and Kerry Blue Terriers, the external ear canal contains hair that may prevent visualization through an otoscope. If the canal is filled with debris, the hair must be removed first. This can usually be accomplished by simple epilation (grab the hair and quickly pull). In dogs and cats with minor infections with only moderate accumulation of debris in the ear, it is recommended that a medical approach be used to treat the ear. Using cotton-tipped applicators in an attempt to remove debris deep in the ear canal is not recommended. Instilling an oil-based product into the external ear canal three to four times daily and massaging will loosen debris and treat the ear infection. Ceruminolytic agents can be irritating and are generally not used. Cotton-tipped applicators may be used to remove debris from the outer part of the external ear canal.

> **Note:** Cotton-tipped applicators are NOT recommended for removing debris deep in the external ear canal.

Deep cleaning of the ear canal should be done in the anesthetized patient using magnification. For all but very simple external cleaning, it is best to use gentle irrigation with warm-water solutions to clean the canal thoroughly and enable a complete otoscopic examination. Cotton-tipped applicators are NOT recommended as they will pack debris deep into the ear canal and, in turn, may result in rupture of the tympanic membrane.

Bacterial culture and sensitivity is indicated in patients with chronic otitis, inflamed tissues, or discharge in the external canal. Before the external canal can be examined visually, debris and discharges must be removed. To clear the ear before examination, a nontoxic cleaning agent should be instilled into the external ear canal. Numerous preparations are commercially available. Most solutions contain dilutions (2%) of acetic or boric acid, propylene glycol, and dioctyl sodium sulfosuccinate (DSS). Tris-EDTA solution is an alkalinization-inducing agent that can be instilled into the external ear canal in 5 mL aliquots to soften and facilitate removal of debris. In the anesthetized patient, the combination of a pulsating water jet (warm water) and an ear loop is recommended for cleaning a chronically infected ear (see Section 4). The irrigation stream is kept parallel to the external ear canal and is applied with a rotating motion. The excess water and debris can be caught in a sink or basin. The canal can then be reinspected and carefully dried with cotton or by using an aspirator. This technique is contraindicated in patients known to have a ruptured tympanic membrane.

Additional Reading

Gotthelf LN: Secondary otitis media: an often overlooked condition, *Canine Pract* 20:14-20, 1995.
Gotthelf LN, Young S: A new treatment for canine otitis externa, *Vet Forum* 14:46-83, 1997.
Radlinsky MG, Mason DE: Diseases of the ear. In Ettinger SJ, Feldman EC, editors: *Textbook of veterinary internal medicine,* ed 6, St. Louis, 2005, Elsevier, pp. 1168-1186.
Taibo RA: Otitis externa. In Taibo RA, editor: *Otology: clinical and surgical issues.* Buenos Aires, 2003, Intermedica.

LYMPH NODES AND THYROID EXAMINATION

CLINICAL HISTORY

Only occasionally does an owner present a dog or cat for evaluation of one or more enlarged lymph nodes. Even less commonly is the dog or cat presented specifically for an enlarged thyroid gland. In fact, an owner's evaluation of the skin is most likely to detect the presence of solitary cutaneous or subcutaneous lumps or masses (e.g., papillomas, sebaceous adenomas, lipomas, mast cell tumors) particularly in older patients. The clinician should therefore be particularly compelled to examine all peripheral lymph nodes *and* the entire ventral neck for evidence of abnormal enlargement in lymph nodes or thyroid glands.

EXAMINATION

Any routine physical examination, at any age, includes assessment of the size, consistency (degree of firmness), symmetry, and location of *all* peripheral lymph nodes and the thyroid glands. It is appropriate to include examination of the lymph nodes and thyroid glands with examination of the skin and hair coat. In the normal patient, this examination will generally be characterized by the ability to palpate small, symmetric submandibular lymph nodes and popliteal lymph nodes. Three additional pairs of peripheral lymph nodes, superficial cervical (also called "prescapular"), axillary, and inguinal lymph nodes, are sufficiently small (or anatomically out of reach: axillary lymph nodes) that palpation frequently is not possible in the normal patient. Considerable *normal* variation in lymph node size (and number) and texture is to be expected among dogs and cats of similar age, weight, and breed. The examination should focus on whether or not there is significant asymmetry or enlargement, *lymphadenomegaly,* of any individual or matched pairs of nodes. When all, some, or even one lymph node is significantly large (by subjective examination), fine needle aspiration and cytology are indicated. There is no known clinical significance attached to lymph nodes that are particularly small or that cannot be palpated during a physical examination.

Examination of the right and left thyroid glands is equally important in both dogs and cats. The preferred examination technique actually begins at the thoracic inlet, on either side of the trachea, rather than the larynx. Enlarged, or hypertrophied, thyroid glands (either individually or together) may migrate ventrally from their normal location adjacent to the larynx. In some cases, one or both enlarged thyroid glands may actually migrate into the cranial thorax and, therefore, may not be palpable. From the thoracic inlet, the examination proceeds by carefully palpating the neck on either side of the trachea, moving from the thoracic inlet to the larynx.

The normal thyroid gland is difficult, or impossible, to delineate on physical examination. Any asymmetric or symmetric enlargement should be noted. Also, the ability to palpate one or both thyroid glands in a location other than on either side of the larynx must be considered abnormal and likely to represent a significant pathologic condition.

Differential Diagnoses

The most serious consideration in any dog or cat with enlargement of one or more lymph nodes is lymphosarcoma, regardless of the patient's age, breed, or gender. However, there are also several nonmalignant causes of lymphadenomegaly that may mimic lymphosarcoma. Examples include generalized skin disease, systemic infection, and recent vaccination. Fine needle aspiration (see Sections 4 and 5 for additional information on collection and interpretation of lymph node aspiration cytology) is generally indicated in any patient with one or more enlarged, asymmetric lymph nodes. Lymph node biopsy (incisional) is strongly recommended in any patient having a lymph node with cytopathologic evidence of neoplasia. Rarely, surgical removal of an entire lymph node (excisional biopsy) is indicated. Feline leukemia virus (FeLV) and feline immunodeficiency virus (FIV) testing is essential in any cat presenting with lymphadenomegaly.

Thyroid gland hyperplasia or enlargement is much more frequently reported in adult and older adult cats (feline hyperthyroidism) than in dogs. Most reported cases in cats are diagnosed as benign hyperplasia, although about 15% are reported to have thyroid adenocarcinoma. Fine-needle aspiration and incisional biopsy in cats with thyroid gland enlargement are rarely performed. Instead, serum is submitted for thyroid hormone (T_4) levels in an attempt to establish a diagnosis of feline hyperthyroidism (see Section 5).

In dogs, thyroid tumors account for less than 4% of all tumors and approximately 10% to 15% of all head and neck tumors. However, most thyroid masses reported in dogs are associated with carcinoma. Therefore, palpation of an enlarged thyroid gland in a dog justifies incisional biopsy to confirm the underlying cause. Hyperthyroidism associated with benign hyperplasia of one or both thyroid glands is reported in dogs but is considerably less common than that reported in cats. Canine hypothyroidism, the most common thyroid disorder of dogs, is not associated with palpable changes in the size, consistency, or symmetry of the thyroid glands.

Additional Reading

Carlotti DN: Cutaneous and subcutaneous lumps, bumps and masses. In Ettinger SJ, Feldman EC, editors: *Textbook of veterinary internal medicine,* ed 6, St. Louis, 2005, Elsevier, pp. 43-46.

MUSCULOSKELETAL (ORTHOPEDIC) EXAMINATION

Examination of the musculoskeletal system is indicated in any patient presenting for lameness, difficulty walking, running, climbing, or jumping, and what the owner perceives is pain. The examination involves methods similar to those used in any other organ system by requiring the clinician to obtain a history, perform a physical examination, and order ancillary tests. Consideration of the patient's body size, breed, age, lameness severity, onset, clinical course, and sometimes sex often provides important insights into the examination (Table 2-11). Certain body sizes and specific breeds are more at risk for particular orthopedic conditions. For example, large, rapidly growing dogs seem to be predisposed to conditions such as osteochondrosis dissecans of the shoulder, elbow, stifle, and tarsal joints and disorders of osteochondrosis in general. Hip dysplasias, fragmented coronoid processes, an ununited anconeal process, and bone tumors are further examples of syndromes seen in larger dogs, whereas small, miniature, and toy breeds are predisposed to conditions such as Legg-Calvé-Perthes disease and medial patella luxation.

Age can determine what conditions are considered likely for diagnosis on the examination. Immature dogs will have a certain differential diagnosis, while mature dogs, older than 1 year, will have others. For example, a grade II forelimb lameness of insidious onset and progressive course may indicate osteochondritis dissecans of the shoulder, whereas the clinician would not initially consider this condition in a mature dog of the same breed with the same history.

TABLE 2-11   **History and Signalment**

Condition	Size predisposition — Dog: Small	Medium	Large	Giant	Cat	Breed	Sex	Lameness grade	Age at onset	Onset	Course
Hip dysplasia	+	2 +	3 +	3 +	+	Several		II	I, M	Slow	Wax and wane, progressive, frequently bilateral
Cruciate syndrome	2 +	2 +	3 +	2 +	+	Rottweiler, Labrador, Newfoundland, Staffordshire Terrier	♂ c ♀s	Any	M	Any	Wax and wane, progressive, frequently bilateral
Medial patella luxation	3 +	2 +	+	+	+	Toy breed	♀	I, II, III	I, M	Slow	Intermittent, progressive, frequently bilateral
Lateral patella luxation	+	2 +	3 +	+	+	Flat-Coated Retriever, Great Dane, Saint Bernard, Irish Wolfhound		I, II, III	I, M	Slow	Intermittent, progressive, frequently bilateral
Bicipital tenosynovitis	+	+	2 +	+				I, II	M	Slow	Intermittent, progressive, sometimes bilateral
Mineralization of supraspinatus tendon	+	+	2 +			Rottweiler, Labrador		I, II	M	Slow	Intermittent, progressive, sometimes bilateral
Neoplasia	+	3 +	3 +	3 +	+			II, III	M	Slow	Progressive

2

				Breed	Sex				Course
Panosteitis	+	3 +	+	German Shepherd Dog	♂	I, M	II	Rapid	Variable, self-limiting, multiple limbs
Osteochondrosis	2 +	3 +	3 +	Rottweiler, Labrador, German Shepherd Dog, Great Dane	♂	I	II	Slow	Wax and Wane, progressive, frequently bilateral
Legg-Calvé perthes disease	3 +			Terrier, toy breed		I	II	Slow	Progressive, sometimes bilateral
Fragmented coronoid process	+	3 +	2 +	Rottweiler, Labrador, Golden Retriever, German Shepherd Dog, Newfoundland, Chow Chow, Bernese Mountain Dog	♂	I, M	I, II	Slow	Wax and wane, progressive
Ununited anconeal process	2 +	3 +	+	German Shepherd Dog, Bassett Hound, English Bulldog	♂	I	II, III	Slow	Wax and wane, progressive
Hypertrophic osteodystrophy	+	3 +	3 +			I	III	Rapid	Variable, self-limiting, multiple limbs, painful, anorectic, febrile

3 +, Frequent; 2 +, sometimes; +, seldom; I, immature; M, mature; ♂ c, male castrate; ♀s, female spayed; ♂, male; ♀, female.
Modified from Schrader SC, Prieur WD, Bruse S: Diagnosis: Historical, Physical, and ancillary examination. *In* Olmstead ML, ed: Small Animal Orthopedics. St Louis, Mosby–Year Book, 1995.

2

EXAMINATION

Sometimes the most difficult aspect of the orthopedic examination is localizing the problem. Lameness, for example, is among the most common reasons a dog is presented for examination. However, it may be as difficult to localize the affected limb as it is to define a muscular or orthopedic cause.

Often it must be determined whether the lameness is due to an orthopedic or neurologic problem. A cursory examination of the spinal column and assessment of the neurologic status of the affected limb should precede orthopedic examination of the extremity. However, one must be careful when performing the neurologic evaluation. Several common orthopedic problems, such as bilateral hip or stifle abnormalities, can appear as neurologic conditions. Animals with these problems can be reluctant to bear full weight on either limb. However, the clinician can be misled by a cursory assessment of the neurologic status when evaluating proprioceptive deficits using the knuckling test. This is because when performing the knuckling test, the animal is reluctant to shift the weight to the contralateral limb to instantaneously correct the paw and continues to bear weight on the dorsum of the overturned digits.

The presence of a "head bob" suggests lameness. The head and neck move upward as the problematic forelimb touches the floor and downward when the affected rearlimb touches down. This action helps to reduce the load carried by the limb. The stride is shortened on the affected side; the animal will offload the abnormal limb more quickly than the normal one. The animal spends less time on the abnormal limb. Audible clicks are sometimes heard in young dogs with hip dysplasia or in dogs that have a meniscus abnormality secondary to rupture of the cranial cruciate ligament.

Palpation and manipulation

It is best to first examine the affected limb without sedation, if possible, to determine the source of discomfort or instability. The limb is palpated and manipulated from the toes proximally. The patient is turned and the procedure repeated on the other side as the contralateral limb can often serve as a normal control when bilateral conditions are not present. An equivocal asymmetric finding requires repeating the examination as many times as necessary to confirm or rule out its presence. Lastly, the animal is walked again, because a subtle lameness is often exacerbated by the manipulation.

- Localized signs of inflammation: pain, swelling, heat, redness, or altered function.
- Muscle atrophy, muscle tremors, muscle atrophy (significant) in the limb/region of the pain.
- Laxity, effusion, crepitation, localized heat, altered range of motion, or decreased joint stability.
- Limited range of motion in joint(s) when compared to same joints on the opposite limb.
- Shift of body weight to unaffected limb.
- Digits of the normal limb spread further apart than digits of the affected limb.
- Arched back as weight is shifted to forelimbs or to hindlimbs.
- Hindlimb stance is wide-based when weight is shift to the hindlimbs.

CARDINAL CLINICAL SIGNS IN THE PATIENT WITH ORTHOPEDIC DISEASE

- Focal or regional inflammation (pain, swelling, heat, redness, and loss of function)
- Muscle atrophy
- Muscle tremors
- Muscle atrophy localized to the muscle group primarily responsible for moving the painful limb
- Laxity, effusion, crepitation
- Localized temperature increase

- Nails of the affected limb are longer than those of the unaffected limbs. (NOTE: Nails that are unusually short or show abrasions on the dorsum of the nail may represent proprioceptive deficits rather than musculoskeletal disorder).
- Self-trauma (licking) of the skin over the affected bone or joint.
- Obvious conformational differences in specific breeds with a known and characteristic conformation or posture.

Often the goal of palpation is only to localize the specific site giving the animal discomfort or pain. Putting together the location of pain with the other known information will frequently lead to a diagnosis. For example, pain on palpation of the elbow joint in an immature German shepherd should lead the clinician to think of an ununited anconeal process rather than fragmentation of the medial coronoid process of the ulna. Fragmentation of the medial coronoid process is more frequently seen in retrievers, rottweilers, basset hounds, and Bernese Mountain Dogs than in German Shepherd Dogs.

Guidelines to use apply when palpating patients for orthopedic or muscular disease

- Digits need to be examined for lacerations, foreign bodies, ingrown nails, or burns, especially with grade III and IV lameness.
- Bite wounds of the limbs are the most common source of lameness in cats.
- In toy and miniature breeds, medial patella luxation results in a toe-in and bowlegged (genu varum) posture. Chronic cases are frequently complicated by rupture of the cranial cruciate ligament due to chronic instability of the stifle. This rupture may lead to an acute-onset presentation following a relatively chronic problem.
- Multiple subluxated joints are often associated with immune-mediated joint disease.
- Abnormal enlargements in diameter of long bones, especially in the metaphyseal regions, may indicate a developmental bone disease such as hypertrophic osteodystrophy or primary bone neoplasia.
- Palpation of the diaphyses of multiple long bones may produce pain in cases of neoplasia, fractures, infection, and panosteitis.
- Pain on palpation of the shoulder with peracute onset of lameness in a large athletic dog may be the result of bicipital tenosynovitis, mineralization of the supraspinatus tendon, or avulsion of the supraglenoid tubercle.
- Pain, lameness, fever, and anorexia are frequently associated with hypertrophic osteodystrophy in large rapidly growing breeds.
- Traumatic injury of the iliopsoas muscle may have a clinical presentation similar to hip dysplasia.

The cruciate syndrome in dogs can have a varied clinical presentation. Onset can be acute or chronically insidious. Any lameness grade is possible; however, grade II progressing to grade III lameness in middle-aged, neutered, obese dogs is very common. Palpation for the cranial drawer test can reveal obvious laxity, but subtle laxity is common with early or late disease. Early, the ligament is degenerating but mostly intact, while late, the ligament is severely degenerated and torn, but there is much fibrosis of the joint preventing gross laxity. Thus, frequently examination of the stifle joint for cruciate syndrome requires either sedation or general anesthesia to appreciate the subtleties. Palpation signs for cruciate ligament disease are a subtle or grossly positive cranial drawer test, increased internal rotation of the tibia on the femur, and medial joint thickening. When palpating for the cranial drawer, position the stifle in different flexion and extension angles while performing the maneuver. The normal joint will give an abrupt endpoint "thud" to the maneuver, as the ligament normally stretches. Minimal cranial translation of the tibia on the femur but with a soft "gushy" feel may indicate early degeneration and partial tearing or advanced degeneration and major tearing with fibrosis.

Hip dysplasia

Clinical signs of hip dysplasia include lameness, gait abnormalities, reluctance to exercise, and pelvic limb muscle atrophy. Specific maneuvers intended to demonstrate Barlow's, Ortolani's, and Barden's signs are useful to evaluate the degree of joint laxity, both when screening young puppies and in performing diagnostics in clinically lame dogs. None of the signs are definitive tests for hip dysplasia, but they should be performed as sequential maneuvers in the examination. Pelvic radiography is mandatory for a definitive diagnosis of hip dysplasia, but it should not be the first step in the examination because other diagnoses or concurrent conditions may be missed.

RADIOGRAPHY

Along with the history and physical examination, radiographs play an important role in the examination of the orthopedic patient. Mostly the two standard views, craniocaudal and lateromedial, are sufficient to define the problem. Proper technique is very important when obtaining radiographs, as it is easy to miss lesions when technique is less than adequate. Less frequently, oblique views or "stress views" are needed to help define the situation. Rarely, special imaging techniques such as tomography, bone scans, and arthrograms are needed. A common error made in veterinary medicine is to use the radiograph as a predictor of the severity of a problem and let it dictate clinical treatment or prognosis. For example, osteochondrosis dissecans of the shoulder joint in the dog may be demonstrated on the radiograph, but surgical exploration is not warranted unless lameness develops. It is difficult and often misleading to predict the severity of degenerative joint disease from radiographs alone; noncartilaginous changes, such as osteophytes, are what can be seen on radiographs. Conversely, inflammatory joint disease, when nonerosive, can be very severe, and the clinician will note minimal or no radiographic changes.

OTHER DIAGNOSTIC TESTS

Besides radiographs, other diagnostic aids are used with the orthopedic examination. Arthrocentesis with joint fluid analysis is a common diagnostic aid (Table 2-12). Other tests include arthroscopy, rheumatoid factor testing, antinuclear antibody testing, *Borrelia burgdorferi* testing, synovial membrane examinations, and other serologic tests and measurement of immune complexes.

Additional Reading

Fox SM, Jones BR: Musculoskeletal disorders. In Schaer M, editor: *Clinical medicine of the dog and cat,* Ames, 2003, Iowa State Press (Blackwell), pp. 538-569.

Goldstein RE: Swollen joints and lameness. In Ettinger SJ, Feldman EC, editors: *Textbook of veterinary internal medicine,* ed 6, St. Louis, 2005, Elsevier, pp. 83-88.

NERVOUS SYSTEM EXAMINATION

Objectively, the neurologic examination is performed to (1) localize a lesion (or lesions) within the peripheral or central nervous system, (2) assess the extent of disease or injury

---

GUIDELINES: RADIOGRAPHY OF THE ORTHOPEDIC PATIENT

- Radiograph the opposite limb whenever necessary to clarify suspected lesions. Consider stress views when suspecting collateral ligament damage to the stifle, elbow, carpus, and tarsus.
- Radiograph both shoulders when considering osteochondrosis dissecans, bicipital tenosynovitis, and mineralization of the supraspinatus tendon.
- Radiograph both elbows when considering elbow dysplasias.
- Radiograph both elbows for dysplasias when considering osteochondrosis of the shoulders.
- Radiograph both shoulders when diagnosing elbow dysplasias.
- Radiograph both stifles when considering cruciate ligament disease.
- Radiograph both hips when considering hip dysplasia or hip degeneration.
- Radiograph both hips when considering cruciate ligament disease.
- Radiograph hips, with or without mechanical aids, while viewing luxation or reduction angles with the animal positioned in dorsal recumbency (helps determine predisposition to hip dysplasia at a young age).

TABLE 2-12 Joint Fluid Analysis

	Normal	Degenerative	Hemarthrosis	Rheumatoid	Lupus erythematosus (LE)	Neoplastic	Aseptic	Septic
Color	None or straw-colored	Pale yellow	Red	Yellow to blood-tinged	Yellow to blood-tinged	Yellow to blood-tinged	Yellow to blood-tinged	Yellow to sanguineous
Turbidity	Clear	Clear to slight	Blood-tinged	Slight to moderate	Slight to moderate	Slight to moderate	Slight to moderate	Turbid to purulent
Viscosity	Normal	Normal	Reduced	Reduced	Reduced	Reduced	Reduced	Reduced
Mucin clot	Good	Good	Fair	Poor	Fair	Good	Fair	Poor
Red blood cells	Rare	Few	Many	Few to moderate	Few to moderate	Few to moderate	Few to moderate	Moderate
White blood cells	$0.1–2.0 \times 10^3$ µL	Few	Moderate	Marked	Marked	Moderate	Moderate to marked	Marked
Neutrophils	1%–10%	Few	Moderate	Many	Many	Moderate	Moderate	Many
Lymphocytes	50%–60%	Moderate	Few	Few	Few to moderate	Few	Few to moderate	Few
Macrophages	Rare	Moderate	Few	Few	Few to moderate	Moderate	Moderate	Few

Continued

TABLE 2-12 Joint Fluid Analysis—cont'd

	Normal	Degenerative	Hemarthrosis	Rheumatoid	Lupus erythematosus (LE)	Neoplastic	Aseptic	Septic
Synovial cells	Moderate	Moderate to many	Rare	Few	Few	Moderate	Few to moderate	Few
Synovial glucose–blood glucose ratio	0.8-1.0	0.8:1.0	1.0	0.5:0.8	0.5 : 0.8	0.5-0.8	0.5:0.8	<0.5
Other	Rare neutrophils and red blood cells unless blood contamination			Phagocytes	LE cells	Neoplastic cells		Toxic changes to cells, micro-organisms
Causes		Conformation, age, osteochondrosis	Trauma, bleeding disorder	Rheumatoid arthritis	Lupus	Synovial, periosteal bone, connective tissue	Trauma, local inflammation, immune mediated Lyme disease, viral, rickettsial, mycoplasmas	Hematogenous, wounds

Modified from Wilkins RJ: Joint serology. In Bojrab MJ, ed: *Disease mechanisms in small animal surgery*. Philadelphia, Lea & Febiger, 1993.

involving the nervous system, (3) assess the nature of the disease/injury affecting the nervous system and, if possible, (4) establish the cause of the neurologic signs.

The challenge of the neurologic exam is to determine whether the presenting sign is, in fact, primarily neurologic in origin or is secondary (e.g., compromised vascularity, neoplasia, immune-mediated, toxic, or infection.)

CLINICAL HISTORY

The breed, sex, and age of the animal should be noted; considered together with the chief complaint, they may help direct the line of questioning in the historical review. Certain breeds are predisposed to specific neurologic ailments, and the age of the animal may reduce the possibility of certain neurologic diseases.

The history should include a summary of all past medical and surgical illnesses and the facts surrounding the present complaint. The line of questioning will be influenced by the chief complaint. However, general questions should include the dosage of and response to medications administered for the condition, the vaccination history, and the health status of littermates or other animals in the household.

EXAMINATION

A comprehensive neurologic examination is divided into five parts: **mental attitude** and **behavior**, **gait**, **postural reactions**, **spinal nerve reflexes**, and **cranial nerve reflexes**. In this description, an intact *reflex* requires the function of only the peripheral nerves being tested and the segments of the spinal cord or brain stem in which the afferent axon enters and the cell bodies and axons of the efferent neurons are located. A *reaction* depends on the same components as the reflex, plus the ascending pathways through the white matter of the spinal cord and brain stem to the cerebellum and sensorimotor cortex of the cerebrum and the descending pathways that return from the cerebrum by way of its internal capsule and the white matter of the brain stem and spinal cord. The lower motor neuron (LMN) has its cell body and dendritic zone in the ventral gray column of the spinal cord or specific cranial nerve nucleus in the brain stem. Its axon leaves the CNS and courses through peripheral nerves to its telodendron in the group of muscle fibers it innervates. The upper motor neurons (UMNs) have cell bodies and dendritic zones in collections of gray matter in the cerebrum (motor cerebral cortex) or brain stem (red nucleus, reticular nuclei). The axons of the UMNs descend in tracts through the white matter in the brain and spinal cord to end in telodendria in the vicinity of the LMN that they ultimately influence (Figure 2-23).

The precise order in which the parts of a neurologic examination are performed varies with the preference of the examiner and the attitude of the patient. An initial assessment should be made of the patient's mental attitude and behavior. If the animal is resting quietly in a cage at the time of examination, the cranial nerve examination may be done first. If the animal is excited or apprehensive, it may be more convenient to perform the cranial nerve examination after the animal has been handled during the examinations of gait, postural reactions, and reflexes.

MENTAL ATTITUDE AND BEHAVIOR

An assessment should be made of the patient's mental attitude, sensorium, and behavior. The owner is usually the best judge of subtle changes in the patient's behavior and should be questioned about this. Is the animal bright, alert, and responsive initially and throughout the examination? The various terms that characterize alterations of this attitude and behavior are depression, lethargy, unresponsiveness, stupor, coma, anxiety, disorientation, hyperactivity, hysteria, propulsion, and aggression.

As a rule, these alterations in the animal's normal sensorium reflect disturbances in the diencephalon and telencephalon and often implicate some portion of the limbic system. It is especially important to evaluate these carefully in the recumbent animal. Cervical spinal cord disease that produces recumbency will not alter the animal's mental attitude, except that some animals may become frantic and hyperexcitable if they are

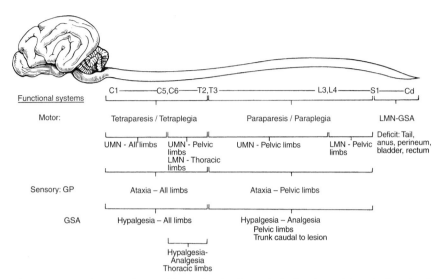

Figure 2-23: Schematic diagram illustrating the four principal regions of the spinal cord and the associated spinal cord segments.

unable to get up. The same degree of tetraplegia can occur with a brain stem lesion that severely alters the animal's responsiveness to its environment. However, cranial nerve abnormalities are generally noted with brain stem lesions.

Gait

The gait should be examined in a place where the animal may be allowed to move freely, unleashed, and where the ground surface is not slippery. The floor of many examining rooms is too slippery for adequate evaluation of the animal's gait. In some patients with vertebral column injury with spinal cord contusion resulting in paresis and ataxia, moving the patient on a slippery floor may cause a fall, and further injury may result. A carpeted room is ideal.

The degree of functional deficit dictates the necessity for further examination of strength and coordination. A patient that is tetraplegic—unable to support its weight or move its limbs when the weight is borne on them—need not have further tests performed for the postural reactions. A grade 0 paraplegic patient need not be examined for postural reactions in the pelvic limbs, but the thoracic limbs should be examined carefully. Occasionally, a patient with progressive myelitis may present as paraplegic because of an extensive thoracolumbar spinal cord location of the lesion; the patient will also have an asymmetric thoracic limb gait because of a less severe focus of the lesion in the cervical spinal cord. An early sign in dogs with ascending myelomalacia associated with an acute severe intervertebral disk extrusion may be a hesitant, stumbling, awkward gait in the

---

GRADING SCALE FOR PELVIC LIMB FUNCTION

5—Normal strength and coordination
4—Can stand to support: *minimal paraparesis and ataxia*
3—Can stand to support, but frequently stumbles and falls: *mild paraparesis and ataxia*
2—Unable to stand to support; when assisted, moves limbs readily but stumbles and falls frequently: *moderate paraparesis and ataxia*
1—Unable to stand to support; slight movement when supported by the tail: *severe paraparesis*
0—Absence of purposeful movement: *paraplegia*

thoracic limbs. The severity of advanced pelvic limb dysfunction is evaluated best by hold-ing the animal suspended at the base of the tail and observing its gait.

POSTURAL REACTIONS

Following observation of the gait for strength and coordination, the postural reactions can be tested, especially to determine whether there are less obvious deficits in strength and coordination when the gait appears to be normal. Each of these reactions requires that all major components of the peripheral and central nervous systems be intact. They are not of localizing value by themselves.

Wheelbarrowing

The thoracic limbs may be tested by supporting the animal under the abdomen, so that the pelvic limbs are off the ground surface, and forcing the animal to walk on its thoracic limbs. The normal animal walks with symmetric movements of both thoracic limbs and with the head extended in normal position. Animals with lesions of the peripheral nerves of the thoracic limbs, cervical spinal cord, or brain stem may have asymmetric movements, with stumbling or knuckling over on the dorsum of the paw of the affected limb. Hypermetria is occasionally observed. With more severe lesions in this area, there is a tendency to carry the head flexed with the nose close to and occasionally reaching the ground surface for support. Animals with neuromuscular disease affecting neck muscles will carry their neck partially flexed and have difficulty with normal extension. If no deficit is observed, extend the neck while the animal is wheelbarrowed. This sometimes reveals a mild deficit, a tendency to knuckle over on the dorsum of the paw, which was not observed previously. This may be helpful to confirm a cervical spinal cord lesion in Great Danes or Doberman pinschers that have a cervical vertebral malformation and show mild pelvic limb paresis and ataxia but no overt thoracic limb signs.

Hopping—thoracic limb

While still supporting the pelvic limbs, hop the animal on one thoracic limb while holding the other off the ground surface so that the limb to be tested supports the entire weight of the body. Move the dog forward and to each side but especially laterally, and observe the strength and coordination of the limb. Repeat this on the other thoracic limb and compare the response. Asymmetry occurs with paresis or ataxia. Hypermetria may be seen with general proprioceptive or cerebellar deficits. This is an effective way of determining minor deficits when the gait appears to be normal, as occurs with contralateral cerebral sensori-motor cortex lesions. An animal with neuromuscular disease that can still move its limbs will usually struggle to hop, but the animal will collapse when all of its weight is borne on the limb being tested. If the weight is held up, the limb to be tested will often respond fairly well, indicating that proprioceptive function is not impaired.

Extensor postural thrust

The same responses to tests can be obtained on the pelvic limbs. The extensor postural thrust reaction is performed by holding the animal off the ground surface by supporting it caudal to the scapulae, lowering it to the ground surface, and observing the animal extend its pelvic limbs to support its weight. Moving the animal forward and backward in this position tests the symmetry of pelvic limb function, strength, and coordination.

Hopping—pelvic limb

Continuing to support the animal by the thorax so that the thoracic limbs are not in contact with the ground surface, hold up one pelvic limb, and force the animal to hop later-ally or forward on the supporting limb. Both pelvic limbs should be tested this way and the responses compared. It is important to compare the pelvic limb hopping responses with each other and not with the ipsilateral thoracic limb. Normally, the hopping response of the pelvic limb seems more stiff or hypertonic, with a slightly larger excursion than that of the thoracic limb.

Hemistanding and hemiwalking

The animal's ability to stand and walk with the thoracic and pelvic limbs on one side can be tested by holding the opposite thoracic and pelvic limbs off the ground surface and forcing the animal to walk forward or to the side. These reactions are referred to as the hemistanding and hemiwalking reactions. With a large dog or uncooperative patient that resists hopping, you may be able to evaluate the hopping responses by observing the responses of the limbs during hemiwalking.

An animal with a unilateral lesion of the sensorimotor cortex or internal capsule may have a normal gait but show deficits in its postural reactions on the side opposite the lesion. Attempts to hemiwalk on the contralateral side are delayed or exaggerated (hypermetric) and spastic, and stumbling may occur. With unilateral cervical spinal cord lesions, the limbs on the same side as the lesion show a deficiency in the gait and are poorly responsive to postural reaction testing, including the animal's inability to respond in the hemiwalking reaction.

Placing

Other postural reactions that can be tested include placing with the thoracic limbs. The animal is supported off the ground surface and its thoracic limbs are brought to the edge of a table or similar surface so that the dorsal surface of the paws makes contact. This test should be performed on both thoracic limbs simultaneously and individually, with and without blindfolding the animal. Vision can compensate for the sense of position when the general proprioceptive system is abnormal, so tactile placing (blindfolded animal) is tested before visual placing.

Tonic neck reaction

The tonic neck reaction involves extension of the head and neck so that the nose is directed dorsally. The normal patient responds by extension of all the joints of both thoracic limbs. An animal with disease of the general proprioceptive system in the cervical spinal nerves, cervical spinal cord, or medulla fails to extend its carpus or digits or both, and these joints passively flex so that the weight is borne on the dorsal surface of the paw. The same response may occur if an animal is paretic as a result of disease of the motor neurons that innervate the thoracic limb or in the white matter of the spinal cord that influences these motor neurons.

Proprioceptive positioning

Proprioceptive positioning tests this afferent system by determining the animal's ability to sense or feel when the paw has been flexed so that the weight is borne on its dorsal surface. With normal proprioception, the animal immediately returns the paw to its usual position. In patients with paresis, this test may also be deficient. Delayed proprioception may also be a manifestation of limb or pelvic pain. Sedatives and analgesics are also likely to delay proprioceptive positioning in otherwise normal animals.

SPINAL NERVE REFLEXES

Spinal nerve evaluation includes assessment of muscle tone and size, spinal reflexes, and cutaneous sensation. Muscle tone and spinal reflexes are evaluated best when the animal is in lateral recumbency and as relaxed as possible. It is important to test muscle tone, tendon reflexes, and the flexor reflex to noxious stimuli, in that order, to maintain the animal's cooperation.

Muscle tone

Muscle tone is evaluated by passive manipulation of the limbs individually. The degree of resistance is determined to be less than normal (hypotonic), normal, or more than normal (hypertonic). The last may be referred to as spasticity. The degree of spasticity varies from a mild increased resistance, to passive manipulation, to rigid extension. Hypotonia usually occurs with LMN disease, whereas UMN disease may be characterized by hypertonia or spasticity. However, normal muscle tone without spasticity can occur in some animals with UMN disease. The functional integrity of the LMN is necessary to cause muscle cell contraction to maintain muscle tone. Functional integrity of the LMN is also necessary to maintain the normal health of the muscle cell it innervates. When denervated, these cells degenerate. The degeneration is observed clinically as neurogenic atrophy and can be detected electromyographically by the production of abnormal potentials in resting muscle. The UMN influences the activity of the LMN to produce voluntary motor activity and to maintain muscle tone for support of the body against gravity. Although the UMN includes both facilitatory and inhibitory functions on the activity of the LMN, when the UMN is diseased the result usually observed is a release of the LMN from inhibition and overactivity of the facilitory mechanism. This release is seen as hypertonia or spasticity.

Dogs that are tetraplegic should be held in a supporting position to observe the muscle tone in the limbs and any voluntary responses. Usually, dogs with cervical spinal cord lesions rostral to the brachial plexus have rigidly extended limbs, and the entire trunk and limbs feel stiff when the dog is held up and the limbs moved along the ground surface. The hypertonia may be severe enough to permit the animal to stand unsupported. Tetraplegic dogs with diffuse neuromuscular diseases such as polyradiculoneuritis are hypotonic or atonic and appear and feel limp when held in a supporting position. There is no reflex tension of the limb, and no support is elicited by placing the paws on the ground. Instead, the limbs buckle under the weight of the body.

Patellar reflexes

The most reliable tendon reflex is the patellar reflex. It is the only tendon reflex that is present in all normal animals. However, the reflex may normally be difficult to detect in older, large-breed dogs. It is obtained by lightly tapping the patellar tendon with the animal in lateral recumbency and as relaxed as possible for proper evaluation. A pediatric neurologic hammer is the most useful instrument, but any hard object such as forceps handles can be used. The reflex can be elicited in all normal dogs and is mediated by the femoral nerve through the L4–6 spinal cord segments. The degree of normal response varies with the breed. Large-breed dogs have a brisker reflex than the short-limbed breeds such as the dachshund. The response should be evaluated as absent (0), hyporeflexic (1), normal (2), hyperreflexic (3), or clonic (4). This reflex should be tested with the animal lying on each side. An absent reflex or hyporeflexia occurs when there is disease of a portion of the reflex arc. Hyperreflexia or clonus is often present as UMN disease.

Biceps and triceps reflexes

In the thoracic limb, the biceps and triceps reflexes can be elicited in many dogs that are relaxed and in lateral recumbency. Lightly tapping the tendon of insertion of the triceps proximal to the olecranon elicits a slight extension of the elbow. The reflex is mediated by the radial nerve through the C7 and C8 and the T1 and T2 spinal cord segments. The biceps reflex is elicited by placing a finger on the distal ends of the biceps and brachialis muscles at the level of the elbow. Tapping this finger with the hammer elicits a slight flexion of the elbow. The muscle contraction can be palpated in some instances when no movement of the joint is seen. The musculocutaneous nerve mediates this reflex through the C6–8 spinal cord segments. The normal animal has a mild reflex response to these stimuli. In a few normal animals, these reflexes are difficult to elicit. They are absent when there is disease of some portion of the reflex arc. They may be hyperactive in some animals with disease of the UMN.

Flexor reflex—pelvic limb

The flexor reflexes to noxious stimuli determine the integrity of the reflex arc as well as the pathway in the CNS that is concerned with the animal's response to noxious stimuli. The most reliable stimulus is pressure exerted on the base of the toenail with hemostats. Many normal animals do not respond to the stimulus of a pin. The pelvic limb is maintained perpendicular to the long axis of the pelvis by placing a hand on the anterior surface of the limb above the stifle when applying the noxious stimuli. The normal animal with UMN lesions will flex the limb at the stifle. The flexor reflex is mediated by the sciatic nerve through the L6 and L7 spinal cord segments and the S1 segment. A depressed or absent flexor indicates a lesion in one of these structures. Abnormality of the motor portion of the sciatic nerve distal to the pelvis causes paralysis, hypotonia, and atrophy of the flexors of the stifle, tarsus, and digits, as well as of the extensors of the hip, tarsus, and digits. There is no resistance to flexion or extension of the tarsus. In the animal walking with a sciatic nerve paralysis, the tarsus is lower on the affected side and the paw may be placed on its dorsal surface; however, the limb is able to support weight as long as the femoral nerve is intact.

Sensory branches of the peroneal nerves supply the dorsal surface of the paw. The plantar surface is supplied by tibial nerve sensory branches. The medial side of the paw is supplied by the saphenous nerve, a branch of the femoral nerve. The saphenous nerve enters the spinal cord through the L4–6 segments. A patient may have a contused sciatic nerve from a pelvic fracture and have no function of the muscles innervated by this nerve and analgesia of the lateral, dorsal, and plantar surfaces of the paw. However, the intact saphenous nerve provides sensation to the medial surface of the paw. If this area is stimulated, the animal will flex the hip with the intact innervation of the iliopsoas muscle, but the stifle, tarsus, and digits fail to flex. For this reason, both the medial and lateral surfaces of the paw should be tested for reflex responses as well as nociception.

Nociception (outward manifestation of pain)

Animals show signs of pain perception by a behavioral response (e.g., crying, biting), not a flexor reflex. The impulses generated by a noxious stimulus enter the spinal cord over the peripheral nerves and dorsal roots and are relayed to tracts in the lateral funiculi of the spinal cord bilaterally. These tracts ascend the spinal cord in the lateral funiculi and continue through the medulla, pons, and mesencephalon to specific nuclei in the thalamus for relay to the somatic sensory cerebral cortex. Pain may be evidenced when the impulses reach the thalamus or cerebrum.

Flexor reflex—thoracic limb

In the thoracic limb, the thoracodorsal, axillary, musculocutaneous, median, ulnar, and radial nerves are responsible for flexion of the shoulder, elbow, carpus, and digits when a noxious stimulus is applied to the paw. These nerves arise from the C6–T2 spinal cord segments. The specific sensory nerve stimulated depends on the location of the stimulus. The median and ulnar nerves innervate the skin of the palmar surface of the paw; the radial nerve supplies the dorsal surface. In the forearm, the radial nerve supplies the skin on the cranial and lateral surfaces. The ulnar nerve supplies the caudal surface, and the musculocutaneous nerve supplies the medial surface. Be aware of the amount of overlap of the cutaneous innervation by these nerves. The thoracic limb is maintained in a position similar to that described for the pelvic limb. Following a noxious stimulus, the normal animal and the animal with a UMN lesion will flex the limb at the elbow. A depressed or absent flexor reflex indicates a lesion in one of the structures that mediate the flexor reflex.

Crossed extensor reflex

In animals with UMN disease and release of the LMN, a crossed extensor reflex may be elicited in the recumbent animal when the flexor reflex is stimulated. The crossed reflex occurs in the limb opposite the one being tested for a flexor reflex. To avoid voluntary extension of the contralateral limb as a response to a noxious stimulus, the flexor reflex first should be elicited with as mild a stimulus as is necessary and the opposite limb observed for extension. When elicited in an animal in lateral recumbency, this is an abnormal reflex, indicative of UMN disease.

Perineal reflex

The perineal reflex is elicited by stimulating the anus with a noxious stimulus and observing contraction of the anal sphincter and flexion of the tail. The reflex is mediated by branches of the sacral and caudal nerves through the sacral and caudal segments of the spinal cord.

Cutaneous reflex

The cutaneous reflex is the contraction of the cutaneous trunci in response to mild stimulation of the skin of the trunk. It can be elicited in normal animals from the thoracic and most of the lumbar region. The regional segmental spinal nerves contain the sensory neurons that are stimulated. The impulses are carried into the related spinal cord segments and then relayed through the white matter of the spinal cord cranially to the C6 spinal cord segment. Here synapse occurs on LMNs of the lateral thoracic nerve that innervate the cutaneous trunci. When the cutaneous response is present, it indicates the spinal cord white matter is intact from the level tested to the C8 spinal cord segment. This reflex may require multiple stimulation to elicit, and occasionally normal animals resist this stimulation; dehydrated animals and animals with advanced generalized muscle atrophy show no reflex.

CRANIAL NERVE EXAMINATION (See Also Table 2-13)

Indications for performing a cranial nerve (CN) examination are based on the initial evaluation of the patient's behavior, attention to the surroundings, ability to see and track objects, ability to hear, posture, and gait. Much of the initial assessment can simply be observed by allowing the animal to walk around inside the exam room or, with larger dogs, outside. When evidence of a deficit or abnormality is present, methodical assessment of the cranial nerves is indicated. Patients with defined cranial nerve deficits are typically manifested ipsilateral to the lesion. Deficits of CN II and IV may be contralateral to the lesion. Figure 2-24 illustrates the point of origin, at the level of the brain and brain stem, for each of the 12 cranial nerves; the nerve type (sensory, motor, or mixed) is also depicted. In the clinical patient, a CN examination entails assessment of the following elements:

Cranial nerve I (olfactory-sensory)

This can be difficult to assess. Passing a strong smelling compound (e.g., canned food) near the patient's nostrils can elicit a response that is sufficient to evaluate whether or not the sense of smell is present. Alcohol-soaked cotton balls also can be used but may actually be sufficiently irritating as to evoke an irritation response in an anosmic patient. Deficits localize to the forebrain and olfactory lobes, but they may also involve damage to the nasal mucosa (e.g., invasive carcinoma with invasion through the cribiform plate into the brain).

Cranial nerve II (ocular-sensory)

Assessment of vision in each eye independently is feasible. The simplest technique is to encourage the patient to track a cotton ball that is tossed across the field of vision. Done first with both eyes unobstructed, the test is repeated with tape covering one eye, then the other. The classic menace response may move sufficient air across the cornea as to cause a blink reflex, which could be interpreted as a visual response. Direct and consensual papillary light reflexes (PLR) should also be performed. However, the PLR may be normal in a blind patient. Unilateral miosis and enophthalmia and prolapse of the third eyelid (classically with ptosis) defines Horner's syndrome, interruption of the sympathetic tract. The lesion in a patient with Horner's syndrome could be anywhere between the hypothalamus and T1-T2 cord segments (central Horner's) or between T1-T2 and the middle ear (peripheral Horner's).

Cranial nerves III (oculomotor-motor), IV (trochlear-motor), and VI (abducens-motor)

Examined as a group, these cranial nerves control eye movement. It is seldom possible to identify discrete CN deficits in dogs and cats. Evidence of divergent or convergent strabismus (unilateral or bilateral) suggests intracranial disease at the level of the midbrain. Furthermore, the absence of physiologic nystagmus as the head is moved left to right and then right to left can also be used to assess function of this nerve group.

2

TABLE 2-13 Evaluation of Cranial Nerves

Nerve	Sign of dysfunction	Test/Responses
I Olfactory	Anosmia	Observe response to smell of food or some mild volatile oils
II Optic	Visual deficit, bumping objects	No menace response–failure to close eyelids or retract head when affected eye is menaced
	Unilateral disease	Light in affected eye–no pupillary response from either eye
	Mild mydrasis in affected eye (slight anisocoria) or none	
	Bilateral disease	Light in affected eye–no pupillary constriction
III Oculomotor	Marked mydriasis bilaterally	Examine with ophthalmoscope
	Marked mydriasis	Light in affected eye–only pupil of normal eye constricts
	Severe anisocoria	Light in normal eye–only pupil of normal eye constricts
	Ventrolateral strabismus	Incompleted adduction of affected eye on moving head side to side
	Ptosis	Inability to elevate upper eyelid completely
IV Trochlear	Slight extorsion (tilting) of eyeball, which may be visualized in the dog only by ophthalmoscopic examination of the position of the retinal veins	
V Trigeminal	Dropped jaw; unable to close mouth if bilateral disease	Hypalgesia can be determined by patient's lack of response to touching nasal septum with forceps
	No motor deficit if unilateral disease	
	Atrophy of muscles of mastication	
	Hypalgesia or analgesia of face	

VI Abducent	Medial strabismus	Incomplete abduction of affected eye on moving head from side to side
VII Facial	Paresis/paralysis of facial muscles–inability to close palpebral fissure, drooped hypotonic lip with drooling of saliva, inability to move ear, but the ears will not droop in all patients (cats and some prick-eared dogs); incomplete dilation of nares on inspiration	
VII Vestibulocochlear		
Cochlear	Deafness (unilateral is difficult to determine)	Lack of response to commands or any noise
Vestibular–Unilateral disease	Head tilt and ataxic toward side of lesion-lean, fall, circle toward side of lesion	Unequal response or postrotatory testing–rapid movement away from side of lesion; extend the neck; eye on affected side will not elevate completely (vestibular strabismus); hold head to side or dorsally and observe for positional nystagmus
	Abnormal resting or positional nystagmus with quick phase away from side of lesion	
Vestibular–Bilateral disease	Crouched gait, stumble to either side	
	No abnormal nystagmus, wide excursions of head	Inability to generate nystagmus on moving head from side to side or spinning–no postrotatory response
IX Glossopharyngeal	Dysphagia, gagging on eating	
X Vagus	Dysphagia, gagging on eating	
	Inspiratory dyspnea	
XI Accessory	None	
XII Hypoglossal	Atrophy of affected side of tongue	
	May deviate toward affected side on protrusion	

2

2

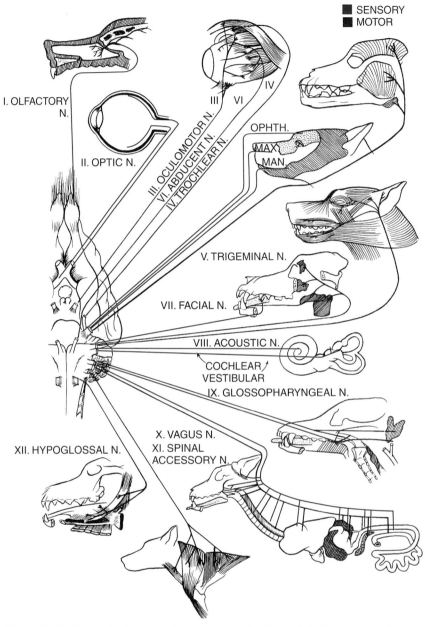

■ SENSORY
■ MOTOR

I. OLFACTORY N.

II. OPTIC N.

III. OCULOMOTOR N.
VI. ABDUCENT N.
IV. TROCHLEAR N.

III VI IV

OPHTH.
MAX.
MAN.

V. TRIGEMINAL N.

VII. FACIAL N.

VIII. ACOUSTIC N.

COCHLEAR
VESTIBULAR

IX. GLOSSOPHARYNGEAL N.

X. VAGUS N.

XII. HYPOGLOSSAL N.   XI. SPINAL ACCESSORY N.

Figure 2-24: Schematic demonstrating the points of origin and the target organs (sensory [green lines] and motor [black lines]) for each of the cranial nerves.
(Modified from Hoerlein BF: *Canine neurology,* ed 3, Philadelphia, 1978, WB Saunders.)

Cranial nerve V (trigeminal-mixed)

A complex nerve, the trigeminal nerve serves a number of sensory and motor functions, making it relatively easy to assess in the clinically affected patient. Sensory function can be assessed by gently touching the cornea or the eyelids (eyelashes in a dog) or gently touching the nasal mucosa of the medial aspect of both nostrils. Ptosis (a component sign of Horner's syndrome) is also a consequence of trigeminal nerve damage. Motor functions are associated with the muscles of mastication. Trigeminal nerve damage may result in a dropped jaw or the inability to prehend (or retain) food. Masseter and temporalis muscle atrophy on the ipsilateral side may be manifest. Swallowing is not affected.

Cranial nerve VII (facial-mixed)

The facial nerve supplies the small muscles of the face. Touching the cornea will elicit a painful response (characterized by movement of the head) but no eyelid blink. The lip and cheek on the affected side may droop and food may be detected between the maxilla and the cheek. Cats are unable to move their whiskers forward. Parasympathetic innervation to the lacrimal gland is carried with CN VII. Some patients may present with keratoconjunctivitis sicca. A Schirmer Tear test is indicated. Futhermore, atropine can be applied with a Q-tip to the tip of the patient's tongue to assess the sensory component of CN VII. Failure to respond indicates facial nerve damage.

Cranial nerve VIII (acoustic and vestibular-sensory)

The dual function of CN VIII allows the clinician to assess the patient for its ability to hear and for its ability to maintain appropriate eye movements and balance. Eliciting a moderately loud noise, away from the patient's line of sight, will generate an alerting response in a dog or cat with normal hearing. Neurogenic hearing deficits not associated with intracranial disease may affect this response in older dogs and some cats. Spontaneous nystagmus, especially horizontal, indicates damage to the vestibular branch of CN VIII. It is usually possible to assess a rapid eye movement (rapid component) in one direction followed by a slower eye movement (slow component). Interesting, the slow component of horizontal nystagmus "points" toward the side of the lesion.

Cranial nerves IX (glossopharyngeal-sensory) and X (vagus-mixed)

Injury to CN IX or X could affect the patient's ability to swallow, but not the ability to prehend food. A gag reflex is conventionally used to assess the ability to swallow; however, unilateral damage to CN IX may not completely impair the patient's ability to swallow.

Cranial nerve XI (spinal accessory-motor)

Spinal accessory nerve function is not specifically assessed during the cranial nerve examination.

Cranial nerve XII (hypoglossal-motor)

Unilateral damage to the hypoglossal nerve will not only compromise swallowing but will cause a visible deviation of the tongue. The tongue will deviate toward the normal (unaffected) side. Bilateral damage is uncommon but will impair tongue movement, the ability to prehend food, and the ability to swallow.

CLINICAL SIGNS ASSOCIATED WITH INTRACRANIAL LESIONS

Medulla and pons

Lesions in the medulla and pons result in spastic tetraparesis and ataxia of all four limbs or tetraplegia, ipsilateral spastic hemiparesis and ataxia (unilateral lesions), central vestibular signs, depression and irregular respirations and heartbeat, and hypalgesia of the trunk and limbs.

Signs of cranial nerve deficit include facial hypalgesia or analgesia (sensory, V); paresis or paralysis of masticatory muscles (motor, V); medial strabismus (VI); facial paresis or paralysis (VII); pharyngeal paresis (IX, X); tongue paresis (XII); and loss of balance, head tilt, and abnormal nystagmus (VIII).

Cerebellum

With diffuse lesions, the signs are symmetric ataxia with preservation of voluntary motor activity, dysmetric gait (hypermetria), truncal ataxia, head tremor, muscle hypertonia, occasional abnormal nystagmus, and bilateral menace deficit. With unilateral lesions, the signs are ipsilateral. The body and the head tilt toward the side of the lesion or occasionally away from the side of the lesion, and there may be ipsilateral menace deficit. With severe rostral lesions, there may be opisthotonus and rigidly extended forelimbs, and the pelvic limbs are extended forward by hip flexion.

Midbrain (mesencephalon)

With lesions in this area, the following signs occur: opisthotonus with rigid extension of all limbs (decerebration); spastic tetraparesis and ataxia of all four limbs; spastic hemiparesis if the lesion is unilateral (usually contralateral); depression; stupor (semicoma) or coma; and hypalgesia of the head, trunk, and limbs. Signs of cranial nerve deficit are ventrolateral strabismus (III) and mydriasis and nonreactive pupil (III). There is deviation of the eye in certain positions of the head, and the head and neck are flexed laterally, with the nose directed toward the shoulder with severe midline or unilateral lesions in the tegmentum. Visual deficits may be observed in acute lesions.

Thalamus and hypothalamus (diencephalon)

Bilateral lesions of the diencephalon produce the following signs: slows postural reactions bilaterally, mild ataxia, bilateral visual deficit with dilated unresponsive pupils (optic tracts), and bilateral hypalgesia.

Unilateral lesions are indicated by contralateral deficient postural reactions, contralateral visual deficit with normal pupils, contralateral hypalgesia (most noticeable in the head), and the adversive syndrome—propulsive circling and head and eye deviation, usually toward the side of the lesion.

With lesions that are either bilateral or unilateral, the manifestations are depression, stupor (semicoma) or coma, behavioral changes, seizures, and hypothalamohypophyseal disorders of body temperature, glucose metabolism, appetite control, autonomic nervous system, water balance, gonadal function, and thyroid and adrenal function.

Cerebrum (telecephalon)

Lesions in this area are evidenced by changes in several ways. Changes in behavior or temperament include depression (lethargy, obtundation); stupor (semicoma); lack of recognition of owner or environment and bewilderment; loss of trained habits; and irritable, hysterical maniacal, or aggressive behavior. In propulsion, the animal often paces and circles in one direction and turns the head and eyes in one direction; this direction is usually toward a unilateral lesion, called the *adversive syndrome* (turn to). This may require a rostral thalamic involvement in the lesion. Seizures are partial (contralateral face or limbs or both) or generalized (grand mal, psychomotor). The gait is usually normal, but contralateral postural reactions are deficient. Bilateral lesions produce blindness. Unilateral lesions produce a contralateral visual deficit with normal pupil responses to light. Occasionally, contralateral facial hypalgesia occurs. Rarely, the hypalgesia is observed in the contralateral trunk and limbs. Acute diffuse lesions may produce bilateral miosis. Pseudobulbar paresis rarely may be observed on voluntary movement: contralateral lower facial paresis (lip and nose), pharyngeal paresis, and tongue paresis.

CLINICAL SIGNS ASSOCIATED WITH SPINAL CORD LESIONS

The objective of the neurologic examination in patients with spinal disorders is to localize the injury/disease. This is accomplished by identifying which of the four major spinal cord divisions are involved:

Cervical region. Spinal cord segments C1 to C5 (Table 2-14).

TABLE 2-14 Representative Disorders Localized to the Cervical Region of the Spinal Cord

Intervertebral disk disease
Discospondylitis
Cervical trauma
Ischemic myelopathy
Neoplasia
Atlantoaxial subluxation
Steroid-responsive meningitis

TABLE 2-15 Representative Disorders Localized to the Cervical Enlargement Region of the Spinal Cord

Intervertebral disk disease
Discospondylitis
Congenital vertebral anomalies
Neoplasia
Spinal trauma

TABLE 2-16 Representative Disorders Localized to the Thoracolumbar Region of the Spinal Cord

Intervertebral disk disease
Discospondylitis
Neoplasia
Degenerative myelopathy
Lumbar trauma

TABLE 2-17 Representative Disorders Localized to the Caudal Segment and Cauda Equina of the Spinal Cord

Intervertebral disk disease
Lumbar vertebral canal stenosis
Discospondylitis
Lumbar/pelvic trauma

Cervical enlargement. Spinal cord segments C6 to T2 (Table 2-15).
Thoracolumbar region. Spinal cord segments T3 to L3 (Table 2-16).
Lumbar enlargement. Spinal cord segments L4 to the caudal segment, including the cauda equine (Table 2-17).

Note: SPINAL CORD SEGMENTS vs. VERTEBRAE It is important to remember that spinal cord segments do not necessarily correspond exactly with individual vertebrae.

Cervical region. This constitutes the critical region of the spinal cord since complete transaction or myelopathy can result in respiratory arrest and death. Injuries involving less than complete myelopathy can spare respirations but still cause ataxia or paresis in all four limbs. Additionally, cervical spinal injuries rarely result in tetraparesis but can cause hind limb paralysis while sparing the thoracic limbs. Injury at this level is likely to result in normal to exaggerated muscle tone and spinal reflexes including normal anal tone. However, distinguishing between cervical myelopathy and lesions in the brain stem and cerebrum can be difficult. Neck pain, for example, can occur in patients with cervical disk disease, but it may also be present in patients with brain tumors or spinal root entrapment (also called *root signature*). (See Table 2-14.)

Cervical enlargement. Ataxia and paresis involving all four limbs characterize lesions at the level of the cervical enlargement (spinal cord segments C6 to T2). Postural reactions and proprioception are depressed. It is possible for some patients to manifest paresis in the thoracic limbs and paralysis in the hind limbs. Spinal reflexes may be normal; however, if spinal reflexes are abnormal, thoracic limb reflexes are likely to be depressed while abnormal hind limb reflexes are expected to be exaggerated; muscle atrophy of the forelimbs can be significant. On the other hand, anal tone remains normal. Evidence of Horner's syndrome (unilateral ptosis, miosis, enophthalmia, and prolapse of the third eyelid) can be a manifestation of injury at the level of the cervical enlargement. (See Table 2-15.)

Thoracolumbar region. Most of the spinal cord injuries/diseases that are manifest in dogs and cats occur in this region. The most striking neurologic feature is that of normal thoracic limb function and gait in a patient with paresis, ataxia, or paralysis of the hind limbs. Proprioception and postural reactions are normal in the thoracic limbs but are expected to be compromised (to absent) in both hind limbs. Spinal reflexes involving the hind limbs are normal to exaggerated. Although voluntary control of defecation may be lost, anal tone is still present. The ability of the patient to perceive pain (significant pressure applied to the toes) will range from normal to absent (usually a poor prognostic sign). Changes in bladder function are not consistent and are determined by the location, type, and severity of the injury. Rarely, however, will patients with significant spinal injury have normal bladder function and be able to voluntarily control urination. Some patients will be incontinent with a flaccid, easily expressed bladder, while others will be difficult (also called an "upper motor neuron" bladder) to express. (See Table 2-16.)

Lumbar enlargement. Injury or disease involving the caudal-most region of the spinal cord will cause variable clinical manifestations ranging from near normal function to paresis, ataxia, and paralysis. While thoracic limb function is normal, the hind limb reflexes and muscle tone can be obviously reduced and in chronic disease, significant muscle atrophy can be apparent. Anal tone is generally reduced and accompanied by fecal incontinence. Some patients may become severely constipated. While the bladder may fill, the patient is unable to voluntarily urinate. The bladder is easily expressed (also called a "lower motor neuron" bladder). (See Table 2-17.)

Neurogenic urinary incontinence

Bladder dysfunction often accompanies severe spinal cord disease. Total LMN paralysis occurs with sacral spinal cord lesions. Severe or total focal thoracolumbar spinal cord lesions produce a UMN type of paralysis. Paralysis is less common with cervical spinal cord lesions unless the lesions are severe. With both LMN and UMN paralysis, retention of urine occurs. Overflow takes place with both but is more constant with LMN disease. Overflow is less frequent in UMN disease, because greater intraluminal pressure is required to overcome the tone in the striated urethral muscle. If the integrity of the bladder wall is retained, reflex urination may follow within a variable period of time. Reflex urination is more efficient in UMN disease, using the intact peripheral nerves and sacral spinal cord segments. In LMN disease, reflex urination must be mediated within the wall of the bladder and is very inefficient.

Additional Reading

Jones BR: Neurologic disorders. In Schaer M, editor: *Clinical medicine of the dog and cat,* Ames, 2003, Iowa State Press (Blackwell), pp. 505-537.

LaCouteur RA, Grandy JL: Diseases of the spinal cord. In Ettinger SJ, Feldman EC, editors: *Textbook of veterinary internal medicine,* ed 6, St. Louis, 2005, Elsevier, pp. 842-887.

O'Brien DP, Axlund TW: Brain disease. In Ettinger SJ, Feldman EC, editors: *Textbook of veterinary internal medicine,* ed 6, St. Louis, 2005, Elsevier, pp. 803-835.

REPRODUCTIVE TRACT EXAMINATION: MALE

CLINICAL HISTORY

In addition to age, breed, history of breedings and breeding problems, body condition, vaccination, and comments on specific disease problems, establish the environmental setting, feeding, management practices, fertility, and breeding data about related animals. The degree of inbreeding may be important in evaluating sexual function. Previous information related to reproduction is particularly important and should include dates and results of all matings (especially for the previous year). Include comments about libido, breeding techniques, previous fertility and therapy, number of pups born, number weaned, and any abortions or deaths.

EXAMINATION

Inspection and palpation of the genital organs is the first procedure. A thickened scrotal wall may produce testicular degeneration from increased temperature. Palpate the spermatic cord and testes for size, symmetry, and consistency (firm resilience), and note whether the testes are both located in the scrotum. Small, soft testes indicate degeneration or hypoplasia; firm masses may be the result of inflammation, fibrosis, or tumors. Testicular tumors are relatively common in dogs over 8 years old and may, depending on tumor type, produce estrogens or testosterone that can cause mammary development, alter reproductive ability/ interest, and may cause life-threatening coagulopathies. The epididymis, palpable dorsal to the testis, may be prominent or firm because of fibrosis or ascending infection. The penis, prepuce, and external urethral orifice should be examined for frenula, hypospadias, phimosis, balanoposthitis, and, in older patients, neoplasia.

The prostate is the only accessory sex gland in the dog. Examine the prostate by rectal palpation. The prostate should be smooth, bilaterally symmetric, nonpainful, and, in most dogs, usually smaller than 3 cm in diameter. Nodules, fixation, and pain are found in carcinomas; nonpainful symmetric enlargements (often so large as to pull the organ into the abdomen) are seen with cysts or benign prostatic hypertrophy. The four major causes of prostatomegaly are benign hypertrophy; prostatitis, including abscessation of the prostate; prostatic cysts; and primary or secondary prostatic tumors. The appearance of an enlarged prostate on survey radiographs, combined with positive contrast retrograde urethrography and prostatic ultrasonography, can be helpful in the differential diagnosis. Hyperplastic and inflammatory prostatic diseases result in more symmetric prostatomegaly than do cystic, neoplastic, or prostatic abscess processes. Signs of acute bacterial prostatitis include urethral discharge, constipation, tenesmus, stilted gait, fever, depression, abdominal pain, dysuria, and leukocytosis. Chronic bacterial prostatitis may include signs associated with recurrent urinary tract infection, and the use of radiography, prostatic fluid evaluation, cultures, and biopsy may be necessary to establish a diagnosis.

Numerous additional testing procedures can be used in evaluating the animal with prostatic disease, including ejaculation and microscopic evaluation, prostatic biopsy, and prostatic aspiration and massage. Techniques for performing these procedures are described in Section 4.

REPRODUCTIVE TRACT EXAMINATION: FEMALE

CLINICAL HISTORY

Disorders associated with breeding, especially failure to conceive, are among the most common female genital presentations. Blood in the urine or frequent urination are the most common presentations involving the female urinary tract. In evaluating the patient, the clinical history is particularly important and should include age, breed, body condition, vaccination status, and comments on specific disease problems. Determine the environmental setting, feeding, breeding, and other management practices concerning the animal and the fertility and breeding data for related animals. The stud dog's records should also be examined. Pedigrees should be examined to determine inbreeding or possible genetic defects. Obtain information about the age at first estrus; number and frequency of estrous cycles; breedings; pregnancies; history of false pregnancies; urogenital problems; litters whelped; and numbers of pups born and weaned, with causes of abortions or deaths, if known. Treatments and prophylactic measures, especially if they involve sex hormones, should be investigated.

EXAMINATION

Inspection and palpation of the external genitalia provide limited but valuable information. The vulva is usually small and wrinkled, with good tone and free of discharge. Obese females may be difficult to examine, particularly when a "hooded" vulva is present. Note the size and condition of the clitoris. The vulva swells during proestrus and has a serosanguineous discharge; during estrus an odorless bloody or mucoid discharge is present. Exudates at other times, especially if fetid, suggest infection (open pyometra), neoplasia, or other endocrine problems. Digital examination of the vestibule and caudal vagina and abdominal palpation of the uterus should be performed in all bitches presenting with a clinical history of vaginal discharge. Contrast vaginography, vaginoscopy, and ultrasonographic examination of the uterus and ovaries may be indicated when disease processes have been localized to these organs. More details about examination of the vagina and vaginal cytology can be found in Section 4.

Individual mammary glands should be palpated and inspected for the presence of infection (mastitis), hypertrophy, or tumors. Acute infections are hot, painful, and swollen; usually involve only one gland; and produce a purulent secretion. Chronic mastitis involves several glands; the glands are enlarged, firm, and nodular on palpation.

Mammary gland tumors constitute about half of all neoplasms in the intact bitch, and about half of these are malignant. The median age of affected bitches is 10.5 years, and mammary gland tumors are multicentric in about 50% of bitches. Of the benign tumor forms, the most frequently recognized histologic patterns are fibroadenomas (benign mixed tumors), 45%; simple adenomas; and benign mesenchymal tumors. Of the malignant tumors in the dog, the most common histologic types are solid carcinomas, tubular adenocarcinomas, papillary adenocarcinomas, anaplastic carcinomas, and sarcomas.

In malignant tumors that metastasize, tumor cells from glands 4 and 5 drain to the inguinal lymph nodes and via the thoracic duct to the lungs. The iliac lymph nodes may also be involved with metastasis. Tumor cells from glands 1 and 2 drain to the axillary lymph nodes and to the lungs and may involve the intrathoracic lymph nodes. Gland 3 appears to drain more commonly to the axillary lymph nodes. Hematogenous spread of mammary tumors with no lymph node involvement is also possible. Many malignant mammary tumors of the bitch metastasize widely and may affect abdominal as well as thoracic organs.

Fine-needle biopsy and cytologic examination may be helpful in distinguishing benign from malignant cell types. Multiple mammary gland tumors, which are present in 50% of dogs, may have different tumor types; thus, all tissues and regional lymph nodes should be sectioned.

Mammary gland neoplasia in the bitch is *almost 100% preventable* if ovariectomy is performed before the first estrous cycle. The incidence of mammary gland neoplasia can be *markedly reduced* if ovariectomy is done before the animal is 2.5 years old or before the first four estrous periods. Pharmacologic doses of progestational compounds have been associated with the development of mixed mammary gland tumors.

Mammary tumors occur more frequently in cats than in any other domestic animal except the dog. Ninety percent of the tumors observed are malignant. The tumors are usually adenocarcinomas and are seen most commonly in cats 7 years of age or older. The tumors usually ulcerate early in their development. The cat normally has four pairs of mammary glands. The cranial two glands on each side have a common lymphatic system and drain into the axillary lymph nodes. The caudal two mammary glands also have a common lymphatic system and drain into the superficial inguinal lymph nodes.

Bacteriologic examination

Bacteriologic examination of mammary secretion, vaginal smear or culture, and intrauterine culture (collected at laparotomy) is very important if infectious processes are suspected. All breeding bitches should be tested for brucellosis; a positive rapid slide test should be confirmed by laboratory tube tests or blood cultures.

Infertility, abortion, premature births, stillbirths, or neonatal deaths can be caused by many infectious agents, such as β-hemolytic streptococci, *E. coli*, *B. canis*, *Staphylococcus*, *Proteus*, *Pseudomonas*, and *Mycoplasma* spp.; canine distemper; adenovirus; and herpesvirus. Fetal resorption, mummification, and abortion may be caused by any of the infectious agents just listed or by numeric chromosomal abnormality, inherited metabolic disease, maternal endocrine abnormality (thyroid insufficiency), lack of uterine space, trauma, placental hemorrhage, hormone deficiency (progesterone), exogenous estrogen, myometrial cysts, hyperplasia, and endometritis. In evaluating these problems, supplement the bacteriologic examination with maternal serology and hormone analysis, pedigree studies of the sire and dam, and, particularly, aggressive diagnostic evaluation of the dead fetus(es) (karyotype, culture, histopathology, metabolic screening).

Radiographic examination

Radiographic examination of the uterus can be performed easily if the organ is enlarged (pyometra, pregnancy, tumors). However, examination is limited to detection of an abnormally enlarged or displace uterus. Radiographic contrast studies, such as injection of a radiopaque dye through the cervix to delineate intrauterine disease (e.g., cystic hyperplasia, myometrial cysts), have been replaced today with abdominal ultrasound. *Peritoneal laparoscopy* is a technique that may be useful for direct observation of abdominal organs such as the uterus. The ovaries are embedded in fatty bursae and thus are difficult to visualize unless the examiner is skilled at incising the bursae. *Exploratory laparotomy* is sometimes necessary to completely examine the female reproductive tract. One can directly view and palpate the uterus, oviducts, and ovaries for malformations and pathologic changes that cannot be delineated in other ways. Placental sites or corpora lutea can be counted to determine embryonic death, and microbiologic samples and biopsy material can be obtained for laboratory evaluation. At the same time, surgical or medical measures may be performed for treatment of abnormalities.

Pregnancy examination

Palpation of the uterus through the abdominal wall is the most practical method of pregnancy examination. At 20 to 22 days following ovulation, the uterus has distinct swellings 2 cm in diameter. After 28 days, these swellings have increased to about 3 to 5 cm in diameter, and this is the optimal time for diagnosis. (Diagnosis in the queen is easiest within 18 to 24 days and is difficult after 30 days.) By 35 days, the uterine swellings become confluent and diagnosis becomes more difficult. As pregnancy continues, individual fetuses may be palpated per rectum or through the abdominal wall.

Mammary glands enlarge at about 35 days of gestation, and the teats become enlarged and turgid. The nipples of a primiparous bitch are often quite red in color. Milk can be expressed from the teats during the last week of pregnancy.

Radiographs first show calcified fetal skeletons between 43 and 54 days after the first breeding in the bitch. Radiographs may be especially helpful if only one or two fetuses are present.

Today, abdominal ultrasonography is routinely performed to confirm a pregnancy diagnosis. Examination may reveal the presence of viable fetuses by the detection of fetal heart beats as early as 24 to 28 days postbreeding.

RESPIRATORY TRACT EXAMINATION: UPPER

ANATOMIC LIMITS

The upper respiratory tract is particularly susceptible to injury and disease. Consequently, dogs and cats are commonly presented with acute-onset and chronic upper respiratory tract signs. While there is no universal agreement stipulating where the upper respiratory tract ends and the lower respiratory tract begins, for this discussion, the term "upper respiratory tract" refers to all air-filled cavities rostral to the first cartilaginous ring of the trachea. This includes the following:

The nasal cavity, external nares, and planum nasale
The frontal sinuses (maxillary sinuses are not usually functional in dogs and cats)
The nasopharynx and posterior nares (choana)
The oral cavity (insofar as it is used for breathing/panting) and the upper dental arcade
The oropharynx including the tonsils
The larynx

LOCALIZING CLINICAL SIGNS OF UPPER RESPIRATORY TRACT DISEASE

Sonorous breathing. Not a localizing sign. This term only refers to loud or noisy breathing.

Sneezing and nasal discharge. Localizes disease to the nasal cavity, frontal sinuses, or the upper dental arcade. In patients with epistaxis, coagulopathy must be ruled out if a nasal, sinus, or dental lesion cannot be identified. Sneezing may occur with or without evidence of nasal discharge. If discharge is present, the character (serous; mucoid, mucopurulent or purulent; hemorrhagic [epistaxis]) should be noted. Indicate whether the discharge is bilateral or unilateral; if unilateral, designate patient's right or left nostril.

Stertor (or snorting). Localizes disease to the oropharynx, the soft palate, or possibly the nasopharynx. THE PATIENT **MUST** BE EXAMINED UNDER GENERAL ANESTHESIA TO ADEQUATELY EVALUATE CAUSES OF STERTOR.

Stridor (or wheezing). Localizes disease to the larynx and occasionally the cervical trachea. This is a **critical sign** in a dog or cat that deserves immediate attention. Restriction of airflow through the larynx is potentially life threatening if not corrected in a timely manner. Tracheal collapse, laryngeal paralysis, laryngeal trauma, and tracheal/larygneal tumor are possible causes that must be ruled out as soon as possible.

Note: Evaluation of the patient presented for chronic, persistent **STERTOR** or **STRIDOR** requires examination under general anesthesia.

EXAMINATION OF THE NOSE AND ORAL CAVITY

External examination of the nose is limited to evaluation for symmetry, pain, nasal discharge (either unilateral [stipulate patient's right or left nostril] or bilateral), and erosions or ulceration of the planum nasale. Further evaluation of the patient presented with a history of sonorous breathing, sneezing, or nasal discharge is indicated. Any additional studies are all special diagnostic procedures (see Section 4) that require general anesthesia to achieve adequate visibility. Additional studies include the following:

Nasal and sinus radiography

Rhinoscopy and biopsy, where indicated

Pharyngoscopy (both of the oropharynx and the nasopharynx) and biopsy, where indicated.

Otic exam (for nasopharyngeal polyps in cats)

Computed tomography (CT) or magnetic resonance imaging (MRI) (*requires access to a veterinary referral center, special equipment, and clinical specialists trained to perform/interpret studies*).

EXAMINATION OF THE NASOPHARYNX AND OROPHARYNX

Stertor, or snorting, is the most common clinical sign associated with disease in the nasopharynx and oropharyrnx. Neither the nasopharynx nor the oropharynx can be properly examined in the awake or sedated patient. ALL dogs and cats presented for stertor or sonorous breathing are candidates for examination under general anesthesia. Examination of the oropharynx can be conducted without the need for special equipment. Even in the anesthetized patient, visual examination of the nasopharynx is limited to what can be observed by retracting the soft palate forward (usually using a spay hook) and by digital palpation of the soft palate. Pharyngeal endoscopy (pharyngoscopy) is a valuable procedure in affected patients as it allows the clinician to visualize the rostral-most aspect of the nasopharynx and the posterior nares, also called the choana.

Commonly encountered disorders include nasopharyngeal foreign bodies (anything goes!), elongated soft palate, nasopharyngeal polyps (feline only), tumor, and parasites (cuterebra larvae).

EXAMINATION OF THE LARYNX

Dogs and cats presenting with clinical signs of laryngeal disease (e.g., stridor or wheezing) should be evaluated immediately for injury or disease that is causing restriction of airflow through the glottis. Assume these patients are emergency cases until proven otherwise. Failing to relieve airway obstruction at the level of the larynx may result in a fatal outcome!

External palpation of the larynx is indicated in the nonsedated patient to determine if change in the character of breathing or the pitch of the stridor can be detected. Patients that are in respiratory distress usually benefit from examination under general anesthesia. The patient should be managed as a critical patient and the clinician should be prepared to place a tracheostomy tube if necessary to sustain anesthesia and provide oxygen to the patient. Once the patient is stable and breathing well, cervical radiographs may be helpful in elucidating certain types of foreign bodies entrapped in laryngeal tissues. Commonly encountered disorders include laryngeal paralysis (dogs and cats), laryngeal edema, laryngeal collapse or compressive trauma, foreign body (e.g., plant material, fish hook), and tumor.

RESPIRATORY TRACT EXAMINATION: LOWER

For purposes of this discussion, the lower respiratory tract extends from the first tracheal ring to the alveoli and includes the parietal and visceral pleura as well as the pleural space. When evaluating an animal with lower respiratory tract disease, it is important to (1) *carefully observe* the animal while listening to the *history*; (2) examine the *whole animal*; and (3) *palpate, percuss,* and *auscultate* the thorax and neck. The completeness of the evaluation is tentative, depending on the animal's condition. Before the animal is disturbed, determine its respiratory rate and pattern. Normally, the dog breathes 10 to 30 times per minute (when not panting) and the cat breathes 20 to 60 times per minute. An increase in the respiratory rate (tachypnea) does not always mean that a respiratory disease is present. Excitement, heat, exercise, pain, shock, or anemia may cause an increased respiratory rate. A decreased respiratory rate may result from narcotic poisoning or metabolic alkalosis.

NORMAL RESPIRATORY RATE (AT REST)
Dog: 10 to 30/min **Cat:** 20 to 30/min

2

An animal may have dyspnea and respiratory disease with a normal respiratory rate. The pattern or rhythm of breathing can help categorize disease.

Labored breathing (dyspnea) can be slow, deep, and deliberate, or rapid and shallow. The dyspneic animal may assume a characteristic posture in a squatting position with abducted elbows. Dyspnea may be principally inspiratory, expiratory, or both. Inspiratory dyspnea is seen as difficulty in expanding the lungs with a relatively easy expiratory effort. Inspiratory dyspnea is observed most frequently in diseases that are restrictive. These diseases include those that restrict expansion of the lung because of disease of the pleura, chest wall, or neuromuscular apparatus or diseases with infiltrate within the lung parenchyma that displace alveolar air. Restrictive diseases are characterized by a reduced vital capacity and a small resting lung volume without an increase in airway resistance relative to lung volume. Elastic recoil is increased, and air is exhaled rapidly. The lung's compliance is decreased. Examples of restrictive pulmonary disorders are pneumothorax, pleural effusions, or diffusely infiltrating diseases such as pneumonias or neoplasia. Inspiratory dyspnea is also observed with upper airway obstructions such as laryngeal paralysis.

Expiratory dyspnea is seen as difficulty in expelling air from the lungs. Normally, expiratory time is shorter than inspiratory time. Expiratory dyspnea is observed most frequently in obstructive lung disease. Airway obstruction due to increased resistance to airflow can be caused by conditions inside the lumen, in the bronchial wall, or in the surrounding bronchial region. A combination of these problems can exist in disease. An airway lumen may be compromised by bronchiectasis, severe pulmonary edema, or aspiration of fluid. Contraction of bronchial smooth muscle (which occurs in bronchial asthma), hypertrophy of mucous glands, or inflammation and edema of the airway wall can cause obstruction. Obstruction outside an airway can be caused by destruction of lung parenchyma that results in loss of radial traction and narrowing, as in emphysema. Narrowing can also be caused by peribronchial edema. With obstructive disease, air can usually get into the lungs, and lung volumes are normal or even elevated. With partial airway obstruction, inspiratory forces open the airway to allow air to enter the lung, but because of dynamic compression, expiratory forces can cause the airway to collapse. Dynamic compression is the narrowing of the airways that occurs during expiration due to increases in intrathoracic pressure and is a normal phenomenon that is exaggerated in situations of increased airway resistance and low lung volume. Inspiratory dyspnea and expiratory dyspnea may be observed together in various diseases, depending on the pulmonary changes present. Frequently, both types of dyspnea are associated with pulmonary edema.

When a dog or cat is dyspneic, the respiratory pattern is one that makes the work of breathing easiest with the least expenditure of energy. With reduced compliance or stiff lungs due to parenchyma or pleural disease, an animal will tend to take small, rapid breaths, whereas an animal with airway obstruction will take deeper, slower breaths. These patterns reflect the altered forces (elastic, viscous resistance) that must be overcome in the breathing process. The cost of an increase in the work of breathing (oxygen consumed) will alter the ability of the animal to exercise.

Cyanosis is the appearance of a bluish tinge to the skin as a result of excess deoxyhemoglobin. For cyanosis to be apparent on physical exam, 5 g of deoxygenated hemoglobin must be present; therefore, marked hypoxemia may be present but not appreciated by observation of mucous membranes.

THE CARDINAL SIGNS OF LOWER RESPIRATORY DISEASE

Cough, dyspnea, production of abnormal secretions or discharges, noisy (or sonorous) breathing, and a change in characteristic airway sounds (either increased or decreased) are principal clinical signs seen in patients with lower respiratory disease. Animals with pulmonary disease may not be presented with clinical signs that direct attention to the lower respiratory tract (e.g., nasal discharge).

Determine the presence or absence of the following:

1. **Nasal discharge.** The discharge may be unilateral or bilateral. Determine the character (blood, mucoid, mucopurulent, purulent, or serous) and duration (acute, chronic) of the discharge.
2. **Abnormal lung sounds.** Carefully auscultate the lungs for evidence of abnormal breath sounds consistent with fluid/mucous in the lower airways.

Note: The absence of normal lung sounds is as important as the presence of abnormal lung sounds.

2

3. *Coughing.* A *true cough* (sudden forced expulsion of air through a closed glottis) is characterized by the animal lowering its head and opening its mouth during expiration. The cough itself may be moist and productive, or dry, nonproductive, and paroxysmal, and it can be accentuated by collar pressure, exercise, or cold air. It should be noted whether the cough is productive or nonproductive. *Caution*: Most dogs swallow expectorated secretions, so the cough may appear to be nonproductive. Examine any expelled secretions for color, consistency, cell content, foreign bodies, and parasites. Hemoptysis (the presence of blood in expectorated secretions) is rare but may indicate tumor, *Paragonimus* spp. infection, injury from smoke inhalation, or pulmonary hypertension (especially heartworm disease).
4. *Dyspnea.* When presented for the chief complaint of intermittent "respiratory distress," the owner should be questioned regarding when the animal has difficulty (e.g., at rest, after exercise) and how severe the distress is (e.g., open-mouth breathing, cyanosis). Animals with dyspnea at rest are critical patients. Stress and excessive handling should be avoided at all costs. In cats, dyspnea can be very subtle and may only be manifest by open-mouth breathing.
5. *Noisy breathing.* Abnormal breathing sounds may be generated from the upper or lower airway. The owner should be questioned about the perceived origin of the abnormal sounds. In general, a noisy airway represents incomplete or partial airway obstruction.

Thoracic percussion

Percussion

Percussion of the thorax entails using the fingers to strike the left and right hemithorax with short, sharp blows as an aid in assessing the presence or absence of air versus fluid in the pleural space and lungs. Subtle changes in the sound produced may reflect excessive air or fluid in the pleural space or lungs. The technique of percussion involves placing the middle finger of the left hand firmly on the chest and using it as a pleximeter. Rap the distal phalanx abruptly with the middle finger of the right hand. Three rules must be applied in percussion:

1. In defining boundaries, always move from the more resonant to the less resonant areas.
2. The long axis of the pleximeter (finger) must be parallel to the boundary of the edges of the organ being percussed.
3. The progression of the line of percussion should be at right angles to the edge of the organ.

Application and interpretation of percussion are more difficult in small animals than in large animals. Differences in sound are slight, and it is helpful to percuss the thorax systematically by tapping the ribs while a stethoscope is held firmly against the opposite chest wall. The percussion tones are thus greatly magnified by the instrument, and differences are more obvious.

Resonance

Resonance is *increased* when the pleural cavity contains air and the lung is collapsed. In this case, the musical "bell sound" may also be heard. Resonance may also be increased by emphysema (rare). Resonance is *decreased* when the lung is more solid than usual, as with edema, pneumonia, or tumor; when the pleura is thickened; when the pleural cavity contains fluid; or when an abdominal viscus is displaced into the thoracic space.

Thoracic radiography

Thoracic radiography is among the most useful and important diagnostic procedures used to characterize lower respiratory tract disease in dogs and cats. Normal radiographic anatomy is depicted for the cat (Figure 2-25).

Thoracic auscultation

The stethoscope

All stethoscopes are not alike. Some are better designed acoustically than others. The bell transmits low-pitched sounds, and the diaphragm transmits soft, high-pitched sounds best. Electronic stethoscopes recently introduced not only include a volume control, but also have specially programmed filters designed to enhance listening to breath sounds versus heart sounds. For best results, do the following:

1. Perform the auscultation in a room as free of noise as possible.
2. Hold the stethoscope firmly against the chest.
3. Do not breathe on the tubing.
4. Avoid hair friction and muscle noises. Wetting the subject's hair may be helpful.
5. Listen with the animal breathing quietly, if possible.
6. Close the mouth of a panting animal; stop the subject from shivering or trembling.
7. Stop cats from purring. Gently blow short bursts of air across the nose and face or turn on a water faucet. And good luck—some cats insist on purring, no matter what!
8. Concentrate on each part of the respiratory or cardiac cycle separately. Listen intently!
9. Repeat the exam. This step is particularly important in dogs/cats suspected of having lower respiratory disease.
10. If using an electronic stethoscope, we have found maximum sound enhancement occurs when a contact medium (ECG or EChG gel) is placed on the diaphragm of the stethoscope, thereby improving the contact between the stethoscope and the patient.

Characterization of breath sounds (see Table 2-4)

There is no clear consensus on the most appropriate terminology to use when describing normal versus abnormal lung sounds in animals. Auscultation of the lung sounds depends not only on the actual intensity of the sounds but also on the reflection and transmission of the sounds of the stethoscope.

Normal breath sounds

Normal breath sounds in dogs and cats include tracheal (very loud, high pitch, harsh), bronchial (loud, high pitch, tubular), and bronchvesicular (moderately loud, medium pitch, rustling). Normal breath sounds ausculted over most of the peripheral lung fields are described as soft, low pitched, and with a gentle rustling quality. Normal breath sounds are usually louder in the cat, kitten, and puppy than in the dog because the transmission of the sounds to the chest wall is greater. Breath sounds may be decreased in intensity with conditions that decrease transmission, such as pleural effusion, pneumothorax, or chest wall thickness. With pleural fluid, the breath sounds are quiet ventrally but loud dorsally. With emphysema or complete airway obstruction, the lungs are too quiet.

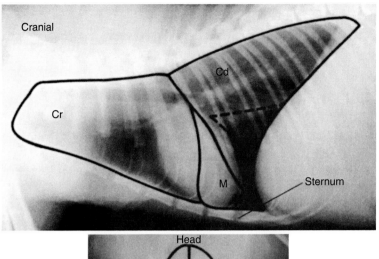

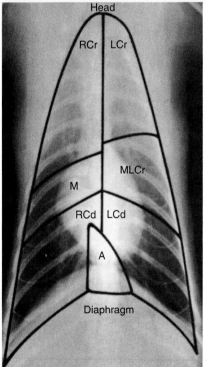

Figure 2-25: **A,** Lateral radiograph of a normal cat with lung lobes identified. Cr, right and left cranial lung lobes; M, right middle lung lobe; Cd, right and left caudal lung lobes. **B,** Dorsoventral radiograph of a normal cat with lung lobes identified. RCr, right cranial lung lobe; M, right middle lung lobe; RCd, right caudal lung lobe; A, accessory lung lobe; LCr, cranial lung lobe; MLCr, middle portion of the left cranial lung lobe; LCd, left caudal lung lobe.

THE FOLLOWING ANATOMIC LANDMARKS SHOULD BE CONSISTENTLY IDENTIFIED AND EVALUATED WHEN REVIEWING THORACIC RADIOGRAPHS

- Trachea (cervical and intrathoracic)
- Tracheal bifurcation (carina)
- RIGHT and LEFT cranial lung lobes
- Middle (RIGHT side only) lung lobe
- RIGHT and LEFT caudal lung lobes

Crackles

Previously called "rales," crackles are discontinuous or interrupted, abnormal breath sounds usually caused by excessive fluid within the airways. This fluid could be due to an exudate, as in pneumonia or other infections of the lung, or a transudate, as can occur in patients with pulmonary edema or decompensated congestive heart failure. Crackles are typically inspiratory and have been subcategorized as "wet" sounding or "dry." Crackles are similar to the sound made when using a thumb and forefinger to rub one's own hair near the ear.

Wheeze

Wheezes are characteristically described as an expiratory sound associated with forced airflow through abnormally collapsed airways with residual trapping of air. In humans, wheeze is commonly associated with asthma. However, in dogs and cats, wheezes are more likely to be associated with other causes such as airway obstruction (tumor) or obstructing foreign bodies.

> **Note:** Stridor, an audible wheeze frequently heard without the need for a stethoscope, is a critical clinical sign commonly associated with laryngeal obstruction (e.g., laryngeal paralysis). In the case of wheeze associated with laryngeal obstruction, the audible sound is likely to be best heard on inspiration.

With restrictive lung diseases, the lung volume is reduced and many airways are collapsed, and the opening of such airways produces crackles. Continuous, musical sounds that are high-pitched, sibilant, or squeaky are called wheezes. Wheezing can occur during inspiration (laryngeal paralysis) or expiration (obstructive bronchial disease). It is important to realize that the absence of abnormal lung sounds does not guarantee that the lungs are normal.

NORMAL BREEDING BEHAVIOR AND PHYSIOLOGY

THE INTACT FEMALE DOG

The puberal estrus in the intact female dog ("bitch") usually occurs between the ages of 6 and 12 months; the reproductive life of the female dog is 8 to 10 years. The canine female is seasonally monestrous and ovulates spontaneously. The interval between estrous cycles ranges from 4 to 12 months, depending on the size and breed of the animal (e.g., basenji, once a year; small breeds, two or three times a year; and large breeds, one or more times a year). For cellular characteristics of vaginal smears, see Section 4.

Proestrus lasts for 3 to 17 (mean = 9) days, during which time serum estradiol concentrations increase. Other characteristics are a bloody discharge from the vagina and a swollen vulva. The bitch attracts males but will not accept mating. Plasma estrogens reach a maximum level at the end of proestrus and then decrease.

Estrus lasts from 3 to 21 (mean = 9) days. Proestrus and estrus periods combined are called the "heat" period. The character of the discharge usually changes from bloody (during proestrus) to straw colored (during estrus) but may remain sanguineous without an adverse effect on fertility. The vulva is less turgid. The bitch is receptive and courts the male through foreplay, jumping, and trying to mount the male. The canine female presents the perineum in a lordosis-like posture and reflexively deviates the tail to one side. The bitch first refuses mating by the male at a variable time after the onset of estrus (usually 6 to 15 days). Ovulation usually occurs early in estrus (within the first 3 days), but some normal bitches may ovulate several days before to 11 days after onset of estrus. The ovum is not ready for fertilization until 48 hours later, after the second polar body has been extruded. The ovum lives 4 to 5 days, the transit time to the uterus being 4 to 10 days. Implantation occurs in 18 to 20 days, and an endotheliochorial deciduate zonary placenta forms. The gestation cycle is 58 to 71 days from a single breeding or 62 to 64 days from ovulation.

Luteinizing hormone (LH) surges within 24 hours of the estrogen peak and causes ovulation. Progesterone increases gradually during estrus and is the cause of "behavioral" estrus. Serum progesterone concentration rises to about 2 ng/mL on the day of the LH surge; best reproductive performance (conception rate and litter size) occurs when the bitch is bred 4 days after the LH surge, which is also 2 days after ovulation. Progesterone reaches a maximum 25 to 30 days after the LH surge and then gradually decreases to less than 1 mg/mL at parturition in the pregnant bitch. The progesterone decline is the cause of the temperature drop just before parturition. After ovum implantation, the hematocrit falls from 40% to 45% to 30%, which is probably a reflection of plasma volume expansion in the pregnant bitch; nonpregnant luteal-phase bitches also show a decline in hematocrit level from anestrous values but do not show the magnitude of decline seen in pregnancy.

Diestrus (2 months) is the period when the corpus luteum produces progesterone, which is present in the bitch's serum in concentrations exceeding 2 ng/mL. Diestrus begins on the first day of a predominantly noncornified vaginal smear and ends when serum progesterone declines to less than 2 ng/mL. Both pregnant and nonpregnant bitches have periods of diestrus lasting approximately 2 months.

Anestrus (approximately 4 months) is the period during which the genital organs are relatively quiescent; the uterine lining regenerates.

THE INTACT MALE DOG

Puberty in the male dog occurs between 6 to 12 months of age. Follicle-stimulating hormone (FSH) initiates spermatogenesis; luteinizing hormone (LH) increases the testosterone secretion of Leydig cells needed to complete spermatogenesis and to maintain accessory sex glands, secondary sex characteristics, and libido. Testosterone has a negative feedback effect on pituitary gonadotropins. Oxytocin and prostaglandins are important in the transport of sperm during ejaculation. Prostaglandins increase LH output and testosterone production and are the reason why sexual foreplay increases ejaculatory output and total number of sperm. Testosterone is of little value in the treatment of infertility, except to increase libido for 2 to 3 days following administration of low doses. Prolonged use causes testicular degeneration and a negative feedback effect on LH release.

In copulation, the male responds to the female in estrus by biting and nuzzling her neck and licking her flanks and perineal region. The male mounts and clasps the female's hindquarters at the rear flank with his forelegs. After pelvic copulatory movement, intromission of the nonerect penis takes place, after which erection of the penis inside the vagina occurs. Ejaculation of the presperm and sperm-rich fractions of semen occurs during the most vigorous pelvic thrusting of the male, after which the male dismounts and, with the engorged penis still entrapped inside the vagina, lifts a hindleg over the rear quarters of the female and stands end to end with her in copulatory lock, or tie. During the tie, which may last from 5 to 60 minutes, the dog ejaculates the third and most voluminous fraction of semen, the prostatic fluid. Some male dogs rebreed within 2 hours of separation.

THE INTACT FEMALE CAT

Puberty in the female cat occurs at 4 to 12 months of age. The reproductive life is 8 to 10 years. The female cat is seasonally polyestrous (January through September in the

Northern Hemisphere, or continuous if 14 hours of light are available daily). Ovulation is induced by coitus or simulated coitus. Estrus occurs every 4 to 30 days. Proestrus lasts 0 to 2 days, during which pheromones increase and a very slight mucoid discharge from the Bartholin glands may occur.

Estrus lasts 6 to 10 days in most queens (range: 2 to 12 days), and estrus length is not influenced by whether ovulation occurs. Following nonfertile induction of ovulation, the corpora lutea last 30 to 40 days, and the cycle averages 6 weeks. The feline female has a characteristic call, rubs the head against objects with affection, purrs, crouches with forelegs, elevates rear quarters and treads, and deflects tail laterally. Ovulation occurs 24 to 50 hours after copulation (sensory nerves stimulate the hypothalamus to release gonadotropin-releasing hormone, which acts on the anterior pituitary to release a surge of LH, causing ovulation). Sperm requires 24-hour capcitation in the uterus to be fertile, and fertilization may occur up to 48 hours after ovulation.

Fertilized ova are in the oviduct for 4 days. Implantation occurs 14 days after breeding, and an endotheliochorial zonary placenta forms. Gestation length is 58 to 70 days (usually 60 to 63 days).

Postestrus occurs if the queen is not induced to ovulate. This stage is 7 to 21 days long; the ova degenerate, and then the queen returns to estrus.

Anestrus lasts 1 to 6 months, depending on photoperiod; during anestrus, the queen does not mate.

THE INTACT MALE CAT

Puberty occurs at about 6 months (depending on age at the beginning of the breeding season) for data about artificial insemination and feline sperm. The tom has depressed sexual activity in the fall. He has rigid territorial and behavioral habits regarding the breeding ritual, and the feline male does much calling and fighting to retain his home territory.

The male approaches the female, makes chattering sounds, and rubs his face over her shoulder and body. Foreplay is limited; the tom grasps the queen's neck skin in his teeth and mounts.

Additional Reading

Feldman EC, Nelson RW: *Canine and feline endocrinology and reproduction,* ed 3. Philadelphia, 2004, WB Saunders.
Grundy SA, Davidson AP: Feline reproduction. In Ettinger SJ, Feldman EC, editors: *Textbook of veterinary internal medicine,* ed 6, St. Louis, 2005, Elsevier, pp. 1696-1707.
Schaefers-Okkens AC: Estrous cycle and breeding management of the healthy bitch. In Ettinger SJ, Feldman EC, editors: *Textbook of veterinary internal medicine,* ed 6, St. Louis, 2005, Elsevier, pp. 1646-1649.
Thomas PGA: Reproductive disorders. In Schaer M, editor: *Clinical medicine of the dog and cat.* Ames, 2004, Iowa State Press (Blackwell), pp. 454-503.

URINARY TRACT EXAMINATION

CLINICAL HISTORY

The history of any patient presenting for urinary tract disorders should include information about onset (acute or gradual), progression (improving, unchanging, or worsening), and response to previous therapy. Information about husbandry includes the animal's immediate environment (indoor or outdoor); use (pet, breeding, show, or working animal); geographic origin and travel history; exposure to other animals; vaccination status; diet; and information about previous trauma, illness, or surgery. A brief review of body systems may be obtained by determining the presence or absence of the following abnormalities: lethargy, anorexia, vomiting, diarrhea, coughing, sneezing, exercise intolerance, polyuria, polydipsia, weight loss, lameness, pruritus, alopecia, and exposure to drugs or toxins.

Questions related to the urinary tract include those about changes in water intake and the frequency or volume of urination. The owner should be questioned about pollakiuria, dysuria, or hematuria. Care must be taken to distinguish dysuria and pollakiuria from polyuria and to differentiate polyuria from urinary incontinence (see Section 3). The distinction between pollakiuria and polyuria is very important because polyuria may be a sign of upper urinary disease, whereas pollakiuria and dysuria usually indicate lower urinary tract disease. Occasionally, an owner will complain that the dog is incontinent because it is urinating in the house when in reality the dog is polyuric but is not allowed outdoors frequently enough. Nocturia may be an early sign of polyuria but also can occur as a result of dysuria.

Note: Normal urine output ranges from 20 to 45 ml/kg/day in dogs and cats.

2

Information about the initiation of urination and diameter of the urine stream may be helpful because animals with partial obstruction may experience difficulty initiating urination or may have an abnormal urine stream. If hematuria is present, question the owner about its timing. Blood at the beginning of urination may indicate a disease process in the urethra or genital tract. Blood at the end of urination or throughout urination may signify a problem in either the bladder or upper urinary tract (kidneys or ureters).

Polydipsia usually is more easily detected by the owner than polyuria. Water intake should not exceed 90 mL/kg/day in dogs and 45 mL/kg/day in cats. It is helpful to describe amounts in quantitative terms familiar to the owner, such as cups (approximately 250 mL per cup) or quarts (approximately 1 L/q). Question the owner about exposure of the animal to nephrotoxins such as ethylene glycol in antifreeze (especially during fall and spring), aminoglycoside antibiotics, amphotericin B, thiacetarsamide, and NSAIDs. Also, determine whether the animal has received any drugs that could cause polydipsia and polyuria, such as corticosteroids or diuretics.

EXAMINATION

Disorders of the upper *and* lower urinary tract can culminate in organ failure and rapid onset systemic illness; hydration should be carefully assessed by evaluating physical parameters such as skin turgor, position of the eyes in the orbits, and moistness of mucous membranes. Pulse rate and character, capillary refill time, and heart rate should also be recorded. The minimal amount of dehydration detectable clinically is approximately 5% of body weight; 15% dehydration is the maximal amount compatible with life. Skin elasticity and subcutaneous fat affect the reliability of skin turgor in the assessment of hydration. Obese animals may be dehydrated yet demonstrate normal skin turgor, whereas emaciated animals may have abnormal skin turgor yet not be dehydrated. Changes in weight can be used to monitor changes in hydration on an acute basis, since 1 L of fluid is equal to 1 kg of body weight. Evaluate the animal for the presence of ascites or subcutaneous edema, which may occur in patients with nephrotic syndrome.

The oral cavity

Examine the oral cavity for ulcers, which may occur in the presence of uremia, especially in dogs. Tongue-tip necrosis occasionally occurs in uremic dogs because of fibrinoid necrosis of vessels in the tongue. Examine the mucous membranes for pallor suggestive of anemia. Vascular injection may be observed in the sclera and soft palate of some uremic dogs. Examine the fundus for evidence of systemic hypertension, which can complicate renal disease: retinal edema, retinal detachment, retinal hemorrhage, and vascular tortuosity.

MAXIMUM NORMAL WATER INTAKE
Dogs: 90 ml/kg/day **Cats:** 45 ml/kg/day

NORMAL SYSTOLIC BLOOD PRESSURE
Dog: 160 to 180 mm Hg **Cat:** 160 to 200 mm Hg

Young growing animals with renal failure may develop marked fibrous osteodystrophy characterized by enlargement and deformity of the maxilla and mandible, but this is uncommon in older dogs with renal failure.

Abdominal palpation

Both kidneys can be palpated in most cats, and the left kidney can be palpated in up to 20% of dogs. Evaluate the kidneys for size, shape, consistency, pain, and location. Unless empty, the bladder can be palpated in most dogs and cats. Note the degree of bladder distention, the presence or absence of pain, and thickness of the bladder wall. Evaluate the bladder for intramural (e.g., tumors) or intraluminal (e.g., stones, clots) masses. In the absence of obstruction, a distended bladder in a dehydrated animal suggests abnormal renal function or administration of drugs that impair urinary concentrating ability (e.g., corticosteroids, diuretics).

Pelvic examination and genitalia

Palpate the prostate gland (males) and pelvic urethra (males and females) by rectal examination. The perianal and sublumbar areas should be palpated carefully during rectal examination to determine the presence of tumors. Evaluate the prostate gland for size, symmetry, pain, and location. Exteriorize and examine the penis and palpate the testes for symmetry, consistency, masses, or pain. In the female dog, perform a vaginal examination to evaluate for abnormal discharge, masses, and the status of the urethral orifice.

Blood pressure measurement

Multiple techniques for diagnostic blood pressure measurement are available. None are consistently perfect and all have advantages, as well as disadvantages. However, measurement and tracking of blood pressure in cats with renal insufficiency, and even in dogs with protein-losing nephropathy, has become an important component of care in the long-term management of these patients. In dogs and cats, blood pressure measurements center on **systolic blood pressure** and the prevention/management of hypertension and mitigate the risk of retinal damage (detachment) and blindness. There is little information known about the clinical significance of **diastolic** hypertension in dogs and cats. Therapeutic intervention (antihypertensives; see Table 6-37) is indicated in patients diagnosed with chronic renal insufficiency and systolic hypertension.

A wide variety of imaging procedures and laboratory tests are used to further assess qualitative and quantitative aspects of renal function, urine production, and micturition. Special diagnostic tests, including renal biopsy and cystoscopy, are described in detail in Section 4.

Laboratory assessment of renal function entails a variety of routine and specialized biochemical analyses, excretory (urinary) studies, and cultures. Laboratory tests and test protocols are described in detail in Section 5.

Additional Reading

DiBartola SP: Renal disease: Clinical approach and laboratory evaluation. In Ettinger SJ, Feldman EC, editors: *Textbook of veterinary internal medicine*, ed 6, St. Louis, 2005, Elsevier, pp. 1716-1730.

Osborne CA, Finco DR, editors: *Canine and feline nephrology and urology.* Baltimore, 1995, Williams & Wilkins.

Senior DF: Urinary disorders. In Schaer M, editor: *Clinical medicine of the dog and cat.* Ames, 2003, Iowa State Press (Blackwell), pp. 409-453.

Stepien RL: Blood pressure assessment. In Ettinger SJ, Feldman EC, editors: *Textbook of veterinary internal medicine*, ed 6, St. Louis, 2005, Elsevier, pp. 470-472.

Clinical Signs

Abdominal Enlargement: With Ascites §, *390*
  Definition
  Associated Signs
  Differential Diagnosis
Abdominal Enlargement: Without Ascites §, *392*
  Definition
  Associated Signs
  Differential Diagnosis
Aggression, *393*
  Definition
  Associated Signs
  Differential Diagnosis
Alopecia (See Hair Loss), *393*
Ataxia (See Incoordination), *393*
Blindness (See Vision Loss), *393*
Blood in Urine: Hematuria, Hemoglobinuria, Myoglobinuria, *393*
  Definition
  Associated Signs
  Differential Diagnosis
Coma: Loss of Consciousness §, *396*
  Definition
  Associated Signs
  Differential Diagnosis
Constipation (Obstipation) (See Also Straining to Defecate), *397*
  Definition
  Associated Signs
  Differential Diagnosis
Cough, *398*
  Definition
  Associated Signs
  Differential Diagnosis
Coughing Blood: Hemoptysis (See Also Difficulty Breathing) §, *401*
  Definition
  Associated Signs
  Differential Diagnosis
Deafness or Hearing Loss, *402*
  Definition
  Associated Signs
  Differential Diagnosis

§ Denotes a clinical sign that poses potential for a life-threatening condition. *IMMEDIATE ASSESSMENT* and *INTERVENTION* is indicated.

Decreased Urine Production: Oliguria and Anuria §, *404*
 Definition
 Associated Signs
 Differential Diagnosis
Diarrhea, Acute-Onset, *405*
 Definition
 Associated Signs
 Differential Diagnosis
Diarrhea, Chronic, *407*
 Definition
 Associated Signs
 Differential Diagnosis
Difficulty Breathing or Respiratory Distress: Cyanosis (See Also Dyspnea) §, *409*
 Definition
 Associated Signs
 Differential Diagnosis
Difficulty Breathing or Respiratory Distress: Dyspnea §, *410*
 Definition
 Associated Signs
 Differential Diagnosis
Difficulty Swallowing: Dysphagia, *411*
 Definition
 Associated Signs
 Differential Diagnosis
Hair Loss: Alopecia, *414*
 Definition
 Associated Signs
 Differential Diagnosis
Hemorrhage (See Spontaneous Bleeding) §, *415*
Icterus (See Yellow Skin) §, *415*
Incoordination: Ataxia, *415*
 Definition
 Associated Signs
 Differential Diagnosis
Increased Urination and Water Consumption: Polyuria and Polydipsia, *417*
 Definition
 Associated Signs
 Differential Diagnosis
Itching or Scratching: Pruritus (See Also Hair Loss), *418*
 Definition
 Associated Signs
 Differential Diagnosis
Jaundice (See Yellow Skin) §, *421*
Joint Swelling: Arthropathy (See Also Lameness), *421*
 Definition
 Associated Signs
 Differential Diagnosis
Loss of Appetite: Anorexia, *422*
 Definition
 Associated Signs
 Differential Diagnosis
Lymph Node Enlargement: Lymphadenomegaly §, *423*
 Definition
 Associated Signs
 Differential Diagnosis
Pain, *424*
 Definition
 Associated Signs
 Differential Diagnosis

§ Denotes a clinical sign that poses potential for a life-threatening condition. *IMMEDIATE ASSESSMENT* and *INTERVENTION* is indicated.

Painful Urination: Dysuria (See Straining to Urinate), *425*
Painful Defecation: Dyschezia (See Straining to Defecate), *425*
Rectal and Anal Pain (See Straining to Defecate), *425*
Regurgitation (See Also Difficulty Swallowing and Vomiting), *425*
   Definition
   Associated Signs
   Differential Diagnosis
Seizures (Convulsions or Epilepsy) §, *426*
   Definition
   Associated Signs
   Differential Diagnosis
Sneezing and Nasal Discharge, *429*
   Definition
   Associated Signs
   Differential Diagnosis
Spontaneous Bleeding: Hemorrhage §, *429*
   Definition
   Associated Signs
   Differential Diagnosis
Straining to Defecate: Dyschezia, *432*
   Definition
   Associated Signs
   Differential Diagnosis
Straining to Urinate: Dysuria §, *434*
   Definition
   Associated Signs
   Differential Diagnosis
Swelling of the Limbs: Peripheral Edema §, *435*
   Definition
   Associated Signs
   Differential Diagnosis
Uncontrolled Urination: Urinary Incontinence, *438*
   Definition
   Associated Signs
   Differential Diagnosis
Vision Loss: Total Blindness, *440*
   Definition
   Differential Diagnosis
Vomiting (See Also Regurgitation), *441*
   Definition
   Associated Signs
   Differential Diagnosis
Vomiting Blood: Hematemesis (See Also Vomiting) §, *444*
   Definition
   Associated Signs
   Differential Diagnosis
Weight Loss: Emaciation/Cachexia, *445*
   Definition
   Associated Signs
   Differential Diagnosis
Yellow Skin or Mucous Membranes: Icterus (or Jaundice) §, *446*
   Definition
   Associated Signs
   Differential Diagnosis

3

§ Denotes a clinical sign that poses potential for a life-threatening condition. *IMMEDIATE ASSESSMENT* and *INTERVENTION* is indicated.

Note: The CLINICAL SIGNS section of the *Handbook* has been designed to facilitate rapid and accurate assessment of individual presenting problems as they are likely to be interpreted by the pet owner and presented to the clinician. Each CLINICAL SIGN is listed by the common name or phrase used by owners to describe the problem. When appropriate, a descripitive medical term for that CLINICAL SIGN follows.

Proper interpretation and assessment of individual CLINICAL SIGNS is fundamental to every patient evaluation and diagnosis. It is the cornerstone of effective therapy. Failing to recognize or interpret clinical signs in patients that are not able to communicate verbally is to fail the diagnostic effort. Interpretation of signs in veterinary medicine remains a critical clinical skill that demands persistent vigilance, experience and intuition. Absolutely no laboratory test, surgical procedure, nor sophisticated imaging technology can empower a clinician more.

ABDOMINAL ENLARGEMENT: WITH ASCITES

DEFINITION

Ascites: In this instance, refers to the abnormal accumulation of fluid in the peritoneal cavity sufficient to cause observable enlargement to the appearance of the abdomen. In this case, abdominal enlargement is observable to the owner. It should be noted, however, that ascites, especially in the early, formative stages, may NOT be associated with abdominal enlargement. Fluid accumulation can result from a variety of inflammatory, infectious, metabolic, degenerative, and neoplastic disorders. Ascites must be distinguished from abdominal enlargement NOT associated with fluid accumulation.

ASSOCIATED SIGNS

Clinical signs associated with abdominal enlargement are common. Once characterized, the associated signs can provide critical information relevant to the underlying diagnosis. The history may include increased water consumption and urination, diarrhea, vomiting, increased or decreased appetite, pain, apparent or real weight gain, and loss of muscle mass.

On physical examination, verify the abdominal enlargement to determine whether or not the enlargement is caused by fluid accumulation. Examine the patient for the presence of a heart murmur and palpable arrhythmia. If fluid is not present, determine the presence or absence of a mass within the abdominal cavity. When fluid is present, analyze the fluid character biochemically and cytologically.

DIFFERENTIAL DIAGNOSIS (Figure 3-1)

DIAGNOSTIC PLANS

1. Physical examination, to establish or rule out cardiopulmonary disease. Evaluate skin and hair coat for signs supporting endocrine disease. Assess abdominal enlargement by palpation and auscultation.
2. Abdominal radiograph and ultrasound, to confirm the presence of fluid, fat, or organomegaly.
3. If fluid *is* present, abdominocentesis, fluid analysis, and, if available, abdominal ultrasound. A laboratory database also is recommended.
4. If fluid *is not* present, contrast radiography of the bowel (barium series), dexamethasone suppression test, abdominal laparotomy, or, if available, abdominal ultrasound (see ABDOMINAL ENLARGEMENT).

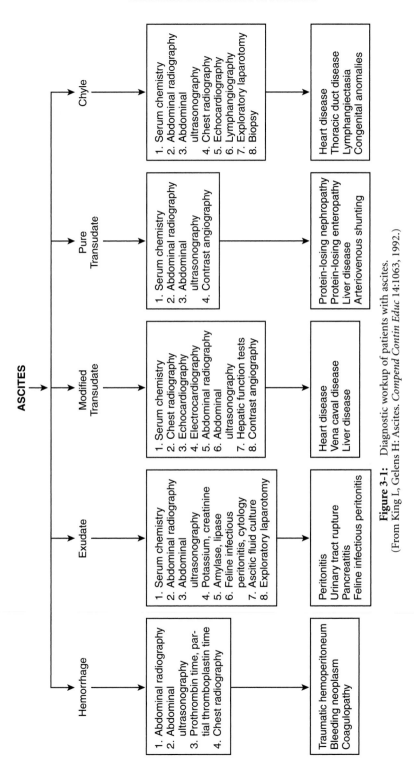

Figure 3-1: Diagnostic workup of patients with ascites.
(From King L, Gelens H: Ascites. *Compend Contin Educ* 14:1063, 1992.)

ABDOMINAL ENLARGEMENT: WITHOUT ASCITES

DEFINITION

Abdominal enlargement (not associated with ascites): Refers to any condition in a dog or cat that causes a real or apparent enlargement of the abdominal cavity as observed during the physical examination. *Real* abdominal enlargement can be physiologic or normal (such as postprandial enlargement in a puppy or kitten or pregnancy) or abnormal (such as that associated with organomegaly).

ASSOCIATED SIGNS

Regardless of the underlying cause, abdominal enlargement is most likely to be associated with increased respiratory effort, usually characterized as tachypnea (increased respiratory rate). Dogs are more likely than cats to vocalize during expiration (grunt). Increased heart rate, lethargy, diminished appetite, and orthopnea (positional breathing) are variably observed.

DIFFERENTIAL DIAGNOSIS (Box 3-1)

DIAGNOSTIC PLANS

1. History. Attempt to establish whether or not a recent meal was consumed or (in the case of adult females) whether or not pregnancy is possible.
2. Abdominal palpation. NOTE: Preferably accomplished with the patient in RIGHT lateral recumbency. Examination is carried out using two hands simultaneously.
3. Abdominal ballottement. Manipulate the abdominal wall in an attempt to determine whether or not an accumulation of fluid exists within the abdomen.
4. Imaging. Abdominal radiograph or abdominal ultrasound.
5. Laboratory profile. Generally conducted to assess patient overall health status. Coagulation profile may be indicated.
6. Fine needle aspiration. May be conducted to remove fluid or aspirate solid organs/masses. Samples are prepared for cytopathology.
7. Exploratory surgery. Laparoscopy may be a suitable alternative but requires experience and special equipment.

BOX 3-1   DIFFERENTIAL DIAGNOSIS OF ABDOMINAL ENLARGEMENT

PHYSIOLOGIC ENLARGEMENT
Postprandial
Pregnancy

WITHOUT FLUID ACCUMULATION
Organomegaly
Neoplasia
Obstipation
Gastric dilation
Hyperadrenocorticism
Ruptured prepubic tendon
Bladder distention
Pneumoperitoneum

WITH FLUID ACCUMULATION
High protein: >2.5 g/dL
   Hepatic failure

Right-sided congestive heart failure
Inflammatory-infectious (e.g., FIP)
Chemical/drug peritonitis
Trauma
Neoplasia
Hepatic vein thrombosis or vascular anomaly
Chyloabdomen
Low protein: <2.5 g/dL
   Hypoproteinemia (renal, hepatic, or gastro-intestinal cause)
   Portal hypertension subsequent to primary liver disease
   Neoplasia

FIP, Feline infectious peritonitis

AGGRESSION

DEFINITION

Aggression: A behavior (either normal or abnormal) in the dog or cat that could lead to the destruction or injury of an animal or person. Furthermore, aggression can be categorized as offensive or defensive. Specific knowledge of the pattern and type of aggression is critical if effective intervention is to be accomplished. To meet the criteria of this definition, it is assumed that organic causes of aggression (e.g., pain or intracranial mass) have been ruled out.

ASSOCIATED SIGNS

Although rare, aggression may be the result of organic disease, particularly disorders affecting the brain. In these patients, the onset of aggressive behavior is usually acute and may be associated with other neurologic signs suggesting cerebral dysfunction (e.g., seizures and circling). However, animals with pain may also manifest aggressive behavior, an apparent secondary response to discomfort. Animals with unilateral or bilateral blindness or deafness may bite or manifest aggressive behavior when approached and touched from the blind, or deaf, side. This behavior is probably the result of the animal's being startled and is far less likely to be representative of abnormal behavior.

DIFFERENTIAL DIAGNOSIS (Boxes 3-2 and 3-3)

DIAGNOSTIC PLANS

1. Thorough laboratory profile and neurologic examination to assess the presence of pain or underlying organic disease (such as brain tumor).
2. The most effective plan for diagnosis and therapy may be for the clinician to make the owners aware of the clinical signs of aggression, alert them to the usual sequelae of early patterns, and direct them to a behavior specialist.
3. NOTE: Administration of a psychotropic drug as empiric therapy for aggression is *not* recommended before determining a possible cause and attempting to modify behavior through training.

ALOPECIA (SEE HAIR LOSS)

ATAXIA (SEE INCOORDINATION)

BLINDNESS (SEE VISION LOSS)

BLOOD IN URINE: HEMATURIA, HEMOGLOBINURIA, MYOGLOBINURIA

DEFINITION

Hematuria: Denotes the presence of blood in the urine; the presence of trace amounts of blood in the urine will not be obvious on gross appearance of a urine sample. Therefore, any noticeable change in the color of urine observed by the owner is likely to be interpreted as "blood in the urine." Further evaluation of the patient is necessary to determine whether or not the discoloration is associated with small blood clots in recently voided urine, blood-tinged urine, or brown or red urine. The presence of blood in the urine, whether gross or occult, is most often indicative of upper or lower urinary tract bleeding, although systemic coagulopathies and reproductive tract disorders may also cause hematuria. The presence of hemoglobin in urine *(hemoglobinuria)* is not necessarily a reflection of urinary tract disease.

BOX 3-2 AGGRESSIVE BEHAVIOR IN THE DOG: DIFFERENTIAL DIAGNOSIS ACCORDING TO ORIGIN

PATHOPHYSIOLOGICALLY BASED AGGRESSIVE BEHAVIOR
Rabies
Intracranial neoplasia
Cerebral hypoxia
Seizure activity
Neuroendocrine disturbances

SPECIES-TYPICAL AGGRESSIVE BEHAVIOR*
Dominance aggression
Possessive aggression

Protective aggression
Predatory aggression
Fear-induced aggression
Intermale and interfemale aggression
Pain-induced, punishment-induced, and
  irritable aggression
Maternal aggression
Redirected aggression

---

*These behavior patterns are not pathologic states. They are typical patterns of the species and are, therefore, normal. Familiarity with normal, species-typical aggressive pattern of the dog enables differentiation of species-typical patterns from pathophysiologically based aggression. Like many animal behavior problems, their species-typically does not lessen their disruptiveness or danger.
From Young MS: Aggressive behavior. *In* Ford RB, (ed): Clinical Signs and Diagnosis in Small Animal Practice. New York, Churchill Livingstone, 1988, p 137.

3

BOX 3-3 AGGRESSIVE BEHAVIOR IN THE CAT: DIFFERENTIAL DIAGNOSIS ACCORDING TO ORIGIN

PATHOPHYSIOLOGICALLY BASED AGGRESSIVE BEHAVIOR
Rabies
Intracranial neoplasia and lesions

SPECIES-TYPICAL AGGRESSIVE BEHAVIOR*
Intermale aggression
Predatory aggression

Play aggression
Territorial aggression
Fear-induced aggression
Pain-induced aggression
Maternal aggression
Redirected aggression

---

*These behavior patterns are not pathologic states. They are typical patterns of the species and are, therefore, normal. Familiarity with normal, species-typical aggressive patterns of the cat enables differentiation of species-typical patterns from pathophysiologically based aggression. Like many animal behavior problems, their species typically does not lessen their disruptiveness or danger.

Systemic disorders (e.g., those leading to intravascular hemolysis) can be associated with significant hemoglobinuria in the presence of a normal urinary system. Owners are likely to interpret this clinical sign to be "blood in the urine." In true hemoglobinuria, without hematuria, microscopic examination will reveal the absence of red blood cells (RBCs).

Distinguishing hemoglobinuria from hematuria is an important diagnostic consideration. Conventional urine test strips (dipsticks) do not differentiate between the two; therefore, microscopic examination of urine sediment for the presence of significant numbers of RBCs is critical.

Myoglobinuria is characterized by brown to dark-red urine, the absence of RBCs in the urine sediment, and a positive test for occult blood. Bilirubinuria can also cause dark-brown to dark-orange urine but alone will not produce a positive test for occult blood. Myoglobinuria is a serious sign and denotes generalized muscle disease.

ASSOCIATED SIGNS

Hematuria associated with the urinary tract may not be associated with any other clinical signs. In patients with significant bleeding of renal origin, evidence of systemic illness may be present but is unlikely to localize the source of hematuria. Hematuria originating from the bladder is more likely to be associated with clinical signs, particularly pollakiuria and dysuria. Reproductive tract disorders (e.g., prostatitis and vaginitis) can also cause significant hematuria. Patients with hematuria or hemoglobinuria should be examined carefully for evidence of systemic bleeding, coagulopathies, and neoplasia.

DIFFERENTIAL DIAGNOSIS (Table 3-1 and Box 3-4)

DIAGNOSTIC PLANS

1. Thorough history and physical examination, with emphasis on examination of the genitalia, palpation of the prostate, and caudal abdominal palpation.

TABLE 3-1   Causes of Hematuria in Dogs and Cats Classified by Anatomical Site of Origin

Site	Dieseases
Kidney	Pyelonephritis
	Glomerulopathy
	Neoplasia
	Calculi
	Renal cysts
	Infarction
	Trauma
	Benign renal bleeding
	Hematuria of Welsh corgis
	Dioctophyma renale infection
	Microfilaria of *Dirofilaria immitis*
	Chronic passive congestion
Bladder, ureter, urethra	Infection
	Calculi
	Inflammation–LUTD
	Neoplasia
	Trauma
	Thrombocytopenia
	Capillaria plica infection
	Cyclophosphamide
Any site	Coagulopathy
	Heatstroke
	DIC
Extraurinary causes (genital tract or spurious hematuria)	Prostate
	Neoplasia
	Infection
	Hypertrophy
	Uterus
	Estrus
	Subinvolution
	Infection
	Neoplasia
	Vagina
	TVT
	Trauma
	Penis
	TVT
	Trauma

DIC, Disseminated intravascular coagulation; *TVT,* transmissible venereal tumor; *LUTD,* lower urinary tract disease.

3

BOX 3-4   DIFFERENTIAL DIAGNOSIS OF HEMOGLOBINURIA

INTRAVASCULAR DESTRUCTION OF RED BLOOD CELLS
Immune-mediated hemolytic anemia
Transfusion hemolysis
Sepsis
Red blood cell parasites (e.g., *Babesia* spp.)
    Chemical-induced
    Phenothiazine
    Acetaminophen
    Methylene blue
    Copper
Hypo-osmolality

EXTRAVASCULAR DESTRUCTION OF RED BLOOD CELLS
Red blood cell parasites
Immune-mediated hemolytic anemia

Pyruvate kinase deficiency (basenji and beagle)
Congenital porphyria (cats)
Hereditary stomatocytosis (malamute)
Microangiopathic disease (e.g., hepatic cirrhosis,
    hemangiosarcoma)

LYSIS OF RED BLOOD CELLS IN URINE
Hematuria combined with very dilute urine
Hematuria in stored urine

---

2. If practical, assessment of urethral patency and the patient's ability to urinate. Attempt to pass a urethral catheter if significant dysuria and evidence of lower urinary tract obstructions are present.
3. Complete urinalysis. Using a fresh sample, include assessment of gross appearance, specific gravity, biochemical reagent strips (dipsticks), and microscopic examination of urine sediment. Ideally, two samples should be collected: a voided urine sample followed by a urine sample collected by cystocentesis.
4. Culture and sensitivity, if bacteria are present.
5. Routine laboratory profile, to include hematology and biochemistry panel.
6. Coagulation profile, if hemoglobinuria is present.
7. Abdominal radiographs, for evidence of calculi, prostatic enlargement, and soft tissue masses.
8. Contrast radiography of the upper and lower urinary tracts.
9. Ultrasound examination of the prostate, urinary bladder, and kidneys.
10. Exploratory laparotomy.

COMA: LOSS OF CONSCIOUSNESS

DEFINITION

Coma: A state of complete reversible or irreversible unconsciousness that can result from neurologic as well as non-neurologic disease. Coma can be a consequence of diffuse or multifocal lesions of the cerebrum or a lesion affecting the rostral brain stem and ascending reticular activating system. A variety of organic central nervous system (CNS) disease leading to metabolic or toxic encephalopathy can also produce coma.

ASSOCIATED SIGNS

Despite the fact that the comatose patient is unconscious, a complete neuro-ophthalmologic examination should be completed. Altered pupil size and pupillary light responses usually indicate brain stem disease. Emergency cardiac assessment of the unconscious patient justifies an electrocardiogram (ECG) and thoracic radiographs. Laboratory assessment of the comatose patient includes hepatic enzymes and, when feasible, hepatic function, electrolytes, and glucose level.

DIFFERENTIAL DIAGNOSIS (Table 3-2)

DIAGNOSTIC PLANS

1. **Critical**: Assessment of vital signs to evaluate airway, breathing, and circulation (pulse, heartbeat, and ECG). Take thoracic radiographs if indicated. If cerebral edema is suspected, administer ventilation support, intravenous hyperosmotic agents (e.g., mannitol 20%, 1 to 2 g/kg of body weight q6h), and glucocorticoids.
2. Conduct careful neurologic examination directed toward evaluation of brain stem function, including motor function, pupillary light responses (or lack thereof), and eye movement.
3. Comprehensive laboratory profile, to include hematology, biochemical profile, and urinalysis.
4. Special diagnostic tests as appropriate:
   a. Metabolic coma. Serum ammonia, bile acids, glucose, blood and urine lead levels.
   b. Neurologic coma. Skull radiographs, cerebral spinal fluid analysis, electroencephalography.
   c. Assessment of response to IV Mannitol.

T A B L E   3 - 2   Differential Diagnosis of Coma

	Neurogenic	Non-neurogenic
Acute, nonprogressive	Intracranial hemorrhage	—
	Brain malformations	—
Acute, progressive	Metastatic lesions	Hypoglycemia
	Epidural, subdural	Diabetic coma
	hemorrhage	Heat stroke
	Meningoencephalitis	Hepatic/uremic
	Cerebral edema	encephalopathy
		Infectious
		Hypoxia
		Thiamine deficiency (cat)
		Heavy metal and drug toxicity
		Carbon monoxide poisoning
Chronic, progressive	Hemorrhage (rare)	Heavy metal toxicity
	Storage diseases	
	Hydrocephalus	
	Encephalitis	

3

CONSTIPATION (OBSTIPATION) (SEE ALSO STRAINING TO DEFECATE)

DEFINITION

Constipation: The infrequent or difficult passage of feces. *Obstipation*: Intractable constipation resulting in fecal impaction through the rectum and possibly the colon. In both dogs and cats, either state is most likely to be acquired.

The act of straining to defecate or painful defecation, the likely manifestation of constipation or obstipation, typically represents the reason for which a constipated dog or cat is presented (see STRAINING TO DEFECATE: DYSCHEZIA).

There is no strict definition of bowel regularity; therefore, there is no "normal" number of daily or weekly bowel movements, deviations from which constitute constipation.

Practically, constipation can be considered to exist when a significant delay in frequency of passing formed stools has been noted or when the stool is observed to be of unusually hard or dry consistency. Constipation is categorized under one of the following headings: Neurogenic; Mechanical (physical); Muscular (smooth muscle); Iatrogenic (drug-induced).

The owner who perceives a pet as straining to defecate may, in fact, be observing a pet that is straining to urinate. This is particularly true among cats with disorders of the lower urinary tract, such as feline urologic syndrome (FUS). In the context of this discussion, dyschezia is discussed only insofar as it is associated with constipation and obstipation (see Figure 3-2).

ASSOCIATED SIGNS

Assessment of the patient presented for constipation/obstipation can represent a significant medical challenge due to the complex and varied pathogenic mechanisms involved. Animals with neurogenic causes of constipation may have significant perianal or rectal pain associated with focal lesions. Other patients may present with nonpainful neurologic disease or long-term complications stemming from previous pelvic or spinal trauma.

Mechanical causes are either extraluminal or intraluminal. Abdominal and rectal palpation is indicated in both male and female dogs and cats. Narrow or blood-tinged feces may signal the presence of an intraluminal lesion, whereas in patients with extraluminal lesions, associated clinical signs may not be manifested.

Muscular causes are the least common and are generally the result of extreme metabolic aberrations. Idiopathic colonic atony is reported, but constipation may also result from severe catabolic states. Laboratory evidence of endocrine disease and electrolyte abnormalities should be assessed (see p. 630).

DIFFERENTIAL DIAGNOSIS (see Box 3-5 on p. 400)

DIAGNOSTIC PLANS (See Figure 3-2)

COUGH

DEFINITION

Cough: A sudden, forceful expiratory response to irritating stimuli (e.g., secretions) situated in the tracheobronchial tree. Cough is the most frequent clinical problem (followed by dyspnea and hemoptysis) that is referable to the lower respiratory tract. At presentation, cough should be characterized as "acute-onset" (duration of only a few days) or "chronic" (duration ≥1 week). It should be noted that attempting to define cough as productive or nonproductive can be difficult in animals and, furthermore, seems to have little value in the overall diagnostic plan.

ASSOCIATED SIGNS

Although cough is a principal sign of lower respiratory tract disease, particularly lower airway (tracheal and bronchial) disease, it may also occur in animals with nonpulmonary disease, particularly cardiac and intrathoracic diseases. Associated signs, therefore, may include a wide spectrum of findings; there may also be no associated signs. Particular attention should be given to determining the character of the cough: it can be paroxysmal and severe, which usually indicates the need for immediate intervention, or mild but persistent. Animals in need of immediate attention are those with cough associated with syncope, dyspnea, or hemoptysis. *Orthopnea*, the inability to breathe without assuming a particular (usually upright) position, is a serious sign that suggests compromised respiratory function

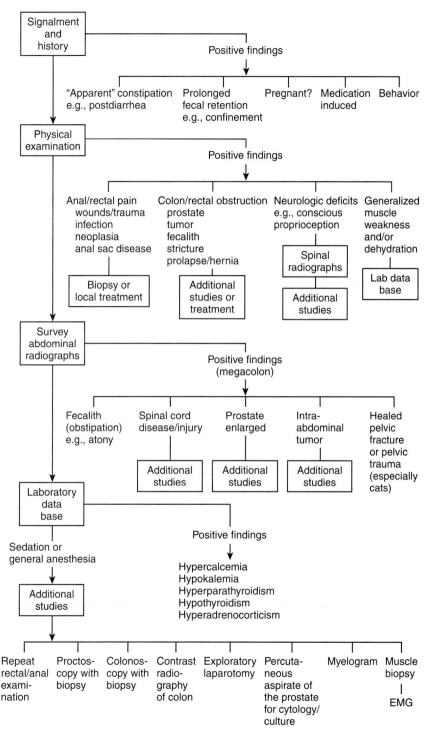

Figure 3-2: Clinical algorithm for constipation in the dog or cat. *EMG,* Electromyogram.

BOX 3-5   DIFFERENTIAL DIAGNOSIS OF CONSTIPATION

NEUROGENIC CAUSES
Cortical (pain-induced)
  Perianal neoplasia
  Anal sac disease
  Perianal fistulas
  Myiasis
CNS disease
  Spinal trauma
  Spinal neoplasia
  Degenerative myelopathy
Peripheral nerve disease (e.g., complication following pelvic trauma)

MECHANICAL CAUSES
Extraluminal
  Prostate (neoplasia or hyperplasia)
  Large intra-abdominal tumors
  Pregnancy (?)
  Pelvic fracture
Intraluminal
  Rectal stricture (e.g., adenocarcinoma)
  Colonic stricture
  Granulomas (e.g., histoplasmosis)
  Benign colorectal tumors
  Fecalith

Rectal-colonic prolapse
Intussusception

MUSCULAR CAUSES
Colonic atony
Severe malnutrition and cachexia
Hypothyroidism
Hypercalcemia
Hyperkalemia
Hyperparathyroidism
Segmental dilation subsequent to surgery

DRUG-INDUCED CAUSES
Anesthetics
Anticholinergics (e.g., atropine)
Anticonvulsants
Barium sulfate
Diuretics
Prolonged laxative therapy
Monoamine oxidase inhibitors
Heavy metal toxicity (e.g., lead)
Behavioral
Soiled or odiferous litter
No litter available

---

and also warrants immediate attention. Nasal discharge, tachypnea, and hyperpnea are less commonly associated with cough.

Cough can be misinterpreted as vomiting, particularly in dogs with tracheobronchitis. Coughing episodes in affected dogs typically terminate in the expectoration of tracheal secretions. The white, foamy phlegm expelled as the dog retches may appear to the untrained eye as vomitus.

DIFFERENTIAL DIAGNOSIS (Box 3-6)

DIAGNOSTIC PLANS

1. History and physical examination. Focus on known breed and age predispositions. Physical examination is particularly valuable in determining the extent of respiratory tract involvement and characterizing the type of cough present, particularly when the cough can be elicited by manipulation of the cervical trachea.
2. Careful thoracic auscultation, to determine the presence or absence of murmur or abnormal lung or airway sounds.
3. Thoracic radiographs, using lateral and ventrodorsal projections. These are critical, particularly when the patient has associated signs compatible with respiratory distress. Oxygen should be available to the dyspneic patient throughout the radiographic procedure. Patients with suspected tracheal collapse should be radiographed twice in the lateral position to assess changes in the intrathoracic tracheal and bronchial diameters between inspiration (open) and expiration (closed). In addition to obtaining a ventrodorsal (VD) projection, patients suspected of having thoracic neoplasia should have LEFT and RIGHT lateral thoracic radiographs assessed.
4. A laboratory profile, to include hematology, biochemistry panel, fecal flotation, urinalysis, heartworm test, and the feline leukemia virus/feline immunodeficiency virus (FeLV/FIV) test in the cat.

BOX 3-6   DIFFERENTIAL DIAGNOSIS OF COUGH

PRIMARY RESPIRATORY TRACT DISEASE
Airway diseases
Tonsillitis and pharyngitis
Tonsillar neoplasm
Pharyngeal polyp (cat)
Laryngeal cyst
Laryngeal neoplasm
Laryngeal paralysis
Tracheobronchitis and tracheitis
Tracheal hypoplasia
Segmental tracheal stenosis
Tracheal collapse—acquired and congenital
Tracheal neoplasia
Tracheal osteochondral dysplasia
Foreign body
Bronchiectasis
Bronchial collapse
Immotile cilia syndrome
Aspiration
Respiratory parasites (e.g., *Capillaria aerophila* in cats; *Filaroides osleri* in dogs)

PULMONARY VASCULAR DISEASE
Pulmonary edema (multiple causes)
Pulmonary hypertension, esp. heartworm disease

PULMONARY PARENCHYMAL DISEASE
Bacterial pneumonia
Systemic mycoses (e.g., histoplasmosis)
Pulmonary neoplasia
Pulmonary abscess
Protozoan pneumonia (e.g., feline toxoplasmosis)
Viral pneumonia
Allergic pneumonitis (e.g., feline asthma)
Metabolic and endocrine (e.g., hyperadrenocorticism)

CARDIOVASCULAR DISEASES
Left heart disease
Left heart failure (cardiogenic pulmonary edema)

INTRATHORACIC DISEASE
Mediastinal abscess
Mediastinal neoplasia

---

5. Special diagnostics:
   a. Primary respiratory disease: transtracheal aspiration, bronchial lavage, bronchoscopy, contrast bronchography, fluoroscopy, and radionuclide assessment of mucociliary transport.
   b. Primary pulmonary disease: fine-needle lung aspiration, arterial blood gases, fungal serology, nuclear studies (perfusion-ventilation), lung biopsy.
   c. Primary cardiac disease: ECG, echocardiogram (M-mode and two-dimensional) and nonselective angiography.

COUGHING BLOOD: HEMOPTYSIS (SEE ALSO DIFFICULTY BREATHING)

DEFINITION

Hemoptysis is the expectoration, during cough, of blood. Seldom is the volume of blood loss sufficient to cause anemia; however, once confirmed, hemoptysis is a severe clinical finding indicative of bleeding into or from the lower airways. Hemoptysis can be attributed to direct injury of the pulmonary or, less commonly, the tracheobronchial blood vessels, pulmonary hypertension, or coagulopathy. Although an uncommon presenting sign, hemoptysis is more prevalent in dogs than in cats.

Since vomiting can be mistaken by the owner for coughing, it becomes essential to differentiate between hemoptysis and hematemesis during the initial examination. Hemoptysis is regarded as an emergency presentation.

ASSOCIATED SIGNS

The most common, and least significant, sign associated with hemoptysis is *melena,* or dark-red or black discoloration of stool that occurs subsequent to swallowing expectorated blood. More serious associated signs include coughing, hyperpnea, orthopnea, and cyanosis. Apparent episodic weakness and collapse may also be reported.

DIFFERENTIAL DIAGNOSIS (Box 3-7)

DIAGNOSTIC PLANS

1. Thorough history and physical examination. In addition, an attempt should be made to determine that the sign for which the patient was presented is, in fact, expectoration of blood during coughing and not bloody vomitus.
2. Routine laboratory profile, to assess the patient's overall health status. Emphasis should be placed on the fecal examination and heartworm tests. Multiple attempts to locate parasite ova in the stool should be made, since lung parasites may be few in number and ova shed intermittently.
3. Thoracic radiographs.
4. Coagulation profile, particularly in those animals with significant bleeding from other sites.
5. Transtracheal aspiration with cytologic studies or bacterial culture and sensitivity tests, or both.
6. Special procedures, including ultrasonography of the lung, particularly when discrete masses are seen on radiographs; echocardiography; blood gas analysis; bronchoscopy; bronchography; and angiography.
7. Radionuclide scans. Although availability is limited, studies may detect areas of pulmonary embolization.

BOX 3-7 DIFFERENTIAL DIAGNOSIS OF HEMOPTYSIS

CARDIOVASCULAR HEMOPTYSIS
Thromboembolic disease
  Heartworm disease (in the dog and cat)
  Hyperadrenocorticism
  Cardiomyopathy
  Renal amyloidosis (in the dog)
  Idiopathic
Acute pulmonary edema
Arteriovenous fistula

PARASITIC HEMOPTYSIS
Lung flukes (e.g., *Paragonimus* spp.)
Lungworms (e.g., *Aelurostrongylus* spp.)

INFLAMMATION-INDUCED HEMOPTYSIS
Chronic bronchitis
Pneumonia
Mycotic lung infection
Lung abscess

NEOPLASIA
Either primary or metastatic

MISCELLANEOUS
Coagulation disorder
Direct injury or trauma
Transtracheal aspirate

DEAFNESS OR HEARING LOSS

DEFINITION

Deafness is the detectable lack or loss, complete or partial, of the sense of hearing. Deafness can result from abnormalities at any one of several levels from the ear to the brain. *Peripheral deafness* is categorized as either *conduction deafness,* involving abnormalities of the transduction apparatus (external ear canal, tympanic membrane, auditory ossicles in the middle ear), or *nerve deafness,* involving the hearing receptors in the cochlea or the auditory branch of the eighth cranial nerve. *Congenital deafness* is usually nerve deafness and is the result of abnormal development of the spiral organ or auditory receptors in the middle ear. Central hearing loss (intracranial cause) is uncommon, since auditory pathways in the brain are multisynaptic.

Loss of hearing, either partial or complete, in one or both ears does occur in both dogs and cats but is particularly difficult to confirm. Partial loss of hearing occurs most commonly in older animals but is rarely confirmed. Deafness is generally first detected by astute owners who observe diminished or absent responses to noise in an animal with no previous history of hearing difficulty.

ASSOCIATED SIGNS

Although rare, invasive lesions or panencephalitis could conceivably cause central hearing loss. However, the associated neurologic signs would be extensive, and hearing loss becomes a secondary or insignificant clinical issue.

Animals with peripheral hearing loss due to acquired unilateral lesions may manifest a variety of signs referable to the vestibular apparatus, particularly head tilt and, less often, circling. Pain or increased sensitivity may be associated with invasive lesions affecting hearing in either ear. Physical evidence of otitis externa is readily detected during routine examinations. Severe swelling associated with a chronic inflammation, a ruptured or damaged tympanic membrane, and infections of the middle ear may effectively decrease hearing acuity. Hypothyroidism may also be associated with degeneration of the cochlea and subsequent decrease in hearing acuity. The clinical history is important and should include any prior exposure to drugs known to be toxic to the cochlear nerve and organ of Corti (e.g., aminoglycosides).

Congenital (hereditary) deafness is associated with a white or merle hair coat in both dogs and cats. In dogs, the highest incidence is in the Dalmatian. However, several breeds are reported to be affected.

DIFFERENTIAL DIAGNOSIS (Box 3-8)

DIAGNOSTIC PLANS

1. Assessment of response to noise while the animal is relaxed or asleep.
2. Thorough physical examination, particularly of the external ear canal and tympanic membrane.
3. Neurologic examination.
4. Assessment of thyroid hormone levels.

BOX 3-8   DIFFERENTIAL DIAGNOSIS OF DEAFNESS

ACQUIRED HEARING LOSS
Degenerative causes
    Neurogenic deafness in the geriatric dog and cat
    Subsequent to chronic inflammatory disease (?)
Metabolic (endocrine) causes
    Hypothyroidism
    Neoplastic causes
    Invasive tumors of the pharynx and retropharyngeal tissue
Infectious-inflammatory causes
    Otitis externa and media
    Canine distemper virus infection

Prototheosis (in the dog)
Toxic
    Aminoglycoside antimicrobials, especially gentamicin, streptomycin, and neomycin
Traumatic
Idiopathic

CONGENITAL HEARING LOSS—BREED PREDISPOSITION
White, blue-eyed cats (may be unilateral or bilateral)
Several breeds affected, particularly those with a white or merle hair coat

5. Radiography of the head, with particular emphasis on the tympanic bullae, for evidence of otitis media.
6. Electrophysiologic studies, including electroencephalography, tympanometry, and brain stem auditory evoked potentials (BAER test).

DECREASED URINE PRODUCTION: OLIGURIA AND ANURIA

DEFINITION

Oliguria: Reduced amount of urine production and output in relation to fluid intake. Patients in which urine production ceases have *anuria* and are considered to be anuric. In contrast to polyuric states, neither oliguria nor anuria is likely to be the primary problem for which a dog or cat is presented to a veterinarian. The metabolic consequences of decreased urine production are severe and generally represent significant compromises in renal blood flow or in the functional status of a critical nephron mass. The daily urine volume at which oliguria begin is a function of solute load and renal concentrating ability. In general, oliguria exists when daily urine production is reduced by 75% or more. Production of 0.5 to 1.0 mL/kg/hr of urine indicates adequate renal perfusion in the dog. Anuria begins or terminates with oliguria; therefore, early detection and treatment of the underlying cause are critical to the overall prognosis.

ASSOCIATED SIGNS

The problem(s) for which an oliguric or anuric patient is presented will likely be related to the metabolic consequences of compromised renal function. Uremia, characterized by vomiting, hematemesis, diarrhea, lethargy, or anorexia, predominates. Any one or a combination of signs may present at the time of initial examination. Some patients may present in a comatose or semiconscious state, in which case it is essential that renal function and urinary output be established immediately.

Since acute renal failure (ARF) is the principal differential diagnosis in oliguria and anuria, once it has been established the clinician must obtain a thorough clinical history and laboratory profile, including urinalysis if possible, in an attempt to determine the cause of renal failure and to institute corrective therapy.

DIFFERENTIAL DIAGNOSIS (Box 3-9)

DIAGNOSTIC PLANS

1. Initiation of fluid therapy and placement of an indwelling urinary catheter, to establish the rate of urine production.
2. History, to address any possible exposure to toxins, particularly antifreeze, as well as recent drug treatment.
3. Radiographs of the abdomen. These may reveal enlarged kidneys, thereby supporting a diagnosis of ARF. Do not rule out the diagnosis of ARF if kidney size appears normal. Ultrasound imaging of kidneys is also helpful in establishing diagnosis.
4. Complete blood count (CBC). The biochemical profile should include electrolytes as well as blood urea nitrogen (BUN) and creatinine levels. Urinalysis (must include urine specific gravity) with microscopic examination of sediment for evidence of crystaluria, RBCs, white blood cells (WBCs), and casts is essential even if only a small volume of urine can be obtained.
5. Blood gases, to assess for metabolic acidosis, which may be severe in ARF.
6. Urine protein-creatinine ratio, to assess proteinuria.
7. If possible, determinations of serum osmolality and serum osmole gap.
8. Special diagnostics: intravenous pyelogram (IVP), renal biopsy, and determinations of lead and other heavy metals in the blood as indicated.

BOX 3-9   DIFFERENTIAL DIAGNOSIS OF ACUTE RENAL FAILURE

INFLAMMATORY-INFECTIOUS CAUSES
Leptospirosis
Pyelonephritis
Immune complex glomerulonephritis
  Systemic lupus erythematosus
  Heartworm disease
  Pyometra
  Endocarditis
  Feline leukemia virus infection
Viral
  Canine distemper virus infection
  Infectious canine hepatitis infection (rare)
  Canine herpesvirus infection (rare)

PRIMARY RENAL CAUSES (NEPHROSES)
Hypoperfusion (ischemia)
Extreme dehydration

Hemorrhage
Trauma
Sepsis
Surgery
Thromboembolic diseases

NEPHROTOXINS
Heavy metals (lead, arsenic, thallium, mercury)
Carbon tetrachloride
Ethylene glycol (antifreeze)
Aminoglycoside antibacterials (amikacin, gentamicin)
Antibiotics (cephaloridine, amphotericin B)
Hypercalcemia
Anesthetics (fluoride metabolites of methoxyflurane)

DIARRHEA, ACUTE-ONSET

3

DEFINITION

Acute diarrhea: A sudden change in bowel pattern, characterized as increased fluidity, frequency, or volume, that is sustained despite empiric or supportive therapy (see also Diarrhea, chronic). Fundamentally, diarrhea occurs when the amount of water and other intestinal contents reaching the colon exceed the ability of the colon to store the feces and adequately remove the excess water. The pathogenesis of acute diarrhea may be categorized:

Osmotic diarrhea: Development of an osmotic gradient in the bowel that favors movement of water into the gut lumen. Disorders of digestion and absorption readily generate such an intraluminal osmotic gradient. In simple osmotic diarrhea, clinical signs should resolve when the patient is fasted and the osmotic gradient equilibrates.

Abnormal gut permeability may be associated with infiltrative disease of the bowel (e.g., inflammatory bowel disease or neoplasia). Inflammatory lesions of the intestine alter mucosal permeability and promote exudation into the gut lumen.

Secretory diarrhea results from the effect of various substances (e.g., enterotoxins, gut hormones) that act as secretagogues. The gut is stimulated to secrete fluids without concurrent changes in permeability, absorptive capacity, motility, or osmotic gradients.

Abnormal bowel motility may occur in several primary disorders of the gastrointestinal (GI) tract, but it appears unlikely that abnormal motility is a primary cause of diarrhea. Normally, peristaltic contractions move chyme aborally, whereas segmental activity retards the movement of chyme, thereby performing the important functions of mixing intestinal contents and maximizing contact with the brush border enzyme systems. As segmental contractions are diminished, intestinal contents flow freely through the flaccid gut.

In the patient with acute diarrhea, it is conceivable that only one of these mechanisms is involved. However, the longer the underlying cause of the diarrhea persists, the more likely that homeostatic and compensatory mechanisms will be overwhelmed. The pathogenesis of the patient's diarrhea is then related to a combination of events.

ASSOCIATED SIGNS

Acute diarrhea is a common presenting sign for which multitudes of diagnostic possibilities exist. The list of associated signs can be, in the clinical setting, extensive. Among the most common signs encountered in an animal presented for acute diarrhea are vomiting, dehydration, slight weight loss, and hematochezia. Abdominal pain, halitosis, flatulence, and borborygmus are other gut-associated signs. However, not all patients with acute diarrhea have primary intestinal disease, such as those with renal or hepatic failure or hypoadrenocorticism. Therefore, icterus, oral ulcers, muscle weakness, and so on may also be encountered. Fever, anorexia, and lethargy may also accompany acute diarrhea in the dog and cat.

DIFFERENTIAL DIAGNOSIS (Box 3-10)

DIAGNOSTIC PLANS

1. History and physical examination, including abdominal palpation. Establish possible exposure to infectious agents and associated signs.
2. Intravenous fluids containing NaCl may be a critical part of the early evaluation (signs associated with hypoadrenocorticism or Addison's disease may resolve within minutes to hours) in severely dehydrated patients presented for acute diarrhea.
3. Laboratory profile (to include routine hematology), biochemistry profile (to include amylase or lipase and sodium and potassium), urinalysis, examination of feces (direct and flotation). Perform several examinations before ruling out parasitic disease. Cats should be tested for both FeLV and FIV. Dogs should be tested for parvovirus antigen in stool.
4. Abdominal radiographs.
5. Special diagnostic tests as indicated: abdominal ultrasound; duodenoscopy and mucosal biopsy; stool culture for viruses or bacteria; serologic studies for rickettsial, viral, and fungal disease; and abdominal laparotomy.

BOX 3-10   DIFFERENTIAL DIAGNOSIS FOR ACUTE-ONSET DIARRHEA

INFECTIOUS CAUSES
Intestinal parasites: nematodes (e.g., ascarids, hookworms, whipworms, *Strongyloides* spp., *Trichinella* spp.); protozoa (e.g., coccidian, giardia, *Cryptosporidium* spp., Pentatrichomas).
Bacterial: *E. coli. Salmonella* spp., *Pseudomonas* spp., *Clostridium* spp., *Campylobacter* spp., *Yersinia entercolitica, Staphylococcus* spp., *Helicobacter* spp (?).
Viral: paramyxovirus (canine distemper), parvovirus (feline and canine), adenovirus-1, (coronavirus and reovirus-minor or insignificant).
Rickettsial: salmon poisoning.

TOXIC CAUSES
Antimicrobials/antibiotics, parasiticides, antineoplastic agents, heavy metals, insecticides, organophosphate-containing compounds, anti-inflammatory drugs.

DIETARY CAUSES
Dietary indiscretion, engorgement, food hypersensitivity, sudden change in diet.

BOWEL OBSTRUCTION
Foreign body, intussusception, volvulus, neoplasia.

EXTRAINTESTINAL CAUSES*
Renal failure, hepatic disease, hypoadrenocorticism (Addison's Disease), pancreatitis (acute and chronic).
Idiopathic Causes

---

*Although characteristically associated with *chronic* disease, the onset of diarrhea may be acute.

DIARRHEA, CHRONIC

DEFINITION

Chronic diarrhea: Persistent or gradual change in bowel pattern—characterized by increased fluidity, frequency, or volume of stool—that is sustained for more than 1 to 2 weeks despite empiric or supportive therapy (see also Diarrhea, Acute-Onset). In the clinical setting, the clinical history and associated signs should be used to further characterize chronic diarrhea as *large bowel* or *small bowel*.

ASSOCIATED SIGNS

Clinical differentiation of small bowel and large bowel diarrhea is fundamentally important for the diagnosis and treatment of chronic diarrhea (Table 3-3).

Less specific signs associated with chronic diarrheal diseases include dehydration, poor-quality hair coat, and fever. On abdominal palpation, discrete masses, thickened bowel loops, pain, or gas may occasionally be detected. Edema, ascites, and pleural effusion in patients with chronic diarrhea suggest substantial protein losses through the bowel. The patient with pallor should be assessed for intestinal bleeding, as well as for an anemia of chronic inflammatory disease.

Hematologic signs of most significance include eosinophilia (allergic or inflammatory) and lymphopenia (lymphangiectasia). Hypoproteinemia is associated with extreme malnutrition, protein-losing enteropathies, and enteric blood loss. Hyperglobulinemia is associated with basenji enteropathy.

DIFFERENTIAL DIAGNOSIS (Table 3-4)

DIAGNOSTIC PLANS

1. Clinical history and physical examination findings, to classify the diarrhea as small bowel or large bowel. Routine patient screening should include hematologic studies, biochemical profile, fecal flotation and direct examination, and urinalysis.

TABLE 3-3 **Clinical Differentiation of Diarrhea of the Small Bowel and Large Bowel Types**

Clinical signs	Small bowel	Large bowel
Fecal volume	Markedly increased daily output (large quantity of bulky or watery feces with each defecation)	Normal or slightly increased daily output (small quantities with each defecation)
Frequency of defecation	Normal or slightly increased	Very frequent: 4–10 times/day
Urgency of tenesmus	Rare	Common
Mucus in feces	Rare	Common
Blood in feces	Dark black (digested)	Red (fresh)
Steatorrhea (malassimilation)	May be present	Absent
Weight loss and emaciation	Usual	Rare
Flatulence	May be present	Absent
Vomiting	Occasional	Occasional

From Sherding RG: Chronic diarrhea. In Ford RB, editor: *Clinical signs and diagnosis in small animal practice.* New York, 1988, Churchill Livingstone, p 466.

TABLE 3-4 **Diagnosis of Specific Chronic Diarrheal Disorders**

Diarrhea	Diagnostic test/procedure
Small Bowel Type	
Exocrine, pancreatic insufficiency	Serum trypsin-like immunoreactivity (TLI)
Chronic inflammatory small bowel disease	
Eosinophilic enteritis	Eosinophilia, biopsy
Lymphocytic-plasmacytic enteritis	Biopsy
	Serum protein electrophoresis
Immunoproliferative enteropathy of basenjis	Radiography, biopsy
Granulomatous enteritis	
Lymphangiectasia	Lymphopenia, biopsy
Villous atrophy	
Gluten enteropathy	Response to gluten-free diet
Idiopathic	Biopsy
Histoplasmosis	Serology, cytology, biopsy
Lymphosarcoma	Biopsy
Small intestinal bacterial overgrowth (SIBO)	Culture intestinal aspirate, folate, response to antibiotics
Giardiasis	Fecal examinations, response to parasiticides
Lactase deficiency	Response to lactose-free diet
Large Bowel Type	
Chronic colitis	Colonoscopy, colon biopsy
Idiopathic	
Histiocytic	
Eosinophilic	
Abrasive colitis	Dietary history, inspection of feces
Whipworm colitis	Fecal flotation, colonoscopy, response to fenbendazole
Protozoan colitis	Saline fecal smears
Amebiasis	
Balantidiasis	
Trichomoniasis	
Histoplasma colitis	Fecal cytology, colon biopsy, serology, culture
Salmonella colitis	Culture
Campylobacter colitis	Culture
Protothecal colitis	Colon biopsy
Rectocolonic polyps	Digital palpation, barium enema
Colonic adenocarcinoma	Colonoscopy, barium enema, possibly abdominal ultrasound
Colonic lymphosarcoma	Barium enema, colonoscopy
Functional diarrhea (irritable colon)	History, diagnostic workup excludes all other diseases

2. Diagnosis of intestinal parasites. Perform a visual examination of the feces and anus for proglottids, a zinc sulfate flotation test for *Giardia* and *Coccidia* cysts, a saline suspension for protozoan trophozoites, and a sedimentation or Baermann determination for *Strongyloides* larvae. Adult whipworms can be seen in the colon on colonoscopy.

3. Additional fecal studies. Beyond routine fecal flotation and direct examination, several other fecal tests are indicated, including microscopic examinations for fat

(Sudan preparation), starch (iodine preparation), and cytologic staining (Gram stain and Wright's stain) to assess for presence of leukocytes and infectious agents. Malassimilation can be assessed through quantitative fecal fat analysis and fecal weight (daily output), although in clinical practice these tests are seldom performed. Several special biochemical and physical tests can also be carried out on feces: fecal water content, nitrogen content (for azotorrhea and malassimilation), electrolytes, pH, osmolality, fecal occult blood, and cultures for both fungi and bacteria.

4. Tests of absorptive and digestive function, such as trypsin-like immunoreactivity (TLI), serum folate, and vitamin B_{12} assay.
5. GI radiography and ultrasonography.
6. GI endoscopy (gastroscopy, duodenoscopy, and colonoscopy), with biopsy of intestinal mucosa. Duodenal intubation and aspiration can be performed to obtain specimens for cytologic examination and culture.
7. Exploratory laparotomy and intestinal biopsy.
8. Response to empiric treatment: Enzyme replacement or treatment of occult parasite infections.

DIFFICULTY BREATHING OR RESPIRATORY DISTRESS: CYANOSIS (SEE ALSO DYSPNEA)

3

DEFINITION

Cyanosis: Bluish discoloration of the skin and mucous membranes resulting from excessive concentration (>5 g/dL) of reduced hemoglobin in the blood. In dogs and cats, cyanosis may develop acutely in hypoxic states or may be chronic. Although cyanosis can develop during hypoxia, the terms are not synonymous.

NOTE: The increased concentration of reduced hemoglobin in blood is the result of either an increase in the quantity of venous blood in the cutaneous tissues (passive venous congestion) or a decrease in oxygen saturation in capillary blood. It is the absolute, rather than the relative, amount of reduced hemoglobin that actually causes the cyanosis to develop. If the concentration of hemoglobin is also reduced, the absolute concentration of *reduced* hemoglobin is also decreased. Therefore, even in severe anemia, cyanosis is not evident. On the other hand, patients with an elevated red blood cell (RBC) mass, or polycythemia, tend to be cyanotic at higher levels of arterial oxygen saturation than patients with a normal RBC mass. Cyanosis also occurs when functional abnormalities of hemoglobin (e.g., methemoglobinemia [dark-brown blood]) exist. In the dog and cat, disorders affecting the oxygen-carrying capacity of hemoglobin are usually drug- or chemical-induced. As little as 1.5 g/dL of methemoglobin or 0.5 g/dL of sulfhemoglobin will produce cyanosis.

ASSOCIATED SIGNS

Cyanosis can result from disorders affecting the cardiovascular system, ventilation, or oxygen-carrying capacity of RBCs. Several cardiovascular diseases, particularly those that compromise cardiac output or are associated with right-to-left vascular shunts, predispose to cyanosis. Therefore, animals with both acquired and congenital cardiac disease are susceptible. Associated signs include cough, respiratory distress, and syncope. The most common congenital heart defects associated with right-to-left shunts are (1) pulmonary valve stenosis as seen in tetralogy of Fallot, stenosis, and ventricular septal defect (VSD) and (2) pulmonary hypertension as seen in patent ductus arteriosus (PDA) and VSD.

Respiratory disorders affecting ventilation predispose to cyanosis. Severe infiltrative lung disease (e.g., neoplasia, pulmonary edema, or generalized pneumonia) can produce cyanosis associated with increased respiratory effort.

Animals that do present with cyanosis not associated with clinical signs other than increased respiratory rate may have abnormal hemoglobin levels, which, if present in sufficient concentration, will cause cyanosis. Associated signs include methemoglobinuria and methemoglobinemia.

Central cyanosis is defined as compromised oxygen saturation or abnormal hemoglobin; *peripheral cyanosis* is compromised blood flow.

DIFFERENTIAL DIAGNOSIS (Box 3-11)

DIAGNOSTIC PLANS

1. Provide 100% oxygen, particularly in patients with respiratory distress. Reassess color of the mucous membranes at 2- or 3-minute intervals. Auscultate the heart and lungs.
2. Thoracic radiographs. Oxygen should be available at all times.
3. Hematology, with particular emphasis on RBC morphology (Heinz bodies in the cat and hematocrit values), biochemical profile, and urinalysis.
4. Special diagnostics: arterial blood gases (with and without 100% oxygen), ECG, echocardiogram, and nonselective angiogram.

BOX 3-11   DIFFERENTIAL DIAGNOSIS FOR CYANOSIS

CARDIOVASCULAR CAUSES
Right-to-left shunting congential heart defect (e.g., R-to-L shunting patent ductus arteriosis)
Pulmonary embolism
Decreased cardiac output
Arterial obstruction

PULMONARY CAUSES
Airway collapse/obstruction (multiple causes)
Hypoxia

Pulmonary edema
Oxygen diffusion-alveolar ventilation abnormalities
Pulmonary arterial-venous shunts/fistulae
Restrictive lung disease (e.g., hydrothorax, diaphragmatic hernia)

TOXIC/DRUG CAUSES
Paraquat poisoning
Acetaminophen (cats)

DIFFICULTY BREATHING OR RESPIRATORY DISTRESS: DYSPNEA

DEFINITION

True *dyspnea:* Pathologic breathlessness ascribed to the unpleasant, distressful sensation of labored breathing most commonly associated with cardiac or pulmonary disease. What actually *is* and *is not* true breathlessness in veterinary medicine is difficult to define in clinical practice. Serious respiratory distress associated with substantive respiratory compromise may appear, to the owner at least, as only a minor problem. Physical examination and patient assessment are critical to the recognition and interpretation of this clinical sign.

Respiratory distress may result from (1) the need for oxygen, (2) metabolic aberrations leading to acidosis (a compensatory mechanism), (3) high environmental temperatures (heat stroke), (4) CNS disease, (5) disorders affecting motor innervation to the muscles of respiration, and (6) pain. In any event, once confirmed, diagnostic evaluation of the patient presented in respiratory distress should not be delayed.

ASSOCIATED SIGNS

The most common respiratory signs that characterize distress or dyspnea include (1) tachypnea (increased respiratory rate), (2) hyperpnea (increased respiratory rate and depth), (3) orthopnea, and (4) cough. In obstructive upper airway diseases, stridor and stertorous breathing may be present on the initial examination.

Fluid accumulation in the thoracic cavity may be accompanied by ascites and hepatomegaly. Physical evidence of hyperadrenocorticism supports thrombolic pulmonary disease. Cyanosis, pallor, evidence of physical trauma, shock, and coma are serious signs often associated with respiratory distress.

DIFFERENTIAL DIAGNOSIS (see Table 3-5 on p. 412)

DIAGNOSTIC PLANS

1. Physical examination. This is justified even before a comprehensive history is completed. Patient stabilization, as required, must be accomplished.
2. History. Historical information relevant to duration, progression, and exposure to noxious substances or trauma is indicated. Knowledge of all current medications, including heartworm preventative, is established.
3. Laboratory profile, to include a CBC, biochemistry panel, urinalysis, heartworm test (in dogs), and FeLV and FIV tests (in cats). Cytologic, bacteriologic, and biochemical assessments of body cavity effusions are indicated.
4. Thoracic and cervical radiographs. Presence of a heart murmur, cardiac arrhythmia, or both, should be further evaluated by electrocardiography and echocardiography.
5. Examination of the upper respiratory tract *in the anesthetized patient* and endoscopy when signs of tracheal and bronchial disease exist.

DIFFICULTY SWALLOWING: DYSPHAGIA

3

DEFINITION

Dysphagia is painful or difficult swallowing. Clinically, dysphagic animals characteristically are presented for making frequent and forced attempts to swallow with or without regurgitation. Signs are most apparent immediately following prehension of food or water.

Swallowing is a complex reflex requiring coordination of multiple muscular and neurologic reactions involving the tongue, palate, pharynx, larynx, esophagus, and gastroesophageal junction. The swallowing reflex is coordinated by cranial nerves V, VII, IX, X, and XI; therefore, neurologic lesions affecting nuclei in the brain stem and reticular formation can alter normal swallowing. Dysphagia may occur as a result of disorders affecting any one of the three swallowing phases: oropharyngeal, esophageal, and gastroesophageal.

Both morphologic as well as functional lesions affecting the oropharynx, esophagus, stomach, and brain or brain stem may result in dysphagia.

Functional or motility disorders that affect swallowing include spasticity, incoordination, or failure of muscular contractions, and they result from neurologic disorders, disorders of neuromuscular transmission, or primary muscle disease. Such disorders may be either congenital or acquired. Disorders affecting the oropharyngeal phase of swallowing are responsible for causing pronounced dysphagia, whereas disorders affecting the esophageal and gastroesophageal phases of swallowing are associated with regurgitation.

ASSOCIATED SIGNS

Dysphagia is observed in young animals, particularly in association with congenital esophageal motility disorders and as an acquired condition in older animals. This is more common as a presenting sign in dogs than in cats. There is no sex predisposition.

Prehension of food in animals presented for dysphagia is characteristically normal. Hypersalivation may occasionally be reported, particularly in animals with nasal discharge associated with regurgitation.

Regurgitation is an inconsistent sign associated with dysphagia that does not necessarily correlate with the severity of the underlying disorder. Generally, regurgitation is a consequence of abnormalities of the esophageal and gastroesophageal phases of swallowing.

3

TABLE 3 - 5   Differential Diagnoses of Dogs and Cats Presented for Dyspnea

Upper Airway	Lower Airway	Restrictive	Miscellaneous
Stenotic nares	Bronchial diseases	Pneumothorax	Anemia
Rhinitis/sinusitis	COPD	Pleural effusion	Methemoglobinemia
Laryngeal diseases	Allergic bronchitis (asthma, PIE)	Right heart failure	Compensation for metabolic acidosis
Nasopharygeal tumor or foreign body	Lungworms	Neoplasia	
Necrotic laryngitis	Pneumonia	Hypoalbuminemia	Heatstroke
Edema	Pulmonary edema	Hemothorax	Damage to respiratory center
Paralysis of vocal folds	Left heart failure	Chylothorax	Head trauma
Everted saccules	Hypoalbuminemia	Pyothorax	Encephalitis
Laryngeal collapse	Others	Feline infectious peritonitis	Neoplasia
Neoplasia	Pulmonary thromboembolism	Pericardial effusion	Neuromuscular weakness
Intraluminal tracheal or bronchial foreign body or mass	Heartworm disease	Diaphragmatic hernia	Polyradiculoneuritis (coonhound paralysis)
	Hyperadrenocorticism	Intrathoracic neoplastic mass	Diaphragmatic paralysis
Extraluminal tracheal or bronchial obstruction	Others	Thoracic wall trauma	Others
	Pulmonary contusions (trauma)	Flail chest	Pain
Mediastinal mass	Pulmonary fibrosis	Extreme obesity	Fractured ribs or vertebrae
Tracheal or bronchial collapse	Pulmonary granulomatosis	Severe hepatomegaly	Pleuritis
Hilar lymphadenopathy	Deep mycosis	Marked ascites	Others
		Large intra-abdominal mass	Paraquat poisoning
		Severe gastric distention (gastric volvulus)	

COPD, Chronic obstructive pulmonary disease; *PIE*, pulmonary infiltrates with eosinophils.

Although most dysphagic patients have a normal to increased appetite (polyphagia), anorexia, weight loss, and coughing may be associated with severe or chronic obstructive esophageal disease or esophageal ulceration.

CAUTION: Assessment of affected patients for evidence of neurologic signs is of paramount importance, since dysphagia is a principal neurologic complication associated with rabies virus infection.

DIFFERENTIAL DIAGNOSIS (Box 3-12)

DIAGNOSTIC PLANS

1. Observation of the patient's attempt to swallow food and water.
2. Hematologic studies, a biochemistry profile, and urinalysis. Findings are usually of little diagnostic value but are important in assessing overall patient status. A fecal flotation test for parasite ova can be diagnostic for *Spirocerca lupi*.
3. Special laboratory tests, including antinuclear antibody (ANA) titer and lupus erythematosus (LE) cell results, to assess for the presence of immune-mediated disease. Serum thyroxine (T_4) and thyroid-stimulating hormone (TSH) tests are indicated to rule out peripheral neuropathy due to primary hypothyroidism.
4. Noncontrast thoracic *and* cervical radiographs.
5. Positive contrast esophogram, both thoracic and cervical.
6. Esophagoscopy, which may be therapeutic if esophageal foreign body can be retrieved. Esophageal endoscopy is not a reliable means for diagnosing megaesophagus.
7. Fluoroscopic evaluation of esophageal motility.
8. Visual examination of the oropharynx in the anesthetized patient. (Findings are of low diagnostic value.)

3

BOX 3-12   DIFFERENTIAL DIAGNOSIS OF DYSPHAGIA

CARDIOVASCULAR
Megaesophagus secondary to congenital persistent fourth aortic arch
Lymphatic and immune
Mandibular, retropharyngeal, and less commonly bronchial lymphadenopathy associated with lymphosarcoma, thymic neoplasia in FeLV-positive cats, and systemic mycoses (histoplasmosis or blastomycosis)
Epidermolysis bullosa-induced esophagitis (rare)

GASTROINTESTINAL
Esophageal obstruction due to foreign body, parasitic granuloma (*Spirocerca lupi*), stricture, esophageal neoplasia
Cricopharyngeal achalasia (young dogs)
Megaesophagus secondary to pyloric obstruction in cats
Esophageal diverticula
Traumatic esophageal rupture
Reflux esophagitis
Doxycycline-induced esophagitis
Feline herpesvirus-induced esophagitis (rare)

NEUROLOGIC
Congenital and acquired megaesophagus
Myasthenia gravis in dogs
Rabies virus infection

FeLV, feline leukemia virus.

HAIR LOSS: ALOPECIA

DEFINITION

Hair loss, also called *alopecia*: Loss or absence of hair in any amounts and any distribution that is the result of one or a combination of disorders affecting the integrity of the hair coat. Therefore, physiologic loss of hair (e.g., normal shedding or hereditary hair loss such as in the Rex cat breed) is excluded from this definition. In clinical practice, hair loss, with and without pruritus, is among the most common reasons a cat, and particularly a dog, is presented. In most cases, the loss of hair is secondary to some underlying disorder rather than being a primary event. The distribution of hair loss is important in that it can be characteristic of the underlying etiology.

Alopecia can be classified on the basis of distribution as (1) diffuse, (2) regional, (3) multifocal, and (4) focal. The causes for hair loss are varied and often complex. Abnormalities of follicular structure may be inherited, ranging from complete absence of hair follicles to selective absence of follicles that produce hair of a specific color. Inflammatory skin diseases that incorporate the hair follicle may disrupt hair growth and maintenance. Bacterial folliculitis, demodectic mange, and follicular hyperkeratosis are examples.

Disorders disrupting the normal follicular cycles can interrupt hair growth without loss or injury to the hair follicle. The cycle is as follows: *Anagen* (growth phase), *Catagen* (transitional phase), *Telogen* (resting phase).

ASSOCIATED SIGNS

The complex pathogenesis of alopecia supports a multitude of associated clinical signs in any animal presented for hair loss. Pruritus is an important associated sign if present. Allergic, inflammatory, and parasitic skin diseases are likely to cause pruritus. Secondary traumatic excoriation of the skin may further provoke cutaneous injury, thereby intensifying the pruritus. Alopecia caused by endocrine, genetic, and metabolic factors is less likely to be associated with pruritus, although pruritus may become a factor if the exposed skin becomes particularly dry or sunburned. Immune-mediated diseases leading to alopecia are variably pruritic, depending on the distribution and type of skin injury. Nutritional alopecia is rarely confirmed but can be a source of dermatitis and associated pruritus.

Alopecia without pruritus may be associated with dramatic physical signs resulting from endocrine or metabolic disorders. Dermatologic signs include thickened skin, hyperpigmentation, and dry and brittle hair coat (hypothyroidism). On the other hand, skin may appear thin and lack elasticity (canine Cushing's syndrome, Sertoli cell tumor). Gynecomastia, skin softness, calcinosis cutis, and pigmented macules are other dermatologic signs associated with alopecia.

DIFFERENTIAL DIAGNOSIS

Virtually all dogs and cats with primary skin disease manifest some degree of alopecia. The pattern of hair loss is typically asymmetric, and primary skin disease can appear to be symmetric (e.g., parasitic dermatoses). In pursuing the diagnosis in dogs or cats presented for hair loss, thorough systemic and skin examinations are indicated. The clinician may find it helpful to characterize a patient's hair loss according to various etiologic categories:

Primary cutaneous causes of hair loss include the following:

- Infectious
- Bacterial
- Ectoparasitic
- Dermatophytoses
- Dermatomycoses
- Neoplastic
- Keratinization

Secondary causes of hair loss include the following:
- Genetic (Box 3-13)
- Nutritional
- Endocrine (e.g., hypothyroidism, hypoadrenocorticism)
- Keratinization
- Atopic (allergenic)/contact hypersensitivity
- Drug therapy (especially corticosteroids and chemotherapeutic agents)
- Environmental factors
- Neoplasia
- Psychogenic

DIAGNOSTIC PLANS

1. History and physical examination, to determine the nature and extent of primary and secondary skin lesions. Distribution, pattern of alopecia, and associated cutaneous lesions should be characterized. Use the physical examination to determine whether or not evidence of systemic disease is present. Time of onset or the seasonal nature of alopecia may be significant, particularly when accompanied by pruritus.
2. Examination (macroscopic and microscopic) of affected and nonaffected hair.
3. Skin scraping (multiple), fungal cultures, and bacterial cultures (particularly of pustules).
    a. Fine-needle aspiration of discrete intracutaneous masses.
    b. Skin biopsy, to include normal and affected skin.
4. Laboratory database, to include hematology, biochemical profile, urinalysis, and fecal flotation. In addition, cats should be tested for FeLV and FIV.
5. Special diagnostics:
    a. Allergic skin disease: Intradermal antigen inoculation, radioallergosorbent test (RAST) (IgE).
    b. Endocrine alopecia: T_4 before and after TSH stimulation, adrenocorticotropic hormone (ACTH) stimulation, dexamethasone suppression, serum testosterone.
6. Implementation of an elimination diet trial (minimum 6 weeks duration).
7. Environmental allergen or irritant.

BOX 3-13 DIFFERENTIAL DIAGNOSIS OF GENETIC DISORDERS CAUSING ALOPECIA

- Hairless breeds (e.g., African Sand Dog, Abyssinian Dog, Chinese Crested, xoloitzcuintli, Turkish Naked Dog; Sphinx Cat, Rex Cat [seasonal alopecial])
- Ectodermal and follicular dysplasias (e.g., Miniature Poodles)
- Hypotrichosis
- Black hair follicular dysplasia
- Color-mutant alopecia
- Pattern baldness
- Feline alopecia universalis
- Demodicosis

HEMORRHAGE (SEE SPONTANEOUS BLEEDING)

ICTERUS (SEE YELLOW SKIN)

INCOORDINATION: ATAXIA

DEFINITION

Ataxia: The loss of coordination *without* spasticity, paresis, or involuntary movement. In practice, however, it is possible for ataxia to be accompanied by additional neurologic signs.

Ataxia is the result of disorders of the conscious or unconscious proprioceptive system, disorders of the cerebellum, or disorders of the vestibular system.

ASSOCIATED SIGNS

In the spectrum of disorders causing ataxia, lesions of the vestibular system predominate. However, vestibular signs may result from other brain disorders and spinal cord syndromes. Associated signs include head tilt, nystagmus, circling, and hemiparesis. Patients with cerebellar lesions typically have symmetric signs: hypermetria, abnormally long range of movement (goose-stepping gait); hypometria, abnormally short range of movement; or tremor, particularly of the head.

DIFFERENTIAL DIAGNOSIS (Box 3-14)

DIAGNOSTIC PLANS

1. Physical examination, with particular attention to the external ear and tympanic membrane.
2. Neurologic examination, to include assessment of the cranial nerves with the intent of localizing the lesion.

BOX 3-14   DIFFERENTIAL DIAGNOSIS OF ATAXIA

CONGENITAL (SIGNS PRESENT BEFORE 3 MONTHS OF AGE)
Reported in Siamese and Burmese cats and several dog breeds. Multiple congenital disorders are present with multiple neurologic signs, including ataxia. Bilateral congenital vestibular disorders have been observed in Doberman Pinschers, Beagles, and Akitas.

INFLAMMATORY
Otitis interna, as an extension of otitis externa and media
Neuritis of the eighth cranial nerve
Infections

TOXIC
Drug-induced aminoglycoside therapy

NUTRITIONAL
Thiamine deficiency (cat only–rare)

METABOLIC
CNS signs secondary to other diseases (e.g., hepatic, renal)

TRAUMATIC-VASCULAR
Head trauma with concussive injury to the cerebellum and brain stem

NEOPLASTIC
Any tumor

DEGENERATIVE
Storage diseases
Demyelinating diseases
Neuropathies
Cerebellar abiotrophy

IDIOPATHIC (PARTICULARLY COMMON CAUSE OF VESTIBULAR SIGNS)
Feline vestibular syndrome
Geriatric canine vestibular syndrome
Acute labyrinthitis

3. Laboratory profile, to assess metabolic or infectious causes.
4. Skull radiographs, to include the tympanic bullae.
5. Collection and examination of cerebrospinal fluid (CSF).
6. Special diagnostics, depending on availability (e.g., electroencephalogram [EEG], computed tomography [CT], or magnetic resonance imaging).

INCREASED URINATION AND WATER CONSUMPTION: POLYURIA AND POLYDIPSIA

DEFINITION

In practice, *polyuria* (PU) and *polydipsia* (PD) are loosely interpreted to mean an increase in urination and water consumption, respectively. The fact that polyuria is an abnormal increase in urine production, usually of low specific gravity, is seldom confirmed in practice. Likewise, although polydipsia is an abnormal or absolute increase in water consumption usually associated with increased thirst, water intake is seldom quantitated. Use of the terms *polyuria* and *polydipsia* is usually justified when a client presents a dog or cat for subjective increases in urination frequency and water intake as the primary problem. When clear evidence of increased urination and increased thirst is not present, actual documentation of 24-hour urinary output and water intake may be necessary.

Polydipsia is a compensatory sign that develops subsequent to polyuria. Primary polydipsia with compensatory polyuria is uncommon.

The pathophysiology behind polyuria is complex in that several renal and nonrenal mechanisms can be involved. Diseases affecting proximal tubules (e.g., primary renal failure, renal glycosuria) or those causing high solute loads overwhelming proximal tubule absorptive capacity (e.g., diabetes mellitus) cause osmotic diuresis. Water conservation is also affected at the level of the loop of Henle (e.g., primary renal disease, diuretics) and in the distal tubules and collecting ducts. Disorders of the distal tubule and collecting duct are frequently responsible for polyuria, including diabetes insipidus, pyometra, hyperadrenocorticism, liver failure, and hypercalcemia.

Polyuria does result in subsequent failure of the sodium chloride pump in the loop of Henle, leading to significant decreases in the renal medullary osmotic gradient. Liver failure resulting in urea depletion and prolonged polyuria can cause medullary washout.

Primary polydipsia subsequent to increased thirst can cause secondary polyuria but is an uncommon clinical finding. Compulsive water drinking (pseudopsychogenic polydipsia) is probably the most important type of primary polydipsia, although the underlying cause is not known. Hypothalamic lesions, hypercalcemia, and increased levels of plasma renin are less common causes of primary polydipsia.

ASSOCIATED SIGNS

Signs associated with PU or PD are varied and dependent on the underlying disease. Generalized signs include weakness, decreased appetite, weight loss, diarrhea, and fever. Polyphagia with weight loss occurs in animals with diabetes mellitus and in cats with hyperthyroidism. Paraneoplastic syndromes, particularly hypercalcemia, may develop in conjunction with PU or PD. A comprehensive physical examination and a laboratory assessment are justified in all patients presented with PU or PD as the primary complaint.

DIFFERENTIAL DIAGNOSIS (Box 3-15)

DIAGNOSTIC PLANS (Figure 3-3)

1. History and physical examination, to facilitate verification of the problem in addition to determining the duration of the problem and associated signs. Of particular importance is knowledge of the recent administration of medication.

BOX 3-15   DIFFERENTIAL DIAGNOSIS OF POLYURIA AND POLYDIPSIA

POLYURIA OF RENAL ORIGIN
Renal failure
  Glomerulonephritis
  Tubular dysfunction
  Renal medullary dysfunction
Postobstructive diuresis (e.g., feline urologic
  syndrome)
Diabetes insipidus (nephrogenic)
Hypercalcemic nephropathy
Fanconi's syndrome
Medullary washout

POLYURIA OF NONRENAL CAUSES
Diabetes insipidus (neurogenic)
Diabetes mellitus

Hyperadrenocorticism
Liver disease (nonspecific)
Pyometra
Pseudopsychogenic polydipsia

DRUG-INDUCED POLYURIA
Glucocorticoids (esp. in dogs)
Mannitol, IV
Dextrose, concentrations >50 mg/dL (5.0%)
Alcohol
Diuretic therapy (e.g., furosemide)
Phenytoin
Vitamin D intoxication

---

2. Laboratory database. The primary focus of the diagnostic plan is interpreting results from a laboratory database, including a CBC, biochemistry profile, urinalysis, fecal culture, heartworm test (in dogs), FeLV and FIV tests (in cats), and urine culture.
3. Collecting urine and measuring water intake over a 24-hour period, to document the problem, if necessary.
4. Abdominal radiographs, if indicated.
5. Special diagnostic tests, if indicated, based on results from a laboratory database:
    a. Water deprivation and modified-water deprivation tests (contraindicated in the presence of azotemia, dehydration, or hypercalcemia).
    b. Antidiuretic hormone (ADH, vasopressin) response test.
    c. Glucose tolerance test.
    d. ACTH stimulation or dexamethasone suppression.
    e. Serum T_4.
    f. Liver function studies (e.g., serum ammonia, bile acids).
    g. Abdominal ultrasound.
    h. Tissue biopsy (e.g., renal and hepatic).
    i. Exploratory laparotomy.

ITCHING OR SCRATCHING: PRURITUS (SEE ALSO HAIR LOSS)

DEFINITION

Pruritus: Abnormally frequent scratching or biting that results from unpleasant, sometimes intense, epidermal stimulation. Histamine, endopeptidases, and other polypeptides liberated from skin cells serve as mediators of pruritus. Histamine is the primary mediator of itch associated with wheal-and-flare reaction. Histamine-mediated itching cannot be completely inhibited by either H_1- or H_2-receptor antagonists (blockers). Other polypeptides (such as bradykinin), β-endorphin, and neuropeptides, such as substance P, can induce itching when applied directly to skin. The close association between itching and inflammation of the skin is attributed to the fact that many of the endogenous mediators and potentiators are released in situ during inflammatory events.

Itching, although a protective response, can become more harmful than helpful. As a feature of dermatitis, itch mediators cannot be removed by the patient. In fact, scratching and biting eventually promote more inflammation and subsequently perpetuate the itching.

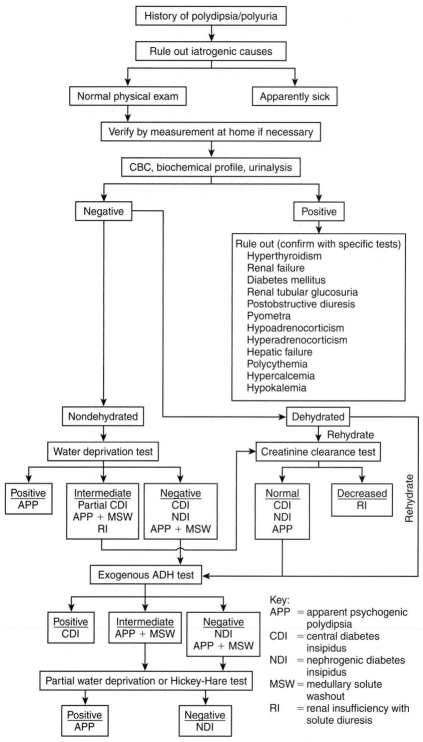

Figure 3-3: Clinical approach to the patient with polydipsia and polyuria. *CBC,* complete blood count; *ADH,* antidiuretic hormone.
(From Fenner WR: *Quick reference to veterinary medicine,* ed. 2, Philadelphia, 1991, JB Lippincott, p. 110.)

ASSOCIATED SIGNS

Skin lesions are commonly associated with pruritus; however, it becomes important to characterize the lesion and to distinguish those that are primary from those that are secondary to scratching or biting. Papules and pustules are characteristic primary lesions that may ultimately develop into secondary lesions, such as crusts, ulcers, scale in collarettes, and pigmented macules. Vesicles and bullae, plaques, and urticaria (wheals) can also occur as primary skin lesions. Linear crusts, irregular ulceration, lichenification, diffuse scaling and pigmentation, and patchy alopecia are characteristic lesions that develop secondary to excoriation.

Pruritus can also occur without primary lesions (i.e., "essential" pruritus). This type of itching is a manifestation of systemic disease, although mediation may be central or cutaneous. Causes include atopy, dry skin, and neurogenic and psychogenic disorders. A spectrum of renal, hepatic, hematopoietic, allergic, and endocrine diseases are associated with essential pruritus.

DIFFERENTIAL DIAGNOSIS (Box 3-16)

DIAGNOSTIC PLANS

1. History and physical examination, to characterize the skin lesion and its distribution, to determine whether or not the condition appears to be contagious, and to determine whether or not systemic disease is present.
2. Laboratory database, if evidence of systemic disease is present.

3

BOX 3-16   DIFFERENTIAL DIAGNOSIS OF PRURITUS

PUSTULAR DERMATITIS
Infectious
   Puppy pyoderma
   Folliculitis and furunculosis
Immune-mediated
   Pemphigus foliaceus
   Vesicle-forming disorders (e.g., drug eruption)
   Linear IgA γ dermatosis
Idiopathic
   Puppy strangles
   Subcorneal pustular dermatosis

VESICULAR/BULLOUS ERUPTION
Bullous dermatoses
Systemic lupus erythematosus (SLE)
Toxic epidermal necrolysis
Drug eruption
Acute contact dermatitis

PLAQUE FORMATION
Infectious dermatitis
Immune-mediated dermatitis
Neoplasia (e.g., mast cell tumor)

PAPULAR ERUPTION (DOG)
Infectious
   Folliculitis (bacterial, fungal, demodectic)

Parasitic (*Sarcoptes*, *Cheyletiella*, lice, fleas)
Vasculitis (Rocky Mountain spotted fever)
Immune
   Allergy (atopy)
   Autoimmune (pemphigus foliaceus, SLE)
   Idiopathic

PAPULAR ERUPTION (CAT)
Infectious (bacterial folliculitis)
Dermatophytosis
Parasitic (otodectic and notoedric mange, *Cheyletiella*, lice)
Immune-mediated (hypersensitivity to food)
Idiopathic military dermatitis

ULCERATIVE DERMATITIS
SLE
Leukocytoclastic vasculitis
Erythema multiforme
Toxic epidermal necrolysis
Mycosis fungoides
Epidermolysis bullosa complex
Dermatomyositis
Acute contact dermatitis
Vogt-Koyanagi-Harada syndrome

3. Skin and coat examination. Perform multiple skin scrapings, and examine skin and hair coat with Wood's light.
4. Microbiologic testing for bacteria and dermatophytes.
5. Immunologic testing, to include intradermal skin testing and direct fluorescent antibody testing of skin (both normal and affected) biopsy specimens.
6. Skin biopsy with dermatohistopathology.
7. Provocative exposure to selected environmental agents, diet, and drugs.

JAUNDICE (SEE YELLOW SKIN)

JOINT SWELLING: ARTHROPATHY (SEE ALSO LAMENESS)

DEFINITION

Joint swelling, or *joint enlargement*: Any abnormal increase in size, either visible or palpable, of any joint that is *not* directly caused by a proliferation of tissue. In practice, joint swelling is the primary presenting sign only occasionally. Pain and associated lameness are more likely causes for presentation, whereas actual enlargement of a joint is detected during physical examination. However, there is not necessarily an association between joint swelling and pain.

Joint swelling, or effusion, occurs subsequent to injury to the synovial membrane in which there is not only an increase in volume of synovial fluid produced, but quantitative biochemical and cellular changes as well. Most joint swelling is attributed to inflammation of the synovial membrane, or synovitis. Abnormal synovial fluid accumulation (effusion) may be classified as serous, fibrinous, purulent, septic, or hemorrhagic.

ASSOCIATED SIGNS

Although lameness is the most common clinical sign associated with joint swelling, it is not consistently present. Joint swelling may also be associated with, or mistaken for, hyperplasia, metaplasia, or neoplasia of the synovium, joint capsule, articular cartilage, or periarticular bone. Hemorrhagic joint effusion (hemarthrosis) may be associated with coagulopathy and spontaneous bleeding from the respiratory, GI, or urinary tract. Subluxation or fracture of a carpus, tarsus, or stifle may also be associated with detectable joint swelling. Arthritis associated with systemic disease (e.g., infectious or immune mediated) can also be accompanied by significant joint swelling.

DIFFERENTIAL DIAGNOSIS (Box 3-17)

DIAGNOSTIC PLANS

1. History. The history generally focuses on associated signs rather than primary joint swelling and should address duration, exposure to ticks, known injury, and evidence of spontaneous bleeding. Physical examination establishes the presence of joint swelling and the number of joints involved. Evidence of inflammation, crepitus, joint laxity, abnormal range of motion, a drawer sign, luxations, or fractures should be determined.
2. Radiography of the affected joint(s).
3. Synovial fluid analysis, including biochemical, cytologic, and culture findings.
4. Coagulation profile in the presence of hemarthrosis.
5. Immune function testing: ANA titer, rheumatoid factor, and LE cell preparation.
6. Contrast arthrography.
7. Joint capsule–synovial membrane biopsy.
8. Periarticular bone biopsy.
9. Surgical exploration of the affected joint.

BOX 3-17 ARTHROPATHIES IN THE DOG AND CAT

NONINFLAMMATORY
Degenerative joint disease (osteoarthritis, osteoarthrosis)
  Primary
  Secondary
  As a sequel to acquired or congenital defects of the joints and supporting structures
Traumatic
Neoplastic involvement
Drug-induced

INFLAMMATORY
Infectious
  Bacterial
  Caliciviral (cat)
  Mycoplasmal
  Fungal
  Protozoal

Rickettsial (neurophilic erlichiosis, Rocky Mountain spotted fever)
  Spirochetal (Lyme disease)
Noninfectious
  Immunologic
    Erosive (deforming)
      Rheumatoid arthritis
    Nonerosive (nondeforming)
      Systemic lupus erythematosus
      Arthritis resulting from chronic infectious disease
      Idiopathic nonerosive arthritis
      Drug reactions (sulfadiazine reaction)
  Nonimmunologic
    Crystal-induced arthritis (gout, pseudogout)
    Chronic hemarthrosis (coagulation defects, congenital or acquired)

LOSS OF APPETITE: ANOREXIA

DEFINITION

Anorexia: Strictly speaking, anorexia is the lack or loss of appetite for food. In veterinary medicine, this term is loosely used to describe *diminished* or *partial*, as opposed to complete loss of, interest in eating. In addition, part of the difficulty in assessing the patient that is presented for loss of appetite is grounded in owner expectation of what is and what is not a normal appetite in a dog or cat. While domesticated pets do tend to eat at regular intervals throughout the day, some do experience transient periods of sustained inappetence that may, in fact, be entirely normal and not associated with underlying disease. When assessing a dog or cat for *partial* loss of appetite, careful history and physical evaluation are indicated to determine whether or not underlying disease may be the cause of this vague clinical sign. In addition, the clinical history must establish the duration of the anorexia and whether the loss of appetite is complete or partial.

Note: What makes *anorexia* such an important clinical sign is the fact that loss of appetite is the very first outward sign the owner may notice when a pet is ill.

ASSOCIATED SIGNS

What makes *anorexia* such an important clinical sign is the fact that loss of appetite is the first outward sign the owner may notice when a pet is ill. *Anorexia* is regarded as a low-yield clinical sign—that is, it is not a discrete sign and, like pain, may be associated with numerous underlying disorders.

Historical evidence of a significant change in the pet's environment (e.g., a new child in the family) or daily routine (e.g., the dog is home alone during the day for the first time) is important to assess. Knowledge of current drug therapy, whether the pet eats sticks or other foreign material, whether or not the pet food type recently changed or may not be fresh (moldy canned and dry food will generally not be consumed) is important.

Physical examination should determine overall body conformation, body weight, extent of weight loss (if present), and any obvious external injuries that might contribute. Age is an important factor in the assessment of anorexia. Diminished sense of smell, neoplasia, joint disease, and dental disease are common age-related disorders that may contribute to anorexia.

DIFFERENTIAL DIAGNOSIS

Differential diagnoses associated with *anorexia* are too numerous to be of assistance in resolving to a diagnosis. The clinician faced with a patient that has only anorexia is faced with a significant clinical challenge in defining the underlying disorder. Even the categories of disease that could be associated with inappetence are wide ranging and include psychologic, metabolic, orthopedic, infectious, inflammatory, and neoplastic causes.

DIAGNOSTIC PLANS

1. Careful observation of the patient on and off the examination table is important.
2. A methodical physical examination.
3. A standard laboratory profile to include hematology, biochemistry, and urinalysis (fecal is optional depending on the presenting signs.
4. Radiography or other imaging study is indicated if the pain can be localized to a discrete region of the body (e.g., abdominal cavity).
5. Special diagnostic tests are indicated if specific abnormalities can be detected (e.g., biopsy, aspiration and cytopathology, myelography).

3

LYMPH NODE ENLARGEMENT: LYMPHADENOMEGALY

DEFINITION

Lymphadenomegaly: Any change in the size or consistency of a lymph node or group of lymph nodes. Lymphadenomegaly refers to those lymph nodes that are larger than expected with or without commensurate changes in consistency. Involved nodes may be unusually soft, firm, or painful, suggestive of inflammation; whereas enlarged, firm, nonpainful lymph nodes suggest neoplasia. Lymphadenomegaly is usually not a presenting problem, with the possible exception of generalized enlargements of all superficial lymph nodes.

Lymph nodes become enlarged as a result of inflammation (pyogenic or granulomatous), reactive lymphoid hyperplasia, or neoplasia (primary or neoplastic). In pyogenic inflammation, neutrophils dilate and engorge the sinuses; whereas in granulomatous inflammation, an infiltrate or macrophages is present (e.g., systemic mycoses). Reactive lymphoid hyperplasia is associated with an increase in the number of germinal centers within the lymph node and an infiltrate of plasma cells. In neoplastic lymph nodes, tumor cells may invade the sinuses (metastatic), gradually destroying the normal node architecture, or the architecture of the lymph node is entirely replaced by malignant lymphocytes (lymphosarsoma)— that is, histologically, the sinuses are obliterated and germinal centers cannot be found.

ASSOCIATED SIGNS

Characterize the consistency and number of affected nodes as well as their location (i.e., generalized or regional). Lymph node pain is an inconsistent finding usually associated with inflammatory disease rather than neoplasia. Associated signs are likely to be regional, as is the lymph node enlargement (i.e., tissue injury or infection). Patients with generalized lymphadenomegaly may not have associated signs, or there may be nonspecific signs, including weight loss, fever, decreased appetite, and lassitude as a result of systemic illness.

DIFFERENTIAL DIAGNOSIS (Box 3-18)

DIAGNOSTIC PLANS

1. History and physical examination, to determine the duration and type of associated signs, if any, and the duration of lymph node enlargement, if known.

BOX 3-18 DIFFERENTIAL DIAGNOSIS FOR LYMPHADENOMEGALY

GENERALIZED

Lymphosarcoma
Diffuse, generalized skin disease
Infectious diseases (numerous infections are known to cause lymph node enlargement)
Parasitic (especially severe ectoparasitism, e.g., demodicosis with secondary pyoderma)
Vaccination

LOCALIZED

Any of the causes of GENERALIZED
Localized infection, especially in the skin or subcutaneous tissues
Cutaneous neoplasia, other than lymphoma

---

2. Laboratory profile, with emphasis on CBC, including platelet count; biochemistry panel; and urinalysis.
3. Specific tests for infectious diseases, as indicated (e.g., FeLV antigen and FIV antibody).
4. Thoracic and abdominal radiographs, as indicated.
5. Fine-needle aspiration of affected lymph node(s).
6. Serum protein electrophoresis.
7. Bone marrow aspirate.
8. Lymph node biopsy and, if indicated, culture.

PAIN

DEFINITION

Pain: The perception of an unpleasant sensation; may be generalized or localized. While *pain* may be the single most common presenting complaint of humans who seek medical attention from a physician, the ability of a dog or cat to communicate pain *and* the ability of the owner to interpret the signs correctly make this a particularly complex clinical sign in animals.

ASSOCIATED SIGNS

As in humans, the actual perception and manifestation of pain varies from one animal to another. Fundamental to the ability to interpret the presence of pain in an animal is the ability to recognize a change in behavior. Acute injury and associated pain is relatively simple to ascertain. However, chronic pain emanating from a specific organ or tissue (e.g., liver or bone) can be extremely difficult to define and localize. Other signs that may be associated with pain include sleeplessness; unusual posture; decreased activity; decreased appetite; reluctance to play, walk, or run; agitation; or altered grooming behavior. Physical findings are also highly varied and may include such findings as hypersalivation, mydriasis, tachycardia, shivering, or increased respiratory rate. Unfortunately, despite efforts to objectively measure pain in animals, there are no tests that clearly define whether or not an individual animal is experiencing pain.

Note: Pain Management has become increasingly recognized as an essential part of clinical practice today. Section 1(Tables 1-17 to 1-22) addresses indications of the drugs and doses most commonly employed in pain management of dogs and cats.

DIFFERENTIAL DIAGNOSIS

Many disorders are associated with pain. Hence, developing a list of differential diagnoses becomes impractical. Since pain is characteristically associated with inflammation or tissue trauma, every effort should be made to localize the source of the pain in order to focus the diagnostic search. Localizing acute-onset pain is generally less problematic than localizing chronic pain. Particularly in the patient with nonlocalizing, chronic pain, developing a clear diagnostic plan is essential in establishing a diagnosis.

DIAGNOSTIC PLANS

1. Careful observation of the patient as it moves, stands, sits, lies down, and so on is critical.
2. A methodical physical examination.
3. A standard laboratory profile to include hematology, biochemistry, and urinalysis (fecal is optional depending on the presenting signs).
4. Radiography or other imaging study is indicated if the pain can be localized to a discrete region of the body (e.g., abdominal cavity).
5. Special diagnostic tests are indicated if specific abnormalities can be detected (e.g., biopsy, aspiration and cytopathology, myelography).
6. In some patients, empiric treatment with anagesics or nonsteroidal antiinflammatory drugs may be indicated. However, utilizing this method for managing pain requires the ability to provide follow-up care to that patient.

3

PAINFUL URINATION: DYSURIA (SEE STRAINING TO URINATE)

PAINFUL DEFECATION: DYSCHEZIA (SEE STRAINING TO DEFECATE)

RECTAL AND ANAL PAIN (SEE STRAINING TO DEFECATE)

REGURGITATION (SEE ALSO DIFFICULTY SWALLOWING AND VOMITING)

DEFINITION

Regurgitation: Retrograde esophageal transport of ingesta subsequent to a mechanical, neurogenic, or myogenic swallowing disorder. Owners most often describe regurgitation as "vomiting." Both regurgitation and vomiting imply a backward flowing of ingesta through the esophagus; however, regurgitation is a relatively effortless act in contrast to the retching and abdominal pressure characteristic of vomiting. Regurgitation localizes the problem to the esophagus.

The pathophysiology of esophageal function is addressed and referenced in the article on dysphagia. Both acquired (e.g., foreign body) and congenital (e.g., familial megaesophagus) forms and esophageal disease can lead to regurgitation. Many esophageal problems remain undiagnosed if regurgitation is not present.

ASSOCIATED SIGNS

Physical signs recognized by owners of dogs or cats with regurgitation include dysphagia characterized by difficulty swallowing food, frequent attempts to swallow food, and hypersalivation. Belching may also be reported subsequent to the entrapment of air in the esophagus. Inappetence and weight loss subsequently develop. Esophageal dilatation may be observed at the level of the lower cervical esophagus or thoracic inlet.

Owners may report expulsion of blood-tinged saliva subsequent to esophageal mucosal injury. Paroxysms of coughing and retching, particularly when eating, may be present along with difficult breathing in animals with significant pneumonia. Nasal discharge may consist of mucoid to mucopurulent exudates or of food and liquid recently consumed.

Rarely, affected animals present with swollen joints, lameness, and severe weakness associated with hypertrophic osteodystrophy subsequent to an intrathoracic lesion. Atypical signs include inspiratory dyspnea, regurgitation unrelated to eating, and recurrent gastric bloating associated with aerophagia.

DIFFERENTIAL DIAGNOSIS (Box 3-19)

DIAGNOSTIC PLANS

1. History and physical examination, to characterize the nature of the problem, to distinguish between vomiting and regurgitation, and to establish the character of the regurgitated material.
2. Laboratory database, to assess patient status, particularly if secondary complications are present.
3. Survey thoracic and cervical radiography, to assess presence of megaesophagus, radiopaque intraesophageal lesion, or both.
4. Contrast esophagram, to confirm any interference with normal bolus transport at the point of obstruction, changes in mucosal integrity or luminal displacement, and the presence of extraluminal gas. (Oral suspension of barium sulfate is recommended over other contrast materials.) NOTE: Contrast medium retention in the esophagus is the hallmark of a motor disorder and often localizes the site of dysmotility.
5. Endoscopy and, as indicated, biopsy, to determine the cause of megaesophagus rather than to diagnose megaesophagus. In some instances, especially foreign body obstruction, endoscopy may be therapeutic.
6. Special procedures, to include contrast esophagram during fluoroscopy, CT, and exploratory laparotomy.

BOX 3-19 DIFFERENTIAL DIAGNOSIS OF REGURGITATION

FUNCTIONAL MEGAESOPHAGUS*
Primary (or congenital)
Secondary (or acquired)
 Foreign body
 Esophageal stricture
 Esophageal diverticula
 Neurogenic (e.g., myasthenia gravis, rabies)
 Myopathy, smooth muscle
 Extraesophageal compressive lesion (e.g., neoplasia)
 Vascular anomaly

ESOPHAGITIS
Gastric reflux
Neoplastic

RESTRICTIVE LESION WITHOUT MEGAESOPHAGUS
Foreign body obstruction
Intrathoracic mass
Vascular ring anomaly
Esophageal stricture

---

*The most prevalent cause.

SEIZURES (CONVULSIONS OR EPILEPSY)

DEFINITION

The terms *seizure, convulsion, epilepsy, epileptic attack,* and *fit* all describe a clinical sign that is characterized by involuntary contraction of a series of voluntary muscles. Seizures result from disorders of the brain that cause spontaneous depolarizations and excitation of cerebral neurons. As a presenting problem, seizures are much more common in the dog than in the cat.

Such disorders may originate from extracranial causes, metabolic or toxic diseases, and intracranial causes (e.g., organic brain disease). When seizures occur in the absence of detectable organic or metabolic CNS abnormalities, the seizures are described as *idiopathic.* Idiopathic epilepsy is the most common type of seizure reported in companion animal species.

A distinction is made between *partial seizures* (also called *focal seizures*) and *generalized seizures.* Three classes of partial seizure are recognized: partial motor seizures (the most common type of seizure in animals), psychomotor seizures, and sensory seizures.

Partial seizures are caused by a cortical lesion or focus that periodically disrupts cerebral function. Generalized motor seizures represent a widespread disorder not referable to any single anatomic or functional system. Clinical manifestations suggest widespread activation of the brain.

Seizures may be repeated frequently in groups of two or three, or they may occur singly. If a series of seizures occurs and the patient fails to regain consciousness during the interictal period, the term *status epilepticus* applies. In contrast to a single seizure, status epilepticus is a serious, life-threatening condition that justifies emergency intervention.

ASSOCIATED SIGNS

Generalized motor seizures are the most prevalent type of seizure encountered in veterinary medicine. Most cases are diagnosed as idiopathic epilepsy on the basis that organic causes of seizure activity cannot be identified. The interictal period in animals with a history of generalized motor seizures is characteristically described by owners as normal. The immediate postictal period, regardless of the cause of the seizure activity, is often associated with transient disorientation, blindness, stumbling, polydipsia, or polyphagia.

The spectrum of possible clinical signs associated with seizure activity is extensive. Before a diagnosis of idiopathic epilepsy is reached, it is important that the patient be evaluated for cardiovascular disease, trauma, toxicity, infectious disease, parasites, neoplasia, and metabolic disorders, particularly those affecting the kidney, liver, and endocrine pancreas.

AGE OF ANIMAL

Seizures in young animals (<1 year old) are commonly caused by developmental abnormalities, hydrocephalus, lissencephaly, encephalitis (infectious), lead poisoning, severe intestinal parasitism, portacaval shunt abnormalities, and juvenile hypoglycemia. Idiopathic epilepsy usually begins when animals are 1 to 3 years of age. Animals over 5 years of age are more likely to have CNS tumors or hypoglycemia from insulin-secreting beta cell pancreatic neoplasms.

BREED PREDISPOSITION

Some basic knowledge about breed predisposition to seizure disorders may be helpful in establishing a diagnosis. Idiopathic epilepsy has been seen in numerous dog breeds, particularly German Shepherd Dogs, Belgian Tervurens, Keeshonds, Saint Bernards, Standard and Miniature Poodles, Beagles, Irish Setters, Cocker Spaniels, Alaskan Malamutes, Siberian Huskies, and Labrador and Golden Retrievers. Juvenile hypoglycemia is most prevalent in toy breeds. Hydrocephalus is common in the toy and brachycephalic breeds. Neoplastic diseases are common in brachycephalic breeds over 5 years of age.

Concerning disorders of CNS metabolism, leukodystrophy is most common in Cairn and West Highland whites; lipodystrophy in German Short-Haired Pointers and English Setters; lissencephaly in the Lhasa Apso; and portacaval shunts and hyperlipoproteinemia in Miniature Schnauzers. A unique, usually fatal, encephalitis occurs in Pugs.

ENVIRONMENT

Exposure to infectious agents or other sick animals may be important, as is exposure to sources of intoxicants, such as lead in paints, linoleum, tar, batteries, or roofing material;

hexachlorophene soap; ethylene glycol (antifreeze); metaldehyde snail bait; and various other insecticides, including chlorinated hydrocarbons, organophosphates, and rodenticides. Dogs and cats on the same premises with swine may be exposed to *Herpesvirus suis* (pseudorabies, or Auzjesky's disease). A high protein diet exacerbates hepatic encephalopathy. Thiamine deficiency may result from long-term consumption of certain fish diets or from cooking pet food.

DIFFERENTIAL DIAGNOSIS (Table 3-6)

DIAGNOSTIC PLANS

1. History, to take into consideration breed predisposition, environmental exposures, past medical illnesses, and medication. Because most seizures are of short duration and the physical (tonic-clonic) manifestations of a seizure are so dramatic, requesting the owner to describe the type and duration of seizure may elicit unreliable information.
2. Thorough physical examination, to include careful neurologic examination, with particular attention to cranial nerves, funduscopic examination, and cardiac auscultation.
3. Laboratory database, essential to rule out metabolic causes. In addition to a CBC, biochemistry profile, urinalysis, and fecal culture, any or all of the following tests are indicated: serum ammonia, bile acids, serum insulin in hypoglycemic patients, blood lead test, and serial blood cultures.
4. Survey radiographs of the skull. These are rarely helpful, as intracranial neoplasms are not detectable on conventional skull radiographs.

3

TABLE 3-6 **Differential Diagnoses for Seizure Disorders**

Intracranial	Extracranial
Congenital	Intoxication
Hydrocephalus	Lead
Lissencephaly	Organophosphates
Other malformations	Chlorinated hydrocarbons
Storage diseases	Strychnine
Vascular anomaly	Drugs
Traumatic	Garbage
Immediate	Metabolic
Post trauma	Hypoglycemia
Inflammatory	Hypocalcemia
Distemper	Hyperkalemia
Rabies	Acid-base
Feline infectious peritonitis	Hepatic encephalopathy
Feline leukemia virus	Uremia
Toxoplasmosis	Hyperlipoproteinemia
Mycosis	Nutritional
Bacteria	Thiamine
Reticulosis	Parasites?
Parasites	Hypoxia
Neoplasia	Cardiovascular disease
Primary	Respiratory disease
Metastatic	Birth
Vascular–cerebrovascular accident	Anesthetic accident
	Hyperthermia

From Russo ME: Seizures. *In* Ford RB, ed: Clinical Signs and Diagnosis in Small Animal Practice. New York, Churchill Livingstone, 1988, p 290.

5. In special circumstances, limited ultrasound examination of the brain may be possible in young dogs through a cranial fontanelle. Evidence of hydrocephalus may be seen.
6. Computed tomography or magnetic resonance imaging (special facilities required).
7. Electrocardiogram or echocardiogram, if indicated.
8. Serologic studies for canine distemper, rabies, feline infectious peritonitis (FIP), FeLV, FIV, toxoplasmosis, and systemic (deep) mycoses.
9. CSF analysis, including biochemistries, antibody titers, and cytologic parameters.
10. EEG. Although limited in availability, the EEG may be useful in detecting inflammatory brain disease and congenital intracranial abnormalities (e.g., hydrocephalus).
11. Contrast studies, requiring special equipment or facilities: radioisotope brain scan, cerebral angiography, pneumoencephalography, and CT scan.

SNEEZING AND NASAL DISCHARGE

DEFINITION

Sneezing: A protective reflex described as a sudden, involuntary, and forceful, even violent, expulsion of air from the upper respiratory tract; may or may not be accompanied by significant nasal discharge. Clients easily recognize sneezing. Although sneezing is a physiologic response to irritating stimuli, increased frequency and paroxysmal sneezing episodes are readily recognized as abnormal. Like sneezing, a nasal discharge, regardless of its consistency, is a clinical sign that clients accurately interpret and reliably describe to the clinician.

Sneezing is the outward manifestation of nasal passage irritation by extraneous (foreign material) or endogenous (antigen-antibody interaction) agents. Afferent impulses travel via the fifth cranial nerve to the medulla, where the initial reflex is triggered. Chronic nasal discharge is a clinical sign that localizes a disorder to the upper respiratory passages, particularly the nasal cavity and frontal sinuses.

ASSOCIATED SIGNS

Important associated signs suggesting systemic involvement include facial asymmetry (neoplasia or fungal infection), atrophy of the masseter and temporal muscles, difficulty prehending or masticating food, conjunctivitis, and ocular discharge. *Epistaxis*, which is distinguished from blood-tinged nasal discharge, is an important associated sign that further supports intranasal disease or coagulopathy. Cleft palate is a common cause of nasal discharge in neonates. Erosion and depigmentation of the planum nasale is often associated with nasal aspergillosis in dogs, whereas cats with nasal cryptococosis may have a detectable granuloma at the rostral aspect of the nose. Occasionally, cough is associated with purulent nasal discharges and sneezing.

DIFFERENTIAL DIAGNOSIS (Box 3-20)
DIAGNOSTIC PLANS (Figure 3-4)

SPONTANEOUS BLEEDING: HEMORRHAGE

DEFINITION

Spontaneous or prolonged bleeding: The visible, abnormal discharge of blood resulting from a failure of one or more hemostatic mechanisms. May result from deficiencies in platelet numbers or function, in the extrinsic or intrinsic coagulation cascades, or in vascular integrity.

3

BOX 3-20 DIFFERENTIAL DIAGNOSIS FOR SNEEZING AND NASAL DISCHARGE

INTRANASAL CAUSES
Serous Nasal Discharge
  Acute viral upper respiratory infection (feline)
  Feline chlamydiosis
  Intranasal parasites
  Oronasal fistula (canine tooth)
  Rhinosporidiosis (canine, rare)
Purulent Nasal Discharge
  Viral upper respiratory infection with secondary bacterial infection (dog and cat)
  Mycotic nasal disease
  Foreign body rhinitis
  Traumatic rhinitis or sinusitis
  Cleft palate
  Neoplasia (several types possible)
  Nasopharyngeal polyps (feline, rare)
  Benign nasal polyps (canine, rare)
  Oronasal fistula
 Mucoid to Mucopurulent Nasal Discharge
  Mycotic nasal disease (e.g., aspergillosis, cryptococcosis, blastomycosis)

Neoplasia (especially adenocarcinoma)
Epistaxis
  Acute nasal trauma
  Oronasal fistula

EXTRANASAL CAUSES
Purulent Nasal Discharge
  Bacterial pneumonia
  Megaesophagus with aspiration pneumonia, congenital or acquired
  Achalasia with nasal reflux of food
  Acquired esophageal stricture
Epistaxis
  von Willebrand's disease (most common canine coagulopathy)
  Factor VIII deficiency (classic hemophilia)
  Other inherited factor deficiencies
  Thrombocytopenia (infectious or immune-mediated)
  Disseminated intravascular coagulation
  Hyperviscosity syndrome

The hemostatic response is a complex defense system that fulfills three basic functions: ensures that blood is confined to the vascular system of the normal animal (vascular integrity), causes the arrest of bleeding at sites of vascular injury, and maintains the patency of the vascular network.

These functions are accomplished through complex interactions between blood platelets, the blood vessel wall, and a variety of plasma enzyme systems. Disorders affecting these interactions can result in spontaneous or prolonged bleeding.

The *primary phase* of hemostasis occurs with platelet aggregation and the formation of the relatively unstable platelet plug. The *secondary phase* of hemostasis, essential to complete hemostasis, reinforces the platelet plug with fibrin. Secondary hemostasis depends on adequate plasma concentration of procoagulant proteins and on their proper interaction. Coagulation can be initiated through an intrinsic pathway, which involves components normally found within the vasculature and which is activated by contact with a foreign surface. The extrinsic pathway is an alternative mechanism through which clotting is initiated.

Secondary hemostasis is regulated by inhibitory products that limit the extent of enzymatic reaction and prevent their dissemination: antithrombin III, a potent inhibitor of kallikrein; factors IXa, XIa, XIIa, and Xa; and thrombin. The fibrinolytic system, another plasma protein-enzyme system, removes the hemostatic plug once its function has been served.

ASSOCIATED SIGNS

Bleeding disorders are most apparent when bleeding develops spontaneously from one or more body orifices and is prolonged. Bleeding from the nose (epistaxis: see Figure 3-4) is perhaps the most commonly reported outward manifestation of a bleeding disorder in dogs. Bleeding into the skin or mucous membranes (e.g., petechiation) may not be immediately apparent to even the most observant owner. Excessive or prolonged bleeding into soft tissues (hematoma) or joints (hemarthrosis) may be seen as physical enlargement of the affected tissues with pain and lameness.

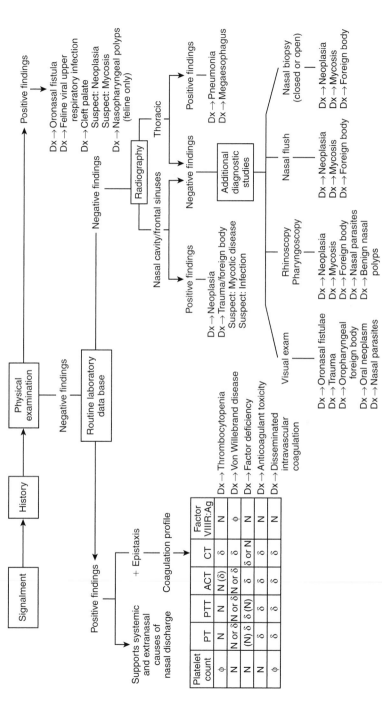

Figure 3-4: Clinical algorithm for the patient presented for sneezing, nasal discharge, or both. *ACT*, activated clotting time; *PT*, prothrombin time; *PTT*, partial thromboplastin time; *CT*, clotting time; Factor VIIIR:Ag, factor VIII-related antigen; φ, decreased (numbers); δ, prolonged (time); N, normal; N (δ), usually normal, occasionally prolonged; ? (N), usually prolonged, occasionally normal.

There may be a history of recurrent minor bleeding episodes in some animals. The severity of clinical signs depends on such factors as type of defect, degree of clotting factor activity, and individual variation. Moderately to severely affected animals are typically young at the time of presentation. Prolonged bleeding subsequent to elective surgical procedures may be the first sign of a bleeding disorder.

DIFFERENTIAL DIAGNOSIS (see Box 3-21 on p. 433)

DIAGNOSTIC PLANS

1. History. Age (inherited versus acquired), sex (sex-linked versus autosomal), and breed (inherited versus acquired) of the bleeding patient must be carefully considered. Bleeding disorders in related animals should also be considered. A detailed history of recent or current drug administration and vaccination is critical.
2. Physical examination. This may be normal. However, evidence of melena, hematuria, epistaxis, and hematoma or hemarthrosis should be pursued. The skin and mucous membranes should be inspected for evidence of petechiae or ecchymoses.
3. Routine laboratory database, indicated in all bleeding patients to assess for the presence of underlying contributory diseases, as well as the possible consequences of bleeding within major organs.
4. Antibody titers for ehrlichiosis and Rocky Mountain spotted fever.
5. Coagulation screening tests:
   a. Peripheral blood smear (for the presence of platelets).
   b. Platelet count followed by buccal mucosal bleeding time (a test of platelet function) is the presence of adequate platelet numbers.
   c. Assessment of clot retraction.
   d. Prothrombin time (PT).
   e. Activated partial thromboplastin time (APTT).
   f. Thrombin clotting time.
   g. Fibrinogen.
   h. Fibrin degradation products.
   i. Clot lysis.
6. Specialized laboratory tests (special facilities required):
   a. Specific factor activity assays.
   b. Platelet function studies (adhesion, aggregation, secretion).
   c. Antiplatelet antibody.
   d. Antithrombin III.
   e. Kallikrein.
   f. Electron microscopic assessment of platelets.

STRAINING TO DEFECATE: DYSCHEZIA

DEFINITION

Dyschezia: Painful or difficult evacuation of feces from the rectum. In the clinical setting, dyschezia may be a difficult problem to ascertain unless the owner is particularly astute and is able to distinguish effort to urinate (see Dysuria) from effort to defecate in cats and female dogs. Therefore, a concerted effort on the part of the clinician is usually necessary to differentiate disorders affecting the urinary outflow tract and micturition from disorders affecting defecation.

The most likely cause for any animal to present with dyschezia is rectal or perianal pain. The origin of the pain may be mucosal, mucocutaneous (anal), or extraluminal lesions. Rectal strictures are uncommon but may contribute to constipation and associated dyschezia. Strictures typically develop subsequent to neoplasia or deep, nonpenetrating injury to the rectum. Although uncommon, dyschezia may also occur subsequent to lesions in the lumbar spinal cord or sacrum.

BOX 3-21   DIFFERENTIAL DIAGNOSIS OF SPONTANEOUS BLEEDING

HEREDITARY DISORDERS—FACTOR DEFICIENCIES
Hypoprothrombinemia (factor II)–Boxers
Hypoproconvertinemia (factor VII)–Beagles, Malamutes
Hemophilia A (factor VIII)–most dog breeds and cats
Hemophilia B (factor IX)–several dog breeds and British short-hair cats
von Willebrand's disease (vWD factor)–most dog breeds
Stuart factor deficiency (factor X)–Cocker Spaniels
Plasma thromboplastin antecedent (PTA) deficiency (factor XI)–Springer Spaniels, Great
    Pyrenees, Kerry Blue Terriers
Hageman factor deficiency (factor XII)–cats

HEREDITARY PLATELET DISORDERS
Thromobocytopenia
Platelet dysfunction
    Thrombasthenia (Glanzmann's disease)*
    Thrombopathia (e.g., osteogenesis imperfecta, Ehlers-Danlos syndrome)*

ACQUIRED CLOTTING FACTOR DISORDERS
Primary hyperfibrinolysis
Disseminated intravascular coagulation (DIC)
Chemical- or drug-induced
    Vitamin K deficiency
    Rodenticide ingestion
    Prolonged enteric antimicrobial therapy*
Circulating anticoagulants
    Heparin
    Warfarin
    Warfarin-like chemical (e.g., diphacinone)
    Plasma expander therapy*
    Antifactor antibody*
Liver disease
    DIC
    Vitamin K deficiency
    Decreased factor synthesis subsequent to severe liver disease*

ACQUIRED PLATELET DISORDERS
Thrombocytopenia (relatively common)
    Decreased or ineffective thrombopoiesis*
    Immunologic destruction: immune-mediated, infectious, drug-induced
    Consumption: DIC, vasculitis
    Sequestration: splenomegaly subsequent to neoplasia*
    Dilutional: IV fluid administration*
Platelet dysfunction
    Secondary to underlying disease: renal failure and uremia, hepatic failure, polycythemia*
    Drug-induced: aspirin, phenylbutazone, estrogen, phenothiazines, plasma expanders*

*These occur rarely.

ASSOCIATED SIGNS

The most common response to dyschezia is constipation, although many owners do not recognize this as a primary problem. Not uncommonly, the pain associated with rectal lesions is intense during attempts to defecate. The animal may cry or turn abruptly and lick the anus in response to the pain. Dogs may circle while assuming the position to defecate. Cats are more likely to make many attempts at defecation or may manifest inappropriate defecation in locations outside of the litter box. Unless attempting defecation, the animal is likely not to manifest pain at all.

Physical examination should include digital examination of the rectum and inspection of the perineum and each anal sac for evidence of lesions. It is important to consider shaving the perineum to assess the integrity of the skin for evidence of lesions, particularly neoplasia.

DIFFERENTIAL DIAGNOSIS (Box 3-22)

DIAGNOSTIC PLANS

1. History and physical examination, to determine the ability of the patient to urinate versus defecate. Physical examination must include the following:
   a. Rectal temperature, as a means of detecting source of pain.
   b. Rectal examination, expressing both anal glands and assessing the character of the discharge (sedation may be required).
   c. Evaluation of the perianal skin (shaving the perineum is recommended).
2. Fecal examination for occult blood.
3. Abdominal radiographs or abdominal ultrasound to assess prostate size (in male dogs), presence of intra-abdominal masses, or presence of fecalith formation.
4. Colonoscopy or proctoscopy, with rigid or flexible endoscope and biopsy of any obvious lesions. Recovered tissues should be examined cytologically and by histopathology. Anesthesia is rarely required for this procedure unless the integrity of the rectal mucosa is substantially compromised or pain is significant.
5. Rarely, exploratory laparotomy, to further elucidate the nature of abnormal intra-abdominal findings.

BOX 3-22   DIFFERENTIAL DIAGNOSIS OF DYSCHEZIA

CONSTIPATION (SEE BOX 3-5)
Idiopathic Ulcerative and Inflammatory Lesions
Colon (colitis)
Rectum (proctitis)
Anal sacs (determined at surgery)

NEOPLASIA
Mucosa (e.g., carcinoma)
Intestinal wall (e.g., carcinoma, sarcoma)
Extramural (intra-abdominal prostate)

Anal glands
Perineum (particularly skin/mucocutaneous tissues)

DIRECT RECTAL INJURY
With stricture formation
Without stricture formation (e.g., linear foreign body)

PERINEAL HERNIA

STRAINING TO URINATE: DYSURIA

DEFINITION

Dysuria: Painful or difficult urination. A relatively common presenting sign in both dogs and cats, dysuria should be regarded as an urgent situation worthy of immediate attention. Owner observations are not entirely reliable in describing dysuria. Therefore, physical examination is usually necessary to differentiate attempts to defecate from attempts to urinate and to distinguish between incontinence and dysuria.

Dysuria generally results from disorders of the lower urinary tract (bladder or urethra), genital tract (prostate or vagina), or both that induce an impediment to urinary outflow resulting in abnormal micturition or inappropriate urination. However, a variety of neurologic lesions, particularly lesions in the caudal lumbar spine and sacrum affecting either parasympathetic or sympathetic innervation to the lower urinary tract, can result in dysuria. Neurologic dysurias are among the most difficult to characterize and to treat.

ASSOCIATED SIGNS

Clinical signs associated with dysuria can often be localized to the point of the primary lesion in the lower genitourinary tract. Dysuria is commonly associated with discolored urine (particularly hematuria), pyuria, or both, subsequent to mucosal inflammation and infection. Certain causes of urinary incontinence may also result in dysuria. The owner may also report frequent attempts at urination by the animal.

Distinguish between two additional clinical signs associated with dysuria: *polyuria* (increased volume) versus *pollakiuria* (increased frequency). Patients with dysuria may also manifest *strangury*, defined as a slow, painful discharge of urine caused by spasm of the bladder and urethra. In male dogs, dysuria caused by an enlarged prostate may also be associated with constipation.

DIFFERENTIAL DIAGNOSIS (Box 3-23)

DIAGNOSTIC PLANS

1. Preliminary measures. The initial diagnostic plan depends on confirmation of dysuria at presentation and whether, on abdominal palpation, the urinary bladder is empty or distended (Figure 3-5).
2. Routine hematology and biochemical profile.
3. Urinalysis, with specific attention to color, specific gravity, protein, glucose, occult blood, and microscopic evaluation of urine sediment.
4. Radiography of the abdomen, including the lower urinary tract. Follow nondiagnostic studies with contrast radiography of the lower urinary tract (contrast urethrography, contrast cystography, and double-contrast cystography).

3

BOX 3-23 DIFFERENTIAL DIAGNOSIS OF DYSURIA

INFECTIOUS AND INFLAMMATORY CAUSES
Bacterial cystitis
Urethritis
Prostatitis/benign prostatic hyperplasia (male dog)
Vaginitis
Feline urologic syndrome

CYSTIC AND URETHRAL CALCULI

NEOPLASIA
Urinary bladder
  Transitional cell carcinoma
  Rhabdomyoma or fibrosarcoma
Prostatic carcinoma

CONGENITAL
Ectopic ureters (esp. female)
Various vaginal malformations

Urethra
  Transitional cell carcinoma
  Transmissible venereal tumor
Vagina and penis
  Transmissible venereal tumor
  Fibroma
  Sarcoma
  Carcinoma

TRAUMA
Ruptured bladder
Urethral laceration (bite wound, calculus)
Urethral stricture

NEUROLOGIC CAUSES
Reflex dyssynergia
Vesicular-urethral asynchronization

SWELLING OF THE LIMBS: PERIPHERAL EDEMA

DEFINITION

Peripheral edema: A pathologic increase in the fluid volume of the interstitium of soft tissue typically affecting the head and neck, forelimbs, or hind limbs. The distribution pattern of peripheral edema can be characterized as generalized, regional, or focal. Peripheral edema

3

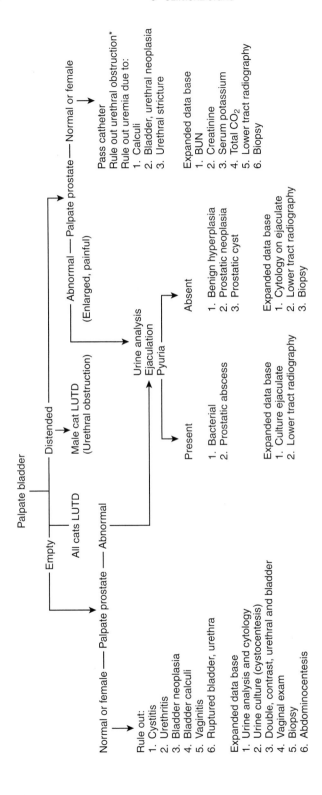

Figure 3-5: Algorithm for the differential diagnosis of dysuria. LUTD: lower urinary tract disease.

*If no obstruction exists, pursue bladder detrusor or neurologic dysfunction.

may or may not be associated with other forms of edema, such as cerebral edema or pulmonary edema.

The distinction between normal and abnormal increases in interstitial fluid volumes is difficult to establish clinically. Moderate to severe increases (30%) in interstitial fluid volume are evident on visual examination of the patient as a result of the physical changes in the tissue caused by the fluid. Any increase in the interstitial fluid volume identified by any means (e.g., histopathology, physical examination) constitutes peripheral edema.

Albumin is the smallest plasma protein and is the primary source of plasma colloidal oncotic pressure. Edema may become clinically evident as the serum albumin concentration falls below 2 g/dL. However, other factors are also involved in the formation of edema, such as decreased plasma volume and increased extracellular space associated with decreased renal excretion of sodium.

ASSOCIATED SIGNS

Patients that are presented with peripheral edema may manifest other signs. Evidence of chronic inflammatory disease, vasculitis, ecchymoses, cardiac disease, allergy, or trauma (including burns) should be considered. Patients with peripheral edema may also have primary protein-losing (renal or GI) disorders. These patients may be presented with increased water consumption or urination or diarrhea and weight loss. Severe hepatic disease may result in diminished synthesis of albumin, thereby contributing to the formation of edema.

DIFFERENTIAL DIAGNOSIS (Box 3-24)

DIAGNOSTIC PLANS

1. History and physical examination, to focus on cardiac, hepatic, GI, and urinary system disease. Particular attention is given to the presence of jugular vein distention or pulsations, tachycardia, and ascites.
2. Clinical pathology.
    a. Routine hematology.
    b. Biochemical profile, including electrolytes, total protein, and albumin.
    c. Urinalysis.
    d. Urine protein-creatinine ratio.
3. Special laboratory testing, as indicated:
    a. Bile acids.
    b. Quantitative urinary clearance studies.
    c. Serology—viral or rickettsial infections.
    d. ANA titer, LE cell preparation, and rheumatoid factor assay.
4. Central venous pressure (CVP).
5. Radiography:
    a. Thorax. Look for evidence of pericardial effusion, pleural effusion, or cardiac disease.
    b. Abdomen. Look for liver or mass lesions in particular, and peritonitis.
    c. Abdominal ultrasound.
6. Contrast radiography. Angiograms or lymphangiograms are indicated to confirm an obstructive lesion or the presence of an arteriovenous fistula.
7. Serologic studies, particularly for ehrlichiosis and Rocky Mountain spotted fever.
8. Edema fluid analysis. Collect by direct insertion of a 22-gauge needle into edematous tissue. A sample is collected into plain and edetic acid (EDTA)-containing tubes. Fluid is analyzed for color, consistency, and turbidity as well as protein and cellularity.
9. Postcapillary venous pressure and oxygen saturation, to confirm proximal obstruction to venous drainage or an arteriovenous fistula. (Normal postcapillary venous pressure = 13 ± 4 mm Hg).
10. Cytology and histopathology. Studies are particularly useful in evaluating mass lesions associated with edematous tissue. Indirect fluorescent antibody (IFA) staining of affected tissue may facilitate detection of immune-mediated disorders.

BOX 3-24 DIFFERENTIAL DIAGNOSIS OF EDEMA

INCREASED CAPILLARY HYDROSTATIC PRESSURE
Functional or structural obstruction to blood flow
   Congestive heart failure
   Venous obstruction
   Compression of a vessel by a mass lesion
Arteriovenous fistula

DECREASED CAPILLARY ONCOTIC PRESSURE (HYPOALBUMINEMIA)
Protein-losing enteropathies
Protein-losing nephropathies
Decreased hepatic synthesis
Decreased dietary intake (protein malnutrition)
Chronic hemorrhage
Exudative lesion with large surface (e.g., burns, peritonitis)

PERMEABILITY
Chronic inflammatory disease
Vasculitis
Vascular trauma
Toxins
Infections
(esp. tick-borne disease, e.g., ehrlichiosis)
Neurogenic, physical, or other vasoactive stimuli

DECREASED LYMPHATIC DRAINAGE (LYMPHEDEMA)
Congenital (primary) lymphedema–an autosomal dominant trait primarily affecting the
   hindlimbs by 3–6 mo of age
Acquired (secondary) lymphedema (focal or regional)
Infectious, granulomatous, neoplastic, traumatic injury, or compression of lymphatics

INCREASED INTERSTITIAL GEL MATRIX
Myxedema (hypothyroidism)–rare

UNCONTROLLED URINATION: URINARY INCONTINENCE

DEFINITION

Urinary incontinence: The lack of normal ability to prevent discharge of urine from the bladder. Urinary incontinence is suspected when an animal that previously exhibited normal control of urination begins passing urine at times or in places that are inappropriate. Determining whether or not the presenting complaint of inappropriate urinary behavior is involuntary can be a formidable task in a dog or cat. Distinguishing between voluntary and involuntary urination is fundamental to the diagnostic plan.

   The normal micturition reflex is a result of the complex interaction of the autonomic and somatic nervous systems. Normal control of micturition can be divided into a series of nervous pathways:

1. Sensory neurons have stretch receptors in the bladder wall that relay information through ascending spinal cord tracts to the brain stem and somesthetic cortex of the frontoparietal lobes. This pathway is the basis for the perception of a full bladder.
2. Frontoparietal motor cortex projects to the brain stem reticular formation centers for micturition that are responsible for storage and evacuation of urine.
3. From these centers, reticulospinal tracts descend the spinal cord to influence gray matter centers responsible for the storage or evacuation of urine. For evacuation, the

visceral efferent neurons in the sacral segments that innervate the detrusor muscle via the pelvic nerves are facilitated. The somatic efferent neurons in the sacral segments that innervate the striate urethralis muscle via the pudendal nerve are inhibited. Facilitation of these pudendal somatic neurons prevents urination.

Urinary incontinence is the physical manifestation of any one of several disorders affecting voluntary urine retention in the bladder. Neurologic lesions involving either upper motor or lower motor neuron segments of the micturition reflex arc result in urinary incontinence. A paralytic bladder usually results in bladder overdistention and urine dribbling. Urine can be easily expressed by manual compression of the bladder in affected patients. A "cord bladder" is caused by a lesion between the brain and the spinal reflex center of micturition. There is usually temporary bladder paralysis followed by involuntary reflex micturition subsequent to manual compression.

Non-neurogenic urinary incontinence may be due to anatomic or functional disorders (e.g., ectopic ureters) affecting the storage phase of micturition. Hormone-responsive incontinence is also a common form of non-neurogenic urinary incontinence. In these patients, the detrusor reflex is normal and the animal exhibits normal urination behavior in addition to urine dribbling.

A number of disorders of micturition are associated with excessive outlet resistance (e.g., urethral calculi, neoplasia) during voiding. Bladder overdistention and urine dribbling are frequently accompanied by dysuria and hematuria.

ASSOCIATED SIGNS

Evidence of urine or blood-tinged urine on the hair coat around the genitalia or on the patient's sleeping surface is frequently the first sign of a micturition disorder that owners recognize. Patients with neurogenic urinary incompetence may show evidence of spinal cord disease with conscious proprioceptive deficits in the hindlimbs, foot drag, and abrasions on the dorsal aspect of the hindfeet. However, lesions involving the cerebral cortex and cerebellum may also be associated with incontinence, as can behavioral disorders.

Obvious straining to urinate, particularly if associated with an enlarged abdomen, may indicate obstructive disease. Affected patients may be uremic, manifesting characteristic signs of lethargy, anorexia, and vomiting.

DIFFERENTIAL DIAGNOSIS (Box 3-25)

DIAGNOSTIC PLANS

1. History and physical examination. The size of the urinary bladder must also be determined.
2. Neurologic examination. A thorough neurologic examination should be performed in an attempt to establish or rule out a neurogenic cause. Particular emphasis is given to the spinal cord and sacral nerve roots. The bulbourethral and perineal reflexes should be assessed.

BOX 3-25 DIFFERENTIAL DIAGNOSIS OF URINARY INCONTINENCE

NEUROGENIC
Cerebral lesions
Cerebellar lesions
Brain stem lesions
Spinal cord lesions
Spinal nerve root lesions

NON-NEUROGENIC WITHOUT DISTENDED BLADDER
Ectopic ureter(s)
Patent urachus
Hormone-responsive incontinence

Urethral incompetence
Neoplasia
Reduced bladder capacity
Cystitis

NON-NEUROGENIC WITH DISTENDED BLADDER
Urethral obstruction, calculi, or neoplasia
Detrusor-urethral dyssynergia
Overflow incontinence (associated with polyuric states)

3. Catheterization of urinary bladder, to determine residual urine (normal=0.2 to 0.4 mL/kg in the dog and cat). Urine collected is submitted for urinalysis and, as indicated, for culture and sensitivity.
4. Laboratory database, to evaluate patient health status.
5. Survey radiographs of the caudal abdomen and spinal cord.
6. Contrast studies, as needed, including, pneumocystogram (only in the absence of hematuria), contrast urethrogram, and excretory urogram (also called intravenous pyelogram).
7. Cystometrogram. Special equipment is required.

VISION LOSS: TOTAL BLINDNESS

DEFINITION

Blindness: The inability to perceive visual stimuli. Because loss of visual function in animals is typically characterized by a change in behavior, the ability of pet owners to detect vision loss depends on their perception of changes in the animal's awareness of and interaction with its surroundings. Vision loss is likely to be apparent to owners only when there is complete loss of vision. An owner is unlikely to detect visual deficits, such as partial vision loss or unilateral blindness, because of the animal's ability to compensate.

Blindness can occur in any of four ways: lesions causing opacification of clear ocular media (e.g., cornea, aqueous humor, or lens); failure of the retina to process visual images; failure of neurologic transmission; and failure in the final image processing (i.e., cortical blindness).

DIFFERENTIAL DIAGNOSIS

When an animal is presented with acute visual loss, the owner is usually describing a bilateral ocular disease problem or the possibility of a CNS problem. Acute unilateral visual loss problems are not often recognized except by the very astute animal owner or observer. For the veterinarian, initial assessment of the animal with acute visual loss depends initially on confirming that the ocular media are clear and allow light to pass from the anterior ocular segment and reach the photoreceptor cells (rods and cones) in the posterior ocular segment. Transillumination should be used to evaluate the ocular media. Such conditions as acute bilateral uveitis, severe corneal edema, bilateral acute keratitis, rapidly developing metabolic cataracts, or acute cyclitis with vitreous involvement may alter the ocular media to interfere with light transmission. Both direct and indirect pupillary responses should be evaluated while evaluating the anterior ocular media. Once it has been determined that light can reach the posterior ocular segment, a fundus evaluation should be done. *Fundic abnormalities associated with acute visual loss* may include acute chorioretinitis, often with exudative retinal detachments; acute choroidal hemorrhages, often associated with abnormal blood pressure in chronic renal disease; and acute optic neuritis.

Acute visual loss in the dog *without accompanying fundic lesions* that can be seen on ophthalmoscopic examination may be associated with a retrobulbar optic neuritis or with the syndrome of sudden acquired retinal degeneration in the dog (SARDS). SARDS is poorly understood. The syndrome appears to involve middle-aged to old female dogs and there is a breed predilection for the dachshund. The visual loss may first start as a nyctalopia and progress over a period of weeks to complete visual loss. In some cases the visual loss is generalized and acute. Associated systemic signs of polydipsia, polyuria, polyphagia, obesity, and hepatomegaly may be present. Laboratory profiles may show abnormal differentials in the WBC count, elevated liver enzymes, an abnormal response to ACTH stimulation testing, or an abnormal response to low-dose dexamethasone suppression testing. The fundus may appear absolutely normal or early signs of retinal thinning and atrophy may be evident. Differential diagnosis with an optic neuritis is based on electroretinography (ERG) testing in which the ERG response is flat in SARDS but the ERG response is normal in optic neuritis. The cause of SARDS is unknown.

Acute visual loss associated with tumors of the CNS, particularly CNS tumors that involve the optic chiasm, are infrequently reported in the dog. Pituitary tumors are most likely to be the source. Pituitary tumors must become macroadenomas before invading and involving midbrain structures and the optic chiasm region. It is not uncommon for macroadenomas to be nonfunctional; thus, the affected animal may not develop any clinical metabolic abnormalities. Papilledema is rarely observed with brain tumors in dogs. Although pituitary macroadenomas that produce chiasmal compression and visual loss are rare in dogs, the differential diagnosis must still be considered.

The availability of CT has provided the ability to diagnose tumors of the hypophysis that may be associated with acute visual loss. Additionally, the use of the same technique has made visualization of the adrenal glands and the ability to diagnose bilateral adrenal gland hyperplasia easier. Pituitary macroadenomas are larger than 1 cm in diameter.

Optic neuritis may present as an acute visual loss problem. There may or may not be observable ophthalmoscopic changes of the optic nerve. Ophthalmoscopic abnormalities are characterized by edema of the disk, hemorrhages in and around the disk, edema, and inflammation of the surrounding retinal tissue. Acute optic neuritis often persists as a retrobulbar lesion without any ophthalmoscopically observable lesions. Pupils are widely dilated and nonresponsive or poorly responsive to light. In suspected acute optic neuritis, a complete physical examination, including a neurologic evaluation, peripheral blood count, and CSF analysis, should be performed, if possible. The presence of pleiocytosis and increased protein content in the CSF is of significance. It may be difficult to specifically diagnose the cause of acute optic neuritis.

DIAGNOSTIC PLANS (Box 3-26)

1. Evaluate pupillary light responses and vision by evaluating the animal's vision in an obstacle course and in altered light conditions.

BOX 3-26 DIFFERENTIAL DIAGNOSIS FOR THE PATIENT PRESENTED FOR SUDDEN ACQUIRED BLINDNESS

OCULAR CAUSES

Cornea
Edema (keratitis, herpesvirus-1 recrudescence [cats], corneal dystrophy)
Infection (bacterial, viral, fungal)
Fibrosis
Neovascularization (keratoconjunctivitis sicca-advanced)
Corneal dystrophy (lipid or congenital)

Anterior Chamber
Anterior uveitis-multiple causes
Hyphema

Lens
Cataract
Subluxation

Vitreal Humor
Hemorrhage
Hyalitis (inflmmation associated with infection [FIP], spontaneous bleeding, trauma)

Retinal Injury
Glaucoma
SARD (sudden acquired retinal degeneration syndrome)

Retinal atrophy-progressive or central progressive
Feline central retinal degeneration
Drug–induced (fluoroquinolone administration in cats)

EXTRAOCULAR CAUSES
Viral infections (canine distemper, FIP)
Fungal infections (deep mycoses)
Intracranial tumor
Brain trauma
Hydrocephalus
Immune-mediated optic neuritis
Sustained hypoxia
Seizure disorder (postictal, transient blindness)
Heat stroke
Granulomatous meningoencephalitis (GME)

RETINAL DETACHMENT
Hypertension, especially in cats with renal failure
Neoplasia
Retinal dysplasia
Congenital detachment (collie eye anomaly)
Infection (FIP)

2. Perform an ophthalmic examination to evaluate the clarity of the ocular media and the ability of light to reach the photoreceptor cells. Evaluate the posterior ocular segment by performing an ophthalmoscopic examination.
3. Evaluate the general physical condition of the animal including a basic neurologic examination:
   a. If acute retinal or vitreal hemorrhage is present, determine if the bleeding involves only the eyes or if there is evidence of bleeding elsewhere in the body. Determine if blood pressure is normal and if there is evidence of chronic renal disease, hyperadrenocorticism, or hyperthyroidism.
   b. If active chorioretinitis with or without exudative retinal detachment is present, determine if the inflammation appears granulomatous; if it does, consider systemic fungal infections and consider performing a vitreal or subretinal aspiration and cytologic examination to look for fungal agents. If inflammation is not granulomatous, perform a complete physical examination, CBC, and chemistry panel, and look for evidence of other systemic inflammatory diseases.
   c. If acute visual loss is *unaccompanied* by any fundus abnormalities, perform a complete physical examination, including a basic neurologic evaluation; if acute retrobulbar optic neuritis is suspected, a CBC and CSF examination should be considered; an ERG may be indicated to distinguish between SARDS and acute optic neuritis.

3

VOMITING (SEE ALSO REGURGITATION)

DEFINITION

Vomiting: Forceful ejection of food or fluid through the mouth from the stomach and, occasionally, the proximal duodenum. The term applies to those animals with overt evidence of effort associated with the expulsion of food and is characterized by vigorous abdominal pressing, arched back, gagging or retching, and hypersalivation. *Projectile vomiting* is the term used to describe the violent ejection of stomach contents without nausea or retching. *Regurgitation*, on the other hand, denotes expulsion of food or fluid from the esophagus and is a considerably more passive act than in vomiting.

Note: Cough-induced gagging associated with tracheitis or tracheobronchitis is often accompanied by the expulsion of mucus from the respiratory tract and can be a forceful act. As such, productive coughs may appear to the owner to be vomiting.

Vomiting is a complex reflex that entails coordination of the GI tract, musculoskeletal system, and nervous system. Although the CNS vomiting center initiates vomiting, it must first be stimulated. Even when vomiting is drug induced, stimulation of the vomiting center is accomplished subsequent to stimulation of a medullary chemoreceptor trigger zone that forwards impulses to the vomiting center. Many sensory nerves can mediate emetic impulses. Therefore, intense pain (especially abdominal); nervous (psychogenic) stimuli; disagreeable odors, tastes, and smells; sensations from the labyrinth and pharyngeal areas; various toxins and drugs; and, presumably, the retention of metabolic waste products all may lead to vomiting. Numerous receptors for vomiting are located in the abdominal viscera, especially the duodenum. Afferent nerve fibers are found in the vagal and sympathetic nerves.

Vomiting can be quite debilitating. When excessive, it causes severe extracellular fluid deficits, particularly of sodium, potassium, and chloride ions and water. Loss of mainly gastric contents results in loss of hydrogen ions, a high serum bicarbonate concentration, and metabolic alkalosis. Vomited material from the proximal intestinal tract contains high concentrations of bicarbonate.

Clinically, vomiting should be addressed as a problem that originates from the GI tract (primary causes) or from causes outside the GI tract (i.e., metabolic causes [secondary]).

ASSOCIATED SIGNS

Depending on the underlying cause, vomiting may be associated with a number of significant clinical signs. Primary causes of vomiting are generally associated with other GI signs, such as diarrhea, abdominal pain, obvious foreign bodies (e.g., a linear foreign body entrapped proximally under the tongue), ingestion of known irritant materials or drugs, hematochezia, or palpable abdominal tumors. Animals with metabolic or secondary causes of vomiting may appear lethargic, anorectic, and weak, particularly when the vomiting episodes have been sustained for several days. In some animals, polyuria or polydipsia, anuria, icterus, cough, and anemia are present.

DIFFERENTIAL DIAGNOSIS (Box 3-27)

DIAGNOSTIC PLANS

1. Verification that the patient is vomiting, not gagging or retching subsequent to tracheal disease. Determine duration, precipitating causes, and current drug therapy. Assess associated signs.
2. Laboratory database, fundamental to the diagnostic plan. It must include CBC, biochemistry profile, urinalysis, and fecal flotation. Cats should also be tested for heartworm disease, FeLV, FIV, and hyperthyroidism. Perform serologic studies, as needed, to rule out systemic infections (e.g., systemic mycoses).
3. Radiographs of the thorax and abdomen; abdominal ultrasound.
4. Contrast radiographic studies of the stomach and small bowel (e.g., barium series).
5. Exploratory laparotomy, depending on patient condition.

BOX 3-27 DIFFERENTIAL DIAGNOSIS OF VOMITING

INFECTIOUS CAUSES
Feline panleukopenia virus infection
Canine parvovirus infection
Canine coronavirus infection
Infectious canine hepatitis
Leptospirosis
Bacterial enteritis
Parasitic enteritis
Heartworm disease (cats)

INFLAMMATORY
Pyometra
Prostatitis
Peritonitis
Acute pancreatitis
Gastritis and enteritis
Gastric ulcers

OBSTRUCTIVE CAUSES
Intestinal foreign body
Gastrointestinal neoplasia
Gastric dilation–volvulus syndrome
Pyloric stenosis
Trichobezoar (hairballs)
Diaphragmatic hernia

METABOLIC CAUSES
Renal failure (uremia)
Hepatic disease
Diabetic ketoacidosis
Hypoadrenocorticism (Addison's disease)
Hypokalemia, regardless of cause
Hyperthyroidism (cats)

CHEMICAL CAUSES
Heavy metals, pesticides, solvents
Digitalis, salicylates, mebendazole, penicillamine, chloramphenicol, morphine, antineoplastic drugs, others

IDIOPATHIC/MISCELLANEOUS CAUSES
Psychogenic, vestibular (car sickness)
Overconsumption of food, especially in puppies
Various CNS diseases
Bilious vomiting syndrome
Autonomic epilepsy
Constipation/obstipation
Ileus, paralytic

6. Special diagnostic procedures: endoscopy, GI biopsy, double-contrast studies of the stomach and small bowel, and gastric motility studies (fluoroscopy).

VOMITING BLOOD: HEMATEMESIS (SEE ALSO VOMITING)

DEFINITION

Hematemesis: The vomiting of blood. An uncommon presentation in the dog and particularly rare in the cat. Although the presence of blood in the vomitus is, by strict definition, hematemesis, repeated episodes of vomiting in which the vomitus is composed of large blood clots, frank, uncoagulated blood, or the so-called coffee-ground appearance of blood denatured by gastric acid represents a serious clinical finding.

ASSOCIATED SIGNS

Hematemesis does not localize the diagnosis to the stomach or GI tract. Since a variety of metabolic and coagulation disorders may result in severe hematemesis, a wide spectrum of physical signs may also be present in affected animals. In addition, blood emanating from the upper respiratory tract may be swallowed and, subsequently, vomited, giving the appearance that bleeding is from the stomach.

Anorexia and vomiting are the most common associated, but nonspecific, signs. Weight loss, weakness, dark stool (melena), dehydration, and inactivity are other related signs having low diagnostic yield. Severe anemia can result from sustained gastric hemorrhage and, if acute, may justify exploratory laparotomy to identify the source of the bleeding.

Increased water consumption and urination may suggest underlying renal or hepatic disease. Intracutaneous or subcutaneous tumors, specifically mast cell tumors, can be associated with severe gastric ulceration and bleeding. Ulcerative lesions in the mouth may indicate recent ingestion of caustic or toxic compounds. The frenulum in the mouth should always be examined to rule out linear foreign bodies.

DIFFERENTIAL DIAGNOSIS (Table 3-7)

DIAGNOSTIC PLANS

1. Comprehensive history. This is critical and should focus on the following:
   a. Recent medications administered, both prescription and nonprescription.
   b. Known and potential exposure to toxic or poisonous substances.

T A B L E 3 - 7   **Differential Diagnosis of Hematemesis**

Primary gastric disorders	Systemic metabolic disorders
Gastritis	Acute pancreatitis
Infectious (e.g., parvovirus)	Adrenocortical insufficiency
Toxic	(Addison's disease)
Bile reflux-bilious vomiting syndrome	Toxins (e.g., lead, ethylene glycol)
Foreign body	Hepatic failure
Gastric ulcers	Renal failure
Drug-induced (e.g., aspirin)	Neoplasia
Idiopathic	
Metabolic (e.g., renal failure)	
Neoplastic	

c. Duration of the primary and associated signs.
d. Physical appearance of the vomitus.
e. Physical status of other pets in the family, if applicable.
2. Laboratory profile, including, as a minimum, hematologic values, particularly in anemic patients; biochemistry findings; urinalysis; and fecal flotation. Emphasis should be placed on renal, adrenal, and hepatic function.
3. Testing of feces for the presence of parvovirus antigen.
4. Activated coagulation time (ACT). A coagulation panel—including partial thromboplastin time (PTT), prothrombin time (PT), fibrin degradation products (FDPs), fibrinogen, and total platelet count—is indicated as appropriate.
5. Fine-needle aspiration of any intracutaneous or subcutaneous tumors.
6. Abdominal and thoracic radiographs; abdominal ultrasound.
7. Gastroscopy and esophagoscopy.
8. Exploratory laparotomy and gastrotomy.
NOTE: In patients with severe hematemesis, surgery may be indicated before obtaining results from the laboratory profile.

WEIGHT LOSS: EMACIATION/CACHEXIA

DEFINITION

Emaciation: A serious, usually chronic and progressive condition characterized by significant (>20%) body weight loss. *Cachexia* is the termed used to describe the end stage of *emaciation*. Significant weight loss, associated with emaciation or cachexia, typically results from catabolism of body fat and protein in excess of caloric intake. Increased metabolism (hypermetabolic), inadequate consumption or assimilation of nutrient, or excessive nutrient loss contributes to significant weight loss.

ASSOCIATED SIGNS

The clinical history should center on diet, appetite, and known health status (i.e., evidence of vomiting, diarrhea, etc). The duration of time over which the owner perceives weight loss occurring is important. Emaciation developing within a month (e.g., neoplasia) may carry a poorer prognosis than animals with emaciation developing over several months. The physical examination should focus on the presence of fever, gastrointestinal disease, and overt changes in size and consistency of internal organs.

DIFFERENTIAL DIAGNOSIS

A spectrum of differential diagnoses must be considered in the patient that presents with emaciation or cachexia. Several categories of illness should be considered evaluating patients with emaciation/cachexia associated with the following:
Malnutrition. Quality and quantity of food, availability of food, evidence of neglect/abuse.
Polyphagia. Malassimilation (i.e., either maldigestion or malabsorption), hypermetabolic states (e.g., hyperthyroidism, pregnancy), excessive nutrient losses (e.g., diabetes mellitus, glomerulonephropathy).
Anorexia. Infectious diseases, neoplasia, neurologic disease, toxicity (e.g., chronic lead poisoning), dental disease (pseudoanorexia).
Gastrointestinal signs. Malassimilation (i.e., either maldigestion or malabsorption); parasitism.
Urinary tract signs. Excess renal loss of fluid and nutrients (polyuric states).
Fever. Infectious diseases.

DIAGNOSTIC PLANS (Figure 3-6)

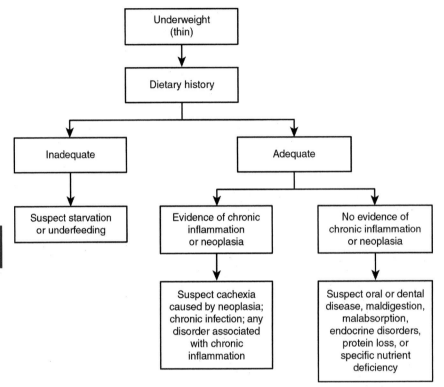

Figure 3-6: Differential diagnosis of weight loss/cachexia.
(From Greco DS: Cachexia. In Ettinger SJ, Feldman EC, editors: *Textbook of veterinary internal medicine,* ed 5, Philadelphia, 2000, WB Saunders, pp. 72-74.)

YELLOW SKIN OR MUCOUS MEMBRANES: ICTERUS (OR JAUNDICE)

DEFINITION

Icterus, or *jaundice*: Yellow discoloration of tissue (especially skin, mucous membranes, and sclera) caused by an increased serum concentration of bilirubin. Is indicative of underlying hepatocellular disease or intravascular hemolytic disease. Hyperbilirubinemia is required for icterus to develop but may not occur concurrently with icterus.

In practice, icterus is an uncommon presenting complaint, since the dense hair coat of cats and dogs precludes early detection of bile pigment in skin. Icteric tissues are most evident in the sclera and in the oral, vaginal, and preputial mucous membranes, particularly in anemic patients. Icterus can occur subsequent to the accumulation of either unconjugated (lipid-soluble) or conjugated (water-soluble) bilirubin in the blood.

Icterus can originate at any of three levels: prehepatic (hemolytic disease), hepatic (hepatocellular disease), posthepatic (obstructive or reduced bile flow).

Unconjugated hyperbilirubinemia results from rapid hemolysis (a common cause in the dog and cat), ineffective erythropoiesis, impaired hepatic uptake of conjugated bilirubin, or impaired conjugation. Conjugated (water-soluble) hyperbilirubinemia is generally the result of disorders intrinsic to the liver that affect bilirubin transport. Cholestatic disease is associated with reduced bile flow and can be characterized by significant bile acidemia and icterus.

ASSOCIATED SIGNS

Icterus can be detected in a dog or cat without overt clinical signs; however, RBC values and hepatic function should be assessed. Prehepatic icterus is characteristically associated with rapid-onset anemia and with generalized weakness, lassitude or acute collapse (caval syndrome), and bright orange urine. Pallor can be difficult to assess in patients with marked icterus. Hepatic icterus and posthepatic icterus are generally associated with lethargy and decreased appetite and are therefore difficult to distinguish clinically. Depending on the type of hepatic injury or the level of obstruction, episodic vomiting or diarrhea, weight loss, abdominal distention, polyuria or polydipsia, peripheral edema associated with hypoproteinemia, and prolonged bleeding (uncommon) may be reported.

DIFFERENTIAL DIAGNOSIS (Box 3-28)

DIAGNOSTIC PLANS

1. Thorough history. This should focus on current and previous drug therapy, including heartworm preventative, as well as duration of illness and associated signs. Physical examination confirms the presence of icterus but is unlikely to reveal the underlying cause. Abdominal palpation may reveal hepatomegaly, a discrete mass, or the presence of fluid.

In obviously anemic patients, when practical, transfusion should be avoided until laboratory test results have been interpreted.

2. Laboratory evaluation of the icteric patient. This is essential and should initially include a CBC, biochemistry panel (to include total and direct bilirubin), fecal analysis, urinalysis, heartworm test (in dogs), serum electrophoresis (in cats), and a test for FeLV antigen and FIV antibody.

BOX 3-28 DIFFERENTIAL DIAGNOSIS OF ICTERUS

PREHEPATIC (HEMOLYTIC)
Immune-mediated hemolytic anemia (Coombs'-positive anemia)
Heartworm disease, especially postcaval syndrome
Hemolytic septicemia
Transfusion-induced hemolysis

HEPATIC (HEPATOCELLULAR)
Cholangitis/cholangiohepatitis
Chronic active liver disease
Copper storage disease (Bedlington terriers and Doberman pinschers)
Drug-induced/vaccine-induced
  Thiacetarsamide–sporadic occurrence
  Imidazole anthelmintics–sporadic occurrence
  Anticonvulsants, especially primidone
  Acetaminophen/methylene blue (in cats)

Hepatic fibrosis
Septicemia
  Gram-negative bacteremia
  Leptospirosis
Viral
  Canine viral hepatitis
  Feline leukemia
  Feline infectious hepatitis
Neoplasia, primary or metastatic

POSTHEPATIC (OBSTRUCTIVE)
Cholangitis/cholangiohepatitis
Hepatic fibrosis
Neoplasia
Acute pancreatitis
Extrahepatic neoplasm (by compression)
Bile duct trauma
Ruptured gallbladder (usually traumatic)
Cholelithiasis

3. Anemic patient. Coombs' test; ANA titer; peripheral blood smear for the presence of parasites; blood cultures, particularly if the patient is febrile; and IFA test on bone marrow for FeLV antigen (in cats).
4. Nonanemic patient. Abdominal radiographs, abdominocentesis with fluid analysis and cytologic study, fine-needle aspiration of liver, plasma ammonia, bile acids, serum amylase, and lipase if not included in the biochemistry panel.
5. Special diagnostic tests. Coagulation profile, followed by liver biopsy (percutaneous or at laparotomy) or exploratory celiotomy with biopsy.
6. Abdominal ultrasound, CT, and perfusion scintigraphy (special facilities required).

Additional Reading

Ettinger SJ, Feldman EC (editors): *Textbook of veterinary internal medicine,* ed 6, vol 1, Section 1: Clinical manifestations of disease. St. Louis, 2005, Elsevier Saunders, pp. 1-240.

Grauer GF: Clinical manifestations of urinary disorders. In Nelson RW, Couto CG, editors: *Small animal internal medicine,* ed 3, St. Louis, 2003, Mosby, pp. 568-583.

Guilford WG, Center SA, Strombeck DR, et al: *Strombeck's small animal gastroenterology,* ed 2, Philadelphia, 1996, WB Saunders.

Hawkins EC: Respiratory system disorders. In Nelson RW, Couto CG, editors: *Small animal internal medicine,* ed 3, St. Louis, 2003, Mosby, pp. 210-343.

Tams TR: Gastrointestinal symptoms. In TR Tams, editor: *Handbook of small animal gastroenterology,* ed 2, St. Louis, 2003, Saunders, pp. 1-50.

Ware WA: The cardiovascular examination. In Nelson RW, Couto CG, editors: *Small animal internal medicine,* ed 3, St. Louis, 2003, Mosby, pp. 1-11.

3

Diagnostic and Therapeutic Procedures

Routine Procedures, *449*
    Administration Techniques for Medications and Fluids, *449*
    Bandaging Techniques, *462*
    Blood Pressure Measurement: Indirect, *462*
    Central Venous Pressure Measurement, *463*
    Diagnostic Sample Collection Techniques, *465*
    Dermatologic Procedures, *489*
    Ear Cleaning: External Ear Canal, *492*
    Endotracheal Intubation, *494*
    Intravenous Catheterization, *495*
    Physical Therapy, *497*
Advanced Procedures, *500*
    Abdominocentesis, *500*
    Biopsy Techniques: Advanced, *501*
    Blood Gas: Arterial, *508*
    Cerebrospinal Fluid Collection, *509*
    Electrocardiography, *511*
    Endoscopy: Indications and Equipment Requirements, *518*
    Fluid Therapy, *523*
    Gastrointestinal Procedures, *526*
    Laparoscopy, *532*
    Ophthalmic Procedures, *535*
    Radiography: Advanced Contrast Studies, *541*
    Reproductive Tract: Female, *549*
    Reproductive Tract: Male, *554*
    Respiratory Tract Procedures, *559*
    Urinary Tract Procedures, *571*

ROUTINE PROCEDURES

ADMINISTRATION TECHNIQUES FOR MEDICATIONS AND FLUIDS

ORAL ADMINISTRATION: TABLETS/CAPSULES—CANINE

Perhaps the simplest and easiest method of administering tablets or capsules to dogs is to hide the medication in food. Offer small portions of *unbaited* cheese, meat, or some favorite food to the dog initially. Then offer one portion that includes the medication.

449

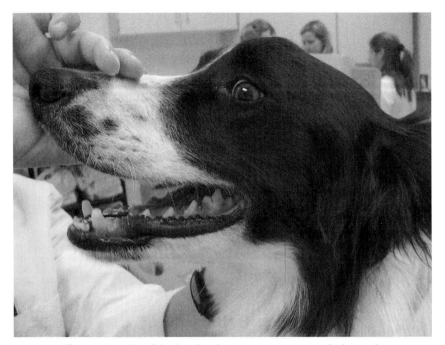

Figure 4-1: Use of the thumb only to open a cooperative dog's mouth.

For anorectic dogs or when pills must be given without food, give medications quickly and decisively so that the process of administering the medication is accomplished before the dog realizes what has happened. With cooperative dogs, insert the thumb of one hand through the interdental space, and gently touch the hard palate. This will cause the dog to open the mouth (Figure 4-1). Using the opposite hand (the one holding the medication), gently press down on the mandibular (lower) incisors to open the mouth further (Figure 4-2). Position the tablet or capsule onto the caudal aspect of the tongue as close to the larynx as possible. Quickly withdraw the hand and close the dog's mouth. When the dog licks its nose, the medication likely has been swallowed.

> **Note:** Oral medication frequently is dispensed to owners without regard for the client's knowledge of how to administer a pill/tablet or without asking whether the client is even physically able to administer medications.
>
> Clear instructions, including a demonstration, and having the client perform the technique in the hospital will improve compliance.

Dogs that offer more resistance can be induced to open their mouths by compressing their upper lips against their teeth. As they open their mouth, roll their lips medially so that if they attempt to close their mouth, they will pinch their own lips.

Dogs that struggle and slash with their teeth are the most difficult, especially if they show aggression toward the individual attempting to administer mediation. They often can be medicated by placing the tablet over the base of the tongue with a 6-inch curved Kelly hemostat or special pill forceps. Cubes of canned food or dried meat often can be "pushed down" a placid but anorectic patient by using the thumb as a lever. The fingers are kept out of the mouth, but the thumb is inserted behind the last molar of the open mouth and pushes the bolus down.

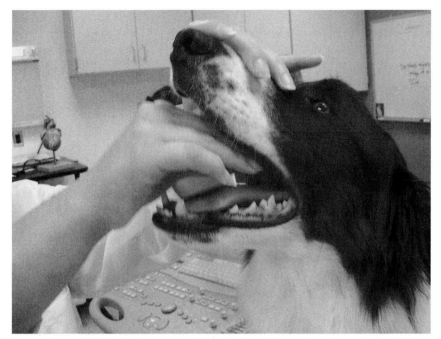

Figure 4-2:   Use of the opposite hand to place a tablet or capsule on the caudal aspect of the tongue.

ORAL ADMINISTRATION: TABLETS/CAPSULES-FELINE

Two methods of pill administration are used in cats. In both methods the cat's head is elevated slightly. Success in administering pills/tables to a cat entails a delicate balance between what works well and what works safely. In cooperative cats, it may be possible to use one hand to hold and position the head (Figure 4-3) while using the opposite hand (the one holding the medication) to open the mouth gently by depressing the proximal aspect of the mandible (Figure 4-4). Press the skin adjacent to the maxillary teeth gently between the teeth as the mouth opens, thereby discouraging the cat from closing its mouth. With the mouth open, drop the medication (try lubricating the tablet or capsule with butter) into the oral cavity as far caudally on the tongue as possible. The cat can be tapped under the jaw or on the tip of the nose to facilitate swallowing if you really think this works. If the cat licks, administration was probably successful.

CAUTION: Only experienced individuals should attempt this technique of administering tablets/capsules to cats. Even cooperative cats that become intolerant will bite. Therefore, this is NOT a technique recommended for inexperienced owners to try at home, even if specific instructions have been given.

Alternatively, some cats will tolerate a specially designed "pilling syringe" in an attempt to administer a tablet or capsule. The pilling syringe works well as long as it is inserted cautiously and atraumatically into the cat's mouth. However, if resistance ensues, the rigid pilling syringe may injure the hard palate during the ensuing struggle. Subsequent attempts to use the syringe may be met with increasing resistance and increasing risk of injury. Success with a pilling syringe depends largely on the cat.

When dispensing oral medications for home administration to cats, do *not* expect clients to force a tablet or capsule into a cat's mouth. Although some clients are remarkably capable and confident with their ability to administer oral medications to cats, the risk of injury to the client can be significant. Whenever feasible, liquid medications or pulverized

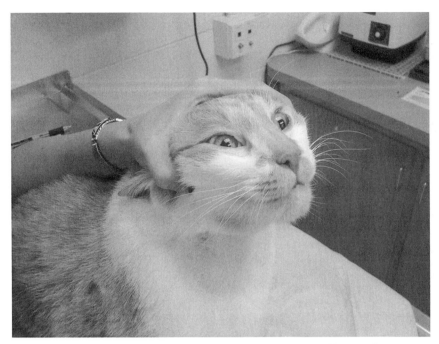

Figure 4-3:   Head restraint technique used while administering a tablet/capsule to a cat.

4

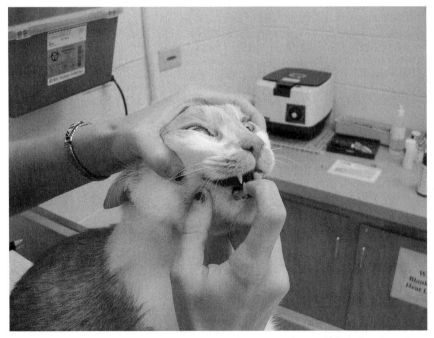

Figure 4-4:   Use of the opposite hand gently to depress a cat's mandible before dropping a tablet into the caudal aspect of the oral cavity.

tablets should be mixed with the diet or an oral treat readily accepted and consumed (see the following discussion).

Oral Administration: Liquids

Without a stomach tube

Small amounts of liquid medicine can be given successfully to dogs and cats by pulling the commissure of the lip out to form a pocket (Figure 4-5). Hold the patient's head level so that the medication will not ooze into the larynx. Deposit the liquid medication into the "cheek pouch" where it subsequently flows between the teeth as the head is held slightly upwards. Patience and gentleness, along with a reasonably flavored medication, are needed for success.

Spoons are ineffective because they measure fluids inaccurately and materials spill easily. A disposable syringe can be used to measure and administer liquids per os. Depending on the liquid administered, disposable syringes can be reused several times, assuming they are rinsed following each administration. In addition, disposable syringes can be dispensed legally to clients for home administration of liquid mediation. Mixing of medications in the same syringe is *not* recommended. However, dispensing of a separate, clearly marked syringe for each type of liquid medication prescribed for home administration is recommended.

With an administration tube

Administration of medications, contrast material, and rehydrating fluids can be accomplished with the use of a feeding tube passed through the nostrils into the stomach or distal esophagus. Today, the general recommendation is to *avoid* passing the tip of a feeding tube beyond the distal esophagus. This is particularly true when a feeding tube is placed for long-term and repeated use (described in Gastrointestinal Procedures in this section). The reason for recommending nasoesophageal intubation *over* nasogastric intubation is based on the additional risk of irritation and even ulceration of the esophageal mucosa at the

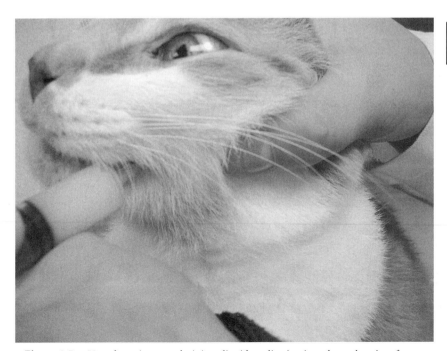

Figure 4-5: Use of a syringe to administer liquid medication into the oral cavity of a cat.

level of the cardia. Reflex peristalsis of the esophagus against a tube passing through the cardia has resulted in significant mucosal ulceration within 72 hours when feeding tubes were left in place. In patients receiving a single dose of medication or contrast material, nasogastric intubation is likely to be as safe as nasoesophageal intubation.

The narrow lumen of tubes passed through the nostril of small dogs and cats limits the viscosity of solutions that can be administered through a tube directly into the gastrointestinal tract. Nasoesophageal intubation can be done with a variety of tube types and sizes (Table 4-1). Newer polyurethane tubes, when coated with a lidocaine lubricating jelly, are nonirritating and may be left in place with the tip at the level of the distal esophagus. When placing the nasogastric tube, instill 4 to 5 drops of 0.5% proparacaine in the nostril of the cat or small dog; 0.5 to 1.0 mL of 2% lidocaine instilled into the nostril of a larger breed dog may be required to achieve the level of topical anesthesia needed to pass a tube through the nostril. With the head elevated, direct the tube dorsomedially toward the alar fold (Figure 4-6). After inserting the tip 1 to 2 cm into the nostril, continue to advance the tube until it reaches the desired length. If the turbinates obstruct the passage of the tube, withdraw the tube by a few centimeters. Then readvance the tube, taking care to direct the tube ventrally through the nasal cavity. Occasionally, it will be necessary to withdraw the tube completely from the nostril and repeat the procedure. In particularly small patients or

4

TABLE 4-1   The French Catheter Scale Equivalents*

| | Size | |
Scale	(mm)	(inches)
3	1	0.039
4	1.35	0.053
5	1.67	0.066
6	2	0.079
7	2.3	0.092
8	2.7	0.105
9	3	0.118
10	3.3	0.131
11	3.7	0.144
12	4	0.158
13	4.3	0.170
14	4.7	0.184
15	5	0.197
16	5.3	0.210
17	5.7	0.223
18	6	0.236
19	6.3	0.249
20	6.7	0.263
22	7.3	0.288
24	8	0.315
26	8.7	0.341
28	9.3	0.367
30	10	0.393
32	10.7	0.419
34	11.3	0.445

*Mutiple types of pediatric polyurethane nasogastric feeding tubes are available in sizes ranging from 8F to 12F that easily accommodate administration of liquids medications and fluids to kittens, cats, and small dogs.

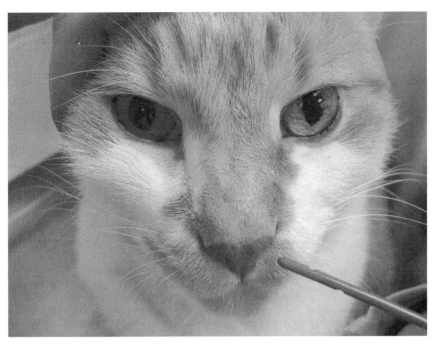

Figure 4-6:   Initial dorsomedial placement of a nasoesophageal tube before complete insertion.

patients with obstructive lesions (e.g., tumor) in the nasal cavity, it may not be possible to pass a tube. Do not force the tube against significant resistance through the nostril.

CAUTION: The tip of the tube possibly can be introduced inadvertently through the glottis and into the trachea. Topical anesthetic instilled into the nose can anesthetize the arytenoid cartilages, thereby blocking a cough or gag reflex. I prefer to check the tube placement with a dry, empty syringe. Attach the test syringe to the end of the feeding tube. Rather than inject air or water in an attempt to auscultate borborygmus over the abdomen, attempt simply to aspirate air from the feeding tube. IF THERE IS NO RESISTANCE DURING ASPIRATION AND AIR FILLS THE SYRINGE, THE TUBE LIKELY HAS BEEN PLACED IN THE TRACHEA. Completely remove the tube and repeat the procedure. However, if repeated attempts to aspirate are met with immediate resistance and NO AIR ENTERS THE SYRINGE, the tube tip is positioned properly within the esophagus. If there is any question regarding placement, a lateral survey radiograph is indicated.

Gavage, or gastric lavage/feeding, in puppies and kittens can be accomplished by passing a soft rubber catheter or feeding tube through the nose and into the stomach. A 12F catheter is of an adequate diameter to pass freely, but it is too large for dogs and cats less than 2 to 3 weeks of age. Mark the tube with tape or a pen at a point equal to the distance from the tip of the nose to the last rib. Merely push the tube into the pharynx and down the esophagus to the caudal thoracic level (into the stomach). Attach a syringe to the flared end, and slowly inject medication or food. Use the same dry syringe aspiration technique to ensure that the tube is positioned in the esophagus/stomach rather than the trachea before administration.

A less desirable but effective technique for one-time tube administration of medications, food, or fluids entails passing the administration tube directly through the oral cavity and into the esophagus or stomach. However, this technique requires the use of a speculum to ensure that the patient does not bite or sever the tube with its teeth. A variety of speculums are available, ranging from hard rubber bite-blocks with a centrally positioned hole

4

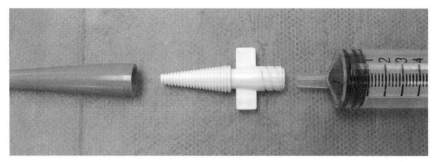

Figure 4-7:   Use of a plastic adaptor ("Christmas tree") to affix a syringe to a nasoesophageal feeding tube.

for passing the tube to improvised speculums such as a roll of 1- to 2-inch adhesive tape positioned between the mandible and maxilla. A well lubricated 22F rubber catheter, up to 30 inches long, is an ideal tube. Attach the catheter to a syringe that delivers the medication.

When the patient swallows, advance the catheter into the esophagus to the level of the eighth or ninth rib. Measure this distance on the tube first, and mark it with a ballpoint pen or a piece of tape. To pass the tube into the trachea in a conscious dog with its head held in a normal position is almost impossible. It may be possible to palpate the neck to feel the tube in the esophagus.

Nasoesophageal intubation in cats is generally much better tolerated that orogastric intubation. The cat can be restrained in a bag or cat stocks or by rolling it in a blanket. The cat is held in a vertical position by an assistant. Position a mouth speculum between the mandible and maxilla. This is where the fun begins. The operator then grasps the cat's head, as for pilling, and quickly passes the prelubricated tube 6 to 10 inches down the esophagus. A 12F to 16F soft rubber catheter, 16 inches long, makes a suitable tube.

Depending on the feeding tube type, the end of the tube may or may not accommodate a syringe. For example, soft, rubber urinary catheters are excellent tubes for single administration use. However, the flared end may not accommodate a syringe. To affix a syringe to the outside end of a tapered feeding tube or catheter, insert a plastic adapter (Figure 4-7) into the open end of the tube.

TOPICAL ADMINSTRATION

Ocular

There are numerous ways to apply medication to the eyes, including the use of drops, ointments, subconjunctival injections, and subpalpebral lavage. The route and frequency of medication depend on the disease being treated.

If more than 2 drops of aqueous material are administered, the fluid will wash out of the conjunctival cul-de-sac and be wasted. Most drops should be applied every 2 hours (or less) to maintain effect. Ointments should be applied sparingly, and their effect may last a maximum of 4 to 6 hours.

Place drops on the inner canthus *without touching the eye with the dropper tip.* Place ointment (1/8-inch-long strip) on the upper sclera or lower palpebral border so that as the lids close, they form a film across the cornea.

Otic

Medicated powders generally are contraindicated in the external ear canal. Thin films of ointments or propylene glycol solutions are more effective vehicles and are recommended. A few drops generally suffice, and the ear should be massaged gently after instillation to spread the medication over the external ear canal.

Nasal

Isotonic aqueous drops are used for nasal application and should be applied without touching the dropper to the nose. Oily drops are not advised because they may damage the nasal mucosa or may be inhaled. There is little indication for routine instillation of medication into the nostrils of dogs and cats.

Dermatologic

Several objectives should be considered when treating dermatologic disorders: (1) eradication of causative agents; (2) alleviation of symptoms, such as reduction of inflammation; (3) cleansing and debridement; (4) protection; (5) restoration of hydration; and (6) reduction of scaling and callus. Many different forms of skin medications are available, but the vehicle in which they are applied is a critical factor (Box 4-1). In all cases, apply topical medications to a clean skin surface in a very thin film, because only the medication in contact with the skin is effective. In most cases, clipping hair from an affected area enhances the effect of medication.

BOX 4-1 VEHICLES USED IN THE ADMINISTRATION OF TOPICAL SKIN MEDICATIONS

Lotions are suspensions of powder in water or alcohol. They are used for acute, eczematous lesions. Because they less easily are absorbed than creams and ointments, lotions need to be applied 2 to 6 times a day.

Pastes are mixtures of 20% to 50% powder in ointment. In general, they are thick, heavy, and difficult to use.

Creams are oil droplets dispersed in a continuous phase of water. Creams permit excellent percutaneous absorption of ingredients.

Ointments are water droplets dispersed in a continuous phase of oil. They are very good for dry, scaly eruptions.

Propylene glycol is a stable vehicle and spreads well. It allows good percutaneous absorption of added agents.

Adherent dressings are bases that dry quickly and stick to the lesion.

Shampoos are usually detergents designed to cleanse the skin. If shampoos are left in contact with the skin for a time, added medications may have specific antibacterial, antifungal, or antiparasitic effects.

4

Note on compounding pharmacies

With the widespread availability of compounding pharmacies, prescribing compounded medications for topical and oral administration recently has become a popular dispensing technique for dogs and cats requiring long-term, daily mediation. Caution is warranted. Some compounding pharmacies that serve the veterinary profession are using inappropriate or ineffective vehicles in which the drug has been compounded, or the drug itself, purchased in bulk, is a lower grade and possibly an ineffective product once compounded. Studies on the quality and efficacy of compounded drugs for use in veterinary patients are limited. However, of those studies that have been performed, serious questions are being raised over the bioavailability of the drug administered.

ADMINISTRATION BY INJECTION (PARENTERAL ADMINISTRATION)

Before aspirating medications from multiple-dose vials, carefully wipe the rubber diaphragm stopper with the same antiseptic used on the skin. Observe this basic rule with all medication vials, even with modified live virus vaccines.

It would be admirable to prepare the skin surgically before making needle punctures to administer medications. Because such preparation is not practical, carefully part the hair and apply a high-quality skin antiseptic such as benzalkonium chloride in 70% alcohol. Place the needle directly on the prepared area, and thrust the needle through the skin. Although the use of antiseptics on the vial and skin is not highly effective, the procedure removes gross contamination and projects an image of professionalism.

Subcutaneous Injection

Dogs and cats have abundant loose alveolar tissue and easily can accommodate large volumes of material in this subcutaneous space. The dorsal neck is seldom used for subcutaneous injections because the skin is somewhat more sensitive, causing some patients to move abruptly during administration. A wide surface area of skin and subcutaneous tissue over the dorsum from the shoulders to the lumbar region makes an ideal site for subcutaneous injections.

Administration of drugs, vaccines, and fluids by the subcutaneous route represents the most commonly used route of parenteral administration in dogs and cats. For small volumes (<2 mL total), such as vaccines, a 22- to 25-gauge needle generally is used. The site most often used is the wide area of skin over the shoulders. The large subcutaneous space and the relative lack of sensitivity of skin at this location make it an ideal injection site. Cleaning of the skin with alcohol or other disinfectant generally is performed before injection. Several injection techniques are used. A common technique entails grasping a fold of skin with two fingers and the thumb of one hand. Gently lift the skin upward. Using the opposite hand, place the needle, with syringe attached, through the skin at a point below the opposite thumb. *Aspiration before injection is not typically necessary when using this route of administration.* Following administration and on removal of the needle from the skin, gently pinch the injection site and hold it for a few seconds to prevent backflow of medication or vaccine onto the skin.

When larger volumes are to be administered—fluids in dehydrated dogs and cats—the skin directly over the shoulders is the injection site most commonly selected. Generally, only isotonic fluids are administered by the subcutaneous route. Depending on the patient's size, needles ranging from 16 to 22 gauge can be used. Because of the larger volumes of fluid involved, warming of the fluids before administration is recommended. Doing so can enhance significantly the patient's tolerance for the displacement of skin during the period of administration. Depending on the rate of administration and breed of dog, relatively large volumes of fluid generally can be given in one location. Cats typically tolerate 10 to 20 mL/kg body mass in a single location. Large dogs can tolerate volumes greater than 200 mL of fluid in a single location. When administering large volumes, it is usually *not* necessary to use *multiple* injection sites for purposes of distributing the total fluid volume. Doing so actually may increase the risk of introducing cutaneous bacteria under the skin. Because the administration time required to deliver larger volumes is longer, and the injection needle will be placed in the skin for extended periods, it is appropriate to cleanse and rinse the skin carefully before actually inserting the needle. Isotonic, warmed fluids may be administered by large syringe or through an administration tube attached to a bag. Monitor skin tension and the patient's comfort tolerance throughout the procedure.

Although fluid absorption begins almost immediately on subcutaneous administration of fluids, significant pressure caused by the bolus of fluid delivered can develop within the fluid pocket. On removal of the needle, firmly grasp the injection site with the thumb and forefinger for several seconds. The procedure is *not complete* until one has verified that back-leakage of fluid from the subcutaneous space onto the skin is not occurring.

Note: Not all parenteral medications can be administered safely by the subcutaneous route. When administering any compound by the subcutaneous route, verify that the product to be administered is approved for subcutaneous administration. Serious reactions, including abscess formation and tissue necrosis, can occur.

Depending on the patient's hydration status and physical condition, fluid absorption may take from 6 to 8 hours.

NOTE: The rate of absorption of fluid administered by the subcutaneous route largely depends on the patient's hydration state and vascular and cardiac integrity. For that reason, the subcutaneous route is not recommended to manage patients in hypovolemic shock. Exceptions to this do exist, for example, when in a life-or-death situation access to a vein is simply not possible. Subcutaneous or intraosseous (see the following discussion) fluid administration may be the only option available.

Implanted subcutaneous fluid ports

In clinical practice, it has become increasingly popular to dispense bags of sterile, isotonic fluids, with appropriate administration tubing and needles, to pet owners for home administration of subcutaneous fluids, such as for especially long-term management of chronic renal failure in cats. Although some owners are comfortable administering subcutaneous fluids through a needle, others are not. Recently, an implantable subcutaneous port* has been introduced for use in patients requiring regular administration of subcutaneous fluids at home. A 9-inch silicon tube is preplaced under the skin and is sutured in place by a veterinarian. Objectively, this offers easy access to the subcutaneous space without need for needle penetration. Owners simply attach a syringe or extension tube tip to the port and administer the appropriate volume of fluids at an appropriate rate and frequency. Because of the usual requirement for long-term placement of an implantable fluid administration tube, there is risk of infection under the skin and around the incision site. Some cats do not tolerate the device.

INTRAMUSCULAR INJECTION

Because the tightly packed muscular tissue cannot expand and accommodate large volumes of injectables without trauma, medications given by this route should be small in volume. These medications are often depot materials that are poorly soluble, and some may be mildly irritating. Never give intramuscular injections in the neck because of the fibrous sheaths there and the complications that may occur. I also believe that injections in the hamstring muscles may cause severe pain, lameness, and occasionally peroneal paralysis because of local nerve involvement. Unless the animal is extremely thin, give injections into the lumbodorsal muscles on either side of the dorsal processes of the vertebral column.

After proper preparation of the skin, insert the needle through the skin at a slight angle (if the animal is thin) or at the perpendicular (if the animal is obese). When injecting any medication by a route other than the intravenous one, it is *imperative* to retract the plunger of the syringe before injecting to be certain that a vein was not entered by mistake. This is especially crucial with oil suspension, microcrystalline suspension, or potent-dose medications.

INTRADERMAL INJECTION

Intracutaneous (or intradermal) injections are used for testing purposes. Prepare the skin by carefully clipping the hair with a No. 40 clipper blade. If the skin surface is dirty, gently clean it with a moist towel. Scrubbing and disinfection are contraindicated because they may produce iatrogenic trauma and inflammation, which interfere with the test. Stretch the skin by lifting a fold, and use a 25- to 27-gauge intradermal needle attached to a 1-mL tuberculin syringe. Insert the point of the needle, bevel up, in a forward lifting motion as if to pick up the skin with the needle tip. Advance the needle while pushing the syringe (levered) downward until the bevel is completely within the skin. Inject a bleb of 0.05 to 0.10 mL of fluid. If the procedure is done correctly, the small bleb will appear translucent. Intradermal injections generally are used in patients subjected to intradermal skin testing for allergenic antigens. Administration of compounds by the intradermal technique is not necessarily simple. Inadvertent administration of medications into the subcutaneous tissues is easy when attempting intradermal injection. For that reason, specific training/experience is recommended before attempting intradermal skin testing of allergic patients.

TRANSDERMAL (NEEDLE-FREE) ADMINISTRATION

Intradermal administration of vaccine and drugs in veterinary and human medicine largely has been limited to the complexities of accurately delivering the desired dose into,

4

---

*GIF-Tube Kit (Greta Implantable Fluid Tube); VSM, Phoenix, Arizona, *www.practivet.com.*

and not under, the skin. In 2004 a transdermal administration system[†] was introduced that was designed after a similar device used in human medicine. This system consistently delivers a precise volume of vaccine into the skin, subcutaneous tissues, and muscle of vaccinated cats. The advantage of delivering vaccine into the skin of animals is the enhanced processing of antigen by the abundant dendritic cells. In addition to using this delivery system for other vaccines, potential application exists for other medications, such as precise delivery of very small quantities of insulin to cats.

INTRAVENOUS INJECTION

Cephalic venipuncture

To restrain a dog or cat for venipuncture of the cephalic vein, place the dog or cat on the table in sternal recumbency. If the right vein is to be tapped or catheterized, the assistant should stand on the left side of the animal and place the left arm or hand under the animal's chin to immobilize the head and neck. The assistant should reach across the animal and grasp the leg just behind and distal to the right elbow joint. The assistant should use the thumb to occlude and rotate the cephalic vein laterally while the palm of the hand holds the elbow in an immobilized and extended position. Make sure that the animal stays on the table if struggling occurs. The person performing the venipuncture then grasps the leg at the metacarpal region and begins the venipuncture on the medial aspect of the leg, just adjacent to the cephalic vein proximal to the carpus.

Jugular venipuncture

For a jugular venipuncture in the dog, place the patient in sternal recumbancy, with the hands of the assistant placed around the patient's muzzle to extend the neck and nose dorsally toward the ceiling. In short-coated dogs, the jugular vein usually can be seen coursing from the ramus of the mandible to the thoracic inlet in the jugular furrow. The vessel may be more difficult to visualize in dogs with long-haired coats or if excessive subcutaneous fat or skin is present. The person performing the venipuncture should place the thumb of the nondominant hand across the jugular vein in the thoracic inlet or proximal to the thoracic inlet to occlude venous drainage from the vessel and allow it to fill. With the dominant hand, the person performing the venipuncture should insert the needle and syringe or Vacutainer (BD, Franklin Lakes, New Jersey) into the vessel at a 15- to 30-degree angle to perform the venipuncture.

For smaller and very large animals, the jugular vein also can be tapped by placing the patient in lateral recumbency. The assistant should pull the animal's front legs caudally and extend the head and neck so that the jugular vein can be visualized. The venipuncture then can be performed as previously described. A jugular venipuncture is contraindicated in patients with thrombocytopenia or vitamin K antagonist rodenticide intoxication.

Place cats in sternal recumbency. The assistant should stand behind the patient so that the patient cannot back away from the needle during the venipuncture. The assistant should extend the cat's head and neck dorsally while restraining the cat's front legs with the other hand. The cat's fur can be clipped or moistened with isopropyl alcohol to aid in visualization of the jugular vein as it stands up in the jugular furrow. The person performing the venipuncture should occlude the vessel at the thoracic inlet and insert the needle or Vacutainer apparatus into the vessel as previously described to withdraw the blood sample. Alternately, place the cat in lateral recumbency as described in the previous paragraph.

Lateral saphenous venipuncture

To perform a lateral saphenous venipuncture, place the patient in lateral recumbency. The lateral saphenous vein can be visualized on the lateral portion of the stifle, just proximal to the tarsus. The assistant should extend the hind limb and occlude the lateral saphenous

---

[†]Vet-Jet Transdermal Administration System for delivery of the recombinant feline leukemia vaccine; Merial Ltd., Duluth, Georgia.

vein just proximal and caudal to the tarsus. The person performing the venipuncture should grasp the distal portion of the patient's limb with the nondominant hand and insert the needle or Vacutainer apparatus with the dominant hand to withdraw the blood sample.

Medial saphenous venipuncture

To perform a medial saphenous venipuncture, place the patient in lateral recumbancy. Move the top hind limb cranially or caudally to allow visualization of the medial saphenous vein on the medial aspect of the tibia and fibula. The assistant should scruff the patient, if the patient is small, or should place the forearm over the patient's neck to prevent the patient from getting up during the procedure. With the other hand, the assistant should occlude the medial saphenous vein in the inguinal region. The person performing the medial saphenous venipuncture should grasp the paw or hock of the limb and pull the skin taught to prevent the vessel from rolling away from the needle. The fur may be clipped or moistened with isopropyl alcohol to aid in visualization of the vessel. The needle or Vacutainer apparatus can be inserted into the vessel at a 15- to 30-degree angle to withdraw the blood sample.

INTRAOSSEOUS ADMINISTRATION

Intraosseous infusion of blood, fluids, or medications is useful whenever rapid, direct access to the circulatory system is required and peripheral or central access is impossible or too time-consuming. This technique can be set up rapidly (3 minutes), is certain, and is especially useful for unusually small patients, especially kittens and puppies. (NOTE: This procedure also is described in Section 1.)

Intraosseous infusion is particularly indicated in shock or circulatory collapse syndromes, edematous states, severe burns, and obesity, and when peripheral veins are thrombosed. This method is contraindicated in birds (because their bones contain air), for infusion into fractured bones, or in cases of sepsis, because osteomyelitis may develop.

Substances injected into the bone marrow reach the general circulation at about the same rate as those injected directly into peripheral veins. Blood and blood components and solutions of colloids, crystalloids, electrolytes, drugs, and nutrients can be given—even in large volumes.

4

Technique

The two easiest and most desirable sites for marrow access are (1) the flat medial side of the proximal tibia but distal to the tibial tuberosity and the proximal growth plate and (2) the trochanteric fossa of the proximal femur.

To perform intraosseous administration, follow this procedure:

1. Prepare the skin site aseptically, and inject 1% lidocaine into the skin and periosteum.
2. Stabilize the leg, and make a small stab incision through the skin. Needles of 18- to 20-gauge are preferred and can be ordinary hypodermic needles (short bevel desired) or special stylet needle sets, such as a spinal needle or an Illinois bone marrow needle (see Fig. 4-10). A needle with a stylet is preferred so that the needle is not occluded with cortical bone or marrow during introduction.
3. Point the needle slightly distally and rotate with firm pressure until it enters the near cortex. A properly seated needle will feel stable and firm. Use a 10-mL syringe to aspirate marrow, fat, and bony debris. Prefill the needle before administering fluids.
4. Attach a regular fluid infusion set, and start fluid administration. The rate should not exceed 11 mL/minute by gravity or 24 mL/minute with pressure up to 300 mm Hg. Gravity flow through a single catheter may be adequate for patients up to 16 lb. For larger animals, multiple catheters in separate bones or pressurized flow, or both, may be needed for rapid infusions.
5. Encase the needle hub in a butterfly tape, and suture the tape in place. Place antibiotic ointment around the skin incision, and protect and immobilize the whole apparatus with a bulky bandage wrap.

6. Manage intraosseous catheters in the same way as intravenous catheters. Flush the catheter every 6 hours with heparinized saline, and place the catheter in a new bone every 72 hours. The same bone can be reused at another location if 25 to 36 hours is allowed for occlusion and healing of the original site.

Complications

Infection is the primary concern. Fat embolism and damage to the growth plates are other concerns. Extravasation of fluid from the bone marrow into the subcutaneous tissue may occur if the needle punctures both cortexes or if more than one hole is made in the cortex. In such cases, remove the needle and select another bone.

Additional Reading

Crow S, Walshaw S: *Manual of clinical procedures in the dog, cat, and rabbit,* ed 2, Philadelphia, 1997, Lippincott-Raven.
Kirby R, Rudloff E: Crystalloid and colloid fluid therapy. In Ettinger SJ, Feldman EC, editors: *Textbook of veterinary internal medicine,* ed 6, St Louis, 2005, Elsevier-Saunders.
Marks S: The principles and practical application of enteral nutrition, *Vet Clin North Am Small Anim Pract* 28:677, 1998.
Wingfield WE: *Veterinary emergency medicine secrets,* Philadelphia, 1997, Hanley & Belfus.

BANDAGING TECHNIQUES (SEE SECTION 1)

BLOOD PRESSURE MEASUREMENT: INDIRECT

Indirect measurement of blood pressure (BP) in dogs and cats is a convenient, noninvasive technique for establishing whether an individual patient's BP is increased (systemic hypertension) or decreased (hypotension). Today, multiple techniques are available; none are perfect. In human medicine, BP measurement is performed routinely and is (relatively) reliable. In veterinary medicine, BP measurement typically is reserved for patient's determined to have diseases most likely to be associated with serious, potentially injurious alterations in BP, such as shock (hypotension) or chronic renal failure (hypertension). Also in veterinary medicine, it is important to note that most of the BP measuring equipment is designed to provide maximum sensitivity in *hypertensive* patients. Sensitivity of the equipment for accurately detecting hypotension is low.

Generally, two techniques are used. Oscillometric BP measurement entails use of an automated recording system. A cuff is applied to the base of the tail or a distal limb for access to an artery. This technique generally is regarded as being most accurate in dogs. When oscillometric BP measurements are performed in dogs, the patient should be in lateral recumbency. This places the cuff at approximately the same level as the heart. In cats the patient generally remains in sternal recumbency (and minimally restrained). Most patients experience a brief acclimation period to the cuff placement. For this reason, at least 3 to 5 separate readings are obtained at 1- to 2-minute intervals. This technique can be used on awake or anesthetized patients (Figure 4-8).

The Doppler-ultrasonic flow detection system is most accurate in cats for measuring systolic BP. Again, the ventral tail base or a dorsal pedal artery (hind limb) or the superficial palmar arterial arch (forelimb) can be used. Apply and inflate an occluding cuff. The readings are obtained by a transducer as the pressure on the cuff is reduced. Caution is recommended in interpreting results from dogs that are reported as hypertensive but have no overt clinical disease. The higher reported occurrence of falsely elevated BP in normotensive dogs measured by this method justifies the additional scrutiny when interpreting Doppler BP results in dogs.

Clinically, the most common use of indirect BP measurement is in assessing cats for the presence (or absence) of systemic hypertension caused by renal insufficiency or hyperthyroidism (thyrotoxicosis). A common finding among untreated hypertensive cats is retinal detachment and blindness. Early detection and therapeutic intervention (e.g., enalapril and or amlodipine) is critical. In dogs, BP measurement is indicated in patients with chronic

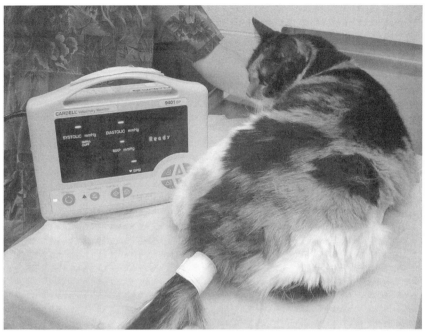

Figure 4-8: Oscillometric blood pressure measurement in a cat.

TABLE 4-2 Systolic Blood Pressure

	Normal	Hypertension	Hypotension
Dog and cat	100-150 mm Hg	>160 mm Hg >180 mm Hg (high risk)	<100 mm Hg

renal insufficiency and/or protein-losing nephropathy, hyperadrenocorticism, and diabetes mellitus. In veterinary medicine, interpretation of BP centers on the *systolic BP reading,* not the diastolic reading (Table 4-2).

Additional Reading

Stepien RL: Blood pressure assessment. In Ettinger SJ, Feldman EC, editors: *Textbook of veterinary internal medicine,* ed 6, St Louis, 2005, Elsevier-Saunders.
Stepien RL: Diagnostic blood pressure measurement. In Ettinger SJ, Feldman EC, editors: *Textbook of veterinary internal medicine,* ed 6, St Louis, 2005, Elsevier-Saunders.

CENTRAL VENOUS PRESSURE MEASUREMENT

Central venous pressure (CVP) is the blood pressure within the intrathoracic portions of the cranial or caudal vena cava. Measurement of CVP in the dog provides an excellent index for determining circulation efficiency. The CVP is controlled by interaction of the circulating blood volume, cardiac pumping action, and alterations in the vascular bed. The CVP is not a measure of blood volume but an indication of the ability of the heart to accept and pump blood brought to it. The CVP reflects the interaction of the heart, vascular tone, and circulatory blood volume. When the heart action and vascular tone remain constant,

CVP reflects blood volume. When blood volume and vascular tone are constant, CVP reflects heart action. When blood volume and heart action are constant, CVP can be used to measure vascular tone.

In addition, the placement of a jugular catheter can be helpful in long-term fluid management and in parenteral alimentation of critically ill animals.

Measurement of CVP is indicated (1) in acute circulatory failure that has not responded to initial treatment; (2) in administration of large volumes of blood or fluids, as may occur in acute shock; (3) as part of the monitoring procedure in poor-risk surgical patients; and (4) in patients with reduced urinary output for which fluids are being administered (e.g., acute renal failure).

For CVP measurement, a catheter must be placed in the external jugular vein such that the catheter is in direct fluid continuity with the right atrium (see Percutaneous Jugular Vein Catheterization). Place the patient in lateral recumbency, and clip the hair over the jugular vein. Surgically prepare the skin in the clipped area.

Make a percutaneous puncture of the jugular vein with the Intracath catheter needle, and advance the tip to approximately the third intercostal space (tip of the catheter at the right atrium). Fasten the catheter securely to the neck of the patient by passing adhesive tape around the neck and the hub of the catheter needle so that the hub of the needle comes to lie at the base of the ear. Connect a three-way stopcock to the catheter. Connect an

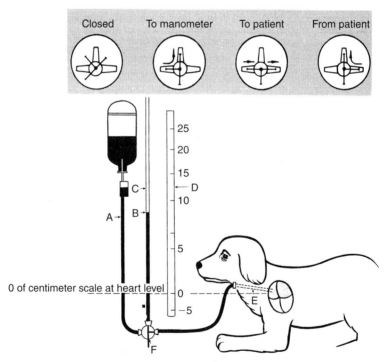

Figure 4-9: Central venous manometer. **A,** Standard intravenous infusion tube. **B,** Central venous pressure level. **C,** Thirty-inch intravenous extension tube. **D,** Centimeter scale. **E,** Plastic tube in great veins in thorax or right atrium via jugular vein. **F,** Three-way stopcock set in measuring position (open from manometer to catheter). Note: This procedure should be performed with the dog in right lateral recumbency.
(From Slatter FP: Shock. In Kirk RW, editor: *Current veterinary therapy III*, Philadelphia, 1968, WB Saunders.)

intravenous setup of isotonic sodium chloride to one end of the stopcock, and to the other end of the stopcock attach a piece of intravenous tubing, which should be taped vertically to a pole or a piece of doweling (Figure 4-9). The metric rule is placed so that the 0 level is aligned with the midpoint of the trachea at the thoracic inlet, and the rule is taped to the vertical pole.

To fill the CVP manometer, turn the three-way stopcock so that fluid will flow from the bottle of saline into the manometer and will exceed the 15-cm mark. Next, turn the stopcock so that a column of fluid exists from the superior vena cava to the manometer. The fluid in the manometer will fall until it reflects the level of the CVP.

It is desirable to allow fluid to flow frequently through the catheter so that the catheter tip does not become plugged with a blood clot. Periodic flushing with heparinized saline will help maintain the patency of the catheter. This setup allows easy intravenous administration of fluids and medication to the patient and collection of blood, if necessary.

There is no absolute value for a normal CVP. The CVP for the normal dog is -1 to $+5$ cm H_2O. Elevations of $+5$ to $+10$ cm H_2O are borderline; however, values greater than 10 cm H_2O may indicate an abnormally expanded blood volume, and those greater than 15 cm H_2O may indicate congestive heart failure. The trend of the CVP is what should be monitored and correlated with the regimen of treatment. One must be aware constantly of the interrelationship between blood volume, cardiovascular function, and vascular tone. If the CVP is at levels of 10 to 15 cm H_2O, the pulmonary venous pressure is approaching 20 to 22 mm Hg, and additional intravenous fluids should not be administered.

Additional Reading

Haskins SC: Monitoring the critically ill patient, *Vet Clin North Am Small Anim Pract* 19:1059-1078, 1989.

Wingfield WE: *Veterinary emergency medicine secrets,* Philadelphia, 1997, Hanley & Belfus.

DIAGNOSTIC SAMPLE COLLECTION TECHNIQUES

BACTERIAL CULTURE

Before actually collecting and submitting a sample for bacterial culture, it is appropriate (whenever feasible to do so) to prepare, stain, and examine a direct smear of the suspect material or tissue. After collecting material on a sterile cotton swab, roll the specimen onto a clear glass slide and allow it to dry completely. Staining with a rapid Romanowsky's-type stain (e.g., Diff-Quik stain) may reveal evidence of neutrophilic inflammation (neutrophilia, especially with a left shift) and occasionally degenerative neutrophils with intracellular bacteria visible. These findings greatly facilitate patient management by documenting the immediate need for interventive empiric antimicrobial therapy until definitive culture and antimicrobial susceptibility results are obtained. The absence of cytologic evidence of bacterial infection does *not* rule out the possibility that the patient is bacteremic.

Routine culture

Inoculate material for culture on blood agar plates or in cystine lactose-electrolyte-deficient (CLED) medium as an acceptable alternative. The CLED medium stimulates growth, detects lactose fermentation, and prevents spreading of *Proteus.* The CLED medium serves as a basis for the isolation of most aerobic microorganisms. Selective media may be necessary for the isolation and identification of specific microorganisms. Biopsy material may be ground in sterile sand and placed in sterile broth.

Multiple-media plates

Multiple-media plates have been developed commercially to facilitate direct antibiotic sensitivity and tentative identification of common pathogenic bacteria. These prepackaged, relatively inexpensive plates help the small laboratory identify pathogenic bacteria by their characteristic behavior on selective media. Some companies have different kits for different suspected infections. In general, kits are most useful for evaluating conjunctivitis, otitis, pyoderma, wound infections, uterine or anterior vaginal infections, fresh necropsy material, and urinary tract infections. Multiple-media plates are not recommended for culturing areas that have a large population of normal microbial organisms (such as the respiratory tract, throat, and vulva), for fecal samples, or for blood cultures to determine bacteremia (Table 4-3).

Direct smears

Cell scrapings taken from conjunctiva during the phase of inflammation (first 10 to 14 days) and stained with Giemsa stain may show typical intracytoplasmic inclusions of initial and elementary bodies accompanied by a polymorphonuclear inflammatory cellular reaction.

TABLE 4-3 Common Bacterial Culture Results

Site	Commensals	Pathogens
External ear canal		
Dog	*Malassezia, Clostridium, Staphylococcus* (a few), *Bacillus* (a few); never *Streptococcus, Pseudomonas,* or *Proteus*	Many *Staphylococcus* and *Malassezia* together; *Pseudomonas, Proteus, Streptococcus, Escherichia coli*
Cat	Not documented	*Staphylococcus aureus,* β-hemolytic streptococcus, *Pasteurella, Pseudomonas, Proteus, E. coli, Malassezia*
Skin		
Dog	*Micrococcus, Clostridium,* diphtheroids, *Staphylococcus epidermidis, Corynebacterium, Malassezia*	*S. aureus* (coagulase positive), *Proteus, Pseudomonas, E. coli*
Cat	*Micrococcus, Streptococcus, S. aureus, S. epidermidis*	*S. aureus, Pasteurella multocida, Bacteroides, Fusobacterium,* haemolytic streptococci
Conjunctiva	*Staphylococcus, Streptococcus, Bacillus, Corynebacterium,* diphtheroids, *Neisseria, Pseudomonas*	*S. aureus, Bacillus, Pseudomonas, E. coli, Aspergillus*
Vagina	*Staphylococcus, Streptococcus, Enterococcus, Corynebacterium, E. coli, Haemophilus, Pseudomonas, Peptostreptococcus, Bacteroides*	*Brucella canis;* pure culture of organisum (esp. *E. coli, Staphylococcus, Pseudomonas*) when accompanied by tissue reaction at vaginal cytology
Urine	*<1000* organisms/mL;* presence of several organisms suggests contamination	More than 100,000* organisms/mL and often pure culture. *E. coli,* enterobacteria, *klebsiella, Proteus, Pseudomonas aeruginosa, Pasteurella multocida, Staphylococcus, Streptococcus*

*Absolute numbers of bacteria depend on the collection technique.

Transport of samples

Because most diagnostic specimens collected for bacterial culture are submitted to commercial laboratories for bacterial isolation, identification, and antimicrobial susceptibility testing, it is important to prepare the sample properly for shipping.

No special transport media are required for routine aerobic culture specimens as long as the sample can remain moist and relatively cool *and* the sample can be inoculated onto culture medium within 3 to 4 hours only. For samples that must be shipped overnight to a laboratory, it is imperative that the specimen be kept cool (not frozen) and moist. Elevated temperatures during shipping contribute to bacterial overgrowth of nonpathogenic bacteria, making isolation and identification of disease-producing organisms difficult. Special transport media may be required. Contact the individual laboratory regarding information pertaining to shipping of specimens for bacterial culture.

Specimens submitted for anaerobic culture need to be inoculated onto culture media within minutes following collection. Although special anaerobic transport media are available, they may not be well suited for extended shipping times (>24 hours).

Isolation and identification

For isolation, obtain columnar epithelial cells (not exudate). Use calcium alginate (not wooden) swabs. Place swabs directly into liquid-holding medium on wet ice. The most commonly used transport medium is 2-SP, composed of 0.2M sucrose and 0.02M phosphate (pH is 7.2) with added antibiotics. This can be supplied by the laboratory that is doing the isolations. Monolayers of McCoy and HeLa cells are best for isolation of *Chlamydophila* spp. Egg (yolk sac) inoculation of embryonated eggs has been abandoned. *Chlamydophila felis* (formerly *Chlamydia psittaci*) inclusions are detected by fluorescent antibody techniques.

Puncture fluids

Aspirate material using aseptic technique. Centrifuge the aspirated material at high speed, and stain a smear of the sediment with Gram stain. Culture the sediment on blood agar, in thioglycolate medium, on Sabouraud dextrose agar, or on one of the multiple-media plates. Also consider anaerobic cultures.

4

Wounds and ulcers

In dealing with an abscess (except those of the eye), clip and clean the abscess site. Aspirate material from the abscess into a sterile syringe and culture in blood agar and thioglycolate broth or on one of the multiple-media plates. In open wounds, use a sterile cotton swab and obtain fresh exudate from the deeper portion of the lesion. Also consider anaerobic cultures.

Spinal fluid

If the spinal fluid is cloudy, make a direct smear and stain with Gram and Giemsa stains. If the fluid is fairly clear, centrifuge for 10 minutes, make a smear, and stain the sediment with Gram stain. Make cultures of the sediment on blood agar, in thioglycolate medium, or on one of the multiple-media plates, and on Sabouraud dextrose agar.

Ear cultures

Collect material on sterile cotton swabs, make a smear, and stain it with Gram stain. Place the swab on blood agar or Columbia colistin-nalidixic acid blood agar and eosin-methylene blue agar. Look for star-shaped colonies (yeasts) after 48 hours on eosin-methylene blue agar.

Eye cultures

Use a sterile cotton swab moistened with sterile saline or broth, and pass it over the conjunctiva of the inferior fornix of each eye. Use one half of a blood agar plate and one half of a mannitol plate for each eye. Also place material into thioglycolate medium.

Alternatively, use one of the commercial multiple-media plates. Make two conjunctival scrapings and stain one with Gram stain and the other with Giemsa stain.

Skin cultures

Cultures made from the surface of the epidermis or open ulcers are of little significance because they usually grow a mixture of nonpathogenic organisms. A culture made from the deep tissue of a biopsy specimen may be helpful in the diagnosis of a bacterial, atypical mycobacterial, or subcutaneous mycotic infection. Diagnostic isolates may be obtained from cultures of tissue sections from ulcers, fistulas, abscesses, enlarged nodes, or granulomatous lesions. Smears and cultures made from exudates of deep fistulas and node aspirates may be useful in some cases.

Intact pustules are satisfactory lesions for making smears and cultures. After the skin surface has been sterilized carefully, gently aspirate the fluid content of the pustule with a sterile needle and syringe for inoculation into appropriate media; alternatively, open the pustule roof and take a culture (by swab) from the fluid inside. In all these procedures, take the utmost care to prevent contamination from tissues outside the area of primary involvement.

When any fluid material or tissue is cultured, it is always desirable to use a portion of the sample to make stained smears. Stained smears often provide immediate clues to the diagnosis (organisms present [yeast, bacteria, or fungi] and indications as to the host response [cell types, phagocytosis, or eosinophils]). Examine the slides for the presence of bacteria and for cell morphology.

Urine culture

Urine, as it is secreted by the kidneys, is sterile unless the kidney is infected. Most urinary tract infections are ascending infections by organisms introduced through the urethra. The most common sites of infection in female animals are the urethra and urinary bladder. Chronic prostatitis is common in male dogs and often is associated with relapsing urinary tract infections.

Urine specimens can be collected by catheterization, by collecting a clean voided midstream sample, or by cystocentesis (Table 4-4). Cystocentesis is the preferred method for qualitative and quantitative bacterial culture. To calibrate bacterial counts in urinary cultures, use a standard platinum milk dilution loop calibrated to deliver 0.001 mL of urine to one half of a blood agar plate. The initial loop of urine is streaked onto the plate. One hundred colonies or more signifies a bacterial count in the original specimen greater than or equal to 10^5 cells/mL. The number of bacteria that is significant varies with the method of collection. With cystocentesis, a bacterial count greater than 10^3 cells/mL of urine is significant; with catheterization, greater than 10^5 cells/mL is significant. A MacConkey agar plate can be used in addition to a blood agar plate.

Cystocentesis samples collected from animals that have received antimicrobial therapy should have 5 mL of urine centrifuged at 2500 rpm for 5 minutes, and the sediment should be streaked onto blood agar and MacConkey agar.

MacConkey agar and eosin-methylene blue agar are selective and differential media that are used to identify urinary tract organisms. MacConkey agar prevents early growth of *Proteus*, inhibits growth of gram-positive bacteria, and allows separation of gram-negative bacteria in lactose-positive and lactose-negative subgroups.

Several commercial methods for urinary culture are available for screening urine for bacterial infection. Bayer Microstix (Fisher Scientific International, Inc., Hampton, New Hampshire) has proved 92% accurate in detecting bacteriuria of greater than 10^5 cells/mL. If urine is collected by cystocentesis, significant bacteriuria may not be observed. Reculture samples that are positive by Microstix using calibrated loop or pour plate techniques.

Use catheterization with aseptic technique or antepubic cystocentesis to collect urine for culture. Refrigerate specimens of urine within a few minutes after collection if culture is not done immediately. Perform bacterial culture of the specimen within 2 hours of collection. Becton Dickinson supplies a Vacutainer urine transport kit for urine culture.

T A B L E 4 - 4 Interpretation of Quantitative Urine Cultures in Dogs and Cats*

| Collection method | Colony-forming units/mL urine | | | | | |
| | Significant | | Suspicious | | Contaminant | |
	Dogs	Cats	Dogs	Cats	Dogs	Cats
Cystocentesis	≥1000	≥1000	100-1000	100-1000	≤100	≤100
Catheterization	≥10,000	≥1000	1000-10,000	100-1000	≤1000	≤100
Voluntary voiding	≥100,000†	≥10,000	10,000-90,000	1000-10,000	≤10,000	≤1000
Manual compression	≥100,000†	≥10,000	10,000-90,000	1000-10,000	≤10,000	≤1000

*The data represent generalities. On occasion, bacterial urinary tract infections may be detected in dogs and cats with the fewer organisms (i.e., false-negative results).
†Caution: Because contamination of midstream samples may result in colony counts of 10,000/mL or more in some dogs (i.e., false-positive results), they should not be used for routine diagnostic culture of urine from dogs.
From Osborne CA, Finco DR: Canine and Feline Nephrology and Urology, Baltimore, Williams & Wilkins, 1995.

4

The Vacutainer tube can hold 5 mL of urine, which can be taken from a midstream catch or cystocentesis. The collection tube has a bacteriostatic fluid that preserves unrefrigerated urine specimens for up to 24 hours for culture.

Prostatic fluid culture

Bacterial infection of the prostate may result in a nidus of infection that can cause recurrent urinary tract infection and prostatomegaly in male dogs. An effective way to evaluate the prostate for bacterial infection is to examine the prostatic fraction (the third fraction) of the male ejaculate; if separation proves to be too difficult, use the whole ejaculate specimen for culture. To better interpret the results of the prostatic culture, obtain urethral cultures before the ejaculate sample (see also Prostatic Wash).

Collect the ejaculate fraction into a sterile side-mouth container (such as a 12-mL sterile plastic syringe container). Make subcultures with 0.1 mL of ejaculate onto differential media as for urethral swabs. The prostatic ejaculate culture shows significant bacterial infection if the number of bacteria in the prostatic culture is greater than 2 logs of growth compared with the bacteria in the urethral culture.

Stool cultures

Acute infectious diarrhea can be caused by bacteria, viruses, and protozoa. The major bacteria in feces are non–spore-forming anaerobic bacilli, but gram-negative facultative anaerobic bacteria such as *Escherichia coli* and other members of the Enterobacteriaceae family are usually present. The clinical picture in acute infectious diarrhea is frequent loose stools containing pus or blood, abdominal pain, and fever. Damage to the intestinal tract may be produced by an enterotoxin, as with *Staphylococcus aureus* or *E. coli*, or by invasion of the mucosa of the small intestine and colon. The most common bacterial pathogens of the intestinal tract in small animals are *E. coli*, *Salmonella* spp., and *Campylobacter jejuni*.

BLOOD CULTURE

Bacteria can enter the blood from extravascular sites by way of the lymphatic circulation. Direct entry of bacteria into the bloodstream can be observed in the presence of endocarditis, suppurative phlebitis, infected intravenous catheters, dialysis cannulas, and osteomyelitis. Bacteremia can be transient, intermittent, or persistent. Transient bacteremia is produced by manipulation of an abscess, dental procedures, urethral catheterization, or surgery on contaminated areas. Intermittent bacteremia is associated with undetected and undrained abscesses. Most dogs with bacteremia, especially gram-negative bacteremia, are febrile and have an abnormal peripheral blood picture with an increased white blood cell count, increased number of band and segmented neutrophils, increased number of monocytes, and lymphopenia. An exception to this is osteomyelitis, in which dogs with bacteremia associated with staphylococci have basically normal hemograms. Large-breed male dogs with valvular insufficiency, congestive heart failure, or thromboembolism should be suspects for infectious endocarditis. The mitral valve most often is involved, followed by the aortic, tricuspid, and pulmonary valve.

The material for culture must be collected under aseptic conditions. Clip and surgically prepare the skin over the cephalic, recurrent tarsal, or jugular vein. Do not draw blood for culture through an indwelling intravenous or intraarterial catheter. Collection vials are available for aerobic and anaerobic bacterial culture. Add the required volume of blood (usually 8 to 10 mL) to the enriched culture medium. Immediately after collection, mix the contents of bottles or tubes to prevent clotting.

Take blood for cultures 1 hour before temperature spikes if intermittent fevers are present (Box 4-2). Take three separate blood culture specimens over a 24-hour-period. With a 1:10 dilution of blood in broth, antibiotics that may have been administered systemically usually are diluted to noninhibitory concentrations. The addition of sodium polyanethole sulfonate to commercial culture media inactivates aminoglycosides present in clinical concentrations.

BOX 4-2   INDICATIONS FOR PERFORMING A BLOOD CULTURE

Any acute illness with fever (fever of unknown origin)
Hypothermia
Leukocytosis, particularly with a left shift
Neutropenia
Unexplained tachycardia
Undiagnosed hypoglycemia
Unexplained tachypnea or dyspnea

Undiagnosed anuria or oliguria
Unexplained icterus
Thrombocytopenia
Disseminated intravascular coagulation
Intermittent shifting leg lameness
Sudden development of, or change in, a murmur

BOX 4-3   INDICATIONS FOR SUBMITTING SPECIMENS FOR ANAEROBIC CULTURE

Any focal pain and swelling with fever
Nonhealing bite or puncture wound
Foul-smelling wounds with persistent discharge
Presence of gas in tissue, especially if associated with a penetrating injury
Abscess, especially if recurrent
Necrotic or devitalized tissue
Dark, discolored discharge from the site of a penetrating injury
Visible sulfur granules in any discharge
Identification of filamentous bacteria during routine microscopy of exudates
Failure to obtain bacterial growth using aerobic techniques

Other media that may be used as selective agents include MacConkey agar, brain-heart infusion agar, mannitol salt agar, Streptosel agar, urea agar, blood agar, and eosin-methylene blue agar. Special techniques make it possible to determine total bacteria counts and whether an organism is coagulase-positive or coagulase-negative.

Anaerobic culture of blood

Because anaerobes may be present in significant numbers in positive cultures from blood, abscesses, wounds, and urine, it may be advisable to make these special examinations. Anaerobes are present in the normal flora in fecal, throat, and bronchial swabs, so the anaerobic culture of these samples may be difficult to evaluate.

Specimens for anaerobic examination should be protected from air, held at room temperature, and inoculated directly onto culture media as soon as possible. Specimens should not be inoculated onto transport or enrichment media. Specimens can be held for short periods in sterile, carbon dioxide–filled, tightly stoppered tubes or bottles. Inoculate the sample onto prereduced anaerobically sterilized medium under oxygen-free gas. Specimens can be inoculated deep into thioglycolate medium for transfer and subculture. With anaerobic organisms, it is especially important to make a smear and a Gram stain and to record all morphotypes present and the relative numbers of each (Box 4-3).

Additional Reading

Dow S: Diagnosis of bacteremia in critically ill dogs and cats. In Bonagura J, editor: *Current veterinary therapy XII. Small animal practice,* Philadelphia, 1995, WB Saunders.

Greene CE: *Infectious diseases of the dog and cat,* ed 3, St Louis, 2006, Elsevier-Saunders.

Osborne C: Three steps to effective management of bacterial urinary tract infections: *Compend Contin Educ Pract Vet* 17:1233-1248, 1995.

Osborne CA, Finco DR: *Canine and feline nephrology and urology,* Baltimore, 1997, Williams & Wilkins.

Scott DW, Miller WH Jr, Griffin CE: *Muller and Kirk's small animal dermatology,* ed 5, Philadelphia, 1997, WB Saunders.

4

FUNGAL CULTURE

Diagnostic fungal cultures depend on selection of the most appropriate culture site, proper collection of specimens, and appropriate use of selective media. Culture specimens from patients suspected of having superficial fungal infections (dermatophytosis) are made from hair, skin, nails, and biopsy tissues. Test patients suspected of having deep mycoses (e.g., blastomycosis and histoplasmosis) by cytopathologic or diagnostic serologic testing (see Section 5).

Hair

If the hair is grossly dirty, clean it with soap and water; if not, wash it carefully with alcohol. Allow the hair to dry thoroughly. Select a site at the edge of an active lesion, and look for broken or stubby hairs. Use a forceps (curved Kelly or mosquito hemostats), and depilate hair from these areas by pulling parallel to the direction of the hair growth. It is important to get the hair root and not break off the hair shaft. Pluck many hairs and implant (push) the roots of the hair into the selected agar. Then gently lay the hair shaft down to contact the surface of the medium. Hairs for inoculation often can be selected by choosing those that fluoresce with a Wood's light.

Examination of some of the plucked hairs with a potassium hydroxide or wet-mount preparation for spores and hyphae is desirable. Never take specimens from areas that have been treated within 1 week. If samples are to be sent to a laboratory, the dry hair can be placed in a clean, tightly sealed envelope and mailed.

Skin

Dermatophyte or yeast infections may affect glabrous skin. If necessary, cleanse culture sites with *alcohol gauze swabs* (cotton will leave excess fibers) and allow to dry. Using a fine scalpel blade, collect superficial scrapings of scales, crusts, and epidermal debris at the periphery of typical lesions. Dermatophytes live in a dry state for several weeks, but yeast infections should be cultured immediately or placed in transport medium to prevent drying.

Nails

Although hard keratin fungal infections are rare in animals, diseased nails should be avulsed, scraped, or ground into fine pieces for collection in a sterile Petri dish. Pieces can be examined directly for arthrospores or hyphae and placed on appropriate media for culture.

Tissue biopsy

Tissue core or excision samples can be sliced and the newly exposed surface used for impression smears or inoculation of medium. Samples also may be chopped or ground and placed in medium. Place small amounts in sterile saline or broth for referral to an appropriate laboratory for further processing.

Dermatophyte media

Sabouraud dextrose agar has been used traditionally in veterinary mycology for isolation of fungi; however, other media are available with bacterial and fungal inhibitors, such as dermatophyte test medium (DTM), potato dextrose agar, and rice grain medium. Mycosel and mycobiotic agar are formulations of Sabouraud dextrose agar with cycloheximide and chloramphenicol added to inhibit fungal and bacterial contaminants. If a medium with cycloheximide is used, fungi sensitive to it will not be isolated. Organisms sensitive to cycloheximide include *Cryptococcus neoformans,* many members of the Zygomycota, some *Candida* spp., *Aspergillus* spp., *Pseudallescheria boydii,* and many agents of phaeohyphomycosis. Dermatophyte test medium is essentially a Sabouraud dextrose agar containing cycloheximide, gentamicin, and chlortetracycline as antifungal and antibacterial agents. The pH indicator phenol red has been added. Dermatophytes use protein in the medium first, and alkaline metabolites turn the medium red. When the protein is exhausted, the dermatophytes use carbohydrates and give off acid metabolites, and the color of the medium returns to yellow. Most other fungi use carbohydrates first and protein later, so they too may produce a red change in DTM, but only after a prolonged incubation (10 to 14 days or more). Consequently, examine DTM cultures daily for the first 10 days. Fungi such as *Blastomyces dermatitidis, Sporothrix schenckii, Histoplasma capsulatum, Coccidioides immitis, P. boydii,* some *Aspergillus* spp., and others may cause a red change in DTM, so microscopic examination is essential to avoid an erroneous presumptive diagnosis. Because DTM may (1) depress development of conidia, (2) mask colony pigmentation, and (3) inhibit some pathogens, fungi recovered on DTM should be transferred to plain Sabouraud dextrose agar for identification.

Potato dextrose agar is useful for promoting sporulation and observing pigmentation. On potato dextrose agar, *Microsporum canis* has a lemon-yellow pigment, whereas *M. audouinii* has a salmon- or peach-colored pigment. Rice agar medium promotes conidia formation in some dermatophytes, especially *M. canis* strains, which produce no conidia on Sabouraud dextrose agar.

Inoculate skin scrapings, nails, and hair onto Sabouraud dextrose agar, DTM, mycosel, or mycobiotic agar. Incubate cultures at 30° C with 30% humidity. A pan of water in the incubator usually will provide enough humidity. Check cultures every 2 to 3 days for fungal growth. Cultures on DTM may be incubated for 10 to 14 days, but cultures on Sabouraud dextrose agar should be allowed 30 days to develop.

Diagnosis should depend on characteristic gross identification of cultures and careful inspection of elements from those cultures using slide preparations and slide cultures for microscopic examination. Cultures of fungi other than dermatophytes should be made by commercial or institutional laboratories with appropriate equipment and special expertise.

The Wood's light

Ultraviolet light filtered through nickel oxide produces a beam called *Wood's light.* If an animal is taken into a dark room and its hair and skin are exposed to a Wood's light, fluorescence may show for several reasons. Hair shafts affected by some species of *Microsporum* fluoresce a bright yellow-green (like the color of a fluorescing watch face). However, iodide medications, petroleum, soap, dyes, and even keratin may produce purple-, blue-, or yellow-colored fluorescence. The positive fungal fluorescence is a valuable aid in selecting affected hairs for culture inoculation. Remember, a negative fluorescence does not preclude a possible diagnosis of fungal infection. False negatives and false positives may occur.

Additional Reading

Dow. S: Diagnosis of bacteremia in critically ill dogs and cats. In Bonagura J, editor: *Current veterinary therapy XII. Small animal practice,* Philadelphia, 1995, WB Saunders.

Greene CE: *Infectious diseases of the dog and cat,* ed 3, St Louis, 2006, Elsevier-Saunders.

Scott DW, Miller WH Jr, Griffin CE: *Muller and Kirk's small animal dermatology,* ed 5, Philadelphia, 1997, WB Saunders.

VIRUS ISOLATION

Several techniques are currently available for the identification of viral infections in dogs and cats. Among the most convenient are antigen-detection systems available as point-of-care tests for feline leukemia virus antigen in blood and canine parvovirus antigen in feces. These tests identify infected patients with excellent accuracy. Additionally, and seldom considered for their value, point-of-care tests for viral infections are especially capable of identifying patients that have not been exposed, allowing the clinician reliably to rule out infection by the organism for which the animal is tested.

In addition, many commercial and point-of-care serologic assays are available that detect antibody to many of the viruses affecting dogs and cats. However, the positive predictive value of antibody tests is considerably lower than that for antigen tests. For example, a single positive antibody titer in a dog for canine distemper is evidence of prior exposure or vaccination. A POSITIVE antibody titer to a particular viral pathogen does *not* constitute a diagnosis of infection, especially in the absence of clinical signs. However, a NEGATIVE antibody titer generally does denote no prior exposure or failure to respond to vaccination. Obtaining acute and convalescent titers in a patient suspected of having an acute viral infection can be a reliable diagnostic tool if a fourfold or greater increase in titer can be demonstrated over 3 to 4 weeks. Acute and convalescent viral titers in individual patients are rarely performed in veterinary medicine.

Virus isolation, however, is a valuable diagnostic tool that is underutilized in veterinary medicine, perhaps because of the limited number of commercial and university laboratories that provide viral isolation services.

Diagnosis of viral upper respiratory infection in cats (herpesvirus-1 and/or calicivirus) is perhaps among the situations for which virus isolation can be most useful, especially in cluster households where many cats and kittens may be at risk. Quickly insert a sterile cotton swab into the oral cavity to the level of the tonsil or oropharynx. By rolling the swab across the epithelium, it is possible to harvest cells and virus from infected cats. Immediately place the swab into a virus transport medium (usually provided by the laboratory). Antibiotics added to the solution prevent bacterial overgrowth of the sample. For short-term transit (5 days or less), hold specimens for viral isolation at 4° C rather than frozen. On reaching the laboratory, the specimen will be inoculated into a suitable tissue culture. Within a few days it is usually possible to establish, based on the cytopathic effect on the tissue culture, whether a virus infection is present. Fluorescent antibody test can be done subsequently to confirm the isolate.

Some laboratories offer direct assessment of specimens (e.g., feces for canine parvovirus or canine coronavirus) by electron microscopy. These methods can be useful for infections in which the virus titer in the specimen reaches 10^6 to 10^7 organisms/mL. Specimens such as feces, vesicle fluid, brain tissue, urine, or serum can be negatively stained for electron microscopy.

Recently, considerable interest has surfaced regarding the availability of virus testing by polymerase chain reaction. Polymerase chain reaction is an exquisitely sensitive test for viral (or bacterial or fungal) DNA in patients known or suspected to have an infection. Objectively, only trace amounts of DNA (or in some cases, RNA) of the infecting virus are required in the specimen. These amounts are amplified millions of times to facilitate identification of the target sequence (and the infecting organism). However, the disadvantages to polymerase chain reaction testing are price (prices are sufficiently high today to preclude routine diagnostic testing for viral infection by polymerase chain reaction) and the sensitivity of the test. So sensitive is polymerase chain reaction, that extraneous, non–target DNA (in the specimen or in the laboratory) may contaminate the sample easily, making diagnosis difficult to impossible.

BLOOD COLLECTION TECHNIQUES

Venipuncture of the dog and cat may be accomplished by using the cephalic, jugular, femoral, or recurrent tarsal veins. In large dogs and cats, the cephalic and jugular veins are preferred. Performance of venipuncture as atraumatically as possible is essential to preserve the integrity of the vein, particularly when multiple venipunctures must be performed and a central venous catheter cannot be placed to facilitate the collection of multiple blood samples. For aesthetic reasons and in show cats and dogs, it is undesirable to clip the fur over the vessels, if this can be avoided. However, clipping the hair can aid in identification and visualization of the vein. After clipping the overlying fur, aseptically scrub the skin or place a quantity of isopropyl alcohol over the vessel. If the fur is not clipped, part the fur with alcohol to improve visualization.

In most instances, a 3- to 5-mL (2-mL minimum according to most commercial laboratories) blood sample is adequate for routine hematologic and biochemical analyses. Plan ahead which samples are required to prevent the need for further venipuncture at a later time, whenever possible. In small dogs and cats, use the jugular veins to allow adequate sample collection. If smaller samples are required, the cephalic, lateral saphenous, or medial saphenous veins can be used for sample collection. Do not use the jugular vein if a coagulopathy is suspected because hemorrhage may be difficult to control following venipuncture.

For successful venipuncture, proper restraint of the animal is important. Details for the proper restraint for various venipuncture locations are discussed with each specific topic throughout this text. The patient must remain comfortable yet relatively motionless to avoid iatrogenic vessel laceration. Stretch the skin tightly over the selected vessel without causing vascular occlusion to help anchor the vessel in place during penetration by the needle.

Use a dry, sterile needle and syringe. Grasp the syringe tightly in between the thumb and forefingers. Place the index finger near the hub of the syringe to help guide it in place. In most cases, it is best to penetrate the skin just lateral to the vessel. Further advance the needle to puncture the vessel from the side. Blood usually will enter the hub of the needle spontaneously but can be encouraged to enter by pulling on the plunger of the syringe. After the skin and underlying fascia have been punctured, some clinicians apply constant gentle negative pressure on the vessel by pulling back on the plunger of the syringe. Too much suction will collapse the vein and cause inadequate flow of blood into the syringe. Decreased blood flow also may be caused by inadequate tissue perfusion, hypothermia, circulatory failure, hematoma formation, and piercing the vessel wall without penetrating into the vessel lumen. Occasionally, the tip of the needle will become snagged on the opposite wall of the vessel, or by a valve within the vessel. Repositioning the needle with slight rotation and retraction from the vessel may correct the problem. The flow of blood can be improved by alternating occlusion and release of the vein, combined with passive motion of the leg. Complications of venipuncture include hematoma formation, minor hemorrhage, vascular trauma, and thrombophlebitis.

The use of a Vacutainer has simplified the collection of blood samples from small animals, particularly when larger vessels are catheterized for blood collection. Do not use the larger-sized Vacutainer containers in small veins because the veins will collapse from the negative pressure within the tube. To ensure that the proper ratio of anticoagulant-to-blood is obtained, fill all tubes that contain anticoagulants until the vacuum is exhausted.

When handling blood samples, use clean and dry syringe, needles, or evacuated blood collection tubes. Avoid hemolysis by using clean, dry equipment and avoiding trauma to the red blood cells. Trauma to the red blood cells occurs because of application of too much or fluctuating suction during aspiration, excessive force when expelling the blood sample into the blood collection tube, or excessive agitation of the sample once within the tube. Hemolysis can interfere with a number of diagnostic tests and should be avoided.

Make an effort to have the animal fast for a minimum of 12 hours before the collection of blood samples to avoid postprandial lipemia. Lipemia is attributable to metabolic disorders (pancreatitis, diabetes mellitus) and to recent meals and adversely and artifactually can affect blood test results. Total protein, albumin, glucose, calcium, phosphorus, and bilirubin are examples of tests that can be affected greatly by sample lipemia. The clinician should be aware of the tests that are affected by lipemia and sample hemolysis and various anticoagulants.

Routine hematologic testing (see also Section 5)

The anticoagulant of choice for hematologic testing is EDTA. Heparin is especially to be avoided if blood films are to be made from blood mixed with anticoagulant because contact with whole blood will distort the morphology of cells significantly. Heparin is acceptable for most procedures requiring blood plasma. The anticoagulant effect of heparin is transitory. Specimens still may clot after 2 to 3 days.

Make blood films immediately after collection because cell morphology rapidly deteriorates after sample collection. Although blood films can be made after introducing blood to EDTA, a better practice is to make blood smears (films) immediately from the collection needle before the blood comes in contact with any anticoagulant. *Never use blood exposed to heparin to make blood smears.*

Incorrect proportions of blood to anticoagulant may result in water shifts between plasma and red blood cells. Such shifts may alter the packed cell volume, especially when small amounts of blood are added to tubes prepared with volumes of anticoagulant sufficient for much larger volumes of blood. Erroneous laboratory results also may be obtained when small volumes of blood are placed in a relatively large container. Evaporation of plasma water and adherence of the cells to the surface of the container can produce artifactual changes in hematologic results.

Refrigerate liquid blood mixed with anticoagulant after collection if there is a delay in making the laboratory determinations. White blood cell (WBC) and red blood cell counts, packed cell volume, and hemoglobin level can be measured within 24 hours of sample collection. Platelet counts, however, should be done within 1 hour of collection. Dried, unfixed blood smears can be stained with most conventional stains 24 to 48 hours after being made. If a considerable delay is anticipated between the time that the blood smear is made and the staining process, the blood smear should be fixed by immersion in absolute methanol for at least 5 minutes. Blood smears fixed by this method are stable indefinitely. Never place unfixed blood smears in a refrigerator because condensation forming after the smear is removed from the refrigerator will ruin the blood smear and make it unusable for cytologic evaluation. Take care to leave unfixed blood smears face down on a countertop or in a closed box. Special stains, such as peroxidase, may require fresh blood films.

Routine biochemistry testing (see also Section 5)

Most clinical chemistry procedures are performed on serum. The serum is obtained by collecting blood without any anticoagulant and allowing the blood to clot in a clean, dry tube. Separate serum from cells within 45 minutes of sample collection (venipuncture). Special vacuum vials are available that produce a strong barrier between the clot and the serum so that it is not necessary to draw off the serum into a separate vial. Clotting of the blood and retraction of the clot occur best and maximum yields of serum are obtained at room or body temperatures. Refrigeration of the sample impairs clot retraction. When the blood is firmly clotted, free the clot from the walls of the container by rimming with an applicator stick or by tapping sharply on the outside of the tube. After the clot is freed, allow clot retraction to occur, and then centrifuge and draw off the clear supernatant serum using a pipette or suction bulb. Serum yield is usually one third of the whole blood volume, unless severe hypovolemia or intravascular dehydration is present.

Many clinical chemistry procedures can be performed on plasma and on serum. The advantage of using plasma is that separation of cells can be accomplished immediately after centrifugation or sedimentation, without the need to wait for clot formation and retraction. The disadvantage of plasma is that the presence of the anticoagulant interferes with many of the chemistry assay procedures. Plasma is less clear than serum, which may be an additional disadvantage for colorimetric assays. Plasma and serum are virtually identical in chemical composition except that plasma has fibrinogen and the anticoagulant. For many procedures in which plasma or whole blood is to be used, heparin is the anticoagulant of choice. Heparinized blood is the only acceptable specimen for blood pH and blood gas analyses. Although blood containing EDTA is acceptable for certain chemical procedures, it cannot be used for determination of plasma electrolytes because it contributes to and sequesters them from the specimen. In addition, EDTA can interfere with alkaline phosphatase levels, decrease total carbon dioxide, and elevated blood nonprotein nitrogen.

Separate serum or plasma and remove it from the cells as soon as possible after blood is collected, because many of the constituents of plasma exist in higher concentrations in red blood cells. With time, these substances leak into the plasma and cause falsely elevated values (positive interference) and falsely lower values (negative interference) (Table 4-5). Under no circumstances should whole blood be sent via the mail; serum derived from such specimens usually is hemolyzed, and results are often inaccurate. Separate serum and transfer it to a clean, dry tube for shipment.

T A B L E 4 - 5 Examples of Positive and Negative Interference on Biochemistry Analytes Induced by Sample Hemolysis

Analyte	Effect of hemolysis*
Alanine transaminase	Minimal effect
Alkaline phosphatase	Increased
Bilirubin	Increased
Chloride	Decreased
Creatinine	Increased
Inorganic phosphate	Increased
Lipase	Decreased
pH	Decreased
Potassium	No detectable effect
Total calcium	Increased
Total protein	Increased
Urea nitrogen	Increased

*Type and degree of interference varies among different testing modalities unique to individual laboratories or in-hospital biochemistry analyzers.

Additional Reading

Meyer DJ, Harvey JW: *Veterinary laboratory medicine,* ed 3, St Louis, 2004, Elsevier-Saunders.

Raskin R, Meyer DJ (eds): Update on clinical pathology, *Vet Clin North Am Small Anim Pract* 26:5, September 1996.

Thomas JS: Introduction to serum chemistries: artifacts in biochemical determinations. In Willard MD, Tvedten H, editors: *Small animal clinical diagnosis by laboratory methods,* ed 4, St Louis, 2004, Elsevier-Saunders.

BONE MARROW ASPIRATION

4

Collection of bone marrow may prove valuable in diseases of the blood in which examination of the peripheral blood reveals abnormal cells or cell counts. Conditions such as leukopenia, thrombocytopenia, nonregenerative anemias, agranulocytosis, pancytopenia, and leukemias may be present because of pathologic changes within the bone marrow.

Bone marrow in the young animal is cellular and exists in the flat bones (sternum, ribs, pelvic bones, and vertebrae) and in the long bones (humerus and femur). As the animal ages, the cellular content of the marrow decreases, especially in the long bones. In older animals, bone marrow cells still exist in the flat bones; however, in conditions of stress in which new blood cells must be produced in large numbers, primitive cells in the bone marrow of the long bones again become active. Interpretation of the bone marrow smear may be limited by (1) technique used to obtain a bone marrow specimen or (2) the specialized knowledge necessary to interpret bone marrow cells.

Bone marrow aspiration is much underused in clinical practice. The procedure does require some degree of skill to obtain high-quality samples, but the procedure is low risk to the patient and can be highly valuable in establishing a diagnosis or prognosis.

Canine

The biopsy techniques that may be used in the examination of bone marrow are aspiration, core, and incisional biopsy. The most frequently used technique is aspiration biopsy. When aspiration biopsy fails to produce bone marrow cells (as in advanced myelofibrosis, neoplasia, or marrow aplasia), a core biopsy of bone marrow is indicated. Bone marrow aspiration needles may be a 16-gauge Rosenthal needle or Illinois needle for medium-sized dogs; an 18-gauge Rosenthal needle for small dogs and cats; or a Jamshidi (pronounced yam-she-dee) bone marrow biopsy needle, 12 gauge for most adult dogs and 14 gauge for small dogs and cats.

The selection of needles for aspiration biopsy of bone marrow is based on the biopsy site, the depth of the biopsy site, and the density of cortical bone. For bone marrow aspiration, the modified disposable Illinois sternal-iliac bone marrow aspiration needle works well (Figure 4-10). For a core biopsy of bone marrow, the Jamshidi bone marrow biopsy-aspiration needle (pediatric, 3.5 inches, 13 gauge) can be used (Figure 4-11).

The iliac crest is a commonly used site for marrow aspiration in dogs. A short-acting anesthetic occasionally may be needed, but tranquilization together with local anesthesia is usually sufficient. Place the animal in lateral recumbency, and clip the hair over the area of the iliac crest. Surgically prepare the site. To aspirate marrow, have the needle enter the widest part of the iliac crest and stop the needle just after penetration of the bone. Remove the stylet, place a 12-mL syringe on the needle, and aspirate 0.2 mL of marrow.

Alternatively, the head of the humerus offers easy access to abundant bone marrow. Sedation may be required. With the patient in lateral recumbency and the humerus flexed (the humerus is positioned parallel to the patient's thorax), instill local anesthetic into the skin and subcutaneous tissues to the level of the head of the humerus. The site of needle insertion is on the most proximal facet of the humoral head (Figure 4-12). Direct the needle into the bone toward the elbow and parallel to the humeral shaft. If the needle is positioned too far medially over the humeral head, it is easy to penetrate the joint capsule. Although this is a common occurrence, it does not pose a risk of injury to the patient (assuming the skin was surgically prepared). However, in the event joint fluid contaminates the bone marrow aspirate, the sample will be rendered useless.

Contamination of the bone marrow with peripheral blood results if (1) the marrow is not aspirated immediately after the needle enters the marrow cavity or (2) if aspiration time is sustained and a large volume of blood enters the syringe subsequent to the rupture of small blood vessels in the bone marrow.

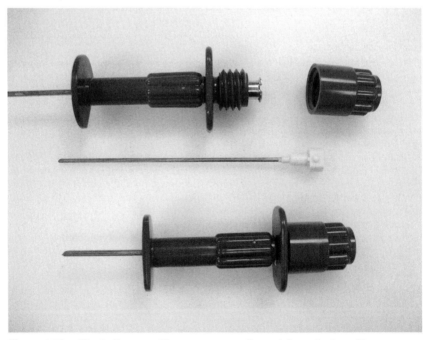

Figure 4-10:   Illinois iliac-sternal bone marrow needle used for aspiration of bone marrow from the humerus, ileum, or femur of dogs and cats.

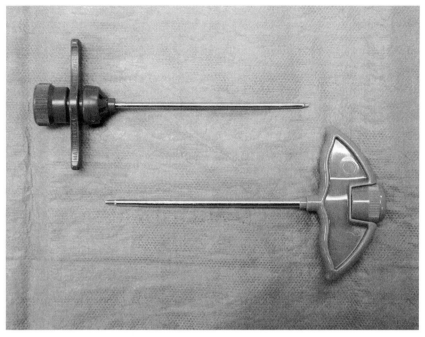

Figure 4-11: Jamshidi bone marrow biopsy needles.

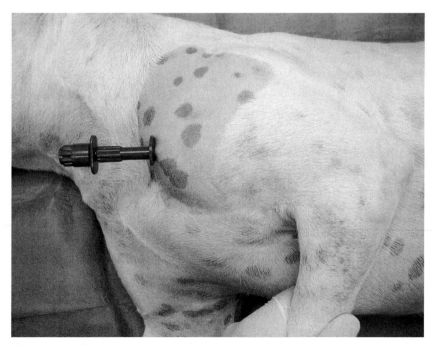

4

Figure 4-12: Illinois bone marrow needle positioned in the humeral head of dog prepared for bone marrow aspiration.

Perhaps the least desired technique is to obtain marrow from the proximal end of the femur by insertion of the bone marrow needle into the trochanteric fossa. Make a small skin incision over the trochanteric fossa just medial to the summit of the trochanter major. Insert the bone marrow aspiration needle medial to the trochanter major, and place the long axis of the needle parallel to the long axis of the femur.

Once the site is selected, grasp the needle firmly. Apply steady, slight pressure while alternately rotating the needle tip against the bone (fast, 180-degree clockwise and then counterclockwise movements). Begin with gentle pressure until the needle begins to seat into the bone. Gradually increase the pressure as the needle penetrates into the bone. Insert the bone marrow needle ½ inch into the femoral canal. Remove the stylet from the needle, and aspirate using a 12- or 20-mL syringe that contains a small volume (approximately 0.1 mL) of 4% EDTA. Use significant negative pressure, for example, by withdrawing the plunger of a 12-mL syringe to the 8- or 9-mL mark. COLLECTION OF MORE THAN 1 ML OF BONE MARROW IS UNNECESSARY. Collection of larger volumes may cause greater amounts of peripheral blood to enter the syringe, leading to hemodilution of the sample. Once collected, immediately transfer the aspirate to a watch glass containing approximately 0.25 mL of 4% EDTA. Immediately mix the sample well using the end of the syringe. This is also a good time to remove the bone marrow needle from the patient.

For accurate bone marrow interpretation, it is important that smears contain marrow particles. Marrow particles (also called spicules) appear as tiny grains within the sample and can be visualized in the watch glass. Prepare slides in a manner similar to that used for peripheral blood smears. Preparation of 5 to 8 quality slides for submission is customary. Smears are air-dried. Slides may be stained using the same stains used for peripheral blood smears.

Feline

Accessible sites for bone marrow sampling in the cat are the iliac crest, the head of the humerus, and the proximal end of the femur via the trochanteric fossa. The techniques described for the dog can be used; however, caution is advised against using vigorous restraint with a severely anemic cat because such restraint may precipitate severe cyanosis, apnea, and cardiac arrest. Adequate sedation with supplemental oxygen administration and local anesthesia may be indicated.

Make smears of bone marrow immediately after aspiration of material. Extrinsic thromboplastin present in bone marrow tissue will cause the marrow to clot within 30 seconds. In addition, small pieces of marrow can be fixed in formalin for histologic preparation. Staining with new methylene blue, Wright's, May-Grünwald, or Giemsa stain may be used. A peroxidase stain may be helpful in differentiating granulocytic elements from lymphocytes.

Another method is to aspirate the bone marrow into a syringe containing 0.25 mL of 4% EDTA solution. Expel the aspirate, up to 1 mL, into a sterile Petri dish, from which the marrow particles can be isolated easily by aspirating an aliquot with a glass pipette, placing an appropriate volume onto several glass slides, making the smear, and then staining.

Additional Reading

Crow S, Walshaw S: *Manual of clinical procedures in the dog, cat, and rabbit,* ed 2, Philadelphia, 1997, Lippincott-Raven.

McSherry LJ: Techniques for bone marrow aspiration and biopsy. In Ettinger SJ, Feldman EC, editors: *Textbook of veterinary internal medicine,* ed 6, St Louis, 2005, Elsevier-Saunders.

Meyer D, Harvey J: *Veterinary laboratory medicine,* ed 3, St Louis, 2004, Elsevier-Saunders.

CYTOPATHOLOGIC SPECIMEN COLLECTION TECHNIQUES

(See also Section 5 for additional information on slide preparation of samples to be submitted for cytopathologic examination.)

Cytopathology involves a simple, direct, and inexpensive technique that can yield significant diagnostic information within a short time at minimal direct cost.

Cytologic examination can be made of material obtained from pustules, vesicles, or the raw, ulcerated, or cut surfaces of a lesion. To make the smear, press a clean microscope slide firmly against a raw or ulcerated lesion to transfer cellular material to the slide. Exudates may be collected by sterile swab or may be aspirated into a sterile syringe. Roll the swab gently across the slide, or place a drop of fluid from the syringe onto the slide and carefully spread the fluid in a uniform film. Transfer material from a block of tissue to the slide by gently pressing the tissue onto the slide in several locations. Use various stains for different conditions.

Rapid stains such as new methylene blue or a quick Romanowsky's-type stain (e.g., Diff-Quik) are useful and convenient for office procedures. Even Wright's and Gram stains for evaluation of bacteria in tissues/fluids are easy to use. The presence of many bacteria, especially mixed types, may mean only surface contamination, whereas single types of bacteria, abundant polymorphonuclear WBCs, and especially phagocytosis support the diagnosis of infection and the host response to it. A *few* acantholytic cells (loose epidermal cells) in the smear may be compatible with infectious processes, but large numbers, or "rafts," of acantholytic cells are highly suggestive of pemphigus and imply the need for more complex tests for positive diagnosis.

Large numbers of eosinophils sometimes are found in stained smears. Contrary to popular opinion, they usually do not mean allergy. These cells are seen most commonly with furunculosis and may be associated with the eosinophilic granulomas, eosinophilic plaques, sterile eosinophilic pustulosis, pemphigus complex, and ectoparasites. Yeasts (usually *Malassezia*, rarely *Candida*) commonly are found as budding cells in masses of wax and debris from ear smears.

Tumor cells may be recognized in some impression or aspiration samples where Giemsa is a preferred stain. Although special expertise is needed, cases of mastocytoma, histiocytoma, and lymphoma are recognized most easily. Always prepare formalin-fixed tissues for histologic diagnosis in tumor evaluations (Box 4-4).

BOX 4-4   CYTOLOGIC FEATURES OF MALIGNANCY

Enlargement of nucleus/nuclei larger than 10 nm	Increase in size and number of nucleoli
Decreased nuclear/cytoplasmic ratio	Increased basophilia of cellular cytoplasm-
Multinucleation because of abnormal mitosis	increased RNA content
Abnormal or frequent mitosis	Anisokaryosis or pleomorphism
Variations in size and shape of nuclei	Multinucleated giant cells

---

Fine-needle aspiration

The ability to aspirate cells from normal and abnormal tissue, apply them to a glass slide, stain the smear, and review the results is among the most useful, cost-effective diagnostic procedures available in clinical practice. The most significant limiting factors are (1) the technical ability to prepare high-quality slides and (2) the ability to interpret the cytologic findings. Some experience is needed to obtain the skills needed to aspirate cells and make diagnostic preparations. Significant training is required to interpret the slides adequately. However, access to cytopathologists affiliated with diagnostic laboratories today makes fine-needle aspiration a highly useful diagnostic tool. The lymph node aspiration technique, described next, illustrates the finer points of the fine-needle aspiration technique.

Lymph node aspiration is a procedure that can, and should, be performed routinely in clinical practice. Follow proper technique to maximize the diagnostic use of this procedure. Lymph node aspiration typically is indicated (1) in patients with generalized lymphadenomegaly, (2) to evaluate abnormally enlarged solitary lymphnodes, and (3) in suspected instances of tumor metastases to lymph nodes. Surgically prepare the skin over the node from which a biopsy specimen is to be taken. With one hand, localize and immobilize the lymph node; with the other hand, guide the aspiration biopsy needle into the affected node. Affix a 6-mL syringe onto a 22- to 20-gauge needle (a 25-gauge needle can be used when the site to be aspirated is particularly small), and advance the needle into the lymph node. Withdrawal of the syringe to approximately 0.5 mL *before inserting it into the tissue* is recommended. Doing so helps to prevent expelling material when removing the sample from the tissue. When the needle is in position in the approximate center of the node, gradually draw negative pressure on the syringe to a level of 4 to 5 mL. Hold the negative pressure in place for a few seconds. Release, and then repeat 2 to 3 times. Before removing the needle from the tissue, release the negative pressure in the syringe (this is why it is recommended to have 0.25 mL of air prepositioned inside). DO NOT REMOVE THE SYRINGE FROM THE TISSUE WHILE MAINTAINING NEGATIVE PRESSURE because this can result in the aspiration of significant amounts of blood from the skin, thereby significantly diluting the sample with peripheral blood. Eject cellular material within the needle onto clean glass slides. Handle all aspirates gently. To make slides, place two slides together and pull the slides apart to avoid shearing the cells. Do not compress or force slides together. In addition, a biopsy of the lymph node can (and usually should) be performed as a means of confirming or supporting diagnostic decisions made on aspirates. Lymph node biopsies can be obtained easily and safely by punch (core) techniques (e.g., 4-mm skin biopsy punch) or Tru-Cut biopsy needle.

Exfoliative cytologic procedure

Also called "touch impression cytology," this technique entails preparing cytologic slides directly from the cut surface of incisional and excisional biopsy samples. Use a scalpel blade to make a full-thickness linear cut through the biopsy specimen. A fresh surface of the tissue of interest is exposed. Using forceps or a sterile needle, gently lay the tissue on a clean glass slide. DO NOT FORCE THE TISSUE ONTO THE SLIDE because this can significantly damage cells. Several imprints can be made from the same surface. As needed, make new cuts to obtain a fresh surface from which to exfoliate cells. Allow the slide to air dry completely. Apply conventional staining, and examine the specimen when it is dry. The remaining tissue, if not significantly damaged, can be submitted for histopathologic examination (recommended).

Scrapings and swabs

Depending on the tissue type and lesion, it may be possible to obtain diagnostic cytologic samples from scrapings (e.g., conjunctival epithelium for virus inclusions), brushes (e.g., material obtained during endoscopy), and swabs (e.g., ear and vaginal swabs). The cells, once harvested, can be applied delicately directly to a clean glass slide by carefully rolling or even by just touching the material to the slide to create a thin layer. Allow the sample to air-dry thoroughly before staining.

Fluids

Cytologic examination of fluids obtained with needle and syringe from body cavities, cysts, and urine typically require additional preparation in obtaining adequate cell concentration to make diagnostic decisions. Analyze fluid specimens with respect to protein and nucleated cell count and a morphologic description of the cells. If overall cell counts are low, centrifugation will be required to concentrate cellular material for analysis. After centrifugation, remove the supranatant (and save it). Resuspend the cells in 2 to 3 drops of the supranatant. Apply a single drop of the mixture to a glass slide and allow it to air dry. I prefer NOT to smear the liquid onto the slide; instead, I allow the liquid to run, by gravity, from one end of the slide to the other. After the liquid is thoroughly air-dried, it can be stained and reviewed.

ECTOPARASITES

Skin scraping

Skin scrapings frequently are obtained to find and identify microscopic parasites or fungal elements in the skin. Material required includes mineral oil in a small dropper bottle, a dull scalpel blade, glass slides, coverslips, and a microscope.

Select undisturbed, untreated skin for a scraping site. The best method is to scrape the periphery of skin lesions and avoid the excoriated or traumatized center areas. In scraping for demodectic mange, pinch a small fold of affected skin firmly and collect the surface material for examination. This procedure forces the mites out of the hair follicles and onto or near the skin surface. For sarcoptic mange, scrape large areas. Select sites on the elbows, hocks, and ear margins when searching for sarcoptic mange. Many or frequent scrapings may be necessary to demonstrate sarcoptic mange mites or their fecal pellets or eggs.

Place the accumulated material on a microscope slide and mix it with mineral oil. Examine the entire area with a ×10 objective thoroughly and carefully. Dry keratin and dead hairs also may be accumulated by scraping without mineral oil for inoculation of fungal cultures.

Acetate tape preparation

This is one of the simplest diagnostic procedures. Use clear (not frosted) acetate tape. Bend the tape into a loop around the fingers with the sticky side facing out. Part the animal's hair coat, and press the tape firmly onto the skin and hair around suspect lesions. The sticky tape picks up loose particles with which it makes contact. Cut the loop of tape and place the strip of tape sticky side down on a clean microscope slide. Use a low-power microscope to look through the tape at the collected particles. This technique is excellent for trapping and identifying biting and sucking lice, *Otodectes* and *Cheyletiella* mites, flea dirt and larvae, fly larvae, or dandruff scales.

Acetate tape also is useful for studying hair abnormalities. Use a strong hemostat to securely clamp and quickly avulse a group of 10 to 20 hair shafts. Press the pointed distal ends onto sticky acetate tape (lined up like pickets in a fence), and cut the hair shafts off in the middle with a scissors. Likewise, press the butt ends with the hair roots onto another piece of tape. Then press the tape holding the hair onto a microscope slide to allow low-power examination of the hairs through the clear tape. The tips of the hairs will be well oriented and controlled; thus, it is easy to evaluate whether the hairs are split, broken, or bitten off and whether the hair roots are in the anagen or telogen growth stage.

Additional Reading

Baker R, Lumsden JH: *Color atlas of cytology of the dog and cat,* St Louis, 2000, Mosby.
Burkhard MJ, Meyer DJ: Invasive cytology of internal organs: cytology of the thorax and abdomen, *Vet Clin North Am Small Anim Pract* 26:1203, 1996.
Cowell R: *Diagnostic cytology of the dog and cat,* St Louis, 1998, Mosby-Year Book.
Ehrhart N: Principles of tumor biopsy, *Clin Tech Small Anim Pract* 13:1998.

4

URINE COLLECTION TECHNIQUES

Urine can be removed from the bladder by one of four methods: (1) naturally voided (aka, the "free catch"), (2) manual compression of the urinary bladder (aka, expressing the bladder), (3) catheterization, or (4) cystocentesis.

For routine urinalysis, collection of urine by natural micturition is often satisfactory. The major disadvantage is the contamination of the sample with cells, bacteria, and other debris located in the genital tract. Discard the first portion of the stream because it contains the most contamination and debris. Voided urine samples are not recommended when bacterial cystitis is suspected.

Manual compression of the bladder may be used to collect urine samples from dogs and cats. Do not use excessive digital pressure; if moderate digital pressure does not induce micturition, discontinue the technique. The technique can be difficult to use in male dogs and male cats.

Urinary catheters are hollow tubes made of rubber, plastic, nylon, latex, or metal and are designed to serve four purposes:
1. To relieve urinary retention
2. To test for residual urine

3. To obtain urine directly from the bladder for diagnostic purposes
4. To perform bladder lavage and instillations

The size of catheters (diameter) usually is calibrated in the French scale; each French unit is equivalent to roughly 0.33 mm. The openings adjacent to the catheter tips are called "eyes." Human urethral catheters are used routinely in male and female dogs; 4F to 10F catheters are satisfactory for most dogs (Table 4-6). Catheters should be individually packaged and sterilized by autoclaving or ethylene oxide gas.

Catheterization of the male dog

Equipment needed to catheterize a male dog includes a sterile catheter (4F to 10F, 18 inches long, with one end adapted to fit a syringe), sterile lubricating jelly, povidine-iodine soap or benzalkonium chloride, sterile rubber gloves or a sterile hemostat, a 20-mL sterile syringe, and an appropriate receptacle for the collection of urine.

Proper catheterization of the male dog requires two persons. Place the dog in lateral recumbency on either side. Pull the rear leg that is on top forward, and then flex it (Figure 4-13). Alternatively, long-legged dogs can be catheterized easily in a standing position.

Next, retract the sheath of the penis and cleanse the glans penis with a solution of povidone-iodine 1%, triclosan (Septisol), benzalkonium chloride, or bichloride of mercury solution diluted 1:1000. Lubricate the distal 2 to 3 cm of the appropriate-size catheter with sterile lubricating jelly. Never entirely remove the catheter from its container while it is being passed because the container enables one to hold the catheter without contaminating it. The catheter may be passed with sterile gloved hands or by using a sterile hemostat to grasp the catheter and pass it into the urethra. Alternatively, cut a 2-inch "butterfly" section from the end of the thin plastic catheter container. This section can be used as a cover for the sterile catheter, and the clinician can use the cover to grasp and advance the catheter without using gloves.

If the catheter cannot be passed into the bladder, the tip of the catheter may be caught in a mucosal fold of the urethra or there may be a stricture or block in the urethra. In small breeds of dogs, the size of the groove in the os penis may limit the size of the catheter that can be passed. One also may experience difficulty in passing the catheter through the urethra where the urethra curves around the ischial arch. Occasionally, a catheter of small diameter may kink and bend on being passed into the urethra. When the catheter cannot be passed on the first try, reevaluate the size of the catheter and gently rotate the catheter while passing it a second time. Never force the catheter through the urethral orifice.

4

TABLE 4-6	Recommended Urethral Catheter Sizes for Routine Use in Dogs and Cats	
Animal	Urethral catheter type	Size (French units*)
Cat	Flexible vinyl, red rubber, or Tom Cat catheter (polyethylene)	3.5
Male dog (≤25 lb)	Flexible vinyl, red rubber, or Polyethylene	3.5 or 5
Male dog (≥25 lb)	Flexible vinyl, red rubber, or Polyethylene	8
Male dog (>75 lb)	Flexible vinyl, red rubber, or Polyethylene	10 or 12
Female dog(≤10 lb))	Flexible vinyl, red rubber, or Polyethylene	5
Female dog (10–50 lb)	Flexible vinyl, red rubber, or Polyethylene	8
Female dog(>50 lb)	Flexible vinyl, red rubber, or Polyethylene	10, 12, or 14

*The diameter of urinary catheters is measured on the French (F) scale. One French unit equals roughly 0.33 mm.
From Crow S, Walshaw S: Manual of Clinical Procedures in the Dog, Cat and Rabbit, ed 2, Philadelphia, Lippincott-Raven, 1997.

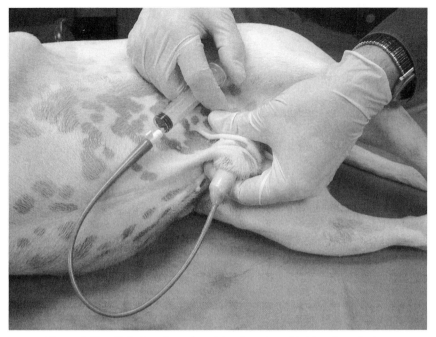

Figure 4-13: Technique for catheterizing the urinary bladder of a male dog.

4

Effective catheterization is indicated by the flow of urine at the end of the catheter, and a sterile 20-mL syringe is used to aspirate the urine from the bladder. Walk the dog immediately following catheterization to encourage urination.

Catheterization of the female dog

Equipment needed to catheterize a female dog includes flexible human ureteral or urethral catheters identical to those used in the male dog. Sterile metal or plastic female catheters also can be used; however, they tend to traumatize the urethra. The following materials also should be on hand: a small nasal speculum, a 20-mL sterile syringe, lidocaine 0.5%, sterile lubricating jelly, a focal source of light, appropriate receptacles for urine collection, and 5 mL of povidone-iodine solution.

Use strict asepsis. Cleanse the vulva with a solution of povidone-iodine, benzalkonium chloride, or bichloride of mercury diluted 1:1000. Instillation of lidocaine 0.5% into the vaginal vault helps to relieve the discomfort of catheterization. The external urethral orifice is 3 to 5 cm cranial to the ventral commissure of the vulva. In many instances, the female dog may be catheterized in the standing position by passing the female catheter into the vaginal vault, despite the fact that the urethral tubercle is not visualized directly.

In the spayed female dog in which blind catheterization may be difficult, the use of an otoscope speculum and light source (Figure 4-14) or an anal speculum with a light source will help to visualize the urethral tubercle on the floor of the vagina. In difficult catheterizations, it may be helpful to place the animal in dorsal recumbency (Figure 4-15 and 4-16). Insertion of a speculum into the vagina almost always permits visualization of the urethral tubercle and facilitates passage of the catheter. Take care to avoid attempts to pass the catheter into the fossa of the clitoris because this is a blind, possibly contaminated cul-de-sac.

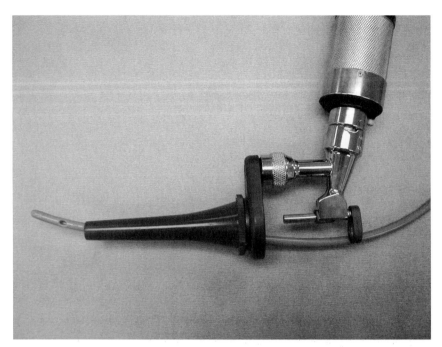

Figure 4-14:   An otoscope speculum with attached light source provides excellent visualization of the urethral orifice in a female dog. Note the position of the otoscope handle (see Figure 4-15).

4

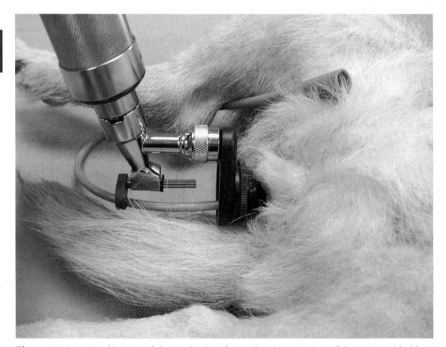

Figure 4-15:   Visualization of the urethral orifice and catheterization of the urinary bladder in a female dog is accomplished using an otoscope with a sterile speculum attached. Note: the patient is in dorsal recumbency with the otoscope handle positioned upwards.

Catheterization of the male cat

Before attempting urinary bladder catheterization of the male cat, administer a short-term anesthetic (e.g., ketamine, 25 mg/kg IM), but only after a careful assessment of the cat's physical status. Males cats with urethral obstruction (partial or complete) may have underlying renal or hepatic disease that precludes the use of a dissociative anesthestic. In such patients, administration of an inhalation anesthetic only may be required. In addition, a topical anesthetic such as a topical ophthalmic anesthetic solution (proparacaine) can be administered directly into the urethral orifice to minimize discomfort. Place the anesthetized patient in dorsal recumbency. Gently grasp the ventral aspect of the prepuce and move it caudally in such a manner that the penis is extruded. Withdraw the penis from the sheath and gently pull the penis backward. Pass a sterile, flexible plastic or polyethylene (PE 60 to 90) catheter or 3- to 5-inch, 3.5F urethral catheter into the urethral orifice and gently into the bladder, keeping the catheter parallel to the vertebral column of the cat. Never force the catheter through the urethra. The presence of concretions within the urethral lumen may require the injection of 3 to 5 mL of sterile saline to back-flush urinary "sand" or concretions so that the catheter can be passed.

Catheterization of the female cat

Urinary bladder catheterization of the female cat is not a simple procedure. However, when indicated, only attempt the technique in the anesthetized cat using the same technique described for the male cat. Take care to assess the health of the patient before administering the anesthetic. Urinary bladder catheterization can be accomplished with the use of a rubber or plastic, side-hole (blunt-ended) urinary catheter. The same catheter type used in male cats is effective in female cats. Instilling lidocaine 0.5% has been recommended as a means of decreasing sensitivity to the required manipulations and catheter insertion. However, if the cat is anesthetized adequately, this additional step is neither helpful nor necessary. Cleanse the vulva with an appropriate antiseptic. Catheterization can be accomplished with the cat in dorsal or ventral recumbency. Experience and size of the cat dictates which technique works best. Because the likelihood of successfully catheterizing a female cat's urinary bladder using a blind technique is low, a speculum is strongly recommended. However, there are only limited types of small-diameter speculums that are suitable. An inexpensive technique entails use of a sterilized otoscope speculum, with attached light source to facilitate visualization of the urethral orifice (Figure 4-16). Insert the catheter through the speculum and into the urethra. The most significant drawback to this technique comes when using the male cat, polyurethane urinary catheter. The diameter of the otoscope speculum may not allow withdrawal of the speculum over the expanded end of the urinary catheter. A soft, rubber catheter, however, can be pulled through even the smallest otoscope speculum and is recommended when necessary to remove the speculum completely and leave the catheter in place. Once the urethral orifice can be visualized, pass the catheter into the orifice until urine flow is established.

Indwelling urethral catheter

For continuous urine drainage, use a closed collection system to help prevent urinary tract infection. A soft urethral or Foley catheter can be used, and polyvinyl chloride tubing should be connected to the catheter and to the collection bottle outside the cage. The collection bottle should be below the level of the animal's urinary bladder. Place an Elizabethan collar on the animal to discourage chewing on the catheter and associated tubing. Apply antibacterial ointment to the urethral orifice. Despite care of the catheter, urinary tract infection still may develop in any patient fitted with an indwelling urinary catheter. Ideally, replace catheters after 48 to 72 hours. Prophylactic antimicrobial therapy is indicated in any dog or cat in which a urinary catheter is in place for more than 48 hours. Observe the animal for development of fever, discomfort, pyuria, or other evidence of urinary tract infection. If infection is suspect, remove the catheter and submit the catheter tip for culture and sensitivity or determination of minimum inhibitory concentration (MIC).

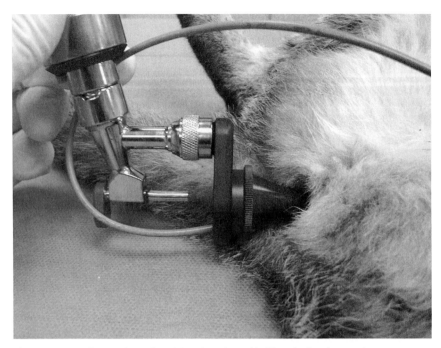

Figure 4-16: Technique for catheterizing the urinary bladder of a female cat using an otoscope speculum and light source.

4

Cystocentesis

Cystocentesis is a common clinical technique used to obtain a sample of urine directly from the urinary bladder of dogs and cats *when collecting a voided, or free-catch, aliquot is not preferred.* The procedure is indicated when necessary to obtain bladder urine for culture purposes. Urine that is collected by free catch has passed through the urethra and may be contaminated with bacteria, thereby making interpretation of the culture results difficult. Cystocentesis also is performed as a convenience when it is desirable to obtain a small sample of urine but the patient is not ready or cooperative.

Generally, cycstocentesis is a safe procedure, assuming the patient is cooperative and the bladder can be identified and stabilized throughout the procedure. However, injury and adverse reactions can occur. In addition to lacerating the bladder with the inserted needle (patient moves abruptly), the needle can be passed completely through the bladder and into the colon (improper technique) risking bacterial contamination of the bladder or peritoneal cavity.

Cystocentesis involves insertion of a needle, with a 6- or 12-mL syringe attached, through the abdominal wall and bladder wall to obtain urine samples for urinalysis or bacterial culture. The technique prevents contamination of urine by urethra, genital tract, or skin and reduces the risk of obtaining a contaminated sample. Cystocentesis also may be needed to decompress a severely overdistended bladder temporarily in an animal with urethral obstruction. In these cases, cystocentesis should be performed only if urethral catheterization is impossible. WARNING: Penetration of a distended urinary bladder with a needle could result in rupture of the bladder.

To perform cystocentesis, clip and surgically prepare the skin over the cystocentesis site on the ventral abdomen. Perform cystocentesis by placing the needle in the ventral abdominal wall slightly (3 to 5 cm) cranial to the junction of the bladder with the urethra. Insert the needle at a 45-degree angle (Figure 4-17). The bladder must contain a sufficient volume

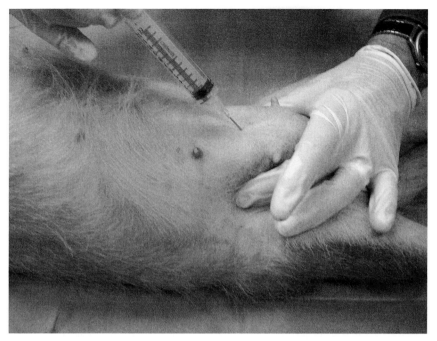

Figure 4-17: Technique for performing cystocentesis in a dog.

of urine to permit palpation through the abdominal wall before cystocentesis. Use one hand to hold the bladder steady within the peritoneal cavity while the other guides the needle.

Although this procedure is relatively safe, the bladder must have a reasonable volume of urine, the procedure should not be made without first identifying and immobilizing the bladder. For the procedure to be performed safely and quickly, the patient *must* be cooperative. If collection of a urine sample by cystocentesis is absolutely necessary, sedation may be indicated to restrain the patient adequately for the procedure.

Additional Reading

Crow S, Walshaw S: *Manual of clinical procedures in the dog, cat, and rabbit,* ed 2, Philadelphia, 1997, Lippincott-Raven.

Osborne CA, Finco DR: *Canine and feline nephrology and urology,* Baltimore, 1995, Williams & Wilkins.

DERMATOLOGIC PROCEDURES

SKIN BIOPSY

Obtaining a skin biopsy from abnormal skin only to receive a nondiagnostic result as reported from a pathologist suggests that improved biopsy technique may culminate in collecting a specimen with higher diagnostic value. The following guidelines apply when performing skin biopsies:

- Consider obtaining multiple samples from multiple sites, which is especially useful when different stages of similar lesions are identifiable.
- Do *not* perform a surgical scrub before collecting the sample; shaving the hair away is fine, but surgically prepared skin removes superficial lesions that, had they been left in place, might have been diagnostic.

- Biopsy of lesions that are *depigmenting* should be done before they have turned white; the absence of color usually denotes absence of active skin lesions; biopsies from completely depigmented skin are less likely to demonstrate active lesions.
- Biopsy of lesions associated with alopecia should be done in the center of the most alopecic area.
- Also, biopsy of lesions associated with alopecia should be done at junctional (between normal- and abnormal-appearing) skin.
- Consider submitting biopsies from completely nonaffect, normal-appearing skin.
- Avoid biopsies from ulcerated skin areas.

Biopsies may be made with a scalpel blade (incisional or excisional) or a dermatologic punch biopsy. Punch biopsy instruments are circular blades available in 4-mm, 6-mm, and 8-mm diameter sizes (Figure 4-18). Hold the punch perpendicular to the skin site of interest. A back-and-forth motion that rotates the circular blade cuts through the skin. When the skin no longer moves as the punch is rotated, the biopsy is complete and the skin sample may be removed (from the skin or from the biopsy instrument). Avoid grasping the dermis/epidermis of the sample with any instrument to prevent crushing of the sample and causing artifact. If the sample must be lifted, use the attached subcutaneous fat only.

If the lesion of interest is deep, the punch biopsy technique may not be effective. In this situation, an incisional or excisional biopsy using a sterile No. 10 or No. 15 surgical blade is indicated. Biopsies of ulcerated skin and solitary nodules are best done by removing a wedge of skin (incisional biopsy). In some cases, it is possible surgically to remove all visible, palpable parts of the lesion (excisional biopsy). Place each sample of skin in buffered formalin, using a volume that is at least 10 times that of the sample size. If particularly large areas of skin are harvested during biopsy, cut these into 1-cm thick pieces before placing them into formalin.

Alternatively, it is possible, and in many cases important, to evaluate a biopsy of skin or subcutaneous tissue at the time of collection. When the lesion of interest is suspected to be neoplastic, quickly differentiating between inflammatory cells and neoplasia may be possible by simply performing an exfoliative cytologic examination (see Section 5) on one of the biopsy samples *in addition to* fixing a separate sample in formalin and submitting it for histopathologic examination. Exfoliated cells on a glass slide are air-dried and stained with a quick Romanowsky's-type stain (e.g., Diff-Quick). Generally, biopsy samples that have been subjected to the additional handling required to make impressions on a glass slide are not good candidates for subsequent fixation and histopathologic examination. One strong

4

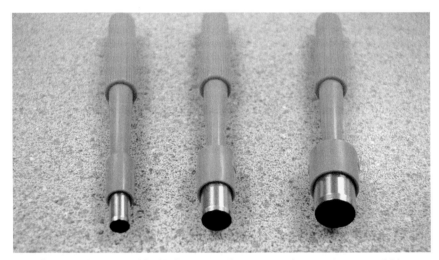

Figure 4-18:   Disposable skin biopsy punches: 4-, 6-, and 8-mm sizes are available.

recommendation is to perform exfoliative cytologic and histopathologic examinations on separate samples.

SKIN SCRAPING

Superficial skin scraping

Among the most common diagnostic procedures carried out on the skin of dogs and cats is a routine skin scraping. Yet despite the frequency this test is used, doing a skin scraping in such a manner that the sample recovered maximizes the opportunity to establish a diagnosis can be anything but routine. A skin scraping, properly done, does require using consistent techniques appropriate to the suspected diagnoses, and as such, superficial or deep scrapings, or both, may be indicated.

Skin scraping is indicated whenever ectoparasite infestation is suspected. Superficial scrapings are appropriate for detecting mites that live on the skin surface, such as *Cheyletiella* spp. and *Otodectes cynotis*, as well as those mites that burrow within the outermost layers of skin (stratum corneum), such as *Sarcoptes* spp. and *Notoedres cati*.

Because the area to be scraped is relatively large (≥ 2 cm^2), shave dogs and cats with long-hair coats before attempting the procedure, unless *Chyletiella* infestation is suspected. Make the scraping over healthy-appearing skin. Do *not* cleanse the skin of superficial scale or crusts. The technique for superficial skin scraping entails the use of mineral oil or pyrethrin ear drops applied to a clean scalpel blade *and* directly onto the area of skin to be scraped. Scraping begins as a gentle motion made in the direction of the hair coat. Gradually increase the pressure of the blade against the skin with repetitive scrapings over the same area. Take care not to lacerate the skin, although minor capillary bleeding at the site is common. Transpose material collected on the edge of the blade to a clean glass slide, cover it with a coverslip, and thoroughly examine the material under low magnification for evidence of ectoparasites. Note that for mites such as *Chyletiella* or scabies, finding just one mite or one egg is diagnostic and justifies implementing treatment.

Deep skin scraping

A slightly different technique is indicated in dogs and cats suspected of having an infestation that includes *Demodex canis* mites. The mites are known to live predominantly in sebaceous glands and hair follicles. They can survive in the skin of animals without manifesting lesions. Hair loss and skin lesions develop where overgrowth of the mite population occurs. *Demodex* infestations can be localized or generalized; infestations can occur in either dogs or cats but the most severe, generalized infestations are much more likely to occur in young dogs.

Although both superficial and deep skin scrapings may reveal the presence of mites on the skin, deep scrapings may reveal *Demodex* mites in some patients when superficial scrapings are negative. The technique for deep skin scraping targets a small area of skin (≤ 2 cm^2). It may be helpful to apply gentle pressure to the skin or actually to squeeze the area of interest between the thumb and a finger in at attempt to force mites from the deeper to the more superficial skin. In some breeds (e.g., Old English Sheepdogs and shar peis) recovering mites on a skin scraping can be particularly difficult. In such cases, where *Demodex* infestation is highly suspected but the results of repeated skin scrapings are negative, a skin biopsy is appropriate. Alternatively, a procedure called a *trichogram* that involves pulling (plucking) a few hairs from the hair follicles using a hemostat may be diagnostic. Once the hairs are plucked from the skin, place them on a glass slide that has been preprepared with a drop of mineral oil, add a coverslip, and examine the hair shaft under low magnification. Half of all dogs with *Demodex* infestation will have a positive trichogram.

Additional Reading

Baker R, Lumsden JH: The skin. In Baker R, Lumsden JH, editors: *Color atlas of cytology of the dog and cat,* St Louis, 2000, Mosby.

Bettenay SV, Mueller RS: Skin scraping and skin biopsies. In Ettinger SJ, Feldman EC, editors: *Textbook of veterinary internal medicine,* ed 6, St Louis, 2005, Elsevier-Saunders.

Campbell KL: Other external parasites. In Ettinger SJ, Feldman EC, editors: *Textbook of veterinary internal medicine,* ed 6, St Louis, 2005, Elsevier-Saunders.

EAR CLEANING: EXTERNAL EAR CANAL

Certainly not all dogs and cats with otitis externa require comprehensive ear flushing and debridement before or as part of the therapy. In many cases, home treatment is sufficient to resolve the problems effectively, assuming the underlying diagnosis has been established. However, in patients with chronic or particularly severe infections, topical treatment administered by the owners at home may not be sufficient. In such cases, the external ear canal requires a careful and comprehensive cleaning before administration of topical medications.

Properly perfomed, flushing and cleaning of the external ear canals is not a quick procedure. Anesthetize the patient. Attempting to perform a thorough ear cleansing under sedation usually will not be successful. Once the animal is anesthetized, perform a careful otoscopic (or videootoscopic) examination to establish the integrity of the ear canal, such as the presence or absence of tumors and mites. In severe cases, the tympanic membrane may not even be visible.

With the patient in lateral recumbency, flush the ear canal (Figure 4-19) or lavage it with warm saline initially, and then aspirate the material from the canal. If this procedure is not successful in removing the debris attached to the epithelium of the ear canal, use ceruminolytic ear solutions to facilitate breakdown and removal of this material. A 5-minute instillation and soak is recommended, followed by thorough flushing to remove debris and the ceruminolytic material. Remove hair growing inside the ear canal with forceps. A suction apparatus is recommended for removal of debris and liquid remaining.

Reintroduce an otoscope to examine the integrity of the skin in the ear canal and to look for any evidence of stenosis, foreign body, or tumor. The flushing process is *not* complete until it is possible to visualize the tympanic membrane. Carefully remove any remaining debris with an otologic loop (Figure 4-20), not a cotton-tipped swab.

4

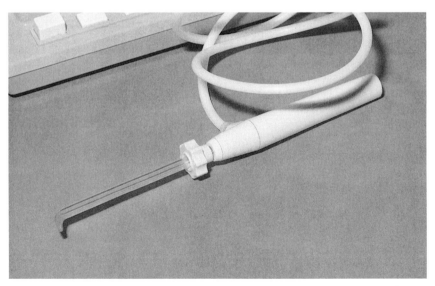

Figure 4-19:   Low-pressure water jet system used to flush the external ear canal in anesthetized patients.

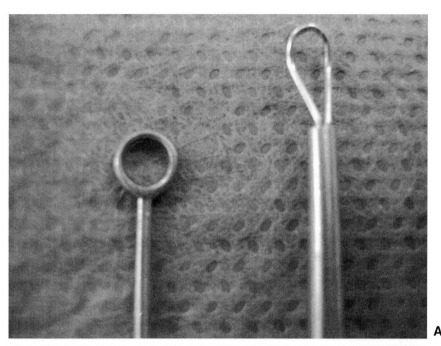

A

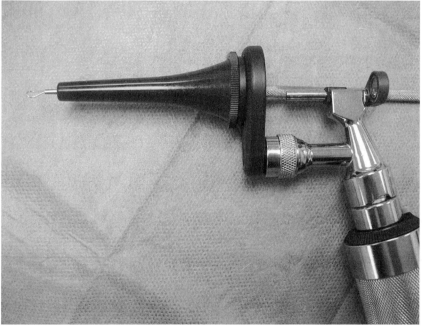

B

Figure 4-20: A, Otologic loops used to remove debris from the external ear canal. **B,** Placement of an otologic loop through the specululm of an otoscope facilitates removal of debris deep in the external ear canal.

Repeat the procedure on the opposite ear as indicated. At the conclusion of the examination, apply appropriate topical medication into the ear canal before allowing the patient to recover from anesthesia. Systemic therapy or surgical intervention may be required in some patients for complete resolution of the problem. However, a thorough examination and cleaning is critical before actually making decisions regarding medical versus surgical intervention.

Additional Reading

Gortel K: Ear flushing. In Ettinger SJ, Feldman EC, editors: *Textbook of veterinary internal medicine,* ed 6, St Louis, 2005, Elsevier-Saunders.

Taibo RA: *Otology: clinical and surgical issues,* Buenos Aires, 2003, Intermedica.

ENDOTRACHEAL INTUBATION

In selecting an appropriate-sized endotracheal tube, consider the size of the animal and select the size of tube that has the largest diameter that can be inserted without force (Table 4-7). The use of high-volume, low-pressure cuffs on endotracheal tubes is better. Overinflation of the endotracheal tube cuff can cause tracheal ulceration, tracheitis, hemorrhage, tracheomalacia, fibrosis, stenosis, and subcutaneous emphysema. Occlusion of high-volume, low-pressure cuffs can be achieved at 25 mm Hg or less.

Always check the cuff of a cuffed tube to ensure that there are no leaks and that the cuff is working properly before intubation. Lubricate the selected endotracheal tube with water or lubricating jelly. Do not intubate the animal until after induction of anesthetic drugs. Intubation in the dog or cat may cause an increase in sympathetic activity or vagal stimulation and result in cardiac dysrhythmias. Administer atropine or glycopyrrolate to canine and feline patients to avoid dysrhythmias associated with intubation.

Following appropriate administration of anesthetic and parasympatholytic drugs, place the patient in lateral or sternal recumbancy and elevate the head. Measure the tube from the mouth to the level of the carina. The person inserting the tube should pull out the tongue, holding the tongue with a piece of gauze to improve handling and stability. Use caution to not lacerate the tongue on the lower incisors. Place the tip of a laryngoscope at the base of the tongue at the glossoepiglottic fold. Use small pediatric blades for cats and small dogs and larger blades for larger dogs. Press the tip of the laryngoscope ventrally to move the epiglottis and expose the glottis. Directly visualize the arytenoid cartilages, and then pass the tube through the arytenoid cartilages into the trachea using a slight twisting motion. If the arytenoid cartilage spasms shut during attempt at intubation, place a drop or two of 2% lidocaine on the arytenoid cartilages to help facilitate passing the tube.

4

TABLE 4-7 Recommended Sizes for Endotracheal Tubes

	Body weight (kg)	Magill size	French size	Internal diameter (mm)
Dogs	2	2	22	6
	4	4–5	26–28	8
	6	6–7	28–30	9
	9	8	32	10
	12	9–10	34–36	11–12
	14	9–10	34–36	11–12
	16	10–11	36–38	11–12
	18–20	11–12	38–44	12
Cats	1	00	13	4
	2	0	16	5
	4	1	20	5

Once inserted into the trachea, never advance the tube farther than the carina, or else one-lung (endobronchial) intubation can occur. Once the tube is in place, secure it in place with a loop of ½-inch white tape or muzzle gauze.

Additional Reading

Muir W, Hubbell J, Skarda R, et al: *Handbook of veterinary anesthesia,* ed 3, St Louis, 2000, Mosby.

INTRAVENOUS CATHETERIZATION

Contamination and infection at the catheterization site are common complications of indwelling venous catheters. Aseptic preparation of the site is therefore paramount. In emergency situations it may be necessary to perform catheterization under less than ideal circumstances and without time for adequate aseptic preparation. When the animal's condition is stabilized, remove the catheter and place it properly elsewhere.

Clip the hair or shave over a wide area to facilitate disinfection of the skin surface. Scrub the skin surface with a detergent solution for 1 to 2 minutes. Then remove the detergent with an iodine or alcohol solution, and spray the skin with an iodine-based solution. If it is necessary to maintain the aseptic conditions of the procedure, wear sterile gloves and drape the field with sterile towels or a fenestrated drape.

When placing the catheter, fix it in position. Do not allow the catheter to move in and out of the skin because this will predispose to mechanical vessel trauma and the introduction of bacteria. When the puncture site is a large flat surface such as the medial femoral area or neck, apply a tag of tape to the catheter at a point close to the puncture site and then suture the tape to the skin. Pass the adhesive tape around the entire circumference of the catheter, and then tape the catheter to the appendage. Additional tape may be applied to isolate the injection site from the underlying skin and to secure the catheter cap. Place an antibiotic-antifungal ointment at the puncture site and incorporate it into the dressing over the skin.

PERCUTANEOUS JUGULAR VEIN CATHETERIZATION

The immobilization procedure for the jugular vein is particularly important because of the tendency of the vein to roll in the loose subcutaneous tissues of the neck. Occlude the vein by digital pressure in the thoracic inlet so that the skin and underlying tissues are retracted toward the body. Extend the head to provide traction on the upper portion of the vein. All of this positioning is accomplished by a second person.

A catheter-inside-the-needle system is easy to maintain sterile, but the needle leaves a larger hole in the vessel than is filled by the remaining catheter, and early postcatheterization hemorrhage may be a problem. Locate the position of the vessel with one hand, and insert the needle subcutaneously with the other hand. Place the needle directly over the jugular vein and below the palpating index finger. Advance the needle steeply at first to secure the superficial wall of the vessel and then more parallel to the vein to allow insertion of the needle into the lumen without penetrating the deep wall of the vessel. Ascertain the position of the needle within the vein by feeling the needle "pop" through the vessel wall and seeing the reflux of blood into the catheter. If, after the initial plunge, the needle is not in the vessel lumen, withdraw the needle slowly. Penetration of the needle into the deep wall of the vein is a common occurrence. Constant traction on the syringe plunger will aspirate blood into the catheter if the needle passes back through the vessel lumen during withdrawal.

When it has been ascertained that the needle is within the lumen, gently thread the catheter into the vein without moving the vein or the needle. Insert the catheter to its full length. If the catheter cannot be advanced fully, consider that (1) the tip of the needle may not have been entirely within the vessel lumen, (2) the vessel and needle may have moved with respect to one another during the initial threading process, (3) the catheter may be caught at the thoracic flexure (change the position of the head), or (4) the catheter may be

4

caught in one of the tributaries to the front legs (change the position of the front leg). Exercise care when withdrawing the catheter through the needle. The catheter can catch on the needle bevel and be cut off, resulting in catheter embolization.

When the catheter has been inserted to the desired length, remove the needle from the skin and place the needle guard. Aspirate air from the catheter, and then flush the catheter with heparinized saline. If blood cannot be aspirated from the catheter, consider that (1) the catheter may be kinked or compressed by the needle guard, (2) the catheter tip may be against a vessel wall (withdraw the catheter slightly), (3) the catheter may be clotted (if the clot cannot be aspirated, remove the catheter), or (4) the catheter may not be in the vein.

Surgical Approach to Jugular Vein Catheterization

Make a skin incision over or next to the jugular vein. The normal jugular vein is superficial and usually rises with venous occlusion. Location of the jugular vein following repeated unsuccessful attempts at percutaneous catheterization is more difficult because of the resultant hematoma. The vein is always located in the middle of the hematoma, and there is a temptation to skirt the hematoma with the dissection procedure. The vein can be identified during blunt dissection by the appearance of an off-white longitudinal structure against the dark background of the hematoma.

Isolate the vein and suspend it by two sutures. Visually introduce the needle into the lumen of the vein, and take care not to penetrate the deep wall of the vessel. Insert the catheter and relax the proximal suture to allow passage of the catheter. Remove both stay sutures (the vein is not tied), and close the incision in a routine manner.

Maintenance of Indwelling Catheters

Re-dress indwelling catheters and inspect them every day. Discard all soiled bandage material. Clean the puncture site with antiseptic solutions and fresh antibiotic-antifungal ointment, and reapply the occlusive wrap. Inspect the skin puncture site and the vessel at each re-dressing. A very small ring of inflammation at the puncture site is normal. Excess inflammation, diffuse tissue swelling, expulsion of exudate from the puncture site upon palpation, and tenderness or pain upon palpation are signs of untoward effects of the indwelling catheter. Phlebitis may be caused by mechanical, chemical, or infectious irritation of the vein. Phlebitis is recognized as warm, erythematous skin overlying a tender, indurated vessel. Purulent thrombophlebitis is heralded by all of the signs of simple phlebitis plus free exudate, which may drain exteriorly with or without palpation or may drain internally and result in a severe septicemia. Thrombotic occlusion of the vessel is recognized by severe hardening (ropiness) of the vessel. Thromboembolic occlusion is associated with inability to infuse fluids by gravity and may result in severe subcutaneous fluid accumulation if the fluids are administered with a pump. Occult infection of the intravenous site may occur in the absence of local inflammatory, thrombotic, or exudative signs. Unexplained fever and leukocytosis may be the only early signs. The diagnosis may be confirmed by obtaining a culture of material from the catheter tip.

Remove the catheter if there is evidence of cellulitis, phlebitis, thrombosis, purulent thrombophlebitis, or catheter-associated bacteremia or septicemia; if the catheter ceases to function properly because of thrombosis or catheter occlusion by a clot or kink; after 3 days if there is another location to which it can be moved; if the patient begins to lick or chew at the bandages; and when it is no longer necessary (Box 4-5).

Infusion fluids and administration tubing must be sterile. Do not disconnect connections unless it is absolutely necessary, and then they must be disconnected aseptically. Clean all injection caps well with an antiseptic solution before needle insertion. Change the fluid bottles and all administration tubing every 1 to 2 days. Change tubing after blood or colloid infusion. Do not use the primary catheter or infusion line for the collection of blood samples except in emergencies. Clearly mark the fluid bottle if any drug or concentrate has been added to the bottle. In-line filters are not necessary for infection control for routine fluid administration.

BOX 4-5   HEPARINIZED SALINE FLUSH
Catheter patency can be maintained with 3-mL syringes preloaded with 2 to 3 mL of heparinized saline kept in a stock solution: Add 100 units of heparin to a single 50-mL bag of sterile saline (2 units heparin/ml saline).

PHYSICAL THERAPY

HYDROTHERAPY

Water baths or soaks are among the easiest and most versatile modes of physical therapy in small animal practice. Wet packs, water soaks, or whirlpool baths can be helpful in adding moisture to (hydrating) or removing moisture from (dehydrating) the skin. Cyclic repetitions of moistening and drying the skin many times a day serve to dehydrate (similar to the chapped lips and hands seen in human beings). Constant moisture hydrates and even macerates the skin.

Whirlpool baths are the most efficient and popular means of applying hydrotherapy and, often, antiseptic medication to the skin. Whirlpool baths combine moist heat, gentle massage, and the solvent properties of water, with or without the mechanical impact of water from a whirlpool, to remove dirt, pus, and necrotic debris. Dry or scaly skin is softened and moisturized. Whirlpools may increase edema and are contraindicated in acute traumatic and inflammatory conditions or in cases of impaired sensation or circulation (unless treated with extreme caution). Whirlpools are particularly beneficial for skin infections, chronic dryness, open or infected wounds, skin grafts, adhesions, arthritis, postsurgical fractures, amputations, muscle spasms, and stiff joints. This modality is especially useful for cleaning and stimulating the skin of patients that are predisposed to decubitus ulcers.

Place the patient in an appropriate water bath at a temperature of 39° to 42° C (102° to 108° F). A low-suds detergent or antiseptic solution (povidone-iodine, chlorine, chlorhexidine) can be added for cleansing or germicidal effects. Allow the water turbine to circulate the water around and against the affected parts for 10 to 15 minutes once or twice daily. Support and reassure the animal during treatment, and never leave an animal unattended. Following therapy, ensure that the tub and turbine are thoroughly cleaned and sanitized.

Commercial whirlpool baths or Jacuzzi-type agitators are a good investment for a busy practice. A less expensive alternative is a variable-temperature bath with agitation provided by a pressure hose.

HEAT THERAPY

NOTE: In the presence of trauma, swelling, and edema, circulation may be impeded and the application of heat may cause necrosis. Cold is more beneficial in the early acute stages of inflammation and edema (Box 4-6).

Superficial heat

Infrared radiation is produced by long-wave generators that glow red and produce heat that penetrates only 1 to 2 mm. Shortwave generators produce invisible light; their heat penetrates 10 to 12 mm and reaches blood-carrying layers of tissue, where the heat is dispersed by the circulation. Because of their penetration, short waves do not produce a burning sensation; however, one should check the skin meticulously during therapy to ensure that it is not overheated. A warm sensation is normal. If the skin feels hot to the touch, the heat is too intense. Shortwave therapy is contraindicated in acute trauma and inflammation. Superficial heat is beneficial for subacute and chronic problems, skin infections, and abscesses. Treat the animal for 15 to 20 minutes once or twice daily.

Hot packs or wet towels can be used to apply mild, gentle heat. The indications are the same as for infrared heat, but additional precautions are needed. Hot packs may spread contagious skin disease, and the weight of the packs in an insensitive area is more likely to cause burns or tissue damage. This modality has the advantage of providing moist heat,

---

BOX 4-6   THE BENEFITS OF HEAT IN PHYSICAL THERAPY

- Hyperemia and dilatation of cutaneous vessels
- Increase in pulse, blood pressure, and pulmonary ventilation
- Increased metabolite transfer across capillary membranes
- General muscle relaxation
- Sedative and analgesic effect
- Improved extensibility of connective tissue

---

which is particularly beneficial for chronic soft tissue problems such as arthritis, myositis, and contractures. Apply hot packs for 10 to 15 minutes several times a day. Check the skin under the packs frequently during therapy.

Whirlpool baths combine moist heat, gentle massage, and the solvent properties of water to remove dirt, pus, and necrotic debris. The moist heat is indicated especially for extensive involvement of musculoskeletal disorders. Warm water baths can be repeated 2 to 3 times daily for 10 to 15 minutes and often can be followed with a gentle massage and passive flexion and extension exercises to improve range-of-motion and soft tissue flexibility.

Deep heat

Shortwave diathermy transmits physical energy deep into tissues; because the body tissues resist the flow of high-frequency current (27 million cps [Hz]), heat is produced. In dissipating heat, there are marked vascular dilatation, sedation, analgesia, and relief of muscle spasm. However, edema may increase. Absolute contraindications are the presence of imbedded metal implants, ischemia, malignancy, and pregnancy. No water can be in the field, and splints and bandages must be removed. This therapy can result in electrical shock to the patient and technician, so all cables, electrodes, and other equipment must be in excellent condition. Safety cannot be overemphasized. Calibrate each unit and adjust units individually to produce only a sensation of warmth. Treatment is applied daily for 15 to 20 minutes.

Microwave techniques produce about the same effects as diathermy except that more localized heating occurs (one side of a joint may be treated at a time). Microwaves are more readily absorbed by water, so great care must be used around the eye or in the presence of edema to ensure that the effects are not excessive.

Ultrasound produces the deepest heat. Ultrasound produces mechanical vibrations (1 million/second) in the elastic media of the body. Ultrasonic waves are reflected from boundaries between different types of tissues. The vibrations produce a micromassage that accelerates fluid absorption by increasing permeability. Ultrasonic therapy can be dangerous if the intensity or application is concentrated too long in a small area. Burn or tissue destruction may result. Ultrasonic therapy is contraindicated in neoplasms, the eye, heart, spine, and brain; near growing bony epiphyses; and in acute infections. Otherwise, its beneficial effects are similar to those of other forms of deep heat. Ultrasound is indicated particularly for softening scar tissue and reducing the pain of neuromas and degenerative joint disease. Ultrasound can be used over and around metal implants.

Ultrasonic waves are applied via a transducer and using coupling medium such as water or contact gel. The transducer is moved constantly over a small area (usually 6 to 8 sq in, depending on the size of the transducer). Shaving of the skin before therapy is best, to enhance contact (or use a water bath).

The dose varies with each patient. Most ultrasonic generators have an output of 700,000 to 1 million Hz at intensities of 0.1 to 1.0 W/cm^2. Use of the lowest intensity possible is best. The maximum dose should be 1.0 W/cm^2 for 5 minutes of application to the affected tissues. This application can be repeated once daily for 5 days and then every other day for five treatments. Then the treatment should not be repeated for at least 1 month. Do not use ultrasonic therapy in acute injuries, inflammations, or infections.

For cervical intervertebral disease, use 0.3 W/cm^2 for 3 minutes daily for 5 days and then every other day for five treatments.

BOX 4-7   THE BENEFITS OF COLD IN PHYSICAL THERAPY

- Decreased tissue temperature
- Decreased blood flow, vasoconstriction
- Decreased tendency to edema
- Decreased delivery of nutrients, phagocytes
- Decreased phagocytic action
- Transient vasoconstriction followed by vasodilation and increased blood flow (brief cold applications)

For arthritis, bursitis, and myositis, use 0.2 W/cm^2 for 3 minutes for joints of the extremities. Repeat 2 times weekly.

Cold therapy

Cold can be applied by blowing cold air on the skin, by evaporation of volatile liquids from the skin, or by direct contact of the cooling substance with the skin surface (Box 4-7).

Cold reduces extravasation of blood and fluid into tissues after trauma, reduces pain and spasticity, and is indicated in acute traumatic and inflammatory conditions. Overtreatment with cold may produce maceration and frostbite. Prolonged cold produces a vascular response with stasis of blood, occlusion of vessels, and tissue anoxia and necrosis.

Cold packs over a damp towel applied to the affected area and covered with a folded dry towel to prevent rapid warming can be used for 15 to 20 minutes. Treatment is repeated several times daily. It is important to keep the rest of the patient's body warm, dry, and comfortable during treatment. Cold treatments are often more effective when alternated with heat treatments (immersion bath or moist warm packs). The combined treatment is most effective when heat for 3 to 4 minutes is alternated with 1 to 2 minutes of cold. This regimen can be repeated for 15 to 20 minutes and should always end with the hot phase.

Cold immersion baths for one or several extremities may be useful. The temperature should be 15.5° to 21° C (60° to 70° F) and can be decreased by adding ice or cold water. Continue treatment until the muscles are relaxed or the animal cannot tolerate the cold, usually 2 to 5 minutes. Modification of this technique can be used for heat stroke, but one must be careful not to overchill such patients.

ELECTROTHERAPY

Medical galvanism is the physiologic use of direct current. This treatment will produce the same effects as heat except that it has no tendency to produce edema. The treatment is beneficial for acute, subacute, or chronic traumatic and inflammatory problems such as arthritis, decubitus sores, neuralgia, tenosynovitis, or postfracture repair. Do not use electricity near the brain, heart, or neoplasms.

Low-intensity therapy (0.5 to 1.0 mA/sq in of electrode) is desirable. Electrodes should be wet and held in firm contact with the skin. No metal should be in or near the area being treated. Halfway through the treatment, reduce the intensity of current to zero, reverse the polarity, and the return the intensity to starting levels.

Electrical stimulation of partially or wholly innervated muscle is possible with alternating current. Intact or denervated muscle will contract when stimulated with interrupted pulses of direct current. These kinds of stimulation improve circulation and nutrition of the muscle, promote venous return, remove lymph, relax spasm, reduce edema, and assist in muscle reeducation. Muscle atrophy and weakness can be retarded or controlled. Each muscle or group of muscles can be stimulated 10 to 20 times for one procedure, depending on the condition. Avoid overtreatment.

MASSAGE THERAPY

Massage is the use of the hands and fingers to manipulate soft tissues. Massage usually is used in combination with heat, cold, or whirlpool treatments. Massage improves circulation, reduces edema, loosens and stretches fibrotic or contracted tissue, and has a soothing

4

or sedative effect. Do not use massage in acute, inflammatory, traumatic, and painful lesions or with tumors, hemorrhages, and perhaps contagious conditions. Massage is indicated for tight or contracted tendons, ligaments, or muscles; chronic traumatic or inflammatory problems; and subacute or chronic edema.

In performing massage, keep the strokes in the direction of venous flow. Firm, rapid pressure tends to be stimulating, whereas slow, light strokes are soothing. Some type of lubricating powder or oil can be used to reduce friction. The massage can be stroking, kneading, or applied with friction. Stroking and kneading assist circulation, whereas friction and kneading tend to loosen adhesions and scars and to stretch tissues. Massage should last 15 or 20 minutes and can be repeated several times daily if desired.

EXERCISE THERAPY

Therapeutic exercise should strengthen musculoskeletal function, improve range-of-motion flexibility, improve endurance or coordination, and increase cardiovascular and respiratory capabilities. Never force exercise, but keep it within safe tolerance of the patient's cardiac and respiratory capacity. Active exercise (such as walking, running, or swimming) is most desirable because endurance and strength increase with repetition. Passive exercise is useful when paralysis or traumatic injuries preclude active exercise.

Never force movements, but use stabilization of parts and controlled pressure to activate only the structures of concern. When attempting to increase range of motion, use smooth, controlled pressure to move the joint slightly beyond its limited range; hold the stretch for a count of five, and slowly release the traction. Several repetitions can be performed 2 or 3 times daily. Gradual improvement can be expected within several weeks.

ADVANCED PROCEDURES

ABDOMINOCENTESIS

Abdominal paracentesis refers to the surgical puncture of the abdominal cavity for the purpose of removing fluids. Always weigh the animal before and after removing abdominal fluid. Any subsequent gain in weight indicates a reaccumulation of abdominal fluid. Place the animal in left lateral recumbency and restrain it in this position. Clip and surgically prepare a 1- to 3-inch square between the bladder and the umbilicus just lateral to the midline. If the bladder is distended, empty it before performing paracentesis. Infiltrate the paracentesis site with lidocaine 0.5% using a 22- to 25-gauge needle. In most cases, local anesthesia is not necessary. Abdominal puncture can be made with an 18- to 20-gauge needle. When the abdominal puncture has been made, allow the animal to rest quietly to facilitate drainage of the fluid. Some clinicians recommend tapping while the patient is in a standing position in the hope of obtaining more complete drainage. Changing the patient's position after the tapping may result in needle-tip laceration of intraabdominal organs. Aspiration may be easier if a specially adapted needle with multiple holes drilled in the shaft is used because it is less likely to become plugged with omentum. Ideally, tap four quadrants of the abdomen. Single-needle taps are not as accurate as instilling a lavage fluid (warmed lactated Ringer's solution) into the abdomen and examining the lavage fluid. Measure the amount of fluid obtained, and examine the fluid to determine whether it is an exudate or a transudate. Cytologic examination and culture also may be performed. Rather than drain the abdominal fluid completely, it may be better to spare protein loss and mobilize the fluids with diuretics. Paracentesis also can be performed by using a sterile intravenous catheter to enter the abdomen. When performing paracentesis, ultrasonographic guidance can prove valuable in placing the needle into the compartmental space desired and in avoiding complications. The major complications in abdominal paracentesis are perforated hollow viscus, laceration of abdominal organs, and iatrogenic peritonitis.

Additional Reading

Meyer DJ, Harvey J: *Veterinary laboratory medicine,* ed 3, St Louis, 2004, Saunders.

Rudloff E: Abdominocentesis and diagnostic peritoneal lavage. In Ettinger SJ, Feldman EC, editors: *Textbook of veterinary internal medicine,* ed 6, St Louis, 2005, Elsevier-Saunders.

BIOPSY TECHNIQUES: ADVANCED

Numerous biopsy techniques are available, and the selection of the appropriate technique is based on the tissue to be examined, the condition of the patient, and the skill of the examiner.

Excisional biopsy refers to the surgical removal of the entire lesion/organ with subsequent histologic examination. Excisional biopsy is used most frequently for skin lesions and cases in which an entire organ may have to be removed (such as an eye or an internal organ that has developed a tumor). *Incisional biopsy* refers to the surgical removal of a *portion* of a lesion with subsequent histologic examination. Choose a representative area of the lesion for biopsy. Include lesion margins, if possible. *Needle aspiration* refers to the use of needle and syringe to remove representative cells from the tissue/organ of interest. Specialized needles are available that allow removal of very small biopsies that can be submitted for histopathologic examination. (See also Cytopathologic Specimen Collection Techniques.)

NEEDLE BIOPSY TECHNIQUES: GENERAL CONSIDERATIONS

Needle biopsy or aspiration techniques refer to a variety of techniques used to obtain diagnostic tissue or cells from internal organs, including the lung, liver, spleen, pancreas, abdominal lymph nodes and mass lesions within the abdomen and thorax. In contrast, fine-needle aspiration is a technique generally used to recover cytopathologic samples (cells only) from skin or subcutaneous tissues (e.g., superficial lymph nodes). The advantage of needle biopsy is related directly to how well the abnormal tissue has been characterized and how easily it can be identified during the procedure. In addition, depending on patient cooperation, most procedures can be performed safely with the patient sedated only. Short-term intravenous anesthesia and general anesthesia eliminate undesired patient movement during the biopsy technique.

Potential lesions or abnormal tissues from which aspirate or biopsy samples are to be taken are located using palpation, radiographs, or ultrasound-guided imaging techniques. Shave the skin over the site of needle penetration and surgically prepare it. The type of sedation or anesthesia depends on the temperament of the animal and the site on which the biopsy will be performed. Attach a 22-gauge needle without stylet to a 12-mL syringe prefilled with 0.5 to 1.0 mL of air. Optionally, affix a flexible extension set to the needle and connect it proximally to the syringe. Needle length may vary from 1 to 3½ inches depending on the required depth of penetration and size of the patient. Guide the needle into the tissue/organ of interest. Stabilize the tip of the needle to avoid random movements through organs, especially highly vascular tissue such as liver and spleen. Once the needle is inserted, the aspiration techniques entails withdrawing the plunger of the syringe to the 7- or 8-mL level. Holding for that position for 1 to 2 seconds, and then releasing. Repeat the procedure. Depending on the nature of the lesion, it may not be indicated to thrust the needle into the tissue at multiple and different angles.

Neutralize the pressure in the syringe, and withdraw the needle rapidly. Expel any material within the needle onto glass slides using the air in the syringe. This same procedure can be repeated with a new needle to obtain an additional three to five samples from alternative sites. This technique allows samples to be obtained without applying negative pressure to the syringe, which may damage cells.

Ultrasound-guided needle aspirations from abdominal tissues greatly enhance the safety of this technique, especially when obtaining samples from smaller animals. Automatic-trigger needles such as Cook or Temno biopsy needles (14 to 18 gauge) are available for use in human beings but are seldom used in veterinary medicine. The risks associated with fine-needle aspiration include rupture of an encapsulated inflammatory process, dissemination of an infectious agent, seeding of neoplastic cells in the needle tract, and hemorrhage.

4

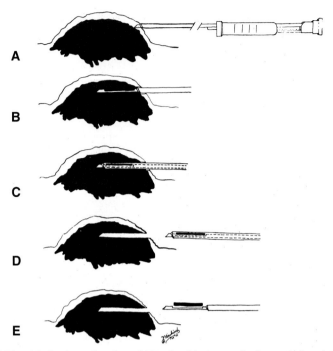

Figure 4-21:   Mechanism of action of Tru-Cut biopsy needle for typical nodular biopsy. A small skin incision is made with a No. 11 blade to allow insertion of the instrument. **A,** With the instrument closed, the outer capsule is penetrated. **B,** The outer cannula is fixed in place, and the inner cannula with specimen notch is thrust into the tumor. Tissue then fills the notch. **C,** The inner cannula now is fixed while the outer cannula is moved forward to cut off the biopsy specimen. **D,** The entire instrument is removed. **E,** The inner cannula is pushed ahead to expose tissue in the specimen notch.
(From Withrow SJ, Lowes N: Biopsy techniques in small animal oncology, *J Am Anim Hosp Assoc* 14:899-902, 1981.)

4

Larger volumes of fluid and cells can be placed directly into a vial containing EDTA to prevent clot formation. Prepare and examine direct and sedimentation specimens.

Needle biopsy of internal organs using the Tru-Cut needle is particularly useful in patients with subcutaneous (Figure 4-21) or cutaneous masses and for localized abdominal and thoracic mass lesions, diffuse liver, kidney, and splenic disease. Serious complications, usually hemorrhage or laceration of the gall bladder (during liver biopsy), can occur when the procedure is performed blindly. Therefore ultrasound-guided needle biopsy is strongly recommended whenever a percutaneous biopsy of internal organs is performed. Additional safety factors provided by ultrasound guidance include the ability to image, and avoid, large aberrant blood vessels.

Risk of complications associated with needle aspiration of the lung is considerably higher than for most abdominal procedures. Pneumothorax can occur following a single, "clean" aspiration attempt. See RESPIRATORY TRACT PROCEDURES for a detailed description of performing fine-needle aspiration of lung.

Additional Reading

Lumsden JH, Baker R: Cytopathology techniques and interpretation. In Baker R, Lumsden JH, editors: *Color atlas of cytology of the dog and cat,* St Louis, 2000, Mosby.

MacNeill AL, Alleman AR: Cytology of internal organs. In Ettinger SJ, Feldman EC, editors: *Textbook of veterinary internal medicine,* ed 6, St Louis, 2005, Elsevier-Saunders.

Menard M, Papgeorges M: Ultrasound-guided liver fine needle biopsies in cats: results of 307 cases, *Vet Pathol* 33:570, 1996.

Menard M, Papgeorges M: Fine needle biopsies: how to increase diagnostic yield, *Compend Contin Educ Pract Vet* 19:738, 1997.

Meyer D, Harvey J: *Veterinary laboratory medicine*, ed 3, St Louis, 2004, Elsevier-Saunders.

SKIN BIOPSY

Histologic examination of diseased skin can serve as a means for diagnosis of cutaneous lesions. The causative agent often is found in acute and chronic skin infections. Punch biopsy of the skin is a quick and accurate means of removing a small sample of diseased skin for histopathologic examination. Select a site that is well developed but not traumatized or excoriated. The sample should include little or no normal tissue. If the lesion (pustule, vesicle) can be identified early in its development and if the biopsy sample is taken only from the lesion, one may obtain a superior specimen. It is best not to take too large a sample that contains much normal skin; by mistake, the technician might take a section that misses the lesion. Proper selection of the biopsy site is crucial to accurate diagnosis. Carefully clip the hair from the lesion. Lightly blot the skin with 70% alcohol. Avoid superficial trauma while cleaning the skin. Inject a small subcutaneous bleb of 2.0% lidocaine to deaden the area. Special equipment needed for the biopsy includes a 4-mm, 6-mm, or 8-mm biopsy punch and 10% buffered formalin solution. After the area has been anesthetized with lidocaine, press and rotate the biopsy punch through the skin until the subcutaneous tissue is penetrated. Remove the biopsy specimen by "spearing" the subcutaneous fat with a fine needle. Do not grasp the specimen with a forceps. Blot the specimen gently between two paper towels. Spread the tissue out gently (like a pancake), place the specimen epidermal side up on a piece of cardboard or tongue depressor, press the specimen gently to cause adhesion, and drop the specimen into the formalin fixative. The skin defect may be closed with one or two simple interrupted sutures. If deep subcutaneous tissue or large biopsy samples are needed, a punch biopsy is inadequate. Use a small (No. 15) scalpel blade to obtain an appropriate sample. In all cases in which skin biopsies are made, take *multiple* samples to increase the odds that at least one will have diagnostic lesions. Specimens submitted to laboratories should be accompanied by extensive, detailed clinical information, including a differential diagnosis. Skin biopsies routinely are stained with hematoxylin-eosin; however, periodic acid–Schiff, Gomori's methenamine silver, and Verhoeff's stains are used for special problems.

LIVER BIOPSY

The diagnosis of liver disease can be made based on clinical signs coupled with clinicopathologic results obtained by laboratory finding, radiography, and abdominal ultrasound. The development of a more specific diagnosis and prognosis in liver disease may be aided greatly by information obtained in a liver biopsy. Percutaneous liver biopsies are of much greater value in generalized liver disease such as cirrhosis, generalized acute hepatic necrosis, or amyloidosis than in focal hepatic disease. The major indications for performing a liver biopsy are (1) to explain an abnormal liver profile, (2) to define reasons for abnormal liver size, (3) to identify a possible liver tumor, (4) to obtain a prognosis and rational approach to management, and (5) to identify the cause of ascites.

The procedures for obtaining liver tissue are numerous; however, needle biopsy of the liver, when performed properly, can be helpful. Careful physical and clinicopathologic examination should precede a liver biopsy. A normal coagulation profile should be documented on every patient undergoing liver biopsy. Detect and correct abnormalities in normal hemostatic mechanisms, if feasible, before needle biopsy of the liver.

> **Note:** The liver biopsy, although a critical diagnostic tool in patients with laboratory evidence of liver disease, can be a fatal event, even in the hands of the experienced clinician. Abdominal ultrasound imaging of the liver before and during biopsy is strongly recommended.

Technique

Percutaneous needle biopsies and fine-needle aspirations of the liver are performed routinely with local anesthesia in the sedated patients. General anesthesia is a reasonable alternative when feasible. Biopsy sites in the liver can be selected best when needle biopsy techniques are used along with laparoscopy or ultrasound techniques. Blind percutaneous needle biopsies of the liver can be performed with relative safety if the liver is significantly enlarged and easily palpated. However, blind biopsies do carry the risk that the operator is unable to determine the impact of penetrating the liver if only an abdominal radiograph and impression of abdominal palpation are available. In cases where the liver is *not* palpable, blind biopsy carries significantly higher risk and should be performed only when no alternative exits.

A modified percutaneous liver biopsy can be performed by the following method. Before biopsy, have the animal fast, and remove any ascitic fluid. Place the animal in dorsal recumbency, and place a local block in the midline of the skin and abdomen at the caudoventral aspect of the left hepatic lobe. The incision into the peritoneal cavity should be large enough to accommodate the gloved index finger. Make a separate skin puncture site in the abdominal wall to accommodate the biopsy needle. Use the index finger manually to fix the left hepatic lobe (or other desired hepatic lobe) against the diaphragm or other adjacent structures, and insert the outer cannula and stylet through the abdominal wall in the isolated hepatic lobe. Remove the stylet, and rapidly insert the cutting prongs. If properly placed, the cutting prongs should not go through the entire hepatic lobe. Advance the outer cannula over the blades of the cutting prongs, thus entrapping the hepatic tissue material within the cutting prongs. Remove the biopsy needle. Using a wooden applicator stick, carefully place the biopsy specimen into fixative. Biopsy samples can be used to prepare slides for cytologic examination, and the biopsy needle may be cultured. Close the abdominal incision in the routine manner.

Another liver biopsy technique uses the Tru-Cut biopsy needle. Place the dog in dorsal recumbency. Clip a 5-cm^2 area over the triangle formed by the xiphoid cartilage and left costal arch, and prepare the area as for aseptic surgery. Make a small paramedian incision large enough to accommodate a sterile otoscope head 7 mm in diameter. Use a halogen-illuminated otoscope head to visualize the liver. Pass a Tru-Cut biopsy needle through the otoscope cone to obtain a biopsy specimen of the liver.

NASAL BIOPSY

Chronic nasal discharge, with or without sneezing, represents the single most common indication for nasal biopsy. Affected patients should have the benefit of nasal radiographs or a computed tomography study of the nose in advance of endoscopy and/or biopsy. Once the justification for biopsy has been established, the clinician can use one of at least two different techniques to obtain samples.

An older technique still in use today entails the use of a polypropylene catheter with an angled (45-degree), pointed cut on the tip to achieve a blind biopsy (Figure 4-22). With the patient anesthetized, measure the distance from the tip of the nose to the eyes externally and mark the catheter at the level of the external nares (this is the "DON'T GO BEYOND HERE" mark). Gently pass the catheter into the nasal cavity until it will not pass further, reaches the "DON'T GO BEYOND HERE" mark, or reaches a depth consistent with that of a lesion demonstrated radiographically. The procedure entails performing a nasal flush and aspiration of fluid for cytopathologic examination or forcing the catheter tip blindly into the tissue, or both. A syringe on the end of the catheter facilitates removal of tissue from the nasal cavity by aspiration. Some of the tissue may be suitable for histopathologic examination.

Alternatively, pass small biopsy forceps (Figure 4-23) into the affected nostril(s). These instruments allow the collection of several small biopsies (usually up to 0.5 cm diameter) from which exfoliative cytologic examination can be performed, or the sample can be submitted for histopathologic examination.

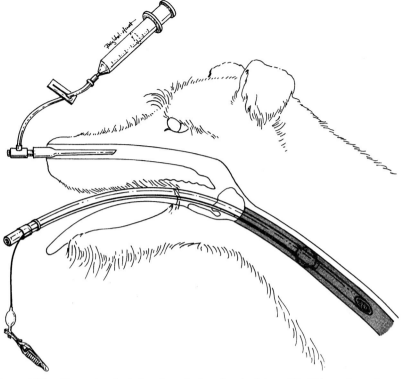

Figure 4-22: Illustration depicting the technique for obtaining a blind biopsy from the nasal cavity of a dog using a polypropylene catheter with an angled tip.

4

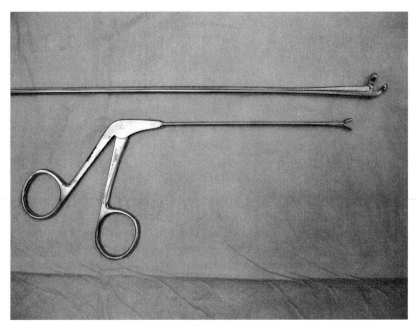

Figure 4-23: Small biopsy forceps used to obtain nasal biopsies.

Rhinoscopy equipment is expensive but does offer the advantage of being able to examine most (sometimes all) of the nasal cavity and actually to visualize an intranasal lesion—sometimes. However, even in the event it is possible to visualize a lesion, simultaneously obtaining the biopsy specimen while observing through the rhinoscope is problematic. Because of the limited amount of working space, most nasal biopsies ultimately are performed blindly.

RENAL BIOPSY

Renal biopsies can be valuable in confirming or eliminating a diagnosis of renal disease that is based on history, physical examination, and radiographic and laboratory data (Box 4-8). In addition, biopsy may be a way of arriving at a prognosis in generalized renal disease and a better means of evaluating the type of treatment to be instituted. Ultrasonographic guidance can prove valuable during renal biopsy for placing the needle into the tissue desired and avoiding complications.

Before renal biopsy, the animal should have a baseline coagulation profile that includes, at the very least, an activated coagulation time and platelet count. A buccal mucosal bleeding time may be indicated if there is any history of spontaneous bleeding in a patient with a normal platelet count. Obtain biopsies from the renal cortex. Administer fluids to patients before and after biopsy.

BOX 4-8   CONTRAINDICATIONS TO RENAL BIOPSY

- Coagulation abnormalities
- A single functional kidney
- Marked hydronephrosis
- Greatly contracted kidneys
- Acute pyelonephritis
- Large cysts

4

Technique

Many patients with generalized renal disease are critically ill and debilitated, and general anesthesia is contraindicated. In these cases, a neuroleptanalgesic agent may be used for sedation. If the animal is a good anesthetic risk and renal function will permit it, use inhalation anesthesia.

When bilateral renal disease is documented, select the LEFT kidney for biopsy because it is more accessible than the right kidney. With the anesthetized patient in right lateral recumbency, surgically prepare the skin behind and below the junction of the costal arch at the level of the second and third lumbar vertebrae. Make a 2-inch paralumbar incision parallel to, but just behind, the costal arch. Dissect muscle and fascia until the peritoneum is visible. Carefully open the peritoneal cavity. Digitally feel for and examine the caudal pole of the left kidney. Guide the needle toward the posterior pole of the kidney with the index finger. Immobilize the kidney against the body wall and insert the Tru-Cut biopsy needle, with the biopsy notch exposed into the parenchyma of the kidney. Capture the biopsy by sliding the outer sleeve of the needle over the (now imbedded in the kidney) biopsy notch. Remove the needle and gently lift the biopsy from the needle and place it into formalin. Evaluate the site for hemorrhage. Once bleeding is controlled, a second biopsy may be collected. Once bleeding from the biopsy site has stopped, the incision can be closed. In dogs, renal biopsy can be performed under ultrasound guidance using probes with channels for biopsy needle insertion.

BONE BIOPSY

Evaluation of bone marrow is indicated in patients with evidence of persistently diminished cell counts of any or all cell lines (white blood cells, red blood cells, platelets) or evidence of morphologically abnormal cells in peripheral blood. Bone marrow aspiration and bone biopsy are extremely helpful but underused diagnostic procedures. The availability of inexpensive, high-quality biopsy needles makes these procedures safe and easy to perform (once experience is gained).

Conventional practice today is to obtain a bone marrow aspirate (cytopathologic examination) *and* a bone biopsy from the same patient during the same procedure when changes in the peripheral blood justify this level of diagnostic testing. Bone marrow aspiration technique is described in this section.

Two types of bone biopsy needles are available. The most commonly described procedure involves use of the Jamshidi biopsy needle, an 11- to 13-gauge needle that ranges in length from 5 to 10 cm (Figure 4-11). The needle contains a stylet that extends beyond the needle tip by 3 to 4 mm. Because of the size of the Jamshidi needle, its use is limited to medium and large dogs. For bone biopsies in cats and small dogs, the author prefers to use the Illinois bone marrow aspiration needle (Figure 4-10), which is a 15- to 18-gauge needle available in lengths ranging from 2.5 to 5.0 cm.

The patient usually is sedated or anesthetized for the procedure. Although some patients will tolerate this procedure when performed under local anesthesia only, the additional manipulation required to obtain a quality sample justifies sedation. In some cases, the patient is sufficiently obtunded that sedation is neither indicated nor required.

The technique is the same regardless of the needle used. Once the site is selected (usually the same sites selected for bone marrow aspiration: head of the humerus, wing of the ileum, ischial tuberosity, proximal femur), clip the hair and surgically prepare the skin. Make a small stab incision in the skin over the site selected. Pass the needle, with stylet in place, through the incision and subcutaneous tissues until the needle tip makes firm contact with bone. Advance the needle using steady, increasing pressure and stable rotation. Rotation, in this case, means rotating the needle back and forth to the left 180 degrees and then to the right 180 degrees. Once the needle is situated in the bone (about 0.5 cm penetration only), STOP. Carefully remove the stylet. Continue the penetration by gradually applying additional pressure and simultaneously rotating the needle.

The usual depth of penetration varies from 1 inch to as much as 3 inches. On reaching the desired depth, remove the needle by continuing to rotate as described but gradually withdrawing the needle from the bone. An obturator is provided to push the sample out of the bone. Place the core of bone directly into buffered formalin and submit it for histopathologic examination (decalicification will be required, which takes a little longer).

Some authors recommend carefully rolling the bone core across a glass slide (for cytopathologic examination) before placing the bone in formalin. I do not recommend this because additional handling of the biopsy sample can sufficiently disrupt the architecture of the tissue and compromise the quality of the biopsy (besides upsetting the pathologist). Note also, the needle can, with a little gentle manipulation, be reinserted into the hole from which the biopsy sample was obtained. Because the Illinois needle and the Jamshidi needle accommodate a syringe, it is possible to obtain (quickly, to prevent clotting) a bone marrow aspirate from the same site. Place that sample directly onto glass slides or (recommended) into 4% EDTA and mix it before making slides.

There are no specific requirements for postbiopsy care of the patient. Clean the blood from the skin using hydrogen peroxide; sutures generally are not required.

PROSTATE BIOPSY (SEE URINARY TRACT PROCEDURES)

Additional Reading

Acierno MJ, Labato MA: Rhinoscopy, nasal flushing, and biopsy. In Ettinger SJ, Feldman EC, editors: *Textbook of veterinary internal medicine,* ed 6, St Louis, 2005, Elsevier-Saunders.

Burkhard MJ, Meyer DJ: Invasive cytology of internal organs: cytology of the thorax and abdomen, *Vet Clin North Am Small Anim Pract* 6:103, 1996.

Crow S, Walshaw S: *Manual of clinical procedures in the dog, cat, and rabbit,* ed 2, Philadelphia, 1997, Lippincott-Raven.

Guilford WG, Center SA, Strombeck DR, et al: *Strombeck's small animal gastroenterology,* ed 3, Philadelphia, 1996, WB Saunders.

Kerwin S: Hepatic aspiration and biopsy techniques, *Vet Clin North Am Small Anim Pract* 25:275, 1995.

Osborne CA, Finco DR: *Canine and feline nephrology and urology,* Baltimore, 1995, Williams & Wilkins.

Stone E: Biopsy: Principles, technical considerations, and pitfalls, *Vet Clin North Am Small Anim Pract* 25:33, 1995.

BLOOD GAS: ARTERIAL

The femoral and dorsal pedal arteries can be punctured to obtain an arterial blood sample for blood gas and electrolyte analyses. To obtain a sample from the femoral artery, place the patient in lateral recumbency and restrain the patient in a manner similar to that for a medial saphenous venipuncture. A 25-gauge needle affixed to a tuberculin syringe is preferred for arterial venipuncture. Prepare the tuberculin syringe by coating it with heparin and forcing all the heparin out except for that left in the hub of the needle. Pull back on the plunger of the syringe slightly to facilitate visualizing the point at which the artery is entered. Arterial blood initially will enter the syringe without the plunger being drawn back. After the proper equipment is assembled and the patient is sufficiently restrained, the individual collecting the arterial blood sample should palpate the medial aspect of the limb over the proximal medial femur until palpating the femoral pulse. Direct the needle at a 30- to 45-degree angle, inserting the needle slowly, watching for a flash of blood in the hub of the needle (Figure 4-24). Gradually withdraw the plunger to facilitate blood entering the syringe. Collect 0.4 to 0.5 mL and immediately submit it for anaylsis.

To obtain blood from a dorsal pedal artery, place the patient in lateral recumbency and extend the rear limb as for a medial saphenous blood sample collection. The person obtaining the blood sample should pull the paw of the down leg in the nondominant hand toward his or her body, rotating the limb slightly in a medial direction to palpate the arterial pulse.

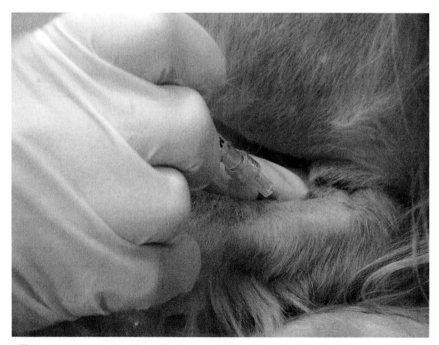

Figure 4-24:   Technique for collecting arterial blood from the dorsal pedal artery of a dog.

Palpate the pulse in the dorsal pedal artery on the dorsomedial aspect of the tarsus. Gently insert the needle on a 30-degree angle into the artery, watching carefully for a flash of blood into the syringe. When the necessary amount of blood has filled the syringe, remove the needle and place pressure over the site of arterial puncture for a minimum of 2 minutes.

Evacuate excess air from the syringe and needle, and cap the needle with a red rubber stopper to prevent air from entering the needle and syringe. Place the sample on ice until analysis, if arterial blood gas analyses cannot be performed immediately.

SURGICAL CUTDOWN

In the event percutaneous access to a peripheral artery is not possible, the femoral artery can be isolated and prepared for surgical cutdown. Following appropriate aseptic skin preparation, make a 4- to 5-cm incision in the skin over the femoral artery. Find the caudal edge of the sartorius muscle by blunt dissection and then reflect it anteriorly to expose the underlying femoral artery, vein, and nerve. Taking care to avoid tearing any vessel branches, gently isolate up to 2 cm of the femoral artery from the surrounding fascia. Visually direct the needle into the artery at this point. Alternatively, catheterize the artery in the event repeated arterial samples are required. Elevate the femoral artery by preplacing two stay sutures beneath the artery and then elevating the vessel to the level of the skin. Insert a long catheter-over-the-needle system into the lumen of the artery without penetrating the deep wall. Gently insert the catheter into the vessel, remove the needle, and cap and flush the catheter. Close the incision and affix the catheter to the skin via a tape tag sutured to the skin.

Additional Reading

Davis H: Venous and arterial puncture. In Ettinger SJ, Feldman EC, editors: *Textbook of veterinary internal medicine,* ed 6, St Louis, 2005, Elsevier-Saunders.

Crow S, Walshaw S: *Manual of clinical procedures in the dog, cat, and rabbit,* ed 2, Philadelphia, 1997, Lippincott-Raven.

Shiroshita Y, Tanaka R, Shibazaki A, et al: Retrospective study of clinical complications occurring after arterial punctures in dogs: 111 cases, *Vet Rec* 146(1):16-19, 2000.

4

CEREBROSPINAL FLUID COLLECTION

In the dog and the cat the preferred site for obtaining a diagnostic sample of cerebrospinal fluid (CSF) is the cerebellomedullary cistern (cisterna magna) at the level of the atlantooccipital articulation (between the back of the skull and the first cervical vertebra). Although the procedure is not commonly done in private practice, a number of infectious and noninfectious conditions justify performing the procedure. Collection of CSF is indicated in any patient suspected of having an infection (bacterial, fungal, viral, rickettsial, protozoal, and [uncommonly] parasitic) suspected of reaching the central nervous system. Several types of noninfectious causes of meningitis are described in dogs and cats. In dogs specifically, most causes of meningitis are idiopathic. Defined diseases include granulomatous meningoencephalitis, breed-specific meningitis (e.g., pug encephalitis), neoplasia, and unexplained seizure disorder, especially in a patient with a history of seizure activity that is increasing in frequency.

CONTRAINDICATIONS

Among the reasons *not* to perform CSF collection, lack of experience perhaps ranks at the top (Box 4-9). Cerebrospinal fluid collection is not without some risk. Inadvertent penetration of the cervical spinal cord can culminate in acute death. Anatomic reasons for *not* performing CSF collection include congenital abnormalities involving malformations of the foramen magnum or suspected neural malformations in the region of the cisterna magna. Patients with fractures, dislocations, or subluxations of the occipital region of the skull or rostral cervical region, resulting in distortion of the brainstem, medulla, cervical cord, and any patient suspected of having brain herniation should not be subjected to the procedure.

BOX 4-9 COMPLICATIONS OF CEREBROSPINAL FLUID COLLECTION

- No cerebrospinal fluid obtained
- Herniation of the brain
- Contamination of the cerebrospinal fluid with blood
- Needle penetration of the medulla or the rostral spinal cord
- Infection of the central nervous system
- Respiratory or cardiac arrest
- Vestibular dysfunction
- Paresis or paralysis

TECHNIQUE

To perform cisternal puncture, intubation and general anesthesia are required. Place the patient in lateral recumbency. Clip and surgically prepare the area of skin at least from the external occipital protuberance to the wings of the atlas and as wide apart as the distance between the ears. Position the animal with the prepared area at the edge of the table. Flex the head ventrally and maintain it at a right angle to the long axis of the neck. Various recommendations have been made regarding how to position the patient with respect to the individual performing the procedure. In the technique described, right-handed persons should position the patient in right-lateral recumbency. Left-handed persons should position the patient in left lateral recumbency.

To identify the site of needle penetration in the skin, the landmarks are a vertical line connecting the *anterior edge* of the first cervical vertebra and a horizontal line from the occipital protuberance that runs parallel to the spine. *The point of intersection of the two lines represents the point of needle penetration.* IMPORTANT: For consistency in performing this technique, as the needle penetrates the skin and muscle overlying the cisterna magna, pass it *perpendicular to the skin* and *parallel to the floor throughout the procedure.*

Using a 2- to 2 ½-inch, 20- to 22-gauge spinal needle (with a stylet), advance the needle methodically and slowly toward the cisterna. The depth of penetration required to reach the cisterna varies considerably among patients of different sizes but can range from less than 1 inch to just over 2 inches. Generally, if the needle hits bone with superficial penetration, the position of the needle is too far caudal. If the needle hits bone after deep penetration (most common), the needle point is on the occipital bone and too far cranial. Only minor changes of a few millimeters generally are required to correct.

On penetration of the cisterna magna, the needle passes through the dura mater. At this point, there is usually a slight degree of resistance felt on the needle, but *not* always. Therefore, checking the position of the needle 3 to 5 times during penetration by withdrawing the sylet to assess for presence of CSF flow is recommended.

Once the flow of CSF is established, collect fluid for analysis by allowing the CSF to *flow freely.* DO NOT ASPIRATE FLUID FROM THE CISTERNA MAGNA BECAUSE THIS MAY CREATE SUFFICIENT NEGATIVE PRESSURE THAT HERNIATION COULD RESULT. Collect aliquots of CSF in two sterile collection tubes (e.g., red-topped blood collection tubes). Collect 0.5 to 2.0 mL in each tube and submit it for fluid analysis. The reason for collecting two aliquots of CSF is that if the cytologic examination of one tube suggests neutrophils (or bacteria), the second sample can be submitted for culture.

The presence of blood contamination is not unusual, particularly when multiple penetrations of the neck muscles have been required. As the flow of CSF is established, if it has a blood-tinged appearance, delay the collection for several drops. If clearing is apparent within a few drops, the blood likely represents contamination. If clearing does not occur after several drops, the blood may represent active bleeding into the central nervous system. Collecting CSF in EDTA is an option if the sample appears to contain significant amounts of blood. If, however, the flow from the spinal needle appears to be pure, dark blood, the needle likely has penetrated one of the large venous sinuses that course outside of and lateral to the spinal cord. This is a consequence of passing the needle perpendicular to the skin but not exactly parallel to the floor. Withdraw the needle and repeat the procedure using a new needle. If the technique is properly performed, clear CSF still can be obtained despite having collected what appears to be pure blood on a previous attempt.

Additional Reading

Anderson SM: Cerebrospinal fluid collection, myelography, and epidurals. In Ettinger SJ, Feldman EC, editors: *Textbook of veterinary internal medicine,* ed 6, St Louis, 2005, Elsevier-Saunders.

Meyer D, Harvey J: *Veterinary laboratory medicine,* ed 3, St Louis, 2004, Elsevier-Saunders.

Oliver J, Lorenz M, Kornegay J: *Handbook of veterinary neurology,* ed 4, St Louis, 2004, Elsevier-Saunders.

ELECTROCARDIOGRAPHY

The electrocardiogram provides a fast, efficient way to obtain considerable data about a patient's cardiovascular status. Electrocardiography is a clinical test and must be correlated with clinical findings (Box 4-10). Keep in mind that an electrocardiogram measures only electrical activity of the heart as seen on the body surface at any one instant. Electrical disorders of the myocardium can be transient or intermittent and, as such, can be missed on a single electrocardiogram.

INTERPRETATION OF THE ELECTROCARDIOGRAM

Read each electrocardiogram using a definite system. Begin by examining the lead II rhythm strip: Is there a P wave for every QRS complex? Is there a QRS complex for every P wave? Do all the P waves look alike? Do all the QRS complexes look alike? Are the P wave and QRS complex consistently related to each other?

If the answer to any of these questions is no, proceed to identify the abnormality. Next, determine the rate, rhythm, and wave character; that is, evaluate measurements of the P wave, PR interval, and QRS complex. Evaluate the ST segment and T wave and the QT interval. Use all leads to determine the axis and any miscellaneous criteria.

HEART RATE

Depending on the type of electrocardiographic equipment used, there are several methods for determining *heart rate* from the electrocardiographic tracing. Many electrocardiographs compute the heart rate and print that on the tracing. However, in patients with a significant dysrhythmia, these calculations can be flawed and should be verified manually when a question exists. Small linear lines or demarcations at the top of the electrocardiogram paper can be used to determine the heart rate. At a paper speed of 50 mm/second, the time between adjacent marks is 1.5 seconds. By counting the number of QRS complexes (or R waves) between just two of these divisions and multiplying by 20 equals the heart rate in beats/minute (Figure 4-25). For those inclined to higher mathematics, the heart rate also may be determined by counting the number of small squares between R waves (at a paper speed of 50 mm/second) and then dividing into 3000 (Box 4-11).

BOX 4-10   INDICATIONS FOR PERFORMING AN ELECTROCARDIOGRAM

- Detect enlargement of any of the cardiac chambers
- Diagnose cardiac arrhythmia
- Identify effects of electrolyte imbalances, especially potassium
- Monitor response to and direct cardiac drug therapy
- Develop prognoses (degree of change in heart function over time)

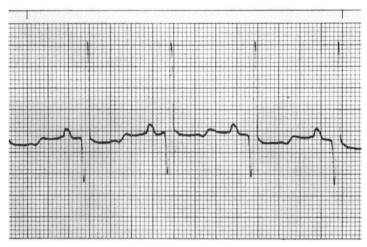

Figure 4-25: Using the electrocardiogram to determine heart rate. The distance between R waves is 20 small boxes: 3000/20 = 150 beats/minute. (Paper speed is 50 mm/second.)

BOX 4-11 NORMAL HEART RATE	
DOG	**CAT**
• Large dogs: 60 to 100 beats/minute	• Domestic cats: 140 to 250 beats/minute
• Medium-size dogs: 80 to 120 beats/minute	
• Small dogs: 90 to 140 beats/minute	
• Puppies: Up to 220 beats/minute	

4

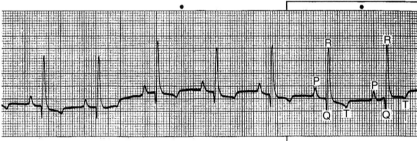

Figure 4-26: Normal lead II QRS complexes in an adult dog.

HEART RHYTHM

The normal heart rhythm is sinus in origin. For every QRS complex there is a P wave (Figure 4-26). The P waves are related to QRS complexes (P-P interval is constant). Sinus arrhythmia, sinus arrest, and wandering pacemaker are normal rhythm variations. In sinus arrhythmia, the P-P interval is irregular. The pauses are never longer than twice the usual P-P interval (Figure 4-27). A *wandering pacemaker* means that the P waves vary in height and may even be negative temporarily (Figure 4-28). *Sinus arrest* is defined as a prolongation of the P-R interval longer than twice the usual P-P interval.

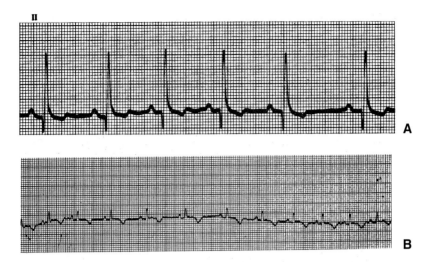

Figure 4-27: **A,** Mild sinus arrhythmia in a dog. There are P waves for every QRS complex, and P waves are related to the QRS complexes, which make this a sinus rhythm. The variation of the R-R intervals also is visible. An irregular sinus rhythm is a sinus arrhythmia. **B,** Sinus arrhythmia in the cat.
(From Edwards NF: *Bolton's handbook of canine and feline electrocardiography,* ed 2, Philadelphia, 1987, WB Saunders.)

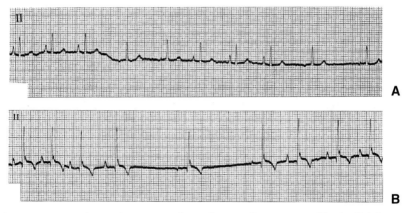

Figure 4-28: **A,** The wandering pacemaker in this recording is suggested by the slightly negative P waves in some of the complexes. Negative P waves of this nature result from vagal depression of the sinoatrial node and the development of a junctional atrioventricular nodal rhythm. **B,** Marked sinus arrhythmia and a wandering pacemaker result in a decreased heart rate (increased R-R interval) and negative P waves in the fifth complex. As the pacemaker returns to the sinoatrial node, the rate increases, and positive P waves of varying amplitude result in the sixth and seventh complexes.

NORMAL ELECTROCARDIOGRAM MEASUREMENTS

P wave

The normal P wave is 0.04 second × 0.4 mV (two boxes wide × four boxes tall) for the dog and 0.04 second × 0.2 mV for the cat. In P mitrale (left atrial enlargement), the P wave is wider than 0.04 second. In P pulmonale (right atrial enlargement), the P wave is taller than 0.4 mV for the dog and 0.2 mV for the cat.

PR interval

The PR interval is measured from the beginning of the P wave to the beginning of the QRS complex. The normal interval is 0.06 to 0.13 second (3 to 6.5 boxes wide) for the dog and 0.06 to 0.08 second for the cat. In first-degree atrioventricular heart block, the PR interval is prolonged. The PR interval is sometimes useful in monitoring the effects of digitalis therapy.

QRS complex

The QRS complex duration is measured from the beginning of the Q wave to the end of the S wave. Normal duration is up to 0.04 second in cats, 0.05 second in small dogs, and 0.06 second in large dogs. A QRS complex that is too wide indicates left ventricular enlargement (Figure 4-29). An R wave that is too tall indicates left ventricular enlargement. The amplitude is measured from the baseline to the top of the R wave (Figure 4-30). The normal R wave can be up to 0.8 mV tall in cats, 2.5 mV in small dogs, and 3.0 mV in large dogs.

ST segment

The ST segment is between the end of the S wave and the beginning of the T wave. Normally, the ST segment lies on the baseline and then dips into the T wave. Slurring of S into T indicates left ventricular enlargement and is seen when the S wave slurs into the T wave and no ST segment is discernible. The ST segment is elevated if it lies more than 0.1 mV (one box) above the baseline (>0.2 mV in CV_6LL and CV_6LU). Elevation of the ST segment may occur with hypercalcemia or myocardial hypoxia. The ST segment is depressed if it lies more than 0.1 mV (one box; >0.2 mV in CV_6LL and CV_6LU) below the baseline. Depression of ST may be seen with myocardial ischemia, hypoxia, or hypocalcemia.

QT interval

The QT interval is measured from the beginning of the Q wave to the end of the T wave. The normal interval is 0.14 to 0.22 second (7 to 11 boxes wide) in dogs and up to

4

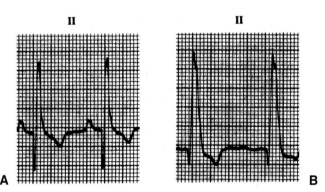

Figure 4-29:   In these two examples of left ventricular enlargement the QRS complexes have normal configuration but are too wide. **A,** This QRS complex from a miniature poodle is 0.07 second (three boxes) wide. **B,** This QRS complex from a Doberman Pinscher is 0.09 second (four boxes) wide. A small dog such as the Poodle should not have a QRS complex wider than 0.05 second (wider), and the larger dog's QRS complex should not exceed 0.06 second (three boxes). Because each dog's QRS complex is too wide, left ventricular enlargement is diagnosed in both cases. The Doberman Pinscher has no P waves because he is in atrial fibrillation. (Paper speed is 50 mm/second; 1 cm equals 1 mV.)
(From Edwards NF: *Bolton's handbook of canine and feline electrocardiography,* ed 2, Philadelphia, 1987, WB Saunders.)

II

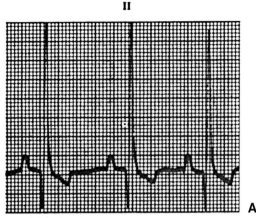

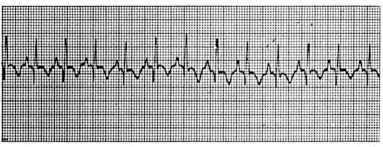

Figure 4-30: **A,** In this tracing the R wave averages 3.8 mV (38 boxes). The R wave should not be taller than 3.0 mV (30 boxes) in any dog. A tall R wave indicates left ventricular enlargement. The measurement is made from the baseline (not from the bottom of the Q wave) to the top of the R wave. Two other criteria that indicate left ventricular enlargement are present. The QRS complex is 0.07 second (three boxes) wide and ST segment slurring is present, because the ST segment moves into the T wave without straightening out along the baseline. (Paper speed is 50 mm/second; 1 cm equals 1 mV.) **B,** Left ventricular enlargement in a cat. This lead II electrocardiogram was recorded from an aged cat suffering from hyperthyroidism. Thyroxine levels were 9.9 mg/dL. Note the tall R waves (>0.9 mV). (Paper speed is 50 mm/seconds; 1 cm equals 1 mV.) ST segment slurring is characterized by the slurring of the downstroke of the R wave into the T wave, with no discernible ST segment. This occurs because of ischemia resulting from wall strain in cardiac enlargement.
(Courtesy of NS Moise, New York State College of Veterinary Medicine, Cornell University, Ithaca, NY. From Edwards NF: *Bolton's handbook of canine and feline electrocardiography,* ed 2, Philadelphia, 1987, WB Saunders.)

0.16 second in cats. A lengthened QT interval may be seen with hypokalemia or hypocalcemia. The QT interval varies with heart rate and tends to be prolonged when bradycardia occurs. A decreased QT interval may be seen with hypercalcemia.

MEAN ELECTRICAL AXIS

The *mean electrical cardiac axis* measures the direction (vector) of the cardiac ventricular impulse during depolarization. Therefore the QRS complex is examined in leads I, II, III, aV_R, aV_L, and aV_F. These six leads determine the axis. They are arranged in a manner known as *Bailey's hexaxial lead system* (Figure 4-31). The procedure is as follows:
1. Find an isoelectric lead; that is, a lead for which the total number of positve (upward) and negative (downward) deflections of the QRS complex is equal to zero (Figure 4-32). When there is no perfectly isoelectric lead, use the one that comes closest.

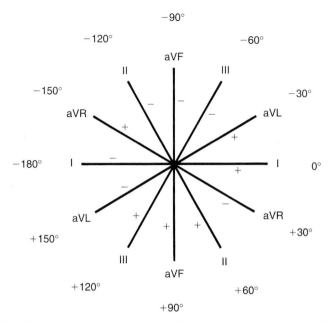

Figure 4-31: Bailey's hexaxial reference system. The lead axes are marked in 30-degree increments from 0 to 180 degrees and from 0 to −180 degrees. The six leads are marked with a plus sign at the positive electrode and a minus sign at the negative electrode. Note that in the leads I, II, III, and aV_F the polarity and the angle of the leads are positive or negative simultaneously. Leads aV_F and aV_L are positive at the positions of −150 degrees and −30 degrees, respectively, because the positive electrodes for those leads lie in the negative 0 to −180 degrees zone. (From Ettinger SJ, Suter PF: *Canine cardiology*, Philadelphia, 1970, WB Saunders.)

4

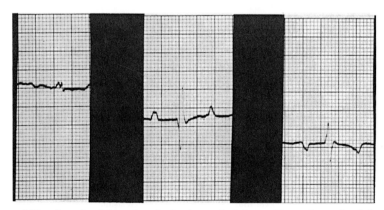

Figure 4-32: In each of these three leads, the total of the positive and negative deflections equals zero. Each is considered an isoelectric lead.

2. Find the lead that is perpendicular to the isoelectric lead: lead I is perpendicular to aV_F; lead II is perpendicular to aV_L; and lead III is perpendicular to aV_R.
3. Determine whether the perpendicular lead is positive or negative on the patient's electrocardiogram. If the perpendicular lead is negative, the axis is at the negative end of that lead (each lead has a plus and a minus pole marked. If the perpendicular lead is positive, the mean electrical axis is at the positive end of the perpendicular lead.

For example, if aVL is isoelectric (normally it is), lead II is its perpendicular. If lead II is positive on the electrocardiogram, the axis is +60 degress. If lead II is negative on the electrocardiogram, the axis is −120 degrees.

Normal mean electrical axis

The normal dog mean electrical axis is +40 to +100 degrees; for the cat it is more variable: ±0 to ±180 degrees. Right axis deviation (axis more than +100) indicates right ventricular enlargement in the dog (Figure 4-33). Left axis deviation (axis 0 to +40 degrees) indicates left ventricular enlargement in the dog. When there is biventricular enlargement, the axis usually remains normal. Axis determinations are of less value in the cat because the normal range is so wide (Boxes 4-12 to 4-14).

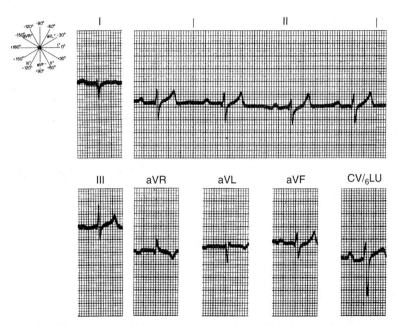

Figure 4-33:   The mean electrical axis in the frontal plane of this electrocardiogram recorded from a wire-haired fox terrier with pulmonic stenosis is approximately +165 degrees.
(From Edwards NJ: *Bolton's handbook of canine and feline electrocardiography,* ed 2, Philadelphia, 1987, WB Saunders.)

BOX 4-12   ELECTROCARDIOGRAM CRITERIA FOR LEFT VENTRICULAR ENLARGEMENT

1. Left axis deviation (dog)
2. QRS complex too wide (but has normal configuration)
3. R wave too tall
4. S-T segment slurring
5. May be associated with P mitrale

BOX 4-13   ELECTROCARDIOGRAM CRITERIA FOR RIGHT VENTRICULAR ENLARGEMENT

1. Right axis deviation (dog and cat)
2. Presence of an S wave in leads I, II, and III (dog only)
3. S wave deeper than 0.7 mV in lead CV_6LU (V_4) in the dog
4. May be associated with P pulmonale

BOX 4-14 ELECTROCARDIOGRAM CRITERIA FOR BIVENTRICULAR ENLARGEMENT

1. Tall R wave
2. Wide QRS complex
3. ST segment slurring
4. Deep Q waves in lead II (deeper than 0.3 mV for the cat, 0.5 mV for the dog)
5. Normal mean electrical axis
6. P mitrale or P pulmonale, or both

ENDOSCOPY: INDICATIONS AND EQUIPMENT REQUIREMENTS

Note: The discussion that follows centers around indications and capabilities of endoscopy in clinical practice. The discussion is not intended to be used as a "How-To" instruction guide on performing endoscopic procedures in dogs and cats. Today, numerous types of endoscopes and accessory materials are available for use in clinical practice. Specific hands-on training and complete familiarity with the equipment package available *is essential* before attempting to perform any of the procedures outlined.

Inappropriate use of endoscopic equipment not only can damage expensive equipment but also can cause serious injury to the patient.

UPPER RESPIRATORY TRACT: LARYNGOSCOPY AND PHARYNGOSCOPY

Endoscopy of the upper respiratory tract is among the most important advanced diagnostic and therapeutic tools used in the evaluation of patients that have stertor (snorting), reverse sneeze, stridor (wheezing), and chronic cough. Laryngoscopy is of value in the diagnosis of upper airway obstructions such as eversion of the lateral ventricles, collapsed arytenoid cartilages, hyperplasia of the vocal cords, nodules on the vocal cords, elongated soft palate, collapsed proximal trachea, and traumatic injuries to the neck. Note also, however, that a careful visual examination of the larynx in the anesthetized patient (only) can be highly valuable even without the use of endoscopic equipment; for example, for assessment of laryngeal movement in patients with laryngeal paralysis. Suspected lesions *inside* the larynx may be difficult to visualize with or without endoscopic equipment. Examination of the trachea and main stem bronchi requires endoscopic evaluation to assess the integrity of the airway for conditions such as collapsed trachea, mediastinal tumors, hilar lymph node enlargement, parasitic nodules *(Filaroides osleri)*, and foreign body aspiration. In addition, tracheobronchoscopy is a valuable technique that permits culturing and cytologic examination of material from bronchi involved in chronic respiratory disease. Upper airway obstruction that is not responsive to conservative therapy is an indication for more extensive diagnostic procedures, such as bronchoscopy.

Endoscopes of varying sizes are appropriate for use in examining the larynx and trachea. However, in cats and small dogs, examination of the trachea using equipment as small as a (human) bronchoscope may limit the examination because the endoscope nearly occludes the tracheal diameter. Additional training and/or experience is recommended when performing tracheoscopy in small patients.

One of the most important endoscopic techniques performed in dogs and cats involves examination of the nasopaharynx, the upper respiratory compartment above the soft palate. Sometimes called pharyngoscopy, examination entails retroflexion of a small-diameter endoscope (e.g., bronchoscope) 170 to 180 degrees to allow visualization of the space between the posterior nares (choana) and the larynx (Figure 4-34). This is a common location for foreign body entrapment and occasional tumor development in cats and dogs (Figure 4-35). Pharyngoscopy is the *only* effective means of examining this portion of the upper respiratory tract in patients that have a history of stertor (snorting) and so-called reverse sneeze.

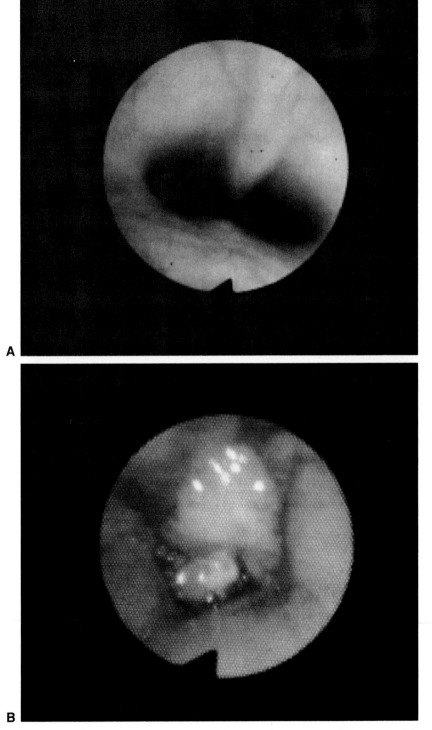

A, 4

Figure 4-34: **A,** The appearance of the normal choana (posterior nares) in a cat. **B,** The appearance of the choana of cat with a posterior nasal mass diagnosed as lymphoma.

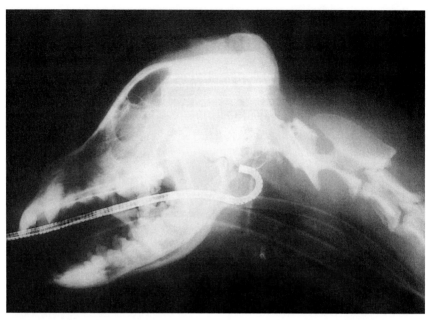

Figure 4-35:   Lateral skull radiograph of a dog depicting the proper endoscopic placement for pharyngoscopy.

LOWER RESPIRATORY TRACT: BRONCHOSCOPY

Endoscopic examination of the bronchi and lower airways is a highly diagnostic, occasionally therapeutic procedure indicated in patients that present for persistent cough. As in all endoscopic procedures, the patient is anesthetized for the examination. However, examination of the lower respiratory tract requires considerable attention to patient oxygenation and respiratory status during the examination. The requirement for oxygen to be administered throughout the procedure may be a significant limiting factor unless special accessories are used. In the ideal situation, the patient is a medium- to large-sized dog and the endoscope can be passed *through* the endoscope using a T adaptor while oxygen and anesthetic are administered simultaneously.

However, in cats and small dogs, it is usually not possible to pass an endoscope through the endotracheal tube. The procedure must be done by passing the endoscope directly into the trachea to the level of the right and left main bronchi and probably not much farther. Supplemental intravenous anesthetic is likely to be required because of the time required to complete the examination. Training and/or experience is essential before performing bronchoscopy, particularly in cats and small dogs.

The greatest advantage in performing bronchoscopy is to visualize the integrity of the trachea and, to a limited extent, the lower airways. Airway collapse, not visible on conventional radiography, can be strikingly apparent. Foreign body entrapment, tumors, respiratory parasites and airway trauma also can be identified with bronchoscopy. Additionally, the bronchoscopic examination allows for collection of cytologic samples from discrete areas (airways) within the lower respiratory tract. The ability to perform bronchoalveolar lavage in patients with reactive airway disease, subclinical or clinical infections, and certain types of tumors can be highly diagnostic.

GASTROINTESTINAL ENDOSCOPY

Flexible fiberoptic endoscopy is a noninvasive, atraumatic means of visualizing the mucosal surfaces of the esophagus, stomach, and colon. Flexible endoscopes are available from several companies at a wide range of prices. To minimize the risk of injury to the animal and to reduce the possibility of damage to the endoscope, place animals undergoing endoscopic examination under general anesthesia after routine preanesthetic preparation. A fast of 12 to 24 hours is recommended for most patients undergoing upper gastrointestinal endoscopy. However, for patients with indications of delayed gastric emptying, a longer fast (24 to 48 hours) may be needed to empty the stomach completely. In preparation for colonoscopy, a 24- to 48-hour fast is recommended. Give a high warm-water enema the evening before and again 2 to 4 hours before the procedure. Give such enemas until the return is clear.

Esophagoscopy

The clinical signs indicating esophageal disease and a potential benefit of esophagoscopy include repeated regurgitation, excessive drooling, ballooning of the esophagus, anorexia or dysphagia, and recurrent pneumonia. Esophagoscopy allows visualization of the mucosal lining of the esophagus and makes it possible to detect inflammation, ulcerations, dilatations, diverticula, strictures, foreign bodies, tumors, and parasite infestations.

Gastroscopy and duodenoscopy

Endoscopic examination of the mucosal aspect of the stomach is indicated when the clinical signs or physical findings suggest the presence of gastric disease or when there is a need for confirmation or clarification of radiographic findings. In most cases, persistent vomiting is the chief complaint. Other clinical signs suggestive of serious gastric disease include hematemesis, melena, weight loss, anemia, and abdominal pain. Gastroscopy allows visualization of the mucosal lining of the stomach and enables detection of inflammation, ulceration, foreign bodies, and tumors. In most dogs and cats the endoscope can be passed into the proximal duodenum. Depending on the patient size and length of the scope, it may be possible to evaluate as much as 12 inches or more of the proximal duodenum.

Colonoscopy

Colonoscopy refers to endoscopic examination of colon, rectum, and anus. The technique is helpful in the definitive diagnosis of lower bowel lesions, such as granulomatous colitis, foreign bodies, tumors, lacerations, and other mucosal abnormalities. The primary indication for colonoscopy is the presence of signs of large bowel disease, which typically include tenesmus and the passage of small, frequent stools containing fresh blood or excess mucus. Endoscopic examination of the colon allows direct visualization of the effects of mucosal inflammation, ulceration, mucosal polyps, malignant neoplasia, and strictures. Histologic examination of mucosal biopsy material will confirm the diagnosis of colonic disease.

The large bowel must be empty for the colonic mucosa to be visualized. The bowel can be emptied by withholding food for 24 hours and performing a colonic irrigation the evening before and again 2 hours before the examination. The material used for the enema must be nonirritating and nonoily. Mildly hypertonic saline solutions such as Fleet enemas work well if given 2 hours before examination so that gas and fluid can be passed completely. However, do not use Fleet enemas in cats or small dogs.

If the general physical condition of the animal is poor and withholding food is not possible, feeding a low-residue diet for 12 to 18 hours preceding colonoscopy can be helpful. This diet could consist of cooked eggs, small amounts of cooked beef or chicken, and small amounts of carbohydrates, such as a slice of toast or ¼ to ½ cup of moist kibble. Maintain good hydration. If all food is contraindicated, oral electrolyte solutions such as Gatorade (PepsiCo, Purchase, New York) can be used to maintain hydration without moving solids through the intestinal tract.

Give the animal a short-acting anesthetic and place the animal on a tilted table in lateral recumbency with the hindquarters elevated. Perform a digital examination of the rectum and pelvic cavity to ensure that there are no strictures, polyps, or other obstructions. Lubricate the proctoscope thoroughly with water-soluble jelly and pass it gently through the anal sphincter. Press the proctoscope forward slowly and carefully with a spiral motion. If any resistance is encountered, stop the motion, remove the obturator, and inspect the bowel to determine the cause of the resistance. If possible, replace the obturator and continue forward motion until the instrument is passed its full length. Withdraw the obturator, and observe the mucosa.

The major portion of the examination is conducted as the instrument is withdrawn. To view the colonic and rectal walls completely, one must move the anterior end of the proctoscope around the circumference of a small circle while withdrawing the proctoscope. Occasional insufflation with the inflating bulb is helpful in smoothing out folds of tissue. Repeated instrumentation may produce petechiae and minor hemorrhages that are not pathologic. For examination of the terminal rectum and anus, the Hirshman anoscope provides adequate, convenient visualization.

Newer techniques for visualizing the upper and lower gastrointestinal tract are being used in dogs. The flexible fiberoptic endoscope enables one to visualize and photograph the esophagus, colon, and stomach. One is able not only to visualize lesions of the gastrointestinal tract directly but also to assess motility, take biopsies of lesions, and remove foreign bodies.

Vaginoscopy

The ability to visualize directly the vestibule, the vagina to the level of the cervix, and the urethral orifice in female dogs is of particular value in evaluating patients with known or suspected congenital urinary tract disorders, such as incontinence or ectopic ureters and vaginal strictures (congenital or traumatic). Numerous vaginal malformations and chronic infections have visual changes that are identified easily during endoscopic examination. Frequently, the procedure can be conducted in the standing awake patient. Sedation or general anesthesia is indicated when extensive manipulation, catheterization of the bladder, or a vaginal biopsy are indicated. Position the sedated or anesthetized patient in dorsal or ventral recumbency to facilitate orientation during the procedure. If catheterization of the urinary bladder is required during the procedure, dorsal recumbency seems to facilitate visualization of the urethral papilla and insertion of the catheter.

Vaginoscopy entails use of a relatively small, flexible endoscope 4 to 6 mm in diameter or a 2- to 3-mm rigid scope. The flexible scope offer the advantage of a larger biopsy channel and the ability to view the lateral vaginal wall easily. Vaginoscopy is considered an invasive procedure and should be conducted under sterile conditions. Before insertion of the sterilized endoscope, the vulva should be free of obvious debris, should be clipped if necessary, and should be cleaned gently with a surgical soap and rinsed. Insert the scope such that initial position of the tip of the scope is directed toward the anus. As insertion proceeds, the tip of the endoscope reaches the horizontal portion of the vestibule and vagina. When feasible, pass the scope to the level of the cervix. Slight insufflation of the vagina may be useful in dilating the vagina, greatly facilitating the examination. Conducting the examination from the level of the cervix caudally is recommended. This maximizes the ability to visualize critical anatomic features.

Cystoscopy

The relatively recent introduction of very small (2-mm diameter) flexible and rigid endoscopes into veterinary medicine allows visual examination of the urethra, trigone, urinary bladder, and the right and left ureterovesicular junctions of female dogs and even cats. Such examinations are most useful when obstructive lesions (tumor or calculi) of the urethra or trigone are suspected. Visual examination of the interior surface of the bladder and the capability of collecting biopsy samples makes this a particularly useful diagnostic tool in the hands of the experienced clinician.

Additional Reading

Guilford WG, Center SA, Strombeck DR, et al: *Strombeck's small animal gastroenterology,* ed 3, Philadelphia, 1996, WB Saunders.

Holt DE: Laryngoscopy and pharnygoscopy. In King LG, editor: *Textbook of respiratory disease in dogs and cats,* St Louis, 2004, Elsevier-Saunders.

Jones B: Incorporating endoscopy in veterinary practice, *Compend Contin Educ Pract Vet* 20:307-313, 1998.

Kuehn NF, Hess RS: Bronchoscopy. In King LG, editor: *Textbook of respiratory disease in dogs and cats*, St Louis, 2004, Elsevier-Saunders.

Tams TR: *Handbook of small animal gastroenterology*, Philadelphia, 1996, WB Saunders.

FLUID THERAPY (SEE ALSO SECTION 1)

MAINTENANCE FLUIDS (MANAGEMENT OF NORMAL FLUID LOSSES)

The volume of fluids required to replace the normal ongoing losses can be determined from predictive charts (Tables 4-8 and 4-9). If a chart is not available, the maintenance volume is assumed to be 40 to 60 mL/kg/day (higher values per kilogram for smaller dogs and cats and lower values per kilogram for larger dogs and cats).

The nature of the fluids used for maintenance is distinctly different from that of fluids used to replace extracellular volume deficits. The average concentration of normal urine and insensible losses is 40 to 50 mEq/L, and the potassium concentration is 15 to 20 mEq/L. Administration of a replacement solution to an animal for its maintenance requirements predisposes to hypernatremia (most animals are able to eliminate the excess sodium) and hypokalemia.

Lactated Ringer's solution or equivalent replacement solutions are poor maintenance solutions because they predispose to hypernatremia and hypokalemia. In one version of a homemade maintenance solution, a replacement solution is supplemented with potassium (15 to 20 mEq/L) to accommodate the potassium losses that normally occur. A further modification is dilution of the replacement solution with one to two parts of 5% dextrose in water per one part of replacement solution. The easiest approach is to use commercial maintenance solutions.

Maintenance solutions also should not be used to replace extracellular volume deficits because they may cause hyponatremia and hyperkalemia when administered in large volumes. If a patient is receiving a maintenance solution and is noted to be dehydrated or hypotensive, administer a replacement solution.

MAINTENANCE FLUIDS (MANAGEMENT OF ABNORMAL FLUID LOSSES)

Ongoing losses that occur via transudation into one of the major body cavities, into the tissues, or through burn wounds are similar in composition to extracellular fluid and should be replaced with lactated Ringer's solution or an equivalent replacement solution. Ongoing losses that occur via vomiting, diarrhea, or diuresis should be replaced with lactated Ringer's solution or an equivalent solution that has been supplemented with potassium (10 to 30 mEq/L). One exception is the patient that has been vomiting stomach contents chronically, a situation in which 0.9% sodium chloride supplemented with potassium (10 to 30 mEq/L) is recommended.

When the fluid therapy plan is being developed, how much fluid the animal will lose over the day is not known. One can leave this category blank initially and then, as losses occur during the day, add equivalent volumes of the appropriate fluid to the fluid therapy regimen. Alternatively, if the patient has a disease that is known to be associated with severe ongoing fluid losses (e.g., parvovirus gastroenteritis), one can fill in an estimated volume initially and then adjust upward or downward as the day progresses.

FLUID THERAPY IN THE NONCRITICAL PATIENT

The fluid therapy prescription is the best guess as to the requirements of the patient. Implementation of a fluid therapy regimen that is as close as possible to the prescription is important; however, considering the inherent inaccuracies in the assumptions used to construct the prescription, it is not imperative to administer exactly what has been prescribed. There are many acceptable ways to administer the prescribed fluids. One way is to mix all of the fluids and additives from each category into one large bottle and administer them throughout the day. Another way is to administer the fluids simultaneously, in

4

TABLE 4-8   Approximate Daily Energy and Water Requirements of Dogs Based on Body Weight*

	Total energy (kcal) or water (mL)		
Body weight (kg)	Per day	Per kilogram	Per hour
1	132	132	5.5
2	222	111	9.5
3	301	100	12.5
4	373	93	15.5
5	441	88	18.5
6	506	84	21
7	568	81	23.5
8	628	78	26
9	686	76	28.5
10	742	74	31
11	797	72	33
12	851	71	35.5
13	904	70	37.5
14	955	68	40
15	1006	67	42
16	1056	66	44
17	1105	65	46
18	1154	64	48
19	1201	63	50
20	1248	62	52
21	1295	62	54
22	1341	61	56
23	1386	60	58
24	1431	60	59.5
25	1476	59	61.5
26	1520	58	63.5
27	1564	58	65
28	1607	57	67
29	1650	57	68.5
30	1692	56	70.5
35	1899	54	79
40	2100	52	87.5
45	2293	51	95.5
50	2482	50	103.5
55	2666	48	111
60	2846	47	118.5
70	3195	46	133
80	3531	44	147
90	3857	43	161
100	4174	42	174

*132 kcal/kg$^{0.75}$.
From Nutritional Requirements of the Dog, National Research Council, Bethesda, MD, 1985.

TABLE 4 - 9 Approximate Daily Energy and Water Requirements of Cats Based on Body Weight*

Body weight (kg)	Total energy (kcal) or water (mL)		
	Per day	Per kilogram	Per hour
1.0	80.0	80	3
1.5	108.4	72	5
2.0	134.5	67	6
2.5	159.1	64	7
3.0	182.4	61	8
3.5	204.7	58	9
4.0	226.3	57	9
4.5	247.2	55	10
5.0	267.5	53	11

*80 $kcal/kg^{0.75}$.
From Nutritional Requirements of the Cat, National Research Council, Bethesda, MD, 1987.

parallel, throughout the day in one administration line. A third way is to administer the fluids in series. Administer the prescribed fluids in a manner that is convenient for your practice situation.

The following are important points to remember in fluid therapy:

1. To determine the rate of intravenous infusion of the fluids and additives, take the total volume of the fluids that have been prescribed and divide the total volume by the total number of hours in the day that are available for safe administration of the fluids. There should be no need to front-load the deficit repair fluid volume as long as the intravascular volume has been stabilized previously.
2. Administer the fluids over as many hours as possible to allow the patient as much time as possible to redistribute and fully use the administered fluids and electrolytes. With faster administration, a diuresis will occur and more of the fluids will be excreted in urine. Do not administer fluids continuously intravenously when the patient cannot be observed periodically to ascertain whether the fluids are continuing to run at an appropriate rate and that the administration line has not become disconnected. If the available time is limited (i.e., less than 12 hours) or if extra time is needed for safe administration of the fluids, an alternative plan (e.g., administering some of the required fluids subcutaneously) is indicated.
3. Intravenous administration of fluids is the preferred route because the fluid is dispersed rapidly and is immediately available to the patient. Intravenous administration may be inconvenient in some practice settings. The prescribed fluid can be administered subcutaneously in several divided doses. The subcutaneous route is usually well tolerated by patients, and therapy often is efficacious. However, the subcutaneous route is slower in onset than the intravenous route, is less efficacious than the intravenous route because some patients (especially those that are severely dehydrated and vasoconstricted) do not absorb the fluids well or at all, and it carries a slight risk of infection. Fluids can be administered orally or via stomach tube, in several divided doses, as long as the gastrointestinal tract is functional. Fluids also can be administered intraperitoneally. The intraperitoneal route is characterized by the same advantages and disadvantages as the subcutaneous route, but in addition there is a danger of injury or perforation of an abdominal organ. Fluids also can be administered via the intramedullary route. Intramedullary administration is more difficult than subcutaneous or intraperitoneal administration but is associated with much more

4

BOX 4-15   RATES OF FLOW AMONG INFUSION SETS

Cutter: 20 drops/mL
Abbott and McGaw: 15 drops/mL
McGaw: 15 drops/mL
Travenol: 10 drops/mL
To calculate drops per minute, use the following formulas:
Fluid volume to be infused (mL)/No. of hours available (hour) = mL/hour
For adult drip sets:
Cutter: mL/hour ÷ 3 = drops/minute
Abbott and McGaw: mL/hour ÷ 4 = drops/minute
Travenol: mL/hour ÷ 6 = drops/minute

---

rapid and reliable systemic uptake. The intramedullary route may be useful when venous access is difficult (e.g., a severely dehydrated kitten or puppy).

4. Fluids may be administered through central or peripheral veins. Indwelling catheters must be introduced and maintained aseptically. All fluids and administration sets must be sterile. Fluids with osmolalities less than 600 mOsm/L can be administered safely via a peripheral vein. Administer fluids with osmolalities greater than 700 mOsm/L via a large central vein because hyperosmolar fluids may cause thrombophlebitis if administered via small peripheral veins.

5. Control of the infusion rate is difficult when fluids are administered by gravity. Eliminate this problem by using an infusion pump (Box 4-15).

Most pediatric drip sets deliver 60 drops/mL (milliliters per hour equals drops per minute). Write fluid orders so that the volume to be administered is recorded as *mL/day, mL/hour,* and *drops/minute.* This will allow personnel to detect major calculation errors more easily. The clinician should not assume that the animal has received the volume of fluid ordered, and nursing personnel should note in the record the volume actually received. Clearly list all additives on the bottle; adhesive labels for this purpose are available. Attach a strip of adhesive tape to the bottle and mark it appropriately to provide a quick visual estimate of the volume of fluid received.

Additional Reading

DiBartola SP: *Fluid electrolyte, and acid-base disorders in small animal practice,* St Louis, 2006, Elsevier-Saunders.

Mathews KA: The various types of parenteral fluids and their indications, *Vet Clin North Am Small Anim Pract* 28:483, 1998.

Phillips S, Polzin D: Clinical disorders of potassium homeostasis: hyperkalemia and hypokalemia, *Vet Clin North Am Small Anim Pract* 28:545, 1998.

Schaer M (ed): Advances in fluid and electrolyte disorders, *Vet Clin North Am Small Anim Pract* 28:3, May 1998.

Wingfield WE: *Veterinary emergency medicine secrets,* Philadelphia, 1997, Hanley & Belfus.

GASTROINTESTINAL PROCEDURES

Numerous techniques are described for administering calories and nutrients to patients that are unable or unwilling to take in, chew, or swallow food. One method, intravenous hyperalimentation, is reserved for patients that are not able to tolerate any food being introduced via the gastrointestinal tract and represents a radical, and ideally transient, departure from normal. However, enteral feeding, which is always preferable to intravenous hyperalimentation, allows the clinician several options for administering food directly into the gastrointestinal tract. However, consideration of several variables is critical when one is initiating enteral feeding programs, such as the patient's diagnosis, attitude, status of the gastrointestinal tract, and the ability of the patient to digest and absorb food once introduced. In addition, consideration of the type and constituency of the diet provided is important. Although the options available for enteral nutrition are much greater that those for intravenous hyperalimentation, the clinician must consider dietary requirements carefully when planning enteral nutritional support.

When evaluating enteral feeding for the individual patient, the clinician has four basic options: nasoesophageal tube, pharyngostomy tube (least recommended), esophagostomy tube, and percutaneous gastroscopy tube (which can be performed using an endoscope or performed using the so-called blind technique). All techniques involve use of polyurethane or silicone feeding tube. The nasoesophageal tube placement technique does not require general anesthesia and may be inserted using a topical anesthetic only. Each of the other techniques described requires the patient to be anesthetized to ensure proper and safe placement.

NASOESOPHAGEAL INTUBATION

For temporary, short-term feeding, nasoesophageal intubation is a simple technique that works well in cats, puppies, and adult dogs. Patients that are comatose; have severe, persistent vomiting; or are unable to swallow are not candidates for this procedure. The objective of the procedure is to place a small-diameter tube (8F to 10F for dogs weighing more than 15 kg and 5F to 8F for small dogs and cats) through the nasal cavity into the distal esophagus. The tube does not have to enter the stomach. When measuring the tube length, measure from the tip of the nose to the eighth or ninth rib (Figure 4-36).

Administer 3 to 5 drops of a topical ophthalmic solution (0.5% proparacaine) directly into one nostril. Hold the head gently upward for a few seconds to allow the solution to reach the back of the nasal cavity. In most patients, it is desirable to wait 1 to 2 minutes and then to repeat the instillation in the same nostril. For larger dogs, 2% lidocaine solution (0.5 to 2.0 mL) gradually instilled into the nostril is an alternative technique to achieve topical anesthesia. Lubricate the tube with a thin coat of a water-soluble lubricant, such a 2% lidocaine lubricating gel. Pass the tube into the nasal cavity while directing the tube tip medial and ventral into the ventral meatus. The anatomic shape of a dog's nostril usually requires directing the tip medially but almost perpendicular to the plane of the nasal cavity

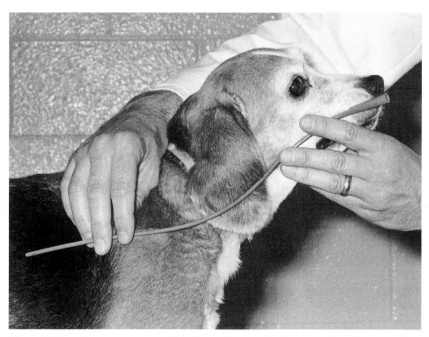

Figure 4-36: Technique for measuring the insertion length of nasoesophageal tube in a dog.

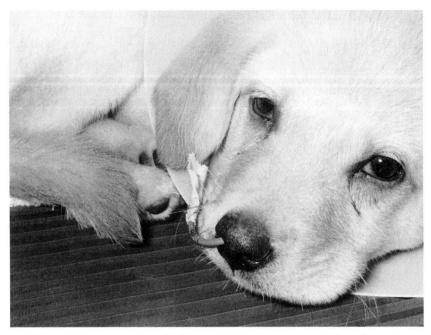

Figure 4-37:   Nasoesophageal tube secured with stay sutures on the face of a puppy.

to facilitate insertion. Initial resistance (pressure, not pain) usually is perceived, and the patient's head as expected quickly retracts, leaving the operator holding the tube tip some inches away from the patient's nose. Be persistent. Repeat the procedure, as necessary, by *quickly* inserting the first inch or more of the tube into the nostril. Once started, the remainder of the technique is relatively straightforward.

As the tube reaches the caudal aspect of the nasopharynx, it should pass directly into the esophagus with little or no resistance. Affix the tube remaining outside the patient to the head or face using a "butterfly" tape, gauze, suture (Figure 4-37), or skin glue (skin glue [Superglue] generally is NOT recommended because this can result in loss of hair and skin pigment when the glue becomes dislodged).

CAUTION: The tip of the tube possibly can be introduced inadvertently through the glottis and into the trachea. Topical anesthetic instilled into the nose can anesthetize the arytenoid cartilages, thereby blocking a cough or gag reflex. I prefer to check the tube placement with a dry, empty syringe. Attach the test syringe to the end of the feeding tube. Rather than inject air or water in an attempt to auscultate borborygmus over the abdomen, simply attempt to aspirate air from the feeding tube (Figure 4-38). IF THERE IS NO RESISTANCE DURING ASPIRATION AND AIR FILLS THE SYRINGE, IT IS LIKELY THAT THE TUBE HAS BEEN PLACED IN THE TRACHEA. Completely remove the tube and repeat the procedure. However, if repeated attempts to aspirate are met with immediate resistance and NO AIR ENTERS THE SYRINGE, the tube tip is positioned properly within the esophagus. If there is any question regarding placement, a lateral survey radiograph is indicated.

Pharyngostomy Tube Placement (Not Generally Recommended)

Originally indicated for use in dogs having long-term enteral feeding requirement, the pharyngostomy tube is associated with a number of complications, including laryngeal obstruction, aspiration, reflux, epiglottic entrapment, ulcerative esophagitis, and tube displacement. This technique generally is not recommended today. The technique entails

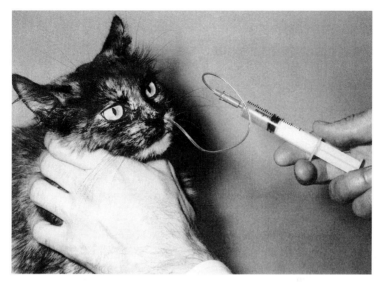

Figure 4-38: Technique for verifying esophageal placement of the tip of a nasoesophageal tube in a cat.

passing a 14F to 20F tube, measured to a length such that the tube tip will not enter the stomach, through the skin overlying the pharynx, caudal to the hyoid apparatus, and into the esophagus. Although the surgery is not particularly complex, the exit point of the tube through the wall of pharynx requires that the skin and tissue of the pharynx be incised in proximity to the external jugular vein, carotid artery, vagosympathetic trunk, and hypoglossal nerve. Alternative options make this technique the least attractive and perhaps highest maintenance.

4

ESOPHAGOSTOMY TUBE PLACEMENT

Less invasive and not requiring endoscopy equipment, esophagostomy tube placement in dogs and cats is an alternative technique to use in patients that have long-term feeding needs. Use a 14F to 20F rubber, polyurethane, or silicone feeding tube placed at the level of the middle of the cervical esophagus to the level of the eighth rib. The technique does require general anesthesia or, in the hands of an experienced individual, short-term intravenous anesthesia. The technique has been described in detail in textbooks (see "Marks SL" under Additional Reading). However, one should observe the technique being performed by someone with experience before attempting to place an esophagostomy tube for the first time. Although postplacement complications generally are limited to local irritation or minor infection at the site of the stoma in the midcervical region, variations to performing the procedure are described, and the placement technique is not intuitive from published descriptions.

PERCUTANEOUS GASTROSTOMY TUBE PLACEMENT

Percutaneous gastrostomy tubes are used routinely to administer nutrients and medications orally over days or weeks to cats and dogs that cannot have nutrients administered by mouth or that will not eat (e.g., because of feline hepatic lipidosis, oropharyngeal neoplasms, maxillary or mandibular fractures, oral reconstructive surgery, esophageal masses or foreign bodies, or severe pharyngitis). The percutaneous gastrostomy tube is placed so that it extends through the skin and left cranial abdominal wall of the abdomen into the body of the stomach.

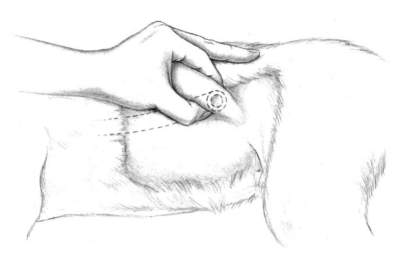

Figure 4-39: Locating the end of the rigid stomach tube at the left lateral abdominal wall. (From Crow S, Walshaw S: *Manual of clinical procedures in the dog, cat, and rabbit,* ed 2, Philadelphia, 1997, Lippincott-Raven.)

Catheter preparation

Catheter preparation for a percutaneous gastrostomy tube is as follows:
1. Use the French-Pezzar mushroom-tipped catheter.
2. Cut off 1.5 cm of the open (distal) end of the catheter with scissors.
3. Cut 3-mm holes on either side of the 1.5-cm piece (outer flange).
4. Cut the distal end of the catheter to form a sharp bevel point.
5. Measure the length of the tube from the mushroom tip to 2 cm below the bevel.

Preparation of the stomach tube

Stomach tube preparation for a percutaneous gastrostomy tube is as follows:
1. Use a smooth-ended vinyl stomach tube.
2. Measure the length of the tube needed to reach the stomach by laying the tube along the animal's side with the rounded end 1 to 2 cm caudal to the last rib.
3. Mark the tube with an indelible marker or adhesive tape at the tip of the muzzle and cut off the excess tube.
4. Put the tube in the freezer for 30 minutes before beginning the procedure to stiffen the tube.

Placement of the percutaneous gastrotomy tube

Placement of a percutaneous gastrostomy tube is as follows:
1. Clip and surgically prepare the skin over the left abdominal wall.
2. Place the mouth speculum between the right canine teeth.
3. Place the stomach tube in the esophagus to the level of the cardia.
4. Rotate the tube counterclockwise while carefully advancing it through the cardia.
5. Turn the tube back clockwise and advance the tube until it can be visualized through the abdominal wall 1 to 2 cm caudal to the last rib (Figure 4-39).
6. Rotate the tube so that the tip lies against the stomach and abdominal wall one third of the distance between the epaxial muscles and the ventral midline.
7. Make a 2- to 3-mm skin incision directly over the lumen of the stomach tube.
8. Use a Sovereign catheter (over the needle) and puncture the abdominal and stomach walls, placing the catheter inside the lumen of the stomach tube. Remove the needle (Figure 4-40).

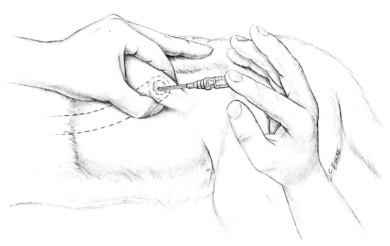

Figure 4-40: Placement of the Sovereign catheter through the abdominal and stomach walls and into the lumen of the somach tube.
(From Crow S, Walshaw S: *Manual of clinical procedures in the dog, cat, and rabbit,* ed 2, Philadelphia, 1997, Lippincott-Raven.)

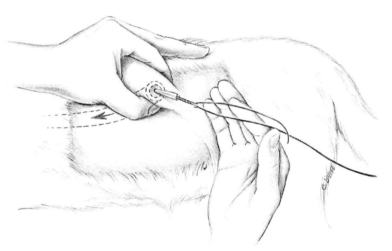

Figure 4-41: Threading the introduction line retrograde through the Sovereign catheter and stomach tube.
(From Crow S, Walshaw S: *Manual of clinical procedures in the dog, cat, and rabbit,* ed 2, Philadelphia, 1997, Lippincott-Raven.)

9. Thread a long, rigid suture through the catheter and advance it through the stomach tube until the end is observed at the mouth end of the tube (Figure 4-41).
10. Carefully remove the plastic catheter from the stomach tube opening and place a hemostat clamp at the end of the suture material.
11. Remove the stomach tube over the oral end of the stiff introduction suture line.
12. Attach the open, beveled end of the French-Pezzar catheter stomach tube to a plastic Sovereign catheter using a mattress suture (Figure 4-42).
13. Force the tip of the rubber stomach tube into the large end of the Sovereign catheter.
14. Advance the catheter-tube through the mouth and esophagus into the stomach by placing traction on the abdominal end of the introduction line.

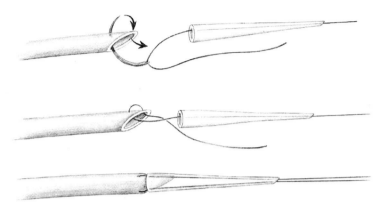

Figure 4-42:   Suturing the introduction line to the beveled end of the gastrostomy catheter. (From Crow S, Walshaw S: *Manual of clinical procedures in the dog, cat, and rabbit,* ed 2, Philadelphia, 1997, Lippincott-Raven.)

15. The catheter will emerge through the skin incision followed by the rubber tube. Grasp the tube with forceps and pull it through the incision opening (Figure 4-43, *A*).
16. Remove the catheter by cutting it off 2 cm below the beveled tip. Pull the rubber tube through the abdominal wall until slight resistance is felt (Figure 4-43, *B*).
17. Slide the outer flange over the end of the tube down to the skin level (Figure 4-44).
18. Apply antimicrobial ointment and a sterile gauze sponge over the skin incision.
19. Bandage the gastrostomy tube in place (Figure 4-45).

Additional Reading

Crow S, Walshaw S: *Manual of clinical procedures in the dog, cat, and rabbit,* ed 2, Philadelphia, 1997, Lippincott-Raven.
Marks SL: Nasoesophageal, esophagostomy, and gastrostomy tube placement techniques. In Ettinger SJ, Feldman EC, editors: *Textbook of veterinary internal medicine,* ed 6, St Louis, 2005, Elsevier-Saunders.
Mazzaferro EM: Esophagostomy tubes: don't underutilize them!, *J Vet Emerg Care* 11(2): 153-156, 2001.

LAPAROSCOPY

Laparoscopy is a procedure for performing a visual examination of the peritoneal cavity and its contents after the establishment of pneumoperitoneum. The advantage of the procedure is that it is minimally invasive, although general anesthesia is required. Laparoscopy does allow limited visualization of several organs, at least in part. Visualization of needle biopsies of kidney, liver, and/or spleen is also possible during the procedure. The disadvantage is that the required equipment can be expensive and specific training and experience are required to become efficient at the procedure. Additionally, insufflation of the abdomen must be monitored in addition to monitoring the patient's quality of respirations and oxygenation (pulse oximetry).

The Dyonics Needlescope (Smith & Nephew, Andover, Massachusetts) is a small fiberoptic laparoscope 1.7 or 2.2 mm in diameter. The device does require a high-intensity light source, but because of its small size, it can be inserted readily into the abdomen. Abdominal insufflation and laparoscopy require general anesthesia, neuroleptanalgesia with local anesthesia, or rarely (in the critically ill animal), regional local anesthesia alone. The depth and type of anesthesia or analgesia depend on the condition of the patient and the skill and experience of the examiner.

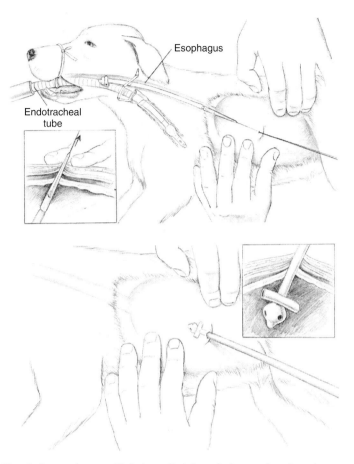

Figure 4-43: Catheter-tube assembly being pulled through the mouth and esophagus and the stomach and abdominal walls.
(From Crow S, Walshaw S: *Manual of clinical procedures in the dog, cat, and rabbit,* ed 2, Philadelphia, 1997, Lippincott-Raven.)

Before laparoscopy, perform a cleansing enema. Surgically prepare the laparoscopy site. To insufflate the abdomen, use a Verees pneumoperitoneum needle. Place the needle 3 to 4 cm below the umbilicus, along the linea alba. Inject 10 mL of saline through the needle, and attempt aspiration to ensure that a blood vessel or hollow viscus has not been penetrated. The intraabdominal pressure created should not be greater than 20 mm Hg. Remove and examine any ascitic fluid that is present.

Inject air into the peritoneal cavity through an in-line filter with the Verees needle. Insufflation should be slow, and vital signs should be monitored. Following effective insufflation, remove the needle, make a small skin incision over the needle entry point, and insert the larger trocar and cannula at a 30-degree angle to the animal's longitudinal plane. Take extreme care when placing the trocar into the abdomen. Move the endoscope (Needlescope) cephalad along the abdominal wall while maintaining good insufflation. Rotate the animal into different positions to enable visualization of various internal organs. Biopsy specimens can be obtained through the Needlescope or through a separate incision while observing through the Needlescope. When endoscopic inspection has been completed, remove the Needlescope, allow the insufflated air to escape, and place the skin sutures.

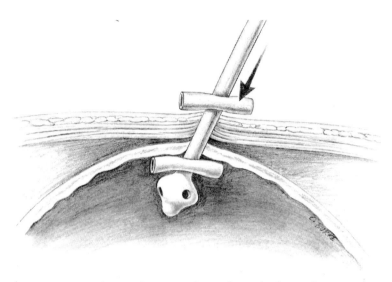

Figure 4-44:   Diagram showing the inner and outer flanges in place against stomach mucosa and skin, respectively.
(From Crow S, Walshaw S: *Manual of clinical procedures in the dog, cat, and rabbit,* ed 2, Philadelphia, 1997, Lippincott-Raven.)

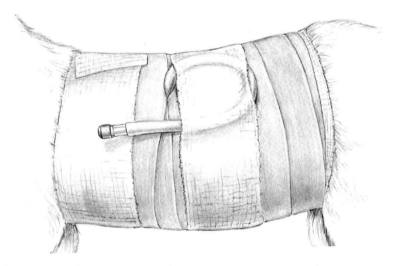

Figure 4-45:   Full abdominal bandage showing the plugged end of the gastostomy tube emerging dorsally.
(From Crow S, Walshaw S: *Manual of clinical procedures in the dog, cat, and rabbit,* ed 2, Philadelphia, 1997, Lippincott-Raven.)

Indications for laparoscopy include biopsy, visual diagnosis, follow-up examinations, and research needs. Contraindications to laparoscopy include peritonitis, hernias, coagulation defects, obesity, abdominal adhesions, and inexperience of the clinician.

Additional Reading

Guilford WG, Center SA, Strombeck DR, et al: *Strombeck's small animal gastroenterology,* ed 3, Philadelphia, 1996, WB Saunders.

Richter K: Laparoscopy. In Ettinger SJ, Feldman EC, editors: *Textbook of veterinary internal medicine,* ed 6, St Louis, 2005, Elsevier-Saunders.

OPHTHALMIC PROCEDURES

EVALUATION OF TEAR PRODUCTION

Tear production comes predominantly from the tarsal and conjunctival glands and from the accessory tarsal glands. The reflex tear secretors are the main lacrimal gland and the accessory lacrimal glands. The production of normal lacrimal secretions can be tested by using Schirmer's tear test, a standardized filter paper (Figure 4-46) that effectively measures the rate of tear production in millimeters per minute. Schirmer's tear strips now are impregnated with a blue dye to facilitate visualization of the distance (in millimeters) that the tear migrates during the 1-minute test.

Each eye can be tested independently, or both eyes can be tested simultaneously in the cooperative patient. Carefully fold the notched end of the test strip before removing it from the plastic package. Insert the folded end into the lower conjunctival cul-de-sac (Figure 4-47) and begin the timing. Maintain the Schirmer's test strip in position by gently holding the eyelids closed but not touching the paper. At the end of 1 minute, note the degree (distance) of wetting that occurred and record it in the medical record. The normal dog and cat should produce wetting over 10 to 25 mm in 1 minute for each eye. Amounts less than that are consistent with keratoconjunctivitis sicca. Amounts greater than 25 mm may be normal or may be consistent with excessive tear production, or epiphora.

FLUORESCEIN STAINING OF THE CORNEA

The cornea is composed of various layers of specialized avascular epithelium and stroma. The outer layer, the corneal epithelium, is a highly sensitive, thin layer overlying the corneal stroma, the thickest layer. Descemet's membrane is a distinct, thin layer of tissue beneath the stroma. The innermost layer of the cornea is the endothelium. Damage to the corneal epithelium occurs frequently in dogs and cats. Clinical presentation typically is characterized by blepharospasm of the affected eye with or without a visible ocular discharge or conjunctivitis.

Whenever superficial corneal injury is suspected, assessment of the integrity of the corneal epithelium is indicated. Fluorescein dye-impregnated test strips can be used to determine whether the epithelial barrier overlying the corneal stroma has been disrupted and, as such, can establish the presence or absence of a corneal ulcer (Figure 4-48).

The test is simple to accomplish. Moisten the dye-impregnated tip of the test strip with a drop of balanced saline solution (or commercial ocular irrigation solution). Gently allow

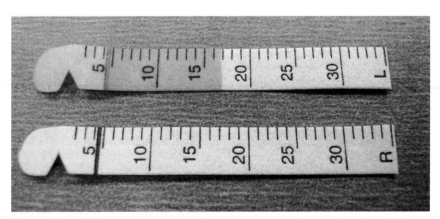

Figure 4-46: Schirmer's tear test strips depicting tear production as a function of distance (millimeters).

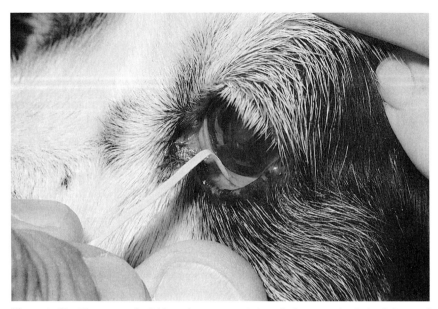

Figure 4-47: Placement of a Schirmer's tear test strip into the lower conjuctival cul-de-sac of a dog; the test strip is held in place for 60 seconds only.

4

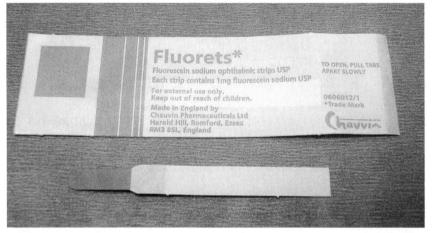

Figure 4-48: Fluorescein sodium–impregnated test strip used to enhance visualization of a corneal ulcer.

the tip of the test paper to touch the cornea, or sclera, of the affected eye. (In patients with particularly painful, sensitive eye, use a topical anesthetic to moisten the test strip or apply the anesthetic directly to the cornea before testing.) Immediately rinse the eye with a sterile irrigation solution to remove the excess dye (the test strip has a lot of dye; be prepared to catch the excess fluid with a 2×2-inch gauze).

Promply examine the eye with a direct, focal light source. Evidence of green dye uptake in the stroma indicates that an ulcer is present. The absence of staining generally indicates that the corneal integrity is intact. One exception exists. Descemet's membrane will not take up fluorescein dye. A patient with a deep corneal ulcer that penetrates through the corneal stroma and allows herniation of Descemet's membrane (descemetocele) will not demonstrate a positive stain. Careful visualization of the cornea, however, is likely to reveal the presence of a such a serious, deep ulcer.

ASSESSMENT OF NASOLACRIMAL DUCT PATENCY

Fluroescein dye can be used to assess patency of the nasolacrimal duct. To perform this examination, place a drop of fluorescein dye from a sterile fluorescein strip into the eye and add 1 to 2 drops of a sterile eye wash. After 2 to 5 minutes, examine the external nares with the aid of a cobalt blue filter or Wood's light for the presence or absence of fluorescence. A clean, 2 × 2-inch white gauze touched against the nasal planum also will pick up the green-colored dye if the duct is patent. If dye is present, the lacrimal excretory system is patent and functioning. If epiphora exists but the primary dye test indicates that the lacrimal excretory system is patent, hypersecretion of tear fluid may be implicated as the cause of the epiphora.

Irrigation of the nasolacrimal system is indicated if the primary dye test is negative. In the dog, the nasolacrimal puncta are located 1 to 3 mm from the medial canthus on the mucocutaneous border of the upper and lower lids. In the dog, use a 20- to 22-gauge (in the cat, a 23-gauge) nasolacrimal cannula (Figure 4-49).Topical anesthesia often is required. Fill a 2-mL syringe with saline, and attach the lacrimal cannula and pass it into the lacrimal puncta of the upper lid.

Several points should be made about evaluating the nasolacrimal system. Brachycephalic breeds of dogs and cats occasionally may have a negative primary dye test, although no blockage in the nasolacrimal system exists. In flushing the nasolacrimal system of some animals, fluid may not appear at the nose; however, the animal may gag and exhibit swallowing movements, indicating that the fluid has entered the mouth and the system is patent.

CONJUNCTIVAL SMEARS, SCRAPINGS, AND CULTURES

In performing conjunctival scrapings, use a platinum spatula (Kimura spatula) the tip of which has been sterilized previously in the flame of an alcohol lamp and has been allowed to cool. Scrape the inferior conjunctival cul-de-sac, preferably without prior topical anesthesia, because anesthetics may distort the cells (Figure 4-50). Place the material on two glass slides. Fix one slide in acetone-free 95% methanol for 5 to 10 minutes; then stain the slide with Giemsa stain. Heat-fix the other slide, and apply Gram stain.

4

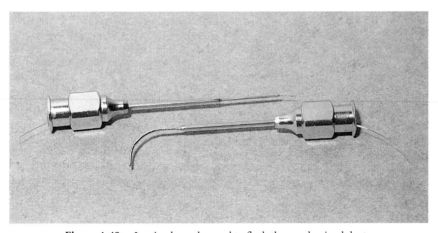

Figure 4-49: Lacrimal canulas used to flush the nasolacrimal ducts.

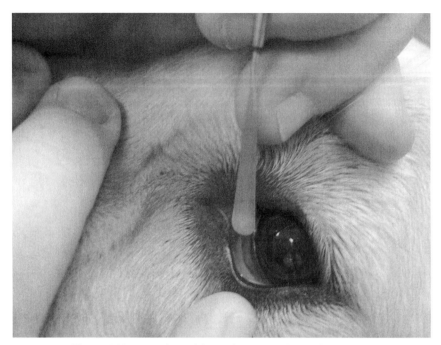

Figure 4-50:   Spatula used for performing conjunctival scrapings.

4

To culture the conjunctiva, use sterile cotton-tipped applicators, fluid thioglycollate medium, and blood agar medium. Evert the palpebral conjunctiva of the lower lid, and pass one side of a sterile cotton applicator, previously moistened with sterile broth or thioglycollate medium, over the palpebral conjunctival surface. Streak the swab onto a sterile blood agar plate; then place the plate in a tube of thioglycollate broth. No topical anesthesia is used before culturing because preservatives present in anesthetics can inhibit the growth of bacteria.

TONOMETRY

Glaucoma is an increase in intraocular pressure incompatible with normal ocular and visual functions. One method used to measure intraocular pressure is tonometry, in which the tension of the outer coat of the eye is assessed by measuring the impressibility, or applanability, of the cornea. Because the measurements based on tonometry involve calculations that have a wide base of variations, tonometry readings are always approximations.

Schiøtz tonometry

The Schiøtz tonometer consists of a corneal footplate, plunger, holding bracket, recording scale, and 5.5-, 7.5-, 10.0-, and 15.0-g weights (Figure 4-51). The principle of the Schiøtz tonometer is that the amount that the plunger protrudes from the footplate is related to the indentability of the cornea, which in turn is related to the intraocular pressure. The plunger is connected to a scale so that 0.05-mm protrusion of the plunger equals 1 scale unit (Table 4-10).

Place the dog in the sitting or dorsal recumbent position. Instill topical anesthesia, and hold open the eyelids with the fingers, which are placed far away from the lid margins. Place the footplate vertically on the central aspect of the cornea (Figure 4-52). Take three readings in each eye and then average the readings. Normal intraocular tension with the Schiøtz tonometer in dogs is 15 to 25 mm Hg.

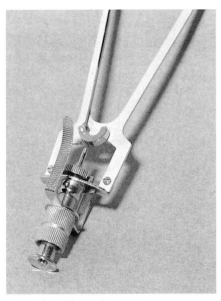

Figure 4-51: Footplate (for corneal contact) of the Schiøtz tonometer.

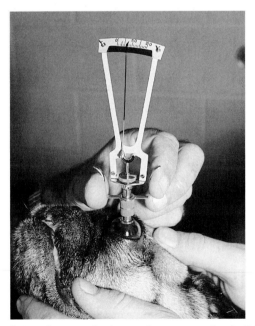

Figure 4-52: Technique for measuring intraocular pressure using the Schiøtz tonometer.

Applanation tonometry

In applanation tonometry, a very small area of the cornea is flattened by a known force, usually a calibrated burst of air. The advantage of this technique over the indentation (Schiøtz) method is that the errors resulting from ocular rigidity and corneal curvature are greatly reduced. Special equipment is required to perform applanation tonometry.

T A B L E 4 - 1 0 Schiøtz Tonometer—Calibration Table for the Canine Eye

Schiøtz scale reading	Intraocular pressure (mm Hg)		
	5.5 g Weight	7.5 g Weight	10.0 g Weight
0.5	52.6	71.2	93.6
1.0	49.3	67.0	88.3
1.5	46.3	63.1	83.3
2.0	43.4	59.4	78.6
2.5	40.8	55.9	74.1
3.0	38.3	52.6	69.6
3.5	36.0	49.6	66.0
4.0	33.9	46.7	62.2
4.5	31.9	44.0	58.7
5.0	30.1	41.6	55.4
5.5	28.4	39.2	52.3
6.0	26.9	37.1	49.4
6.5	25.5	35.1	46.7
7.0	24.2	33.2	44.2
7.5	23.0	31.5	41.8
8.0	21.9	29.9	39.6
8.5	21.0	28.5	37.5
9.0	20.1	27.1	35.6
9.5	19.3	25.9	33.8
10.0	18.6	24.8	32.1
10.5	18.0	23.8	30.6
11.0	17.4	22.8	29.1
11.5	17.0	22.0	27.8
12.0	16.6	21.3	26.6
12.5	16.3	20.6	25.5
13.0	16.0	20.0	24.5
13.5	15.8	19.5	23.6
14.0	15.7	19.1	22.8
14.5	15.7	18.8	22.0
15.0	15.7	18.5	21.4
15.5	15.8	18.3	20.8
16.0	15.9	18.1	20.3
16.5	16.1	18.0	19.9
17.0	16.4	18.0	19.5
17.5	16.8	18.1	19.2
18.0	17.2	18.2	19.0
18.5	17.7	18.4	18.8
19.0	18.3	18.7	18.7
19.5	19.0	19.0	18.6
20.0	19.7	19.4	18.7

GONIOSCOPY

Glaucoma can be caused by many different disorders that elevate intraocular pressure. In many types of glaucoma, there is an abnormality in the anterior angle of the eye (filtration angle). Gonioscopy permits one to visualize and examine the iridocorneal angle, which cannot be seen without the use of a special contact lens.

The Koeppe gonioscopic lens seems to be well-suited to dogs and cats. The lens is available in 17-, 19-, and 21-mm sizes. The lens can be inserted into the eye following the application of topical anesthesia. The gonioscopic lens can be filled with 1% methylcellulose or saline. The inside of the lens is illuminated with a Barkan lamp, otoscope head, or binocular indirect ophthalmoscope. Magnification suitable for visualization of the angle can be provided by an otoscope head, indirect ophthalmoscope, or Haag-Streit goniomicroscope.

Additional Reading

Barnett KC, Sansom J, Heinrich C: *Canine ophthalmology*, Philadelphia, 2002, WB Saunders.
Barnett KC, Crispin SM: *Feline ophthalmology*, Philadelphia, 1998, WB Saunders.

RADIOGRAPHY: ADVANCED CONTRAST STUDIES

GASTROINTESTINAL STUDIES

When considering a contrast study of the gastrointestinal tract, it is not unreasonable to question the value of doing this procedure. At issue is the fact that abdominal ultrasound and/or gastrointestinal endoscopy have largely replaced contrast radiography of the gastrointestinal tract and for good reason. Diagnostic modalities such as ultrasound (in the hands of an experienced individual) and endoscopy have a much greater diagnostic yield than the less sensitive contrast study. So, why even try? Endoscopes are not available in every practice, and access to an ultrasound, much less someone who is qualified to use the equipment, puts routine use of advanced diagnostic modalities out of reach for many practices. However, it must be appreciated that the diagnostic value of a radiographic contrast study of the gastrointestinal tract is a far less sensitive diagnostic modality than abdominal ultrasound or endoscopy. However, the procedure for gastrointestinal radiographic contrast study is outlined next.

Contrast agents available for gastrointestinal studies include barium suspension preparations or Micropaque (Guerbet, Villepente, France); and water-soluble agents (Gastrografin [Bracco Diagnostics Inc., Princeton, New Jersey], which is 60% meglumine and 10% sodium diatrizoate). Water-soluble agents are used if bowel perforation is suspected. Undiluted water-soluble agents are hypertonic and should be diluted at a ratio of one part Gastrografin to two parts water. No single procedure is appropriate for all gastrointestinal cases. The clinician must select procedures based on the clinical history and physical findings, apparent location of the lesion within the gastrointestinal tract, endoscopic findings, and results from other imaging studies, such as abdominal ultrasound.

Contrast esophagram

The contrast esophagram also is called barium swallow. The decision to perform a contrast esophagogram is based on physical evidence of dysphagia (difficulty or pain while attempting to swallow) and/or persistent regurgitation (reflux of swallowed food without effort). The procedure necessitates that the animal fast for 12 hours before radiography. Remove all leashes from around the animal's neck, and obtain survey radiographs of the thorax. In esophageal contrast studies, administer barium suspension contrast medium, 2 to 5 mL/kg body mass. *Administration of barium as a contrast material is contraindicated if a perforation of the esophagus is suspected.* When the esophagus has been coated with radiopaque material, take lateral, ventrodorsal, and right ventrodorsal oblique thoracic radiographs to visualize the esophagus.

Properly prepared, the barium should be thick and pasty (like marshmallow fluff). Position the patient and cassette, and have the radiographic technique set up. Give a table-spoonful of barium orally. Make the exposure when the animal takes its second swallow after the barium has been given.

For esophageal studies and barium swallows, sedation with acepromazine 0.1 mg/kg and buprenorphine 0.015 mg/kg will produce no adverse alteration in gastrointestinal motility.

4

For cats, ketamine 10 mg and midazolam 0.2 mg/kg (combined) can be administered intramuscularly with no significant effect in esophageal motility.

In some cases of incomplete esophageal stricture, barium liquid will pass through the esophagus unobstructed, whereas food will not. Veterinarians have to be particularly helpful in these patients to mix kibbled food with the barium and allow the patient to eat the mixture just before making the radiograph.

Ideally, however, contrast esophagrams are performed using fluoroscopy, rather than conventional radiographs. In this manner, it is possible not only to identify strictures and dilatations, if present, but also to obtain a dynamic study of the esophagus that provides valuable information pertaining to swallowing and esophageal motility and function and an opportunity to evaluate sphincter activity at the level of the cardia.

Upper gastrointestinal tract (stomach, pylorus, and small intestine)

Contrast studies of the upper gastrointestinal tract are used to facilitate diagnosis of persistent vomiting, hematemesis, unexplained and chronic diarrhea, suspected enteric foreign bodies, suspected neoplasms and obstructions, and for confirmation of displaced intestinal organs, as may be seen in diaphragmatic hernias.

That said, the availability of abdominal ultrasound has largely replaced the upper gastrointestinal series. At the hands of an experienced ultrasonographer, the diagnostic value of abdominal ultrasound far exceeds that derived from evaluating sequential radiographs of a patient after oral administration of contrast medium such as barium. In the event ultrasound capability is *not* available, contrast study of the upper gastrointestinal tract still can be used. However, the clinician must appreciate that a barium contrast study of the stomach, duodenum, jejunum, and ileum has a low sensitivity as a diagnostic test. That is, negative findings are not expected to correlate well with the absence of clinical disease. A negative study does not rule out disease. Likewise, a contrast study of the upper gastrointestinal tract is not recognized for its ability to confirm a diagnosis gastrointestinal tract disease, even when disease is present. Perhaps the greatest value in performing the upper gastrointestinal series in a dog or cat today centers on the need to identify a displacement of the stomach and/or small intestine because of an extraluminal mass lesion or congenital defect in the patient. In addition, the use of a microfine barium suspension may facilitate identification of intestinal ulcers, irregularities (e.g., intraluminal neoplasia), and radiolucent foreign bodies. However, variable-diameter, solid-phase radiopaque markers called BIPS (barium-impregnated polyethylene spheres) can be used to assess gastric emptying time, gastrointestinal transit times, and to some extent, obstructive disorders.

Technique for upper gastrointestinal study

If an upper gastrointestinal study is indicated, follow the technique described:

1. Ensure that the hair of the animal is free from dirt, paint, and foreign material. Bathe the animal if necessary.
2. Withhold food for 18 to 24 hours.
3. If the colon is filled with feces, administer a cleansing (Fleet) enema the evening before performing the procedure. In dogs, give a second enema 3 to 5 hours before the start of the gastrointestinal series.
4. At the start of an upper gastrointestinal series, obtain survey radiographs of the abdomen. Administer a barium sulfate (micropulverized) preparation by stomach tube, or induce the animal to swallow the fluids. Flavored, prepared barium suspensions are available, but they taste bad (personal experience). Dosage levels vary, but for barium suspensions, give approximately 10 mL/kg. As an alternative to barium, use an organic iodide liquid preparation. Administer 0.5 mL/kg by stomach tube. Obtain lateral and dorsoventral radiographs of the abdomen immediately following administration of the contrast material and at 30-minute, 1-hour, and 2-hour intervals. Water-soluble contrast material passes through the gastrointestinal tract in

30 to 90 minutes. Barium suspensions take 60 to 180 minutes to traverse the intestine. The colon usually is filled with barium 6 hours after oral administration and may contain barium for 2 to 3 days following administration.

Barium contrast radiography is contraindicated if perforation of the stomach or upper gastrointestinal tract is suspected. In these cases, use water-soluble contrast media such as the oral diatrizoates because leakage into the abdomen will produce no foreign body granuloma. In addition, do not administer barium sulfate when an obstruction of the lower bowel may be present. In these cases, barium may only contribute to the obstipation.

The following radiographic views are recommended following administration of radiographic contrast material:

1. Immediately following administration of contrast material obtain a ventrodorsal, right lateral, and left lateral views. The right lateral view shows the pylorus of the stomach filled with barium, and the left lateral view shows the cardia and fundic portion filled with barium. The objective is to evaluate the distended stomach and initial gastric emptying.
2. Twenty to 30 minutes following administration of contrast material, obtain ventrodorsal and right lateral views to assess the stomach, pyloric emptying, and the proximal duodenum.
3. Sixty minutes following administration of contrast material, repeat the ventrodorsal and right lateral recumbency views to assess the small intestine.
4. Two hours following administration of contrast material, repeat the ventrodorsal and right lateral views to evaluate passage of contrast material into the colon and complete emptying of the stomach; contrast material should be in the terminal portion of the small intestine.

Guidelines for passage of contrast material through the gastrointestinal tract

The passage of contrast material through the normal gastrointestinal tract is variable; however, the following guidelines have been suggested:

1. Contrast material is in the duodenum within 15 minutes in most patients. Excitement can delay gastric emptying time to 20 to 25 minutes.
2. Contrast material reaches the jejunum within 30 minutes and is within the jejunum and ileum at 60 minutes.
3. Contrast material reaches the ileocecal junction in 90 to 120 minutes.
4. At 3 to 5 hours after administration, contrast material has cleared the upper gastrointestinal tract and is within the ileum and the large intestine.

In evaluation of gastrointestinal contrast studies, consider the following criteria: (1) the size of the intestinal mass, (2) the contour of the mucosal surface, (3) thickness of the bowel wall, (4) flexibility and motility of the bowel wall, (5) position of the small intestine, (6) continuity of the opaque column, and (7) transit time.

The barium enema

Clinical disorders for which the barium enema is indicated in dogs include ileocolic intussusception and cecal inversion (intussusception), mechanical and functional large bowel obstruction, invasive lesions of the large bowel, a mass outside the large bowel compressing the bowel, and inflammation of the lower intestinal tract. Barium sulfate enemas are contraindicated in suspected obstruction of the colon and rupture or perforation of the colon. However, these same disorders also can be identified by ultrasonic examination or colonoscopy, either of which is the preferred diagnostic modality over a barium enema.

Use the following procedure when giving barium enemas:

1. Twenty-four hours preceding radiographs, administer a liquid diet only, preferably water or broth.
2. During the 18 to 24 hours before the radiographs, administer a mild high colonic enema or give a saline laxative orally.
3. Do not give any irritating enemas within 12 hours of the scheduled radiographic examination; however, administer isotonic saline solution or plain water enemas before the examination to ensure that the bowel is clear.

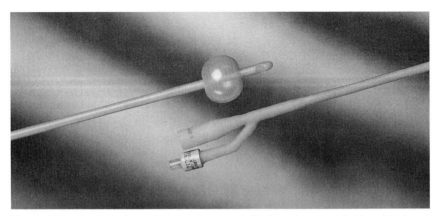

Figure 4-53: Bardex catheter depicting the expanded balloon tip used to facilitate infusion of barium into the colon.

4. Obtain survey radiographs of the abdomen, and examine the colon to ensure that this portion of the bowel is clear.
5. Do not force barium into the colon under pressure. Do not elevate the enema bag more than 18 inches above the animal.
6. Do not perform a proctoscopic examination on the same day that the barium enema is given.

Cuffed rectal catheters (Bardex cuffed rectal catheters, 24F to 38F, and the Bardex cuffed pediatric rectal catheter, 18F [C.R. Bard, Inc., Murray Hill, New Jersey]) can be used in dogs (Figure 4-53). For very small dogs and cats, use smaller catheters. A plastic catheter adapter and a three-way stopcock are needed. Various barium sulfate preparations can be used; however, the final concentration should be 15% to 20% w/v. A commercially available barium enema kit is helpful.

To perform a barium enema effectively, sedate or anesthetize the animal. Place the cuffed rectal catheter so that the inflated bulb is cranial to the anal sphincter. Place the animal in right lateral recumbency and fill the colon with contrast material at a dose of 20 to 30 mL/kg body mass. Take the radiographs after infusion of a two-thirds dose of barium. If the colon is not filled, infuse more contrast agent. Obtain radiographs in the ventrodorsal and lateral positions, and determine whether the colon is distended adequately. Remove as much of the contrast material as possible from the colon, and repeat the radiographs. Then insert air at 2 mL/kg into the colon, and repeat the radiographs. Deflate the cuff on the catheter, and remove the catheter from the rectum. Throughout the procedure of filling the colon with contrast material or air, take care not to overdistend the colon, which may lead to rupture.

When reviewing individual radiographs, look for the following radiographic lesions: (1) irregularity of the barium-mucosal interface; (2) spasm, stricture, or occlusion of the bowel lumen; (3) filling defects; (4) outpouching of the bowel wall caused by diverticulum or perforation; and (5) displacement of the bowel.

Additional Reading

Burk RL, Ackerman N: *Small animal radiology and ultrasonography: a diagnostic atlas and text,* ed 3, St Louis, 2003, Saunders.
Hall EJ, German AJ: Diseases of the small intestine. In Ettinger SJ, Feldman EC, editors: *Textbook of veterinary internal medicine,* ed 6, St Louis, 2005, Elsevier-Saunders.
Thrall DE: *Textbook of veterinary diagnostic radiology,* ed 4, Philadelphia, 2002, Saunders.
Washabau RJ, Holt DE: Diseases of the large intestine. In Ettinger SJ, Feldman EC, editors: *Textbook of veterinary internal medicine,* ed 6, St Louis, 2005, Elsevier-Saunders.

Excretory Urography

Intravenous administration of organic iodinated compounds in high concentrations permits visualization in four phases: (1) the arteriogram, (2) the nephrogram, (3) the pyelogram, and (4) the cystogram (Box 4-16). The arterial phase demonstrates renal blood flow; the nephrogram demonstrates the accumulation of contrast agent in the renal tubules and is used to evaluate renal parenchyma; the pyelogram phase evaluates the urinary collecting system, including the ureters; and the cystogram reveals the collection of contrast agent in the urinary bladder. Excretory urography does not result in any quantitative information about renal function and is not a substitute for renal function tests. The degree of visualization of contrast material within the renal excretory system depends on the concentration of iodine in the contrast medium, the technique of excretory urography performed, the state of hydration of the patient, renal blood flow, and the functional capacity of the kidneys.

The contrast medium most commonly used is a diatrizoate or iothalamate compound. Rapidly administer 850 mg/kg of an iodine compound intravenously. Obtain a ventrodorsal radiograph at 10 seconds after injection, and repeat ventrodorsal and lateral radiographs 1, 3, 5, 15, 20, and 40 minutes following injection. This method is the current standard technique. If the patient's blood urea nitrogen level is greater than or equal to 50 mg/dL or the creatinine level is greater than 4 mg/dL, double the dose rate.

Lesions that can be detected by using intravenous urography are renal mass lesions; neoplasia; renal cysts; renal and ureteral traumatic lesions; pyelonephritis; hydroureter; hydronephrosis; renal agenesis; hypoplasia; pelvic and ureteral obstructions (calculi, blood clots); renal parasites; ectopic ureter; and duplication of the collecting system.

BOX 4-16 PATIENT PREPARATION FOR EXCRETORY UROGRAPHY

1. Have the patient fast for 12 to 18 hours.
2. Administer a cleansing enema or give a saline laxative orally 12 to 18 hours before radiography.
3. Ensure that the animal's hair is free of dirt and debris.
4. Try to limit the animal's fluid intake in the 12 hours preceding radiography.
5. Empty the animal's bladder immediately before taking radiographs.
6. Take survey radiographs before administering contrast media.

4

Retrograde Contrast Urethrography

Retrograde urethrography is a diagnostic tool used to localize diseases of the lower urinary tract of dogs and cats. This method can reveal conditions such as urethral neoplasms, strictures, trauma, calculi, or other anomalies.

The technique involves the injection of an aqueous iodine contrast medium into the urethra through a ureteral or balloon-tipped catheter. The radiopaque contrast material is mixed to a three- to fivefold dilution with sterile lubricating jelly to increase the viscosity. A dilution of 1:3 contrast medium with sterile distilled water or saline also can be used. Before retrograde contrast urethography is performed, give the animal a cleansing enema. Sedation or anesthesia may be necessary. Inject 5 to 10 mL of contrast medium. Near the end of the injection, while the urethra is still under pressure, obtain a lateral radiograph.

If the urinary bladder is to be distended with contrast material or air, remove urine from the bladder. In the male dog, position the catheter so that the tip of the catheter is distal to the os penis. Inject lidocaine 1 to 2 mL into the urethral lumen to anesthetize the urethra adjacent to the balloon-tipped catheter. Take extreme care in the amount of fluid placed in the bladder if the urethra is occluded by a balloon catheter. Overdistention of the bladder results in hematuria, pyuria, urinary bladder rupture, and mild to severe bladder inflammation. Palpate the bladder carefully during distention, and note the backpressure on the syringe used in filling the bladder.

Retrograde contrast urethrography is a definite aid in defining the extent of urethral damage (stricture) or in demonstrating urethral calculi in male cats. In male cats, use a 4F balloon catheter or a 3.5F Tomcat open-ended urethral catheter. Insert the catheter 1.5 cm into the penile urethra. If the urethra is patent, 2 to 3 mL of contrast material will enable visualization of the urethra, but increased amounts of contrast material (2 to 3 mL/lb) injected into the bladder are needed for maximum distention of the preprostatic urethra. A voiding positive contrast urethrogram is necessary to visualize the distal (penile) urethra. Apply external pressure to the bladder (using a wooden spoon or other external compression device), and radiograph the distal urethra.

CYSTOGRAPHY

Cystography refers to contrast radiographic procedures that facilitate visualization of the lumen and/or contents of the urinary bladder and trigone (Box 4-17). Three procedures can be used to image the urinary bladder: positive contrast cystography, negative contrast cystography (also called pneumocystography), and double contrast cystography (combination of positive and negative cystography performed in the same patient). NOTE: Many of the indications for performing contrast cystography are also indications for ultrasound examination. Contrast cystography is most useful for characterizing congenital and acquired alternations in the normal anatomy and function of the ureters and lower urinary tract, such as ectopic ureter. Abdominal ultrasound, when available, remains the preferred method for imaging abnormalities within the bladder lumen (e.g., calculi and tumors) and changes within the bladder wall.

BOX 4-17   INDICATIONS FOR CYSTOGRAPHY

- Incontinence unresponsive to medical treatment, especially in young dogs
- Persistent hematuria (WARNING: *Pneumocystography is contraindicated.*)
- Stranguria
- Pyuria
- Persistent crystalluria
- Significant proteinuria
- Dysuria
- Persistent or recurrent urinary tract infection

Pneumocystography

Pneumocystography, also called negative-contrast cystography, involves the insufflation of a soluble gas into the lumen of the urinary bladder to facilitate imaging of any material or tissue within the bladder lumen that otherwise would be obscured by the presence of urine or positive contrast material. Prepare the patient as described previously. Once a urinary catheter is placed and the urethra is occluded, use a syringe and a three-way valve to inject 4 to 10 mL/kg of carbon dioxide or nitrous oxide. Palpate the bladder while filling it with gas to avoid overdistention or rupture. Inject air until there is pressure on the syringe barrel or leakage of air around the catheter. Replace any air that escapes during the procedure. Take lateral and ventrodorsal views of the abdomen.

Note: Room air is the most accessible contrast material and generally can be found in most practices. *However,* an increased risk of air emboli is associated with the placement of room air into the bladder under positive pressure.

Pneumocystography is not an innocuous procedure; fatal venous air emboli have occurred in dogs and cats. This complication is seen most commonly in cases of severe hematuria. Ultrasound or positive contrast cystography is preferred over pneumocystography in such cases if a soluble gas is not available. If possible, use a gas that is readily soluble in blood (such as carbon dioxide or nitrous oxide) for bladder insufflation.

Positive contrast cystography

The injection of radiographic contrast material into the urinary bladder is referred to as contrast cystography or positive contrast cystography. When ultrasound examination is not available or not feasible, the clinical and radiographic findings noted in Box 4-18 justify the use of a contrast radiography to image the bladder.

The same principles of preparation apply as for performing a pneumocystogram. Use a urethral catheter with a three-way valve or a small Foley catheter with an inflatable cuff. Organic iodides are the contrast material of choice and should be used in 5% to 10% concentrations.

Double contrast cystography

Double contrast cystography also can be performed in patients for which a positive contrast study is not diagnostic, yet there is reasonable indication for an intraluminal lesion. In this case, using the same urinary catheter as used for the contrast study, remove all remaining urine and contrast material. If necessary, inject 2 to 5 mL of an aqueous organic iodine contrast material into the bladder. Gently roll the patient over in an attempt to coat the bladder with contrast material. Then distend the bladder with air in the same manner as described for pneumocystography.

Some of the routine lesions diagnosed with the aid of cystography are calculi (Table 4-11); neoplasia; cystitis, if proliferative changes are present; muscle hypertrophy; bladder diverticula; duplications; adhesions, especially uterine stump infection; persistent urachus; ruptures; and atonic bladder.

Additional Reading

Burk RL, Ackerman N: *Small animal radiology and ultrasonography: a diagnostic atlas and text,* ed 3, St Louis, 2003, Saunders.

BOX 4-18   INDICATIONS FOR PERFORMING CONTRAST CYSTOGRAPHY

- Frequent urination
- Intermittent or chronic hematuria or small volumes of voided urine
- Hematuria that is seen throughout or in the later stages of voiding
- Dysuria
- Persistent posttraumatic hematuria
- Areas of increased or decreased density associated with the urinary bladder
- Nonvisualization of the urinary bladder after trauma
- Evaluation of abnormal caudal abdominal masses and structures adjacent to the urinary bladder
- Evaluation of abnormal bladder shape or location

4

TABLE 4-11   Radiopacity of Cystic Calculi on Plain Abdominal Radiographs

Calculus composition	Density
Calcium oxalate	Radiopaque
Calcium carbonate	Radiopaque
Triple phosphate	Radiopaque—small calculi may be nonradiopaque
Cystine	Variable density—may have radiopaque stippling
Uric acid and urates	Nonradiopaque
Xanthine	Nonradiopaque
Matrix concretions	Nonradiopaque

From Park RD: Radiology of the urinary bladder and urethra. In O'Brien TR, ed: *Radiographic diagnosis of abdominal disorders in the dog and cat.* Philadelphia, WB Saunders, 1978.

Osborne CA, Finco DR: *Canine and feline nephrology and urology,* Baltimore, 1995, Williams & Wilkins.

Thrall DE: *Textbook of veterinary diagnostic radiology,* ed 4, St Louis, 2002, Saunders.

Myelography

Myelography is the study of the spinal cord and vertebral canal made possible by the use of contrast media in the subarachnoid space. Ideally, the contrast material should be relatively nontoxic and absorbable, should provide good contrast, and should be distributed evenly throughout the subarachnoid space. Indications for myelography are progressive neurologic disease in which survey radiographs have failed to reveal substantive findings.

The nonionic water-soluble agents currently are preferred for myelography. The agents are iopamidol, iohexol, and ioxaglate. These agents are stable in solution and much more convenient than metrizamide and have low toxicity and low epileptogenic activity, are inert to nervous tissue, have no long-term side effects, and are resorbed and excreted rapidly from the CSF. These agents can be injected into the subarachnoid space at the cerebellomedullary cistern or at the caudal lumbar spine (preferred) at a dose level of 0.22 mL/kg. Five minutes after cisternal injection, if there is no obstruction, the cervical and thoracic cord segments are outlined, and after 10 to 15 minutes the entire cord is outlined.

Patients undergoing myelography can be pretreated with diazepam at a dose of 0.25 mL/kg, not to exceed 10 mL in larger patients. Diazepam has a short biologic half-life of 30 to 45 minutes and may be better used after myelography if seizures do occur.

Myelography is a relatively high-risk procedure and should be performed only by individuals with additional training and experience. The following steps are involved:

1. Have the patient fast for 18 to 24 hours preceding myelography if the procedure is elective.
2. Anesthetize the patient with a short-acting anesthetic agent, and maintain the animal on the gas anesthetic of choice. Maintain an intravenous catheter and good hydration through fluid support.
3. Clip and surgically prepare the skin over the cisterna magna or in the lumbosacral area, depending on where one wishes to enter the spinal canal. When fluoroscopic visualization is available, myelograms can be done for all animals from a lumbar subarachnoid tap. Lumbar puncture can be made between L1 and L6 or between L4 and L5. Use a short-bevel spinal needle (1.5-inch, 22-gauge needle for dogs under 20 lb, and a 2.5-inch, 22-gauge needle for larger dogs). The average dose for any of the four agents is 0.22 mL/kg. More is needed per kilogram for small dogs and less per kilogram for large dogs (for cisterna magna puncture).
4. Inject the contrast medium through a flexible extension tube attached to the needle. The recommended dose of iohexol 300 mg/mL is for cervical myelogram (lumbar tap), 0.45 mL/kg; for cervical tap, 0.30 mL/kg; for thoracolumbar myelogram (lumbar tap), 0.30 mL/kg; for thoracolumbar myelogram (cervical tap), 0.30 mL/kg; and for cervicothoracolumbar myelogram (cervical or lumbar), 0.45 mL/kg.

Additional Reading

Burk RL, Ackerman N: *Small animal radiology and ultrasonography: a diagnostic atlas and text,* ed 3, St Louis, 2003, Saunders.

Thrall DE: *Textbook of veterinary diagnostic radiology,* ed 4, St Louis, 2002, Saunders.

Cholecystography

Cholecystography refers to the use of contrast material to facilitate imaging of the gall bladder and the common bile duct. Use of this technique depends on the ability of selected radiopaque compounds to be removed from the blood and excreted via active transport by hepatocytes. Contrast agents for cholecystography can be administered either orally or intravenously. Oral cholecystographic examination requires that the contrast agent (1) enter the small bowel, (2) be absorbed and enter the portal circulation, and (3) be excreted into the bile and concentrated in the gallbladder. Intravenous cholecystography eliminates some of the variables within the digestive tract and may be a more reliable technique in dogs and cats. For that reason, and others, cholecystography is *not* a particularly popular procedure. The reality is that abdominal ultrasound, in the hands of an experienced ultrasonographer, will provide more reliable diagnostic information on the liver and biliary tract than will contrast radiography.

REPRODUCTIVE TRACT: FEMALE

CULTURE OF THE VAGINA

Vaginal examination is indicated for collection of material from the mucosal wall for culture and exfoliative cytologic examination and for vaginoscopic examination of vaginal and cervical mucosa (Box 4-19).

Examination of the vagina for culture and cytologic or vaginoscopic examination occasionally can be performed in the cooperative patient without the use of sedation or anesthesia. An assistant is used to restrain the patient on an examination table. Bitches that can be restrained for other minor examinations (ears, teeth, toenails, anal sacs, and blood samples) often will tolerate vaginal examinations. Those that need further restraint may require sedation or administration of a short-acting barbiturate anesthetic.

If the vulva appears clean, no preparation before examination is needed. If the vulva is soiled or vulvar hair is matted or soiled, trim the hair and wash the area with a germicidal or surgical scrub such as povidone-iodine, or give a general grooming and bath a few hours before examination. Water and germicidal soap usually will not control surface contamination by *Pseudomonas* and *Proteus* spp., which frequently contaminate culture swabs. Bitches with long hair should have the leg hair pinned to one side with clips and the tail bandaged before examination.

Obtain a deep vaginal culture FIRST to avoid contamination during the general examination. Pass a sterile, warm vaginal speculum with only a thin coating of lubricating gel into the posterior vagina while an assistant spreads the vulva. Guide the speculum into the vagina by placing the speculum into the vulva just at the dorsal commissure of the vulva and applying pressure up and out against the commissure. Direct the speculum *dorsally* toward the rectum until meeting resistance, and then direct it horizontally into the cranial vagina. This procedure bypasses the clitoral fossa and enables visualization of the urethral opening and pelvic arch.

Take a guarded culture swab (swab covered by a protective plastic pipette) from its individual sterile bag and pass it inside the vaginal speculum to the anterior vagina or cervical area. Then expose the swab from the protective plastic tubing and rotate it against the mucosa. Retract the swab into the protective plastic tubing and carefully remove it from the vagina. The protected swab then may be placed back in its original sterile bag until it is processed for culture (30 minutes) or placed in Amies transport medium with charcoal. Amies transport medium with refrigerator packs and a styrofoam-insulated mailing box

---

BOX 4-19 EQUIPMENT TO USE FOR EXAMINATION OF THE CANINE VAGINA

Sterile vaginal speculum (e.g., adjustable-spreading, stainless steel, or disposable plastic; cylindric; glass, plastic, stainless steel, or nylon)
Sterile otoscope heads of variable size for small dogs
Sterile protected culture swabs (Tiegland type or other)
Sterile culture swabs (Culturettes)
Amies transport medium with charcoal
Viral transport media
Glass slides and coverslips
Sterile proctoscope (Welch Allyn, human pediatric type) or other endoscope, flexible or rigid
Sterile offset biopsy punch

will retain fastidious organisms for 72 to 96 hours. Process bacterial, *Mycoplasma,* and *Ureaplasma* cultures for potential infectious agents. Viral transport medium can be used for a separate sterile swab if viral agents such as the genital form of canine herpesvirus are suspected.

Immediately after the swabbing for culture, while the vaginal speculum is still in place, advance a clean or sterile swab moistened with sterile physiologic saline solution carefully into the anterior vagina to make a smear for cytologic examination. Gently scrape vaginal epithelial cells from the ceiling of the vagina at or cranial to the region of the external urethral orifice. Collect samples from the region of the clitoral fossa, which is lined by stratified squamous epithelium at all stages of the estrous cycle. Gently rub the swab on the vaginal mucosa. Remove the swab and roll it smoothly onto two or three clean glass slides. The smears may be fixed immediately in 95% alcohol, sprayed with a commercial fixative or hair spray, or left to dry in air.

A drop of new methylene blue stain placed on a coverslip and inverted on the smear can be used to examine a wet mount preparation immediately. This stain is not permanent and precipitates when it dries, and new methylene blue–stained smears cannot be used for comparison with other smears made later in the cycle. A better and quick method that provides a permanent record is the use of the Diff-Quik or Leukostat stain. Giemsa stain, toluidine blue, Wright's stain, Shorr's stain, or phase-contrast microscopy also can be used. Examine the smear for stage of estrous cycle and evidence of active inflammation. Compare these findings with culture results and vaginoscopic findings to interpret evidence for an active genital tract infection, a carrier state of a potential infectious agent, or a possible contaminant at culture. A diagnostic laboratory with the ability to isolate specific infectious agents should indicate the number of organisms (few, moderate, many, or heavy) and report whether the isolates are pure or mixed and their significance.

EXAMINATION OF THE VAGINA

The vagina of the bitch is long in comparison to that of other domestic animals, hence digital examination of the cervix, and in many cases, the urethral orifice, is simply not possible. The mucosa forms longitudinal folds. The clitoris is in a well-developed fossa in the floor of the vestibule. The vagina can be visualized completely with a small, sterile proctoscope or flexible endoscope. Lubricate the warmed, sterile instrument, and pass it to the region of the cervix. Examine first without insufflation for true color and vaginal fluids or discharge. When insufflation is performed while the vulva is compressed around the sterile proctoscope, the vagina expands and its entire wall can be viewed completely as the instrument is withdrawn.

The normal canine vagina has a uniform light pink color and longitudinal folds. During proestrus and estrus, the folds become more prominent and cross-striations give the surface a cobblestone appearance. This cobblestone appearance remains smooth when estrogen levels are high but quickly becomes angular (worn cobblestone appearance) when estrogen levels drop during the luteinizing hormone peak (ovulation), and progesterone levels increase. This change can be used to indicate ovulation and the ideal time for breeding. The hyperemia causes the vagina to appear reddish and congested. The pressure of air insufflation balances the mucosa. The canine vulva has a large cranial dorsal median fold that may obscure the cervix. In fact, ridges near the dorsal fold may give a false impression that this fold is the cervix. During estrogen stimulation, the cervix may be open and uterine blood may be escaping. In the management of dystocia, the vaginoscope can be used to detect puppies in the birth canal and to diagnose malpositions and aid in the correction of these conditions.

During the endoscopic examination, small tumors or polyps can be removed or large masses can be sampled with the biopsy punch. Ulcers or erosions can be cauterized, and foreign bodies can be removed.

A complete vaginal examination must include careful palpation of the vaginal wall and pelvic canal. This palpation is accomplished by digital examination through the vulva (using a sterile glove) and is assisted by palpation through the posterior abdominal wall. Incomplete hymen rings, vaginal fibrous stenotic rings, or pelvic malformation can be diagnosed. A digital rectal examination may be needed for vaginal masses or pelvic deformities.

ESTROUS CYCLE: STAGING AND CYTOLOGIC FINDINGS—CANINE

The canine reproductive cycle begins at the age of 6 to 12 months and repeats at intervals of 4 to 12 months. In the average bitch, ovulation occurs spontaneously 1 to 3 days after the onset of estrus; in normal bitches ovulation may occur between 3 days before and 11 days after the onset of estrus. Sperm live in the uterus of the estrous bitch up to 11 days, and the ovum lives up to 5 days after ovulation. The fertilized ovum takes 4 to 10 days to reach the uterus, and implantation takes place 18 to 20 days after ovulation. The gestation period from the first breeding is 57 to 72 days and from the luteinizing hormone peak is 64 to 66 days.

Anestrus

Anestrus is characterized by dryness of the mucosa and a thin vaginal wall with stratified squamous epithelial cells a few cells to several layers thick but without cornification. Noncornified epithelial cells and WBCs are present in a ratio of 1:5 in the vaginal smear. The WBCs are polymorphonuclear. The noncornified epithelial cells are 15 to 51 nm in diameter and have round free edges, granular cytoplasm, and large nuclei with distinct chromatin granules. The period of anestrus is 2 to 3 months or longer in some breeds.

Proestrus

In proestrus the vaginal wall is thicker than in anestrus, and the mucosa shows prominent cornified squamous epithelium (20 to 30 cells thick) with rete pegs. The longitudinal and transverse vaginal folds are thick, smooth, and round. The vaginal wall becomes impervious to WBCs, but there is extravasation of red blood cells to the surface epithelium. The red blood cells are discharged. Vaginal smears show predominantly red blood cells and noncornified epithelial cells, which become cornified as proestrus progresses. White blood cells are present, but their numbers decrease as estrus approaches. Debris and bacteria are abundant for 7 to 10 days.

Estrus

The vagina is thick with longitudinal and transverse folds that become angular as estrogen levels decrease and progesterone levels increase. Fluid is abundant, often tinged with blood. Noncornified epithelial cells and WBCs are absent. Cornified epithelial cells, which are polyhedral and contain pyknotic nuclei or no nucleus, are predominant; their presence seems to be related to the appearance of flirting by the bitch and acceptance of the stud. White blood cells reappear about 36 to 96 hours after ovulation. Bacteria and debris are absent during estrus, but they are seen again in the smears after ovulation when WBCs reappear 7 to 10 days later.

Diestrus

The number of WBCs increases rapidly, the number of cornified epithelial cells decreases, and the number of noncornified epithelial cells increases. After 5 to 7 days, the number of WBCs may decrease to 10 to 30 per field.

Following parturition, much cellular debris, WBCs, red blood cells, and a few epithelial cells are present for several days, until placental sloughing is complete. The presence of masses of degenerate WBCs (and bacteria) indicates metritis or endometritis. The continued presence of blood-tinged fluids containing abundant red blood cells, a few noncornified epithelial cells, and occasional WBCs (nontoxic) plus necrotic cells for months postpartum is evidence of subinvolution of placental sites.

ESTROUS CYCLE: STAGING AND CYTOLOGIC FINDINGS—FELINE

Most of the characteristics just discussed that apply to bitches also pertain to queens. However, the small size of the feline vagina precludes palpation and early vaginoscopy. A sterile, warm, small-animal otoscope speculum enables fairly good visualization of the vaginal mucosa and can be used with a small, 4-mm-diameter sterile swab to obtain smears for culture procedures. Use of the speculum is easiest following parturition or during estrus.

Vaginal cells for cytologic examination can be obtained with a moistened 3-mm cotton swab (Calgiswab) inserted 2 cm into the vagina. In some cases, flushing the vagina with sterile saline injected and aspirated with a clean glass eyedropper is more successful. Use of an eyedropper may trigger ovulation, as it simulates coitus.

Unlike the bitch, the queen shows no diapedesis of red blood cells during proestrus or throughout the estrous cycle. Cytologic examination of feline vaginal smears reveals the following by stage of the estrous cycle.

Anestrus or prepuberty

Cytologic examination reveals scarce debris and numerous small, round epithelial cells with a high nuclear/cytoplasmic ratio, frequently in groups (seasonal: from September to January in the Northern Hemisphere).

Proestrus

Cytologic examination reveals increased debris and fewer but larger nucleated epithelial cells with a low nuclear/cytoplasmic ratio (0 to 2 days).

Estrus

Cytologic examination reveals markedly less debris and numerous large polyhedral cornified cells with curled edges and small dark pyknotic nuclei or loss of nuclei (6 to 8 days) following coitus or induced ovulation.

Early diestrus

Cytologic examination reveals hazy, ragged-edged cornified cells and zero to numerous WBCs with numerous bacteria and increased debris.

Late diestrus

Cytologic examination reveals increasing numbers of small basophilic cells with WBCs still present (total period of metestrus, 7 to 21 days). If ovulation does not occur, the smear will return to an anestrous stage with few to no WBCs.

The feline estrous cycle is continuous every 14 to 36 days if 12 to 14 hours of light is present daily. Ovulation is induced 24 to 30 hours after coitus. Sperm require 2 to 24 hours for capacitation in the uterus. Implantation is expected 13 to 14 days after coitus.

Additional Reading

Baker R, Lumsden JH: The reproductive tract: vagina, uterus, protate, and testicle. In Baker R, Lummsden JH, editors: *Color atlas of the cytology of the dog and cat,* St. Louis, 2000, Mosby. (NOTE: Textbook contains exceptional color plates of normal and abnormal reproductive tract cytologic findings of the dog and cat.)

Feldman EC, Nelson RW: *Canine and feline endocrinology and reproduction,* ed 3, St Louis, 2004, Elsevier-Saunders.

Grundy SA, Davidson AP: Feline reproduction. In Ettinger SJ, Feldman EC, editors: *Textbook of veterinary internal medicine,* ed 6, St Louis, 2005, Elsevier-Saunders.

Schaefers-Okkens AC: Estrous cycle and breeding management of the healthy bitch. In Ettinger SJ, Feldman EC, editors: *Textbook of veterinary internal medicine,* ed 6, St Louis, 2005, Elsevier-Saunders.

BOX 4-20   MATERIALS USED FOR PERFORMING ARTIFICIAL INSEMINATION

- Dry, warm, sterile 5- or 10-mL syringes
- Rubber adapter tubing, ¾ inch long
- A 6- to 9-inch plastic or polypropylene inseminating pipette
- A sterile examination glove
- Alcohol
- Cotton

  Do not use lubricating materials.

ARTIFICIAL INSEMINATION: CANINE

The procedure for artificial insemination in dogs includes the following steps:

1. Determine the correct time to inseminate by test-teasing with a stud, by cytologic examination of vaginal smears, or by vaginoscopic examination to determine the day when vaginal folds change from round to angular. Breed the day after the bitch first stands staunchly to accept service and "flags" her tail or during cytologic indications of estrus (complete cornification of vaginal epithelial cells) but before WBCs reappear in the smears. Breed at 48-hour intervals until the female dog goes out of heat or for three or four inseminations.
2. If the vulva is soiled, clean it thoroughly with alcohol swabs (Box 4-20).
3. Gently aspirate semen through the inseminating pipette into the warm syringe.
4. Using a gloved left index finger (not lubricated) as a guide, insert the pipette through the vulva and dorsally into the vagina and forward to the cervix. Elevate the bitch's rear quarters to a 45-degree angle by having an assistant pick up the bitch by holding the hock region so that no pressure is applied to the ventral abdomen and uterus. Eject the semen gently and slowly. Eject a bubble of air to push all the semen through the pipette. Deposit the semen in the anterior vagina.
5. Remove the pipette, and hold the bitch in an elevated position for 5 minutes. During this time, use the finger encased in a sterile glove to "feather" the ceiling of the vagina to stimulate constrictor activity. This may be important to simulate a "tie" and transport semen into the uterus.
6. Lower the bitch to the normal position, and immediately walk her for 5 minutes so that she does not sit down or jump up on a person and allow semen to run back out of the vagina.
7. For best conception, inseminate undiluted fresh semen immediately.
8. Refrigerated extended semen is best used within 24 to 48 hours if possible. However, refrigerated semen has been kept viable for up to 9 days with proper care.

   Skim milk has been used as an economical and adequate extender. Heat milk to 92° to 94° C for 10 minutes, cool it, and skim it at room temperature. To each milliliter, add 1000 units of crystalline penicillin. If *Pseudomonas* spp. affect the semen, polymyxin B may be added at 200 units/mL of extender. Dilute semen with extender at a semen/extender ratio of 1:1 to 1:4. Extend canine semen for freezing with a diluent containing 11% lactose, 4% glycerin, and 20% egg yolk. Refrigerate the 1:4 diluted semen; then pipette 0.05-mL portions into depressions in a block of dry ice and hold them for 8 minutes to freeze. Store the frozen pellets in liquid nitrogen. Frozen semen can be thawed in buffered saline at 30° to 37° C. Good semen may be stored in liquid nitrogen for many years without significant loss of motility. Conception is best when large numbers of thawed motile sperm are deposited in the cervix or uterine cavity. Conception is poor when thawed semen is placed in the anterior vagina, as done in artificial breeding with raw semen.

Additional Reading

Memon MA, Sirinarumitr K: Semen evaluation, canine male infertility, and common disorders of the male. In Ettinger SJ, Feldman EC, editors: *Textbook of veterinary internal medicine,* ed 6, St Louis, 2005, Elsevier-Saunders.

REPRODUCTIVE TRACT: MALE

SEMEN COLLECTION: CANINE

Semen is collected for examination for breeding soundness, for investigation of infertility or prostatic disease, and for artificial insemination (Box 4-21).

The following steps outline the procedure for collecting semen from a male dog:

1. Take the stud and an estrous teaser bitch (if available) to a quiet room where there will be no distractions and where there is good traction (rubber mats or rug) for mounting by the stud.
2. Hold the bitch, and allow the stud to "flirt" (become aroused) for several minutes. If the bitch is in heat, a brief period of foreplay (I am not really certain if "foreplay" is an appropriate word to use when describing the mating behavior of dogs, but you get the point) with both dogs unrestricted will help the process.
3. If necessary, have assistants restrain the muzzled bitch and control the stud by a collar and leash. Bring the stud up to the rear end of the bitch, and allow him to mount her or keep his nose in the region of her perineal area.
4. Attach the artificial vagina to the semen collection tube, and apply a scant amount of lubricant to the opening of the artificial vagina.
5. If mounting occurs, allow the stud to grasp the bitch and start to thrust his pelvis in an attempt to copulate. Gently, from the side of the sheath, grasp the penis by the prepuce and move the prepuce back over the engorged bulbus glandis; while applying the artificial vagina to the shaft of the penis, apply pressure with the thumb and forefinger proximal to the exposed glandis. This usually can be done with one motion as the stud is thrusting. If the stud is shy and not interested, massage the penis slightly in the prepuce or in the artificial vagina to cause erection. When erection of the bulbus is felt, reflect the prepuce posteriorly to free the bulbus. Apply pressure with the thumb and forefinger behind the bulbus, circling the shaft of the penis. After completion of the most rapid pelvic thrusting and ejaculation of the sperm-rich fractions of semen (1 to 3 mL), twist the penis 180 degrees backward in a horizontal plane, between the hind legs, so that the penis remains in the same plane as in the forward position with the thumb and forefinger still applying pressure around the circumference of the penis proximal to the bulbus. The penis cannot be twisted unless the prepuce is reflected posterior or proximal to the bulbus glandis. Twisting the penis in this position simulates a natural "tie" and allows the person collecting the semen to better visualize the collection (artificial vaginas are widely available now and are much preferred because they simulate the natural pressure of the vagina). The first drops of ejaculate may be discarded, especially if any urine is present. Collect the sperm-rich fraction separately. A clear ejaculate is prostatic fluid, which may be collected separately for examination.

4

BOX 4-21 EQUIPMENT USED TO COLLECT SEMEN FROM A MALE DOG

STERILE
Sterile rubber cone (artificial vagina) connected to a semen collection tube
Glass, polytef (Teflon), or plastic test tubes
Saline solution, 0.9%
Sterile aqueous lubricant

NONSTERILE
Microscope slides and coverslips (warmed)
A quick Romanowsky's stain, buffered formalin
Hemocytometer-counting chamber and 1:100 white blood cell dilutor pipette or Unopette
Microscope with oil immersion objective (×1000) and light
Muzzle gauze

6. After semen collection, place the penis in the forward position, straighten out the prepuce to avoid paraphimosis, and remove the bitch from the room. Allow the stud to lick the erect penis and lose the erection. Check the stud for evidence of paraphimosis before he is released or caged. The ejaculate consists of three fractions:

   First fraction: Urethral secretion (usually clear fluid)—0.1 to 2 mL within 50 seconds, pH 6.3. If evidence of urine is present, discard this fraction and do not add it to the sperm-rich fraction. In most ejaculates collected from dogs, the first and second semen fractions are collected together.

   Second fraction: Sperm-containing secretion (milky opaque fluid)—0.5 to 3 mL within 1 to 2 minutes, pH 6.1.

   Third fraction: Prostatic secretion (usually clear fluid)—2 to 20 mL within 30 minutes, pH 6.5. The total specimen is 0.3 to 20 mL, pH 6.4. Because the first and third fractions are clear, waterlike material and the second fraction is milky-opaque, the clinician can separate them by changing collecting tubes as each fraction is ejaculated. Collection of only enough prostatic fluid to rinse the sperm fraction into the test tube is best. Too much prostatic fluid may be detrimental to the longevity of sperm in storage. Collecting individual fractions may be important in determining the site of an inflammatory reaction, but for artificial insemination only the sperm-rich, low-volume ejaculate is needed for insemination, dilution, or freezing.

7. Return the stud to his cage. Retain the bitch until the semen is examined, if insemination is to be performed.

EVALUATION OF SEMEN

Immediately after semen collection, slowly invert the tube several times to mix the semen gently. Determine the *motility of sperm* by placing 1 drop of semen on a warmed microscope slide. Cover the slide with a coverslip, and observe the specimen under low power for progressive motility. There will be no "waves," but general vigorous forward motion should be evident. If the sample is too concentrated for individual sperm to be found, mix 1 drop of semen with 1 drop of saline at body temperature on a warmed microscope slide. Using high power, count 10 different groups of 10 sperm, observing the numbers of motile and nonmotile sperm. Total motility for a suitable sample should be 80% or greater. Motility less than 60% is not satisfactory.

Determine the *number of sperm* in the total ejaculate. Sperm concentration may be determined in a hemocytometer with a 1:100 blood cell dilutor kit (Unopette), and concentration then is multiplied by volume to determine sperm numbers per ejaculate. Remember that more dilute samples will be obtained when prostatic fluid is collected, but total sperm numbers in the ejaculate will be only marginally influenced by dilution with prostatic fluid. Total sperm per ejaculate should exceed 300 million in a normal male dog and may approach 2 billion in large dogs. A minimum number of 200 million sperm per insemination is needed on average for conception.

Determine morphology. Make a smear of a drop of semen like a blood smear and allow it to air dry. Then stain the smear with Diff-Quik stain; dip the slide into the fixative and solutions 1 and 2 for 2 to 3 minutes each. Then count 100 sperm at ×1000 magnification, noting normal and abnormal sperm. If there is any question about abnormality, examine 500 sperm cells.

Normal canine sperm are 63 nm long; the heads are 7 nm long. The percentage of abnormal sperm should be less than 20%. Differential abnormality is important, and the following abnormalities should not be exceeded in any sperm count: abnormality of the head, 10% to 12%; midpiece abnormalities, 3% to 4%; tail abnormalities, 3% to 4%; and retained protoplasmic droplets, 3% to 4%. Figure 4-54 shows abnormalities that should be counted and recorded. The presence and location of distal or proximal protoplasmic droplets, which may indicate cell immaturity, is important to note.

Defects of the cells within the testes are generally more serious than defects that occur in the sperm during epididymal transport or after ejaculation (such as fractured heads, retained protoplasmic droplets, or bent tails). Usually, a biopsy should not be done on

SPERM

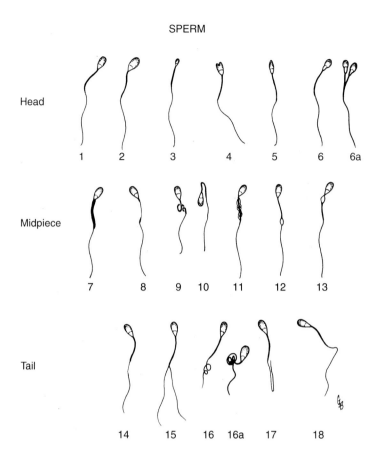

Head	Midpiece	Tail
1. Normal	7. Thickened	14. Thinned
2. Giant	8. Thinned	15. Double
3. Small	9. Coiled	16., 16a. Coiled
4. Indented	10. Bent	17. Folded
5. Pointed	11. Extraneous	18. Kinked
6. Pear-shaped	12. Distal cytoplasmic	
6a. Double	droplet	
	13. Proximal cytoplasmic	
	droplet	

Figure 4-54:   Chart of abnormal sperm.

material from testes unless the testes are azoospermic. Damage produced after the sperm have left the testes may indicate epididymal disease or may be the result of cold, trauma, or osmotic or urinary contamination. When abnormalities are found, it is wise to obtain two or three semen samples within a few days for baseline evaluation and then repeat the studies in 4 to 6 weeks to determine whether there is a healing or regressing trend. There are usually 64 days from the date of sperm formation to the date of ejaculation: 54 days in the testes and 10 days in transport and maturation in the epididymis.

Normal male dogs can be used at stud once every other day indefinitely or once every day for 7 to 9 days, after which sperm numbers in the ejaculate will decline but not to less than the numbers needed to achieve conception.

Semen Collection: Feline

Semen can be collected by means of electroejaculation in the anesthetized male cat (and, after reviewing the following procedures for use of an artificial vagina, this technique may be preferred). For semen collection with an artificial vagina, the male cat must be trained for several weeks and even then, not all male cats will effectively ejaculate; thus the artificial vagina method generally is not used except in larger catteries. Teaser queens can be produced by injecting spayed females with 0.25 mg of estradiol cyclopentyl propionate, or normal queens in heat can be used.

An artificial vagina can be made by cutting off the bulb end of a 2-mL rubber bulb pipette and inserting a 3 × 44-mm test tube into the cut end. Place the apparatus into a 60-mL plastic bottle filled with warm water (52° C). Stretch the rolled end of the rubber pipette over the rim of the bottle. Sparingly lubricate the opening of the pipette ("vagina") with sterile aqueous lubricant. Place a teaser queen in a quiet cage with the tom. As the tom mounts the queen and develops an erection, place the artificial vagina over the penis. The ejaculation takes 1 to 4 minutes, the semen volume is 0.05 mL (range is 0.03 to 0.3 mL), and the semen contains 50 million to 100 million sperm. Motility is normally 80% to 90%, and pH is 7.4. There should be less than 10% abnormal sperm. The semen can be diluted for insemination to contain 10 million sperm in 0.1 mL of saline; then each 0.1 mL is an adequate insemination volume. With such small samples, microequipment is essential to avoid losing semen by surface absorption. Toms can undergo this collection procedure 3 times weekly and maintain excellent semen quality and libido.

Queens can be detected in estrus by stroking their backs and necks daily and noting the arching of the back and the extended and treading action of the rear feet when they are in receptive heat. Estrus is verified by examination of vaginal smears, which show epithelial cell cornification with pyknotic nuclei. Insemination is carried out with a 0.25-mL syringe and a bulb-tipped 9-cm spinal needle. Ovulation is induced by intramuscular injection of 25 µg of gonadotropin-releasing hormone or 250 IU of human chorionic gonadotropin. If insemination is repeated 24 hours later, the conception rate improves from 60% to 75%.

Additional Reading

Baker R, Lumsden JH: The reproductive tract: vagina, uterus, protate, and testicle. In Baker R, Lummsden JH, editors: *Color atlas of the cytology of the dog and cat,* St Louis, 2000, Mosby. (NOTE: This textbook contains exceptional color plates of normal and abnormal reproductive tract cytologic findings of the dog and cat.)

Feldman EC, Nelson RW: *Canine and feline endocrinology and reproduction,* ed 3, St Louis, 2004, Elsevier-Saunders.

Memon MA, Sirinarumitr K: Semen evaluation, canine male infertility, and common disorders of the male. In Ettinger SJ, Feldman EC, editors: *Textbook of veterinary internal medicine,* ed 6, St Louis, 2005, Elsevier-Saunders.

Wright PJ, Parry BW: Cytology of the canine reproductive system, *Vet Clin North Am Small Anim Pract* 19:851-874, 1989.

4

Prostatic Wash

Although castration is a common first recommendation for any male dog with known or suspected prostatic disease, a number of prostatic disorders are recognized for which cytopathologic and histopathologic examination, rather than castration, is indicated. Benign prostatic hyperplasia is recognized as the most common prostatic disorder of male dogs. In half of the dog population, changes consistent with benign prostatic hyperplasia are present by 4 to 5 years of age, especially older intact dogs. Because benign prostatic hyperplasia is androgen dependent, routine castration is the recommended treatment. However, at least three differential diagnoses justify additional diagnostic tests: prostatic neoplasia (usually adenocarcinoma), acute and chronic bacterial prostatitis, and prostatic cysts (septic and nonseptic).

In male dogs presenting with prostatomegaly and associated signs (dysuria and/or dyschezia), further evaluation of the prostate is indicated. Several techniques have been described. Abdominal ultrasonography is the preferred technique for evaluating prostate size, shape, and consistency. Distention retrograde contrast urethrocystogram has been described as a means for evaluating the internal integrity of the prostate and is moderately effective in distinguishing normal from abnormal. However, this technique is not known to distinguish among various types of prostate disease.

Cytologic examination and quantitative bacterial culture of the ejaculate (especially the third fraction) of a male dog is recommended in any patient with prostatomegaly. However, sample collection can be difficult and is frequently not successful. In addition to lumbar radiographs and abdominal ultrasonography, performing a prostatic wash is a simple, noninvasive technique that may yield diagnostic information.

Using aseptic technique, place a conventional urinary catheter into the bladder and remove all urine. Lavage of the urinary bladder with up to 5 mL of sterile saline is recommended. Recover the saline and save it (sample No. 1). Subsequently, retract the catheter tip, but only to the level of the prostate gland (immediately caudal to the trigone). Position of the tip usually can be verified by tactile placement and the detection of increased resistance to catheter movement during retraction. Position can be confirmed with a lateral radiograph of the pelvis.

With the catheter in place, identify the prostate on a digital rectal examination and gently massage for approximately 1 minute to force prostatic fluids into the urethra. Infuse 5 mL of sterile saline through the catheter. The objective is to wash prostatic fluids and cells into the urinary bladder and recover the saline from the bladder (sample No. 2).

Examine fluid from both samples cytologically by distributing a drop of fluid across a glass slide, air drying, and staining; submit a small aliquot (0.5 mL) for bacterial culture. Cytologic examination is used to detect the presence of inflammatory cells versus neoplastic cells. Low numbers of neutrophils (<5 cells per high power field) are present in ejaculates and prostatic washes from normal dogs. Quantitative bacterial culture, with a yield of greater than 2 $\log_{10}$ of one or more bacterial species in sample No. 2 confirms bacterial prostatitis.

Complications from this procedure are unlikely, but conceivably a patient with septic prostatitis and prostatic abscesses could become bacteremic following this procedure, which in some patients could lead to sepsis.

PROSTATE BIOPSY AND FINE-NEEDLE ASPIRATION

Ultrasound examination is an important first step, when available, in assessing the size, shape, and internal integrity of the canine prostate gland and for detecting any changes in structures adjacent to the prostate. However, ultrasonography generally will *not* distinguish between different types of prostatic disease. Further diagnostic tests are especially indicated in castrated, middle-aged to older male dogs with evidence of prostatomegaly. Percutaneous fine-needle aspiration and/or prostatic biopsy are indicated.

Fine-needle aspiration of the prostate is performed through a ventral abdominal approach. Use aseptic technique, and surgically prepare the skin at the level of needle insertion. Because needle movement, once the needle inserted, could damage the urethra or adjacent structures, perform the procedure in the sedated or anesthetized patient. Use an approach similar to that used for cystocentesis in a male dog with the exception that needle entry is at a point caudal to that used to enter the urinary bladder but is cranial to the pubis. The procedure can be performed with or without ultrasound guidance. In the absence of ultrasound guidance, determine needle position by tactile placement and detection of resistance as the needle enters the prostate. Multiple needle penetrations and aspirations are attempted without withdrawing the needle from the skin. Relieve negative pressure in the syringe before removing the needle. Apply any material collected to a glass slide and allow it to air dry before staining. Any conventional stain used for peripheral blood is appropriate.

A transrectal approach to fine-needle aspiration of the prostate has been used in dogs and is performed routinely in men. However, the distance from the anus to the prostate, visualization, and the risk of infection generally are cited as reasons for not performing this technique in dogs.

Fine-needle aspiration may not be diagnostic, particularly in patients with isolated, discrete lesions (cysts or neoplastic nodules) within the prostatic parenchyma. In such cases, ultrasound-guided needle (Tru-Cut) biopsy of the prostate is indicated. Specific training and experience are indicated when performing this procedure because significant complications can result.

Complications associated with prostate biopsy and fine-needle aspiration are not insignificant. Hematuria and periprostatic hemorrhage are described. Postaspiration/biopsy abscess also is described. Consider the risk of urethral penetration and subsequent stricture at the site of penetration.

Additional Reading

Kutzler MA, Yeager A: Prostatic diseases. In Ettinger SJ, Feldman EC, editors: *Textbook of veterinary internal medicine,* ed 6, St Louis, 2005, Elsevier-Saunders.

RESPIRATORY TRACT PROCEDURES

UPPER RESPIRATORY TRACT

For purposes of this discussion, the anatomic limits of the upper respiratory tract of the dog and cat extend caudally from the nasal planum to the first tracheal ring. Key anatomic structures that principally can cause clinical signs include the anterior (external) nares, nasal cavity, nasal turbinates, frontal sinuses, maxillary recesses, upper dental arcade (especially the roots of the maxillary canine teeth), the choana (posterior nares), nasopharynx, soft palate, arytenoid cartilages, glottis, larynx, and the vocal folds.

Clinical signs related to the upper respiratory tract in dogs and cats are among the most common presenting complaints encountered in small animal practice and interestingly are frequent reasons for referral to specialty practices and veterinary teaching hospitals. The oral and nasal cavities are important portals of entry for foreign body entrapment and infectious agents. In addition to the occurrence of nasal neoplasia and trauma, it is not surprising that upper respiratory tract diseases in dogs and cats are common presentations. However, upper respiratory signs can be associated with significantly different underlying causes. Localizing the problem amid a variety of clinical signs in an anatomically complex area represents significant diagnostic and therapeutic challenges to even the most astute clinician. The presentation addresses upper respiratory disease in the dog, with specific emphasis on clearly defining the presenting clinical signs, localizing the problem, and establishing the diagnosis.

4

Anatomic limits

Strictly speaking, the anatomic limits of the upper respiratory tract are not defined. For this presentation, the upper respiratory tract begins at the level of the external nares and ends at the level of the first tracheal ring. In the clinical setting, however, it is practical to establish anatomic limits, or compartments, around the various clinical signs attributable to upper respiratory disease. For example, using the foregoing anatomic limits, the upper respiratory tract can be categorized into three distinct compartments. EACH compartment is associated with a defining clinical sign (Table 4-12). The importance of this categorization is to facilitate the search for the underlying problem and to establish a diagnosis quickly. Properly characterizing the clinical signs is the first step in establishing the cause and defining the diagnosis of upper respiratory tract disease.

Clinical signs

The first and most important step in establishing a diagnosis of canine upper respiratory disease is to define the presenting sign. Experience has shown that an owner's ability to

TABLE 4-12 **Anatomic Limits of the Upper Respiratory Tract and Defining Clinical Signs**

Compartment	Anatomic limits	Defining clinical sign(s)
I	Nose, nasal cavity, and paranasal sinuses	Sneezing and/or nasal discharge
II	Nasopharynx, posterior nares (choana), and soft palate	Stertor (snort) and reverse sneeze
III	Larynx	Stridor (wheeze)

describe the patient's clinical signs accurately, particularly when signs are *not* present at the time of examination, is usually inconsistent and inaccurate, although it can be most entertaining. The four localizing clinical signs characteristically associated with upper respiratory diseases are sneezing and/or nasal discharge, stertor, stridor, and cough. Each sign, considered independently, will focus the examination to the appropriate anatomic region of the upper respiratory tract.

Sneezing and/or nasal discharge

Definition of the clinical signs sneezing and nasal discharge may seem intuitive. This is the most common presenting sign in dogs with upper respiratory disease. Owners that present a dog for *sneezing* are likely to be accurate in their description of the problem. However, the presence or absence of a nasal discharge may be more difficult to establish. Volume, character, and frequency of the discharge ultimately determine whether the owner will have even observed this sign. The astute owner will report whether the discharge is unilateral or bilateral. In the patient that has a history of sneezing and nasal discharge, instillation of a topical nasal decongestant into each nostril occasionally will provoke sneezing and elicit the nature of any discharge that is present.

Sneezing and/or nasal discharge localize the problem to the nose, nasal cavity, and paranasal sinuses. However, thorough examination of the nose and nasal cavity can be difficult, even with the availability of appropriate endoscopy equipment. In addition to careful examination of facial symmetry, the first part of the examination begins in the oral cavity, with emphasis on the maxilla, the hard palate, and the canine teeth. Examine the hard palate for evidence of trauma (penetrating or nonpenetrating) and congenital cleft palate (puppies). Carefully probe the medial aspect of the maxillary canine teeth for evidence of oronasal fistulas. Despite normal-appearing teeth and gingiva, severe, occult periodontal disease with resulting necrosis of bone does result in a septic communication between the oral and nasal cavity. The owner characteristically describes paroxysms of sneezing associated with a sanguineous nasal discharge or spray.

If these findings are negative, radiographs of the skull are indicated. Three views, obtained in the anesthetized patient, are indicated: lateral, ventrodorsal, and occlusal (open mouth) view. Radiographic interpretation of the nasal cavity and sinuses dictates that the clinician has a thorough understanding of the anatomy of the upper respiratory tract. Subsequently, with the patient still anesthetized, attempt a visual examination of the nasal cavity. Radiographs are always performed before visual examination of the nasal cavity. Manipulation of the tissue may result in intranasal bleeding, which will significantly complicate radiographic interpretation. A simple otoscope speculum placed into each nostril allows an adequate examination of the proximal 20% to 25% of the nasal cavity in most dogs. Visual examination of the caudal 75% of the nasal cavity can be attempted only with a small-diameter endoscope. Flexible and rigid scopes are available; each has advantages and disadvantages that will be discussed. Computed tomography and magnetic resonance imaging are important alternative diagnostic tools; however, expense and availability are significant limiting factors.

Understanding the most commonly diagnosed causes of sneezing and nasal discharge is especially helpful in patient management. In no particular order, the most common differential diagnoses for sneezing and/or nasal discharge include the following:

1. *Oronasal fistulas:* Especially common in middle-aged to older dogs, despite a history of recent dental prophylaxis. Empiric treatment with an orally administered antibiotic typically results in rapid and complete resolution of clinical signs, but only during the time the patient is receiving the antibiotic. Diagnosis is confirmed by probing the gingival sulcus of the upper canine teeth.

2. *Nasal neoplasia:* Most commonly reported in dogs between 8 and 10 years of age (range: 1 to 15 years of age). No breed is predisposed, but the condition is uncommon in brachycephalic breeds. Persistent nasal discharge, sneezing, and intermittent epistaxis are common presenting signs. Nasal radiographs may demonstrate lytic bone lesions. Lysis of the vomer strongly supports neoplasia versus mycotic rhinitis. Exposure to tobacco smoke has been associated with 2.5 times greater risk in long-nosed dogs. No or minimal response of the discharge to antibiotics occurs. Eighty percent of nasal tumors are malignant. Adenocarcinoma is most common, followed by squamous cell carcinoma. Sarcomas account for small number of nasal tumors.

3. *Mycotic rhinitis:* Difficult to distinguish from neoplasia. Persistent and voluminous mucoid nasal discharge, with or without sneezing, and nasal pain are reported. Erosion of external nares is an important physcial finding. Discharge is NOT responsive to antimicrobial treatment. Occlusal view radiographs of the nasal cavity may demonstrate evidence of turbinate destruction and/or increased fluid density on the affected side. Forty percent of patients are 3 years or younger; 80% are 7 years and younger. The diagnosis is uncommon in brachycephalic breeds. Localized *Aspergillus fumigatus* infection is reported most commonly.

4. *Lymphoplasmacytic rhinitis:* Poorly described clinical syndrome associated with chronic sneezing and nasal discharge (bilateral or unilateral). Affected dogs are typically young to middle-aged, large-breed dogs. Signs are NOT usually responsive to antibiotics or steroids (topical or systemic). Diagnosis is based on ruling out other causes and nasal biopsy.

Stertor

4

The second most common clinical sign associated with upper respiratory disease in dogs, stertor refers to intermittent, yet persistent, or continuous snorting, also called stertorous breathing. Paroxysms of stertor, typically called reverse sneezing, characterize rapid, consecutive inspiratory bursts through the nose. Seldom actually seen during examination, reverse sneezing is likely to result from the patient's attempt to displace matter trapped in the nasopharynx and move it into the oropharynx, where it can be swallowed.

Visualization of the nasopharynx and choana is essential in the patient that has chronic or persistent stertor. The examination can be accomplished only in the anesthetized patient. Sedation is NOT sufficient to conduct the examination. A flexible endoscope with the ability to flex approximately 170 to 180 degrees is recommended. Examination allows visualization of the nasopharynx and associated mucosa, the choana (posterior nares), and the top of the soft palate (see Figure 4-34).

Nasopharyngeal foreign bodies are by far the most common finding. Sticks, plant material (grass and juniper twigs), peas, cotton balls, and thread are just a few examples. Neoplasia is the second most common finding. In cats, lymphoma (feline leukemia virus–related) obstructing the choana most commonly is observed (see Figure 4-35). In dogs, neoplasia is uncommon, but (in my experience) sarcomas in young dogs have been seen most frequently.

Stridor

The least commonly encountered of the upper respiratory signs is stridor, or stridulous breathing. Stridor is audible wheezing and is associated with restriction to airflow, usually at the level of the larynx. Therefore stridor is *the most critical and potentially life-threatening upper respiratory sign.* This is especially true when stridor is continuous. The patient that has continuous stridor deserves immediate attention. Make every effort to discern the cause once the clinical sign is characterized. In obtaining the history, owners generally describe wheezing accurately; however, some patients actually may present for severe dyspnea or orthopnea. Careful questioning of the client is indicated to determine whether wheezing is associated with the additional effort to breath. The clinician also should make an effort to discern whether the owner has observed any change in the ability of the dog to vocalize or bark.

Simply listening to the patient breath in a quiet room is the first step in assessing stridor. A stethoscope is not required to hear wheezing but should always be used to examine the cervical trachea, the larynx, and the lungs. Any restriction to airflow in the larynx or cervical trachea can cause stridor. However, in the majority of cases, the stridor will be significantly louder at the level of the larynx, indicating a restrictive lesion at that level.

If any indication of respiratory distress is reported or is manifest during the examination, subject the patient to a visual examination under general anesthesia. Sedation is NOT sufficient to conduct the examination. Be prepared. These patients are NOT routine. Emergency resuscitation may be required on induction of anesthesia, including the need to perform a tracheostomy.

On induction, *carefully* place an endotracheal tube. If there are no complications associated with inserting the tube, once anesthesia is effectively induced and the patient is stable, a lateral and dorsoventral radiographs of the larynx and cervical trachea are indicated. Metallic objects (e.g., fish hooks) can become buried in the mucosa and may not be observed during a visual examination.

Remove the endotracheal tube in order to conduct a visual examination. A focal, hands-free light source directed into the oropharynx is strongly recommended. Carefully examine the epiglottis, arytenoid cartilages, glottis and vocal folds using a cotton-tipped applicator. Careful observation of the symmetry and function of the arytenoid cartilages is essential. The left and right cartilages normally respond to tactile stimuli when the patient is in a light plane of anesthesia; both sides should move to the medial plane rapidly and at the same time. They may not close, depending on the depth of anesthesia. It should be possible to visualize the cartilage on the inside of the tracheal rings while looking through the glottis.

In large breed, middle-aged and older dogs, laryngeal paralysis is the most common cause of stridor. Associated signs may include exercise intolerance and collapse during exertion. Laryngeal paralysis and stridor also may be observed in young breeds as a congenital disorder (Dalmatian, Rottweiler, Bouvier des Flandres, Siberian Husky, and Bull Terrier). Foreign body penetration of the laryngeal tissues can cause serious and life-threatening obstruction because of infection and swelling. Neoplasia may cause obstructive mass lesions involving the larynx, especially squamous cell carcinoma and lymphoma. Granulomatous laryngeal disease and fungal mycetoma have been reported.

The presence of a mass lesion, assuming there is no foreign body detected, warrants biopsy of the lesion. Additional effort to control postbiopsy bleeding is important. I use a cotton-tipped applicator saturated with a 1:10,000 dilution of epinephrine held against the biopsy site for 30 to 60 seconds. This is time well spent. Postbiopsy administration of systemically effective dexamethasone has been suggested to control laryngeal swelling, but I have not found this to be effective or important.

Additional Reading

Holt DE: Upper airway obstruction, stertor, and stridor. In King LG, editor: *Textbook of respiratory disease in dogs and cats,* St Louis, 2004, Elsevier-Saunders.

Van Pelt DV, McKiernan BC: Pathogenesis and treatment of canine rhinitis, *Vet Clin North Am Small Anim Pract* 24:789, 1994.

Van Pelt DV, Lappin MR: Pathogenesis and treatment of feline rhinitis, *Vet Clin North Am Small Anim Pract* 24:807, 1994.

Withrow SJ: Tumors of the gastrointestinal system: cancer of the oral cavity. In Withrow SJ, MacEwan EG, editors: *Small animal clinical oncology,* ed 3, Philadelphia, 2001, Saunders.

LOWER RESPIRATORY TRACT

NOTE: Cats and dogs with acute, severe dyspnea must be regarded as having a life-threatening condition until proved otherwise. Immediate therapeutic and diagnostic intervention is indicated. Section 1 describes appropriate interventive procedures for the management of these patients.

The following diagnostic procedures are elective and are indicated in patients with chronic disorders of the lower respiratory tract that are not considered life-threatening.

Transtracheal aspiration

Transtracheal aspiration is a safe and clinically useful method for obtaining material for cytologic and bacteriologic examination from the lower respiratory tract of medium-sized to large dogs without invading the oval cavity. This procedure is *not* indicated in cats. The technique can be performed on the unanesthetized animal, although some sedation may be necessary in fractious animals. In small dogs and cats, tracheal aspirates are collected by passing the catheter through sterile tracheal tubes. Light levels of anesthesia are used to accommodate coughing and tracheal intubation.

Place the animal in sternal recumbency, and elevate and extend the head. Clip the area around the larynx, and surgically prepare the skin. Locate the cricothyroid membrane by moving the finger cranially along the trachea until the large ventral ridge of the cricoid cartilage is felt. Use a 16-gauge, $\frac{1}{2}$-inch intravenous catheter to collect material through the trachea (Figure 4-55). Puncture the cricothyroid membrane with the 16-gauge needle, and pass the catheter into the trachea until it reaches the distal trachea or main stem bronchus. (Alternatively, in large dogs, insert the catheter between the tracheal rings at the junction of the middle third and distal third of the cervical trachea.) Withdraw the needle, and leave the catheter in place. Attach a 12-mL syringe containing sterile saline solution to the catheter. Expel 1 to 2 mL of saline from the syringe. When the animal coughs, aspirate with the syringe to collect cells and mucus for bacteriologic and cytologic examination. When material has been collected, remove the catheter and bandage the animal's neck. Culture material present in the syringe in blood agar and in thioglycollate medium. Prepare material from aspiration for cytologic examination. Press large plugs of mucus between two clean glass slides, and stain thin smears with Wright's or Giemsa stain.

Complications of transtracheal aspiration biopsy include catheter trauma to the lower airway or needle trauma to the larynx, resulting in bleeding, subcutaneous emphysema, pneumomediastinum, pneumothorax, or airway obstruction.

Endotracheal wash

In cats and small dogs and in dogs for which general anesthesia is *not* contraindicated, tracheal aspiration (or tracheal wash) is a relatively safe, easy-to-perform procedure that can yield excellent diagnostic cytologic and culture specimens. The procedure has some advantages over transtracheal aspiration in that it allows sample collection from airways beyond the bifurcation of the trachea (carina) and avoids complications associated with patient discomfort and movement during the procedure. However, cough reflexes are eliminated completely, thereby decreasing potential sample yields from deep in the airway structure. In either case, transtracheal and tracheal aspirations provide the best diagnostic material from large airways, not small airways and alveoli.

The anesthetized dog or cat usually is placed in sternal recumbency. Lateral recumbency (affected side down) may facilitate recovery of specimens from patients with focal or regional lung disease. Use a sterile endotracheal tube to administer the anesthetic and oxygen. Introduce a sterile red rubber catheter (long enough to extend beyond the carina) through the endotracheal tube (Figure 4-56). (NOTE: Disposable adapters for use with endotracheal tubes are available that allow continuous administration of anesthetic gases while passing the rubber catheter through the tube [Figure 4-57].) Introduce the catheter blindly until resistance is met as the tube attempts to enter smaller airways.

Use aliquots of warmed, sterile saline in prepared syringes to wash and retrieve samples. Aliquots of 3 to 5 mL can be used per collection attempt in small dogs and cats, whereas

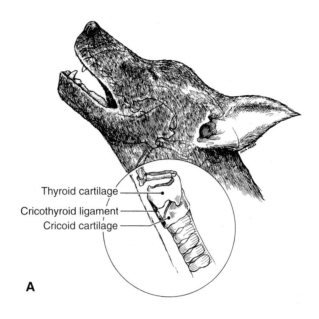

Thyroid cartilage

Cricothyroid ligament

Cricoid cartilage

A

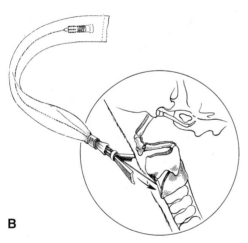

B

Figure 4-55: **A,** Diagramatic representation of anatomic structures involved with transtracheal aspiration technique. The best landmark for percutaneous puncture is the cricothyroid ligament of the larynx, although the tracheal lumen also can be entered between cervical tracheal rings. **B,** The needle is advanced and directed slightly caudad until the trachea is entered. Once the needle is positioned within the tracheal lumen, the catheter is advanced through the needle and down the trachea.
(From Kirk RW: Current veterinary therapy VIII: Small Animal Practice, Philadelphia, 1983, WB Saunders.)

volumes up to 10 and 20 mL are appropriate for larger dogs. With the catheter positioned as deep as practical in the airway, infuse the entire volume of saline. *Gentle agitation* (intermittent aspiration/injection) may facilitate sample collection. If 10 mL is infused, retrieval of only 1 to 2 mL as a final volume per collection attempt is not unusual. The remaining fluid is rapidly (seconds) absorbed into the pulmonary vasculare. IMPORTANT: When

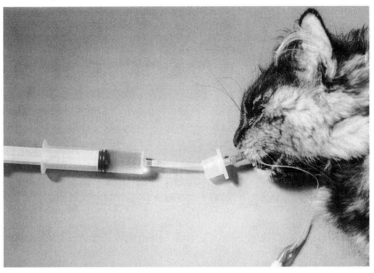

Figure 4-56: Endotracheal wash performed directly through a prepositioned endotracheal tube in a cat.

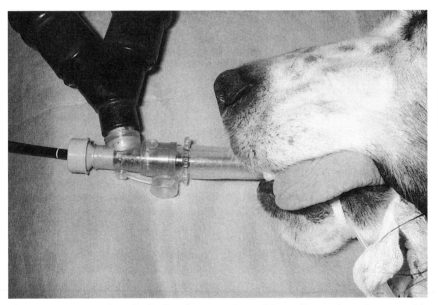

Figure 4-57: An endotracheal tube adapter can be used in medium to large dogs to enable administration of anesthetic gases and oxygen throughout the endotracheal wash procedure.

performing this procedure, DO NOT withdraw the rubber catheter while maintaining a high negative pressure on the syringe. Doing so actually may tear mucosa away from the airway and could lead to pneumothorax or pneumomediastinum.

The procedure can be repeated safely in the same patient several times. Collection of three to five samples is routine. More samples may be indicated depending on the patient's condition and response to the procedure. Monitoring of patients undergoing a tracheal wash procedure for oxygen saturation (pulse oximetry) throughout the procedure is recommended. In some patients with reactive airways, infusion of saline may cause significant bronchoconstriction, detected by a rapid decline in oxygen saturation.

Process samples collected immediately. Submit at least one sample of liquid (*not* a swab of the liquid) for bacterial culture and sensitivity or MIC. Quantitative cultures are impractical because specimens will be diluted. If the sample appears to be highly cellular (characterized by turbidity), place aliquots into tubes containing EDTA.

Additional Reading

Syring RS: Tracheal washes. In King LG, editor: *Textbook of respiratory disease in dogs and cats,* St Louis, 2004, Elsevier-Saunders.

BRONCHOALVEOLAR LAVAGE

Bronchoalveolar lavage (BAL) is an alternative diagnostic procedure to transtracheal aspiration and endotracheal wash. Bronchoalveolar lavage has the advantage of retrieving fluid samples from distal airways and alveoli. This is a highly diagnostic procedure indicated in patients with generalized lung and regional (interstitial and/or airway) disease that are *not* in respiratory distress. Patients suspected of having allergic or infectious respiratory disease or neoplasia are candidates for BAL. Although BAL is used as a therapeutic procedure in human beings with chronic lung disease associated with accumulations of surfactant in the alveoli, there is no therapeutic indication for BAL in dogs or cats.

The technique for BAL entails instilling sufficiently large volumes of fluid into the distal airways to reach, and recover, reasonable cytological samples representative of small airways and alveoli. Several variations on the technique are described, but all recommend blind or visual placement of a catheter or bronchoscope into an airway of a lung lobe such that the airway is occluded. Sterile, nonbacteriostatic 0.9% saline, warmed to approximately body temperature and drawn into prepared syringes, is the fluid of choice. The volume of fluid varies with the size of the patient. Defined doses of saline per kilogram of body mass have not been described. In large dogs, two 25-mL aliquots (50 mL total) can be infused into each lobe sampled. In small dogs and cats, total volumes per lobe generally are restricted to 10-mL aliquots. Recovery may be as low as 2 to 5 mL with each attempt.

For dogs undergoing BAL, particularly when reactive (allergic) airway disease is suspected, pretreatment with a bronchodilator is appropriate and is recommended. Aminophylline can be administered at 5 mg/kg (cats) or 11 mg/kg (dogs) orally 1 to 2 hours before the procedure. Alternatively, terbutaline, 0.01 mg/kg, can be administered subcutaneously to cats 30 minutes before the procedure.

Bronchoscopic BAL allows direct visualization of the airway/lobe of interest. In medium to large dogs, place the bronchoscope directly through a sterile endotracheal tube. Use of an inexpensive, disposable endotracheal tube adaptor permits simultaneous administration of oxygen and anesthetic throughout the procedure. Saline can be infused from a syringe directly through the biopsy channel of the endoscope. The bronchoscope serves as the infusion catheter. Using this technique, samples can be collected effectively from multiple lobes. Blind placement (nonbronchoscopic) BAL using a rubber end-hole catheter is required in cats and small dogs. Blind placement is also appropriately used in patients with generalized lung or airway disease when discrete placement of bronchoscope cannot be accomplished reliably.

As with the endotracheal wash procedure described before, *gentle agitation with the syringe* (intermittent aspiration/injection) may facilitate sample collection. DO NOT withdraw the bronchoscope or catheter while maintaining significant negative pressure because this may lacerate the airway, leading to pneumothorax or pneumomediastinum.

Bronchoalveolar lavage is an invasive diagnostic procedure that is not without risk of injury or death. Following completion of BAL, administration of 100% oxygen for 5 to 10 minutes via endotracheal tube is recommended for all patients. Evaluate the patient carefully for breathing effort and oxygen saturation (pulse oximetry) during recovery.

Although significant quantities of fluid remain in the airways following BAL, most of the volume is absorbed rapidly. Residual amounts of fluid, however, can be retained for 24 to 48 hours after the procedure. During this time, some patients will manifest cough. Crackles may be auscultated.

Additional Reading

Hawkins EC: Bronchoalveolar lavage. In King LG, editor: *Textbook of respiratory disease in dogs and cats*, St Louis, 2004, Elsevier-Saunders.

Hawkins EC, DeNicola DB, Plier ML: Cytological analysis of bronchoalveolar lavage fluid in the diagnosis of spontaneous respiratory tract disease in dogs, *J Vet Intern Med* 9:386-392, 1995.

FINE-NEEDLE ASPIRATION OF LUNG

Percutaneous aspiration needle biopsy can be helpful in establishing a diagnosis in conditions such as (1) chronic inflammatory disease of the lung—for example, granulomatous lung disease caused by mycotic organisms; (2) chronic inflammatory disease; (3) metastases to the lung; and (4) primary lung tumors. The biopsy may provide enough diagnostic information to preclude performing an exploratory thoracotomy. Lung biopsy is contraindicated in animals with hemorrhagic disease or thoracic disease that produces forceful breathing and coughing.

Clip and surgically prepare the biopsy site. Infiltrate the skin, subcutaneous tissue, muscle, and parietal pleura with 1% to 2% lidocaine.

In diffuse parenchymal lung disease, taking biopsy material from the diaphragmatic lobes is recommended. The dorsal portions of the seventh to ninth intercostal spaces are preferred for percutaneous biopsies. In diffuse lesions, take biopsy material from the right or left thorax.

Understanding of the risks associated with performing fine-needle aspiration of lung is important. Lung aspirates will yield only cells, fluid, and trace amounts of tissue, yet there is a significant risk of inducing pneumothorax following the procedure, even when performed without difficulty or complications.

When performing the procedure, a 22- to 25-gauge disposable needle (such as a 1-inch spinal needle) with stylet is preferred. Leave the stylet within the needle until the lung has been penetrated. Then quickly remove the stylet and immediately attach a sterile 6- to 12-mL syringe. The amount of air that might enter the lung between the time the stylet is removed and the syringe attached is negligible. Holding the syringe carefully and steadily against the patient's thorax, establish negative pressure in the same manner as when obtaining an aspiration from a lymph node. As much as the patient will permit, attempt three to four aspirations without withdrawing the needle.

Alternatively, insert a conventional 25-gauge needle, attached to a 6-mL syringe, *subcutaneously* over the area of interest. Then establish significant negative pressure while the tip of the needle is still positioned in the subcutaneous tissues *outside the parietal pleura*. While maintaining the same amount of negative pressure in the syringe, direct the needle into the lung, leave it in place for 1 to 2 seconds, and withdraw it completely. Apply any material collected directly to glass slide. This procedure is best conducted in patients that are awake. Attempting the procedure in anesthetized dogs or cats could result in an unsuccessful aspirate or, if the lungs were under positive pressure (ventilation or bagging), the risk of causing pneumothorax could be increased. Other reported complications include hemothorax (always exciting), lung laceration caused by patient movement during the procedure, pulmonary hemorrhage, and hemoptysis. Contraindications to fine-needle aspiration include patients with a known bleeding diathesis and coagulopathy, thrombocytopenia, uncontrolled coughing, pulmonary hypertension, pulmonary cysts, and bullous emphysema.

Ultrasound guided techniques for fine-needle aspiration or biopsy of lung recently have been described and generally are associated with fewer procedural complications. However, additional training and experience, in addition to having access to the proper size and type of ultrasound probe, is critical.

4

Additional Reading

Cole SG: Fine needle aspirates. In King LG, editor: *Textbook of respiratory disease in dogs and cats,* St Louis, 2004, Elsevier-Saunders.

NEBULIZATION AND AEROSOL THERAPY

Inhalation therapy can be defined as nebulization (humidification of the inspired air) and aerosol therapy (the process whereby drugs are vaporized in a solution and delivered directly into the respiratory tract). In companion animals, inhalation therapy is most useful for humidifying air in the respiratory tract and moistening the mucous membranes (nebulization). Sustained inspiration of dry air/gases causes irritation to the respiratory epithelium, which in turn results in swelling, bronchial gland hypertrophy, goblet cell proliferation, and loss of ciliary epithelium over time. Respiratory secretions become thick and tenacious, and efficient bronchial drainage is impaired.

The objectives of inhalation therapy include the following:

1. Humidification of bronchial mucous membranes
2. Deposition of miniscule amounts of potent drugs in smaller airways to obtain optimal topical therapeutic effects with minimal systemic side effects (e.g., bronchodilators)
3. Deposition of moderate amounts of potent agents or agents that are only effective topically (e.g., antibiotics and mucolytics)
4. Deposition of relatively large quantities of bland substances that promote bronchial drainage with minimal irritation (e.g., saline, propylene glycol, glycerine, and detergents)

Nebulization is used (1) in combination with oxygen therapy; (2) in tracheostomy care; (3) in acute respiratory diseases such as tracheobronchitis, bronchiolitis, upper respiratory disease of cats, pneumonia, and postoperative atelectasis and pneumonia; and (4) in chronic respiratory diseases such as chronic bronchitis, bronchopneumonia, collapsed trachea with secondary tracheobronchitis, emphysema, and bronchiectasis.

Aerosol therapy, however, is a limited-use therapeutic technique used in dogs and cats to administer antimicrobials, bronchodilators (aminophylline, 100 mg), or corticosteroids. The advantage of doing so is to achieve relatively high levels of drug in the respiratory tract in patients with *defined* lower respiratory tract disease. In addition, administration of potentially toxic antimicrobials (aminoglycosides) by this route has been shown to be associated with minimal or insignificant uptake into the general circulation, thereby minimizing (or eliminating) any risk of renal toxicity.

Principles of action

Large water particles (10 to 60 μm) in the high-velocity air flow of the nose and throat settle on the mucosa of the larynx, nose, and throat. Particles smaller than 10 μm (2 to 10 μm) are deposited in the bronchi, but only the smallest particles reach the bronchioles. Ultrasonic aerosol generators are the most effective machines for nebulization. The mists can be directed into a cage or a face mask. If nebulization is used with an endotracheal or tracheostomy tube, warm inspired gases to body temperature.

Dense mist from an unheated jet nebulizer (Figure 4-58) contains only slightly more water than is needed to humidify air with temperature increasing from 22° to 37° C. Evaporation of the aerosol solution can be prevented by stabilization; that is, by heating it to 35° C or by reducing the vapor pressure by adding 10% propylene glycol. Because distilled water and hypertonic solutions are irritating to the mucosa, use only isotonic or half-strength isotonic saline.

Although continuous, low-level humidification of the oxygen tent atmosphere is necessary, periodic medication by aerosol spray is permissible. High levels of water can be introduced several times daily for 10 to 15 minutes per treatment, or drugs can be added to the solution during these times. Many drugs have been used; isoproterenol, epinephrine, and phenylephrine are some of the drugs that may cause bronchodilation and decreased airway resistance.

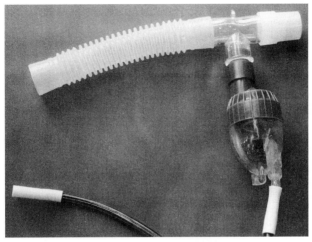

Figure 4-58: Disposable jet nebulizer used to administer humidified air and/or medication directly into the respiratory tract.

Differentiation of obstruction of the bronchi caused by pulmonary edema from that caused by bronchial secretions is important. In both cases the patient cannot breath because of fluids or semifluid liquids in the bronchi. In pulmonary edema, the fluid turns to a frothy, bubbly material that produces a rattling sound in the trachea.

Thick, inflammatory exudates, however, must be thinned by detergent materials that liquefy bronchial secretions. However, these agents increase frothing and, indirectly, anoxia if used in pulmonary edema. In patients with acute, severe bronchial inflammation, mucolytic agents such as acetylcysteine have been administered *intravenously* to dogs at doses as high as 144 mg/kg followed by 70 mg/kg 12 hours later. Aerosolization of acetylcysteine currently is used in human medicine but has not been validated in dogs.

Heated aerosol units (vaporizers) produce large water droplets that do not penetrate small bronchioles and may overheat the patient. These units should not be used for intensive therapy.

Drug delivery by aerosolization

Drugs that can be applied by jet nebulizer (Figure 4-59 and 4-60) include the following:
1. *Bronchodilators:* Always use bronchodilators when administering drugs that may be irritating and constricting, such as isoetharine hydrochloride 1% and phenylephrine 0.25%, 0.5 to 1.0 mL in 2 to 3 mL of saline 3 to 4 times daily.
2. *Antibiotics:* Antibiotics are poorly absorbed from the respiratory mucosa. Systemic administration of most antibiotics produces adequate pulmonary concentration for antibacterial effect. For *Bordetella* spp. that are located at the tips of bronchial cilia, topical contact via nebulization may be useful. Antibiotics that have been used successfully and safely include kanamycin (250 mg in 5 mL saline twice daily); gentamicin (50 mg in 5 mL saline twice daily); and polymyxin B (333,000 IU in 5 mL saline twice daily).
3. *Bland solutions:* Use these in large volume for prolonged mist effect: 0.9% sterile saline (5 to 200 mL as needed); glycerine (5% in saline); and propylene glycol (10% to 20% solution in saline).
4. *Detergents and mucolytics:* These compounds are irritating and currently are not recommended by most authors.
5. *Antifoaming agents:* Administer ethyl alcohol (70% solution 5 to 10 mL twice daily).

4

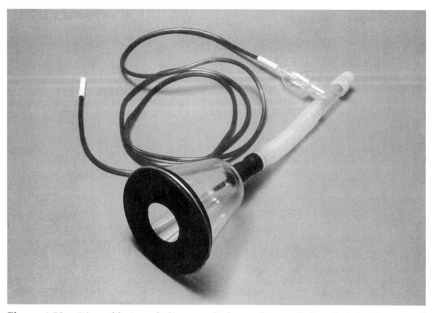

Figure 4-59: Disposable jet nebulizer attached to a face mask for administering aerosol therapy to dogs.

4

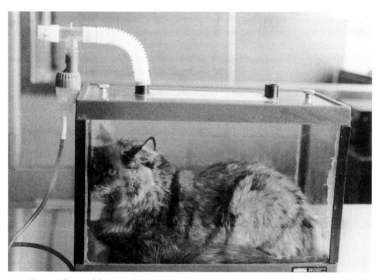

Figure 4-60: A disposable jet nebulizer attached to a Plexiglas anesthesia induction box for administration of aerosol therapy to cats.

Additional Reading

Boothe DM: Drugs affecting the respiratory system. In King LG, editor: *Textbook of respiratory disease in dogs and cats*, St Louis, 2004, Elsevier-Saunders.

Tseng LW, Drobatz KJ: Oxygen supplementation and humidification. In King LG, editor: *Textbook of respiratory disease in dogs and cats*, St Louis, 2004, Elsevier-Saunders.

URINARY TRACT PROCEDURES

UROHYDROPROPULSION

Removal of uroliths from dogs and cats is a commonly performed, yet critically important, clinical procedure. Several techniques are available for removal of calculi and obstructive concretions in male and female animals. Cystotomy is performed routinely to remove calculi from the lumen of the bladder but especially in male dogs may not be an effective approach for removing obstructing urethral calculi. Advanced and expensive techniques recently have been described: laparoscopic-assisted cystotomy, Ellik evacuator, use of stone "baskets" (through a cystoscope), and lithotripsy are examples. However, for removal of uroliths from dogs and cats with partial or complete urinary obstruction, urohydropulsion is among the more effective yet inexpensive techniques available.

Urohydropulsion is a therapeutic procedure for removal of foreign material, namely, uroliths, from the bladder and/or urethra of dogs. Two techniques are described: *voiding* urohydropulsion and *retrograde* urohydropulsion. Both procedures have advantages and disadvantages.

Voiding urohydropulsion

The objective of voiding urohydropulsion is to induce forceful voiding of urine by manually compressing the bladder to facilitate removal of cystic uroliths in *female* dogs. Do not perform this procedure until it can be confirmed by catheterization or cystoscopy that the urethra is patent. With the bladder filled with urine or saline (via catheterization), lift the patient (preferably sedated or anesthetized, although this procedure can be done in the awake patient) into a position such that the tail and perineum are ventral and head is upright. The spine should be approximately perpendicular to the working surface. Using one or both hands, gradually increase pressure on the bladder to induce and maintain a forceful stream of urine. Objectively, small uroliths will be extruded. If the procedure is only partially successful, it can be repeated as necessary. Obviously, voiding urohyropulsion has limitations and cannot be used in male dogs or in dogs with urethral obstructions or strictures.

Retrograde urohydropulsion

This procedure is indicated for male dogs and cats with partial or complete urethral obstruction caused by uroliths or accumulations of "sand." Preferably perform the procedure in the anesthetized patient.

NOTE: There are discrepancies in the literature regarding whether to empty the urinary bladder of urine before performing this procedure. Because patients with urethral obstructions may have a significant volume of urine in the bladder at the time of presentation, some authors recommend performing cystocentesis to relieve the internal pressure before attempting urohydropulsion. However, in patients that have had a profoundly distended bladder for several hours (even days), penetrating the urinary bladder with a needle presents significant risk of rupturing a fragile bladder. The next step, of course, is abdominal surgery. I recommend avoiding cystocentesis whenever possible. The volume of saline required to flush uroliths into the bladder is inconsequential considering the total volume already present.

With the patient positioned in lateral recumbency, retract the prepuce and expose the penis as for conventional bladder catheterization technique. Use sterile technique to pass an appropriately sized flexible catheter, which is advanced to the point of obstruction. Attach a catheter-tipped 60-mL syringe filled with warmed (my preference) sterile saline and a water-soluble lubricant mixture (approximately 2 parts saline to 1 part lubricant) to the urinary catheter. An assistant places a gloved (always preferred) finger into the rectum to identify and occlude the lumen of the pelvic urethra at the level of the pubis. Subsequently, infuse saline forcefully into the catheter to dilate the urethra proximal to the obstructing urolith. At that point, release the digital pressure on the proximal urethra while the solution continues to be infused through the catheter. Objectively, the pressure within the urethra forces small stones retrograde into the urinary bladder, thereby relieving the obstruction.

NOTE: The objective of this procedure is NOT to push the calculi into the bladder with the catheter, because this can substantially injure the urethral mucosa, nor to force the calculi around the catheter and move it antegrade.

Additional Reading

Adams LG, Syme HM: Canine lower urinary tract diseases. In Ettinger SJ, Feldman EC, editors: *Textbook of veterinary internal medicine,* ed 6, St Louis, 2005, Elsevier-Saunders.

Osborne CA, Finco DR: *Canine and feline nephrology and urology,* Baltimore, 1995, Williams & Wilkins.

4

SECTION 5

Laboratory Diagnosis and Test Protocols

Common Reference Range Values, *576*
Sample Handling, *576*
    Sample Identification, *576*
    Sample Collection Tubes, *576*
    Sample Storage and Transport, *580*
    Patient Preparation, *581*
    Minimizing Hemolysis, *581*
    Avoiding Clots and Platelet Clumps, *581*
Submission Requirements for Rabies Suspects, *582*
    Sample Submission for Rabies Testing, *582*
    Packaging Requirements for Authorized Samples, *583*
    Information Requested on the Rabies Specimen History Form, *583*
    Submission Guidelines, *583*
    Packing and Shipping Directions, *583*
Histopathology and Cytopathology, *584*
    Histopathology, *584*
    Cytopathology, *585*
Biochemistry—Routine, *589*
    Analyte or Test Name (Synonyms), *590*
Routine Diagnostic Tests, *591*
    Alanine Aminotransferase (ALT; Formerly SGPT), *591*
    Albumin, *591*
    Albumin/Globulin Ratio (A:G), *591*
    Alkaline Phosphatase (SAP or Alk Phos), *591*
    Amylase, *592*
    Anion Gap, *592*
    Aspartate Aminotransferase (Formerly SGOT), *592*
    Bicarbonate (HCO_3^-), *592*
    Bilirubin, *592*
    Blood Urea Nitrogen (BUN), *593*
    Calcium (Ca), *593*
    Chloride (Cl), *593*
    Cholesterol (CH), *593*
    Creatine Kinase (CK; Formerly CPK), *594*
    Creatinine (Cr), *594*
    Gamma Glutamyltransferase (GGT; Gamma GT [GGT]), *594*
    Globulin, *594*
    Glucose, *594*

Lipase, *595*
Phosphorus (P), *595*
Potassium (K⁺), *595*
Sodium (Na⁺), *595*
Total Protein (TP), *595*
Triglyceride (TG), *596*
Special Diagnostic Tests and Test Protocols, *596*
  ACTH Stimulation Test: See Endocrinology, *596*
  Adrenocorticotropic Hormone (ACTH), Endogenous: See Endocrinology, *596*
  Aldosterone: See Endocrinology, *596*
  Ammonia (NH₃) (Fasting Ammonia), *596*
  Ammonia Tolerance Test, *597*
  Antinuclear Antibody (ANA): See Immunology, *597*
  Bile Acids, *597*
  Blood Gases (Arterial and Venous), *598*
  Body Fluids (Submitted for Chemistry Analysis), *599*
  Calcium, Ionized (iCa), *599*
  Cerebrospinal Fluid (CSF), *599*
  Cobalamin (Vitamin B₁₂), *600*
  Ethylene Glycol, *600*
  Fecal Fat, 72-Hour Quantitative Collection, *601*
  Fecal Occult Blood, *601*
  Folate, *601*
  Fructosamine, *602*
  Glycosylated Hemoglobin (Glycated Hemoglobin; Gly Hb), *602*
  Iron, *602*
  Lactic Acid (Lactate), *603*
  Lead, Blood, *603*
  Lipoprotein Electrophoresis, *604*
  Magnesium (Mg), *604*
  Osmolality, Estimated (Serum), *604*
  Pancreatic Lipase Immunoreactivity (PLI), *605*
  Protein Electrophoresis (Serum), *605*
  Trypsin-Like Immunoreactivity, Canine (Canine TLI), *606*
  Trypsin-Like Immunoreactivity, Feline (Feline TLI), *606*
Hemostasis and Coagulation, *606*
  Initial In-Office Screening Tests, *607*
  Ancillary Tests of Hemostasis, *608*
  Submission of Samples for Coagulation Testing, *609*
  Activated Coagulation (Clotting) Time (ACT), *610*
  Activated Partial Thromboplastin Time (APTT), *610*
  Antiplatelet Antibody: See Immunology, *610*
  Blood Typing, Feline, *610*
  Blood Typing for Complete Dog Erythrocyte Antigen (DEA), *611*
  Buccal Mucosal Bleeding Time (BMBT), *611*
  Clot Retraction Test, *611*
  Coagulation Factor Activity (Factor Assay), *611*
  Cross-Match: Major and Minor, *612*
  D-Dimer (Fragment D-dimer; Fibrin Degradation Fragment), *613*
  Fibrinogen, Qualitative (Estimated), *613*
  Fibrinogen, Quantitative, *613*
  Fibrin Degradation Products (FDPs; Fibrin Split Products [FSPs]), *614*
  Partial Thromboplastin Time (PTT): See Activated Partial Thromboplastin Time (APTT), *614*
  PIVKA Test (Proteins Induced by Vitamin K Antagonists Test; "Thrombotest"), *614*
  Platelet Count, *615*
  Prothrombin Time (PT), *615*
  Von Willebrand Factor (vWD Factor), *615*
Endocrinology, *616*
  Adrenocorticotropic Hormone (ACTH), Endogenous, *616*
  ACTH Stimulation Test; "Stim"), *617*
  Aldosterone (Serum), *617*

5

Cobalamin (Vitamin B$_{12}$), *618*
Cortisol, Resting (Basal): See ACTH Stimulation Test, *618*
Dexamethasone Suppression Test, Low-Dose (LDDS Test; Dexamethasone Screening Test), *618*
Dexamethasone Suppression Test, High-Dose (HDDS Test), *619*
Estradiol (Baseline), *620*
Folate, *620*
Fructosamine, *620*
Gastrin, *621*
Glucagon Stimulation Test (IVGS Test), *621*
Glucose Curve, 12-Hour, *621*
Glucose Tolerance Test, Intravenous (IVGT Test), *622*
Glucose Tolerance Test, Oral (OGT Test), *622*
Insulin, *623*
Parathyroid Hormone (PTH), *623*
Parathyroid Hormone-Related Protein (PTHrP), *623*
T$_3$(3,5,3'-Triiodothyronine), *624*
Reverse T$_3$ (rT$_3$; 3,3',5'-Triiodothyronine), *624*
T$_3$ Suppression, *624*
Free T$_4$ (fT$_4$), *625*
Total T$_4$, (Thyroxine or Tetraiodothyroinine), *625*
Thyrotropin, Canine (Thyroid-Stimulating Hormone [TSH]; Baseline TSH), *626*
Thyroid-Stimulating Hormone, Canine: See Thyrotropin, Canine, *626*
Thyrotropin Response (TSH Response Test), *626*
Immunology, *626*
Allergen-Specific IGE Antibody Test (Radioallergosorbent Test [RAST]; Allergy Screen), *626*
Antibody Titers for Infectious Disease Diagnosis: See Infectious Disease Serology and
Microbiology, *627*
Antinuclear Antibody (ANA), *627*
Antiplatelet Antibody, *627*
Coombs Test (Direct Coombs Test; Direct Antiglobulin Test [DAT]), *627*
Rheumatoid Factor, Canine, *628*
Infectious Disease Serology And Microbiology, *628*
Anaplasma phagocytophila Antibody (formerly *Ehrlichia equi*), *628*
Aspergillus spp. Antibody titer (Non-avian), *628*
Babesia Antibody Titer, Canine, *629*
Bartonella spp. (*Bartonella henselae* Titer), *629*
Blastomycosis Antibody Titer, *629*
Blood Culture (Bacteria), *630*
Borrelia burgdorferi: See Lyme Borreliosis, *630*
Brucella canis Antibody, *630*
Canine Distemper Antibody, *631*
Cerebrospinal Fluid (CSF) (IgG or IgM), *631*
Serum (IgG or IgM), *631*
Coccidioidiomycosis Antibody Titer (AGID), *632*
Cryptococcal Antigen (Serum or CSF), *632*
Ehrlichia canis Antibody, *633*
Ehrlichia equi Antibody: See *Anaplasma phagocytophila* Antibody, *633*
Ehrlichia spp.: See Polymerase Chain Reaction (PCR) For Test Method, *633*
Feline Coronavirus Antibody (FeCoV Ab), *633*
Feline Infectious Anemia: See *Haemobartonella (Mycoplasma haemofelis)*, *633*
Feline Leukemia Virus Antigen (FeLV Ag; P27 Test), *633*
Feline Immunodeficiency Virus Antibody (FIV Ab), *634*
GIARDIA Antigen, *635*
Heartworm Antibody, Feline, *635*
Heartworm Antigen, Feline, *636*
Heartworm Antigen,Canine, *636*
Haemobartonella (Feline Infectious Anemia; *Mycoplasma haemofelis, M. haemominutum*), *636*
Leptospirosis Antibody Titer, *637*
Lyme Borreliosis *(Borrelia burgdorferi)*, *637*
Rabies Titer (By RFFIT), *639*
Rocky Mountain Spotted Fever (RMSF), *639*

5

Toxoplasmosis Titers (IgG and IgM), *640*
Vaccine Titers: See Specific Pathogen, *640*
Urine, *641*
    Cortisol, Urine. See Urine Cortisol:Creatinine Ratio (UC:CR; Urinary C:C Ratio), *641*
    Microalbuminuria Test (Early Renal Disease [ERD] In-Hospital Test Kit), *641*
    Urine Cortisol:Creatinine Ratio (UC:CR, Urinary C:C Ratio), *641*
    Urine Protein-Creatinine Ratio (UPCr; P:Cr; UPC), *641*

COMMON REFERENCE RANGE VALUES*

SAMPLE HANDLING

SAMPLE IDENTIFICATION

Identification of specimens is critical if the right result on a given patient is to get back to the right clinician in a timely manner. The following steps are recommended:

1. Write the animal/client name on *each* specimen container.
2. Write the animal and client name, species, breed, gender, and date on the test requisition form.
3. Make sure that the originating clinic name and account number are clearly identified on the form.
4. Clearly mark or write down the needed tests on the form. (NOTE: Commercial laboratories receive hundreds of samples each day with no test marked!)
5. Indicate the source, if other than a blood sample, on the form.
6. Identify the tissue or fluid source and clinic ID on all slides submitted for cytology (use a lead pencil to write on the frosted side).

SAMPLE COLLECTION TUBES

Most practices utilize a variety of **glass** vacuum tubes (Vacutainer)[†] to collect and submit blood, serum, or plasma from individual patients. The tubes are actually designed for collecting blood samples from humans. A variety of tube sizes, each of which maintains a pre-determined negative pressure (vacuum) inside, are available. The vacuum facilitates collection of an appropriate volume of the patient's blood to nearly fill the tube. Additionally, most of the blood collection tubes contain an additive that will either accelerate or prevent clot formation.

Adult (human) tubes are available in 5-mL, 7-mL, 10-mL, and 15-mL sizes. Pediatric (human) tubes, appropriate for use in companion animal patients, are available in 2-mL, 3-mL, and 4-mL sizes. For tubes containing an additive, filling the tube with an appropriate volume of blood is important. *Underfilling* any tube that contains an additive may sufficiently alter the sample such that the test results are adversely affected and may not accurately represent the patient's status.

The color of the stopper in the top of the tube indicates the type of additive, if any, and the specific type of tests that can be performed with that sample. For example, do not send serum when plasma is required!

---

*NOTE: Reference Range values listed throughout this section are for general reference *only*. Test results from individual patients *must be compared to the Reference Range Values* for the laboratory that performs the test.

[†]Vacutainer® is the registered trademark of Becton, Dickenson and Company (B-D).

Reference range values listed for Tables 5-1 to 5-5 are representative values only and will vary among individual laboratories.

TABLE 5-1 Hematology Reference Range Values

Test	Adult canine	Adult feline	Units
Red Blood Cell (total)	5.32-7.75	6.68-11.8	$\times 10^6$ cells/mm^3
Hemoglobin (Hgb)	13.5-19.5	11.0-15.8	grams
Hematocrit (Hct)	39.4-56.2	33.6-50.2	%
Mean Corpuscular Volume (MCV)	65.7-75.7	42.6-55.5	fL
Mean Corpuscular Hemoglobin (MCH)	22.57-27.0	13.4-18.6	pg
Mean Corpuscular Hemoglobin Concentration (MCHC)	34.3-36.0	31.3-33.5	g/dL
Platelet Count	194-419	198-405	$\times 10^3$ cells/mm^3
Mean Platelet Volume (MPV)	8.8-14.3	11.3-21.3	fL
White Blood Cell (Total)	4.36-14.8	4.79-12.52	$\times 10^3$ cells/mm^3
Segmented Neutrophils (Segs)	3.4-9.8	1.6-15.6	$\times 10^3$ cells/mm^3
Non-Segmented Neutrophils (Bands or Non-Segs)	0-0.01	0-0.01	$\times 10^3$ cells/mm^3
Lymphocytes (Lymphs)	0.8-3.5	1.0-7.4	$\times 10^3$ cells/mm^3
Monocytes (Monos)	0.2-1.1	0-0.7	$\times 10^3$ cells/mm^3
Eosinophils (Eos)	0-1.9	0.1-2.3	$\times 10^3$ cells/mm^3
Basophils (Basos)	0	0	$\times 10^3$ cells/mm^3

TABLE 5-2 Biochemistry Reference Range Values

Test	Adult canine	Adult feline	Units
Glucose	73-116	63-150	mg/dL
Blood Urea Nitrogen (BUN)	8-27	15-35	mg/dL
Creatinine (Cr)	0.5-1.6	0.5-2.3	mg/dL
Phosphorus (P)	2.0-6.7	2.7-7.6	mg/dL
Calcium (Ca)	9.2-11.6	7.5-11.5	mg/dL
Ionized Calcium (iCa)	1.15-1.39	—	mg/dL
Total Protein (TP)	5.5-7.2	5.4-8.9	g/dL
Albumin (Alb)	2.8-4.0	3.0-4.2	g/dL
Globulin (Glob)	2.0-4.1	2.8-5.3	g/dL
Cholesterol (Ch)	138-317	42-265	mg/dL
Bilirubin (Total)	0-0.2	0.1-0.5	mg/dL
Alkaline Phosphatase (SAP or Alk Phos)	15-146	0-96	IU/L
Alanine Aminotransferase (ALT)	16-73	5-134	IU/L
Gamma Glutamyltransferase (GGT)	3-8	0-10	IU/L
Creatine Kinase (CK; formerly CPK))	48-380	72-481	IU/L
Sodium (Na)	147-154	147-165	mEq/L
Potassium (K)	3.9-5.2	3.3-5.7	mEq/L
A:G ratio	0.6-2.0	0.4-1.5	—
Na/K ratio	27.4-38.4	30-43	—
Chloride (Cl)	104-117	113-122	mEq/L
Bicarbonate (Venous)	20-29	22-24	mEq/L
Anion Gap	16.3-28.6	15-32	—
Osmolality (Calculated)	292-310	290-320	mOsm/kg
Amylase	347-1104	489-2100	IU/L
Lipase	22-216	0-222	IU/L
Triglyceride (TG)	19-133	24-206	mg/dL

5

TABLE 5-3   Urinalysis (Voided Sample) Reference Range Values

Test	Canine	Feline
Specific Gravity (SpGr)	variable	variable
Color	pale to dark yellow	pale to dark yellow
pH	5.0 to 8.5	5.0 to 8.5
Protein	negative to + 1	negative to + 1
Glucose	negative	negative
Ketones	negative	negative
Bilirubin	negative to trace	negative
Blood	negative	negative
Microscopic:		
Red Blood Cell (RBC) Count	<5 RBCs/hpf	<5 RBCs/hpf
White Blood Cell (WBC) Count	<3 WBCs/hpf	<3 WBCs/hpf
Epithelial Cells	negative	negative
Casts	negative	negative
Bacteria	negative	negative
Special: Urine Protein:Creatinine	<0.3	<0.6

TABLE 5-4   Hemostasis Reference Range Values

Test	Canine	Feline
Platelet Count	$166\text{-}600 \times 10^3/\mu L$	$230\text{-}680 \times 10^3/\mu L$
Prothrombin Time (PT)	5.1-7.9 sec	8.4-10.8 sec
Activated Partial Thromboplastin Time (APTT)	8.6-12.9 sec	13.7-30.2 sec
Fibrin Degradation Products (FDP)	$< 10\ \mu g/mL$	$< 10\ \mu g/mL$
Fibrinogen	100-245 mg/dL	110-370 mg/dL
Activated Clotting Time (ACT)	60-110 sec	50-75 sec

TABLE 5-5   Blood Gas Analysis—Arterial Reference Range Values

Test	Canine	Feline	Units
pH	7.36-7.44	7.36-7.44	-
P_{O_2}	90-100	90-100	mmHg
P_{CO_2}	36-44	28-32	mmHg
HCO_3^-	24-26	20-22	mEq/L
T_{CO_2}	25-27	21-23	mEq/L

Note: Most commercial laboratories recommend collecting a minimum volume of 2.0 whole blood for routine biochemical analyses; 2.0 mL of whole blood will yield close to 1.0 mL of serum. Dehydrated patients are expected to have a higher hematocrit, and therefore a larger volume of whole blood may be required in order to obtain a 1.0-mL sample of serum.

Note: When collecting blood from a patient, it is critical to use:
1. The appropriate sized tubes
2. Tubes that contain the proper additive for the test(s) being requested

Types of commercial blood collection tubes used in veterinary medicine are discussed in Tables 5-6 to 5-14. Interpretation of the in-office coagulation screen is discussed in Table 5-15.

TABLE 5-6 Red-Topped Tube

Additive	None
Effect	Allows blood to clot naturally; centrifugation is required to separate serum
Tests	Routine biochemistry, serology; cross-match; most liquid samples collected by centesis or aspiration for biochemistry or cytopathology— e.g., CSF, abdominal fluid

---

TABLE 5-7 Red and Gray Mottled Top ("Tiger-Topped Tube"); Also Called Serum Separator Tube (SST)

Additive	Serum separator gel with clot activator
Effect	Gel at the bottom of tube acts to separate cells (lower fraction) and serum (upper fraction); sample should be centrifuged to stabilize
Tests	Routine biochemistry, serology

TABLE 5-8 Lavender-Topped Tube; Also Called "Purple-Topped Tube"

Additive	EDTA (liquid)
Effect	Anticoagulant; removes calcium
Tests	Routine hematology; cross-match. NOTE: Invert eight times to prevent clotting and platelet clumping

---

TABLE 5-9 Dark Green-Topped Tube

Additive	Sodium heparin or lithium heparin
Effect	Anticoagulant; inactivates thrombin and thromboplastin, allowing isolation of plasma; sample must be centrifuged to isolate plasma
Tests	Ammonia, lactate, and other tests requiring plasma (see under **Sample** and **Submit** for individual tests listed in this section)

TABLE 5-10 Light Blue-Topped Tube

Additive	Sodium citrate
Effect	Anticoagulant; removes calcium; NOTE: EDTA anticoagulated samples do NOT substitute for samples requiring citrated plasma
Tests	Most coagulation profiles; NOTE: Tube must be filled to the capacity allowed by the vacuum

5

TABLE 5 - 1 1   Dark Blue-Topped Tube

Additive	Sodium heparin or Na EDTA
Effect	Anticoagulant; tube is designed to contain no contaminating metals
Tests	Toxicology and trace element testing (e.g., zinc, copper, lead, mercury) and certain drug level testing (consult with laboratory prior to submitting)

TABLE 5 - 1 2   Gray-Topped Tube

Additive	Sodium fluoride and potassium oxalate
Effect	Antiglycolytic agent that serves to preserve glucose for up to 5 days
Tests	Glucose and 12- hour glucose curves; NOTE: Inadequate volume may result in sample hemolysis

TABLE 5 - 1 3   Yellow-Topped Tube

Additive	Acid-Citrate-Dextrose (ACD)
Effect	Inactivates complement
Tests	DNA testing

TABLE 5 - 1 4   Brown-Topped Tube

Additive	Sodium heparin
Effect	Inactivates thrombin and thromboplastin
Tests	Lead determination (consult with individual laboratory regarding alternative handling)

TABLE 5 - 1 5   Interpretation of the In-Office (or Point-of-Care) Coagulation Screen

Platelet (estimate)	Low	Thrombocytopenia
ACT	Rapid, prolonged	Intrinsic or common clotting pathway defect
APTT	Rapid, prolonged	Intrinsic or common clotting pathway defect
BMBT	Prolonged	Thrombocytopenia, thrombocytopathia

5

SAMPLE STORAGE AND TRANSPORT

Several types of sample collection/sample submission storage tubes are available. It is critical that the type of blood collection and/or storage tube used meets the requirements of the test as defined by the laboratory.

To prepare a sample for storage and transport:

1. Stabilize serum from serum separator tubes (SSTs) by centrifuging the specimen before submission. If being mailed, it is preferable to transfer the separated serum to a labeled plain red-topped tube (RTT).

> **Note:** Depending on the test requested, the tube used to *COLLECT* the sample is frequently *NOT* the same tube used to *SUBMIT* the sample. Sample collection and sample submission requirements are provided for ALL tests listed in this section.

2. Centrifuge the blood samples in a plain RTT and transfer the serum to another RTT.
3. Refrigerate and transport all blood specimens, cytology fluids, tissues, viral cultures, and urines for urinalysis or culture with ice packs.
4. Keep all routine microbial cultures (except urine) and blood cultures at room temperature.
5. If a specimen must remain frozen for transport, dry ice is required. It is usually the responsibility of the individual practice to package frozen samples correctly. Most laboratories do not provide dry ice for shipping.

PATIENT PREPARATION

Fasting the patient for 8-12 hours (an overnight fast with free access to water) is often helpful to reduce the likelihood of lipemia, which may interfere with several tests by falsely increasing or decreasing the results. When applicable, comments about the presence and influence of lipemia and/or hemolysis should appear on the laboratory reports. For special tests, patient preparation may include restriction of food *as well as* water and certain drugs. It is important to follow the guidance provided in this section regarding patient preparation or to contact the laboratory for specific instructions.

MINIMIZING HEMOLYSIS

Hemolysis during blood drawing can be minimized by adhering to the following recommendations.

Procure a nonlipemic (fasted) sample, because lipemia can increase red cell fragility. During phlebotomy, negative pressure created by the vacuum tube or syringe may collapse the lumen of the vein against the needle, thereby crushing numerous red cells. The flutter of the lumen against the needle can be stopped by reducing the negative pressure exerted during collection and by repositioning the needle with slight rotation or deeper insertion.

Excessive negative pressure exerted as the blood enters the vacuum tube or syringe can create hemolysis. This occurs during a slow or difficult collection, because the natural tendency is to use more negative force to enhance blood flow. More patience and "milking" the vein by alternating gentle negative pressure with a short release of all pressure usually solves the problem.

Hemolysis often occurs during the transfer of blood from a syringe into vacuum or other tubes. If a small-gauge needle is used, transfer of blood to specimen tubes is slowed, especially if small clots are present. Forcing the blood through a small-bore needle contributes to hemolysis. This problem can be avoided by removing the needle and top of the specimen tube, and transferring the blood directly into the open tube. Recapping the tube and aspirating a small amount of air to reestablish negative pressure helps to avoid having caps coming off in transit.

AVOIDING CLOTS AND PLATELET CLUMPS

The presence of clots and clumped platelets in anticoagulated blood is most commonly caused by a slow blood draw and the resulting delay in mixing it with the appropriate anticoagulant. If the venipuncture was traumatic, tissue fluid (thromboplastin), activated clotting factors, and hemolysis will quickly promote clot formation. The slight transfer delay when using a syringe for collection can also contribute to this problem. To avoid the formation of clots:

1. Select a vein with good blood flow—the larger the better.
2. Minimize the trauma of venipuncture.
3. Collect blood directly into anticoagulated vacuum tubes (e.g., blue-topped tube [citrated] or lavender-topped tube [EDTA]).
4. Mix the tube well by inverting several times *immediately* after filling.

If the syringe method is selected and a difficult draw is anticipated, the potential for clotting can be minimized by first rinsing the needle and syringe with a small quantity of liquid citrate (blue-topped tube) or EDTA (lavender-topped tube). However, the anticoagulant must be emptied from the syringe before proceeding, and care must be taken to match the anticoagulant chosen with the tests to be performed. Even trace amounts of heparin or EDTA will invalidate coagulation testing, whereas EDTA or citrate will alter the accuracy of several chemistry assays. A small amount of heparin contamination is acceptable in most chemistry assays and complete blood count parameters.

Platelet clumping in samples from cats is very common and is caused by contact aggregation. An effective method to prevent this clumping has not been found. Applying fresh blood directly to the slide from the syringe and making the blood smear immediately after collection is an effective method of assessing platelet numbers in cats.

SUBMISSION REQUIREMENTS FOR RABIES SUSPECTS

Guidelines for submitting tissue from dead dogs or cats for rabies diagnostic testing vary somewhat from state to state. It is always important to contact your State Veterinary Diagnostic Laboratory or Dept of Public Health *prior to shipping any* samples. Most public health authorities require advance notification about impending submission of samples for rabies testing. Veterinarians should verify the address, paper work requirements and shipping requirements prior to submitting any samples for rabies testing.

Note: CAUTION: Care must be taken during sample preparation to avoid direct personal contact with specimens. Pre-exposure rabies vaccination is recommended for persons preparing rabies specimens.

SAMPLE SUBMISSION FOR RABIES TESTING

1. Laboratories may limit acceptance of tissue from dead animals for rabies testing to those for which there is a documented reason for considering that animal a **rabies-suspect mammal.** Generally this includes animals for which there has been a **reported bite, scratch, or other possible saliva or nervous tissue exposure to a human.**
2. Most laboratories will accept any bat as long as there is reasonable likelihood that a human was exposed.
3. Brain tissue from a rabies-suspect mammal reported to have bitten (or otherwise had "intimate" contact with) a domestic animal will likely be acceptable (e.g., brain tissue from a stray dog or cat that bit a pet dog or cat).
4. **Highly suspect surveillance specimens** (with no reported contacts) include
   a. A rabies vector species (e.g., skunk or raccoon) showing clear signs of rabies infection
   b. A mammal **not commonly recognized as a rabies vector, but showing clear signs of rabies infection**
   c. A domestic animal that dies or is euthanized under the care of a veterinarian for which rabies is **part of the differential diagnosis of a neurologic disorder.**
5. Most laboratories will not accept live animals as rabies suspects. The intact head only of authorized specimens will be accepted. Exceptions include bats, which should be

submitted whole, and livestock, for which a cross-section of the brainstem and representative sections of brain (as defined by the laboratory) may be removed by a veterinarian and submitted. Special livestock instructions may apply.

PACKAGING REQUIREMENTS FOR AUTHORIZED SAMPLES

In the case of a suspect dog or cat, the entire brain must be properly packaged in a standard rabies shipping container (these are often provided at County Health Departments). Specimens must be accompanied by a completed **rabies specimen history form.** Forms can often be downloaded from a website designated by the State Public Health authorities or the diagnostic laboratory.

INFORMATION REQUESTED ON THE RABIES SPECIMEN HISTORY FORM

1. Name and address of veterinarian submitting the specimen.
2. Name and address of owner (if known).
3. Indicate whether or not human exposure occurred and the type of exposure (e.g., bite, scratch). Also note whether exposure to a rabid animal is known or highly suspect.
4. Specimen:
   a. Type of specimen.
   b. Age/breed/gender/pet versus stray versus wildlife.
   c. Cause of death (euthanasia, killed, natural causes).
   d. Medical history of the animal (if known), including date of last rabies inoculation.
   e. Health status of the animal at the time of death.
5. Location: describe the geographic location (exact address) of the animal when the specimen was collected.

SUBMISSION GUIDELINES

1. Diagnostic testing of the specimen is generally performed by a designated laboratory within the state. Prior authorization to submit a rabies-suspect specimen is generally required; it is always recommended.
2. If the submission is an emergency, or made over a weekend/holiday, most laboratories will provide specific instructions to accommodate a veterinarian's request.
3. Do not submit live animals.
4. If the suspect animal is alive, it should be humanely euthanized without damaging the head. The head must then be removed from the body and submitted intact for examination. Brain tissue that is damaged may not be accepted by the laboratory. Dead suspect bats can usually be submitted with the head intact.
5. Specimens must be preserved by refrigeration. Freezing should be avoided. Only if refrigeration is not available can the tissue be submitted frozen.
6. Tissues must not be fixed with chemical preservatives.
7. Tools, cages, and other surfaces potentially contaminated with infectious saliva or blood can be disinfected with a solution of sodium hypochlorite (1 part household bleach to 10 parts water) in water.
8. Properly packaged specimens may be shipped directly to the rabies laboratory (verify correct address) by parcel post or commercial mail carrier. Special arrangements are likely to be required for samples arriving over weekends or holidays.

PACKING AND SHIPPING DIRECTIONS

An acceptable rabies suspect shipping set may include any of the following:
1. One pre-assembled shipping container, including outer cardboard box, insulated cooler, and two gallon-sized cans with lid-locking plastic seal. Packing instructions for package are printed on top inner flaps.

5

2. Two gel packs of refrigerant (store the pack—*not the specimen*—frozen until needed).
3. Two plastic bags (13 × 20 inches × 4 mil) in which the animal head, brain of livestock or other large animal, or intact bat is to be sealed before placing in can.
4. Two plastic bags (13 × 20 inches × 4 mil) in which to place the cans.
5. One large plastic bag that surrounds the closed insulated cooler.
6. Two absorbent pads to be placed in the cans, surrounding the specimen.
7. Two blank rabies history forms and directions for collection and submission of specimens.

To prepare the specimen for shipping:
1. Remove the head from the body of the animal (except bats) and place the head in a small plastic bag. Cool specimen in a refrigerator or freezer before packaging, to enhance preservation.
2. When shipping samples consisting of only cerebellum and brainstem, first place the brain tissue in a small plastic container, then place the container in the small plastic bag. If sharp objects protrude from the specimen (e.g., bone fragments, porcupine quills) wrap specimen in several layers of newspaper before putting head in the plastic bag. Wrap bagged specimen in provided absorbent material and place inside the metal can.
3. Place the lid on the metal can and secure with a mallet. Place a plastic pressure ring (provided) on the can and secure with a mallet. The plastic ring will be seated more easily if a hard surface is placed on top of the ring before using the mallet. This will allow even pressure to be applied to the ring. **CAUTION! Infectious splashes can occur when hammering the lid in place if the groove is contaminated with blood or body fluids in the specimen.**
4. Wash hands well with soap and water. Disinfect or burn all materials contaminated in specimen preparation.
5. Complete the rabies specimen history form provided with the package. Answer all questions as accurately as possible; the history form will be used to report results to the local health authority. Place form on the outside of the plastic bag that surrounds the EPS cooler. When shipping more than one specimen in the container (e.g., bats), be certain that: **each** specimen is individually bagged to prevent cross contamination; **each** is clearly identified, and a separate history included for **each** specimen.
6. CAUTION: Do not use glass, wire, or other packaging materials capable of causing wounds or injuring skin.

HISTOPATHOLOGY AND CYTOPATHOLOGY

Histopathology and cytopathology are among the most important diagnostic tools available for use in clinical practice. Generally, diagnostic specimens are submitted to a commercial laboratory or university where specially trained technologists can prepare and stain the cells/tissue to be interpreted by a pathologist. One critical limiting factor in obtaining diagnostic cytology or histopathology is the quality of the specimen submitted. *It is the responsibility of the practice to not only obtain, but also prepare, specimens properly before submission and interpretation.* This part of Section 5 describes standards for preparing and submitting specimens for cytologic or histopathologic interpretation. Sample collection techniques are described in Section 4.

HISTOPATHOLOGY

BIOPSY TISSUE

Tissue specimens for histology must be preserved and transported in formalin (10 parts formalin to 1 part tissue). The ideal tissue specimen is less than an inch thick. OSHA and transportation safety regulations limit the size and quantity of formalin containers that can be shipped. It is strongly recommended to use containers supplied by the laboratory or the FAA-approved airline, place the container in a ziplock plastic bag, and then in a second outer bag that contains the requisition. Samples packaged inappropriately may not be picked up by the courier. **CAUTION:** Do not enclose cytology samples in bags containing formalin-fixed tissues because this may alter the cytologic appearance and staining of the cells of interest.

Very Large Specimens

Several (preferably three or more) representative sections of large tissues or organs should be selected, preserved, and transported for histology. The remainder should be placed in a large plastic container of formalin, refrigerated, and retained in case additional samples are needed.

Tissue Orientation and Information

Knowing the orientation and other facts about the tissue mass is critical for the pathologist. A diagram may be included on the requisition form. Borders and areas of interest on the mass can be marked with colored or numbered sutures. State whether the entire mass has been excised, if all is being submitted, or if the tissue had to be divided into sections before submission.

Very Small Specimens

Tiny samples, such as endoscopic biopsy specimens, are best preserved if they are first placed in a labeled tissue cassette holder (usually available from the laboratory) and then dropped into formalin. Small biopsies should not be placed in a container with large tissue, because they are easily lost.

CYTOPATHOLOGY

Used alone, as a diagnostic screening test for underlying disease, or used in conjunction with the surgical biopsy to facilitate rapid assessment of a potentially serious lesion, cytopathology is among the most fundamental and important diagnostic tools used in clinical practice. Cytopathology is not a clinical discipline restricted to the realm of board-certified clinical pathologists. Several continuing education short courses and laboratories on diagnostic cytopathology are offered at major conferences throughout the U.S. In addition, excellent textbooks, with abundant color plates, are available to facilitate cytologic interpretation of specimens collected from dogs and cats.

Cytologic preparations are perhaps most useful for distinguishing details between cell types (e.g., mesenchymal vs. epithelial) and cellular activity (e.g., inflammation vs. neoplasia). Detection of intracellular vs. extracellular organisms can provide immediate clues, without waiting for organisms to be cultured, about the nature of the disease. Noninflammatory lesions can generally be distinguished as benign or neoplastic (Box 5-1).

Although it is the responsibility of the individual clinician to understand personal limitations, there is one special advantage that the clinician does have over the pathologist— familiarity with the patient's health status and the nature of the lesion/disease under consideration. Described here are guidelines for *preparing and submitting* samples for cytologic interpretation (see Section 4 for sample collection techniques). Whether samples are sent to a commercial laboratory or a university, or are interpreted within the practice, the following recommendations are important when preparing a high-quality specimen.

5

Note: The accuracy of interpreting cytopathologic specimens is dependent on four key variables:

- Experience and training of the clinician
- Selection of the appropriate case/lesion
- Cellular quality of the specimen selected
- Techniques used to collect, prepare, and stain the sample

FINE NEEDLE ASPIRATION (FNA)

Indications

FNA Involves the use of a syringe and needle to extract cells from a palpable lesion. Most commonly, FNA is performed on cutaneous and subcutaneous lesions. However, with the increasing use of ultrasound in private practice, it may not be necessary to actually "palpate" a lesion in order to extract diagnostic cytology (e.g., ultrasound-guided hepatic or splenic aspirates). Additional experience and training are essential when attempting to perform ultrasound-guided FNA.

Sample preparation

Because sample size ("harvest") typically is small, the cells collected are discharged directly onto a dry, clean slide and allowed to *rapidly* (within 5 to 10 seconds) air-dry. It is recommended that the needle tip actually contact the slide as the aspirate is discharged *rather* than blowing the sample over the slide. If fluid is inadvertently recovered, the FNA should be reattempted from the peripheral limits of the lesion.

Extremely small harvest of cells can be sprayed directly on the slide, remain untouched, and allowed to air-dry. If the volume recovered allows placement of a formed drop onto the slide, the sample should be spread over the surface of the slide, prior to air-drying, in the same way that a peripheral blood smear is prepared.

Staining options

Once the sample has air-dried (rapidly), use of a quick Romanowsky-type (Wright's) stain is appropriate. Alcohol fixation is *not* recommended if the specimen is to be reviewed/ interpreted immediately. Alternative stains, such as new methylene blue (wet mount), Gram stain, Giemsa stain, or Wright-Giemsa stain, can be used in practice as dictated by cytologic objectives.

FNA specimens mailed to an outside laboratory typically are air-dried and left unstained. Some laboratories recommend that the specimen be immersed in methyl alcohol for a few minutes prior to sending, although this additional step seems to be optional.

Common mistakes

Low cell harvest, high cellular density on the slide (e.g., the result of making a "bad" slide or failing to adequately disperse the sample), and obtaining nondiagnostic material are the three most common mistakes when obtaining samples for diagnostic cytopathology. Contamination of the "wet" (not yet air-dried) sample with water, alcohol, or stain can create artifacts that will compromise the diagnostic value of the specimen. Excessive blood or tissue fluids may profoundly dilute the diagnostic sample, making interpretation difficult or impossible.

EXFOLIATIVE CYTOLOGY ("IMPRESSION SMEAR")

Indications

Exfoliative cytology is made from a clean surface of exposed lesions or from the surface of tissue collected during biopsy. Preparations made from the cut surface of fresh biopsy specimens or post-mortem tissues provide the greatest diagnostic yield.

Sample preparation

To avoid one of the most common mistakes, excessive tissue fluid or blood is absorbed from the cut surface (using a scalpel blade) of the specimen before attempting to exfoliate cells on a slide. Clean, high-quality absorptive paper (such as filter paper) works well, and fragments of paper will not be left on the specimen.

Once excess fluid has been absorbed from the surface, the specimen is gently grasped and allowed to make *gentle* contact with a clean slide. The actual weight of the specimen is usually sufficient; it is usually not necessary to press the specimen onto the slide. After multiple contacts with the slide have been made, the sample is rapidly air-dried.

Staining options

Once the sample has air-dried (rapidly), use of a quick Romanowsky-type (Wright's) stain is appropriate. Alcohol fixation is not recommended if the specimen is to be reviewed/interpreted immediately. Alternative stains, such as new methylene blue and Gram stain (wet mounts), Giemsa stain, or Wright-Giemsa stain, can be used in practice as dictated by cytologic objectives.

Common mistakes

Excessive or rough handling of the specimen before attempting exfoliation will compromise the quality of the specimen. In addition, excessive blood or tissue fluid on the cut surface of the tissue may effectively "dilute" the diagnostic cells in the specimen, making interpretation difficult. When additional pressure is used to exfoliate cells or specimen is rubbed across the slide, individual cells are likely to rupture and smear, rendering the sample nondiagnostic. Failure to obtain adequate numbers of diagnostic cells is more likely to be the consequence of the type of tissue being examined than poor technique. Epithelial tissues (liver/spleen/adenoma/carcinoma) tend to exfoliate abundant numbers of cells when applied to a slide. In contrast, mesenchymal cell tissues (fibrosarcoma/chondrosarcoma) tend *not* to exfoliate well. Diagnostic yield of cells from mesenchymal tissue may be so low as to warrant submission of fixed tissue for histopathologic examination.

SWABS, SCRAPINGS, WASHINGS, OR BRUSHINGS

Indications

A variety of techniques are available to collect cytologic specimens from the upper and lower respiratory tract, conjunctiva, ear canals, and vaginal mucosa. In most cases, cytologic objectives focus on the recovery and identification of infectious organisms (mites, bacteria, etc). Section 4 describes the various techniques of sample collection from these locations.

Sample preparation

Skin scrapings and ear swabs for diagnosis of infectious agents, and occasionally neoplasia, are perhaps the most common samples used in practice to collect diagnostic specimens. Gentle handling of the specimen once collected is the rule when attempting to exfoliate diagnostic cells or organisms. In addition, it may not be necessary to air-dry or apply a stain depending on the samples collected (e.g., skin scrapings or ear swabs for mites).

Samples collected from washings vary considerably in the cell harvest, the consistency of the fluid recovered, and the quality of the diagnostic specimen. In some cases, fluid recovered from washings (e.g., bronchoalveolar lavage, transtracheal aspiration) will require centrifugation to acquire sufficient numbers of diagnostic cells. The supernatant (fluid portion) of the sample is discarded. The cells recovered may be re-suspended in 1 or 2 drops of sterile saline or a volume of saline equal to the volume of specimen remaining in the centrifuge tube. A pipette is used to apply a sample of the fluid to a slide. The sample is distributed over the slide in the same way that a peripheral blood smear is prepared. The slide is air-dried and stained. In other cases, the sample collected from cytologic washings will be highly cellular and may be applied directly to a slide, air-dried, and stained.

Samples collected from brushings normally are obtained with specially made cytology brushes designed for use during endoscopy. Although small "pinch" biopsies are preferred, occasionally the use of a brush may be the only practical option. Cytologic specimens collected by brushing tend to be especially low in yield. Furthermore, the additional manipulation required to extract cells from the brush and onto a slide for examination tends to yield specimens of poorer quality. Cells obtained during brushing may be applied directly to a clean slide, air-dried, and stained. In other cases, it may be preferable to wash the brush in a centrifuge tube containing a small volume (<1.0 mL) of sterile saline. The suspended cells may be applied directly to a slide, distributed, and then air-dried and stained. It may be necessary to centrifuge the sample (as described for washings previously) before preparing the sample.

5

Staining options

Generally, the same staining options previously described apply to specimens collected from washings or brushings. Samples collected from skin scrapings typically are suspended in oil or hydrogen peroxide on the slide and examined "wet" without the use of additional stain. Swabs, especially from ears, may be stained with a quick Romanowsky-type stain or a Gram stain (wet mount) to facilitate identification of organisms.

Common mistakes

Samples collected from skin scrapings and swabs tend to be relatively high in yield when diagnostic cells or organisms are present. Cells collected from washings and brushings are usually collected during endoscopic procedures; the yield of diagnostic cells can vary, depending on the extent of the lesion as well as the skill of the individual performing the procedure.

BODY FLUIDS

Indications

The accumulation of fluid in either the pleural space or the abdomen, or in both, justifies attempts to remove fluid for diagnostic cytology. The volume of sample can be difficult to determine, but ideally would be 2-3 mL of fluid collected by needle and syringe (centesis) under sterile conditions. Smaller samples of joint fluid and CSF are also collected for chemical and cytologic analysis. Any fluid recovered should be examined for color, consistency, total nucleated cell count, and protein concentration as well as for morphology of the cells recovered. Other chemistries (creatinine, amylase, etc.) can be determined depending on the nature of the fluid recovered and the patient's condition.

Sample preparation

Because the volume of fluid obtained may be large and the concentration of cells in the fluid recovered may be low, centrifugation is indicated to concentrate cells in small aliquots of fluid. After centrifugation and removal of the supernatant, cells can be resuspended in 1-2 drops of sterile saline/supernatant. Suspended cells should be distributed directly on a slide, allowed to air-dry, and stained.

Note: It is important not to delay processing of cytologic samples recovered from body fluid. The longer cells are allowed to remain in suspension, the greater is the opportunity for morphologic changes of cells to occur.

Spinal fluid must be processed within 30 minutes of collection because of the fragility of cells in CSF. Furthermore, conventional centrifuges may damage any cells collected. Because of the complexities associated with processing of CSF for cytopathology, most samples are evaluated within specialty or referral hospitals.

Staining options

Air-dried cytologic preparations can be stained in the same manner described previously.

Common mistakes

Attempting to evaluate uncentrifuged cytologic specimens collected from body fluids can result in a low yield of diagnostic cells and may compromise the study. Allowing the cells to remain in the fluid for an extended period of time before making the cytologic preparations may significantly alter the morphology of individual cells, making interpretation difficult or impossible. Furthermore, the presence of peripheral blood in any sample collected from a body cavity must be distinguished from contamination associated with the sampling technique versus a primary bleeding disorder.

Bone Marrow

Indications

Cytologic examination of a bone marrow aspirate is an especially valuable tool in the assessment of patients with persistent anemia, particularly nonregenerative anemia, abnormal numbers (either high or low) of leukocytes, thrombocytopenia, any blood dyscrasia detected in peripheral blood, and any combination of these findings. Bone marrow specimens will yield the most information if *both* a core biopsy and aspirate slides are submitted. The biopsy should be cut first, and the core placed in a tissue-processing cassette, labeled, and dropped into a formalin container. The aspirate needle can then be placed into the same puncture site as the biopsy needle. (Bone marrow biopsy and aspiration collection techniques are described in Section 4.)

Thrombocytopenia is *not* necessarily a contraindication to performing bone marrow aspiration. Assuming normal platelet function, bone marrow aspiration is indicated even when platelet counts are extremely low (e.g., 5000 platelets/mm^3). The author has observed persistent bleeding and large hematoma formation at the site of aspiration in dogs with platelets counts <3000 platelets/mm^3 in peripheral blood.

Sample preparation

In most patients undergoing bone marrow aspiration, sufficient numbers of platelets will be present in the sample to justify routine use of an anticoagulant. *Before* collecting the sample, a few drops of 4% EDTA are placed in the center of a watch glass. The same 12-cc syringe used to draw the EDTA is used to collect the sample. This syringe will contain a small amount of EDTA. Collection of marrow is typically limited to 0.5 mL. Larger volumes may cause hemodilution of the sample, making interpretation difficult. On withdrawing the appropriate volume, the sample is *immediately* added directly to the EDTA and mixed thoroughly. A glass pipette can be used to transfer the aspirated marrow onto a clean, dry slide. Other techniques are described in Section 4. Using the same technique to distribute peripheral blood for a differential count will suffice. The sample is allowed to air-dry.

Staining options

Bone marrow staining routinely entails use of a quick Romanowsky-type stain. Special staining, usually performed by a commercial or university laboratory, may be indicated when looking for the presence of iron stores or specific types of organisms.

Common mistakes

If the bone marrow contains functional platelets, failing to quickly transfer the aspirate into the EDTA can result in clot formation. The presence of clots is likely to entrap diagnostic cells, making interpretation difficult or impossible. Hemodilution and an excessive volume of EDTA are also common mistakes that can compromise the quality of the smears. Other complications usually are caused by errors in the technique of making the slide. For example, failing to adequately distribute the sample across the slide can result in a unusually thick preparation. Bone marrow aspirates taken from the head of the humerus can become contaminated with joint fluid, making the sample completely unusable.

5

BIOCHEMISTRY—ROUTINE

The ability to obtain a comprehensive biochemical profile, and to do so quickly and inexpensively, has become a routine part of the clinical work-up for the companion animal patient. Clearly, the biochemistry profile greatly expands the clinician's ability to assess the patient presenting with a history of clinical illness. Additionally, it is now feasible to obtain a biochemical profile on seemingly healthy patients as part of a routine "wellness examination."

This section discusses those analytes offered by most clinical laboratories performing companion animal (dog and cat) biochemistry profiles. Although specific analytes included on panels vary among laboratories, any individual test not discussed here can probably be found in the following section entitled Special Diagnostic Tests and Test Protocols.

The following criteria are applicable to *all* samples in which blood/serum/plasma is collected for which a routine biochemisty profile or special laboratory test is requested.

ANALYTE OR TEST NAME (SYNONYMS)

The name of the individual chemical analyte being measured (e.g., alkaline phosphatase) is followed in parentheses by common abbreviations used by laboratories when reporting results (e.g., SAP or Alk Phos). In some cases the name of the test is presented rather than the actual chemical being tested for (e.g., ACTH stimulation, in which cortisol is the actual analyte measured).

NORMAL

Representative reference range values for normal adult dogs and cats are listed with each analyte. In addition, Tables 5-1 to 5-6 summarize reference ranges for dogs and cats.

> **Note:**   Reference range values listed throughout this section are for general reference *only*. Test results from individual patients *must be compared with the reference range values of* the laboratory that performs the test.

PATIENT PREPARATION

Any unique patient preparation parameters should be followed *before* collecting the sample. For routine biochemistry profiles, an 8- to 10-hour fasting period is recommended when feasible. When performing routine profiles on normal patients, it is preferable to collect samples in the morning. Owners are instructed to withhold food and water after midnight on the day the blood sample is to be collected.

COLLECT

This section stipulates the type and volume of sample to be collected, as well as the type of collection tube to be used. For routine biochemistry, collecting at least 2.0 mL of whole blood in a red-topped tube (or serum separator tube) is required to obtain the minimum 1.0 mL of serum required for sample analysis. Dehydrated patients have a higher hematocrit, and a larger volume of whole blood may be required to obtain 1.0 mL of serum.

SUBMIT

This section stipulates the type and volume of sample that is to be submitted for analysis. Also, the type of vial/container in which the sample should be shipped is specified. Unless specified in the protocol, do not store or ship samples as whole blood; instead, separate whole blood from serum before shipping unless using an appropriate serum separator tube. Serum samples should be shipped in a sterile red-topped tube. Freezing of the sample is not required for routine biochemistry profiles.

INTERPRETATION

Each analyte and test procedure is described separately.

INTERFERENCE

This section stipulates common interfering substances/factors and indicates, when known, if the interference will falsely elevate or lower test results. Samples that are lipemic, icteric, and/or hemolyzed may cause test interference with individual analyte assays, resulting in unreliable test results. Interference may be positive (false increased test results) or negative (false decreased test results). The degree and type of interference vary depending on the test methodology used. Most laboratories provide details in final reports pertaining to known or potential interfering factors.

PROTOCOL

If indicated, the protocol stipulates specific test procedures or shipping requirements necessary to obtain the most valid results. For routine biochemistry profiles, other than recommended fasting of the patient, no specific test protocol is indicated. For special laboratory diagnostic tests for which patient preparation is required or a defined protocol is available, a detailed description is provided.

ROUTINE DIAGNOSTIC TESTS

ALANINE AMINOTRANSFERASE (ALT; FORMERLY SGPT)

Normal:
16-73 IU/L (dog); 5-134 IU/L (cat).
Interpretation:
Used in the assessment of liver disease (*not a test of liver function*). Increased values indicate hepatocyte injury and leakage of intracellular enzymes, such as could occur in acute hepatitis, hepatic trauma, neoplasia (occasionally), and cirrhosis. Decreased values may be noted in end-stage liver disease.

ALBUMIN

Normal:
2.8-4.0 g/dL (dog); 3.0-4.2 g/dL (cat).
Interpretation:
Evaluated with total protein and globulin. This test is important in the assessment of hydration status, renal disease, gastrointestinal disease, liver function, and selected chronic infectious diseases. Increased values generally support dehydration; a commensurate increase in globulin and total protein should be expected. Decreased values suggest abnormal loss (gastrointestinal tract or renal) and decreased production (protein-restricted diet, malnutrition, liver disease). Values in healthy young dogs and cats (<3 months of age) are normally lower than those in adult animals.

ALBUMIN/GLOBULIN RATIO (A:G)

Normal:
0.6-2.0 (dog); 0.4-1.5 (cat).
Interpretation:
The A:G should NOT be interpreted without consideration of the concentration (g/dL) of both albumin and globulin. Further characterization of serum proteins can be obtained with serum protein electrophoresis. An increased A:G is considered to be clinically insignificant because it represents either elevated albumin and/or decreased globulin. Alternatively, a decreased A:G indicates either decreased albumin and/or increased globulin and may indicate renal or gastrointestinal loss of albumin, certain neoplasms, or chronic infections.

ALKALINE PHOSPHATASE (SAP OR Alk Phos)

Normal:
15-146 IU/L (dog); 0-96 IU/L (cat).

5

Interpretation:
This test is routinely used to assess obstructive liver and/or biliary tract disease *(not a test of liver function)*. Increased values are normal in young dogs and cats (<3 months of age) (reflecting bone growth). In adults, increased values may indicate biliary obstruction/cholestasis, hepatitis, hepatic lipidopathy, destructive bone lesions (osteosarcoma), hyperphosphatemia, and acute pancreatitis. NOTE: Corticosteroid therapy will induce SAP, causing significant elevations in the absence of cholestasis.

AMYLASE

Normal:
347-1104 IU/L (dog); 489-2100 IU/L (cat).
Interpretation:
Increased value indicates pancreatitis, especially in patients with evidence of vomiting and abdominal pain. Amylase clearance is dependent on normal renal function; patients with compromised renal function (chronic renal failure) are likely to have abnormally elevated amylase not associated with pancreatic disease. Pancreatic lipase immunoreactivity (PLI) may be helpful in assessing pancreatitis in dogs and cats (see under Special Diagnostic Tests and Test Protocols).

ANION GAP

Normal:
16.3-28.6 (dog); 12-24 (cat).
Interpretation:
The anion gap is a laboratory calculation ($Na - [Cl + HCO_3^-]$ = anion gap) used to assess quantities of unmeasured cations (Ca, Mg) and anions (proteins, sulfates, phosphates, and certain organic acids). A high anion gap suggests metabolic acidosis (ketoacidosis, lactic acidosis). Other causes of metabolic acidosis (e.g., renal tubular acidosis) may have a normal anion gap. Hypoalbuminemia is the most common cause of a low anion gap. Other causes include hypernatremia, certain gammopathies (myeloma), and severe hypercalcemia. There are numerous causes for false high and low anion gap results.

ASPARTATE AMINOTRANSFERASE (FORMERLY SGOT)

Although sometimes reported in companion animal laboratory profiles, these values are NOT considered to have clinical significance in either the dog or cat.

BICARBONATE (HCO_3^-)

Normal:
24-26 mEq/L (dog); 22-24 mEq/L (cat).
Interpretation:
Bicarbonate measurement usually is included as a component with of blood gas and/or electrolyte panel. Levels are increased with metabolic alkalosis (and with compensated respiratory acidosis) and decreased with metabolic acidosis (and with compensated respiratory alkalosis).

BILIRUBIN

Normal:
0-0.2 mg/dL (dog); 0.1-0.5 mg/dL (cat).
Interpretation:
Increased value (hyperbilirubinemia) may be associated with icterus or jaundice, reflects accumulation of bilirubin in serum, and may indicate intravascular hemolysis, compromised

bile excretion, biliary tract obstruction (intrahepatic or extrahepatic), and primary hepatic disease affecting bile excretion.

BLOOD UREA NITROGEN (BUN)

Normal:
8-27 mg/dL (dog); 15-35 mg/dL (cat).
Interpretation:
NOTE: abnormally elevated BUN (azotemia) does not define "uremia." Increased BUN indicates decreased renal clearance of nitrogenous waste (dehydration, renal failure, urinary tract obstruction). An elevated BUN is NOT indicative of renal disease unless interpreted in light of other parameters (e.g., urine specific gravity, serum creatinine, history of increased water consumption or increased urination). Decreased BUN indicates increased renal excretion of nitrogenous waste (diuresis) or decreased protein intake (malnutrition, low-protein diet) or decreased production (portosystemic shunt).

CALCIUM (Ca)

Normal:
9.2-11.6 mg/dL (dog); 7.5-11.5 mg/dL (cat).
Interpretation:
WARNING: Levels ≤7 mg/dL dogs and cats may result in tetany; sustained levels >12 mg/dL may cause renal damage subsequent to calcium deposition. Increased levels are associated with primary hyperparathyroidism, pseudohyperparathyroidism (paraneoplastic syndrome associated with neoplasia, especially lymphosarcoma and perianal carcinoma), metastatic bone disease or primary bone tumors, hypervitaminosis D (chronic), hyperthyroidism (in cats), Addison's disease (hypoadrenocorticism), and acromegaly. Hypercalcemia may be idiopathic in some animals. Decreased values are associated with any condition causing low total protein and albumin levels (most serum calcium is albumin-bound). Serum ionized calcium is indicated in assessing any patient with significant, unexplained hyper- or hypocalcemia. Other causes of decreased calcium include conditions causing elevated phosphorus levels (e.g., renal insufficiency, hypoparathyroidism), acute pancreatitis, intravenous fluid administration, renal tubular acidosis. See also Calcium, Ionized (iCa).

CHLORIDE (Cl)

Normal:
104-117 mEq/L (dog); 113-122 mEq/L (cat).
Interpretation:
Increased Cl is associated with dehydration as well as intravenous saline administration. Decreased Cl can be associated with overhydration, Addison's disease (hypoadrenocorticism), burns, metabolic alkalosis, syndrome of inappropriate secretion of ADH, and certain types of diuretic therapy.

5

CHOLESTEROL (CH)

Normal:
138-317 mg/dL (dog); 42-265 mg/dL (cat).
Interpretation:
Increased CH (hypercholesterolemia) is most commonly found in hyperlipidemic patients and reflects extreme elevations of triglyceride rather than a primary underlying metabolic disorder affecting CH metabolism. In dogs, hypercholesterolemia is inconsistently associated with hypothyroidism and hyperadrenocorticism (Cushing's syndrome). Hypercholesterolemia has limited diagnostic significance. Decreased CH (hypocholesterolemia) has not been found to be of diagnostic significance in the dog and cat, but has been observed with hypoadrenocorticism.

CREATINE KINASE (CK; FORMERLY CPK)

Normal:
48-380 IU/L (dog); 72-481 IU/L (cat).
Interpretation:
Increased CK indicates increased skeletal muscle activity or destruction (myopathy or rhabdomyolysis), inflammation or infection (myositis), or widespread muscle trauma. No diagnostic significance has been associated with a decreased CK.

CREATININE (Cr)

Normal:
0.5-1.6 mg/dL (dog); 0.5-2.3 mg/dL (cat).
Interpretation:
Increased Cr is an important indicator of glomerular filtration and occurs with renal insufficiency and urinary tract obstruction; shock, severe dehydration, and untreated congestive heart failure may result in increased Cr due to decreased renal blood flow. Rhabdomyolysis will also cause increased Cr. Pathologic causes of decreased Cr are uncommon but may occur in severe debilitation or disease causing extreme decreases in muscle mass. Cr is less influenced by diet than by BUN.

GAMMA GLUTAMYLTRANSFERASE (GGT; GAMMA GT [GGT])

Normal:
3-8 IU/L (dog); 0-10 IU/L (cat).
Interpretation:
Parameters causing increased and decreased GGT typically parallel alkaline phosphatase (SAP) in the presence of underlying liver pathology, especially cholestasis, but *not* in patients with destructive bone disease. GGT is commonly elevated in cirrhosis and (obstructive) hepatic/biliary tract disease. Extreme elevations of GGT have been associated with metastatic liver disease in humans; a similar association has not been reported in animals.

GLOBULIN

Normal:
2.0-4.1 g/dL (dog); 2.8-5.3 g/dL (cat).
Interpretation:
Globulin is a component of total protein that must be interpreted with albumin. Increased value (hyperglobulinemia) may reflect dehydration (albumin and total protein also increased), chronic inflammation, chronic infection, or myeloid neoplasia (albumin may be abnormally decreased). Serum protein electrophoresis is indicated to characterize the nature of the globulin increase. Decreased value (hypoglobulinemia) typically indicates decreased protein intake (low protein diet or malnutrition) or decreased globulin production (neoplasia).

GLUCOSE

Normal:
73-116 mg/dL (dog); 63-150 mg/dL (cat).
Interpretation:
Increased value (hyperglycemia) indicates decreased glucose metabolism (insulin deficiency or diabetes mellitus). NOTE: normal cats may experience transient "stress hyperglycemia" with values as high as 350 mg/dL (typically, glycosuria is absent). Decreased value (hypoglycemia) indicates excessive utilization of glucose (insulin secreting tumor) or severe illness (sepsis).

LIPASE

Normal:
22-216 IU/L (dog); 0-222 IU/L (cat).
Interpretation:
Increased lipase is most commonly associated with acute pancreatitis. Certain neoplasms have been reported to cause extreme elevations of lipase in the absence of pancreatic disease. There is no clinical significance associated with decreased lipase.

PHOSPHORUS (P)

Normal:
2.0-6.7 mg/dL (dog); 2.7-7.6 mg/dL (cat).
Interpretation:
Increased P is normally present in young, growing dogs and cats (associated with increase SAP activity). Abnormal elevations are most likely to occur in patients with chronic renal failure or hypoparathyroidism. Improper sample handling (hemolysis) can cause elevations in P. Decreased P is expected in patients with primary hyperparathyroidism (with increased calcium), renal tubular acidosis and Fanconi syndrome. Several systemic illnesses may be associated with decreased P. WARNING: Values ≤1 mg/dL may be associated with neuromuscular abnormalities and cardiac arrhythmia.

POTASSIUM (K⁺)

Normal:
3.9-5.2 mEq/L (dog); 3.3-5.7 mEq/L (cat).
Interpretation:
Increased value (hyperkalemia) may indicate mineralocorticoid deficiency (Addison's disease or hypoadrenocorticism) but must be interpreted with serum sodium and an ACTH stimulation test. Numerous causes of decreased potassium are recognized. GI and renal losses are the most common and most significant. Persistent hypokalemia warrants significant efforts to determine the underlying cause(s).
WARNING: Potassium levels >7.5 mEq/L may cause cardiac arrhythmias (profound bradycardia) and death. Potassium levels <2.5 mEq/L may cause profound weakness.

SODIUM (Na⁺)

Normal:
147-154 mEq/L (dog); 147-165 mEq/L (cat).
Interpretation:
Increased value (hypernatremia) may result from excess dietary consumption or severe dehydration. Decreased value (hyponatremia) may indicate mineralocorticoid deficiency (Addison's disease or hypoadrenocorticism) but must be interpreted in light of other tests (e.g., serum osmolality, potassium, ACTH stimulation test). Persistent diuresis caused by drugs (furosemide) or an inherent medical disorder (nephrotic syndrome) can deplete serum sodium to significantly low levels. Depending on the laboratory methodology, pseudohyponatremia may occur in patients with profoundly lipemic serum.

TOTAL PROTEIN (TP)

Normal:
5.5-7.2 g/dL (dog); 5.4-8.9 g/dL (cat).
Interpretation:
TP must be evaluated with constituent proteins albumin and globulin. Increased TP (hyperproteinemia) may indicate dehydration (elevated albumin and globulin) or extreme

5

elevations in globulin (chronic inflammation, infection, neoplasia, especially myeloma). Decreased TP may indicate increased protein loss (especially albumin), chronic malassimilation/maldigestion, starvation, or chronic illnesses (tumor cachexia).

TRIGLYCERIDE (TG)

Normal:
19-133 mg/dL (dog); 24-206 mg/dL (cat).
Interpretation:
Increased TG is normally increased in any animal during the postprandial state (with 6 hours following a meal). TG is the cause of gross lipemia when concentrations exceed ~500 mg/dL. Increased TG (in the fasted patient) is associated with familial hypertriglyceridemia, a condition most often reported in Miniature Schnauzers (other breeds and mixed breeds may be affected) born in the U.S. (the condition has not been described in Miniature Schnauzers in Europe or the United Kingdom) and certain lines of mixed-breed cats. There is no clinical significance associated with decreased TG in either the dog or cat.

SPECIAL DIAGNOSTIC TESTS AND TEST PROTOCOLS

This section includes advanced biochemical laboratory tests not typically included in routine companion animal medicine laboratory profiles. These tests are selected on the basis of abnormal findings revealed during routine physical examination and laboratory profiling. Additional special laboratory tests and test procedures can be found in the organ system-specific sections that follow (see Chapter Outline).

Note: Throughout the Special Diagnostic Test section, the following information is provided, where appropriate, for each laboratory test described:

- Test or analyte name (abbreviations or common names)
- Normal (representative reference range value for normal adult dogs and cats)
- Patient preparation (includes any special requirements before sample collection)
- Sample (type of sample and recommended minimum volume to be collected)
- Submit (component of sample to submit for analysis, store, or mail)
- Interpretation (basic interpretation of test results that are outside the reference range)
- Interference (variables that may falsely elevate or decrease test results)
- Protocol (as applicable, accepted procedures for performing the test are outlined)

5

ACTH STIMULATION TEST: See ENDOCRINOLOGY

ADRENOCORTICOTROPIC HORMONE (ACTH) ENDOGENOUS: See ENDOCRINOLOGY

ALDOSTERONE: See ENDOCRINOLOGY

AMMONIA (NH$_3$) (FASTING AMMONIA)

Normal:
45-120 µg/dL (dog); 30-100 µg/dL (cat).
Patient Preparation:
Overnight fast.
Collect:
Whole blood, 2.0 mL minimum, in EDTA (purple-topped tube) or in heparin.
Submit:
Plasma, 1.0 mL minimum.

Interpretation:
Decreased levels of ammonia are not considered clinically significant. Elevated ammonia levels support the diagnosis of underlying, significant liver disease. This test generally is considered a liver function test and usually is performed to support a diagnosis of hepatic encephalopathy. Fasting ammonia and ammonia tolerance tests are *uncommonly performed today* because of sample instability and specimen handling requirements. These tests have largely been replaced by pre– and post–bile acid assay.

Interference:
Hemolysis; elevated BUN; glucose values >600 mg/dL. NH_3 is unstable if not frozen at −20° C. LIMITING FACTORS: ideally, blood should be collected in a sealed, cold *glass* collection tube, centrifuged immediately, and plasma analyzed within 20 minutes of collection. Alternatively, plasma can be stored for up to 48 hours if frozen immediately after collection and kept frozen until time of analysis.

AMMONIA TOLERANCE TEST

Normal Resting Values:
45-120 μg/dL (dog); 30-100 μg/dL (cat).
NOTE: Minimal change should be detected following oral challenge because clearance is nearly 100% following a single pass through the liver.

Patient Preparation:
Overnight fast.

Collect:
Whole blood, 2.0 mL minimum, in EDTA (purple-topped tube) or in heparin.

Submit:
Plasma, 1.0 mL minimum, for each pre- and post challenge sample.

Interpretation:
Elevated ammonia levels support the diagnosis of underlying, significant liver disease. This generally is considered a liver function test and is usually performed to support a diagnosis of hepatic encephalopathy. Fasting ammonia and ammonia tolerance tests are *uncommonly performed today* because of sample instability and specimen handling requirements. These tests have largely been replaced by pre– and post–bile acid assay.

Interference:
Hemolysis; elevated BUN; glucose values >600 mg/dL. NH_3 is unstable if not frozen at −20° C. LIMITING FACTORS: Ideally, blood should be collected in a sealed, cold *glass* collection tube, centrifuged immediately, and plasma analyzed within 20 minutes of collection. Alternatively, plasma can be stored for up to 48 hours if frozen immediately after collection and kept frozen until time of analysis.

Protocol:
Two plasma samples are required. The first is a baseline sample. The second sample is collected 30 to 45 minutes following administration of ammonium chloride (NH_4Cl) at 100 mg/kg body weight as an oral 5% solution in approximately 20-50 mL of saline. NH_4Cl is also available as a powder that can be administered orally, at the same dose, which lowers the risk of vomiting/aspiration.

5

ANTINUCLEAR ANTIBODY (ANA): SEE IMMUNOLOGY

BILE ACIDS

Normal (dog and cat):
Pre-feeding, ≤7 μmol/L; Post-feeding, ≤15 μmol/L.

Patient Preparation:
12-hour or overnight fast before collecting the pre-feeding sample.

Collect:
Whole blood, 2.0 mL minimum, in red-topped tube for each sample collected.

Submit:
Serum, 1.0 mL minimum, for each sample submitted.

Interpretation:
Bile acids are indicated for the assessment of hepatobiliary disease in *non-icteric* patients. There is no value in performing this test in patients that are icteric. Hepatobiliary disease (e.g., portosystemic shunt) is supported with *either* a pre-feeding sample >7 μmol/L or a post-feeding sample >15 μmol/L. NOTE: Reference range values may vary among different laboratories.

Interference:
Lipemia; icterus; hemolysis. Results in patients that vomit the meal prior to collecting the 2-hour post-feeding sample cannot be expected to be reliable. Individual variations in gastric emptying and absorption can result in discordant results (e.g., the pre-feeding sample is higher than the post-feeding sample). Such results are not reliable and the test should be repeated.

Protocol:
1. The pre-feeding (or fasting) blood sample is collected following a 12-hour fast. Label the tube accordingly.
2. Feed a relatively high-fat meal (to stimulate gallbladder contraction). A protein-restricted diet with corn oil added is appropriate for those patients with protein intolerance and signs of hepatic encephalopathy.
3. Two hours following consumption of the meal, collect the post-feeding sample. Label the tube accordingly.

BLOOD GASES (ARTERIAL AND VENOUS)

NOTE: values represented below are expected from patients breathing room air.

Normal:

Value	Arterial		Venous	
	Dog	**Cat**	**Dog**	**Cat**
pH	7.36-7.44	7.36-7.44	7.34-7.46	7.33-7.41
P_{CO_2}	36-44	28-32	32-49	34-38
P_{O_2}	90-100	90-100	24-48	35-45
T_{CO_2}	25-27	21-23	21-31	27-31
HCO_3^-	24-26	20-22	20-29	22-24

Patient Preparation:
Patients breathing 100% oxygen at the time of sample collection are expected to have different results than those of patients that are breathing room air during sample collection. Note the conditions under which the sample was collected.

Collect:
Whole blood, either arterial or venous, depending on the assessment required.

Submit:
Sample cannot be stored. Immediate testing is required to obtain reliable results.

Interpretation:
T_{CO_2} is synonymous with HCO_3^- in patients breathing room air. The overall interpretation of venous and/or arterial blood gas results will vary considerably depending on the patient's health status. Several variations in test results are possible. The clinician should consult appropriate references to interpret results of individual patients (see Section 1).

Interference:
The test should be performed immediately on collecting the sample. Delays could cause significant abnormalities in actual results. Exposure of the sample to room air (bubbles within the sample) may cause P_{CO_2} to decrease, whereas pH and P_{O_2} may increase.

BODY FLUIDS (SUBMITTED FOR CHEMISTRY ANALYSIS)

Normal:
Not applicable.

Patient Preparation:
When feasible, the skin over the site selected for centesis should be shaved and surgically prepared prior to attempting sample collection to avoid contamination of either the sample or the body cavity from which the sample is collected.

Collect:
1-2 mL, minimum, by direct centesis of body cavity or fluid-filled compartment.

Submit:
Centrifugation of whole blood contamination is indicated to remove particulate material (e.g., blood cells, cellular debris) when prompt evaluation of specimen is not possible.

Interpretation:
Any biochemical analyte determined in serum or plasma may be assayed in body fluid—e.g., amylase, lipase (pancreatitis), urea nitrogen, creatinine (ruptured bladder), glucose, lactate

Interference:
Interference from blood and blood components, bilirubin, bile, and urine may significantly interfere with test results. Centrifugation of the sample (blood contamination) may be necessary before performing any biochemistry test.

CALCIUM, IONIZED (iCa)

Normal:
1.12-1.42 mmol/L (dog); 1.12-1.42 mmol/L (cat)

Patient Preparation:
None.

Collect:
Whole blood, 2.0 mL.

Submit:
Serum, 1.0 mL.

Interpretation:
Results reflect the concentration of the biologically active, ionized fraction of calcium without the influence of plasma proteins (e.g., albumin).

Interference:
The reported values of iCa can vary with patient's blood pH; iCa decreases as pH increases.

CEREBROSPINAL FLUID (CSF)

Normal:

5

Value	Dog	Cat
WBCs ($\times 10^3$/L)	≤3	≤2
RBCs ($\times 10^6$/L)	≤30	≤30
Protein (mg/dL)	≤33	≤36
Cytology (%)		
Monocytes	87	69-100
Lymphocytes	4	0-27
Neutrophils	3	0-9
Eosinophils	0	0
Macrophages	6	0-3

Patient Preparation:
General anesthesia is required. For a description of the technique for collecting spinal fluid from dogs and cats, see Section 4, Advanced Procedures. Specific training and/or experience is strongly recommended before collecting CSF from the cisterna magna (between the head and C1). Fatalities can result from improper technique.

Collect:
Usually, two 0.5- to 1.0-mL samples are collected in red-topped tube (no additives).

Submit:
Samples collected.

Interpretation:
If one sample contains excessive numbers of neutrophils, the second sample is submitted for culture and sensitivity; treatment recommendations should include use of an antibiotic (preferably intravenous) that will penetrate the blood-brain barrier.

Interference:
Blood contamination is the most common interfering factor. An RBC count greater than $30 \times 10^6/L$ is consistent with peripheral blood contamination. Immediate analysis is recommended. It is not recommended to submit CSF via mail for assessment.

Protocol:
Proper patient preparation and collection technique is critical (see Section 4).

COBALAMIN (VITAMIN B$_{12}$)

Normal:
Results vary considerably among laboratories; consult individual laboratory.

Patient Preparation:
Fasted.

Collect:
Whole blood, 2.0 mL minimum (red-topped tube).

Submit:
Serum, 1.0 mL.

Interpretation:
Test usually is performed with folate and trypsin-like immunoreactivity (TLI). It is used in the assessment of chronic small bowel diarrhea with associated weight loss. Significantly decreased cobalamine supports the need to measure TLI (exocrine insufficiency) and also supports mucosal disease, and may be indicative (in cats) of hepatic disease (hepatic lipidosis).

Interference:
Hemolysis; lipemia.

ETHYLENE GLYCOL*

Normal:
Negative. "Trace" amounts may be detected in normal patients.

Patient Preparation:
None.

Collect:
Urine (within 3-6 hours of ingestion), whole blood, or serum. Collect volume of sample in accordance with manufacturer's directions.

Submit:
Not applicable. Procedure is an in-hospital test kit for emergency use.

Interpretation:
Values >20-50 mg/dL indicate exposure to ethylene glycol. Immediate treatment is indicated. Supporting laboratory documentation of ethylene glycol exposure is based on

---

*Ethylene Glycol Test Kit, PRN Pharmacal Inc., Pensacola, Fla.

results of serum osmolality (increased), demonstration of an osmolar gap, and anion gap (increased). Blood gas analysis may reveal severe metabolic acidosis. In addition, urine examined under polarizing light microscopy may detect calcium oxalate crystals if examined within 3-6 hours post ingestion.

Interference:
Some drugs (pentobarbital and diazepam) will cause false elevations of ethylene glycol in the test kit results but will not induce calcium oxalate crystalluria.

Protocol:
Follow manufacturer's recommendations for use of the test kit.

FECAL FAT, 72-HOUR QUANTITATIVE COLLECTION

NOTE: No one wants to either collect or analyze a pound of feces. Better tests are available. See Trypsin-Like Immunoreactivity (TLI) in this section.

FECAL OCCULT BLOOD

Normal:
Negative for blood (dog and cat).

Patient Preparation:
Discontinue all red meat and orally administered drugs at least 3 days before collecting the sample for analysis (see Interference).

Collect:
Fresh feces.

Submit:
1 g of fresh feces is sufficient. NOTE: Sample may be stored for up to 4 days at 2° to 8° C.

Interpretation:
Guaiac test methodology is used to detect the presence of occult blood. Animals with two positive consecutive test results 48 hours apart are likely to have a primary lesion in the gastrointestinal tract. Benign ulcerative lesion and neoplasia are the two principal rule-outs.

Interference:
Thrombocytopenia; known platelet disorder; recent aspirin administration; corticosteroid therapy (oral or parenteral); oral iron supplementation; diet containing red meat.

FOLATE

Normal:
Results vary considerably among laboratories; consult individual laboratory.

Patient Preparation:
Overnight fast.

Collect:
Whole blood, 4.0 mL (red-topped tube); separate serum from cells immediately.

Submit:
Serum, 2.0 mL.

Interpretation:
Test usually is performed in conjunction with TLI and serum cobalamin (vitamin B_{12}). Decreased levels of folate support the diagnosis of small intestinal mucosal disease. Increased levels of folate support exocrine pancreatic insufficiency and/or small intestinal bacterial overgrowth.

Interference:
Hemolysis; lipemia.

5

FRUCTOSAMINE

Normal:
225-375 μmol/L (dog and cat).
NOTE: consult individual laboratory because test results may vary.
Patient Preparation:
None.
Collect:
Whole blood, 2.0 mL (red-topped tube).
Submit:
Serum, 1.0 mL; sample must be frozen and shipped on cold packs for overnight delivery.
Interpretation:
This is a single-sample test representing mean blood glucose over the last 1 to 3 weeks. Increased fructosamine indicates poor glycemic control (hyperglycemia); declining fructosamine indicates improved or adequate glycemic control. Values >500 μmol/L suggest inadequate glycemic control over the past 1 to 3 weeks. Values less than the lowest reference range value suggest that the patient has sustained significant periods of hypoglycemia over the past 1 to 3 weeks. Values <400 μmol/L *and* clinical signs of polyuria/polydipsia (PU/PD) and polyphagia are suggestive of a Somogyi phenomenon. Fructosamine levels should *not* be used to make specific adjustments in daily insulin therapy.
Interference:
The assay is a colorimetric procedure; therefore, significant hemolysis or icterus could affect results. Hypoproteinemia and/or hypoalbuminemia will cause falsely low values. Hyperlipidemia and azotemia may also alter results similarly.

GLYCOSYLATED HEMOGLOBIN (GLYCATED HEMOGLOBIN; Gly Hb)

Normal:
1.7% to 4.9% (dog and cat).
NOTE: consult individual laboratory because test results may vary.
Patient Preparation:
None.
Collect:
Whole blood, 2.0 mL in EDTA (purple-topped tube).
Submit:
Plasma, 1.0 mL; separate plasma and refrigerate until assayed.
Interpretation:
This is a single-sample test representing mean blood glucose over the lifespan of red blood cells (~3-4 months). This test is used less in veterinary medicine than the fructosamine assay. In dogs, values consistently between 4% and 6% are associated with adequate glycemic control and owner satisfaction.
Interference:
Storage at room temperature and for longer than 7 days will decrease values; patients with a hematocrit (Hct) <35% may have lower than expected values. NOTE: laboratories must use an assay that has been validated for dogs and for cats. Human assays performed on animal plasma may not be valid.

IRON

Normal:
NOTE: Consult individual laboratory because test results may vary.
Patient Preparation:
None.
Collect:
Whole blood, 2.0 mL (red-topped tube).

5

Submit:
Serum, 1.0 mL.
Interpretation:
Results should be interpreted with total iron-binding capacity (TIBC) and ferritin. Decreased values reflect chronic, not acute, blood loss (e.g., hookworms, intestinal ulceration, bleeding from neoplasia). In cases of iron deficiency, expect TIBC to be normal or high, whereas serum ferritin will be low. Patients with anemia associated with chronic inflammatory disease are expected to have normal to low TIBC, whereas serum ferritin will be normal to high.
Interference:
Hemolysis; lipemia.

LACTIC ACID (LACTATE)

Normal:
2-13 mg/dL (0.22-1.44 mmol/L) (dog); results not reported for cats.
Patient Preparation:
Avoid venous stasis when collecting sample. Clean venipuncture and rapid draw of sample is important.
Collect:
Whole blood, 2.0 mL, in lithium heparin plasma or in iodoacetate tubes. Some laboratories will accept samples collected in fluoride tubes.
Submit:
Plasma, which should be rapidly separated from blood. If this is not possible, the sample may be refrigerated immediately at 4° C, but only for 2 hours, at which time the plasma must be separated from blood.
Interpretation:
Resting values >6.0 mmol/L indicate severe acidosis and a poor prognosis. Test is also used to assess metabolic myopathies, especially in Labrador Retrievers.
Interference:
Aspirin, phenobarbital, and epinephrine may alter lactate values. Also, allowing the sample to sit at room temperature will result in increased level of lactate.
Protocol:
To diagnose metabolic myopathy in Labrador Retrievers: two samples are recommended; the first blood sample is collected at rest. A second sample is collected following 10-15 minutes of brisk walking/running.

LEAD, BLOOD

Normal:
Results vary considerably among laboratories; consult individual laboratory. Usually, values <0.05 ppm in whole blood (or <3 ppm in liver or kidney) are within the range of normal.
Patient Preparation:
None.
Collect:
Whole blood, 2.0 mL, in EDTA (lavender-topped tube) or heparin.
Submit:
Entire sample.
Interpretation:
Refer to the individual laboratory for specific interpretation of the values reported. Values >0.3 ppm suggest exposure. Values >0.4 ppm are generally considered diagnostic of toxicosis.
Interference:
Incorrect tube used for collection/storage of whole blood.

5

LIPOPROTEIN ELECTROPHORESIS

Normal:
Normal values have not been established for the dog and cat.
Patient preparation:
12-hour fast.
Collect:
Whole blood, 1.0 mL (red-topped tube).
Submit:
Serum, 0.5 mL.
Interpretation:
Test consists of electrophoretic separation of various lipoprotein categories in serum. It may qualitatively identify various categories of lipoproteins, including chylomicrons, very-low-density lipoproteins (VLDLs), low-density lipoproteins (LDLs), and high-density lipoproteins (HDLs). Standards have not been established for the dog or cat.
Interference:
Lipemia is not an interfering factor because electrophoresis will separate various lipid fractions.

MAGNESIUM (Mg)

Normal:
1.5-2.5 mg/dL (dog and cat).
Patient Preparation:
None.
Collect:
Whole blood, 2.0 mL, in red-topped tube.
Submit:
Serum, 1.0 mL.
Interpretation:
Increased Mg may reflect renal failure or insufficiency. Decreased Mg is observed in many gastrointestinal disorders (malabsorption, pancreatitis, chronic diarrhea), renal disease (glomerulonephritis, diuresis, tubular necrosis), and multiple endocrine diseases, as well as with sepsis, blood transfusion, and parenteral nutrition.
Interference:
Mg-containing drugs (oral antacids and laxatives) will falsely elevate test results. Some intravenous fluids contain Mg, which also may falsely elevate test results. Falsely decreased values may result from diuretic therapy or intravenous fluid therapy–induced diuresis.

OSMOLALITY, ESTIMATED (SERUM)

Normal:
290-310 mOsm/kg (dog); 308-335 mOsm//kg (cat).
Patient Preparation:
None.
Collect:
Whole venous blood, 2.0 mL, in a red-topped tube or serum separator tube.
Submit:
Serum, 1.0 mL.
Interpretation:
Osmolality of extracellular fluid (ECF) is determined predominantly by electrolytes, especially sodium, and small molecules (glucose and urea) and is reflective of fluid shifts between the vascular space and the interstitium. Increased ECF osmolality (>350 mOsm/L), or hyperosmolality, is likely to be associated with clinical signs (especially neurologic) because of the shift of water from the interstitial space into the vascular space.

NOTE: Direct laboratory measurement of serum osmolality can be performed but is expensive. Serum osmolality is usually calculated according to the following formula:

$$mOsm/kg = 1.86 \ (Na^+ + K^+) + (glucose \div 18) + (BUN \div 2.8) + 9$$

PANCREATIC LIPASE IMMUNOREACTIVITY (PLI)

Normal:
2.2-102.1 µg/L (dog); 2.0-6.8 µg/L (cat)
Patient Preparation:
Fasted for 12 hours before collecting blood.
Collect:
Whole blood, 3.0 mL minimum in red-topped tube or serum separator tube.
Submit:
Serum,1.0 mL minimum. *Immediately* separate serum from clot. Ship serum only. Do not ship whole blood.
Interpretation:
NOTE: PLI is species-specific; samples must be labeled "DOG" (cPLI) or "CAT" (fPLI).
Interference:
Anticoagulant, hemolysis; moderate or greater lipemia.
Protocol:
Serum should be separated *immediately* following clot formation and retraction.

PROTEIN ELECTOPHORESIS (SERUM)

Normal:

Value	Dog	Cat
Total protein (g/dL)	6.0-7.6	7.3-7.8
Albumin (g/dL)	2.7-3.7	2.8-4.2
α1-Globulin (g/dL)	0.25-0.60	0.3-0.65
α2-Globulin (g/dL)	0.72-1.40	0.40-0.68
β1-Globulin (g/dL)	0.63-0.89	0.77-1.25
β2-Globulin (g/dL)	0.60-1.0	0.35-0.50
γ1-Globulin (g/dL)	0.50-0.83	1.39-2.22
A:G ratio	0.8-1.0	0.63-1.15

Patient Preparation:
Fasted for 12 hours (overnight) to prevent postprandial lipemia.
Collect:
Whole blood, 2.0 mL (red-topped tube).
Submit:
Serum, 1.0 mL (most laboratories will accept a volume of serum from 0.5 to 1.0 mL).
Interpretation:
Multiple interpretations are possible, depending on the patient's condition. Test usually is performed to assess degree of loss of albumin or increases in one or more globulin fractions (e.g., hypergammaglobulinemia associated with FIP, canine ehrlichiosis, multiple myeloma). The test is NOT used to confirm a diagnosis.
NOTE: Most clinical assessments are made from the shape of the curve in a densitometer tracing of the electrophoresis rather than specific numbers. When requesting serum protein electrophoresis, it is important to request a copy of the curve as well as the quantitated results for each protein fraction.
Interference:
Lipemia; hemolysis.

5

TRYPSIN-LIKE IMMUNOREACTIVITY, CANINE (CANINE TLI)

Normal:
5.0-35.0 µg/L.
Patient Preparation:
Fasted.
Collect:
Whole blood, 2.0 mL in red-topped tube.
Submit:
Serum, 1.0 mL. Separate serum from clot. Ship serum only. Do not ship whole blood.
Interpretation:
NOTE: TLI is species-specific; samples must be labeled "DOG". It is a sensitive and specific test for the diagnosis of exocrine pancreatic insufficiency in dogs and cats. Values <2.5 µg/L, in the presence of clinical signs, support the diagnosis. Values >50 µg/L have been used to diagnose pancreatitis in dogs. However, TLI has been replaced by the canine pancreatic lipase immunoreactivity (cPLI) assay to diagnose pancreatitis in dogs.
Interference:
Hemolysis; moderate or greater lipemia.

TRYPSIN-LIKE IMMUNOREACTIVITY, FELINE (FELINE TLI)

Normal:
12-82 µg/L.
Patient Preparation:
Fasted.
Collect:
Whole blood, 2.0 mL (red-topped tube).
Submit:
Serum, 1.0 mL. Separate serum from clot. Ship serum only. Do not ship whole blood.
Interpretation:
NOTE: TLI is species-specific; samples must be labeled "CAT". This is a sensitive and specific test for the diagnosis of exocrine pancreatic insufficiency in dogs and cats. Values <2.5 µg/L in the presence of clinical signs supports the diagnosis. Values >100 µg/L have been used to diagnose pancreatitis in cats. However, TLI has been replaced by the feline pancreatic lipase immunoreactivity (fPLI) assay to diagnose pancreatitis in cats.
Interference:
Hemolysis; moderate or greater lipemia.

Note: Serum for PLI and TLI assays may be submitted to the Gastrointestinal Laboratory Department of Small Animal Medicine and Surgery, Texas A & M University, 4474 TAMU, College Station, Texas, 77843-4474.

5

HEMOSTASIS AND COAGULATION

Tests of hemostasis are directed at determining platelet numbers and function, activation and abnormalities of the intrinsic and extrinsic clotting cascade, and quantitation of breakdown products of thrombosis and fibrinolysis. Obtain blood samples for evaluation of coagulation abnormalities by careful venipuncture, and insert samples into plastic or silicone-coated glass syringes.

Because tissue thromboplastin can activate the clotting cascade, some authors advocate using two syringes and two needles to obtain blood for coagulation tests. First, carefully insert the needle into the vein and withdraw 1 mL of blood. Leave the needle in the vessel, and remove the first syringe. Attach a second syringe and obtain the appropriate volume of blood; then remove the needle from the vessel. Rapidly replace the needle on the second syringe with a fresh needle and then inject the blood sample into the appropriate tubes for later analyses.

Platelet tests should be performed on fresh samples within 2 hours of collection. Plasma samples can be spun down and frozen at −20°C for several days, and at −40° C for several months to a year for later analyses.

INITIAL IN-OFFICE SCREENING TESTS

The initial in-office screening tests for coagulation defects include a hematocrit (Hct), peripheral blood smear, activated coagulation test (ACT) or activated partial thromboplastin time (APTT), prothrombin time (PT), and, if indicated, buccal mucosal bleeding time assay.

HEMATOCRIT

The patient's hematocrit and total protein should be evaluated to determine whether anemia is present. The color of the plasma in the spun-down microhematocrit tube can aid in making a diagnosis if intravascular hemolysis (red) or icterus (yellow) is present. The buffy coat from a microhematocrit tube can be evaluated microscopically for the presence of microfilaria in heartworm disease or mast cells in systemic mastocytosis.

PERIPHERAL BLOOD SMEAR

The peripheral blood smear should be evaluated for RBC morphology, RBC fragments (schizocytes), platelet count, large platelets, WBC count and morphology, and blood parasites.

PLATELET COUNT

One of the most simple cage-side tests when determining the cause of a coagulopathy is the platelet count. To perform this test:
1. Obtain an anticoagulated (trisodium citrate or sodium oxalate are the anticoagulants of choice for platelet and coagulation testing) sample of peripheral blood, and make a stained blood smear.
2. Scan the slide, including the peripheral edge, for platelets and platelet clumps. If platelet clumps are present, the platelet estimate cannot be accurately measured; also, it is unlikely that thrombocytopenia is the cause of the patient's hemorrhage.
3. If no platelet clumps are present in the feathered edge of the blood smear, scan multiple areas of the slide on 100× (oil) magnification. Count the number of platelets per high-power field (hpf) and then multiply the value by 15,000 to give an approximate estimation of platelet number.

Hemorrhage secondary to thrombocytopenia occurs when platelet numbers decrease to <40,000/uL (<2-3 platelets/hpf). If there are signs of superficial hemorrhage and more than 4-5 platelets/hpf, a thrombocytopathia (platelet function problem) such as von Willebrand's disease, DIC, or aspirin-induced coagulopathy may be present.

ACTIVATED COAGULATION (CLOTTING) TIME (ACT)

The ACT measures the function of the intrinsic and common coagulation pathway (factors II, V, VIII, IX, X, XI, and XII). The ACT can be used reliably to screen for disorders of secondary hemostasis. Severe thrombocytopenia (<10,000-20,000 platelets/µL) and decreased fibrinogen, in addition to decreases in activated clotting factors listed previously, can cause prolongation in the ACT. An ACT tube contains diatomaceous earth that stimulates blood clotting on contact.
To perform the ACT:
1. Warm the ACT tube to 37° C in a heating block or water bath.
2. Use a 3-mL syringe without any anticoagulant to obtain 3.0 mL of blood. The venipuncture should be atraumatic. Because tissue factor stimulates the clotting cascade, quickly change the needle and push 2.0 mL of the blood sample into the ACT tube, inverting the tube several times to mix the contents, and then place the tube in

5

the water bath or heat source. Start counting the time at the moment you inject the blood into the tube. (The remaining blood can be used to fill microhematocrit tubes and make peripheral blood smears.)
3. To check the tube for clots, quickly invert the tube and then return it to the heat source at 60 seconds and then every 5 seconds thereafter. Record the time that the first signs of a clot (gel) is observed.
   Normal ACT time is 90-120 seconds for dogs, and 80-100 seconds for cats.
Activated partial thromboplastin time (APTT) is another, more sensitive test to detect defects in the intrinsic clotting cascade. It is more sensitive than the ACT in that it will become prolonged earlier than the ACT. Point-of-care coagulation analyzers (SCA-2000, Symbiotics, Inc., San Diego) are available that require less blood than an ACT, and thus may be the preferred test.

PROTHROMBIN TIME (PT)

PT is a test to determine abnormalities in the extrinsic (factor VII) coagulation pathway. Because factor VII is the most labile clotting factor and has the shortest half-life, PT will become prolonged before any changes in ACT or APTT (intrinsic pathway). The prothrombin-complex clotting factors are II, VII, and X; these factors interact with factor V and fibrinogen in the presence of tissue thromboplastin and calcium chloride.

BUCCAL MUCOSAL BLEEDING TIME (BMBT)

The BMBT measures the time required for platelets to become activated and interact with damaged vascular endothelium to form a primary platelet plug. It is a test of primary hemostasis. The BMBT becomes prolonged with thrombocytopenia (<100,000/μL) and platelet dysfunction syndromes such as von Willebrand's disease. The BMBT is usually performed without any sedation in dogs and with ketamine in cats.
To perform the BMBT:
1. When performing the BMBT in dogs, place a loose tie of gauze around the dog's muzzle to lift the lip so that the buccal mucosa is exposed and the veins slightly engorged. It is important to not tie the gauze too tightly, as vasoconstriction can artifactually change test results.
2. Use a BMBT template (Simplate R) to make two small nick incisions in the buccal mucosa. Gently wick the blood away from the site with a piece of filter paper (if you don't have filter paper, a coffee filter works well). Allow the blood to wick into the filter paper without touching the incisions or the clot.
3. Note the time from making the initial incision to the time that hemorrhage stops (i.e., a platelet plug has formed). Normal BMBT is less than 3 minutes in dogs and cats.
   If the BMBT is prolonged, von Willebrand's disease, NSAID influence, congenital thrombopathies (Bassett and Otter Hounds), and systemic illness (azotemia, hepatic failure, malignancy) should be ruled out. If the BMBT is normal in the face of a normal platelet count and clinical bleeding, tests of the coagulation cascade (APTT, PT, ACT) should be considered.

ANCILLARY TESTS OF HEMOSTASIS

THROMBIN TIME

The thrombin time is a measure of the amount of functional fibrinogen in plasma. The test is used in the diagnosis of DIC when fibrinogen levels are low. Fibrinogen levels may also be normal in DIC, but thrombin time will still be altered because of in vivo fibrinolysis. This test is now rarely used, because since more sensitive and specific tests such as D-dimer concentration are available for the diagnosis of DIC.

FIBRINOGEN

Fibrinogen levels are used in the detection of DIC. In DIC, fibrinogen levels can *decrease* as a result of the activation of thrombin and fibrin formation and the activation of plasmin, which causes degradation of fibrin and fibrinogen. Fibrinogen levels can be decreased, normal, or increased in cases of chronic DIC due to a compensatory overproduction. Because of the variability in fibrinogen levels, this test alone is not conclusive to make a diagnosis of DIC.

FIBRIN(OGEN) DEGRADATION PRODUCTS (FDPs)

FDPs (also called fibrin split products [FSPs]) are formed when the enzyme plasmin acts on fibrin monomers, cross-linked fibrin, and fibrinogen. Because fibrinogen can *increase* during periods of inflammation without DIC, the presence of FDPs alone does not allow a diagnosis of DIC. FDPs are cleared by the hepatic reticuloendothelial system. In cases of hepatic insufficiency or hepatic failure, FDPs can be elevated without concurrent DIC.

D-DIMERS

D-dimers are used in the diagnosis of DIC. D-dimers are released as the result of the breakdown of cross-linked fibrin by plasmin. Because D-dimers occur as a result of a stable fibrin clot, elevated levels are more sensitive and specific for a diagnosis of DIC.

THE PIVKA TEST

The PIVKA (proteins induced by vitamin K absence or antagonism) test is most useful in diagnosing vitamin K deficiencies. Moderate deficiencies in Vitamin K–dependent coagulation factors (II, VII, IX, and X) will cause abnormal PIVKA test results. The PIVKA test becomes prolonged 12-24 hours after the PT test becomes prolonged.

SALINE AGGLUTINATION

The saline agglutination test is simple to perform in-house and aids in the diagnosis of immune-mediated hemolytic anemia. To perform a saline agglutination test:
1. Place one drop of 0.9% saline on a microscope slide. Mix the drop of saline with one drop of the patient's anticoagulated blood and observe for the presence of agglutination under the microscope.
2. If agglutination is present, mix a second drop of saline with the blood-saline mixture on the slide and review under the microscope a second time.

If the "agglutination" disperses, it is likely caused by rouleaux secondary to inflammation. If the agglutination remains, autoagglutination of red blood cells is occurring due to interaction with antibodies directed against glycoprotein moieties on the surface of the RBC membranes.

Note: Management of patients with a confirmed coagulopathy involves correcting any underlying cause, replenishing oxygen-carrying capacity in the form of red blood cells or purified hemoglobin, replacing clotting factors and antithrombin in the form of fresh frozen plasma, and maintaining end-organ perfusion. The management of specific conditions and coagulopathies is listed under their subheadings. A more thorough approach to transfusion management is listed in Section 1.

5

SUBMISSION OF SAMPLES FOR COAGULATION TESTING

1. Draw blood sample into a blue-top tube (BTT) that contains sodium citrate. Fill the BTT to at least 75%, but preferably 90% or more, because results will be affected by excess citrate anticoagulant.
2. Centrifugation and separation of plasma from cells is *strongly recommended* if transportation to the laboratory may require more than 12 hours.
3. Use a plastic pipette or small syringe to transfer the plasma to a clean plastic tube. Cap the tube and keep cold or freeze at −20° C or lower. Freezing the plasma is not necessary unless testing will be delayed for more than 24 hours, but it should always stay cold. Repeated freezing and thawing of plasma denatures coagulation proteins.
4. If samples will be mailed, ship overnight with frozen cold packs.

ACTIVATED COAGULATION (CLOTTING) TIME (ACT)

Normal:
90-120 seconds (dog); 80-100 seconds (cat).
Patient Preparation:
Direct penetration of the vein is important.
Collect:
Venous blood in an ACT Vacutainer tube. Fill to maximum allowed by vacuum.
Submit:
Blood sample in collection tube per protocol.
Interpretation:
ACT is a convenient in-hospital screening test that evaluates both the intrinsic and common coagulation pathways. Prolonged clotting time implies coagulation factor deficiency. A specific coagulation factor deficiency must be less than 5% to increase the ACT. NOTE: hemophiliac patients may have factor VIII or IX activity only 40% to 60% of normal and yet would have a normal ACT (and a normal APTT).
Interference:
The presence of tissue thromboplastin in sample (e.g., failing to obtain blood from a "clean" venipuncture) will activate the extrinsic pathway.
Protocol:
A two-tube technique is recommended to eliminate any chance of tissue thromboplastin contaminating the sample. Fill two tubes from the same draw. Use the second tube only. Pre-warm the tubes in a water bath or heating block (37° C). Place the filled sample tubes in the water bath or heating block and begin timing. Incubate the sample in the collection tube for 60 seconds for dogs, and 45 seconds for cats. Invert sample every 5 seconds to assess for evidence of clot formation. Stop procedure at first sign of clot formation.

ACTIVATED PARTIAL THROMBOPLASTIN TIME (APTT)

Normal:
8.6-12.9 seconds (dog); 13.7-30.2 seconds (cat).
Patient Preparation:
None (atraumatic venipuncture is recommended).
Collect:
Venous blood in citrate (blue-topped tube); fill Vacutainer tube to the maximum allowed by the vacuum.
Submit:
Citrated plasma only (plasma must be separated from cells) in red-topped tube.
Interpretation:
APTT is the most sensitive and specific test of coagulation factor activity. Prolonged APTT implies anticoagulant therapy (heparin) or specific coagulation factor deficiency.
Interference:
Clotted sample, failure to use citrate as the anticoagulant; incorrect ratio of citrate to whole blood.
Protocol:
On collection of blood, invert tube several times to assure adequate mixing of sample and anticoagulant. Centrifuge IMMEDIATELY. Transfer plasma to red-topped tube and label as Citrated Plasma.

ANTIPLATELET ANTIBODY: SEE IMMUNOLOGY

BLOOD TYPING, FELINE

Normal:
Results reported as positive or negative for blood type A, B, or AB.
Patient Preparation:
None.

Collect:
Venous blood, 1.0 mL, in EDTA (lavender-topped tube).
Submit:
Entire sample.
Interpretation:
The majority of blood donors should be type A. However, blood typing and cross-matching blood prior to transfusion in cats is highly recommended, because some type B cats are present in the U.S. NOTE: it is reported that as little as 1.0 mL of type A blood transfused into a type B cat was fatal.

BLOOD TYPING FOR COMPLETE DOG ERYTHROCYTE ANTIGEN (DEA)

Normal:
Results are reported as positive or negative for DEA-1.1, DEA-1.2, DEA-3, DEA-4, DEA-5, and DEA-7.
Patient Preparation:
None.
Collect:
Venous blood, 1.0 mL, in EDTA (lavender-topped tube).
Submit:
Entire sample.
Interpretation:
Universal or A-blood donors should be NEGATIVE for DEA-1.1, DEA-1.2, and DEA-1.7.

BUCCAL MUCOSAL BLEEDING TIME (BMBT)

Normal:
2.6 ± 0.48 minutes (dog); results not reported in cats.
Patient Preparation:
None.
Collect:
Not applicable.
Submit:
Not applicable. This is an in-hospital screening test for platelet function.
Interpretation:
BMBT is a sensitive and specific test of platelet function. Prolonged BMBT is expected in patients with von Willebrand's disease and uremia. Test is NOT generally recommended for thrombocytopenic patients.
Interference:
Improper technique thrombocytopenia.
Protocol:
The test entails a standardized cut into the buccal mucosa with subsequent "capture" of blood onto filter paper until bleeding ceases.

CLOT RETRACTION TEST

Not generally recommended.
NOTE: Because of the insensitivity of this test, the clot retraction test is NOT recommended for the assessment of patients with suspected disorders of hemostasis.

COAGULATION FACTOR ACTIVITY (FACTOR ASSAY)

The following inherited coagulation factor deficiencies have been reported in dogs and cats:
    Hemophilia A (factor VIII deficiency)—the most common factor deficiency
    Hemophilia B (factor IX deficiency)
    Factor XII deficiency (Hageman trait)—of minor significance in affected cats

Vitamin K–dependent factor deficiency— occurs in Devon Rex cats, with severe bleeding Other, rare deficiencies have been reported.

DIAGNOSIS OF COAGULATION FACTOR DEFICIENCY

Coagulation factor deficiency usually is suggested in the individual dog or cat on the basis of initial test results from routine coagulation profiles (see ACT, APTT, and PT in this section). occasionally, It is possible to measure activity of specific factors in individual patients. Specialized laboratories experienced in performing these assays should be consulted regarding sample, sample size, submission requirements, and interpretation.

CROSS-MATCH: MAJOR AND MINOR

Normal:
Results (in dogs and cats) are reported as "compatible" ("no agglutination") or "incompatible" ("agglutination and/or hemolysis") in either major or minor cross-match tubes.
Patient Preparation:
None.
Donor Preparation:
None.
Collect (Patient):
Venous blood, 2 mL, in red-topped tube PLUS anticoagulated venous blood, 2.0 mL, in lavender-topped tube.
Collect (Donor):
The same (this is where it's important to label the tubes!).
Submit (Patient):
Serum, 1 mL, PLUS anticoagulated whole blood, 1.0 mL.
Submit (Donor):
The same.
Interpretation:
  No agglutination and/or hemolysis in either tube indicates that the match is
     compatible and the donor's blood may be used.
  The presence of agglutination and/or hemolysis in the *major* cross-match tube
     indicates that the donor's blood should not be used.
  The presence of agglutination and/or hemolysis in the *minor* cross-match tube
     suggests that the compatibility is not ideal; if another donor cannot be found, the
     blood can be used—although with caution.
  The presence of agglutination and/or hemolysis in the *donor control* (donor cells
     mixed with donor serum) suggests incompatibility; the donor's blood should not
     be used.
  The presence of agglutination and/or hemolysis in the *patient control* (patient cells
     mixed with patient serum) likely reflects the patient's diagnosis. Transfusion is
     indicated.
Interference:
In vitro hemolysis associated with difficulty collecting a sample or inappropriate handling of the blood; profound lipemia (lactescence).
Protocol:
1. Wash RBCs from patient and donor in 0.9% SALINE solution three times; add 4.8 mL
   of saline to 0.2 mL of RBCs from patient and donor. Mix accordingly:
   a. Major cross-match: Mix 0.1 mL (2 drops) of donor RBCs + 0.1 mL (2 drops)
      of patient serum
   b. Minor cross-match: Mix 0.1 mL (2 drops) of patient RBCs + 0.1 mL (2 drops)
      of donor serum
   c. Patient control: Mix 0.1 mL (2 drops) of patient RBCs + 0.1 mL (2 drops)
      of patient serum

    d. Donor control: Mix 0.1 mL (2 drops) of donor RBCs + 0.1 mL (2 drops) of donor serum
2. Incubate for 15 minutes at 37° C. Centrifuge for 1 minute.
3. Observe the supernatant in all tubes for evidence of hemolysis in the test samples. Examine the suspension of RBCs for agglutination (macroscopically and microscopically).

D-DIMER (FRAGMENT D-DIMER; FIBRIN DEGRADATION FRAGMENT)

Normal:
Consult laboratory reference range (dog); studies in cats are lacking.
Patient Preparation:
None.
Collect:
Anticoagulated venous blood, 2 mL, in EDTA or heparin.
Submit:
Plasma, 1.0 mL.
Interpretation:
D-dimer is the proteolytic fragment of fibrinogen degradation. D-dimer concentration is used in the assessment of DIC in dogs. Elevated levels represent a marker of clot lysis and therefore support a diagnosis of DIC; a negative test result has a high negative predictive value and reliably rules out a diagnosis of DIC. The test also has the potential to identify patients with pulmonary thromboembolic disease, although results are not reliably predictive.
Interference:
None reported.

FIBRINOGEN, QUALITATIVE (ESTIMATED)

Normal:
Refer to laboratory reference range (dog and cat).
Patient Preparation:
None.
Collect:
Whole venous blood, 2.0 mL, in EDTA (lavender-topped tube).
Submit:
Plasma, 1.0 mL.
Interpretation:
Fibrinogen levels can be estimated as the difference between plasma protein concentrations before and after heating. An increased value correlates with clot lysis and supports the diagnosis of DIC.
Interference:
Clots in sample.
Protocol:
Invert tube several times to assure adequate mixing of venous blood and anticoagulant.

FIBRINOGEN, QUANTITATIVE

Normal:
100-245 mg/dL (dog); 110-370 mg/dL (cat).
Patient Preparation:
None.
Collect:
Completely fill a citrated (blue-topped) tube with whole blood. *Mix thoroughly. Centrifuge immediately.* Transfer plasma to a red-topped tube.

5

Submit:
Plasma, 1.0 mL, in a red-topped tube; label as CITRATED PLASMA.
Interpretation:
Increased concentration is associated with DIC. However, there is no single test for the diagnosis of DIC. The clinician must also assess fibrin degradation products (increased), APTT (prolonged), PT (prolonged), and platelet count (decreased).
Interference:
Incorrect ratio of citrate (anticoagulant) to whole blood; clots in sample; use of anticoagulants other than citrate.
Protocol:
On collection of blood, invert tube several times to assure adequate mixing of sample and anticoagulant. *Centrifuge immediately.* Transfer plasma to a red-topped tube; (label as CITRATED PLASMA). NOTE: Sample is stable for only 24 hours if held at 2° to 8° C; for extended storage, sample must be frozen.

FIBRIN DEGRADATION PRODUCTS (FDPs; FIBRIN SPLIT PRODUCTS [FSPs])

Normal:
<10 μg/mL (dog); <10 μg/mL (cat).
Patient Preparation:
None.
Collect:
Venous blood, 2.0 mL, in EDTA or in a red-topped tube.
Submit:
1.0 mL serum or plasma, 1.0 mL.
Interpretation:
Assay is used to document breakdown of fibrin clots. Increased concentration is associated with DIC (see also D-Dimer). However, there is no single test for DIC diagnosis. The clinician must also assess fibrinogen (increased), APTT (prolonged), PT (prolonged), and platelet count (decreased).
Interference:
Clots in sample.

PARTIAL THROMBOPLASTIN TIME (PTT): SEE ACTIVATED PARTIAL THROMBOPLASTIN TIME (APTT)

PIVKA TEST (PROTEINS INDUCED BY VITAMIN K ANTAGONISM TEST; "THROMBOTEST")

5

Normal:
Refer to laboratory reference range (dog and cat).
Patient Preparation:
Atraumatic venipuncture is recommended.
Collect:
Completely fill a citrated (blue-topped) tube with whole blood. *Mix thoroughly. Centrifuge immediately.* Transfer plasma to a red-topped tube.
Submit:
Plasma, 1.0 mL, in red-topped tube; label as CITRATED PLASMA.
Interpretation:
Test is used in conjunction with prothrombin time in the assessment of patients suspected of warfarin toxicosis.
Interference:
Incorrect ratio of citrate (anticoagulant) to whole blood; clots in sample; use of anticoagulants other than citrate.

Protocol:

On collection of blood, invert tube several times to assure adequate mixing of sample and anticoagulant. *Centrifuge immediately.* Transfer plasma to a red-topped tube; label as CITRATED PLASMA. NOTE: Sample is stable for only 24 hours if held at 2° to 8° C; for extended storage, sample must be frozen.

PLATELET COUNT

Normal:

$166\text{-}600 \times 10^3/\mu L$ (dog); $230\text{-}680 \times 10^3/\mu L$ (cat).

Patient Preparation:

Atraumatic collection is recommended.

Collect:

Venous blood, 1.0 mL, in EDTA (lavender-topped tube).

Submit:

Entire sample.

Interpretation:

Decreased platelet count is indicative of many disorders, including immune-mediated thrombocytopenia (extremely low platelet count), infection, sepsis, and DIC, and therefore must be assessed in light of other physical, hematologic, and biochemical parameters. Elevated platelet counts (up to 1 million cells/μL) can be normal for some patients. Cats with extreme thrombocytosis should be tested for feline leukemia virus.

Interference:

Slow draw of blood from the vein, transfer of blood from syringe to tube, and traumatic venipuncture may falsely decrease platelet count.

PROTHROMBIN TIME (PT)

Normal:

5.1-7.9 seconds (dog); 8.4-10.8 seconds (cat).

Patient Preparation:

None.

Collect:

Collect whole blood in a citrated (blue–topped) tube. Fill the tube to the capacity allowed by the vacuum. Invert immediately to mix. Centrifuge immediately and collect plasma. Transfer to a sterile *plastic* tube, using *plastic* pipette. Freeze. NOTE: label as CITRATED PLASMA.

Submit:

Citrated plasma, 1.0 mL. Ship sample with dry ice. Store frozen.

Interpretation:

PT is used to assess extrinsic and common coagulation pathways. Prolonged PT is used to assess patients with suspected vitamin K antagonism (warfarin toxicosis).

Interference:

Incorrect ratio of citrate to whole blood; clots in specimen; use of a non-citrated anticoagulant (e.g., EDTA in lavender-topped tube). NOTE: If the citrated plasma sample contacts glass, clotting factor activation may occur.

Protocol:

On collection of blood, invert tube several times to assure adequate mixing of sample and anticoagulant. *Centrifuge immediately.* Transfer plasma to a red-topped tube. (Label as CITRATED PLASMA). NOTE: sample is stable for only 24 hours if held at 2° to 8° C; for extended storage, sample must be frozen.

5

VON WILLEBRAND FACTOR (vWD FACTOR)

Normal:

Results reported are specific for the laboratory performing the test.

Patient Preparation:
None.
Collect:
Collect whole blood in a citrated (blue-topped) tube. Fill the tube to the capacity allowed by the vacuum. Invert immediately to mix. *Centrifuge immediately* and collect plasma. Transfer to a sterile *plastic* tube, using a *plastic* pipette. Freeze. Label tube as CITRATED PLASMA. Although EDTA (lavender-topped tube) may be accepted by some laboratories, sodium citrated samples are preferred when submitting samples for vWD factor.
Submit:
Citrated plasma, 1.0 mL. Ship sample with dry ice. If storing longer than 24 hours, store frozen.
Interpretation:
vWD is the most common inherited hemostatic disorder reported in dogs. This test is usually performed to confirm the diagnosis of vWD, in conjunction with the BMBT. Although the condition is inherited, variable degrees of expression are recognized. Dogs with vWD levels ≤30% have a tendency to bleed spontaneously (e.g., epistaxis).
Interference:
Recent transfusion may falsely elevate vWD levels. Incorrect ratio of citrate to whole blood, a clotted specimen, and use of a non-citrated anticoagulant (e.g., EDTA in lavender-topped tube) can also affect results. Do NOT use a glass pipette or glass tube. If the citrated plasma sample contacts glass, clotting factor activation may occur.

ENDOCRINOLOGY

ADRENOCORTICOTROPIC HORMONE (ACTH), ENDOGENOUS

Normal:
10 to 70 pg/mL (dog); results not reported for cat.
Patient Preparation:
Patient should be hospitalized overnight.
Collect:
Whole blood, 2.0 mL, in EDTA (chilled, lavender-topped tube); *Immediately* transfer plasma to plastic tube (ACTH adheres to glass) and freeze. Samples should be stored frozen until assayed. Maximum storage time: 1 month at −20° C.
NOTE: Contact laboratory directly before collecting samples for ACTH. Some laboratories request plasma samples be submitted in aprotonin and will provide specially prepared tubes for this purpose. Aprotonin (protease inhibitor) is added to a lavender-topped tube to stabilize ACTH. Freezing the sample is not necessary. The treated plasma should be separated immediately by centrifugation, transferred to a plastic tube, capped, and refrigerated. Transport sample to the lab with cold packs.
Submit:
Plasma, 1.0 mL; sample should NOT be allowed to sit at room temperature even for a short period.
Interpretation:
Adrenal tumors and iatrogenic Cushing's syndrome are expected to suppress ACTH secretion; pituitary-dependent Cushing's syndrome is characterized by excessive plasma concentration of ACTH.
Interference:
Recent or current corticosteroid administration; "stress" at or around the time of blood collection. NOTE: samples *must* be handled quickly because ACTH disappears quickly from whole fresh blood.
Protocol:
Following overnight hospitalization, the sample is collected between 8 and 9 AM the following morning.

ACTH STIMULATION TEST (ACTH "Stim")

Normal:

	Dog	**Cat**
Pre-test:	0.5 to 6.0 µg/dL	0.5 to 5.0 µg/dL
Post-test:	6 to 17 µg/dL	≤ 13 µg/dL

NOTE: 17-22 µg/dL is considered "borderline" for dogs; 13-16 µg/dL is considered "borderline" for cats.

Patient Preparation:
No prior treatment with corticosteroids for at least 5-7 days before testing.

Collect:
Heparinized whole blood, 2.0 mL (green-topped tube). NOTE: Do NOT submit blood collected in EDTA.

Submit:
Plasma, 0.5 mL minimum for each sample submitted; sample should be refrigerated if shipped. Sample is assayed for cortisol.

Interpretation:
This is the most commonly used screening test for hyperadrenocorticism in dogs and cats. Patients with pituitary-dependent hyperadrenocorticism or adrenal tumor are expected to have an exaggerated cortisol response following stimulation with ACTH, assuming that the adrenal glands have retained ACTH responsiveness. Post-stimulation values ≥22 µg/dL are considered diagnostic for hyperadrenocorticism in dogs (>16 µg/dL in cats) in the presence of clinical signs (especially polydipsia) and supporting laboratory data and abdominal ultrasound. NOTE: ACTH stimulation does NOT differentiate between pituitary-dependent hyperadrenocorticism and adrenal tumor. An alternative test to use when screening for canine Cushing's syndrome is the low-dose dexamethasone test (see following entry).

The ACTH stimulation test is the *only* reliable test for monitoring patients undergoing o,p'-DDD (Lysodren) treatment of pituitary-dependent hyperadrenocorticism. Dogs with adequate pharmacologic suppression of adrenal function should have unchanged pre- and post-stimulation values (typically <2.0 µg/dL for both).

Interference:
Concurrent or recent treatment with corticosteroids. Anticonvulsant medications may adversely affect test results.

Protocol:
Several protocols are available; the following are representative.

Collect pre-test sample; then administer ACTH gel at 2.2 IU/kg IM (dog). Collect post-test sample 2 hours after ACTH administration;

or

Collect pre-test sample; then administer synthetic (expensive) ACTH (tetracosactrin, cosyntropin [Cortrosyn]) at 0.25 mg (dog) or 0.125 mg (cat) IM or IV. Collect post-test sample 1 hour after ACTH administration (dogs).

or

Collect pre-test sample; then administer ACTH at 125 µg IM (cat). Collect two post-test samples 30 minutes and 60 minutes after ACTH administration (cats).

ALDOSTERONE, SERUM

Normal:
Pre-test, 49 pg/mL (mean); post-test, 306 pg/mL (mean); reported range, 146 to 519 pg/mL (dogs). Results not reported for cats.

Patient Preparation:
None.

Collect:
Venous blood, 2.0 mL, in EDTA (lavender-topped tube) as baseline (pre-test); and repeat in 1 hour.

5

Submit:
Plasma, 1.0 mL, for each of the two samples collected.

Interpretation:
Low baseline and minimal or no increase in aldosterone levels support a diagnosis of hypoaldosteronism. The test is designed to distinguish dogs with primary hypoadrenocorticism from those with secondary hypoadrenocorticism. However, the sensitivity of the test in dogs is such that the positive predictive value is relatively low.

Interference:
Clots in sample.

Protocol:
In dogs, the pre-test and post-test samples are collected at 1-hour intervals following administration of ACTH. Follow the same protocol used to test for hyperadrenocorticism (see ACTH Stimulation).

COBALAMIN (VITAMIN B$_{12}$)

See Also TLI and Folate.
Normal:
249-733 ng/L (dog); 290-1500 ng/L (cat).

Patient Preparation:
Overnight fast.

Collect:
Whole blood, 4.0 mL (red-topped tube); separate serum from cells immediately.

Submit:
Serum, 2.0 mL.

Interpretation:
The test usually is performed in conjunction with TLI and serum folate. Decreased levels of cobalamin (vitamin B$_{12}$) support the diagnosis of small intestinal mucosal disease, small intestinal bacterial overgrowth, and exocrine pancreatic insufficiency. There is no significance attached to levels above the reported reference range.

Interference:
Hemolysis; lipemia.

CORTISOL, RESTING (BASAL):See ACTH STIMULATION TEST

Not Generally Recommended.
Normal:
0.5-6.0 µg/dL (dog); 0.5-5.0 µg/dL (cat)
Resting plasma cortisol in dogs is not routinely recommended because of the wide range of values in healthy animals. Although dogs with hyperadrenocorticism are expected to have increased values, reported values may still be within the limits of the reference range listed for normal dogs.

DEXAMETHASONE SUPPRESSION TEST, LOW-DOSE (LDDS TEST; DEXAMETHASONE SCREENING TEST)

Normal:

	Dog	**Cat**
Pre-test:	0.5 to 6.0 µg/dL	0.5 to 5.0 µg/dL
4-hr Post-test:	Usually <1.0 µg/dL	Same
8-hr Post-test:	Usually < 1.0 µg/dL	Same

Patient Preparation:
No prior treatment with corticosteroids for at least 5-7 days before testing.

Collect:

Heparinized whole blood, 1.0 mL to 2.0 mL at each collection (green-topped tube). NOTE: Do NOT collect blood in EDTA.

Submit:

Plasma, 0.5 mL minimum for each sample submitted; sample should be refrigerated if shipped. Sample is assayed for cortisol.

Interpretation:

This a screening test for hyperadrenocorticism in dogs and cats. Administration of dexamethasone decreases plasma cortisol to <1.0 or 1.4 µg/dL (depending on the laboratory) within 2-3 hours in normal dogs. An 8-hr post-test sample >1.4 µg/dL is consistent with Cushing's syndrome in dogs and cats with clinical signs (especially polydipsia) and supporting laboratory data and abdominal ultrasound. NOTE: LDDS does NOT differentiate between pituitary-dependent hyperadrenocorticism and adrenal tumor.

The 4-hr post-test sample is not interpreted as part of the screening test but is considered an aid in differentiating pituitary-dependent hyperadrenocorticism from adrenal-dependent disease. Demonstrating a transient cortisol suppression (4-hour post-tests sample) supports pituitary-dependent disease and rules out adrenal-dependent disease.

Interference:

Recent or concurrent corticosteroid administration. Anticonvulsant medications may adversely affect test results.

Protocol:

Collect pre-test sample of plasma; administer dexamethasone (either in sodium phosphate or polyethylene glycol) at **0.01 mg/kg IV** in dogs, or **0.1 mg/kg IV** in cats; then collect a 4-hr post-test plasma sample, followed by an 8-hr post-test plasma sample. Submit the three plasma samples. (NOTE the higher dose of dexamethasone used in cats vs. dogs.)

DEXAMETHASONE SUPPRESSION TEST, HIGH-DOSE (HDDS TEST)

Normal:

	Dog	**Cat**
Pre-test:	0.5 to 6.0 µg/dL	Same
4-hr Post-test:	Usually <1.0 µg/dL	Same
8-hr Post-test:	Usually <1.0 µg/dL	Same

Patient Preparation:

No prior treatment with corticosteroids for at least 5-7 days before to testing.

Collect:

Heparinized whole blood, 1.0 mL to 2.0 mL at each collection (green-topped tube). NOTE: Do NOT collect blood in EDTA.

Submit:

Plasma, 0.5 mL minimum for each sample submitted; sample should be refrigerated if shipped; sample is assayed for cortisol.

Interpretation:

The HDDS test is used in dogs with abnormal ACTH stimulation or LDDS test results to distinguish between pituitary-dependent disease and adrenal tumor. Administration of dexamethasone decreases plasma cortisol to <1.0 or 1.4 µg/dL (depending on the laboratory) within 2-3 hours in normal dogs. Dogs with an adrenal tumor or pituitary-dependent hyperadrenocorticism are not expected to demonstrate suppression of cortisol following administration of dexamethasone at the dose prescribed.

NOTE: "Suppression" is defined as:

Plasma cortisol concentration <50% of baseline at 4 hours or at 8 hours following dexamethasone administration.

or

Plasma cortisol concentration <1.4 µg/dL at 4 hours or at 8 hours following dexamethasone administration.

Interference:
Recent or concurrent corticosteroid administration. Anticonvulsant medications may adversely affect test results.

Protocol:
Collect pre-test sample of plasma; administer dexamethasone (either in sodium phosphate or in polyethylene glycol) at **0.1 mg/kg IV** in dogs, or **1.0 mg/kg IV** in cats; then collect a 4-hour post-test plasma sample, followed by an 8-hour post-test plasma sample. Submit the three plasma samples. (NOTE the higher dose of dexamethasone used in cats vs. dogs.)

ESTRADIOL (BASELINE)

Normal:
Not normally detectable (dog and cat).

Patient Preparation:
None.

Collect:
Venous blood, 2.0 mL, in a red-topped tube.

Submit:
Serum, 1.0 mL.

Interpretation:
This assay is not commonly requested for dogs and cats. Elevated levels have been used to detect testicular tumors and ovarian remnant syndrome. However, better tests are available.

Interference:
Variations in results occur with different methodologies used.

FOLATE: See also TLI AND COBALAMIN

Normal:
6.5-11.5 µg/L (dog); 9.7-21.6 µg/L (cat).

Patient Preparation:
Overnight fast.

Collect:
Whole blood, 4.0 mL (red-topped tube); separate serum from cells *immediately*.

Submit:
Serum, 2.0 mL.

Interpretation:
Assay usually is performed in conjunction with TLI and serum cobalamin. Elevated levels of folate support the diagnosis of small intestinal bacterial overgrowth in the upper small intestine. Values below the reference range support the diagnosis of proximal small intestinal disease.

Interference:
Hemolysis; lipemia.

FRUCTOSAMINE

Normal:
225-375 µmol/L (dog and cat).
NOTE: refer to laboratory reference range; ranges vary depending on methodology used.

Patient Preparation:
Fasted.

Collect:
Whole blood, 2.0 mL, in a red-topped tube (serum), lavender-topped tube (plasma in), or green-topped tube (plasma in heparin). CAUTION: sample must be non-hemolyzed.

Submit:
Serum or plasma, 1.0 mL.
Interpretation:
Test reflects glycemic levels over the preceding 1 to 3 weeks; it generally is used in assessing quality of glycemic control in patients with diabetes mellitus.
Interference:
Hemolysis; icterus.

GASTRIN

Normal:
Varies according to individual laboratory (dog); results not established for cat.
Patient Preparation:
None.
Collect:
Venous blood, 2.0 mL, in red-topped tube.
Submit:
Serum, 1.0 mL; sample should be kept frozen until assayed.
Interpretation:
Test is not commonly performed. Levels will be elevated in patients with functional gastrinoma, pyloric obstruction, renal failure, and gastric ulcers. There is no significance associated with decreased values.
Interference:
Concurrent administration of H_2 antagonist drugs (e.g., cimetidine).

GLUCAGON STIMULATION (IVGS TEST)

This is a complex test protocol to perform and yields results that are not generally reliable in distinguishing patients with type 1 diabetes from those with type 2 diabetes. It has been used to diagnose patients with insulin-secreting tumor. However, risk is associated with performing this test in patients with insulin-secreting tumor. Administration of glucagon will elevate serum glucose, which, in turn, promotes secretion of excessive amount of insulin; subsequent hypoglycemic crisis is a potential consequence.

GLUCOSE CURVE, 12-HOUR

Normal:
Glucose concentration ranges between 100 mg/dL and 250 mg/dL for the entire sampling period (dog and cat).
Patient Preparation:
Ideally, a venous catheter should be placed 1 hour before starting serial collections. Patient attitude during testing is important, because stressed or unusually aggressive animals may not be appropriate subjects for this test.
Collect:
Venous blood, approximately 1 mL per collection; plan on drawing as many as seven samples.
Submit:
Serum from each sample for routine glucose determination.
Interpretation:
This test is used to evaluate glucose levels in diabetic patients receiving insulin, particularly those that may experience recurrence of clinical signs as a result of under-treatment. Objectively, sufficient numbers of samples should be collected to establish a true nadir (lowest point) during the day. For example, if the nadir is >450 mg/dL, each dose of insulin might be increased by 1 to 2 units. When increasing insulin dose, it is appropriate to increase the dose by the same units for each administration throughout the day.

5

Interference:
Stress. Also, use of portable glucose meters to measure serial glucose levels in individual patients tends to result in lower values than actually are occurring.

Protocol:
The patient is given the usual dose of insulin and fed at home in the morning. On arrival at the hospital, a short intravenous catheter is placed in a suitable vein and secured appropriately. Serial samples are collected at 2-hour intervals over a 10-12 hour period. At the conclusion of the sampling period, the patient is usually fed and given a second daily dose of insulin, as appropriate. Then you, and the patient, can go home.

GLUCOSE TOLERANCE TEST, INTRAVENOUS (IVGT TEST)

Not Generally Recommended.

Normal:
By 60 minutes post-injection, serum insulin should be within 1 standard deviation of the baseline, and serum glucose should be within normal reference range for both dogs and cats.

Patient Preparation:
24-hour fast. Pre-placement of an intravenous catheter is recommended.

Collect:
Whole blood, 2.0 mL in a red-topped tube, *for each sample submitted.*

Submit:
Serum, 1.0 mL, for each sample submitted.

Interpretation:
Uncommonly performed, the IVGT test is an "insulin secretagogue test" used to distinguish type 1 diabetes from type 2 in cats. (NOTE: It is appropriate to consider all diabetic dogs as having type 1 [insulin-dependent] diabetes.) Patients with a mean serum insulin level >15 µg/mL by 60 minutes following injection are likely to have type 2 (non–insulin-dependent) diabetes. However, in cats, results are inconsistent and rarely diagnostic—another reason why this is NOT a popular test.

Interference:
Hemolysis. Prolonged contact of serum with RBCs will cause a false decrease in glucose concentration. (NOTE: Do NOT use gray-topped tubes to collect samples.) The IVGT test can be adversely influenced by diet, certain drugs (steroids, insulin), stage of estrus, underlying illness or infection (sepsis), and stress.

Protocol:
1. Fast the patient overnight.
2. Place an intravenous catheter.
3. Collect venous blood in a red-topped tube. Submit 1.0 mL serum for a baseline glucose.
4. Administer 0.5 g/kg of 50% glucose solution IV over 30 seconds.
5. Collect approximately 2.0 mL of whole blood each: 1 minute, 5 minutes, 15 minutes, 25 minutes, 35 minutes, 45 minutes, 1 hour, and 2 hours following administration of glucose. (times may vary slightly depending on author and/or reference used).
6. Submit 0.5-1.0 mL of serum for each sample. NOTE: Centrifuge and separate each serum sample as soon as practical after clot formation.
   Each sample is submitted for *both* insulin and glucose determination.

GLUCOSE TOLERANCE TEST, ORAL (OGT TEST)

Not Generally Recommended.
The OGT test, although commonly performed in humans, is rarely performed in dogs and cats because of the difficulty associated with reliably administering the required volume of glucose orally.

An oral glucose absorption test has previously been described in the literature as a means of assessing patients with malabsorptive gastrointestinal disorders. Today, considering that superior tests are available, this test is no longer recommended for the assessment of malassimilation in dogs and cats.

INSULIN

Normal:
5-20 µU/mL (dog and cat).
Patient Preparation:
Overnight fast.
Collect:
Whole blood, 2.0 mL, in red-topped tube.
Submit:
Serum, 1.0 mL.
Interpretation:
Test is indicated for the diagnostic assessment of patients suspected of having an insulin-secreting tumor (e.g., insulinoma). If the patient has profound hypoglycemia at the time the test sample is collected, test results for insulin may be reported as normal. Simultaneous testing of serum glucose is recommended. Low glucose (<60 mg/dL) and an insulin level >20 µU/mL are consistent with insulin-secreting tumor.
Interference:
Hemolysis; blood collected in EDTA (plasma).
Protocol:
Most laboratories recommend that the patient's insulin level be determined in conjunction with blood glucose. Profound hypoglycemia may result in a normal insulin level being reported. A recent meal as well as several drugs can influence insulin concentrations.

PARATHYROID HORMONE (PTH)

Normal:
2-13 pmol/L (dog and cat). Results vary among laboratories.
Patient Preparation:
12-hour fast.
Collect:
Whole blood, 2.0 mL, in red-topped tube.
Submit:
Serum (FROZEN), 1.0 mL, in sterile plastic tube.
Interpretation:
PTH levels will be increased in patients with primary hyperparathyroidism, secondary renal or nutritional hyperparathyroidism, and other disorders causing hypocalcemia. No measurable PTH level is consistent with primary hypoparathyroidism. PTH testing should always include ionized calcium (iCa) assay.
Interference:
Hemolysis; thawing of sample for extended periods.
Protocol:
Serum should be separated from cells within 1 hour following collection; serum should be frozen and shipped on ice. Deliver to laboratory via overnight delivery. Keep frozen.

5

PARATHYROID HORMONE-RELATED PROTEIN (PTHrP)

Normal:
Refer to laboratory reference range values (dog and cat).
Patient Preparation:
12-hour fast.
Collect:
Whole blood, 2.0 mL, in red-topped tube.

Submit:
Serum (FROZEN), 1.0 mL, in sterile plastic tube.
Interpretation:
Interpretation of PTHrP entails simultaneous testing for calcium (or iCa) and PTH. PTHrP levels are low to undetectable in patients with primary hyperparathyroidism. Patients with hypercalcemia associated with lymphosarcoma or chronic renal insufficiency will have increased levels of PTHrP.
Test Interference:
Hemolysis; thawing of sample for extended periods.
Protocol:
Serum should be separated from cells within 1 hour following collection; serum should be frozen and shipped with ice in plastic tube. *Deliver to laboratory via overnight delivery. Keep frozen.*

T_3 (3,5,3′-TRIIODOTHYRONINE)

Normal:
0.8-1.5 mg/dL by radioimmunoassay (RIA) (dog); 0.8-1.5 ng/mL (by RIA) (cat).
NOTE: results will vary among different laboratories.
Patient Preparation:
None (patient should not be receiving exogenous thyroid hormone supplementation).
Collect:
Whole blood, 1-2 mL, in red-topped tube.
Submit:
Serum, 0.5 mL minimum. NOTE: Storage/shipment of samples in *plastic,* rather than glass, containers is recommended. Sample should be frozen and shipped with cold packs.
Interpretation:
T_3 is a *poor indicator* of thyroid function and generally provides little reliable diagnostic information pertaining to thyroid-related disease; baseline T_3 does NOT reliably distinguish between hypothyroid and euthyroid states. Test results for T_3 include both free T_3 (fT_3) and protein-bound T_3. RIA is the preferred test method.
Interference:
Patients receiving exogenous thyroid supplementation can have positive or negative test interference, depending on the dose of drug administered and the time the last dose was given. T_3 autoantibody, if present, may falsely lower test results. NOTE: Storage of serum or plasma *in glass* can cause a significant false increase in serum T_3 concentration.

REVERSE T_3 (RT_3; 3,3′,5′-TRIIODOTHYRONINE)

There are currently no established diagnostic guidelines associated with baseline reverse T_3 values in dogs and cats.

T_3 SUPPRESSION

Normal:
Suppression of T_4 to 1.5 µg/dL following seven doses of synthetic T_3 (in cats).
Patient Preparation:
None.
Collect:
Whole blood, 3.0 mL, in red-topped tube, for each sample (pre-test and post-test).
Submit:
Serum, 1.0 mL minimum for each sample.
Interpretation:
This test measures T_4 and T_3 following sequential administration of seven doses of synthetic T_3; it may distinguish between euthyroid and slightly hyperthyroid cats. Hyperthyroid cats

demonstrate minimal or no decrease in serum T_4, which remains at 2.0 μg/dL or more. T_4 values between 1.5 and 2.0 g/dL are nondiagnostic. T_3 values should increase in all cats (normal as well as hyperthyroid). NOTE: If T_3 values do NOT increase, test results are considered invalid.

Interference:
Hemolysis; lipemia; icterus; blood collected in EDTA.
Protocol:
Pre-test sample is collected (to be submitted for T_3 and T_4).

FREE T_4 (fT_4)

Normal:
0.8-3.5 ng/dL (dog); 1.0-4.0 ng/dL (cat).
Patient Preparation:
None.
Collect:
Venous blood, 2.0 mL, in red-topped tube.
Submit:
Serum, 1.0 mL minimum; freeze and store in plastic tubes rather than glass; ship samples with cold packs to arrive for analysis within 5 days of collection.
Interpretation:
Free T_4 is used in preference to conventional T_4 to confirm hypothyroidism in dogs and hyperthyroidism in cats. Results <0.8 ng/dL (and *especially* <0.5 ng/dL) are consistent with a diagnosis of hypothyroidism in dogs. As with conventional T_4 levels, free T_4 levels in cats that exceed 4.0 ng/dL are consistent with the diagnosis of hyperthyroidism.
Interference:
Storing/shipping serum in glass container may alter test results; circulating thyroid autoantibody does NOT interfere with test results. Results determined by RIA alone may be significantly lower than those determined by the MED method. Severe illness may cause low fT_4 values in dogs with normal thyroid function (sick, euthyroid). T_4 autoantibody does NOT interfere with the assay for free T_4.

TOTAL T_4, (THYROXINE OR TETRAIODOTHYRONINE)

Normal:
1.5-3.5 μg/dL (dog); 1.0-4.0 μg/dL (cat).
NOTE: A point-of-care ELISA test kit for in-hospital assessment of T_4 is available. However, it is recommended that ELISA test results be confirmed by RIA.
Patient Preparation:
None (patient should not be receiving exogenous thyroid hormone supplementation).
Collect:
Whole blood, 1-2 mL, in red-topped tube.
Submit:
Serum, 0.5 mL minimum. NOTE: storage/shipment of samples in *plastic,* rather than glass, containers is recommended. Sample should be frozen and shipped with cold packs.
Interpretation:
T_4 is produced within the thyroid gland, and therefore the total T_4 is the preferred test of thyroid function. The test combines measurement of free T_4 (fT_4) plus protein-bound T_4. Dogs with T_4 levels <2.0 μg/dL are likely to have hypothyroidism (if associated clinical signs are present); cats with T_4 levels >4.0 μg/dL are likely to have hyperthyroidism.
Dogs: Decreased values suggest hypothyroidism (dogs); however, dogs with underlying illness NOT related to abnormal thyroid function may still have abnormally decreased T_4 concentration (sick, euthyroid). A comprehensive physical examination and laboratory profile are indicated in establishing a diagnosis of hypothyroidism in dogs.

5

Cats: In middle-aged and old cats, hyperthyroidism becomes an important differential diagnosis when T_4 levels exceed 4.0 µg/dL in the presence of clinical signs. Most cases are caused by a functional multinodular adenoma. Less than 5% of cases are associated with thyroid adenocarcinoma.

Interference:
Patients receiving exogenous thyroid supplementation can have positive or negative test interference, depending on the dose of drug administered and the time the last dose was given. Underlying illness and T_4 autoantibody, if present, may falsely lower test results. NOTE: Storage of serum or plasma *in glass* can cause a significant false increase in serum T_4 concentration.

THYROTROPIN, CANINE (THYROID-STIMULATING HORMONE [TSH]; BASELINE TSH)

Normal:
Up to 0.6 ng/mL (dog); values not established for cats.
NOTE: Lower limits of normal (~ 0.1 ng/mL) for methodologies used are below the sensitivity of the assay.
Patient Preparation:
None, if patient is not receiving exogenous thyroid hormone supplementation.
Collect:
Venous blood, 1-2 mL, in red-topped tube.
Submit:
Serum, 0.5 mL minimum. NOTE: Storage/shipment of samples in *plastic,* rather than in *glass,* containers is recommended. Sample should be frozen and shipped with cold packs.
Interpretation:
This is a reasonable test for the assessment of hypothyroidism in dogs; however, TSH fluctuations can produce normal results in 20% to 40% of hypothyroid dogs. TSH should not be interpreted without having same-sample results for T_4 or fT_4. A low T_4 or fT_4 and increased TSH in a dog are consistent with the diagnosis of hypothyroidism. Normal T_4 or fT_4 and TSH effectively rule out hypothyroidism. Clinical signs and a routine laboratory profile must be part of the diagnostic assessment of any patient suspected of having thyroid disease.
Interference:
The same interfering factors that influence T_4 assays are likely to affect TSH.

THYROID-STIMULATING HORMONE, CANINE: See THYROTROPIN, CANINE

THYROTROPIN RESPONSE (TSH RESPONSE TEST)

Not Generally Recommended.
Initially believed to be useful in diagnosing hyperthyroidism, the TSH response test has been shown in subsequent studies to be limited in the ability of abnormal thyroid tissue to respond to stimulation. Other test limitations, including the removal of bovine TSH from the market, have resulted in the current recommendation against its use.

IMMUNOLOGY

ALLERGEN-SPECIFIC IGE ANTIBODY TEST (RADIOALLERGOSORBENT TEST [RAST]; ALLERGY SCREEN)

Normal:
Refer to laboratory for interpretation of results reported.
Patient Preparation:
None.

Collect:
Venous blood, 2.0 mL, in red-topped tube,
Submit:
Serum, 1.0 mL.
Interpretation:
This in vitro assay is used to identify causative allergens in atopic animals. The RAST has also been suggested for evaluation of patients with suspected food-related hypersensitivity. At this time, results are inconclusive.
Interference:
Concurrent corticoid therapy.

ANTIBODY TITERS FOR INFECTIOUS DISEASE DIAGNOSIS: See INFECTIOUS DISEASE SEROLOGY AND MICROBIOLOGY

ANTINUCLEAR ANTIBODY (ANA)

Normal:
Results are reported as a titer (ratio); refer to the laboratory reference range (dog and cat).
Patient Preparation:
None.
Collect:
Venous blood, 2.0 mL, in red-topped tube.
Submit:
Serum, 1.0 mL.
Interpretation:
This is an adjunctive (arguably the most important) test in the assessment of patients suspected of having systemic lupus erythematosus (SLE). Results must be interpreted after considering other underlying disorders in the individual patient. Low positive titers will be reported in patients having any of several disorders, including inflammatory disease, neoplasia, and infectious diseases. A high positive titer, in the presence of associated clinical and laboratory findings, supports a diagnosis of SLE.
Interference:
Concurrent illness or infection.

ANTIPLATELET ANTIBODY

No Commercially Available Test.
To date, a sensitive and specific test for the diagnosis of immune-mediated thrombo-cytopenia (ITP) by determination of antiplatelet antibody has not been developed. Generally, *extreme* thrombocytopenia (<30,000 platelets/mm³) is managed with immunosuppressive doses of corticosteroids on the assumption that the condition is immune-mediated.

5

COOMBS TEST (DIRECT COOMBS TEST; DIRECT ANTIGLOBULIN TEST [DAT])

Normal:
Negative (dog and cat).
Patient Preparation:
None.
Collect:
Anticoagulated venous blood, 2.0 mL, in EDTA (lavender-topped tube).
Submit:
Entire sample.
Interpretation:
The Coombs test detects presence of antibody and/or complement on the surface of RBCs and supports the diagnosis of immune-mediated hemolytic anemia (IMHA). It is generally

reported by degree of positivity: +1 to +4. Strength of the reaction does not predict severity of the disease or prognosis. A negative test result does not rule out the diagnosis of IMHA. The test is reported to be positive only 60% to 70% of the time.

Interference:
Concurrent steroid therapy; severe autoagglutination.

RHEUMATOID FACTOR, CANINE

Normal:
Negative (dog); values not established for cats.
Patient Preparation:
None.
Collect:
Venous blood, 2.0 mL, in red-topped tube.
Submit:
Serum, 1.0 mL.
Interpretation:
This assay detects the presence of circulating autoantibody directed against IgG. It is an adjunctive test used in the diagnostic assessment of patients suspected of having rheumatoid arthritis or SLE. Results are reported as "positive" or "negative." A positive test result does not confirm a diagnosis of rheumatoid arthritis. Several other immune-mediated disorders, especially if chronic, can cause positive test results.
Interference:
Osteoarthritis; fibrositis; polyarteritis nodosa.

INFECTIOUS DISEASE SEROLOGY AND MICROBIOLOGY

ANAPLASMA PHAGOCYTOPHILA ANTIBODY (FORMERLY *EHRLICHIA EQUI*)

Normal:
Negative (dog)
Patient Preparation:
None.
Collect:
Venous blood, 2.0 mL, in red-topped tube.
Submit:
Serum, 1.0 mL.
Interpretation:
Limited studies are available about antibody responses to infection with *A. phagocytophila*; refer to the laboratory test results for information on interpretation.
Interference:
Cross-reactivity with *A. platys* is expected.

ASPERGILLUS SPP. ANTIBODY TITER (NON-AVIAN)

Not Generally Recommended.
The high rate of false-positive and false-negative test results (depending on test methodology) limits the value of serology in establishing a diagnosis of aspergillosis in dogs without clinical signs.
Normal:
Negative (dog and cat).
Patient Preparation:
None.
Collect:
Venous blood, 2-3 mL, in red-topped tube.

5

Submit:
Serum, 1.0 mL minimum.
Interpretation:
It is recommended to concurrently request *Penicillium* spp. titer. A positive antibody titer in a dog that is not responsive to empirical antibiotic therapy and with persistent nasal discharge, masseter muscle atrophy, and erosions of the nasal planum is highly suspect for aspergillosis.
Interference:
A positive test result may simply denote exposure.

BABESIA ANTIBODY TITER, CANINE

Normal:
B. canis, <80; *B. gibsoni*, <320 .
Patient Preparation:
None.
Collect:
Venous blood, 2-3 mL, in red-topped tube.
Submit:
Serum, 1.0 mL minimum.
Interpretation:
Titers >80 for *B. canis* or >320 for *B. gibsoni* are consistent with the diagnosis of infection in patients with corresponding clinical symptoms.
Interference:
There can be considerable cross-reactivity between serologic assays for *B. canis* and *B. gibsoni*. Negative results in patients suspected of being infected should be followed with a convalescent sample 4 weeks following the initial test.

BARTONELLA SPP. (*BARTONELLA HENSELAE* TITER)

Normal:
Negative (cat).
Patient Preparation:
None.
Collect:
Venous blood, 2.0 mL, in red-topped tube.
Submit:
Serum, 1.0 mL.
Interpretation:
Different test methodologies are used commercially, including IFA (immunofluorescent assay), ELISA (enzyme-linked immunosorbent assay), and Western blot analysis. Although there is cross-reactivity with other *Bartonella* species, the test is reported to be relatively sensitive and specific for infection in cats. At issue, however, is whether all cats that test positive are, in fact, clinically ill and whether treatment is indicated on the basis of one positive test result. Results on positive cats may be reported as Serum, +1 to +4.
Interference:
None reported.

5

BLASTOMYCOSIS ANTIBODY TITER

Normal:
Negative (dog and cat).
Patient Preparation:
None.

Collect:
Venous blood, 2.0 mL, in red-topped tube.
Submit:
Serum, 1.0 mL minimum.
Interpretation:
A positive serologic test in a dog with clinical signs consistent with blastomycosis does correlate with infection. Many cats with known blastomycosis infection, however, will have negative serologic results.
Interference:
None reported.

BLOOD CULTURE (BACTERIA)

Normal:
Negative at 10+ days following incubation (dog and cat).
Patient Preparation:
Ideally, sample should be collected while patient is febrile. The peripheral vein must be surgically prepared prior to venipuncture. Use at least two veins. Do not collect blood via a catheter.
Collect:
Venous blood, 6-10 mL, in a syringe (with no anticoagulant added).
Submit:
Transfer blood directly to a suitable (commercially prepared) vial containing a blood culture medium. NOTE: special media designed to remove certain antibiotics are available for patients that are concurrently receiving antibacterial therapy at the time of sample collection.
Interpretation:
The laboratory will report identification of any growth and minimum inhibitory concentration (MIC) susceptibility test results.
Interference:
Contaminating bacteria obtained during the collection process.
Protocol:
Samples from a separate vein, when feasible, should be collected. Generally, three samples are submitted from the same patient taken at approximately 1-hour blood intervals, collected by venipuncture (syringe and needle) from different sites.

BORRELIA BURGDORFERI: See LYME BORRELIOSIS

BRUCELLA CANIS ANTIBODY

Preliminary Assessment by RSAT OR TAT

(RSAT = rapid slide agglutination test; TAT = tube agglutination test)
Normal:
Negative (dog).
Patient Preparation:
None.
Collect:
Venous blood, 2.0 mL, in red-topped tube.
Submit:
Serum, 1.0 mL.
Interpretation:
Dogs with a negative test result are likely not to be infected. Follow-up testing is recommended for dogs with a negative test result but high likelihood of infection. Dogs with a positive test result should be retested by agar gel immunodiffusion (AGID) (see following entry) to confirm infection.

Interference:
Because of the nature of the screening tests, the frequency of false-positive test results can be high.
Protocol:
Both the RSAT and the TAT should be performed with 2-mercaptoethanol (2-ME) to eliminate interference caused by heterologous IgM (responsible for most false-positive reactions). NOTE: optional testing by IFA is commercially available. Consider using IFA to compare with the RSAT and TAT.

CONFIRMATORY TEST BY AGID (AGAR GEL IMMUNODIFFUSION)

Normal:
Titers <50 are considered negative (dog).
Patient Preparation:
None.
Collect:
Venous blood, 2.0 mL, in red-topped tube.
Submit:
Serum, 1.0 mL.
Interpretation:
Titers >200 are generally consistent with positive results on blood culture.
Interference:
None reported.

CANINE DISTEMPER ANTIBODY

CEREBROSPINAL FLUID (CSF) (IgG or IgM)

Normal:
Negative (refer to laboratory reference range).
Patient Preparation:
Fluid should be collected from the cisterna magna; sample is collected with the patient under general anesthesia and an endotracheal tube placed; sterile technique is required.
Collect:
CSF.
Submit:
CSF, 1.0 mL.
Interpretation:
The presence of any titer for canine distemper virus antibody (IgG or IgM) in CSF is consistent with infection, provided there is no contamination of the sample with blood or plasma. CSF titers should be assessed in conjunction with serum antibody titer.
Interference:
Blood or plasma contamination of sample during collection may cause false-positive results in vaccinated dogs. Vaccine-induced antibody is not expected to cross into CSF.
NOTE: when assessing individual patients for distemper antibody, various laboratory methods are used to perform serology. The virus neutralization (VN) test method for CDV antibody is recommended.

SERUM (IgG or IgM)

Normal:
IgG (single sample titer is inconclusive). Uninfected dogs have no evidence of a rising titer when results of the acute and convalescent titers are compared. A single IgM titer will be negative. Vaccination will affect results. Refer to laboratory reference range.
Patient Preparation:
None.

5

Collect:
Whole blood, 2.0 mL.
Submit:
Serum, 1.0 mL.

Virus Neutralization (VN) Test

Normal:
Vaccination will affect results. Refer to laboratory reference range.
Patient Preparation:
None.
Collect:
Whole blood, 2.0 mL, in red-topped tube.
Submit:
Serum, 1.0 mL.
Interpretation:
Actual test results may vary from one laboratory to another. Individual laboratories will provide interpretation information.
NOTE: Serum virus neutralization is the preferred test to use when assessing antibody response subsequent to vaccination.

COCCIDIOIDOMYCOSIS ANTIBODY TITER (AGID)

Normal:
Negative (dog and cat).
Patient Preparation:
None.
Collect:
Whole blood, 2.0 mL, in red-topped tube.
Submit:
Serum, 1.0 mL.
Interpretation:
Commercial laboratories may perform an initial screening test on samples. False positive rates on these tests may be high. Any patient having a positive test result on screening should be subjected to an antibody titer by AGID.
Interference:
Cross-reactivity in patients with histoplasmosis or blastomycosis can occur with all test methods used to detect *C. immitis* antibody.

CRYPTOCOCCAL ANTIGEN (SERUM OR CSF)

Normal:
Negative (dog and cat).
Patient Preparation:
None.
Collect:
Venous blood, 2.0 mL, in red-topped tube; CSF, 0.5 mL.
Submit:
Serum, 1.0 mL; CSF, 0.5 mL.
Interpretation:
Any titer to *C. neoformans* is consistent with infection and justifies treatment. Antibody titers for cryptococcosis are not valid.
Interference:
None reported.

EHRLICHIA CANIS ANTIBODY

Normal:
Refer to laboratory reference range (dog and cat).
A point-of-care test for in-hospital use in dogs will be negative in the non-exposed patient.
Patient Preparation:
None.
Collect:
Venous blood, 2.0 mL, in red-topped tube.
Submit:
Serum, 1.0 mL.
Interpretation:
Interpretation varies among laboratories and methodologies used to detect antibody. The clinician must consider test results with clinical signs and results of routine laboratory profiles when making the decision to treat a patient with a positive titer. Dogs with confirmed infections may continue to have a positive antibody titer for *E. canis* for several months following recovery.
NOTE: Correlation between antibody titer and active infection is poor with *all available antibody tests* on the market today.
Interference:
None reported.

EHRLICHIA EQUI ANTIBODY: See *ANAPLASMA PHAGOCYTOPHILA* ANTIBODY

EHRLICHIA SPP.: See POLYMERASE CHAIN REACTION (PCR) FOR TEST METHOD

FELINE CORONAVIRUS ANTIBODY (FeCoV Ab)

Inappropriately called the "FIP Ab test"; not generally recommended.
Coronavirus titer is not a diagnostic test for feline infectious peritonitis (FIP). In fact, at this time there is no diagnostic test for FIP. The only value in submitting serum for a coronavirus titer is to identify cats that have a truly negative antibody titer (titered to zero). A negative antibody titer, although exceptionally rare among domestic cats, may denote no prior exposure to coronavirus (FIP).

EHRLICHIA spp (by Polymerase Chain Reaction [PCR])

Normal:
Negative (dog and cat).
Patient Preparation:
None.
Collect:
Venous blood, 2.0 mL, in EDTA (lavender-topped tube).
Submit:
Entire sample.
Interpretation:
Reported as positive or negative; positive samples should be subjected to further testing in order to confirm infection.
Interference:
PCR tests are subject to false-positive results because of minute traces of cross-reacting DNA in the sample.

5

FELINE INFECTIOUS ANEMIA: See *HAEMOBARTONELLA (MYCOPLASMA HAEMOFELIS)*

FELINE LEUKEMIA VIRUS ANTIGEN (FeLV Ag; p27 TEST)

NOTE: ALL commercial and in-hospital FeLV tests detect antigen, *not* antibody.

Normal:
Negative (denotes absence of virus).
Patient Preparation:
None.
Collect:
IFA: Whole blood, 1.0 mL, in EDTA (lavender-topped tube).
ELISA: Whole blood, 2.0 mL, in red-topped tube.
Submit:
IFA: buffy coat smear or 1.0 mL anticoagulated whole blood collected in EDTA; NOTE: IFA is the preferred method for assessing bone marrow aspiration samples for FeLV Ag.
ELISA: Serum, 1.0 mL.
Interpretation:
Both the IFA and the ELISA detect the presence of the core protein p27.
IFA: a positive test result identifies the presence of FeLV cell–associated antigen (in WBCs and/or platelets) and defines "persistent infection," especially in cats with clinical and/or laboratory signs consistent with FeLV infection.
ELISA: a positive test result identifies the presence of soluble, circulating FeLV antigen; healthy cats with a positive test result should be retested 1 to 2 months later to reassess virus status OR be subjected to corroborative testing by IFA.

　　NOTE: The AAFP/AFM Task Force on Feline Retrovirus Testing stresses that healthy cats with positive test results may have false-positive test results (by either method). Corroborative testing is indicated using a different test method. A positive test result in a cat with clinical signs suggestive of chronic illness, lymphoid neoplasia, or significant hematologic abnormalities is highly indicative of infection. Negative test results are highly accurate.
Interference:
FeLV vaccination will not interfere with test results, regardless of test method used.
IFA: Thrombocytopenia and/or leukopenia may cause false-negative test results. Poor slide quality, eosinophilia, and hemolysis may influence ability to accurately read stained slides.
ELISA: Hemolysis.

　　NOTE: The AAFP/AFM Task Force on Feline Retrovirus Testing no longer stipulates that the IFA for FeLV Ag is the "confirmatory test" for cats with positive ELISA results. In fact, the ELISA is more sensitive than the IFA in detecting the presence of FeLV antigen.

FELINE IMMUNODEFICIENCY VIRUS ANTIBODY (FIV Ab)

Normal:
Negative (negative test results indicate no prior FIV exposure).
Patient Preparation:
None.
Collect:
Whole blood, 2.0 mL, in red-topped tube.
Submit:
Serum, 1.0 mL each for IFA (or ELISA) and Western blot analysis.
Interpretation:
Cats with a positive test result by IFA (or ELISA) should be subjected to confirmatory testing by Western blot analysis.
Interference:
Any cat having received at least 1 inoculation with the FIV vaccine (killed, adjuvanted product) will produce interfering antibody that is detected by all commercially available FIV Ab tests (IFA, ELISA, Western blot analysis). False-positive test results are expected to persist for at least 1 year following vaccination. Currently, there is NO test that will reliably and consistently distinguish between infected and vaccinated cats, including polymerase

chain reaction (PCR). Also, kittens that have nursed from vaccinated queens are expected to have a false-positive test result for FIV Antibody associated with maternally derived antibody. Duration of the false-positive results is unknown.

Kittens less than 6 months of age are expected to have maternally derived antibody if the queen is infected and may have a false positive test result when tested by IFA or ELISA. Subsequent testing of positive kittens at 6 months of age or older is indicated to determine true infection status.

NOTE: The AAFP/AFM Task Force on Feline Retrovirus Testing stresses that healthy cats with a positive test result (by IFA or ELISA) may have false-positive test results, especially in populations in which the prevalence of infection is low. Confirmatory testing is indicated using the Western blot analysis. Negative test results are highly accurate.

GIARDIA ANTIGEN

Normal:
Negative for antigen (dog and cat).
Patient Preparation:
None.
Collect:
2 to 5 grams of fresh feces.
Submit:
Entire sample in a sterile container; sample can be stored for 24 hours at 2° to 8° C. Frozen feces may be stored for slightly longer periods.
Interpretation:
Test results are reported as either positive or negative for antigen; positive test results are expected in dogs or cats during active cyst and trophozoite shedding. The zoonotic potential of canine and feline giardiasis is controversial.
Interference:
Extended or improper storage of the sample could result in false-negative results.

HEARTWORM ANTIBODY, FELINE

NOTE: See also Heartworm Antigen, Feline.
Normal:
Negative.
Patient Preparation:
None.
Collect:
Whole blood, 1.0 mL, in red-topped tube.
Submit:
Serum, 1.0 mL.
Interpretation:
Test results should be interpreted in conjunction with a heartworm antigen test performed on the same sample. Because diagnostic confirmation of heartworm infection in cats is problematic (for several reasons), serologic test results must be considered in light of other laboratory and radiographic assessments.

A negative heartworm antibody (HW-Ab) test result suggests that there has been no exposure to *Dirofilaria immitis*. A negative result typically is used to rule out feline heartworm infection.

A positive HW-Ab test result only supports prior exposure. It does NOT confirm infection. Cats that are positive for HW-Ab should be subsequently tested for heartworm antigen (see below).
Interference:
Marked hemolysis or lipemia.

5

HEARTWORM ANTIGEN, FELINE

NOTE: See also Heartworm Antibody, Feline.
Normal:
Negative.
Patient Preparation:
None
Collect:
Whole blood, 2.0 mL, in a red-topped tube.
Submit:
Serum, 1.0 mL.
Interpretation:
Test results should be interpreted in conjunction with a heartworm antibody test performed on the same sample. Because diagnostic confirmation of heartworm infection in cats is problematic (for several reasons), serologic test results must be considered in light of other laboratory and radiographic assessments.

A negative heartworm antigen (HW-Ag) test result is not diagnostically useful; heartworm infection is still possible. A positive HW-Ag test result is highly specific; infection is likely.
Interference:
Marked hemolysis may cause a false-positive test result. A cat with male heartworm infection only will not have a positive result. Low worm burdens (common) may result in false-negative test results.

HEARTWORM ANTIGEN, CANINE

Normal:
Negative.
Patient Preparation:
None.
Collect:
Whole blood, 2.0 mL, in red-topped tube.
Submit:
Serum, 1.0 mL.
Interpretation:
A negative (HW-Ag) test result implies no infection; a positive HW-Ag test result strongly supports active infection.
Interference:
Marked hemolysis may cause a false-positive test result. A dog with a small worm burden may have a false-negative test result. NOTE: the canine HW-Ag test may remain positive for up to 16 weeks following adulticide therapy.

HAEMOBARTONELLA (FELINE INFECTIOUS ANEMIA; *MYCOPLASMA HAEMOFELIS, M. HAEMOMINUTUM*)

Normal:
Negative.
Patient Preparation:
None.
Collect:
Whole blood, 1.0 mL in EDTA (lavender-topped tube).
Submit:
Submit entire sample; see Polymerase Chain Reaction (PCR) for test method.
Interpretation:
A positive test result is supportive of the diagnosis of infection; a negative test result implies no exposure.

Interference:
Sample contamination; improper handing; extended storage times. Samples are stable for 48 hours if refrigerated at 2° to 8° C.

LEPTOSPIROSIS ANTIBODY TITER

Normal:
Negative.
Patient Preparation:
None.
Collect:
Whole blood, 4.0 mL, in red-topped tube.
Submit:
Serum, 2.0 mL
Interpretation:
Laboratories in the U.S. provide titers for some or all of the following serovars: *L. canicola, L. icterohemorrhagica, L. grippotyphosa, L. pomona, L. bratislava, L. hardjo, and L. autumnalis.* A positive test result may indicate infection (high titers in the presence of clinical signs), prior exposure, or recent vaccination. A negative titer indicates no recent exposure. CAUTION: interpretation of Ab titer results for leptospirosis on the basis of *a single serum sample* in previously vaccinated dogs is difficult and may not be indicative of infection. A single positive antibody titer for *any* serovar in a healthy, recently vaccinated dog is not diagnostic for infection. Documentation of a rising titer, based on test results of two samples 3 to 4 weeks apart, is strongly recommended to establish a diagnosis.
Interference:
Recent vaccination (regardless of the titer and the number of vaccine serovars administered). NOTE: when submitting samples for leptospirosis serology, it is important to provide information regarding date of last vaccination (if known), key clinical signs, and known laboratory abnormalities.

LYME BORRELIOSIS (*BORRELIA BURGDORFERI*)

C6 PEPTIDE AB BY ELISA (SNAP 3DX TEST)

Normal:
Negative (dog).
Patient Preparation:
None.
Collect:
Venous blood, 1.0 mL, in a syringe or red-topped tube (for submission).
Submit:
Use collected sample for the point-of-care (SNAP) test. Submit a minimum of 0.5 mL of serum if test is being sent to a commercial laboratory.
Interpretation:
A positive test result denotes exposure to *B. burgdorferi*; the presence of C6 antibody has a high correlation with infection. Infection is not always associated with clinical signs. The decision to treat or not to treat a healthy dog with a positive test result is based on the clinician's assessment of the individual patient and supporting laboratory data.
NOTE: Occasionally, a dog will have a negative test result subsequent to treatment. However, this an inconsistent finding. Use the quantitative C6 antibody test to monitor response to treatment.
Interference:
None; prior vaccination (regardless of vaccine used) will NOT cause false-positive test results.
Protocol:
Sample may be submitted to a commercial laboratory or can be rapidly assessed in the hospital as a point-of care (SNAP) test; follow manufacturer's procedure outline.

5

Quantitative C6 Antibody Test

Normal:
Usually <30 antibody units (dog); refer to the laboratory reference range.
Patient Preparation:
None.
Collect:
Venous blood, 2.0 mL, in red-topped tube.
Submit:
Serum, 1.0 mL.
Interpretation:
Patients with antibody levels >30 antibody units by the quantitative assay may be at risk of developing clinical disease. Patients with an initial positive test that undergo treatment for Lyme borreliosis infection can be monitored for response (decline in antibody level) to treatment over time.
Interference:
None; prior vaccination (regardless of vaccine used) will NOT cause false-positive test results.
Protocol:
The quantitative test generally is indicated for patients that have (1) tested *positive* by the SNAP test and/or (2) are undergoing treatment for Lyme borreliosis.

Borrelia burgdorferi Antibody (IFA and Western Blot Analysis)

Not Generally Recommended
The sensitivity and specificity data on C6 antibody support the recommendation that routine laboratory testing of patients suspected of having Lyme borreliosis be based on either the C6 antibody (SNAP test) or the quantitative C6 antibody test.

Indirect Fluorescent Antibody (IFA)

Normal:
Values vary among laboratories. A negative titer is normal and indicates no exposure to *B. burgdorferi* or recent vaccination.
Patient Preparation:
None.
Collect:
Whole blood, 2.0 mL, in red-topped tube.
Submit:
Serum, 1.0 mL.
Interpretation:
Titers performed by IFA may not distinguish between vaccinated and infected dogs. Lyme borreliosis titers performed by IFA are only indicated in dogs that have NOT been vaccinated against Lyme disease. Lyme borreliosis vaccination can result in a positive titer. Dogs with a positive test result should be subjected to either the Western blot analysis or the quantitative C6 antibody test (preferred).
Interference:
Prior vaccination against Lyme disease can result in a positive test result.

Western Blot Analysis

Normal:
Values vary among laboratories. A negative test result is normal and indicates NO exposure to *B. burgdorferi*.
Patient Preparation:
None.
Collect:
Whole blood, 2.0 mL, in red-topped tube.

Submit:
Serum, 1.0 mL.
Interpretation:
Titers may distinguish between vaccinated and infected dogs. Western blot analysis is indicated for dogs that have a positive IFA titer, as an alternative test.
Interference:
Prior vaccination with a whole-cell, killed *B. burgdorferi* vaccine may complicate interpretation of the Western blot analysis.

RABIES TITER (BY RFFIT)

RFFIT= rapid fluorescent focus inhibition test.
Normal:
Dog and cat: A titer of 0.5 IU/mL or higher is usually required for animals exported to most rabies-free areas. NOTE: it may to necessary to contact individual countries for current import requirements prior to shipping animals.
Patient Preparation:
None.
Collect:
Whole blood, 4.0 mL, in red-topped tube.
Submit:
Serum, 2.0 mL (minimum is 500 µL), in a leak-proof container (e.g., with screw-on cap). Place sample container should be placed inside a second container with gel packs or dry ice. Overnight shipping is recommended.
Interpretation:
As stipulated by the laboratory. NOTE: Values for a "protective titer" in animals have not been established.
Interference:
Gross hemolysis; lipemia; samples other than serum (e.g., plasma is NOT acceptable). **NOTE:** Other causes for sample to be rejected include insufficient quantity of serum, bacterial contamination of sample, and unlabeled sample.
Protocol:
Samples may be sent to: Rabies Laboratory/RFFIT, Mosier Hall, Kansas State University, 1800 Denison Avenue, Manhattan, KS 66506-5600 (Tel. 785-532-4483).
NOTE: For samples sent to Kansas State University:
1. All specimen tubes must be labeled with the patient's name and/or identification number. Samples submitted without labels will not be accepted.
2. All samples must have an accompanying RFFIT submission form.
3. All animals being tested for export must have a microchip number (or tattoo) included.
   Forms may be downloaded from the KSU Rabies Laboratory website: www.vet.ksu. edu/rabies

5

ROCKY MOUNTAIN SPOTTED FEVER (RMSF)

Normal:
Negative (dog and cat).
Patient Preparation:
None.
Collect:
Whole blood, 2.0 mL, in red-topped tube.
Submit:
Serum, 1.0 mL.

Interpretation:
Generally, two samples are recommended ("acute" and "convalescent"), obtained 2 to 3 weeks apart. Titers reported vary among laboratories. The laboratory performing the titer will provide recommendations for interpreting results.
Interference:
None.

TOXOPLASMOSIS TITERS (IgG AND IgM)

Normal:
See Interpretation.
Patient Preparation:
None.
Collect:
Whole blood, 2.0 mL, in red-topped tube.
Submit:
Serum, 1.0 mL.

Interpretation:
A positive titer denotes exposure, not active infection. IgG and IgM titers typically are reported individually. A titer >1:256 for IgM is consistent with active infection in patients with clinical signs (e.g., pneumonia in cats, myositis in dogs). It is recommended that two samples for IgG titer be submitted; samples should be collected 2 to 3 weeks apart. A fourfold or greater rise in titer within 2 to 3 weeks is supportive of the diagnosis of active infection. Cats seropositive on a single titer are unlikely to be shedding oocysts.
Interference:
Hemolysis; lipemia.

VACCINE TITERS: SEE LISTING UNDER SPECIFIC PATHOGEN

Laboratories providing vaccine titers typically limit these services to canine parvovirus, canine distemper, and feline panleukopenia. A limited number of laboratories offer titers for feline herpesvirus-1 and feline calicivirus.

Note: Several university and commercial laboratories now provide antibody titers for selected canine and feline viruses as a means of assessing immunity to prior vaccination.

Note: National laboratory standards for determining serum antibody titers against these pathogens have not been established. Because methods for performing titers vary among laboratories, titer results and ranges also can vary dramatically.
It is recommended that samples be analyzed by laboratories using the virus neutralization test (for canine distemper) and hemagglutination inhibition (for canine parvovirus and feline panleukopenia).

Note: A "positive" antibody titer usually will equate with "PROTECTIVE IMMUNITY"
A "negative" antibody titer does NOT necessarily equate to "SUSCEPTIBILITY"

URINE

A red-topped tube is the preferred collection tube for urinalysis. A Copan swab can be used for urine culture, but this precludes quantitation of bacteria, if present. Urine for culture is best collected by cystocentesis and transported with a cold pack to prevent bacterial overgrowth.

CORTISOL, URINE. SEE URINE CORTISOL:CREATININE RATIO (UC:CR; URINARY C:C RATIO)

MICROALBUMINURIA TEST (EARLY RENAL DISEASE (ERD) IN-HOSPITAL TEST KIT)

Normal:
Negative test strip indication (dog and cat).
Patient Preparation:
None.
Collect:
2-mL (minimum) aliquot of urine in a clean container.
Submit:
Same.
Interpretation:
Test strip indicator grades the approximate degree of microalbuminuria. The manufacturer of the test kit provides recommendations for interpreting test results. However, it should be noted that a positive test result in clinically normal dogs is NOT known to be predictive of impending renal disease. In various studies, it has been shown that a significant percentage of healthy dogs and certain breeds (soft-coated Wheaten Terriers) will have positive test results. Until more information is available about the clinical utility of this test, its use should be restricted to monitoring urine protein loss in patients with known or suspected glomerular disease.
Interference:
Blood contamination of urine sample.

URINE CORTISOL:CREATININE RATIO (UC:CR, URINARY C:C RATIO)

Normal:
Varies according to individual laboratory and test methodology used (dog and cat).
Patient Preparation:
Owner should collect urine at home on the day (morning is preferable) that the test is submitted, thereby reducing stress-induced artifact.
Collect:
3.0- to 5.0-mL aliquot of pooled urine in a sterile container.
Submit:
Same; sample should be refrigerated during transport to the laboratory.
Interpretation:
The UC:CR is reported to have high sensitivity (negative predictive value) and therefore has been recommended *to rule out the diagnosis of hyperadrenocorticism in dogs.*
Controversy exists regarding the diagnostic value of the UC:CR to diagnose canine Cushing's syndrome. Reference values for the cat are not reported. The test currently is NOT recommended as a single diagnostic test. In SERIAL UC:CR studies performed in hyperthyroid cats, elevated ratios were observed; successful treatment (medical and surgical) did result in a significant decrease in UC:CR in cats.
Interference:
The effect of urine collected from hospitalized dogs (stress) vs. urine collected from dogs at home remains an arguable variable. Owners should be advised to collect urine at home on the scheduled day of examination/testing.

5

Protocol:
Instruct the owner to collect urine in a single, clean container over 2 consecutive hours on the same day that the urine sample is to be submitted to the laboratory. A 3.0- to 5.0-mL aliquot of pooled urine is submitted for analysis. NOTE: Not all commercial laboratories offer this test. Check before submitting.

URINE PROTEIN-CREATININE RATIO (UPCr; P:Cr; UPC)

Normal:
Ratio <0.3 (dog); ratio <0.6 (cat).
Patient Preparation:
None.
Collect:
2- to 3-mL aliquot of randomly collected urine in a clean container.
Submit:
Same.
Interpretation:
UP:Cr titer >1.0 is consistent with the diagnosis of pathologic proteinuria. The ratio does not confirm the source of the protein loss. However, in patients with consistent hypoalbuminemia and significantly elevated urine P:Cr, loss of protein through the glomerulus is likely (e.g., glomerulonephritis).
Interference:
Blood contamination (cystitis, cystocentesis).

5

Charts and Tables

Emergency Hotlines, *644*
Dog Breeds Recognized by the American Kennel Club (AKC), *645*
Cat Breeds Recognized by the Cat Fanciers' Association (CFA), *647*
Useful Information for Rodents and Rabbits, *648*
Determination of the Sex of Mature and Immature Rodents and Rabbits, *650*
Blood Values and Serum Chemical Constituents for Rodents and Rabbits, *651*
Ferrets—Physiologic, Anatomic, and Reproductive Data, *652*
Hematologic Values for Normal Ferrets, *652*
Serum Chemistry Values for Normal Ferrets, *653*
Electrocardiographic Data for Normal Ferrets, *653*
Conversion of Body Weight in Kilograms to Body Surface Area in Meters Squared for Dogs, *654*
Conversion of Body Weight in Kilograms to Body Surface Area in Meters Squared for Cats, *654*
French Scale Conversion Table, *655*
International System of Units (SI) Conversion Guide, *656*
Units of Length, Volume, and Mass in the Metric System, *659*
Annualized Vaccination Protocols and Criteria Defining Risk for the Dog and Cat, *660*
Types of Vaccines Licensed for Use in Dogs in the United States, *661*
Types of Vaccines Licensed for Use in Cats in the United States, *662*
Annualized Vaccination Protocol for Dogs at Moderate Risk, *663*
Annualized Vaccination Protocol for Dogs at Low Risk, *665*
Annualized Vaccination Protocol for Dogs at High Risk, *667*
Annualized Vaccination Protocol for Cats at Moderate Risk, *669*
Annualized Vaccination Protocol for Cats at Low Risk, *670*
Annualized Vaccination Protocol for Cats at High Risk, *671*
Compendium of Animal Rabies Prevention and Control, 2005, National Association Of State
   Public Health Veterinarians, Inc. (NASPHV), *674*
Prescription Writing Reference…Do's and Don'ts, *684*
Common Drug Indications and Dosages, *685*

TABLE 6-1   Emergency Hotlines

Need	Agency	Phone number
To obtain information regarding the treatment of a known or suspected poisoning/toxicosis case.	ASPCA Animal Poison Control Center ($50 fee for service may apply)	888-426-4435
To report known or suspected adverse drug *(not vaccine)* reactions.	Food & Drug Administration (FDA) Center for Veterinary Medicine (CVM)	888-332-8387 (voice messages accepted)
To report shortages of medically necessary veterinary drugs.	Food & Drug Administration (FDA) Center for Veterinary Medicine (CVM)	301-827-4570 or 888-463-6332
To report known or suspected adverse vaccine reactions.	US Dept of Agriculture (USDA) Center for Veterinary Biologics (Also, contact vaccine manufacturer directly. NOTE: this is for reporting purposes *only*; adverse event information on a specific product is usually not provided.)	800-752-6255
For inquiries on transfusion medicine (no charge).	Animal Blood Bank HOTLINE	800-243-5759 (24-hour)
For inquiries on transfusion medicine and purchase of blood and blood components.	Eastern Veterinary Blood Bank	800-949-3822 (24-hour)
For inquiries on access to blood and blood products for all species.	Midwest Animal Blood Services	517-851-8244 (24 hour)
For inquiries on transfusion medicine—a full-service, nonprofit blood bank and educational network for animals	HEMOPET	714-891-2022 (24-hour)
Access to a commercial blood bank and purchase of blood and blood components.	Veterinarians' Blood Bank	812-358-8500
For inquiries on pesticides, pesticide products, poisonings and toxicities.	National Pesticide Information Center	800-858-7378 npic@ace.orst.edu
For inquiries on pet shipping regulations and regulations for shipping pets on airlines	US Dept of Agriculture (USDA) (voice response service)	800-545-8732
To contact the Office of Diversion Control of the DEA	Drug Enforcement Agency	800-882-9539

6

TABLE 6-2 Dog Breeds Recognized by the American Kennel Club (AKC)

The American Kennel Club (AKC) currently recognizes 150 dog breeds, each of which is assigned to one of 7 breed groups. The AKC maintains an excellent website offering considerable information on individual breeds (see http://www.akc.org/breeds/index.cfm)

Sporting group
American Water Spaniel
Brittany Spaniel
Chesapeake Bay Retriever
Clumber Spaniel
Cocker Spaniel
Curly-Coated Retriever
English Cocker Spaniel
English Setter
English Springer Spaniel
Field Spaniel
Flat-Coated Retriever
German Shorthaired Pointer
German Wirehaired Pointer
Golden Retriever
Gordon Setter
Irish Setter
Irish Water Spaniel
Labrador Retriever
Nova Scotia Duck Tolling Retriever
Pointer
Spinone Italiano
Sussex Spaniel
Vizsla
Weimaraner
Welsh Springer Spaniel
Wirehaired Pointing Griffon

Hound group
Afghan Hound
American Foxhound
Basenji
Basset Hound
Beagle
Black and Tan Coonhound
Bloodhound
Borzoi
Dachshund
English Foxhound
Greyhound
Harrier
Ibizan Hound
Irish Wolfhound
Norwegian Elkhound
Otterhound
Petit Basset Griffon Vendéen
Pharaoh Hound
Rhodesian Ridgeback

Saluki
Scottish Deerhound
Whippet

Working group
Akita
Alaskan Malamute
Anatolian Shepherd Dog
Bernese Mountain Dog
Black Russian Terrier
Boxer
Bullmastiff
Doberman Pinscher
German Pinscher
Giant Schnauzer
Great Dane
Great Pyrenees
Greater Swiss Mountain Dog
Komondor
Kuvasz
Mastiff
Neapolitan Mastiff
Newfoundland
Portuguese Water Dog
Rottweiler
Saint Bernard
Samoyed
Siberian Husky
Standard Schnauzer

Terrier group
Airedale Terrier
American Staffordshire Terrier
Australian Terrier
Bedlington Terrier
Border Terrier
Bull Terrier
Cairn Terrier
Dandie Dinmont Terrier
Irish Terrier
Kerry Blue Terrier
Lakeland Terrier
Manchester Terrier (Standard)
Miniature Bull Terrier
Miniature Schnauzer
Norfolk Terrier
Norwich Terrier
Parson Russell Terrier
Scottish Terrier

6

Continued

TABLE 6-2 Dog Breeds Recognized by the American Kennel Club (AKC)—cont'd

Sealyham Terrier
Skye Terrier
Smooth Fox Terrier
Soft Coated Wheaten Terrier
Staffordshire Bull Terrier
Welsh Terrier
West Highland White Terrier
Wire Fox Terrier

Toy group
Affenpinscher
Brussels Griffon
Cavalier King Charles Spaniel
Chihuahua
Chinese Crested
English Toy Spaniel
Havanese
Italian Greyhound
Japanese Chin
Maltese
Manchester Terrier (Toy)
Miniature Pinscher
Papillon
Pekingese
Pomeranian
Pug
Shih Tzu
Silky Terrier
Toy Fox Terrier
Yorkshire Terrier

Non-sporting group
American Eskimo Dog
Bichon Frise
Boston Terrier
Bulldog
Chinese Shar-pei
Chow Chow

Dalmatian
Finnish Spitz
French Bulldog
Keeshond
Lhasa Apso
Löwchen
Poodle
Schipperke
Shiba Inu
Tibetan Spaniel
Tibetan Terrier

Herding group
Australian Cattle Dog
Australian Shepherd
Bearded Collie
Belgian Malinois
Belgian Sheepdog
Belgian Tervuren
Border Collie
Bouvier des Flandres
Briard
Canaan Dog
Cardigan Welsh Corgi
Collie
German Shepherd Dog
Old English Sheepdog
Pembroke Welsh Corgi
Polish Lowland Sheepdog
Puli
Shetland Sheepdog

Miscellaneous class
Beauceron
Glen of Imaal Terrier
Plott
Redbone Coonhound

6

TABLE 6-3 Cat Breeds Recognized by the Cat Fanciers' Association (CFA)

The Cat Fanciers' Association (CFA) presently recognizes 37 pedigreed breeds for showing in the Championship Class, and 4 breeds as Miscellaneous. For additional information on individual breeds on the CFA website, see http://www.cfainc.org/breeds.html.

Championship class
- Abyssinian
- American Curl
- American Shorthair
- American Wirehair
- Balinese
- Birman
- Bombay
- British Shorthair
- Burmese
- Chartreux
- Colorpoint Shorthair
- Cornish Rex
- Devon Rex
- Egyptian Mau
- European Burmese
- Exotic
- Havana Brown
- Japanese Bobtail
- Javanese
- Korat
- Maine Coon
- Manx
- Norwegian Forest Cat
- Ocicat
- Oriental
- Persian
- Ragdoll
- Russian Blue
- Scottish Fold
- Selkirk Rex
- Siamese
- Singapura
- Somali
- Sphynx
- Tonkinese
- Turkish Angora
- Turkish Van

Miscellaneous
- American Bobtail
- LaPerm
- RagaMuffin
- Siberian

6

POCKET PETS - PHYSIOLOGICAL DATA (TABLES 6-4 TO 6-10)

T A B L E   6 - 4   Useful Information for Rodents and Rabbits

	Hamster	Rabbit	Mouse	Rat	Gerbil	Guinea pig
Weight at birth	2 g	100 g	1.5 g	5.5 g	3 g	100 g
Puberty	(F) 28–31 days (M) 45 days (best to breed 70 days)	4–9 mo	35 days	50–60 days	(F) 3–5 mo (M) 10–12 wk	(F) 20–30 days (M) 70 days
Duration of estrous cycle*	4 days	Ovulation not spontaneous; stimulated by copulation; doe ovulates 10–13 hr after	4 days	4 days	4 days	16 days
Gestation (days)	16	28–36	19–21	21–23	24	62–72
Separation of adults during parturition and weaning	Yes	Yes	No	No	No (mates for life)	No
Number per liter	4–10	7	10	8–10	1–12	1–4
Eyes open	15 days	10 days	11–14 days	14–17 days	16–20 days	Prior to birth
Wean at	25 days	42–56 days	21 days	21 days	21 days	14–21 days or 160 g
Postpartum estrus	Within 24 hr	14 days	Within 24–48 hr	Within 24–48 hr	Within 24–72 hr	Within 24 hr
Breeding life	11–18 mo	1–3 years (max. 6 yr)	12–18 mo	14 mo	15–20 mo	3–4 yr
Adult weight	(F) 120 g (M) 108 g	(F) 4.0 kg (M) 4.3 kg	(F) 30 g (M) 39 g	(F) 300 g (M) 500 g	(F) 75 g (M) 85 g	(F) 850 g (M) 1000 g
Life span (yr)	2–3	5–7	3.0–3.5	3	4	4–5
Body temperature	97°–101°F (36.1°–38.3°C)	101°–103.2°F (38.3°–39.5°C)	96.4°–100°F (35.8°–37.7°C)	99.5°–100.6°F (37.5°–38.1°C)	100.8°F (32.8°C)	100.4°–102.5°F (38–39.2°C)

6

Daily adult water consumption	8–12 mL/day	80 mL/kg body weight	3–3.5 mL/day	20–30 mL/day	4 mL/day	10 mL/100 g body weight
Daily adult food consumption (varies with age and condition)	7–12 g/day	100–150 g/day	2.5–4.0 g/day	20–40 g/day	10–15 g/day	30–35 g/day
Diet	Commercial rat, mouse, or hamster chow supplemented with kale,† cabbage,† apples, milk	Commercial rabbit pellets, greens in moderation	Commercial mouse chow	Commercial rat or mouse chow	Commercial mouse or rat chow (lowest fat possible); sunflower seeds	Commercial guinea pig chow, good-quality hay, kale, cabbage, fruits (cannot rely on vitamin C levels of commercial ration)
Room temperature	65°–75°F (18.3°–24°C)	62°–68°F (17°–20°C)	70°–80°F (21°–27°C)	76°–18°F (24.5°–25.5°C)	65°–80°F (18.3°–26.6°C)	65°–75°F (18.3°–24°C)
Humidity (%)	50	50	50	50	<50	50

* All species listed except rabbits are seasonally polyestrous.
† Better source of vitamin C than lettuce.
From Schuchman SM: Individual care and treatment of rabbits, mice, rats, guinea pigs, hamsters, and gerbils. *In* Kirk RW, ed: Current Veterinary Therapy X. Philadelphia, WB Saunders, 1989, p 739.

6

T A B L E   6 - 5   Determination of the Sex of Mature and Immature Rodents and Rabbits

Mature hamsters, mice, rats, guinea pigs, and gerbils

Male	Female
1. Anogenital distance longer in the male	1. Anogenital distance shorter in the female.
2. Manipulate "genital papilla" (prepuce) to protrude penis.	2. Look for the three external openings in the inguinal area:
3. Palpate for testicles either in a scrotal sac (if present) or subcutaneous in inguinal region.	a. Anus (most caudal opening).
	b. Vaginal orifice (middle opening) – look carefully.
4. Males have only two external openings in the inguinal area:	c. Urethral orifice at tip of urethral papilla (most anterior opening).
a. Anus	In these animals the urethral papilla is located
b. Urethral orifice at tip of penis.	outside the vagina (unlike dogs and cats).
In very fat males there may be a depression between the penis and anus. This depression can be obliterated by manipulating the skin in this area.	In very fat females or young females, the vaginal orifice may be either hidden by folds of skin (the former) or sealed (latter). Gentle manipulation of the skin in this area will divulge the orifice.

Mature rabbits

Male	Female
1. Protrude penis by manipulating skin of prepuce.	1. There is a common orifice for both the vagina and urethra (like dogs and cats).
2. Palpate for testicles.	2. No. structure like a "penis" can be protruded from the urogenital orifice.
3. Anogenital distance is longer.	3. Anogenital distance is shorter

From Schuchman SM: Individual care and treatment of rabbits, mice, rats, guinea pigs, hamsters, and gerbils. *In* Kirk RW, ed: Current Veterinary Therapy X. Philadelphia, WB Saunders, 1989, p 740.

6

TABLE 6-6 Blood Values and Serum Chemical Constituents for Rodents and Rabbits

Laboratory test	Rats	Mice	Hamsters	Guinea pigs	Rabbits	Mangolian gerbils
AST (Sigma-Frankel units)	25–42	32–41	22–36	10–25	14–27	–
Alkaline phosphatase (Bodansky units)	4.1–8.6	2.4–4.0	2.0–3.5	1.5–8.1	2.1–3.2	–
BUN (mg/dL)	10–20	8–30	10–40	8–20	5–30	18–24
Sodium (mEq/L)	144	114–154	106–185	120–155	100–145	144–158
Potassium (mEq/L)	5.9	3.0–9.6	2.3–9.8	6.5–8.2	3.0–7.0	3.8–5.2
Bilirubin, total (mg/dL)	0.42	0.18–0.54	0.3–0.4	0.24–0.30	0.15–0.20	–
Blood glucose (mg/dL)	50–115	108–192	32.6–118.4	60–125	50–140	69–119
RBCs (10^6 cells/mm³)	7.2–9.6	9.3–10.5	4.0–9.3	4.5–7.0	3.2–7.5	8.3–9.3
Hemoglobin (g/dL)	14.8	12–14.9	9.7–16.8	11–15	10–15	10–16
Hematocrit (%)	40–50	35–50	40–52	35–50	35–45	35–45
WBCs (10^3 cells/mm³)	8–14	8–14	7–15	5–12	8–10	9–14
Segmented (%)	30	26	16–28	42	30–50	10–20
Nonsegmented (%)	0	0	8	0	0	
Lymphocytes (%)	65–77	55–80	64–78	45–81	30–50	70–89
Eosinophils (%)	1	3	1	5	1	1
Monocytes (%)	4	5	2	8	9	0
Basophils (%)	0	0	0	2	0	0

AST, aspartate aminotransferase; *BUN*, blood urea nitrogen; *RBCs*, red blood cells; *WBCs*, white blood cells.
*These are values found in healthy-appearing animals and can be used as guides but should not be interpreted as physiologic norms for the species listed. Modified from Schuchman SM: Individual care and treatment of rabbits, mice, rats, guinea pigs, hamsters, and gerbils. *In* Kirk RW, ed: Current Veterinary Therapy X. Philadelphia, WB Saunders, 1989, p 746.

6

TABLE 6-7 Ferrets—Physiologic, Anatomic, and Reproductive Data

Data	Range or value
Physiologic data	
Life span	5–9 yr (average 5–7)
Commercial breeding life	2–5 yr
Body temperature	101°–104°F (38°-40°C)
Respiratory rate	32–36 breaths/min
Heart rate	220–250 bpm (average 240)
Water consumption	75–100 mL/day
Chromosome number	2n = 40
Anatomical data	
Dental formula	2 (I3/3, C1/1, P3/4, M1/2)
Vertebral formula	C-7, T-14, L-6, S-3, Cd-14–Cd-18
Reproductive data	
Gestation	39–46 days (average 42)
Litter size	2–17 kits (average 8)
False pregnancy	40–42 days
Placentation	Zonal
Implantation time	12–31 days
Weaning	5–6 wk
Ovulation	30–40 hr post coitus

From Randolph RW: Medical and surgical care of the pet ferret. *In* Kirk RW, ed: Current Veterinary Therapy X. Philadelphia, WB Saunders, 1989, p 766.

TABLE 6-8 Hematologic Values for Normal Ferrets*

Laboratory test	Mean	Range
Hematocrit (%)	52.3	42–61
Hemoglobin (g/dL)	17.0	15–18
RBCs (10^6 cells/mm^3)	9.17	6.8–12.2
WBCs (10^3 cells/mm^3)	10.1	4.0–19
WBCs		
Lymphocytes (%)	34.5	12–54
Neutrophils (%)	58.3	11–84
Monocytes (%)	4.4	0–9.0
Eosinophils (%)	2.5	0–7.0
Basophils (%)	0.1	0–2.0
Reticulocytes (%)	4.6	1–14
Platelets (10^3 cells/mm^3)	499	297–910
Total protein (g/dL)	6.0	5.1–7.4

*Values are for both sexes.
From Ryland L, Bernard S, Gorham J: A clinical guide to the pet ferret. Compend Contin Educ Pract Vet 5:25, 1983, which was adapted from Thornton, et al: Lab Anim 13:119, 1979.

6

TABLE 6-9 Serum Chemistry Values for Normal Ferrets*

Analyte	Unit	Mean	Range
Glucose	mg/dL	136	94–207
BUN	mg/dL	22	10–45
Albumin	mg/dL	3.2	2.3–3.8
Alkaline phosphatase	IU/L	23	9–84
AST	IU/L	65	28–120
Total bilirubin	mg/dL	<1.0	
Cholesterol	mg/dL	165	64–296
Creatinine	mg/dL	0.6	0.4–0.9
Sodium	mEq/L	148	137–162
Potassium	mEq/L	5.9	4.5–7.7
Chloride	mEq/L	116	106–125
Calcium	mg/dL	9.2	8.0–11.8
Phosphorus	mg/dL	5.9	4.0–9.1

BUN, blood urea nitrogen; *AST*, aspartate aminotransferase.
*Values for both sexes.
From Ryland L, Bernard S, Gorham J: A clinical guide to the pet ferret. Compend Contin Educ Pract Vet 5:25, 1983, which was adapted from Thornton, et al: Lab Anim 13:119, 1979.

TABLE 6-10 Electrocardiographic Data for Normal Ferrets*

Parameter	Mean	Range
Rate rhythm	224 ± 51	150–340
Normal sinus rhythm		
Sinus arrhythmia		
Measurements		
P wave		
Width	0.03 ± 0.009	0.015–0.04 s
Height	0.106 ± 0.03	0.05–0.20 mV
P–R interval		
Width	0.05 ± 0.01	0.04–0.08 s
QRS complex		
Q wave	Usually none	
R wave		
Width	0.049 ± 0.008	0.04–0.06 s
Height	1.59 ± 0.63	0.6–3.15 mV
S wave		
Height	0.166 ± 0.101	0.1–0.25 mV
S–T segment		
Width	0.030 ± 0.016	0.01–0.06 s
Q–T interval		
Width	0.13 ± 0.027	0.10–0.18 s
T wave		
Width	0.06 ± 0.01	0.03–0.1 s
Height	0.24 ± 0.12	0.10–0.45 mV
Mean electrical axis (frontal plane)		+65–100 degrees

6

*Ferrets in right lateral recumbency; sedation with ketamine and xylazine.

TABLE 6-11 Conversion of Body Weight in Kilograms to Body Surface Area in Meters Squared for Dogs

Kg	M²	Kg	M²
0.50	0.06	26.00	0.88
1.00	0.10	27.00	0.90
2.00	0.15	28.00	0.92
3.00	0.20	29.00	0.94
4.00	0.25	30.00	0.96
5.00	0.29	31.00	0.99
6.00	0.33	32.00	1.01
7.00	0.36	33.00	1.03
8.00	0.40	34.00	1.05
9.00	0.43	35.00	1.07
10.00	0.46	36.00	1.09
11.00	0.49	37.00	1.11
12.00	0.52	38.00	1.13
13.00	0.55	39.00	1.15
14.00	0.58	40.00	1.17
15.00	0.60	41.00	1.19
16.00	0.63	42.00	1.21
17.00	0.66	43.00	1.23
18.00	0.69	44.00	1.25
19.00	0.71	45.00	1.26
20.00	0.74	46.00	1.28
21.00	0.76	47.00	1.30
22.00	0.78	48.00	1.32
23.00	0.81	49.00	1.34
24.00	0.83	50.00	1.36
25.00	0.85		

TABLE 6-12 Conversion of Body Weight in Kilograms to Body Surface Area in Meters Squared for Cats

Kg	M²
0.50	0.06
1.00	0.10
1.50	0.12
2.00	0.15
2.50	0.17
3.00	0.20
3.50	0.22
4.00	0.24
4.50	0.26
5.00	0.28
5.50	0.29
6.00	0.31
6.50	0.33
7.00	0.34
7.50	0.36
8.00	0.38
8.50	0.39
9.00	0.41
9.50	0.42
10.00	0.44

6

TABLE 6-13 French Scale Conversion Table

The standard French, or Charrière, scale (abbreviated F or Fr) is generally used in the size calibration of catheters and other tubular instruments. It is based on the metric system, with each unit being approximately 0.33 mm, with a difference of 0.33 mm in diameter between consecutive sizes. Example: 27F indicates a diameter of 9 mm; 30F, a diameter of 10 mm.

A convenient conversion table from the French scale to the English and American scales that is sometimes used for certain instruments is given below.

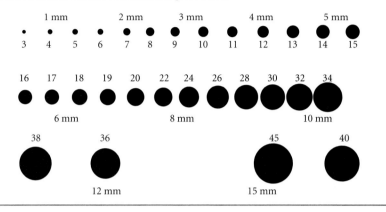

TABLE 6-14 International System of Units (SI) Conversion Guide*

Analyte	Fluid	Traditional units	Conversion Factor Multiply (×)→ ←Divide (÷)	SI units
ACTH (adrenocorticotropin; corticotropin)	Plasma	pg/mL	0.2202	pmol/L
ALT (alanine aminotransferase; SGPT)	Serum	mg/dL	1	U/L
Albumin	Serum	g/dl	10	g/L
Aldosterone	Serum	ng/dL	27.74	pmol/L
Ammonia (NH_3)	Plasma	μg/dL	0.5872	μmol/L
Ammonium (NH_4^+)	Plasma	μg/dL	0.5543	μmol/L
Amylase	Serum	units/L	1	U/L
Antibodies	Serum	Highest possible dilution	1	Highest possible dilution
AST (aspartate aminotransferase; SGOT)	Serum	units/L	1	U/L
Bile acids (total)	Serum	μg/mL	2.547	μmol/L
Bilirubin (total)	Serum	mg/dL	17.1	μmol/L
Blood gases:	Arterial blood			
P_{CO_2}		mm Hg	0.1333	kPa
pH		pH units	1	pH units
P_{O_2}		mm Hg	0.1333	kPa
BUN (blood urea nitrogen)	Serum	mg/dL	0.357	mmol/L of urea
Calcium	Serum	mg/dL	0.250	mmol/L
Calcium, ionized (iCa)	Serum, plasma	mEq/L	0.500	mmol/L
CBC (complete blood count):	Whole blood			
Hematocrit		%	0.01	as a fraction of 1
Hemoglobin		g/dL	10	g/L
MCH (mean corpuscular hemoglobin)		pg	1	pg
MCHC (mean corpuscular hemoglobin concentration)		g/dL	10	g/L
			1	

Test	Specimen	Conventional Units	Conversion Factor	SI Units
MCV (mean corpuscular volume)		um²	1	fL
Platelet count		10³/mm³	1	10⁹/L
Reticulocyte count		No. per 1000 RBCs	0.001	as a fraction of 1
Reticulocyte count		As a %	0.01	as a fraction of 1
Differential cell count				
Neutrophils (segmented)		cells/mm³ (µL)	1	10⁶ cells/L
Neutrophils (band)		cells/mm³	1	
Lymphocytes		cells/mm³	1	
Monocytes		cells/mm³	1	
Eosinophils		cells/mm³	1	
Basophils		cells/mm³	1	
Cholesterol (total)	Serum	mg/dL	0.02586	mmol/L
CK (creatine kinase)	Serum	Units/L	1	U/L
Cortisol	Serum, plasma	µg/dL	27.59	nmol/L
Cortisol (free)	Urine	µg/24 hours	2.759	nmol/day
Creatinine	Serum	mg/dL	88.4	µmol/L
Electrolytes				
Chloride	Serum	mEq/L	1	mmol/L
CO_2 (bicarbonate)	Whole blood	mEq/L	1	mmol/L
Potassium	Serum	mEq/L	1	mmol/L
Sodium	Serum	mEq/L	1	mmol/L
Fibrinogen (coagulation factor I)	Plasma	g/dL	29.41	µmol/L
		or mg/dL	0.01	g/L
Fibrin (fibrin degradation products)	Serum	µg/mL	1	mg/L
GGT (gamma glutamyl transferase)	Serum	Units/L	1	U/L
Glucose	Serum	mg/dL	0.05551	mmol/L
Insulin	Serum	µU/ml	7.175	pmol/L
		mU/L	7.175	pmol/L
		µg/L	172.2	pmol/L

6

Continued

TABLE 6-14   International System of Units (SI) Conversion Guide*—cont'd

Analyte	Fluid	Traditional units	Conversion Factor Multiply ($\times$)$\rightarrow$ $\leftarrow$Divide ($\div$)	SI units
Lead	Plasma	µg/dL	0.04826	µmol/L
		mg/dL	48.26	µmol/L
Lipase	Serum	units/L	1	U/L
Magnesium	Serum	mg/dL	0.4114	mmol/L
		mEq/L	0.500	mmol/L
Phosphorus	Serum	mg/dL	0.3229	mmol/L
Plasminogen	Plasma	%	0.01	as a fraction of 1
Protein (total)	Serum	g/dL	10	g/L
Protein (spinal fluid)	CSF	mg/dL	0.01	g/L
PT (prothrombin time)	Plasma	seconds	1	seconds
PTT (partial thromboplastin time)	Plasma	seconds	1	seconds
Thyroid tests:				
TSH (thyroid-stimulating hormone)	Serum	µU/mL	1	mU/L
T_4 (thyroxine)	Serum	µg/dL	12.87	nmol/L
Thyroxine, free T_4	Serum	ng/dL	12.87	pmol/L
T_3 (triiodothyronine)	Serum	ng/dL	0.01536	nmol/L

*Presented in alphabetical order.

TABLE 6-15 Units of Length, Volume, and Mass in the Metric System

Prefix	Multiply by	Factor
milli-	0.001 (1/1000)	$\times 10^{-3}$
centi-	0.01 (1/100)	$\times 10^{-2}$
deci-	0.1 (1/10)	$\times 10^{-1}$
deka-	10	$\times 10$
hecto-	100	$\times 10^{2}$
kilo-	1000	$\times 10^{3}$

Parameter	Unit	Abbreviations
The standard unit of **volume** in the metric system is the liter.	1 milliliter = 0.001 liter	1 milliliter = 1 mL = 1 cc[1]
	1 centiliter = 0.01 liter	1 centiliter = 1 cL
	1 deciliter = 0.1 liter	1 deciliter = 1 dL
	1 liter	1 liter = 1 L
	1 kiloliter = 1000 liters	1 kiloliter = 1 kL
The standard unit of **mass** in the metric system is the gram.	1 milligram = 0.001 gram	1 milligram = 1 mg
	1 centigram = 0.01 gram	1 centigram = 1 cg
	1 decigram = 0.1 gram	1 decigram = 1 dg
	1 gram	1 gram = 1 g
	1 kilogram = 1000 grams	1 kilogram = 1 kg
The standard unit of **length** in the metric system is the meter.	1 millimeter = 0.001 meter	1 millimeter = 1 mm
	1 centimeter = 0.01 meter	1 centimeter = 1 cm
	1 meter	1 meter = 1 m
	1 decimeter = 0.1 meter	1 decimeter = 1 dm
	1 kilometer = 1000 meters	1 kilometer = 1 km

[1]1 cc (or cubic centimeter) = 1 cm^3 = 1 mL.

6

ANNUALIZED VACCINATION PROTOCOLS AND CRITERIA DEFINING RISK FOR THE DOG AND CAT

The fact that the canine and feline criteria recommend triennial vaccination for certain vaccines in no way stipulates that adult dogs and cats should *only* be vaccinated every 3 years. In fact, annual vaccination does represent a high standard of medical care, *as long as the vaccination appointment incorporates a thorough health/wellness examination.* Considering the large population of pet dogs and cats and the remarkable spectrum of risk factors for exposure to infectious pathogens, it is quite unreasonable to assume that a single vaccination protocol would be applicable in all patients seen in practice. Two of the most important variables to consider when assessing risk are the *age* of the patient and the patient's *"lifestyle."* In implementing a vaccination protocol in clinical practice, it is critical that the clinician consider these factors when recommending core, or non-core, vaccines for an individual patient.

The following tables exemplify *annualized* vaccination protocols for dogs and cats at *moderate risk* (applies to most), *high risk*, and *low risk* of exposure to infectious agents while also taking into consideration the recommendations set forth in the canine and feline criteria.

6

TABLE 6-16   Types of Vaccines Licensed for Use in Dogs in the United States

Vaccine type	Core vs. non-core	Recommended vaccination interval for administration of booster inoculations	Minimum duration of immunity
Distemper: modified live (parenteral)	Core	3 years	5+ to 7+ years (depending on strain)
Recombinant distemper (parenteral)	Core	3 years	3 years+
Distemper-measles: modified live (parenteral)	Non-core	Not indicated	Not applicable
Parvovirus: modified live (parenteral)	Core	3 years	7+ years
Parvovirus: killed (parenteral)	Non-core	Annual	1 year (studies are not available)
Coronavirus: modified live (parenteral)	NR	Not indicated	Cannot be determined
Coronavirus: killed (parenteral)	NR	Not indicated	Cannot be determined
Canine adenovirus-2: modified live (parenteral)	Core	3 years	7+ years
Canine adenovirus-2: modified live (topical)	Core	3 years	7+ years
Canine adenovirus-2: killed (parenteral)	Non-core	Annual	Unknown
Canine adenovirus-1: modified live & killed (parenteral)	NR	DO NOT USE	Unknown
Parainfluenza virus: modified live (parenteral)	Non-core	3 years	5 + years
Parainfluenza virus: modified live (topical)	Non-core	3 years	5 + years (preferred)
Bordetella bronchiseptica: killed (parenteral)	Non-core	Annual	~12 months
Bordetella bronchiseptica: avirulent live (topical)	Non-core	Annual	~12 months
Bordetella bronchiseptica: antigen extract (parenteral)	Non-core	Annual	1 year
Leptospira var. canicola	Non-core	Annual	Not definitively established (antibody titers persist for approximately
Leptospira var. icterhemorrhagiae	Non-core	Annual	3 months in dogs that seroconvert
Leptospira var. pomona	Non-core	Annual	following an initial vaccination series)
Leptospira var. grippotyphosa	Non-core	Annual	
Recombinant Lyme (parenteral)	Non-core	Annual	1 year
Lyme: killed (parenteral)	Non-core	Annual	1 year
Crotalus arrox (Rattlesnake vaccine)	Non-core	Annual or as recommended by manufacturer based on risk	Unknown (license is conditional at this writing—challenge studies in dogs have not been performed)
Giardia lamblia: killed (parenteral)	NR	Not applicable	Is not known to prevent infection
Rabies, 1-year: killed (parenteral)	Core	As defined by local/state law	3+ years
Rabies, 3-year: killed (parenteral)	Core	As defined by local/state law	3+ years

NR, Not Generally Recommended.

6

TABLE 6-17 Types of Vaccines Licensed for Use in Cats in the United States

Vaccine type	Adjuvanted vs. non-adjuvanted	Core vs. non-core	Recommended vaccination interval for administration of booster inoculations	Minimum duration of immunity
Panleukopenia: modified live (parenteral)	Non-adjuvanted	Core	3 years	7+ years
Panleukopenia: killed (parenteral)	Adjuvanted	Non-core	Annual	5+ years
Panleukopenia: modified live (topical)	Non-adjuvant	Non-core	3 years	Not known to be more than 1 year…but is likely
Herpesvirus-calicivirus: modified live (parenteral)	Non-adjuvanted	Core	3 years	5+ years
Herpesvirus-calicivirus: killed (parenteral)	Adjuvanted	Non-core	Annual	5+ years
Herpesvirus-calicivirus: modified live (topical)	Non-adjuvanted	Non-core	Annual (3 year duration of immunity is likely)	Not known…but expected to be at least 2 years
Chlamydophilia felis: killed	Adjuvanted	Non-core	Annual	1 year (maximum)
Chlamydophilia felis: live, avirulent	Non-adjuvanted	Non-core	Annual	
Recombinant feline leukemia	Non-adjuvant	Non-core*	Annual	1 year
Feline leukemia virus: killed	Adjuvanted	Non-core*	Annual	1 year
Feline immunodeficiency virus: killed	Adjuvanted	Non-core†	Annual	1 year
Feline infectious peritonitis: modified live (topical)	Non-adjuvanted	NR	Not applicable	Does not confer protective immunity
Bordetella bronchiseptica: modified live (topical)	Non-adjuvanted	Non-core	Annual	1 year
Giardia lamblia: killed (parenteral)	Adjuvanted	NR	Not applicable	Is not known to prevent infection
Microsporum canis: killed	Adjuvanted		Vaccine has been discontinued	
Recombinant rabies (parenteral)	Non-adjuvanted	Core	Annual	3 years
Rabies, 1-year: killed (parenteral)	Adjuvanted	Core	Annual	3+ years
Rabies, 3-year: killed (parenteral)	Adjuvanted	Core	3 years (as required by law)	3+ years

*Because of the high susceptibility for infection in kittens, several authors have recommended FeLV vaccine be classified as *core* through the first year of life, then *non-core* thereafter.
†The Recombinant (Transdermal) FeLV vaccine and FIV vaccine were not licensed in 2000 when the latest iteration of the feline vaccine guidelines was published. The "Non-Core" classification is the author's recommendation.

6

TABLE 6-18 **Annualized Vaccination Protocol for Dogs at Moderate Risk***

Age at vaccination	Vaccine
6-8 weeks	Distemper (MLV or recombinant)
	Parvovirus
	Adenovirus-2
	Optional:
	+ Parainfluenza virus
10-12 weeks	Distemper (MLV or recombinant)
	Parvovirus
	Adenovirus-2
	Rabies (1 dose at 12, 14, or 16 weeks)[†]
	Optional:
	+ Parainfluenza virus
	+ *B. bronchiseptica* (killed parenteral, 2 doses required, 3-4 weeks apart)[‡]
	+ Leptospirosis (serovars as indicated at 12 weeks or older)
14-16 weeks	Distemper (MLV or recombinant)
	Parvovirus
	Adenovirus-2
	Rabies (now or at 12 weeks)
	Optional:
	+ Parainfluenza virus
	+ *B. bronchiseptica* (Live-intranasal, 1 dose or the 2nd killed-parenteral dose)
	+ Leptospirosis (serovars as indicated)
+1 year	Distemper (MLV or recombinant)
	Parvovirus
	Adenovirus-2
	Rabies (booster required)
	Optional:
	+ *B. bronchiseptica* (intranasal or parenteral)
	+ Parainfluenza
	+ Leptospirosis (serovars as indicated)
+2 years	*Optional*:
	+ *B. bronchiseptica* (intranasal or parenteral)
	+ Leptospirosis (serovars as indicated)
+3 years	*Optional*:
	+ *B. bronchiseptica* (intranasal or parenteral)
	+ Leptospirosis (serovars as indicated)
+4 years	Distemper (MLV or recombinant)
	Parvovirus
	Adenovirus-2
	Rabies
	Optional:
	+ *B. bronchiseptica* (parenteral)
	+ Parainfluenza
	+ Leptospirosis (serovars as indicated)
+5 years	*Optional*:
	+ *B. bronchiseptica* (parenteral)
	+ Leptospirosis (serovars as indicated)
+6 years	*Optional*:
	+ *B. bronchiseptica* (parenteral)
	+ Leptospirosis (serovars as indicated)

6

TABLE 6-18   Annualized Vaccination Protocol for Dogs at Moderate Risk*—cont'd

Age at vaccination	Vaccine
+7 years	Distemper (MLV or recombinant)
	Parvovirus
	Adenovirus-2
	Rabies
	Optional:
	+ *B. bronchiseptica* (parenteral)
	+ Parainfluenza
	+ Leptospirosis (serovars as indicated)
Beyond 7 years	Cycle repeats as indicated

Defining criteria for MODERATE RISK-canine (applies to most dogs)

1. *B. bronchiseptica* vaccination is indicated if:
   - Dog is ever boarded in a commercial kennel, or
   - Dog requires occasional grooming, or
   - Dog regularly has supervised walks/runs outside with likelihood of contact with other dogs.
2. Parainfluenza vaccination is indicated if:
   - Dog is ever boarded in a commercial kennel, or
   - Dog requires occasional grooming, or
   - Dog regularly has supervised walks/runs outside with likelihood of contact with other dogs.
   - NOTE: Parainfluenza vaccine is combined with all intranasal *B. bronchiseptica* vaccines.
3. *Leptospira* vaccination is indicated if:
   - The dog is 12 weeks of age or older, and
   - Dog has opportunities for unsupervised outdoor activities, or
   - Cases of leptospirosis are known to have been confirmed in the area, or
   - Dog has access (supervised or otherwise) to areas inhabited by "reservoir" hosts (eg: opossum, skunk, raccoon, vole) or other domestic animals such as cattle or pigs (horses).
   - NOTE: risk of exposure is *not* limited to rural areas.
4. Lyme borreliosis vaccination is not indicated unless:
   - Dog will travel to known endemic areas (Northeastern US or upper Midwest) and will spend time outside, or
   - Lyme borreliosis cases have been diagnosed (via IDEXX Snap 3Dx or Western Blot analysis) in the community, or
   - Dog is not receiving any form of topical tick preventative (eg, fipronil).

*For any vaccine preceded by "+," see defining criteria.
†In some states or municipalities, annual rabies vaccination may be required.
‡All intranasal *B. bronchiseptica* vaccines also contain parainfluenza virus; some also contain canine adenovirus-2.
MLV, modified live virus.

6

TABLE 6-19 Annualized Vaccination Protocol for Dogs at Low Risk*

Age at vaccination	Vaccine
6-8 weeks	Distemper (MLV or recombinant) Parvovirus Adenovirus-2 *Optional:* + Parainfluenza virus

10-12 weeks	Distemper (MLV or recombinant)
	Parvovirus
	Adenovirus-2
	  Rabies (1 dose at 12, 14, or 16 weeks)[†]
	Optional:
	  + Parainfluenza virus

14-16 weeks	Distemper (MLV or recombinant)
	Parvovirus
	Adenovirus-2
	  Rabies (now or at 12 weeks)
	Optional:
	  + Parainfluenza virus

+1 year	Distemper (MLV or recombinant) Parvovirus Adenovirus-2 Rabies (required in most states) *Optional:* + Parainfluenza
+2 years	Health examination Non-core vaccines considered if risk assessment changes
+3 years	Health examination Non-core vaccines considered if risk assessment changes
+4 years	Distemper (MLV or recombinant) Parvovirus Adenovirus-2 Rabies (required in most states) *Optional:* + Parainfluenza
+5 years	Health examination Non-core vaccines considered if risk assessment changes
+6 years	Health examination Non-core vaccines considered if risk assessment changes

+7 years	Distemper
	Parvovirus
	Adenovirus-2
	  Rabies (required in most states)
	Optional:
	  + Parainfluenza

Beyond 7 years	Cycle repeats as indicated

6

TABLE 6-19 **Annualized Vaccination Protocol for Dogs at Low Risk*—cont'd**

Defining criteria for LOW RISK-canine
(only CORE vaccines need be administered)

1. *B. bronchiseptica* is NOT indicated because:
   - Dog is never boarded in a commercial kennel.
   - Grooming is not an issue.
   - Dog lives exclusively indoors.
   - Dog has no exposure to other dogs (does occur...but is rare)

2. Parainfluenza vaccination is indicated if:
   - Dog is ever boarded in a commercial kennel, or
   - Dog requires occasional grooming, or
   - Dog regularly has supervised walks/runs outside with likelihood of contact with other dogs.
   - NOTE: Parainfluenza vaccine is combined with all intranasal *B. bronchiseptica vaccines.*

3. *Leptospira canicola, L. icterohemorrhagiae, L. pomona, and L. grippotyphosa* are NOT indicated because:
   - There is NO exposure to other dogs.
   - There is NO opportunity for unsupervised outdoor activities.
   - The dog lives exclusively indoors.
   - Leptospirosis is not known to occur in the area.

3. **Lyme borreliosis is NOT indicated because**:
   - Dog does not reside in a known Lyme borreliosis endemic area.
   - Dog does not travel to known endemic areas.
   - Dog neither lives in or travels into a known tick-vector area.
   - Dog is reliably treated with topical flea/tick preparation.
   - Dog has never known a tick and never will.

---

*For any vaccine preceded by "+,"see defining criteria.
†All intranasal *B. bronchiseptica* vaccines also contain parainfluenza virus; some also contain canine adenovirus-2.
‡In some states or municipalities, annual rabies vaccination may be required.
MLV, modified live virus.

6

TABLE 6-20 Annualized Vaccination Protocol for Dogs at High Risk*

Age at vaccination	Vaccine
6-8 weeks	Distemper (recombinant) Parvovirus Adenovirus-2 Parainfluenza *B. bronchiseptica* [intranasal recommended]†
10-12 weeks	Distemper (recombinant) Parvovirus Adenovirus-2 Parainfluenza Rabies (at 12, 14, or 16 weeks)‡ *B. bronchiseptica* [*intranasal* recommended] *Optional*: + Leptospirosis + Lyme borreliosis (recombinant)
14-16 weeks	Distemper (recombinant) Parvovirus Adenovirus-2 Parainfluenza *B. bronchiseptica* [intranasal recommended] Rabies (now or at 12 weeks) *Optional*: + Leptospirosis + Lyme borreliosis (recombinant)
+1 year	Distemper (MLV or recombinant) Parvovirus Adenovirus-2 Parainfluenza *B. bronchiseptica* (intranasal or parenteral) Rabies (required) *Optional*: + Leptospirosis + Lyme borreliosis (recombinant)
+2 years	*B. bronchiseptica* (intranasal or parenteral) *Optional*: + Leptospirosis + Lyme borreliosis (recombinant)
+3 years	*B. bronchiseptica* (intranasal or parenteral) *Optional*: + Leptospirosis + Lyme borreliosis (recombinant)
+4 years	Distemper (MLV or recombinant) Parvovirus Adenovirus-2 Parainfluenza *B. bronchiseptica* (intranasal or parenteral) Rabies (required) *Optional*: + Leptospirosis + Lyme borreliosis (recombinant)
+5 years	*B. bronchiseptica* (intranasal or parenteral)

6

T A B L E 6 - 2 0 Annualized Vaccination Protocol for Dogs at High Risk*—cont'd

Age at vaccination	Vaccine
	Optional:
	+ Leptospirosis
	+ Lyme borreliosis (recombinant)
+6 years	*B. bronchiseptica* (intranasal or parenteral)
	Optional:
	+ Leptospirosis
	+ Lyme borreliosis (recombinant)
+7 years	Distemper (MLV or recombinant)
	Parvovirus
	Adenovirus-2
	Parainfluenza
	B. bronchiseptica (intranasal or parenteral)
	Rabies (required)
	Optional:
	+ Leptospirosis
	+ Lyme borreliosis (recombinant)
Beyond 7 years	Cycle repeats as indicated

Defining criteria for HIGH RISK-canine

1. **B. bronchiseptica booster is indicated because:**
   - Dog is regularly boarded in a commercial kennel.
   - Dog is routinely groomed at a facility where other dogs are maintained.
   - Dog is regularly allowed outdoors and is unsupervised.
   - Dog has regular exposure to other, unknown dogs.
   - Dog is on a first-name basis with animal control officers.
2. **Annual *Leptospira* spp booster is indicated if:**
   - Dog lives outside and is not constrained to a gated kennel.
   - Dog lives on a farm and has ample outdoor activity.
   - Dog is regularly allowed to roam freely.
   - Dog is exclusively outdoors.
   - Dog is used for hunting or other extended outdoor activity.
   - Cases of leptospirosis are known to have been confirmed in the area.
   - Dog has access (supervised or otherwise) to areas inhabited by "reservoir" hosts (e.g., opossum, skunk, raccoon, vole) or other domestic animals such as cattle or pigs (horses?).
3. **Annual Lyme borreliosis booster is indicated if:**
   - Dog resides in a known Lyme borreliosis endemic area (eg: Northeastern US or Upper Midwest).
   - Dog resides outside most or all of the time and does have tick exposure.
   - Dog regularly travels to known endemic areas.
   - Cases of Lyme borreliosis have been identified by serologic testing (IDEXX Snap 3Dx or Western Blot) among dogs in the patient population.
   - Dog is inconsistently treated with topical flea/tick preparation.
   - Dog is only treated with OTC tick preparations.
   - Ticks are known to be constant companions for this dog.

---

*For any vaccine preceded by "+," see defining criteria.

†All intranasal *B. bronchiseptica* vaccines also contain parainfluenza virus; some also contain canine adenovirus-2.

‡In some states or municipalities, annual rabies vaccination may be required.

MLV, modified live virus.

TABLE 6-21 Annualized Vaccination Protocol for Cats at Moderate Risk*

Age at vaccination	Vaccine
9-10 weeks	Panleukopenia (MLV)
	Herpesvirus-1 and calicivirus (MLV)
	Optional:
	+ FeLV (recombinant, transdermal)
12-14 weeks	Panleukopenia (MLV)
	Herpesvirus-1 and calicivirus (MLV)
	+ Rabies (recombinant)†
	Optional:
	+ FeLV (recombinant, transdermal)
+1 year	Panleukopenia (MLV)
	Herpesvirus-1 and calicivirus (MLV)
	+ Rabies (recombinant)
	Optional:
	+ FeLV (recombinant, transdermal)
+2 years	+ Rabies (recombinant, transdermal)
+3 years	+ Rabies (recombinant)
	Panleukopenia (MLV)
+4 years	Herpesvirus-1 and calicivirus (MLV)
	+ Rabies (recombinant)
+5 years	+ Rabies (recombinant)
+6 years	+ Rabies (recombinant)
	Panleukopenia (MLV)
+7 years	Herpesvirus-1 and calicivirus (MLV)
	+ Rabies (recombinant)
+8 years	+ Rabies (recombinant)
+9 years	+ Rabies (recombinant)
+10 years	Panleukopenia (MLV)
	Herpesvirus-1 and calicivirus (MLV)
	+ Rabies (recombinant)
Beyond 10 years	Cycle repeats as indicated

Defining criteria for MODERATE RISK-feline (applies to most cats)
1. **FeLV vaccine is indicated if:**
   - The cat lives indoors predominantly, but *not* exclusively ... *and*
   - The cat is less than 6 months of age ... *and*
   - The cat is known to occasionally have contact with other cats of unknown health status ... *or*
   - Other cats in the household are known to be FeLV infected
   - Other cats live in the household but are of unknown FeLV status ... *or*
   - Other cats in the household are known to roam at will, or
   - Owner may bring stray cats into the houshold.
2. ***Bordetella bronchiseptica*** **and** ***Chlamydophila felis*** **vaccines are not indicated because:**
   - The cat is an adult (current literature suggests that clinical *B. bronchiseptica* infections are most likely to occur in kittens), ... *and*
   - The cat does not have exposure to other cats, ... *and*
   - Any other cats in the household are known to be strictly indoor cats ... *and*
   - Owner is unlikely to bring stray cats into the household.
3. **Rabies vaccination in cats**
   - Is NOT required by many states and municipalities; however, in accordance with the Feline Vaccination Guidelines, rabies is a CORE vaccine and is highly recommended for all cats.

*For any vaccine preceded by "+," see defining criteria.
†Although administration of rabies vaccine to cats may not be required by state or local statutes, it is recommended for all cats, regardless of risk.
MLV, modified live virus.

6

TABLE 6-22 Annualized Vaccination Protocol for Cats at Low Risk*

Age at vaccination	Vaccine
9-10 weeks	Panleukopenia (MLV)
	Herpesvirus-1 and calicivirus (MLV)
12-14 weeks	Panleukopenia (MLV)
	Herpesvirus and calicivirus (MLV)
	+ Rabies (recombinant)†
+1 year	Panleukopenia (MLV)
	Herpesvirus-1 and calicivirus (MLV)
	+ Rabies (recombinant)
+2 years	+ Rabies (recombinant)
+3 years	+ Rabies (recombinant)
+4 years	Panleukopenia (MLV)
	Herpesvirus-1 and calicivirus (MLV)
	+ Rabies (recombinant)
+5 years	+ Rabies (recombinant)
+6 years	+ Rabies (recombinant)
+7 years	Panleukopenia (MLV)
	Herpesvirus-1 and calicivirus (MLV)
	+ Rabies (recombinant)
+8 years	+ Rabies (recombinant)
+9 years	+ Rabies (recombinant)
+10 years	Panleukopenia (MLV)
	Herpesvirus-1 and calicivirus (MLV)
	+ Rabies (recombinant)
Beyond 10 years	Cycle repeats as indicated

Defining criteria for low risk-feline (protocol centers around CORE vaccines)
1. **FeLV and FIV vaccines are not indicated because:**
   - Cat is known to be a strictly indoor cat, *and*
   - Any other cats in the household are known to be both FeLV and FIV-free and were tested within the last 12 months, *and*
   - Other cats in the household are known to be strictly indoor cats.
   - Owner does not bring stray cats into the household.
2. ***Bordetella bronchiseptica* and *Chlamydophila felis* vaccines are not indicated because:**
   - The cat is an adult (current literature suggests that clinical *B. bronchiseptica* infections are most likely to occur in kittens), *and*
   - The cat does not have exposure to other cats, *and*
   - Any other cats in the household are known to be strictly indoor cats.
   - Owner does not bring stray cats into the household.
3. **Rabies vaccination in cats**
   - Is NOT required by many states and municipalities; however, in accordance with the Feline Vaccination Guidelines, rabies is a CORE vaccine and is highly recommended for all cats.

*For any vaccine preceded by "+," see defining criteria.
†Although administration of rabies vaccine to cats may not be required by state or local statutes, it is recommended for all cats, regardless of risk.
MLV, modified live virus.

6

TABLE 6-23 Annualized Vaccination Protocol for Cats at High Risk*

Age at vaccination	Vaccine
9-10 weeks	Panleukopenia (MLV)
	Herpesvirus-1 and calicivirus (MLV)
	Optional:
	+ FeLV (recombinant, transdermal)
	+ *B. bronchiseptica*
	+ *Chlamydophila* (non-adjuvanted)†
	+ FIV
12-14 weeks	Panleukopenia (MLV)
	Herpesvirus-1 and calicivirus (MLV)
	+ Rabies (recombinant)‡
	Optional:
	+ FeLV (non-adjuvanted)
	+ *B. bronchiseptica*
	+ *Chlamydophila* (non-adjuvanted)
	+ FIV
+1 year	Panleukopenia (MLV)
	Herpesvirus-1 and calicivirus (MLV)
	+ Rabies (recombinant)
	Optional:
	+ FeLV (recombinant, transdermal)
	+ *B. bronchiseptica*
	+ *Chlamydophila* (non-adjuvanted)
	+ FIV
+2 years	+ Rabies (recombinant)
	Optional:
	+ FeLV (recombinant, transdermal)
	+ *B. bronchiseptica*
	+ *Chlamydophila* (non-adjuvanted)
	+ FIV
+3 years	+ Rabies (recombinant)
	Optional:
	+ FeLV (recombinant, transdermal)
	+ *B. bronchiseptica*
	+ *Chlamydophila* (non-adjuvanted)
	+ FIV
+4 years	Panleukopenia (MLV)
	Herpesvirus-1 and calicivirus (MLV)
	+ Rabies (recombinant)
	Optional:
	+ FeLV (recombinant, transdermal)
	+ *B. bronchiseptica*
	+ *Chlamydophila* (non-adjuvanted)
	+ FIV
+5 years	+ Rabies (recombinant)
	Optional:
	+ FeLV (recombinant, transdermal)
	+ *B. bronchiseptica*
	+ *Chlamydophila* (non-adjuvanted)
	+ FIV

6

Continued

TABLE 6-23 Annualized Vaccination Protocol for Cats at High Risk*—cont'd

Age at vaccination	Vaccine

+6 years	+ Rabies (recombinant)
	Optional:
	  + FeLV (recombinant, transdermal)
	  + *B. bronchiseptica*
	  + *Chlamydophila* (non-adjuvanted)
	  + FIV

+7 years	Panleukopenia (MLV)
	Herpesvirus-1 and calicivirus (MLV)
	+ Rabies (recombinant)
	Optional:
	  + FeLV (recombinant, transdermal)
	  + *B. bronchiseptica*
	  + *Chlamydophila* (non-adjuvanted)
	  + FIV

+8 years	+ Rabies (recombinant)
	Optional:
	  + FeLV (recombinant, transdermal)
	  + *B. bronchiseptica*
	  + *Chlamydophila* (non-adjuvanted)
	  + FIV

+9 years	+ Rabies (recombinant)
	Optional:
	  + FeLV (recombinant, transdermal)
	  + *B. bronchiseptica*
	  + *Chlamydophila* (non-adjuvanted)
	  + FIV

+10 years	Panleukopenia (MLV)
	Herpesvirus-1 and calicivirus (MLV)
	+ Rabies (recombinant)
	Optional:
	  + FeLV (recombinant, transdermal)
	  + *B. bronchiseptica*
	  + *Chlamydophila* (non-adjuvanted)
	  + FIV

Beyond 10 years	Cycle repeats as indicated

Defining criteria for HIGH RISK-feline
1. **Both FeLV and FIV vaccines are indicated because:**
   - Cat is known to roam at will and engage in fighting (risk of FIV in male cats is 4X greater than in female cats), *or*
   - There is likely exposure to other cats with unknown health status, or
   - There are other cats in the household that are known to roam at will and engage in fighting...*or*
   - Owner regularly adopts (or hoards) cats.
2. ***Bordetella bronchiseptica* and *Chlamydophila felis* vaccines are indicated because:**
   - The cat is a kitten and resides within a cluster household (current literature suggests that clinical *B. bronchiseptica* infections are most likely to occur in kittens), *or*
   - The cat has regular exposure to other cats of unknown health status, *or*

6

T A B L E 6 - 2 3 Annualized Vaccination Protocol for Cats at High Risk*—cont'd

- There are other cats in the household known to roam at will and have contact with other cats ... *or*
- Owner regularly adopts (or hoards) cats.
3. **Rabies vaccination in cats:**
   - Is NOT required by many states and municipalities; however, in accordance with the Feline Vaccination Guidelines, rabies is a CORE vaccine and is highly recommended for all cats.

---

*For any vaccine preceded by "+," see defining criteria.
†*Chlamydia psittaci* has been renamed *Chlamydophila felis* (the name on vaccine label may not reflect the new classification).
‡Although administration of rabies vaccine to cats may not be required by state or local statutes, it is recommended for all cats, regardless of risk.
MLV, modified live virus.

Additional Reading

Richards J, Rodan I, Elston T, et al: 2000 Report of the American Association of Feline Practitioners and Academy of Feline Medicine Advisory Panel on Feline Vaccines, Nashville, Tenn.

Report of the American Animal Hospital Association (AAHA) Canine Vaccine Task Force: 2003 Canine and Recommendations. *J Am Anim Hosp Assoc* 39:119-131, 2003. (The complete report, including supporting literature, is available to AAHA members at www.aahanet.org.)

Ford RB (ed): Veterinary Clinics of North America: Small Animal Practice. WB Saunders, Philadelphia, May 2001.

6

TABLE 6-24 Compendium of Animal Rabies Prevention and Control, 2005*, National Association of State Public Health Veterinarians, Inc. (NASPHV)[†]

Rabies is a fatal viral zoonosis and a serious public health problem.[1] The recommendations in this compendium serve as the basis for animal rabies prevention and control programs throughout the United States and facilitate standardization of procedures among jurisdictions, thereby contributing to an effective national rabies-control program. This document is reviewed annually and revised as necessary. Principles of rabies prevention and control are detailed in Part I; Part II contains recommendations for parenteral vaccination procedures. All animal rabies vaccines licensed by the United States Department of Agriculture (USDA) and marketed in the United States are listed in Part III.

Part I: Rabies prevention and control
A. Principles of rabies prevention and control

1. **Rabies exposure.** Rabies is transmitted only when the virus is introduced into bite wounds, open cuts in skin, or onto mucous membranes from saliva or other potentially infectious material such as neural tissue.[2] Questions about possible exposures should be directed to state or local health authorities.
2. **Human rabies prevention.** Rabies in humans can be prevented either by eliminating exposures to rabid animals or by providing exposed persons with prompt local treatment of wounds combined with the administration of human rabies immune globulin and vaccine. The rationale for recommending preexposure and postexposure rabies prophylaxis and details of their administration can be found in the current recommendations of the Advisory Committee on Immunization Practices (ACIP).[2] These recommendations, along with information concerning the current local and regional epidemiology of animal rabies and the availability of human rabies biologics, are available from state health departments.
3. **Domestic animals.** Local governments should initiate and maintain effective programs to ensure vaccination of all dogs, cats, and ferrets and to remove strays and unwanted animals. Such procedures in the United States have reduced laboratory-confirmed cases of rabies in dogs from 6949 in 1947 to 117 in 2003.[3] Because more rabies cases are reported annually involving cats (321 in 2003) than dogs, vaccination of cats should be required. Animal shelters and animal control authorities should establish policies to ensure that adopted animals are vaccinated against rabies. The recommended vaccination procedures and the licensed animal vaccines are specified in Parts II and III of the compendium.
4. **Rabies in vaccinated animals.** Rabies is rare in vaccinated animals.[4] If such an event is suspected, it should be reported to state public health officials; the vaccine manufacturer; and USDA, Animal and Plant Health Inspection Service, Center for Veterinary Biologics (Internet: http://www.aphis.usda.gov/vs/cvb/ic/adverseeventreport.htm, telephone: 800-752-6255, or e-mail: CVB@usda.gov). The laboratory diagnosis should be confirmed and the virus characterized by a rabies reference laboratory. A thorough epidemiologic investigation should be conducted.
5. **Rabies in wildlife.** The control of rabies among wildlife reservoirs is difficult.[5] Vaccination of free-ranging wildlife or selective population reduction might be useful in some situations, but the success of such procedures depends on the circumstances surrounding each rabies outbreak (see Part I. C. Control Methods in Wildlife). Because of the risk of rabies in wild animals (especially raccoons, skunks, coyotes, foxes, and bats), AVMA, NASPHV, and CSTE strongly recommend the enactment and enforcement of state laws prohibiting their importation, distribution, and relocation.
6. **Rabies surveillance.** Laboratory-based rabies surveillance is an essential component of rabies control and prevention programs. Accurate and timely information is necessary to guide human postexposure prophylaxis decisions, determine the management of potentially exposed animals, aid in emerging pathogen discovery, describe the epidemiology of the disease, and assess the need for and effectiveness of oral vaccination programs for wildlife.

Continued

TABLE 6-24	Compendium of Animal Rabies Prevention and Control, 2005*, National Association of State Public Health Veterinarians, Inc. (NASPHV)†—cont'd

7. **Rabies diagnosis.** Rabies testing should be performed by a qualified laboratory that has been designated by the local or state health department[6] in accordance with the established national standardized protocol for rabies testing (http://www.cdc.gov/ncidod/dvrd/rabies/ Professional/publications/DFA_diagnosis/DFA_protocol-b.htm). Euthanasia[7] should be accomplished in such a way as to maintain the integrity of the brain so that the laboratory can recognize the anatomic parts. Except in the case of very small animals, such as bats, only the head or brain (including brainstem) should be submitted to the laboratory. Any animal or animal specimen being submitted for testing should be kept under refrigeration (not frozen or chemically fixed) during storage and shipping.

8. **Rabies serology.** Some "rabies-free" jurisdictions may require evidence of vaccination and rabies antibodies for importation purposes. Rabies antibody titers are indicative of an animal's response to vaccine or infection. Titers do not directly correlate with protection because other immunologic factors also play a role in preventing rabies, and our abilities to measure and interpret those other factors are not well developed. Therefore, evidence of circulating rabies virus antibodies should not be used as a substitute for current vaccination in managing rabies exposures or determining the need for booster vaccinations in animals.[8]

B. Prevention and control methods in domestic and confined animals

1. **Preexposure vaccination and management.** Parenteral animal rabies vaccines should be administered only by or under the direct supervision of a veterinarian. Rabies vaccinations may also be administered under the supervision of a veterinarian to animals held in animal control shelters prior to release. Any veterinarian signing a rabies certificate must ensure that the person administering vaccine is identified on the certificate and is appropriately trained in vaccine storage, handling, and administration and in the management of adverse events. This practice ensures that a qualified and responsible person can be held accountable to ensure that the animal has been properly vaccinated.

    Within 28 days after primary vaccination, a peak rabies antibody titer is reached and the animal can be considered immunized. An animal is currently vaccinated and is considered immunized if the primary vaccination was administered at least 28 days previously and vaccinations have been administered in accordance with this compendium.

    Regardless of the age of the animal at initial vaccination, a booster vaccination should be administered 1 year later (see Parts II and III for vaccines and procedures). No laboratory or epidemiologic data exist to support the annual or biennial administration of 3-year vaccines following the initial series. Because a rapid anamnestic response is expected, an animal is considered currently vaccinated immediately after a booster vaccination.

    a. **Dogs, cats, and ferrets.** All dogs, cats, and ferrets should be vaccinated against rabies and revaccinated in accordance with Part III of this compendium. If a previously vaccinated animal is overdue for a booster, it should be revaccinated. Immediately following the booster, the animal is considered currently vaccinated and should be placed on an annual or triennial schedule depending on the type of vaccine used.

    b. **Livestock.** Consideration should be given to vaccinating livestock that are particularly valuable or that might have frequent contact with humans (e.g., in petting zoos, fairs, and other public exhibitions).[9,10] Horses traveling interstate should be currently vaccinated against rabies.

    c. **Confined animals.**

    1) **Wild.** No parenteral rabies vaccines are licensed for use in wild animals or hybrids (the offspring of wild animals crossbred to domestic animals). Wild animals or hybrids should not be kept as pets.[11-14]

6

2) **Maintained in exhibits and in zoological parks.** Captive mammals that are not completely excluded from all contact with rabies vectors can become infected. Moreover, wild animals might be incubating rabies when initially captured; therefore, wild-caught animals susceptible to rabies should be quarantined for a minimum of 6 months before being exhibited. Employees who work with animals at such facilities should receive preexposure rabies vaccination. The use of pre- or postexposure rabies vaccinations for employees who work with animals at such facilities might reduce the need for euthanasia of captive animals. Carnivores and bats should be housed in a manner that precludes direct contact with the public.

3) **Stray animals.** Stray dogs, cats, and ferrets should be removed from the community. Local health departments and animal control officials can enforce the removal of strays more effectively if owned animals have identification and are confined or kept on leash. Strays should be impounded for at least 3 business days to determine if human exposure has occurred and to give owners sufficient time to reclaim animals.

2. **Importation and interstate movement of animals.**

   a. **International.** The CDC regulates the importation of dogs and cats into the United States. Importers of dogs must comply with rabies vaccination requirements (42 CFR, Part 71.51[c] [http://www.cdc.gov/ncidod/dq/animal.htm]) and complete CDC form 75.37 (http://www.cdc.gov/ncidod/dq/pdf/cdc7537-05-24-04.pdf). The appropriate health official of the state of destination should be notified within 72 hours of the arrival into his or her jurisdiction of any imported dog required to be placed in confinement under the CDC regulation. Failure to comply with these requirements should be promptly reported to the Division of Global Migration and Quarantine, CDC (telephone: 404-498-1670).

   Federal regulations alone are insufficient to prevent the introduction of rabid animals into the country.[15,16] All imported dogs and cats are subject to state and local laws governing rabies and should be currently vaccinated against rabies in accordance with this compendium. Failure to comply with state or local requirements should be referred to the appropriate state or local official.

   b. **Interstate.** Before interstate (including commonwealths and territories) movement, dogs, cats, ferrets, and horses should be currently vaccinated against rabies in accordance with the compendium's recommendations (see Part I. B.1. Preexposure Vaccination and Management). Animals in transit should be accompanied by a currently valid NASPHV Form 51, Rabies Vaccination Certificate (http://www.nasphv.org/83416/106001.html). When an interstate health certificate or certificate of veterinary inspection is required, it should contain the same rabies vaccination information as Form 51.

   c. **Areas with dog-to-dog rabies transmission.** The movement of dogs from areas with dog-to-dog rabies transmission for the purpose of adoption or sale should be eliminated. Rabid dogs have been introduced into the United States from areas with dog-to-dog rabies transmission.[15,16] This practice poses the risk of introducing canine-transmitted rabies to areas where it does not currently exist.

3. **Adjunct procedures.** Methods or procedures which enhance rabies control include the following:

   a. **Identification.** Dogs, cats, and ferrets should be identified (e.g., metal or plastic tags or microchips) to allow for verification of rabies vaccination status.

   b. **Licensure.** Registration or licensure of all dogs, cats, and ferrets may be used to aid in rabies control. A fee is frequently charged for such licensure, and revenues collected are used to maintain rabies- or animal-control programs. Evidence of current vaccination is an essential prerequisite to licensure.

6

Continued

TABLE 6-24 Compendium of Animal Rabies Prevention and Control, 2005*, National Association of State Public Health Veterinarians, Inc. (NASPHV)†—cont'd

    c. **Canvassing.** House-to-house canvassing by animal control officials facilitates enforcement of vaccination and licensure requirements.

    d. **Citations.** Citations are legal summonses issued to owners for violations, including the failure to vaccinate or license their animals. The authority for officers to issue citations should be an integral part of each animal-control program.

    e. **Animal control.** All communities should incorporate stray animal control, leash laws, and training of personnel in their programs.

4. **Postexposure management.** Any animal potentially exposed to rabies virus (see Part I. A.1. Rabies Exposure) by a wild, carnivorous mammal or a bat that is not available for testing should be regarded as having been exposed to rabies.

    a. **Dogs, cats, and ferrets.** Unvaccinated dogs, cats, and ferrets exposed to a rabid animal should be euthanized immediately. If the owner is unwilling to have this done, the animal should be placed in strict isolation for 6 months. Rabies vaccine should be administered upon entry into isolation or 1 month prior to release to comply with preexposure vaccination recommendations (see Part I.B.1.a.). Protocols for the postexposure vaccination of previously unvaccinated domestic animals have not been validated, and evidence exists that the use of vaccine alone will not prevent the disease.[17] Animals with expired vaccinations need to be evaluated on a case-by-case basis. Dogs, cats, and ferrets that are currently vaccinated should be revaccinated immediately, kept under the owner's control, and observed for 45 days. Any illness in an isolated or confined animal should be reported immediately to the local health department.

    b. **Livestock.** All species of livestock are susceptible to rabies; cattle and horses are among the most frequently infected. Livestock exposed to a rabid animal and currently vaccinated with a vaccine approved by USDA for that species should be revaccinated immediately and observed for 45 days. Unvaccinated livestock should be slaughtered immediately. If the owner is unwilling to have this done, the animal should be kept under close observation for 6 months. Any illness in an animal under observation should be reported immediately to the local health department.

    The following are recommendations for owners of livestock exposed to rabid animals:

      1) If the animal is slaughtered within 7 days of being bitten, its tissues may be eaten without risk of infection, provided that liberal portions of the exposed area are discarded. Federal guidelines for meat inspectors require that any animal known to have been exposed to rabies within 8 months be rejected for slaughter.

      2) Neither tissues nor milk from a rabid animal should be used for human or animal consumption.[18] Pasteurization temperatures will inactivate rabies virus; therefore, drinking pasteurized milk or eating cooked meat does not constitute a rabies exposure.

      3) Having more than one rabid animal in a herd or having herbivore-to-herbivore transmission is uncommon; therefore, restricting the rest of the herd if a single animal has been exposed to or infected by rabies might not be necessary.

    c. **Other animals.** Other mammals bitten by a rabid animal should be euthanized immediately. Animals maintained in USDA-licensed research facilities or accredited zoological parks should be evaluated on a case-by-case basis.

5. **Management of animals that bite humans**

    a. **Dogs, cats, and ferrets.** Rabies virus may be excreted in the saliva of infected dogs, cats, and ferrets during illness and/or for only a few days prior to illness or death.[19-20] A healthy dog, cat, or ferret that bites a person should be confined and observed daily for 10 days[22]; administration of rabies vaccine to the animal is not recommended during the observation period to avoid confusing signs of rabies with possible side effects of vaccine administration.

6

T A B L E   6 - 2 4   **Compendium of Animal Rabies Prevention and Control, 2005*, National Association of State Public Health Veterinarians, Inc. (NASPHV)[†]—cont'd**

Such animals should be evaluated by a veterinarian at the first sign of illness during confinement. Any illness in the animal should be reported immediately to the local health department. If signs suggestive of rabies develop, the animal should be euthanized and the head shipped for testing as described in Part I.A.7. Any stray or unwanted dog, cat, or ferret that bites a person may be euthanized immediately and the head submitted for rabies examination.

  b. **Other biting animals.** Other biting animals that might have exposed a person to rabies should be reported immediately to the local health department. Management of animals other than dogs, cats, and ferrets depends on the species, the circumstances of the bite, the epidemiology of rabies in the area, and the biting animal's history, current health status, and potential for exposure to rabies. Prior vaccination of these animals may not preclude the necessity for euthanasia and testing.

C. Prevention and control methods related to wildlife

The public should be warned not to handle or feed wild mammals. Wild mammals and hybrids that bite or otherwise expose persons, pets, or livestock should be considered for euthanasia and rabies examination. A person bitten by any wild mammal should immediately report the incident to a physician who can evaluate the need for antirabies treatment (see current rabies prophylaxis recommendations of the ACIP[2]). State-regulated wildlife rehabilitators may play a role in a comprehensive rabies control program. Minimum standards for persons who rehabilitate wild mammals should include rabies vaccination, appropriate training, and continuing education. Translocation of infected wildlife has contributed to the spread of rabies[23,24]; therefore, the translocation of known terrestrial rabies reservoir species should be prohibited.

  1. **Terrestrial mammals.** The use of licensed oral vaccines for the mass vaccination of free-ranging wildlife should be considered in selected situations, with the approval of the state agency responsible for animal rabies control.[5] The distribution of oral rabies vaccine should be based on scientific assessments of the target species and followed by timely and appropriate analysis of surveillance data; such results should be provided to all stakeholders. In addition, parenteral vaccination (trap-vaccinate-release) of wildlife rabies reservoirs may be integrated into coordinated oral rabies vaccination programs to enhance their effectiveness. Continuous and persistent programs for trapping or poisoning wildlife are not effective in reducing wildlife rabies reservoirs on a statewide basis. However, limited population control in high-contact areas (e.g., picnic grounds, camps, suburban areas) may be indicated for the removal of selected high-risk species of wildlife.[5] State agriculture, public health, and wildlife agencies should be consulted for planning, coordination, and evaluation of vaccination or population-reduction programs.

  2. **Bats.** Indigenous rabid bats have been reported from every state except Hawaii and have caused rabies in at least 40 humans in the United States.[25-29] Bats should be excluded from houses, public buildings, and adjacent structures to prevent direct association with humans.[30,31] Such structures should then be made bat-proof by sealing entrances used by bats. Controlling rabies in bats through programs designed to reduce bat populations is neither feasible nor desirable.

Part II: Recommendations for parenteral rabies vaccination procedures

A. Vaccine administration

All animal rabies vaccines should be restricted to use by, or under the direct supervision of a veterinarian[32] except as recommended in Part I.B.1. All vaccines must be administered in accordance with the specifications of the product label or package insert.

Continued

TABLE 6-24 Compendium of Animal Rabies Prevention and Control, 2005*, National Association of State Public Health Veterinarians, Inc. (NASPHV)[†]—cont'd

B. Vaccine selection

Part III lists all vaccines licensed by USDA and marketed in the United States at the time of publication. New vaccine approvals or changes in label specifications made subsequent to publication should be considered as part of this list. Any of the listed vaccines can be used for revaccination, even if the product is not the same brand previously administered. Vaccines used in state and local rabies control programs should have a 3-year duration of immunity. This constitutes the most effective method of increasing the proportion of immunized dogs and cats in any population.[33] No laboratory or epidemiologic data exist to support the annual or biennial administration of 3-year vaccines following the initial series.

C. Adverse events

Currently, no epidemiologic association exists between a particular licensed vaccine product and adverse events, including vaccine failure.[34,35] Adverse events should be reported to the vaccine manufacturer and to USDA, Animal and Plant Health Inspection Service, Center for Veterinary Biologics (Internet: http://www.aphis.usda.gov/vs/cvb/ic/adverseeventreport.htm; telephone: 800-752-6255; or e-mail: CVB@usda.gov).

D. Wildlife and hybrid animal vaccination

The safety and efficacy of parenteral rabies vaccination of wildlife and hybrids have not been established, and no rabies vaccines are licensed for these animals. Parenteral vaccination (trap-vaccinate-release) of wildlife rabies reservoirs may be integrated into coordinated oral rabies vaccination programs as described in Part I. C.1. to enhance their effectiveness. Zoos or research institutions may establish vaccination programs, which attempt to protect valuable animals, but these should not replace appropriate public health activities that protect humans.[9]

E. Accidental human exposure to vaccine

Human exposure to parenteral animal rabies vaccines listed in Part III does not constitute a risk for rabies infection. However, human exposure to vaccinia-vectored oral rabies vaccines should be reported to state health officials.[36]

F. Rabies certificate

All agencies and veterinarians should use NASPHV Form 51, Rabies Vaccination Certificate, which can be obtained from vaccine manufacturers or from NASPHV(http://www.nasphv.org). It is also available from CDC (http://www.cdc.gov/ncidod/dvrd/rabies/professional/professi.htm). The form must be completed in full and signed by the administering or supervising veterinarian. Computer-generated forms containing the same information are also acceptable.

---

*The material in this report originated at the National Center for Infectious Diseases (Anne Schuchat, MD, Acting Director), and the Division of Viral and Rickettsial Diseases (James W. LeDuc, PhD, Director).

[†]The NASPHV Committee: Suzanne R. Jenkins, VMD, MPH, Co-Chair; Mira J. Leslie, DVM, MPH, Co-Chair; Michael Auslander, DVM, MSPH; Lisa Conti, DVM, MPH; Paul Ettestad, DVM, MS; Faye E. Sorhage, VMD, MPH; and Ben Sun, DVM, MPVM.

Consultants to the Committee: Donna M. Gatewood, DVM, MS, Center for Veterinary Biologics, U.S. Department of Agriculture (USDA); Ellen Mangione, MD, MPH, Council of State and Territorial Epidemiologists (CSTE); Lorraine Moule, National Animal Control Association (NACA); Greg Pruitt, Animal Health Institute; Charles E. Rupprecht, VMD, MS, PhD, CDC; John Schiltz, DVM, American Veterinary Medical Association (AVMA); Charles V. Trimarchi, MS, New York State Health Department; and Dennis Slate, PhD, Wildlife Services, USDA.

This compendium has been endorsed by AVMA, CDC, CSTE, and NACA. Corresponding author: Mira J. Leslie, DVM, MPH, Washington Department of Health, Communicable Disease Epidemiology, 1610 NE 150th Street, MS K17-9, Shoreline, WA 98155-9701.

6

Continued

T A B L E   6 - 2 4   Compendium of Animal Rabies Prevention and Control, 2005*, National Association of State Public Health Veterinarians, Inc. (NASPHV)†—cont'd

Rabies vaccines licensed and marketed in the United States, 2005

Product name	Produced by	Marketed by	For use in	Dosage (mL)	Age at primary vaccination*	Booster recommended	Route of inoculation
MONOVALENT (inactivated)							
Defensor 1	Pfizer, Inc. License No. 189	Pfizer, Inc.	Dogs	1	3 mos†	Annually	IM‡ or SC§
			Cats	1	3 mos	Annually	SC
Defensor 3	Pfizer, Inc. License No. 189	Pfizer, Inc.	Dogs	1	3 mos	1 year later and triennially	IM or SC
			Cats	1	3 mos	1 year later and triennially	SC
			Sheep	2	3 mos	Annually	IM
			Cattle	2	3 mos	Annually	IM
Rabdomun	Pfizer, Inc. License No. 189	Schering-Plough	Dogs	1	3 mos	1 year later and triennially	IM or SC
			Cats	1	3 mos	1 year later and triennially	SC
			Sheep	2	3 mos	Annually	IM
			Cattle	2	3 mos	Annually	IM
Rabdomun 1	Pfizer, Inc. License No. 189	Schering-Plough	Dogs	1	3 mos	Annually	IM or SC
			Cats	1	3 mos	Annually	SC
Rabvac 1	Fort Dodge Animal Health Licence No. 112	Fort Dodge Animal Health	Dogs	1	3 mos	Annually	IM or SC
			Cats	1	3 mos	Annually	SC
Rabvac 3	Fort Dodge Animal Health License No. 112	Fort Dodge Animal Health	Dogs	1	3 mos	1 year later and triennially	IM or SC
			Cats	1	3 mos	1 year later and triennially	IM or SC
			Horses	2	3 mos	Annually	IM
Rabvac 3 TF	Fort Dodge Animal Health License No. 112	Fort Dodge Animal Health	Dogs	1	3 mos	1 year later and triennially	IM or SC
			Cats	1	3 mos	1 year later and triennially	IM or SC
			Horses	2	3 mos	Annually	IM
Prorab-1	Intervet, Inc. License No. 286	Intervet, Inc	Dogs	1	3 mos	Annually	IM or SC
			Cats	1	3 mos	Annually	IM or SC
			Sheep	2	3 mos	Annually	IM

Product	Produced by	Marketed by	For use in	Doses	Age at primary	Booster recommended	Route
Prorab-3F	Intervet, Inc. License No. 286	Intervet, Inc.	Cats	1	3 mos	1 year later and triennially	IM or SC
Imrab 3	Merial, Inc. License No. 298	Merial, Inc.	Dogs	1	3 mos	1 year later and triennially	IM or SC
			Cats	1	3 mos	1 year later and triennially	IM or SC
			Sheep	2	3 mos	1 year later and triennially	IM or SC
			Cattle	2	3 mos	Annually	IM or SC
			Horses	2	3 mos	Annually	IM or SC
			Ferrets	1	3 mos	Annually	SC
Imrab 3 TF	Merial, Inc. License No. 298	Merial, Inc.	Dogs	1	3 mos	1 year later or triennially	IM or SC
			Cats	1	3 mos	1 year later or triennially	IM or SC
			Ferrets	1	3 mos	Annually	SC
Imrab Large Animal	Merial, Inc. Licence No. 298	Merial, Inc.	Cattle	2	3 mos	Annually	IM or SC
			Horses	2	3 mos	Annually	IM or SC
			Sheep	2	3 mos	1 year later or triennially	IM or SC
Imrab 1	Merial, Inc. License No. 298	Merial, Inc.	Dogs	1	3 mos	Annually	SC
			Cats	1	3 mos	Annually	SC
Monovalent (Rabies glycoprotein, live canary pox vector)							
Purevax feline Rabies	Merial, Inc. Licence No. 298	Merial, Inc.	Cats	1	8 wks	Annually	SC
Combination (Inactivated rabies)							
Equine Potomavac + Imrab	Merial, Inc. License No. 298	Merial, Inc.	Horses	1	3 mos	Annually	IM
Mystique 11 Potomavac +	Intervet, Inc. License No. 286	Intervet, Inc.	Horses	1	3 mos	Annually	IM
Combination (Rabies glycoprotein, live canary pox vector)							
Purevax feline 3/Rabies	Merial, Inc. License No. 298	Merial, Inc.	Cats	1	8 wks	Annually	SC
Purevax Feline 4/Rabies	Merial, Inc. Licence No. 298	Merial, Inc.	Cat	1	8 wks	Annually	SC
Oral (Rabies glycoprotein, live vaccinia vector) - RESTRICTED TO USE IN STATE AND FEDERAL RABIES-CONTROL PROGRAMS							
Raboral V-RG	Merial, Inc. Licence No. 298	Merial, Inc.	Racoons Coyotes	N/A	N/A	AG determined by local authorities	Oral

*Minimum age (or older) and revaccinated 1 year later.
†1 month = 28 days.
‡Intramuscularly.
§Subcutaneously.

6

References

1. Rabies. In: Chin J, ed. Control of communicable diseases manual. 17th ed. Washington, DC: American Public Health Association; 2000:411-9.
2. CDC. Human rabies prevention—United States, 1999. Recommendations of the Advisory Committee on Immunization Practices (ACIP). MMWR 1999;48:(No. RR-1).
3. Krebs JW, Mandel EJ, Swerdlow DL, Rupprecht CE. Rabies surveillance in the United States during 2003. J Am Vet Med Assoc 2004;225:1837-49.
4. McQuiston J, Yager PA, Smith JS, Rupprecht CE. Epidemiologic characteristics of rabies virus variants in dogs and cats in the United States, 1999. J Am Vet Med Assoc 2001;218: 1939-42.
5. Hanlon CA, Childs JE, Nettles VF, et al. Recommendations of the Working Group on Rabies. Article III: Rabies in wildlife. J Am Vet Med Assoc 1999;215:1612-8.
6. Hanlon CA, Smith JS, Anderson GR, et al. Recommendations of the Working Group on Rabies. Article II: Laboratory diagnosis of rabies. J Am Vet Med Assoc 1999;215:1444-6.
7. American Veterinary Medical Association. 2000 Report of the AVMA Panel on Euthanasia. J Am Vet Med Assoc 2001;218:669-96.
8. Tizard I, Ni Y. Use of serologic testing to assess immune status of companion animals. J Am Vet Med Assoc 1998;213:54-60.
9. National Association of State Public Health Veterinarians. Compendium of measures to prevent disease and injury associated with animals in public settings. Available at http://www.nasphv.org/83416/84501.html.
10. Bender J, Schulman S. Reports of zoonotic disease outbreaks associated with animal exhibits and availability of recommendations for preventing zoonotic disease transmission from animals to people in such settings. J Am Vet Med Assoc 2004;224:1105-9.
11. Wild animals as pets. In: Directory and resource manual. Schaumburg, IL: American Veterinary Medical Association; 2002:126.
12. Position on canine hybrids. In: Directory and resource manual. Schaumburg, IL: American Veterinary Medical Association; 2002:88-9.
13. Siino BS. Crossing the line. American Society for the Prevention of Cruelty to Animals, Animal Watch 2000;Winter:22-9.
14. Jay MT, Reilly KF, DeBess EE, Haynes EH, Bader DR, Barrett LR. Rabies in a vaccinated wolf-dog hybrid. J Am Vet Med Assoc 1994;205:1729-32.
15. CDC. An imported case of rabies in an immunized dog. MMWR 1987;36:946,101.
16. CDC. Imported dog and cat rabies—New Hampshire, California. MMWR 1988;37: 59-60.
17. Hanlon CA, Niezgoda MN, Rupprecht CE. Postexposure prophylaxis for prevention of rabies in dogs. Am J Vet Res 2002;63:1096–100.
18. CDC. Mass treatment of humans who drank unpasteurized milk from rabid cows—Massachusetts, 1996–1998. MMWR 1999;48:228-9.
19. Vaughn JB, Gerhardt P, Paterson J. Excretion of street rabies virus in saliva of cats. J Am Med Assoc 1963;184:705.
20. Vaughn JB, Gerhardt P, Newell KW. Excretion of street rabies virus in saliva of dogs. J Am Med Assoc 1965;193:363-8.
21. Niezgoda M, Briggs DJ, Shaddock J, Rupprecht CE. Viral excretion in domestic ferrets (Mustela putorius furo) inoculated with a raccoon rabies isolate. Am J Vet Res 1998;59: 1629-32.
22. Tepsumethanon V, Lumlertdacha B, Mitmoonpitak C, Sitprija V, Meslin FX, Wilde H. Survival of naturally infected rabid dogs and cats. Clin Infect Dis 2004;39:278-80.
23. Jenkins SR, Perry BD, Winkler WG. Ecology and epidemiology of raccoon rabies. Rev Infect Dis 1988;10:Suppl 4:S620-5.
24. CDC. Translocation of coyote rabies—Florida, 1994. MMWR 1995;44:580-7.
25. Messenger SL, Smith JS, Rupprecht CE. Emerging epidemiology of bat-associated cryptic cases of rabies in humans in the United States. Clin Infect Dis 2002;35:738-47.
26. CDC. Human rabies—California, 2002. MMWR 2002;51:686-8.
27. CDC. Human rabies—Tennessee, 2002. MMWR 2002;51:828-9.
28. CDC. Human rabies—Iowa, 2002. MMWR 2003;52:47-8.
29. CDC. Human death associated with bat rabies—California, 2003. MMWR 2003;53:33-5.
30. Frantz SC, Trimarchi CV. Bats in human dwellings: health concerns and management. In: Decker DF, ed. Proceedings of the first eastern wildlife damage control conference. Ithaca, NY: Cornell University Press; 1983:299-308.

6

31. Greenhall AM. House bat management. US Fish and Wildlife Service, Resource Publication 143; 1982.

32. Model rabies control ordinance. In: Directory and resource manual. Schaumburg, IL: American Veterinary Medical Association; 2002:114-6.

33. Bunn TO. Canine and feline vaccines, past and present. In Baer GM, ed. The natural history of rabies. 2nd ed. Boca Raton, FL: CRC Press; 1991:415-25.

34. Gobar GM, Kass PH. World wide web-based survey of vaccination practices, postvaccinal reactions, and vaccine site-associated sarcomas in cats. J Am Vet Med Assoc 2002;220: 1477-82.

35. Macy DW, Hendrick MJ. The potential role of inflammation in the development of postvaccinal sarcomas in cats. Vet Clin North Am Small Anim Pract 1996;26:103-9.

36. Rupprecht CE, Blass L, Smith K et al. Human infection due to recombinant vaccinia-rabies glycoprotein virus. N Engl J Med 2001;345:582-6.

6

TABLE 6-25 Prescription Writing Reference . . . Do's & Don'ts

Veterinarian information	Owner information

Always include:

Prescribing veterinarian's name	Patient's name (in "quotes")
Practice address	Patient's age or date of birth
Practice telephone number	Owner's name (or that of an owner representative)
DEA # (if written for a controlled substance)	Owner's address
Current date	Owner's phone number
Rx	

- **Drug Name:** (Print FULL brand name or generic name... NEVER abbreviate)
- **Dosage Form:** (specify tablet, capsule, suspension, other)
- **Strength:** (mg, g, μg, etc.) or concentration (mg/ml)... use metric units
- **Total Quantity:** (# 10 [for 10 tablets]; 60 ml)
- **Sig:** *Include the following:* Dose (individual); route; frequency; duration; indication or use
- **Number of Refills:** define the number permitted
- **Designate:** whether or not generic substitution is permissible
- **Signature:**

Common prescription writing errors

- Always use metric units: e.g., **g** (gram) for solids; **ml** or **mL** (milliliter) for liquids.
- Use **per** instead of a slash (**/**), which can be interpreted as the number **1**.
- Use **units** instead of the abbreviation **u**, which can be interpreted as **0** or **4** or **μ**.
- Use **once daily** instead of **sid**, which has been interpreted as **5/d** or **5 per day!** (NOTE: "sid" is *not* a conventional prescription abbreviation.)
- Use **three times daily** instead of **tid,** and **four times daily** instead of **qid.**
- Use **every other day** instead of **qod.**
- REMEMBER—abbreviations like **qd, qid,** and **qod** are easily confused with each other
- When writing numbers:
  - Use a **leading zero** with decimals: e.g., use **0.5 ml** rather than **.5 ml**.
  - Avoid using a **trailing zero:** e.g., use **3** rather than **3.0**.
- And FINALLY—**When in doubt ...spell it out.**

6

TABLE 6-26   Common Drug Indications and Dosages†

Drug	Proprietary names	Action/Use	Formulation	Recommended dosage
Acepromazine	Many generic products	Tranquilizer and antiemetic	5-, 10-, and 25-mg tablets and 10-mg/mL injection	Dog: 0.56-1.13 mg/kg IM, SC, IV; 0.56-2.25 mg/kg PO q6-8h Cat: 1.13-2.25 mg/kg IM, SC, IV
Acetaminophen	Tylenol and other generic brands	NSAID/analgesia	120-, 160-, 325-, and 500-mg tablets	Dog: 15 mg/kg PO q8h Cat: DO NOT USE
Acetaminophen with codeine	Tylenol with codeine; other generic products	NSAID + opioid/ analgesia	Oral solution and tablets. Many forms (e.g., 300 mg acetaminophen plus either 15, 30, or 60 mg codeine)	Follow dosing recommendations for codeine Dog: (analgesia) 0.5-1 mg/kg PO q4-6h Cat: DO NOT USE
Acetazolamide	Diamox	Diuretic/management of glaucoma	125- and 250-mg tablets	Glaucoma: 5-10 mg/kg PO q8-12h Diuretic: 4-8 mg/kg PO q8-12h
◆ Acetylcysteine	Mucomyst	Antidote/acetamin-ophen toxicosis in cats	20% solution (200 mg/mL)	Cat: (acetaminophen toxicosis) 140 mg/kg (initial loading dose; then 70 mg/kg PO or IV q4h for 5 doses
ACTH Gel	See Corticotropin			
Activated charcoal	See Charcoal, activated			
Albendazole	Valbazen	Antiparasitic/especially respiratory parasites and Giardia spp.	113.6-mg/mL suspension and 300 mg/mL paste	General antiparasitic: 25-50 mg/kg PO q12h for 3 days Respiratory parasites: 50 mg/kg, q24h PO for 10-14 days Giardia: 25 mg/kg q12h for 2 days; 2 to 5 puffs four times daily
Albuterol	Proventil; Ventolin	Bronchodilator	2-, 4-, and 5-mg tablets; 2 mg/5 mL syrup; aerosol (metered inhaler @ 90 mcg/dose)	20-50 µg/kg four times/day; up to maximum of 100 µg/kg four times/day

Note: Listings preceded by ◆ are for rapid reference and denote drug/dosage used in the emergency or critical care setting.

6

TABLE 6-26   Common Drug Indications and Dosages†—cont'd

Drug	Proprietary names	Action/Use	Formulation	Recommended dosage
Allopurinol	Lopurin; Zyloprim	Antiinflammatory/ adjunct therapy for Leishmaniasis; urolith prevention	100- and 300-mg tablets	Urolith prevention: 10 mg/kg q8h; then reduce to 10 mg/kg q24h Leishmaniasis: 10 mg/kg, q12h PO for 4 months or more.
Aluminum carbonate gel	Basalgel	Antacid/GI phosphate binder (uncommonly used today)	Capsules (equivalent to 500 mg aluminum hydroxide)	10-30 mg/kg PO q8h (with meals)
Aluminum hydroxide gel	Amphogel	Antacid/GI phosphate binder (uncommonly used today)	64 mg/mL oral suspension; 600-mg tablet	10-30 mg/kg PO q8h (with meals)
Amikacin	Amiglyde-V (veterinary); Amikin (human)	Antibacterial	50- and 250-mg/mL injection	Dog and cat: 6.5 mg/kg IV, IM, SC q8h or 20 mg/kg IV, IM, SC q24h
Aminophylline	Many generic brands	Bronchodilator/ chronic bronchitis and asthma	100- and 200-mg tablets; 25 mg/mL injection	Dog: 10 mg/kg PO, IM, IV q8h Cat: 6.6 mg/kg PO q12h
◆ Amiodarone	Cordarone	Antiarrhythmic/life-threatening arrhythmias	200 mg tables and 50 mg/mL injection	Dog: 10-15 mg/kg, PO, q12h, up to 1 wk; then 5-7.5 mg/kg PO q12h for 2 wk; then 7.5 mg/kg q24h as maintenance Cat: no dosage recommendation
Amitraz	Mitaban	Antiparasitic/especially ectoparasites: Demodex and Sarcoptes	10.6 mL concentrated dip (19.9%)	10.6 mL per 7.5 L water (0.025% solution); apply three to six topical treatments every 2 weeks for refractory cases, this dose has been exceeded to produce increased efficacy. Doses that have been used include 0.025%, 0.05%, and 0.1% concentration applied twice a week and 0.125% solution applied to one-half body every day for 4 weeks to 5 months.

6

Amitriptyline	Elavil	Behavior modifier/ *separation anxiety and (in cats) chronic idiopathic cystitis*	10-, 25-, 50-, 75-, 100-, and 150-mg tablets; 10 mg/mL injection	Dog: 1-2 mg/kg PO q12-24h (range: 0.25-4 mg/kg q12-24h) Cat: 2 mg/kg or approx 5-10 mg per cat per day PO
Amlodipine	Norvasc	Calcium channel blocker/ *vasodilator for systemic hypertension*	2.5-, 5-, and 10-mg tablets	Dog: 2.5 mg/dog or 0.1 mg/kg PO once daily Cat: 0.625 mg/cat/day PO initially; then increase if needed to 1.25 mg/cat/day (average is 0.18 mg/kg once daily)
Ammonium chloride	Generic	Urinary acidifier/*acidify urine and treat metabolic alkalosis*	Available as crystals	Dog: 100 mg/kg PO q12h Cat: 800 mg/cat (approximately ⅓ to ¼ tsp) mixed with food daily
Amoxicillin trihydrate	Amoxi-Tabs; Amoxi-drops; Amoxil; others	Broad-spectrum antibacterial	50-, 100-, 200-, and 400-mg tablets; 50 mg/mL oral suspension	6-20 mg/kg PO q8-12h
Amoxicillin/ clavulanate	Clavamox	Broad-spectrum antibacterial	62.5-, 125-, 250-, and 375-mg tablets; 62.5 mg/mL suspension	Dog: 12.5-15 mg/kg PO q12h Cat: 62.5 mg/cat PO q12h; consider administering these doses q8h for gram-negative infections
Amphotericin B	AmBisome (new formulation; less toxic but expensive)	Antifungal (liposomal formulation)/*deep, systemic fungal infection & leishmaniasis*	50-mg injectable vial	3-5 mg/kg/day IV administered over 60-120 min
	Fungizone (traditional formulation)	Antifungal/*deep systemic fungal infection & leishmaniasis*	50-mg injectable vial	0.5 mg//kg IV (slow infusion) q48h; cumulative dose is 4-8 mg/kg CAUTION: Monitor renal function
Ampicillin	Omnipen; Principen; others	Broad-spectrum antibacterial	250- and 500-mg capsules; 125-, 250-, and 500-mg vials of ampicillin sodium	10-20 mg/kg IV, IM, SC q6-8h (ampicillin sodium); 20-40 mg/kg PO q8h

Continued

Note: Listings preceded by ◆ are for rapid reference and denote drug/dosage used in the emergency or critical care setting.

6

TABLE 6-26 **Common Drug Indications and Dosages†—cont'd**

Drug	Proprietary names	Action/*Use*	Formulation	Recommended dosage
◆ Ampicillin + sulbactam	Unasyn	Broad-spectrum antibacterial	1.5- and 3-g vials in 2:1 combination for injection	10-20 mg/kg IV, IM q8h
Ampicillin trihydrate	Polyflex	Broad-spectrum antibacterial	10- and 25-mg vials for injection	6.5-10 mg/kg IM, SC q12h
Amprolium	Amprol, Corid	Thiamine analog/ *treatment of coccidia*	9.6% (9.6 g/dL) oral solution; soluble powder	1.25 g of 20% amprolium powder to daily feed, or 30 mL of 9.6% amprolium solution to 3.8 L of drinking water for 7 days
◆ Antiserum, snakebite	Antivenin	Antivenin/*concentrated serum globulin from horses immunized with multiple types of venom*	10-mL vials	Dose varies from 10 to 50 mL (1 to 5 vials) initially; additional doses may be administered 2 h following initial treatment
Apomorphine hydrochloride	Generic	Emetic (potent)	6-mg tablet	0.02-0.04 mg/kg IV, IM, 0.1 mg/kg SC, or instill 0.25 mg in conjunctiva of eye (dissolve 6-mg tablet in 1-2 mL of saline)
Ascorbic acid	Vitamin C	Vitamin supplement	Various forms	100-500 mg/animal/day (diet supplement) or 100 mg/animal q8h (urine acidification)
L-Asparaginase	Elspar	Antineoplastic/*lymphoid malignancies*	10,000 U per vial for injection	Dog: 10,000 to 20,000 IU/m² IV once weekly Cat: 400 U/kg SC or IM (as part of a protocol) *Pretreatment with antihistamine* (diphenhydramine), 2 mg/kg (dog) and 1 mg/kg (cat) 30 minutes earlier is recommended
Aspirin	Many generic and brand name products (e.g., Bufferin, Ascriptin)	NSAID; anticoagulant	81- and 325-mg tablets	Dog: *Mild analgesia:* 10 mg/kg q12h *Antiinflammatory:* 20-25 mg/kg q12h *Antiplatelet:* 5-10 mg/kg q24-48h Cat: 10-20 mg/kg q48h *Antiplatelet:* 80 mg q48h

6

Atenolol	Tenormin	*Beta-blocker/hypertension and tachyarrhythmias*	25-, 50-, and 100-mg tablets; 25 mg/mL oral suspension; and 0.5 mg/mL ampule for injection	Dog: 6.25-12.5 mg/dog q12h (or 0.25-1.0 mg/kg q12-24h) Cat: 6.25-12.5 mg/cat q12h
Atracurium	Tracrium	*Neuromuscular blocking agent/adjunct to general anesthesia for muscle relaxation*	10-mg/mL injection	0.2 mg/kg IV initially; then 0.15 mg/kg q30min (or IV infusion at 3-8 µg/kg/min) (approx. 3 mg/kg)
◆ Atropine	Many generic products	*Antimuscarinic-anticholinergic/preanesthetic agent and treatment of some bradyarrhythmias*	400-, 500-, and 540 µg/mL injection; 15 mg/mL injection	0.02-0.04 mg/kg IV, IM, SC q6-8h or 0.2-0.5 mg/kg (as needed) for organophosphate and carbamate toxicosis
Auranofin (triethylphosphine gold)	Ridaura	*Gold compound/immune-mediated skin disease*	3-mg capsule	0.1-0.2 mg/kg PO q12h
Aurothioglucose	Solganol	*Gold compound/immune-mediated skin disease*	50 mg/mL injection	Dog <10 kg: 1 mg IM 1st wk, 2 mg IM 2nd wk, and then 1 mg/kg/wk maintenance; >10 kg: 5 mg IM 1st wk, 10 mg 2nd wk, and then 1 mg/kg/wk maintenance Cat: 0.5-1 mg/cat IM q7days
Azathioprine	Imuran	*Purine antagonist/immunosuppressive agent*	50-mg tablet; 10 mg/mL injection	Dog: 2 mg/kg PO q24h initially; then 0.5-1 mg/kg q48h Cat (use cautiously): 1 mg/kg PO q48h *Monitoring patient CBC is indicated during therapy*
Azithromycin	Zithromax	*Antibacterial/broad-spectrum activity with very long tissue half-life*	250-mg capsule; 250- and 600-mg tablets; 20 mg/mL oral suspension	Dog: 5-10 mg/kg PO once daily for 3-5 days (treatment may be extended for up to 10 days of consecutive treatment) Cat: 5-10 mg/kg PO daily for 3-5 days.

Note: Listings preceded by ◆ are for rapid reference and denote drug/dosage used in the emergency or critical care setting.

Continued

6

TABLE 6-26 Common Drug Indications and Dosages†—cont'd

Drug	Proprietary names	Action/Use	Formulation	Recommended dosage
BAL	*See* Dimercaprol, Lotensin			
Benazepril		ACE inhibitor/chronic heart failure, hypertension, first choice in treating protein-losing nephropathies	5-, 10-, 20-, and 40-mg tablets	Dog: *Heart failure*: 0.25-0.5 mg/kg PO q24h *Hypertension*: 0.25 mg/kg PO q12h Cat: *Heart failure*: 0.25-0.5 mg/kg PO once or twice daily *Hypertension*: 0.25-1.0 mg/kg PO once or twice daily
Betamethasone	Celestone	Potent glucocorticoid/antiinflammatory and immune-mediated disease	600-µg (0.6-mg) tablet; 3 mg/mL sodium phosphate injection	Dog and cat: *Antiinflammatory*: 0.1-0.2 mg/kg PO q12-24h *Immunosuppressive*: 0.2-0.5 mg/kg once or twice daily
Bethanechol	Urecholine	Muscarinic-cholinergic/enhance urinary bladder contraction	5-, 10-, 25-, and 50-mg tablets; 5 mg/mL injection	Dog: 5-15 mg/dog PO q8h Cat: 1.25-5 mg/cat PO q8h
Bisacodyl	Dulcolax	Stimulant laxative	5-mg tablet	5 mg/animal PO q8-24h
Bismuth subsalicylate	Pepto-Bismol	GI protectant/treatment of simple (uncomplicated) diarrhea	Oral suspension; 262 mg/15 mL or 525 mg/mL in extra strength formulation; 262-mg tablet	1-3 mL/kg/day (in divided doses) PO
Bleomycin	Blenoxane	Antineoplastic/used in multiple cancer protocols	15-U vials for injection	Dog: 10 U/m² IV or SC for 3 days; then 10 U/m² weekly (maximum cumulative dose 200 U/m²)
Bromide	*See* Potassium bromide			
Bromocriptine mesylate	Parlodel	Dopamine agonist and prolactin inhibitor/pregnancy termination or pseudopregnancy (pseudocyesis) in dogs	2.5-mg tablets and 5.0-mg capsules	*Pseudocyesis*: 10 µg/kg PO for 10 days, or 30 µg/kg PO for 16 days *Pregnancy termination*: 50-100 µg/kg PO for 4-7 days; begin treatment from day 35-45 after LH surge CAUTION: Vomiting is a common side effect
Bunamidine hydrochloride	Scolaban	Antiparasitic/tapeworms	400-mg tablet	20-50 mg/kg PO per treatment

Continued

Drug	Brand/Generic	Classification/Indication	Available Forms	Dosage
Bupivacaine	Marcaine; generic	Local anesthetic (parenteral)	2.5- and 5-mg/mL solution injection	1 mL of 0.5% solution/10 cm for an epidural
Buprenorphine	Buprenex	Partial opiate agonist *analgesic*	0.3 mg/mL solution	Dog: 0.005-0.02 mg/kg IV, IM, SC q6-12h; Cat: 0.005-0.01 mg/kg IV, IM q6-12h; Buccal administration is well tolerated in cats and lasts ~6 hours
Buspirone	BuSpar	Non-benzodiazepine anxiolytic/*control urine spraying*	5- and 10-mg tablets	Cat: 2.5-5 mg/cat PO daily (may be increased to twice daily for some cats)
Busulfan	Myleran	Oral antineoplastic/*chronic granulocytic leukemia*	2-mg tablet	3-4 mg/m^2 PO q24h
Butorphanol	Torbutrol; Torbugesic	Opioid analgesic/ *perioperative analgesia*	1-, 5-, and 10-mg tablets; 0.5 or 10 mg/mL injection	Dog: *Antitussive*: 0.055 mg/kg SC q6-12h or 0.55 mg/kg PO; *Preanesthetic*: 0.2-0.4 mg/kg IV, IM, SC (with acepromazine); *Analgesic*: 0.2-0.4 mg/kg IV, IM, SC q2-4h or 0.55-1.1 mg/kg PO q6-12h; Cat: *Analgesic*: 0.2-0.8 mg/kg IV, SC q2-6h or 1.5 mg/kg PO q4-8h
Calcitriol	Rocaltrol; Calcijex	*Calcium supplement/ increases calcium absorption in the GI tract; used in management of hypoparathyroidism*	Available as injection (Calcijex) and capsules (Rocaltrol): 0.25- and 0.5-µg capsules; 1- or 2-µg/mL injection	Dog: 0.25 to 0.5 µg/dog/day PO q24h; Cat: 0.25 µg/cat PO q48h
Calcium carbonate	Generic and many brand name products (e.g., Tums)	Calcium supplement	Many tablets or oral suspension (e.g., 650-mg tablet contains 260 mg calcium ion)	5-10 mL oral solution PO q4-6h; *For phosphate binder*: 60-100 mg/kg/day PO in divided doses
◆Calcium chloride	Generic	Calcium supplement	10% (100 mg/ml) solution	0.1-0.3 mL/kg IV (slowly)
Calcium citrate (OTC)	Citrical	Calcium supplement	950-mg tablet (contains 200 mg calcium ion)	Dog: 20 mg/kg/day PO (with meals); Cat: 10-30 mg/kg q8h PO (with meals)
◆Calcium gluconate	Kalcinate and generic	Calcium supplement	10% (100 mg/mL) injection	0.5-1.5 mL/kg IV (slowly)
Calcium lactate (OTC)	Generic	Calcium supplement	Available as a powder and various-sized tablets	Dog: 0.5-2.0 g/dog/day PO (in divided doses); Cat: 0.2-0.5 g/cat/day PO (in divided doses)

Note: Listings preceded by ◆ are for rapid reference and denote drug/dosage used in the emergency or critical care setting.

6

TABLE 6-26 Common Drug Indications and Dosages†—cont'd

Drug	Proprietary names	Action/*Use*	Formulation	Recommended dosage
Captopril	Capoten	ACE inhibitor (vasodilator)/ *hypertension and congestive heart failure*	25-mg tablet	Dog: 0.5-2 mg/kg PO q8-12h Cat: 3.12-6.25 mg/cat PO q8h
Carbenicillin	Geopen; Pyopen	Antibacterial	1-, 2-, 5-, 10-, and 30-g vials for injection	40-50 mg/kg and up to 100 mg/kg IV, IM, SC q6-8h
Carbenicillin indanyl sodium	Geocillin	Antibacterial	500-mg tablet	10 mg/kg PO q8h
Carboplatin	Paraplatin	Antineoplastic/*multiple tumor types*	50- and 150-mg vials for injection	Dog: 300 mg/m² IV q3-4 wk Cat: 200 mg/m² IV q4wk
◆ Carprofen	Rimadyl	NSAID	25-, 75-, and 100-mg tablets 50 mg/mL in 20-mL vials for injection	Dog: 2.2 mg/kg PO q12h Cat: Not approved for use in cats
Cascara sagrada (OTC)	Many brand name products	Laxative	100- and 325-mg tablets	Dog: 1-5 mg/kg/day PO Cat: 1-2 mg/cat/day
Castor oil (OTC)	Generic	Laxative	Oral liquid (100%)	Dog: 8-30 mL/day PO Cat: 4-10 mL/day PO
Cefaclor	Ceclor	Antibacterial	250- and 500-mg capsules and 25 mg/mL oral suspension	4-20 mg/kg PO q8h
◆ Cefadroxil	Cefa-Tabs; Cefa-Drops	Antibacterial	50 mg/mL oral suspension; 50-, 100-, 200-, and 1000-mg tablets	Dog: 22-30 mg/kg PO q12h Cat: 22 mg/kg PO q24h
Cefepime	Maxipime	Antibacterial	500-mg, 1-g, and 2-g vials for injection	40 mg/kg IV q6h
Cefixime	Suprax	Antibacterial	20 mg/mL oral suspension; 200- and 400-mg tablets	10 mg/kg PO q12h *For cystitis:* 5 mg/kg PO q12-24h
Cefotaxime	Claforan	Antibacterial	500-mg and 1-, 2-, and 10-g vials for injection	Dog: 50 mg/kg IV, IM, SC q12h Cat: 20-80 mg/kg IV, IM q6h
Cefotetan	Cefotan	Antibacterial	1-, 2-, and 10-g vials for injection	30 mg/kg IV, SC q8h
◆ Cefoxitin sodium	Mefoxin	Antibacterial	1-, 2-, and 10-g vials for injection	30 mg/kg IV q6-8h

Drug	Trade/Generic	Category	Formulation	Dosage
Ceftazidime	Fortaz; Ceptaz; Tazicef	Antibacterial	0.5-, 1-, 2-, and 6-g vials reconstituted to 280 mg/mL	Dog and cat: 30 mg/kg IV, IM q6h *CRI:* Loading dose 4.4 mg/kg; then 4.1 mg/kg/h with IV fluids
Ceftiofur	Naxcel (ceftiofur sodium); Excenel (ceftiofur HCl)	Antibacterial	50 mg/mL injection	Dog: 30 mg/kg, SC, q4-6h 2.2-4.4 mg/kg SC q24h (for urinary tract infections)
◆ Cephalexin	Keflex; generic	Antibacterial/*especially skin, urinary, respiratory tract infections*	250- and 500-mg capsules; 250- and 500-mg tablets; 100 mg/mL or 125 and 250 mg/5 mL oral suspension	10-30 mg PO q6-12h *Pyoderma:* 22-35 mg/kg PO q12h
Cephalothin sodium	Keflin	Antibacterial	1- and 2-g vials for injection	10-30 mg/kg IV, IM q4-8h
Cephapirin	Cefadyl	Antibacterial	500-mg and 1-, 2-, and 4-g vials for injection	10-30 mg/kg IV, IM q4-8h
◆ Charcoal, activated	ActaChar; Charcodote; Toxiban; generic	GI adsorbent	Oral suspension	1-4 g/kg PO (granules) 6-12 mg/kg (suspension)
Chlorambucil	Leukeran	Antineoplastic/*has also been used to treat eosinophilic granuloma complex in cats*	2-mg tablet	2-6 mg/m² q24h initially; then q48h PO Cat: 0.1-0.2 mg/kg q24h initially; then q48h PO
Chloramphenicol and chloramphenicol palmitate	Chloromycetin; generic	Antibacterial	30 mg/mL oral suspension (palmitate); 250-mg capsule; and 100-, 250-, and 500-mg tablets	Dog: 40-50 mg/kg PO q8h Cat: 12.5-20 mg/kg PO q12h
Chloramphenicol sodium succinate	Chloromycetin; generic	Antibacterial	100 mg/mL injection	Dog: 40-50 mg/kg IV, IM q6-8h Cat: 12.5-20 mg/cat IV, IM q12h
Chlorothiazide	Diuril	Diuretic/*also used as an antihypertensive*	250- and 500-mg tablets; 50 mg/mL oral suspension and injection	20-40 mg/kg PO q12h

Continued

Note: Listings preceded by ◆ are for rapid reference and denote drug/dosage used in the emergency or critical care setting.

6

TABLE 6-26   Common Drug Indications and Dosages†—cont'd

Drug	Proprietary names	Action/Use	Formulation	Recommended dosage
Chlorpheniramine maleate (OTC)	Chlor-Trimeton; Phenetron; others	Antihistamine (H$_1$-blocker)/ *weak antipruritic agent in allergic animals*	4- and 8-mg tablets	Dog: 4-8 mg/dog PO q12h (up to maximum of 0.5 mg/kg q12h) Cat: 2 mg/cat PO q12h
Chlorpromazine	Thorazine	Tranquilizer/antiemetic	25-mg/mL injection solution	0.5 mg/kg IM, SC q6-8h *Before cancer chemotherapy:* 2 mg/kg SC q3h
Chlortetracycline	Generic	Antibacterial	Powdered feed additive	25 mg/kg PO q6-8h
Chorionic gonadotropin	*See* Gonadotropin			
Cimetidine	Tagamet	Antihistamine (H$_2$ blocker)/ *treatment and prevention of gastric ulcer*	100-, 150-, 200-, and 300-mg tablets; 60 mg/mL injection	10 mg/kg IV, IM, PO q6-8h *In renal failure:* 2.5-5 mg/kg IV, PO q12h
Ciprofloxacin	Cipro	Antibacterial	250-, 500-, and 750-mg tablets, 2 mg/mL injection	5-15 mg/kg PO, IV q12h
Cisapride	Propulsid	Prokinetic/stimulates *GI tract motility*	10-mg tablet	Dog: 0.1-0.5 mg/kg PO q8-12h (doses as high as 0.5-1.0 mg/kg have been used in some dogs) Cat: 2.5-5 mg/cat PO q8-12h (doses as high as 1 mg/kg q8h have been used in cats)
Cisplatin	Platinol	Antineoplastic/*multiple tumor types*	1-mg/mL injection; 50-mg vials	Dog: 60-70 mg/m² IV q3-4wk (administer fluid for diuresis with therapy) Cat: DO NOT USE.
Clemastine	Tavist; Contac 12 Hour; generic	Antihistamine (H$_1$-blocker)/ *antipruritic in allergic dogs*	1.34-mg tablet (OTC); 2.64-mg tablet (Rx); 0.134 mg/mL syrup	Dog: 0.05-0.1 mg/kg PO q12h
◆ Clindamycin	Antirobe; Cleocin	Antibacterial/*especially gram-positive infections.* Recommended for toxoplas-mosis (controversial).	25 mg/mL oral liquid; 25-, 75-, and 150-mg capsule; and 150-mg/mL injection (Cleocin)	Dog: 11 mg/kg PO q12h or 22 mg/kg PO q24h Cat: 5.5 mg/kg q12h, or 11 mg/kg q24h (staphylococcal infections); 11 mg/kg q12h or 22 mg/kg q24h (anaerobic infections) PO *Toxoplasmosis:* 12.5 mg/kg PO q12h for 4 wk
Clofazimine	Lamprene	Antibacterial	50- and 100-mg capsules	Cat: 1 mg/kg PO up to maximum of 4 mg/kg/day
Clomipramine	Anafranil (human); Clomicalm (veterinary)	Tricyclic antidepressant/ *behavior modification*	10-, 25-, and 50-mg tablets (human); 5-, 20-, and 80-mg tablets (veterinary)	Dog: 1-2 mg/kg PO q12h up to maximum of 3 mg/kg PO q12h Cat: 1-5 mg/cat PO q12-24h

Clonazepam	Klonopin	Anticonvulsant/also used to manage certain types of behavior disorders	0.5-, 1-, and 2-mg tablets	0.5 mg/kg PO q8-12h
Clorazepate	Tranxene	Anticonvulsant/also used to manage certain types of behavior disorders	3.75-, 7.5-, 11.25-, 15-, and 22.5-mg tablets	2 mg/kg PO q12h
Clotrimazole (CTL)	Many generic products, including lotrimazole topical solution, USP 1%	Antifungal (topical only)/nasal aspergillosis	1% topical solution in 30 mL	*For nasal aspergillosis in dogs:* Infuse 1% solution in each nasal cavity for 1 h in anesthetized dog. *NOTE: patient preparation is required*
Cloxacillin	Cloxapen; Orbenin; Tegopen	Antibacterial	250- and 500-mg capsules; 25 mg/mL oral solution	20-40 mg/kg PO q8h
Codeine	Generic	Opioid analgesic	15-, 30-, and 60-mg tablets; 5 mg/mL syrup; 3 mg/mL oral solution	*Analgesia:* 0.5-1 mg/kg PO q4-6h *Antitussive:* 0.1-0.3 mg/kg PO q4-6h
Colchicine	Generic	Antiinflammatory/hepatic failure	500- and 600-µg tablets; 500 µg/mL ampule injection	0.01-0.3 mg/kg PO q24h
Colony-stimulating factor	Neupogen	Hormone/stimulate granulocyte production in bone marrow	300 µg/mL injection	2.5 µg/kg SC q12h
◆ Corticotropin (ACTH Gel)	H.P. Acthar Gel (*expensive*)	Hormone/diagnostic test drug for the diagnosis of hyper- and hypoadrenocorticism	5 mL (multiple dose) 80 USP units/mL	*Response test:* Collect pre-ACTH sample and inject 2.2 IU/kg IM; Dog: Collect post-ACTH sample in 2 h Cat: Collect post-ACTH samples at 1 and 2 h
◆ Cosyntropin	Cortrosyn	Hormone/diagnostic test drug for the diagnosis of hyper- and hypoadrenocorticism	250 µg per vial (can be stored in freezer for 6 months)	*Response test:* Dog: Collect pre-sample and inject 5 µg/kg IV Cat: Collect pre-sample and inject 0.125 mg/kg IV Dog and cat: Collect post sample 1 h post-administration.

Note: Listings preceded by ◆ are for rapid reference and denote drug/dosage used in the emergency or critical care setting.

Continued

6

TABLE 6-26   Common Drug Indications and Dosages†—cont'd

Drug	Proprietary names	Action/use	Formulation	Recommended dosage
Cyanocobalamin	*See* Vitamin B$_{12}$			
Cyclophosphamide	Cytoxan; Neosar	Antineoplastic/multiple tumor types and adjunctive in immune-mediated disorders	25 mg/mL injections; 25- and 50-mg tablets	*Anticancer:* 50 mg/m^2 PO once daily 4 days/wk or 150-300 mg/m^2 IV and repeat in 21 days *Immunosuppressive therapy:* 50 mg/m^2 (approx 2.2 mg/kg) PO q48h or 2.2 mg/kg once daily for 4 days/wk *Cat:* 6.25-12.5 mg/cat once daily 4 days/wk
Cyclosporine (cyclosporin A)	Neoral, Sandimmune; Optimmune (ophthalmic)	Immunosuppressant (CMI)/ multiple uses ranging from atopic dermatitis to hemolytic anemia to perianal fistulas Consult additional references before prescribing	Neoral: 25-mg and 100-mg microemulsion capsules; 100-mg/mL oral solution (for microemulsion) Sandimmune: 100-mg/mL oral solution; 25- and 100-mg capsules Optimmune: 0.2% ointment	*Dog:* 3-7 mg/kg, PO, q12-24h (adjust dose based on condition being treated and by monitoring blood levels) *Hemolytic anemia:* Up to 10 mg/kg PO q12h (as adjunctive therapy) *Cat:* 4-6 mg/kg PO q12h NOTE: *multiple products are available but all are NOT bioequivalent*
Cyproheptadine	Periactin	Antihistamine/appetite stimulant in cats	4-mg tablet; 2 mg/5 mL syrup	*Antihistamine:* 1.1 mg/kg PO q8-12h *Appetite stimulant:* 2 mg/cat PO
Cytarabine (cytosine arabinoside)	Cytosar-U	Antineoplastic/lymphoma and leukemia	100-mg vial	*Dog* (lymphoma): 100 mg/m^2 IV, SC once daily or twice daily for 4 days *Cat:* 100 mg/m^2 once daily for 2 days
Dacarbazine	DTIC	Antineoplastic/lymphoreticular neoplasms and soft tissue sarcomas	200-mg vial for injection	200 mg/m^2 IV for 5 days q3wks; or 800-1000 mg/m^2 IV q3wks
◆ Dalteparin	Fragmin	Low molecular weight heparin/management of thromboembolic disease	Multiple injectable preparations	*Prophylaxis:* 70 IU/kg q24h SC *Treatment:* 200 IU/kg q24h SC
Danazol	Danocrine	Anabolic steroid/adjunctive therapy for immune-mediated disease	50-, 100-, and 200-mg capsules	5-10 mg/kg PO q12h

6

Drug	Brand/Forms	Use	Dosage Forms	Dosage
Dantrolene	Dantrium	Muscle relaxant/urethral obstruction and prevention of malignant hyperthermia	100-mg capsules; 0.33 mg/mL injection	*Malignant hyperthermia: 2-3 mg/kg IV Muscle relaxation:* Dog: 1-5 mg/kg PO q8h Cat: 0.5-2 mg/kg PO q12h
Dapsone	Generic	Antibacterial/ *Mycobacterium* spp.	25- and 100-mg tablets	1.1 mg/kg PO q8-12h
◆ Deferoxamine	Desferal	Antidote/iron toxicosis	500-mg vial for injection	10 mg/kg IV, IM q2h for two doses; then 10 mg/kg q8h for 24 h
Deprenyl (L-deprenyl)	*See Selegiline (Anipryl)*			
◆ Desmopressin acetate	DDAVP	Hormone/*used in the clinical management of patients with diabetes insipidus and patients with von Willebrand's disease*	100 µg/mL injection and desmopressin acetate nasal solution (0.01% metered spray); 0.1- and 0.2-mg tablets	Diabetes insipidus: 2-4 drops (2 µg) q12-24h intranasally or in eye; animal oral dose not established, but dose extrapolated from humans is 0.05 mg/animal q12h PO with increase to 0.1 or 0.2 mg/animal as needed. *von Willebrand's disease:* 1 µg/mL (0.01 mL/kg) SC, IV diluted in 20 mL saline administered over 10 min
Desoxycorticosterone pivalate	Percorten-V; DOCP; DOCA pivalate	Mineralocorticoid/ *hypoadrenocorticism*	25 mg/mL suspension for injection	1.5-2.2 mg/kg IM q25days
◆ Dexamethasone (dexamethasone solution and dexamethasone sodium phosphate)	Azium solution in polyethylene glycol; sodium phosphate forms include Dexaject SP, Dexavet, and Dexasone; tablets include Decadron and generic	Glucocorticoid/multiple *uses as antiinflammatory and immunosuppressive agent; also used in the diagnosis of hyperadrenocorticism*	Azium solution, 2 mg/mL; sodium phosphate forms are 3.33 mg/mL; 0.25-, 0.5-, 1-, 1.5-, 2-, 4-, and 6-mg tablets.	Antiinflammatory: 0.07-0.15 mg/kg IV, IM, PO q12-24h *For shock, spinal injury:* 2.2-4.4 mg/kg IV (of sodium phosphate form) *Diagnostic testing use:* See Dexamethasone Suppression in Section 5.
◆ Dextran	Dextran 70; Gentran-70	Replacement fluid	Injectable solution: 250, 500, and 1000 mL	10-20 mL/kg IV to effect

Continued

Note: Listings preceded by ◆ are for rapid reference and denote drug/dosage used in the emergency or critical care setting.

6

TABLE 6-26 Common Drug Indications and Dosages†—cont'd

Drug	Proprietary names	Action/Use	Formulation	Recommended dosage
Dextromethorphan	Benylin and others	Antitussive/weak cough suppressant	Available in syrup, capsule, and tablet; many OTC products	0.5-2 mg/kg PO q6-8h
◆ Dextrose solution 5% in water	D5W	Replacement fluid	Fluid solution for IV administration	40-50 mL/kg IV q24h
◆ Diazepam	Valium; generic	Anticonvulsant/multiple neurotropic effects ranging from behavior disorders to seizure control	2- and 5-mg tablets; 5 mg/mL solution for injection	Preanesthetic: 0.5 mg/kg IV Status epilepticus: 0.5 mg/kg IV, 1.0 mg/kg rectal; repeat if necessary Appetite stimulant (cat): 0.2 mg/kg IV
◆ Dichlorphenamide	Daranide	Diuretic/management of glaucoma	50-mg tablet	3-5 mg/kg PO q8-12h
Dichlorvos	Task	Antiparasitic/roundworms, hookworms, whipworms	10- and 25-mg tablets	Dog: 26.4-33 mg/kg PO Cat: 11 mg/kg PO
Dicloxacillin	Dynapen	Antibacterial	125-, 250-, and 500-mg capsules; 12.5 mg/mL oral suspension	25 mg/kg IM q6h Oral doses not absorbed
Diethylcarbamazine (DEC)	Caricide; Filaribits	Antiparasitic/prevention of heartworm disease in dogs; treatment of ascarids in cats	Chewable tablets; 50-, 60, 180-, 200-, and 400-mg tablets	Heartworm prophylaxis: 6.6 mg/kg PO q24h Cat: (for ascarids) 55-110 mg/kg PO once
Diethylstilbestrol (DES)	Limited availability; compounding required	Hormone/estrogen replacement and urinary incontinence; induce abortion in dogs	Tablets (prepared through compounding pharmacies)	Dog: 0.1-1.0 mg/dog PO q24h Cat: 0.05-0.1 mg/cat PO q24h
Difloxacin	Dicural	Antibacterial	11.4-, 45.4-, and 136-mg tablets	5-10 mg/kg/day PO
Digitoxin	Crystodigin	Cardiac inotrope/congestive heart failure and management of various tachyarrhythmias	0.05- and 0.1-mg tablets	0.02-0.03 mg/kg PO q8h

Drug	Trade name	Indication/use	Available forms	Dosage
Digoxin	Lanoxin; Cardoxin	*Cardiac inotrope/congestive heart failure and management of various tachyarrhythmias*	0.0625-, 0.125-, 0.25-mg tablets; 0.05 and 0.15 mg/mL elixir	Dog: <20 kg, 0.01 mg/kg q12h; >20 kg, 0.22 mg/m² PO q12h (subtract 10% for elixir) Dog (rapid digitalization): 0.0055-0.011 mg/kg IV q1h to effect Cat: 0.08-0.01 mg/kg PO q48h (approximately ¼ of a 0.125-mg tablet/cat)
Dihydrotachysterol (DHT)	*See* Vitamin D analog			
◆ Diltiazem	Cardizem; Dilacor	*Calcium channel blocker/hypertension; also supraventricular tachycardia and hypertrophic cardiomyopathy*	30-, 60-, 90-, and 120-mg tablets; 50 mg/mL injection	Dog: 0.5-1.5 mg/kg PO q8h; 0.25 mg/kg over 2 min IV (repeat if necessary) Cat: 1.75-2.4 mg/kg PO q8h; for *Dilacor XR* or *Cardizem CD*, dose is 10 mg/kg PO once daily
◆ Dimenhydrinate	Dramamine	*Antihistamine/prevention of motion sickness*	50-mg tablets; 50 mg/mL injection	Dog: 4-8 mg/kg PO, IM, IV q8h Cat: 12.5 mg/cat IV, IM, PO q8h
◆ Dimercaprol (BAL)	BAL in Oil	*Chelating agent/bind heavy metals (lead, mercury) and arsenicals*	100 injection	4 mg/kg IM q4h
Dinoprost tromethamine	*See* Prostaglandin F$_{2a}$			
Dioctyl calcium sulfosuccinate	*See* Docusate calcium			
Dioctyl sodium sulfosuccinate	*See* Docusate sodium			
◆ Diphenhydramine	Benadryl	*Antihistamine/weak sedative, prevents motion sickness*	Available OTC: 2.5 mg/mL elixir; 25- and 50-mg capsules and tablets; 50 mg/mL injection	2-4 mg/kg PO q6-8h or 1 mg/kg IM, IV (for dogs, administer 25-50 mg/dog IV, IM, PO q8h)

Continued

Note: Listings preceded by ◆ are for rapid reference and denote drug/dosage used in the emergency or critical care setting.

6

TABLE 6-26   Common Drug Indications and Dosages†—cont'd

Drug	Proprietary names	Action/use	Formulation	Recommended dosage
Diphenoxylate	Lomotil	Meperidine congener/*treatment of diarrhea*	2.5 mg tablets	Dog: 0.1-0.2 mg/kg PO q8-12h Cat: 0.05-0.1 mg/kg PO q12h
Diphenylhydantoin	*See* Phenytoin			
Diphosphonate disodium etidronate	*See* Etidronate disodium			
Dipyridamole	Persantine	Anticoagulant/*prevention of thromboembolism*	25-, 50-, 75-mg tablets; 5 mg/mL injection	4-10 mg/kg PO q24h
Disopyramide	Norpace	Antiarrhythmic in dogs/*oral treatment or prevention of ventricular arrhythmias (dog only)*	100- and 150-mg capsules	Dog: 6-15 mg/kg, PO, q8h
Divalproex sodium	*See* Valproic acid			
◆ Dobutamine	Dobutrex	Rapid acting cardiac inotrope (beta-agonist)/*short-term treatment of heart failure*	250 mg/20 mL vial for injection (12.5 mg/mL)	Dog: 5-20 µg/kg/min IV infusion Cat: 0.5-2 µg/kg/min IV infusion WARNING: may induce arrhythmias, facial twitching, or seizure (cats)
Docusate calcium	Surfak; Doxidan	Stool softener	60-mg tablet (and many others)	Dog: 50-100 mg/dog PO q12-24h Cat: 50 mg/cat PO q12-24h
Docusate sodium	Colace; Doxan; Doss; many OTC products	Stool softener	50- and 100-mg capsules; 10 mg/mL liquid	Dog: 50-200 mg/dog PO q8-12h Cat: 50 mg/cat PO q12-24h
◆ Dolasetron	Anzemet	5-HT$_3$ receptor antagonist/*antiemetic*	50- and 100-mg tablets; 20 mg/mL injection	*Prevention:* 0.6 mg/kg, PO or IV q24h *Treatment:* 1 mg/kg, PO or IV q24h
◆ Dopamine	Intropin	Cardiac inotrope (beta-agonist)/*vasodilation (lower doses); adjunctive treatment of acute heart failure and oliguric renal failure*	40-, 80-, or 160-mg/mL	2-10 µg/kg/min by IV infusion; treatment limited to the critical care setting.

Generic	Trade name	Indication/Use	Formulation	Dosage
◆ Doxapram	Dopram	CNS stimulant/*stimulate respiration, especially in neonates*	20-mg/mL injection	5-10 mg/kg IV Neonate: 1-5 mg SC, sublingual, or via umbilical vein
Doxepin	Sinequan	Tricyclic antidepressant/*psychogenic dermatoses*	Various capsules; 10 mg/mL oral solution	0.5-1.0 mg/kg PO q12h (*especially lick granuloma*)
Doxorubicin	Adriamycin	Antineoplastic (antibiotic)/*used in treatment protocols for multiple tumor types*	2 mg/mL injection	30 mg/m^2 IV q 21 days; or >20 kg, 30 mg/m^2; <20 kg, 1 mg/kg Cat: 1 mg/kg IV q3wk
Doxycycline	Vibramycin; generic	Antibacterial	10 mg/mL oral suspension; 100-mg tablet; 100-mg injection vial	3-5 mg/kg PO, IV q12h; or 10 mg/kg PO q24h *For Rickettsia* in dogs: 5 mg/kg q12h
◆ EDTA (edetate calcium disodium)	Calcium disodium versenate	Chelates heavy metals/*treatment of lead or zinc toxicosis*	20 mg/mL injection	25 mg/kg SC, IM, IV q6h for 2-5 days
Edrophonium	Tensilon; others	Short-acting cholinergic/*administered as a test agent for myasthenia gravis*	10 mg/mL injection	Dog: 0.11-0.22 mg/kg IV Cat: 2.5 mg/cat IV
Enalapril	Enacard	ACE inhibitor/vasodilator *used in the treatment of heart failure and/or hypertension; also used in the treatment of patients with protein-losing nephropathies and chronic renal failure*	2.5-, 5-, 10-, and 20-mg tablets	Dog: 0.5 mg/kg PO q12-24h Cat: 0.25-0.5 mg/kg PO q12-24h
Enflurane	Ethane	Inhalation anesthetic	Available as solution for inhalation	*Induction: 2-3%* *Maintenance: 1.5-3%*

Note: Listings preceded by ◆ are for rapid reference and denote drug/dosage used in the emergency or critical care setting.

Continued

6

TABLE 6-26   Common Drug Indications and Dosages†—cont'd

Drug	Proprietary names	Action/use	Formulation	Recommended dosage
Enilconazole	Imaverol; ClinaFarm-EC	Antifungal (topical only)/ infusion for treatment of nasal aspergillosis and topical uses in certain dermatophytoses	10% or 13.8% emulsifiable concentrate	*Nasal aspergillosis:* 10 mg/kg q12h instilled into nasal sinus via surgically implanted tubes for 14 days (10% solution diluted 50/50 with water)... this is nasty! NOTE: generally replaced by clotrimazole soak (see Clotrimazole). *Dermatophytes:* dilute 10% solution to 0.2% and wash lesion with solution four times at 3- to 4-day intervals
◆ Enoxaparin	Lovenox	Low molecular weight heparin/ thromboembolic disease	Multiple preparations	*Prevention:* 0.5 mg/kg SC q24h *Treatment:* 1-2 mg/kg SC q12h
◆ Enrofloxacin	Baytril	Antibacterial	68-, 22.7-mg, and 5.7-mg tablets; Taste Tabs are 22.7 and 68 mg; 22.7 mg/mL injection	5-10 mg/kg/once daily (or divided twice daily) PO or IM; Parenteral solution for IM use has been administered by the IV route...administer slowly if indicated. WARNING: Doses of 10 mg/kg and higher are not recommended in cats because of risk of drug-induced retinal damage and blindness
◆ Ephedrine	Ephedrin sulfate	Sympathomimetic/*primarily for urinary incontinence* EMERGENCY USE: *Hypotension associated with anesthesia*	25-mg capsules and 50 mg/mL in 1-mL ampules for injection	Urinary incontinence: Dog: 4 mg/kg, or 12.5-50 mg/dog (total) PO q8-12h; Also, 1.2 mg/kg PO q8h, or 5 to 15 mg/dog (total) q8h Cat: 2-4 mg/kg, PO q8-12h *Hypotension:* 0.03-0.1 mg/kg IV bolus NOTE: dilute 5 mg in 10 mL saline; give the lower dose first; may repeat in 5 minutes after first dose if hypotension does not improve
◆ Epinephrine	Adrenalin; generic products (adrenaline)	Alpha- and beta-adrenergic agonist/*anaphylaxis and cardiac arrest*	1 mg/mL (1:1,000) injection solution	*Cardiac arrest:* 10-20 μg/kg IV or 200 μg/kg intratracheal (may be diluted in saline) *Anaphylaxis:* 2.5-5 μg/kg IV or 50 μg/kg intratracheal (may be diluted in saline)

Drug	Brand/Generic	Classification/Use	Formulation	Dosage
Epsiprantel	Cestex	Oral cesticide/tapeworms	Coated tablet	Dog: 5.5 mg/kg PO given once Cat: 2.75 mg/kg PO given once
Ergocalciferol	*See Vitamin D$_2$*			
Erythromycin	Many brand name and generic products	Antibacterial/also used as a prokinetic (increases gastric emptying in dogs and cats)	250-mg capsule or tablet	*Antibacterial dose:* 10-20 mg/kg PO q8-12h *Prokinetic dose:* 0.5-1.0 mg/kg PO q8h
Erythropoietin, human recombinant (rHuEPO)	Epogen; Epoetin alfa; Procrit	Hormone/*induction of erythropoiesis in anemia associated with chronic renal failure*	Various preparation as U/mL in single-dose and multidose vials for injection	Doses range from 35 or 50 U/kg three times/wk to 400 U/kg/wk IV, SC (adjust dose to hematocrit of 0.30-0.34)
Esmolol	Brevibloc	Ultrashort-acting beta-1 blocker/*short-term treatment of cardiac arrhythmias, especially supraventricular tachycardia*	10 mg/mL injection	500 μg/kg IV, which may be given as 0.05-0.1 mg/kg slowly every 5 minutes or 50-200 μg/kg/min infusion
Estradiol cypionate	ECP; Depo-Estradiol; generic	Hormone/*previously used to prevent pregnancy following an unplanned breeding WARNING: NOT recommended for use as an abortifacient in dogs or cats*	2 mg/mL injection	*Pregnancy Avoidance:* Dog: 22-44 μg/kg IM (total dose not to exceed 1.0 mg) Cat: 250 μg/cat IM between 40 h and 5 days of mating WARNING: may cause bone marrow suppression; in some cases, may cause aplastic anemia.
Etidronate disodium	Didronel	Bisphosphonate/*reduced calcium resorption from bone in hypercalcemic patients*	200- and 400-mg tablets; 50 mg/mL injection	Dog: 5 mg/kg/day PO Cat: 10 mg/kg/day PO
Etodolac	Etogesic	Oral NSAID/*pain management in dogs*	150- and 300-mg tablets	Dog: 10-15 mg/kg PO once daily Cat: DO NOT USE

Continued

Note: Listings preceded by ◆ are for rapid reference and denote drug/dosage used in the emergency or critical care setting.

6

TABLE 6-26 Common Drug Indications and Dosages†—cont'd

Drug	Proprietary names	Action/Use	Formulation	Recommended dosage
◆ Famotidine	Pepcid	H₂-receptor antagonist/ reduces gastric acid production; used to treat or prevent gastric ulcer	10-mg tablet; 10 mg/mL injection	0.5 mg/kg IM, SC, IV, or PO q12-24h WARNING: may cause intravascular hemolysis when given IV to cats
Felbamate	Felbatol	Dicarbamate anticonvulsant/ management of seizures in dog only	400- and 600-mg tablets; 120 mg/mL oral flavored suspension	Dog: Start with 15 mg/kg PO q8h and increase gradually to maximum of 65 mg/kg q8h
Fenbendazole	Safe-Guard; Panacur	Anthelmintic/effective against a variety of internal parasites	Panacur granules 22.2% (222 mg/kg) (222 mg/kg); 100 mg/mL liquid	25 to 50 mg/kg/day PO for 3 days (NOTE: for some parasites, recommended treatment duration may be longer)
◆ Fentanyl	Sublimaze; generic	Analgesic (opiate)/ parenteral pain control	250 mg/5 mL injection	0.02-0.04 mg/kg IV, IM, SC q2h; or 0.01 mg/kg IV, IM, SC (with acetylpromazine or diazepam) For analgesia: 0.01 mg/kg IV, IM, SC q2h
Fentanyl transdermal	Duragesic	Analgesic (opiate)/ transdermal pain control	25-, 50-, 75-, and 100-μg/h patch	Dog: 10-20 kg, 50 μg/h patch q72h Cat: 25 μg/h patch every 3 days NOTE: when administering fentanyl by the transdermal route, dosing regimens can vary among patients; consult individual sources to match patient size with patch size and patch placement. Do not cut the patch to achieve lower doses.
Ferrous sulfate (OTC)	Generic	Oral iron supplement/iron deficiency anemia	Many oral preparations available	Dog: 100-300 mg/dog PO q24h Cat: 50-100 mg/cat PO q24h
Finasteride	Proscar	5-alpha-reductase inhibitor/benign prostatic hyperplasia in dogs	5-mg tablets	Dog: 0.1 mg/kg PO q24h or 5 mg/10-50 kg dog PO q24h
Fipronil	Frontline	GABA-regulated chloride channel inhibitor/ topical control of ticks and fleas	Topical solution only	Applied topically once each month as recommended by the manufacturer; approved for use in both dogs and cats

6

Firocoxib	Previcox	*NSAID/for management of inflammation and pain associated with osteoarthritis in dogs.*	57 mg and 227 mg chewable tablets	Dogs only: 5 mg/kg, PO, once daily.
Florfenicol	Nuflor	*Antibacterial (primarily used in cattle)*	300 mg/mL (available only as a cattle preparation)	Dog: 25-50 mg/kg q8h SC or IM Cat: 25-50 mg/kg q12h SC or IM
Fluconazole	Diflucan	*Antifungal/oral (dog and cat) or parenteral (dog only) treatment for systemic deep mycoses or nasal fungal infection*	50-, 100-, 150-, and 200-mg tablets; 10 or 40 mg/mL oral suspension; 2 mg/mL IV injection	Dog: 2.5-5.0 mg/kg once daily PO or IV Cat: 2.5-10 mg/cat PO q12h; or 25 mg/cat/day PO
Flucytosine	Ancobon	*Antifungal/treatment of systemic mycoses*	250-mg capsule; 75 mg/mL oral suspension	25-50 mg/kg PO q6-8h (up to a maximum dose of 100 mg/kg PO q12h)
Fludrocortisone	Florinef	*Mineralocorticoid/treatment of hypoadrenocorticism*	100-μg (0.1-mg) tablet	Dog: 0.2-0.8 mg/dog or 0.02 mg/kg PO q24h (13-23 μg/kg) Cat: 0.1-0.2 mg/cat PO q24h
◆ Flumazenil	Romazicon	*Benzodiazepine antagonist/antidote: reverse therapeutic effects or overdose*	100 μg/mL (0.1 mg/mL) injection	0.01 -0.02 mg (total dose) IV as needed CAUTION: may cause significant hypotension
Flumethasone	Flucort	*Oral glucocorticoid/antiinflammatory*	0.5 mg/mL injection	Dog: 0.0625-0.25 mg/day in divided doses IV, IM, SC Cat: 0.03-0.125 mg/day IV, IM, SC
Flunixin meglumine	Banamine	*NSAID/pain management*	250-mg packet granules; 10 and 50 mg/mL injection	Intra-articular: 0.166 to 1.0 mg total dose mg/kg IV, IM, SC once or 1.1 mg/kg/day PO 3 days/wk Ophthalmic: 0.5 mg/kg IV once
5-Fluorouracil (5-FU)	Fluorouracil	*Antineoplastic/used in treatment protocols for multiple tumor types*	50-mg/mL vial	Dog: 150 mg/m² IV once/week Cat: DO NOT USE
Fluoxetine	Prozac	*Selective-serotonin reuptake inhibitor (SSRI)/treatment of behavior disorders*	10- and 20-mg capsules; 4 mg/mL oral solution	Dog: 0.5 mg/kg day initially PO; then increase to 1 mg/kg/day PO (10-20 mg/dog) Cat: 0.5-4 mg/cat PO q24h

Continued

Note: Listings preceded by ◆ are for rapid reference and denote drug/dosage used in the emergency or critical care setting.

6

TABLE 6-26 **Common Drug Indications and Dosages†—cont'd**

Drug	Proprietary names	Action/Use	Formulation	Recommended dosage
Fluvoxamine	Luvox	Selective serotonin reuptake inhibitor (SSRI)/*treatment and diagnosis of behavior disorders*	25-, 50-, and 100-mg tables	Dog: 0.5-2.0 mg/kg, PO, bid Cat: 0.25-0.5 mg/kg PO once daily
◆ Fomepizole (4-Methylpyrazole; 4-MP)	Antizol-Vet	Antidote/*ethylene glycol poisoning*	1.5-mL single-use vials; reconstitute in 30 mL of 0.9% NaCl for a 5% solution (50 mg/mL)	20 mg/kg IV initially within 8 h of ingestion; then 15 mg/kg IV at 12- and 24-h intervals; then 5 mg/kg IV at 36 h
Furazolidone	Furoxone	Antibacterial and antiprotozoal/*generally a second-choice drug*	100-mg tablet	4 mg/kg PO q12h for 7-10 days
Furosemide	Lasix, generic	Diuretic/*multiple uses; commonly used to treat congestive heart failure and pulmonary edema*	12.5-, 20-, and 50-mg tablets; 10 mg/mL oral solution; 50 mg/mL injection	Dog: 2-6 mg/kg IV, IM, SC, PO q8-12h (or as needed); 0.6-1.0 mg/kg/h IV Cat: 1-4 mg/kg IV, IM, SC, PO q8-24h
Gemfibrozil	Lopid	Antilipemic/*treatment of hypertriglyceridemia in patients that do not respond to dietary fat restriction*	300-mg capsules; 600-mg tablets	7.5 mg/kg PO q12h
Gentamicin	Gentocin	Antibacterial (aminoglycoside)	50 and 100 mg/mL solution for injection	Dog: 2-4 mg/kg q6-8h or 6-10 mg/kg IV, IM, SC q24h Cat: 3 mg/kg q8h or 9 mg/kg IV, IM, SC q24h WARNING: Do NOT administer to patients that are dehydrated or acidotic; can cause acute renal failure
Glipizide	Glucotrol	Oral hypoglycemic/*variably effective control of type 2 diabetes in cats*	5- and 10-mg tablets	2.5-7.5 mg/cat PO q12h; usual dose is 2.5 mg/cat initially; then increase to 5 mg/cat q12h

Drug	Other names	Use	Formulation	Dosage
Glucosamine + chondroitin sulfate	Cosequin and other brands	Neutraceutical/adjunctive treatment of nonseptic arthritis; may be useful in treating cats with lower urinary tract disease (FLUTD)	Regular (RS) and double-strength (DS) capsules	Dog: 1-2 RS capsules per day (2-4 capsules of DS for large dogs) Cat: 1 RS capsule daily
Glyburide	Diabeta; Micronase; Glynase	Oral hypoglycemic/variably effective control of type 2 diabetes in cats	1.25-, 2.5-, and 5-mg tablets	0.625 mg per cat once daily (represents one half of 1.25-mg tablet)
Glycerin (OTC)	Generic	Oral osmotic/reduces intraocular (and CSF) pressure	Oral solution	1-2 mL/kg PO q8h
Glycopyrrolate	Robinul-V	Antimuscarinic/multiple uses: pre-anesthetic medication, antidote	0.2 mg/mL injection	0.005-0.011 mg/kg IV, IM, SC
Gold sodium thiomalate	Myochrysine	Gold salt/treatment of immune-mediated skin disorders	Injection	1-5 mg IM 1st wk, then 2-10 mg IM 2nd wk, then 1 mg/kg IM once/wk maintenance
Gold therapy	See Aurothioglucose			
GoLYTELY	See Polyethylene glycol electrolyte solution			
Gonadorelin	Factrel; GnRH; LHRH	Hormone/diagnosis and treatment of various reproductive disorders	50-µg/mL injection	Therapeutic doses: Dog: 50-100 µg/dog IM q24-48h Cat: 25 µg/cat IM once
Gonadotropin, human chorionic (hCG)	Profasi; Pregnyl; APL; generic	Hormone/induce luteinization	5000, 10,000 and 20,000 U injection	Dog: 22 U/kg IM q24-48h or 44 U IM once Cat: 250 U/cat IM once WARNING: Do NOT use in pregnant animals
Gonadotropin-releasing hormone	See Gonadorelin			
Granisetron	Kytril	Antiemetic/prevent emesis associated with chemotherapy	1 mg/mL injection; 1-mg tablet	0.01 mg/kg (10 µg/kg) IV

Note: Listings preceded by ◆ are for rapid reference and denote drug/dosage used in the emergency or critical care setting,

Continued

6

TABLE 6-26   Common Drug Indications and Dosages†—cont'd

Drug	Proprietary names	Action/Use	Formulation	Recommended dosage
Griseofulvin (microsize)	Fulvicin U/F	Antifungal (fungistatic antibiotic)/ treatment of dermatophytes (especially M. canis)	125-, 250-, and 500-mg tablets; 25 mg/mL oral suspension; 125 mg/mL oral syrup	50 mg/kg PO q24h (up to a maximum dose of 110-132 mg/kg/day in divided treatments)
Growth hormone (hGH)	Humatrope; Nutropin; Protropin; Somatotropin; Somatrem	Hormone/replacement hormone in patients with confirmed deficiency.	5 and 10 mg/vial	0.1 U/kg SC, IM three times per wk for 4-6 wk WARNING: Is diabetogenic
Halothane	Fluothane	Inhalation anesthetic	250 mL liquid	Induction: 3% Maintenance: 0.5-1.5%
Hemoglobin glutamer	Oxyglobin	Blood substitute	13 g/dL in 125 mg single-dose bags	10-30 mL/kg, IV; or up to 10 mL/kg/hour.
◆ Heparin sodium	Liquaemin	Anticoagulant/treat DIC and treatment and prevention of thromboembolic disease	1000 and 10,000 U/mL injection	100-200 units/kg IV loading dose; then 100-300 units/kg SC q6-8h Low-dose prophylaxis (dog and cat): 70 U/kg SC q8-12h
◆ Hydroxyethyl starch (HES)	Hetastarch	Volume expander/used when colloidal therapy is indicated	Injection	10-20 mL/kg IV to effect, 20-30 mL/kg/day
◆ Hydralazine	Apresoline	Vasodilator/hypertension and adjunctive treatment of heart failure	10-mg tablet; 20 mg/mL injection	Dog: 0.5 mg/kg (initial dose); titrate to 0.5-2 mg/kg PO q12h Cat: 2.5 mg/cat PO q12-24h
Hydrochlorothiazide	HydroDIURIL; generic	Diuretic/hypertension, congestive heart failure, and nephrogenic (ADH-resistant) diabetes insipidus	10 and 100 mg/mL oral solution; 25-, 50-, and 100-mg tablets	2-4 mg/kg PO q12h
Hydrocodone bitartrate	Hycodan (contains atropine)	Analgesic (opiate)/pain management	5-mg tablet	Dog: 0.22 mg/kg PO q4-8h Cat: no dose available
Hydrocortisone	Cortef; generic	Glucorticoid/antiinflammatory and replacement therapy in adrenal insufficient conditions	5-, 10-, and 20-mg tablets	Replacement therapy: 1-2 mg/kg PO q12h Antiinflammatory: 1.5-5 mg/kg PO q12h
◆ Hydrocortisone sodium succinate	Solu-Cortef	Glucorticoid/antiinflammatory and shock treatment	Various size vials for injection	Shock: 50-150 mg/kg IV Antiinflammatory: 5 mg/kg IV q12h

Drug	Trade name	Use	Forms available	Dosage
◆ Hydromorphone	Dilaudid	*Analgesic (opiate)/pain management and restraint*	Tablets, oral solution, and injectable (IM) forms available	Dog: 0.22 mg/kg, IM, SC, q4-6h as needed for pain.
Hydroxyurea	Hydrea	*Antineoplastic/polycythemia vera, mastocytoma, leukemias*	500-mg capsule	Dog: 50 mg/kg PO once daily, 3 days/wk; Cat: 25 mg/kg PO once daily, 3 days/wk
Hydroxyzine	Atarax	*Antihistamine/antipruritic and sedative effects, especially in atopic patients*	10-, 25-, and 50-mg tablets; 2 mg/mL oral solution	Dog: 1-2 mg/kg q6-8h IM, PO; Cat: DO NOT USE
Ifosfamide	Ifex	*Antineoplastic/lymphomas and other sarcomas*	1 gram powder for IV infusion in single-dose vials	Dogs and cats: Dose ranges from 300 to 500 mg/m² IV CAUTION: Consult treatment protocol before administering
Imidacloprid	Advantage	Topical flea treatment for dogs and cats	Topical solution	Apply topically once monthly as directed by the manufacturer for the treatment of fleas
Imidacloprid + permethrin	K9 Advantix	Topical flea treatment and tick repellent for DOGS ONLY	Topical solution	Apply topically once monthly as directed by the manufacturer for the treatment of fleas; Cat: DO NOT USE; contains permethrin
Imipenem + cilastin	Primaxin	Antibacterial	250- or 500-mg vials for injection	5-10 mg/kg IV, IM q6-8h; has been administered to dogs at 10 mg/kg q8h SC
Imidocarb dipropinate	Imizol	*Antiprotozoal/treatment of babesia, ehrlichiosis (not regarded as effective), Cytauxzoon felis, and related infections*	Parenteral solution for IM or SC injection; 120 mg/mL in 10-mL multi-dose vials	Dog: 5 mg/kg IM or SC once; repeat in 2 wk; For babesiosis: 6.6 mg/kg IM or SC once; repeat in 2 wk); Cat: (cytauxzoonosis) 5 mg/kg IM q2wk as needed
Imipramine	Tofranil	*Tricyclic antidepressant/ treatment of behavior disorders*	10-, 25-, and 50-mg tablets	2-4 mg/kg PO q12-24h

Continued

Note: Listings preceded by ◆ are for rapid reference and denote drug/dosage used in the emergency or critical care setting.

6

TABLE 6-26 Common Drug Indications and Dosages†—cont'd

Drug	Proprietary names	Action/Use	Formulation	Recommended dosage
Indomethacin	Indocin			Safe dose has not been established
Interferon (interferon alpha-2a, HuIFN-alpha)	Roferon	Cytokine/immunomodulation in cats with FeLV and/or FIV infection (clinical value of treatment is not established)	3 million U/vial	Cat: 30 U/cat/day, PO; or 15-30 U/cat IM or SC once daily for 7 days and repeated every other wk
Ipecac syrup (OTC)	Ipecac	Oral emetic		NO LONGER RECOMMENDED: can cause fatal arrhythmias
Ipodate	Bilivist; Oragrafin	Organic iodine/treatment of hyperthyroidism (especially in cats)	500-mg capsules (should be formulated for cats as 50-mg ampules)	Dog: 15 mg/kg, PO, q12h Cat: 100-200 mg (total dose)/cat once daily; dose may be reduced if the 2-wk response is judged satisfactory
Iron	See Ferrous sulfate			
◆ Isoflurane	Isoflurane; Forane; Aerrane; others	Inhalation anesthetic	100-mL bottle	Induction: 5% Maintenance: 1.5-2.5%
◆ Isoproterenol	Isuprel	Beta-agonist/uncommonly used to treat acute bronchoconstriction and certain cardiac arrhythmias	0.2 mg/mL ampules for injection	10 μg/kg IM, SC q6h; or dilute 1 mg in 500 mL of 5% dextrose or Ringer's solution and infuse IV 0.5-1 mL/min (1-2 μg/min) or to effect
◆ Isosorbide dinitrate	Isordil; Isorbid; Sorbitrate	Vasodilator/congestive heart failure	2.5-, 5-, 10-, 20-, 30-, and 40-mg tablets; 40-mg capsules	2.5-5 mg/animal PO q12h (or 0.22-1.1 mg/kg PO q12h)
◆ Isosorbide mononitrate	Monoket	Vasodilator/congestive heart failure	10- and 20-mg tablets	5 mg/dog PO, two doses/day 7 h apart
Isotretinoin	Accutane	Synthetic retinoid/treatment of dermatologic diseases associated with epithelial cell proliferation (e.g., ichthyosis, cutaneous lymphoma)	10-, 20-, and 40-mg capsules	1-3 mg/kg/day (up to maximum recommended dose of 3-4 mg/kg/day PO)
Itraconazole	Sporanox	Antifungal/treatment of systemic mycoses	100-mg capsules	Dog: 2.5 mg/kg PO q12h or 5 mg/kg PO q24h Cat: 1.5-3.0 mg/kg PO up to 5 mg/kg PO q24h

Generic Name	Trade Names	Application	Formulations	Dosage
Ivermectin	Heartgard; Ivomec; Eqvalan liquid	*Antiparasiticide/multiple applications*	1% (10 mg/mL) injectable solution; 10 mg/mL oral solution; 18.7 mg/mL oral paste; 68-, 136-, and 272-μg tablets	Heartworm preventative: Dog: 6 μg/kg (range: 3 to 12 μg/kg) PO q30 days Cat: 24 μg/kg PO q30days *Microfilaricide:* 50 μg/kg PO 2 wk after adulticide therapy *Ectoparasite therapy* (dog and cat): 200-300-μg/kg IM, SC, PO *Endoparasites* (dog and cat): 200-400 μg/kg SC, PO weekly *Demodex therapy:* 600 μg/kg/day PO for 60-120 days
Kanamycin	Kantrim	Antibacterial	200- and 500-mg/mL injection	10 mg/kg IV, IM, SC q6-8h
Kaopectate (kaolin + pectin) (OTC)	Kaopectate	*GI adsorbent/management of acute, simple diarrheal disorders, especially result of dietary indiscretion*	12 oz oral suspension	1-2 mL/kg PO q2-6h
◆ Ketamine	Ketalar; Ketavet; Vetalar	Dissociative anesthetic	100 mg/mL injection solution	Dog: 5.5-22 mg/kg IV, IM (recommend adjunctive sedative or tranquilizer treatment) Cat: 2-25 mg/kg IV, IM (recommend adjunctive sedative or tranquilizer treatment)
Ketoconazole	Nizoral	*Antifungal/systemic mycoses, Malassezia canis infection; limited application in the treatment of canine hyperadrenocorticism*	200-mg tablet; 100 mg/mL oral suspension (only available in Canada)	Dog: 10-15 mg/kg PO q8-12h *Malassezia canis:* 10 mg/kg PO q24h or 5 mg/kg PO q12h) Cat: 5-10 mg/kg PO q8-12h *Hyperadrenocorticism:* Dog: 15 mg/kg PO q12h

Continued

Note: Listings preceded by ◆ are for rapid reference and denote drug/dosage used in the emergency or critical care setting.

6

TABLE 6-26   Common Drug Indications and Dosages†—cont'd

Drug	Proprietary names	Action/Use	Formulation	Recommended dosage
◆ Ketoprofen	Orudis-KT (OTC); Ketofen	NSAID/*pain management*	12.5-mg tablet (OTC); 100 mg/mL injection	Dog and cat: 1 mg/kg PO q24h for up to 5 days or 2.0 mg/kg IV, IM, SC for one dose
Ketorolac tromethamine	Toradol	NSAID/*pain management*	10-mg tablet; 15 and 30 mg/mL injection in 10% alcohol	Dog: 0.5 mg/kg PO, IM, IV q12h for not more than two doses Cat: DO NOT USE
L-Dopa	See Levodopa			
◆ Lactated Ringer's solution	Generic	Fluid replacement	250-, 500-, and 1000-mL bags	*Maintenance:* 40-50 mL/kg/day IV *Shock therapy:* Dog: 90 mL/kg IV Cat: 60-70 mL/kg IV
Lactulose	Chonulac; generic	Disaccharide laxative/*limit bowel absorption of protein and facilitate lowering of blood ammonia levels in patients with hepatic encephalopathy*	10 g/15 mL	*Constipation:* 1 mL/4.5 kg PO q8h (to effect) *Hepatic encephalopathy:* Dog: 0.5 mL/kg PO q8h Cat: 2.5-5 mL/cat PO q8h
◆ Leucovorin (folinic acid)	Wellcovorin; generic	Antidote/*folic acid antagonism; application in dogs and cats is not established*	5-, 10-, 15-, and 25-mg tablets; 3 and 5 mg/mL injection	*With methotrexate administration:* 3 mg/m^2 IV, IM, PO *Antidote for pyrimethamine toxicosis:* 1 mg/kg PO q24h
Levamisole	Levasole, Tramisol Injectable	Antiparasitic/*treatment of nematode infection; also proposed to be a non-specific immunostimulant*	0.184-g bolus; 11.7-g/13-g packet; 50-mg tablet	Dog: *Hookworms:* 5-8 mg/kg PO once (up to 10 mg/kg PO for 2 days) *Microfilaricide:* 10 mg/kg PO q24h for 6-10 days *Immunostimulant:* 0.5-2 mg/kg PO 3 times/wk Cat: 4.4 mg/kg once PO (for *lungworms:* 20-40 mg/kg PO q48h for five treatments)
Levodopa	Larodopa; l-Dopa	Dopamine agonist/*hepatic encephalopathy*	100-, 250-, and 500-mg tablets or capsules	*Hepatic encephalopathy:* 6.8 mg/kg initially; then 1.4 mg/kg q6h

6

Drug	Trade names	Indication	Supplied	Dosage
Levothyroxine sodium (T₄)	Soloxine; Thyro-Tabs; Synthoid	Hormone/hypothyroidism	0.1- to 0.8-mg tablets (in 0.1-mg increments)	Dog: 18-22 µg/kg, PO, q12h (adjust dose via monitoring T₄ levels) Cat: 10-20 µg/kg/day, PO (adjust dose via monitoring T₄ levels)
◆ Lidocaine (without epinephrine)	Xylocaine; generic	Anesthetic and anti-arrhythmic/ventricular arrhythmias; also local and regional anesthetic; has been used systemically for pain	5-, 10-, 15-, and 20-mg/mL injection	Dog (antiarrhythmic): 2-4 mg/kg IV (to a maximum dose of 8 mg/kg over 10-min period); 25-75 µg/kg/min IV infusion Cat (antiarrhythmic): 0.25-0.75 mg/kg IV slowly; for epidural (dog and cat): 4.4 mg/kg of 2% solution
Lincomycin	Lincocin	Antibacterial	100-, 200-, and 500-mg tablets	15-25 mg/kg PO q12h For pyoderma: Doses as low as 10 mg/kg q12h have been used
Liothyronine (T₃)	Cytomel	Hormone (active form of T₃)/replacement therapy in patients with hypothyroidism that fail to respond to T₄	60-µg tablet	4.4 µg/kg PO q8h For T₃ suppression test (cats): Collect presample for T₄ and T₃; administer 25 µg q8h for 7 doses; then collect post samples for T₃ and T₄ after last dose
Lisinopril	Prinivil; Zestril	ACE inhibitor/vasodilator for treatment of hypertension or heart failure	2.5-, 5-, 10-, 20-, and 40-mg tablets	Dog: 0.5 mg/kg PO q24h Cat: No dose established
Lithium carbonate	Lithotabs	Nonspecific immunostimulant/adjunctive treatment to increase neutrophil counts in patients with chemotherapy-induced neutropenia	150-, 300-, and 600-mg capsules; 300-mg tablet; 300 mg/5 mL syrup	Dog: 10 mg/kg PO q12h Cat: Not recommended
Loperamide	Imodium; generic	Analgesic (opiate)/nonspecific management of diarrhea	2-mg tablet; 0.2 mg/mL oral liquid	Dog: 0.1 mg/kg PO q8-12h Cat: 0.08-0.16 mg/kg PO q12h

Note: Listings preceded by ◆ are for rapid reference and denote drug/dosage used in the emergency or critical care setting.

Continued

6

TABLE 6-26   Common Drug Indications and Dosages†—cont'd

Drug	Proprietary names	Action/Use	Formulation	Recommended dosage
Lufenuron	Program	Antiparasitic/flea control	45-, 90-, 135-, 204.9- and 409.8-mg tablets; 135 and 270 mg suspension per unit pack	Dog: 10/mg/kg PO q30days Cat: 30 mg/kg PO q30days; 10 mg/kg SC q6mo
Lufenuron + milbemycin oxime	Sentinel tablets; Flavor Tabs	Antiparasitic/flea control plus heartworm preventative effective against certain intestinal parasites	Milbemycin/lufenuron ratio is as follows: 2.3/46-mg Sentinel tablets; 5.75/115-, 11.5/230-, and 23/460-mg Flavor Tabs	Dog: Administer 1 tablet q30days as recommended by manufacturer (each tablet formulated for size of dog) Cat: DO NOT USE
Luteinizing hormone	See Gonadorelin			
l-Lysine (OTC)	l-Lysine (multiple preparations)	Amino acid/prevention of feline herpesvirus-1 recrudesence	250- 500-mg capsules	Cat (empiric dose): Mix 250 mg with food once daily NOTE: Efficacy studies have not been performed; no known effect on feline calicivirus carrier cats
◆ Magnesium chloride	Generic	Elemental salt/ventricular dysrhythmias, refractory hypokalemia, and ventricular fibrillation	200 mg/mL in 50-mL vials for injection	0.15–0.3 mEq/kg IV over 2-10 min; or 0.75 mEq/kg/day IV by CRI
Magnesium citrate	Citroma; Citro-Nesia (Citro-Mag in Canada)	Laxative	Oral solution	2-4 mL/kg PO
Magnesium hydroxide (OTC)	Milk of Magnesia	Laxative	Oral liquid	Antacid: 5-10 mL/kg PO q4-6h Cathartic: Dog: 15-50 PO mL/kg Cat: 2-6 mL/cat PO q24h
Magnesium sulfate (OTC)	Epsom salts	Laxative/also used for oral magnesium supplementation	Crystals; many generic preparations	Dog: 8-25 g/dog PO q24h Cat: 2-5 g/cat PO q24h
◆ Mannitol	Osmitrol	Diuretic (osmotic)/management of anuric and/or oliguric renal failure; applications in management of glaucoma and cerebral edema	5-25% solution for injection	Diuretic: 1 g/kg 5-25% solution IV to maintain urine flow Glaucoma or CNS edema: 0.25-2 g/kg 15-25% solution IV over 30-60 min (repeat in 6 h if necessary)

6

Drug	Trade name	Indication	Supplied	Dosage
Marbofloxacin	Zeniquin	Antibacterial	25-, 50-, 100-, 200-mg tablets	Dog: 2.75-5.55 mg/kg PO q24h Cat: dose not established
MCT oil	MCT oil (many sources)	Medium-chain triglyceride/lipid supplement used in patients with GI absorptive disorders	Oral liquid	1-2 mL/kg/day in food
Mebendazole	Telmintic	Antiparasitic/multiple applications for treatment of endoparasites	40 mg/powder	22 mg/kg (with food) q24h for 3 days
◆ Meclizine	Antivert; generic	Antihistamine/antiemetic, especially when nausea is associated with vertigo	12.5-, 25-, and 50-mg tablets	Dog: 25 mg PO q24h (for motion sickness, administer 1 h before traveling) Cat: 12.5 mg PO q24h
Meclofenamate	Arquel; Meclomen	NSAID/pain management	50- and 100-mg capsules	Dog: 1 mg/kg/day PO for up to 5 days
◆ Medetomidine	Domitor	Analgesic/adjunct for anesthesia; restraint	1.0 mg/mL injection	750 µg/m² IV or 1000 µg/m² IM
Medium-chain triglycerides	See MCT oil			
Medroxyprogesterone acetate	Depo-Provera (injection); Provera (tablets)	Hormone/management of certain dermatologic and behavior disorders, including urine spraying in cats; benign prostatic hyperplasia;	150 and 400 mg/mL suspension injection; 2.5-, 5-, and 10-mg tablets	1.1-2.2 mg/kg IM q7days Behavior disorders: 10-20 mg/kg SC Prostatic hyperplasia: 3-5 mg/kg SC, IM
Megstrol acetate	Ovaban; Megace	Hormone/management of certain dermatologic and behavior disorders, including urine spraying in cats	5-mg tablet	Dog: Proestrus: 2 mg/kg PO q24h for 8 days Anestrus: 0.5 mg/kg PO q24h for 30 days Behavior disorders: 2-4 mg/kg q24h for 8 days (reduce dose for maintenance) Cat (NOTE: Any use in cats is EXTRA-LABEL): Dermatologic therapy or urine spraying: 2.5-5 mg/cat PO q24h for 1 wk; then

Continued

Note: Listings preceded by ◆ are for rapid reference and denote drug/dosage used in the emergency or critical care setting.

6

TABLE 6-26 Common Drug Indications and Dosages†—cont'd

Drug	Proprietary names	Action/Use	Formulation	Recommended dosage
				reduce to 5 mg once or twice/wk *Estrus suppression:* 5 mg/cat/day for 3 days; then 2.5-5 mg once/wk for 10 wk
Melarsomine	Immiticide	Antiparasitic (arsenical)/ *treatment of canine heartworm disease*	25 mg/mL injection; after reconstitution retains potency for 24 h	Administer via deep IM injection Class 1-2 dogs: 2.5 mg/kg/day for 2 consecutive days Class 3 dogs: 2.5 mg/kg once, then in 1 mo two additional doses 24 h apart Cat: DO NOT USE
◆ Meloxicam	Metacam	NSAID/*pain management*	1.5 mg/mL oral solution	0.2 mg/kg PO, initial loading dose; then 0.1 mg/kg PO q12h
Melphalan	Alkeran	Antineoplastic/*used in treatment protocols for multiple tumor types*	2-mg tablet	1.5 mg/m^2 or 0.1-0.2 mg/kg PO q24h for 7-10 days; repeat every 3 wk
Meperidine	Demerol	Analgesic (opiate)/*pain management*	50- and 100-mg tablets; 10 mg/mL syrup; 25, 50, 75, and 100 mg/mL injection	Dog: 5-10 mg/kg IV, IM as often as q2-3h (or as needed) Cat: 3-5 mg/kg IV, IM q2-4h (or as needed)
Mepivicaine	Carbocaine-V	Local anesthetic	2% (20 mg/mL) injection	Variable dose for local infiltration *For epidural,* 0.5 mg of 2% solution q30sec until reflexes are absent.
6-Mercaptopurine	Purinethol	Antineoplastic/*used in treatment protocols for multiple tumor types*	50-mg tablet	50 mg/m^2 PO q24h Caution: Consult treatment protocol before administering.
Meropenem	Merrem	Antibacterial/*especially in treating resistant infections caused by Pseudomonas, E. coli, and Klebsiella*	500 mg in 20-mL vial, or 1 g in 30-mL vial for injection	20 mg/kg IV q8h *For meningitis:* 40 mg/kg IV q8h

Drug	Trade Names	Use	Form	Dose
Mesalamine	Asacol; Mesasal; Pentasa	*Antidiarrheal/alternative use in patients unable to tolerate sulfasalazine in treatment of colitis*	400-mg tablet; 250-mg capsule	Veterinary dose has not been established. The usual human dose is 400-500 mg q6-8h (also see Sulfasalazine, Olsalazine)
Metaproterenol	Alupent; Metaprel	*Beta-agonist/bronchodilator therapy*	10- and 20-mg tablets; 5 mg/mL syrup; inhalers	0.325-0.65 mg/kg PO q4-6h
Metaformin	Glucophage	*Oral hypoglycemic/ management of type 2 diabetes in cats*	500- and 800-mg tablets	Cats: 2 mg/kg PO q12h
Methazolamide	Neptazane	*Carbonic anhydrase inhibitor/ treatment of open-angle glaucoma*	25- and 50-mg tablets	2-4 mg/kg (up to maximum dose of 4-6 mg/kg) PO q8-12h
Methenamine hippurate	Hiprex; Urex	*Urinary antiseptic/of questionable value*	1-g tablet	Dog: 500 mg/dog PO q12h Cat: 250 mg/cat PO q12h
Methenamine mandelate	Mandelamine; generic	*Urinary antiseptic/of questionable value*	1-g tablet; granules for oral solution; 50 and 100 mg/mL oral suspension	10-20 mg/kg PO q8-12h
Methimazole	Tapazole	*Antithyroidal/management of feline hyperthyroidism*	5- and 10-mg tablets	Cat: 2.5 mg/cat q12h PO for 7-14 days; then 5-10 mg/cat PO q12h and adjust by monitoring T_4
Methionine (DL)	Uroeze; DL-methionine powder	*Urinary acidifier*	500-mg tablets and powders added to animal's food; 75 mg/5 mL pediatric oral solution; 200-mg capsule	Dog: 150-300 mg/kg/day PO Cat: 1-1.5 g/cat PO (added to food each day)
Methionine (S-adenosyl)	See SAMe			
◆ Methocarbamol	Robaxin-V	*Muscle relaxant/adjunctive therapy for trauma, acute inflammation of skeletal muscle and/or tremorigenic toxins*	500- and 750-mg tablets; 100 mg/mL injection	44 mg/kg PO q8h on the first day; then 22-44 mg/kg PO q8h

Continued

Note: Listings preceded by ◆ are for rapid reference and denote drug/dosage used in the emergency or critical care setting.

6

TABLE 6-26 Common Drug Indications and Dosages†—cont'd

Drug	Proprietary names	Action/Use	Formulation	Recommended dosage
Methohexital	Brevital	Ultra-short-acting barbiturate/anesthetic induction	0.5-, 2.5-, and 5-gram vials for injection	3-6 mg/kg IV (give slowly to effect)
Methotrexate	MTX; Mexate; Folex; Rheumatrex; generic	Antineoplastic/used in treatment protocols for multiple tumor types, especially lymphomas	2.5-mg tablet; 2.5 or 25 mg/mL injection	2.5-5 mg/m² PO q48h (dose depends on specific protocol) or: Dog: 0.3-0.5 mg/kg IV once/wk Cat: 0.8 mg/kg IV q2-3wk
◆ Methoxamine	Vasoxyl	Vasopressor/used in critical care setting to increase blood pressure	20 mg/mL injection	200-250 μg/kg IM or 40-80 μg/kg IV
Methoxyflurane	Metofane	Inhalation anesthetic/uncommonly used today	4-oz bottle for inhalation	*Induction:* 3% *Maintenance:* 0.5-1.5%
◆ Methylene blue 0.1%	Generic; also called new methylene blue	Antidote/emergency treatment of methemoglobinemia	1% solution (10 mg/mL)	1.5 mg/kg IV slowly; use once.
Methylprednisolone	Medrol	Glucocorticoid/antiinflammatory and immunosuppressive	1-, 2-, 4-, 8-, 18-, and 32-mg tablets	In cats, Use With Caution 0.22-0.44 mg/kg PO q12-24h NOTE: Methylprednisolone is 1.25 times more potent than prednisolone
Methylprednisolone acetate	Depo-Medrol	Repository glucocorticoid/antiinflammatory (extended duration of activity)	20 and 40 mg/mL suspension for injection	Dog: 1 mg/kg (or 20-40 mg/dog) IM q1-3wk Cat: 10-20 mg/cat IM q1-3wk NOTE: Actual dose may vary, depending on use and effect
◆ Methylprednisolone sodium succinate	Solu-Medrol	Glucocorticoid/adjunctive treatment for patients in shock or with spinal cord trauma/swelling	1- and 2-g and 125- and 500-mg vials for injection	*For emergency use:* 30 mg/kg IV; repeat at 15 mg/kg IV in 2-6 h For replacement therapy or antiinflammatory therapy; see also Prednisolone
◆ 4-Methylpyrazole (4-MP)	*See* Fomepizole			

6

Methyltestosterone	Android; generic	Hormone/replacement therapy; also an anabolic agent used to induce erythropoiesis	10- and 25-mg tablets	Dog: 5-25 mg/dog PO q24-48h Cat: 2.5-5 mg/cat PO q24-48h
◆ Metoclopramide	Reglan: Maxolon; others	Antiemetic/especially in patients with vomiting associated with gastroparesis	5- and 10-mg tablets; 1 mg/mL oral solution; 5 mg/mL injection	0.2-0.5 mg/kg IV, IM, PO q6-8h; or 1-2 mg/kg/day IV by CRI (approx 0.1-0.2 mg/kg/h)
Metoprolol	Lopressor	Beta blocker/management of tachycardia	50- and 100-mg tablets; 1 mg/mL injection	Dog: 5-50 mg/dog (0.5-1.0 mg/kg) PO q8h Cat: 2-15 mg/cat PO q8h
◆ Metronidazole	Flagyl; generic	Antiparasitic and antibacterial/effective against anaerobic bacteria; somewhat effective against Giardia (fenbendazole is preferred)	250- and 500-mg tablets; 50 mg/mL suspension; 5 mg/mL injection	*Anaerobic infection:* Dog: 15 mg/kg PO q12h or 12 mg/kg q8h; Cat: 10-25 mg/kg PO q24h; *Giardia:* Dog: 12-15 mg/kg PO q12h for 8 days; Cat: 17 mg/kg (1/3 tablet per cat) q24h for 8 days
◆ Mexiletine	Mexitil	Antiarrhythmic/ventricular arrhythmias	150-, 200-, and 250-mg capsules	Dog: 5-8 mg/kg PO q8-12h (USE CAUTIOUSLY) Cat: No dose established
Mibolerone	Cheque Drops	Hormone (androgenic)/suppression of estrus and treatment of false pregnancy (pseudocyesis)	55 μg/mL oral solution	Dog: 0.45-11.3 kg, 30 μg; 11.8-22.7 kg, 60 μg; 23-43.3 kg, 120 μg; >45.8 kg, 180 μg; or approximately 2.6-5 μg/kg/day PO Cat: DO NOT USE WARNING: Multiple adverse effects are possible when used in prepubertal females
◆ Midazolam	Versed	Benzodiazepine/pre-anesthetic medication	5 mg/mL injection	0.1-0.25 mg/kg IV, IM (or 0.1-0.3 mg/kg/h IV infusion) NOTE: May cause excitement in cats

Continued

Note: Listings preceded by ◆ are for rapid reference and denote drug/dosage used in the emergency or critical care setting.

6

TABLE 6-26 Common Drug Indications and Dosages†—cont'd

Drug	Proprietary names	Action/Use	Formulation	Recommended dosage
Milbemycin oxime	Interceptor; Interceptor Flavor Tabs	GABA inhibitor/prevention of canine heartworm disease, microfilaricide; also used to treat demodicosis	23-, 11.5-, 5.75-, and 2.3-mg tablets	Dog: *Microfilaricide:* 0.5 mg/kg *Demodex:* 2 mg/kg PO q24h for 60-120 days *Heartworm prevention:* 0.5 mg/kg PO q30days
Milk of Magnesia (OTC)	*See* Magnesium hydroxide			
Mineral oil (OTC)	Generic	Laxative (lubricant)	Oral liquid	Dog: 10-50 mL/dog PO q12h Cat: 10-25 mL/cat PO q12h
Minocycline	Minocin	Antibacterial	50- and 100-mg tablets; 10 mg/mL oral suspension	5-12.5 mg/kg PO q12h
◆ Misoprostol	Cytotec	Prostaglandin E₁ analog/treatment of gastric ulcers, especially those associated with NSAID use	0.1-mg (100-µg) and 0.2-mg (200-µg) tablets	Dog: 2-5 µg/kg PO q6-8h Cat: Dose not established
Mitotane (o,p′-DDD)	Lysodren	Cytotoxic agent/treatment of hyperadrenocorticism associated with adrenal hyperplasia; less effective if treating adrenal gland neoplasia	500-mg tablet	Dog: *Pituitary-dependent hyperadrenocorticism:* 50 mg/kg/day (in divided doses) PO for 7-10 days; then 25 mg/kg/wk PO *Adrenal neoplasia:* 50-75 mg/kg/day for 10 days; then 75-100 mg/kg/wk PO
Mitoxantrone	Novantrone	Antineoplastic/used in treatment protocols for multiple tumor types	2 mg/mL injection	Dog: 6 mg/m² IV q21days Cat: 6.5 mg/m² IV q21days
◆ Morphine	Generic	Analgesic (opiate)/pain management	1 and 15 mg/mL injection; 30- and 60-mg delayed-release tablets	Dog: 0.1-1 mg/kg IV, IM, SC (dose is escalated as needed for pain relief) q4-6h *Epidural:* 0.1 mg/kg Cat: 0.1 mg/kg q3-6h IM, SC (or as needed)
◆ Naloxone	Narcan	Opiate antagonist/opiate reversal	20 and 400 µg/mL injection	0.01-0.04 mg/kg IV, IM, SC as needed to reverse opiate

Naltrexone	Trexan	Opiate antagonist/*management of certain behavioral disorders (e.g., tail chasing, self-mutilation)*	50-mg tablet	Dog: 2.2 mg/kg PO q12h
Nandrolone decanoate	Deca-Durabolin	Anabolic steroid/*appetite stimulant; also used to stimulate erythropoiesis*	50, 100, and 200 mg/mL injection	Dog: 1-1.5 mg/kg/wk IM Cat: 1 mg/cat/wk IM
Naproxen	Naprosyn; Naxen; Aleve (naproxen sodium)	NSAID/*pain management*	220-mg tablet (OTC); 25-mg/mL suspension liquid; 250-, 375-, and 500-mg tablets (Rx)	Dog: 5 mg initially, then 2 mg/kg q48h
Neomycin	Biosol	Antibacterial/*management of hepatic encephalopathy (gut "sterilization")*	500-mg bolus; 200 mg/mL oral liquid	10-20 mg/kg PO q6-12h
Neostigmine bromide and neostigmine methylsulfate	Prostigmin; Stiglyn	Anticholinesterase/*diagnosis of myasthenia gravis; antidote for anticholinergic intoxication and massive ivermectin overdose in cats*	15-mg tablet (neostigmine bromide); 0.25 and 0.5 mg/mL injection (neostigmine methylsulfate)	2 mg/kg/day PO (in divided doses, to effect) *Injection:* antimyasthenic: 10 µg/kg IM, SC, as needed; antidote for nondepolarizing neuromuscular block: 40µg/kg IM, SC; diagnostic aid for myasthenia gravis: 40 µg/kg IM or 20 µg/kg IV
Nitrofurantoin	Macrodantin; Furalan; Furatoin; Furadantin; generic	Antibacterial/*especially in susceptible urinary tract infections*	*Macrodantin and generic:* 25-, 50-, and 100-mg capsules *Furalan, Furatoin, and generic:* 50- and 100-mg tablets *Furadantin:* 5 mg/mL oral suspension	10 mg/kg/day divided into four daily treatments; then 1 mg/kg PO at night

Note: Listings preceded by ◆ are for rapid reference and denote drug/dosage used in the emergency or critical care setting.

Continued

6

TABLE 6-26 Common Drug Indications and Dosages†—cont'd

Drug	Proprietary names	Action/Use	Formulation	Recommended dosage
◆ Nitroglycerin ointment	Nitrol; Nitro-Bid; Nitrostat	Venodilator/management of congestive heart failure	0.5, 0.8, 1, 5-, and 10 mg/mL injection; 2% ointment; transdermal (0.2 mg/h systems patch)	Dog: 4-12 mg (up to 15 mg) topically q12h Cat: 2-4 mg topically q12h (or ¼ inch of ointment per cat)
◆ Nitroprusside	Nitropress	Vascular and smooth muscle relaxant/acute hypertension; acute heart failure secondary to mitral regurgitation	50-mg vial for injection	1-5 mg, up to maximum of 10 μg/kg/min IV infusion
Nizatidine	Axid	H₂ receptor antagonist/reduce gastric acid production and prevention of gastric ulcers	150- and 300-mg capsules	2.5-5.0 mg/kg, PO once daily
Norfloxacin	Noroxin	Antibacterial	400-mg tablet	22 mg/kg PO q12h
Olsalazine	Dipentum	Antidiarrheal/alternative drug to sulfasalazine for management of colitis in dogs (expensive)	500-mg tablet	Dosage in animals is not established Dog: 5-10 mg/kg, PO q8h is recommended
Omeprazole	Prilosec (formerly Losec); Gastrogard (equine paste)	Proton pump inhibitor/gastric ulceration and erosion	20-mg capsule	Dog: 20 mg/dog PO once daily (or 0.7 mg/kg q24h) Cat: DO NOT USE
◆ Ondansetron	Zofran	5-HT₃ receptor antagonist/antiemetic for patients with severe vomiting NOTE: Is well tolerated in dogs	4- and 8-mg tablets; 2 mg/mL injection	0.1-1.0 mg/kg PO 30 min before cancer chemotherapy For intractable vomiting: 0.11 to 0.176 mg/kg, IV slow push
Orbifloxacin	Orbax	Antibacterial	5.7-, 22.7-, and 68-mg tablets	2.5 to 7.5 mg/kg PO once daily
Ormetoprim + Sulfadimethoxine	Primor	Antibacterial	Combination tablet: 120-, 250-, 600-, and 1200-mg tablets.	27 mg/kg on 1st day followed by 13.5 mg/kg PO q24h
Oxacillin	Prostaphlin; generic	Antibacterial	250- and 500-mg capsules; 50 mg/mL oral solution	22-40 mg/kg PO q8h
Oxazepam	Serax	Benzodiazepine/appetite stimulant	15-mg tablet	Cat: appetite stimulant: 2.5 mg/cat PO

Drug	Brand	Indication	Formulation	Dosage
Oxtriphylline	Choledyl-SA	*Bronchodilator/chronic bronchitis (feline asthma?)*	400- and 600-mg tablets (oral solutions and syrup available in Canada but not U.S.)	Dog: 47 mg/kg (equivalent to 30 mg/kg theophylline) PO q12h Cat: Dose Not Available
Oxybutynin	Ditropan	*Urinary antispasmodic/adjunctive treatment of detrusor hyperreflexia (includes FeLV-positive cats)*	5-mg tablet	Dog: 0.2 mg/kg PO q8-12h (or 1.25 to 3.75 mg/dog q12h) Cat: 0.5-1.0 mg/kg PO q8-12h
Oxymetholone	Anadrol	*Hormone (anabolic steroid)/may stimulate erythropoiesis*	50-mg tablet	1-5 mg/kg/day PO
Oxymorphone	Numorphan	*Analgesic (opiate)/pain management*	1.5 and 1 mg/mL injection	*Analgesia:* 0.1-0.2 mg/kg IV, SC, IM (as needed); redose with 0.05-0.1 mg/kg q1-2h. *Preanesthetic:* 0.025-0.05 mg/kg IM, SC
Oxytetracycline	Terramycin	*Antibacterial*	250-mg tablets; 100 and 200 mg/mL injection	7.5-10 mg/kg IV q12h; 20 mg/kg PO q12h
Oxytocin	Pitocin; Syntocinon (nasal solution); generic	*Hormone/induction of labor or parturition*	10 and 20 U/mL injection; 40 U/mL nasal solution	Dog: 5-20 U/dog SC, IM (repeat every 30 min for primary inertia) Cat: 3-5 U/cat SC, IM (repeat every 30 min)
2-PAM	*See* Pralidoxime chloride			
Pancreatic enzyme	Viokase	*Digestive enzymes/management of exocrine insufficiency*	16,800 U lipase, 70,000 U protease, and 70,000 U amylase per 0.7 g; also capsules and tablets	Mix 2 tsp powder with food/20 kg; or 1-3 tsp/0.45 kg of food 20 min before feeding
Pancuronium bromide	Pavulon	*Neuromuscular blocker/muscle relaxation as an adjunct to anesthesia*	1 and 2 mg/mL injection	0.1 mg/kg IV, or start with 0.01 mg/kg and additional doses of 0.01 mg/kg q30min

Continued

Note: Listings preceded by ◆ are for rapid reference and denote drug/dosage used in the emergency or critical care setting.

6

TABLE 6-26   Common Drug Indications and Dosages†—cont'd

Drug	Proprietary names	Action/Use	Formulation	Recommended dosage
Paregoric	Corrective mixture	Antidiarrheal/management of simple diarrhea	2 mg morphine per 5 mL of paregoric	0.05-0.06 mg/kg PO q12h
Paromomycin	Humatin	Antiparasitic/cryptosporidiosis in cats	250-mg capsules	Cat: 125-165 mg/kg, PO, q12h for 7 days. WARNING: toxicity and renal damage have been reported at these doses
Paroxetine	Paxil	Selective serotonin reuptake inhibitor (SSRI)/management of behavior disorders	10-, 20-, 30-, and 40-mg tablets	Dog and Cat: 2.5-5.0 mg (total dose) PO once daily Cat (alternative): 1/8 to 1/4 of 10-mg tablet daily PO
D-Penicillamine	Cuprimine; Depen	Chelating agent/treatment of lead poisoning; also for cystine urolithiasis	125- and 250-mg capsules and 250-mg tablets	10-15 mg/kg PO q12h
Penicillin G benzathine	Benza-Pen; others	Antibacterial	150,000 U/mL, combined with 150,000 U/mL procaine penicillin G	24,000 U/kg IM q48h
Penicillin G potassium; penicillin G sodium	Multiple	Antibacterial	5 million– to 20 million–unit vials	20,000-40,000 U/kg IV, IM q6-8h
Penicillin G procaine	Generic	Antibacterial	300,000 U/mL suspension	20,000-40,000 U/kg IV, IM q12-24h
Penicillin V	Pen-Vee	Antibacterial	250- and 500-mg tablets	10 mg/kg PO q8h
Pentazocine	Talwin-V	Analgesic (opiate)/pain management	30 mg/mL injection	Dog: 1.65-3.3 mg/kg IM q4h Cat: 2.2-3.3 mg/kg IV, IM, SC; 25-30 mg/kg IV for anesthesia
◆ Pentobarbital	Nembutal; generic	Anesthetic/sedative or injectable anesthetic	50 mg/mL NOTE: This formulation is NOT to be used for euthanasia.	
Pentoxifylline	Trental	Antiinflammatory effects/has been used to treat immune-mediated skin disorders (e.g., associated with vasculitis) in dogs	400-mg tablet	Dog: For use in canine dermatology and for vasculitis, 10 mg/kg PO q12h

6

◆ Phenobarbital	Luminal; generic	*Barbiturate/sedation and anticonvulsant*	15-, 30-, 60-, and 100-mg tablets; 30, 60, 65, and 130 mg/mL injection; 4 mg/mL oral elixir solution	Dog: 2-8 mg/kg PO q12h Cat: 2-4 mg kg PO q12h Dog and cat: Adjust dose by monitoring plasma concentration *Status epilepticus:* Administer in increments of 10-20 mg/kg IV to effect
Phenoxybenzamine	Dibenzyline	*Alpha-adrenergic blocker/ reduces internal urethral sphincter tone associated with detrusor areflexia; also hypertension associated with pheochromocytoma*	10-mg capsule	Dog: *Urinary:* 0.25 mg/kg PO q8-12h or 0.5 mg/kg q24h *Hypertension:* 0.2-1.5 mg/kg, PO bid for 10-14 days before surgery Cat: 2.5 mg/cat q8-12h or 0.5 mg/cat PO q12h NOTE: In cats, doses as high as 0.5 mg/kg IV have been used to relax urethral smooth muscle
Phentolamine	Regitine	*Vasodilator/hypertension*	5-mg vial for injection	0.02-0.1 mg/kg IV
Phenylbutazone	Butazolidin; generic	*NSAID*	100-, 200-, 400-mg and 1-g tablets; 200 mg/mL injection	NOT recommended for use in dogs and cats (better drugs are available)
◆ Phenylephrine	Neo-Synephrine	*Alpha-adrenergic/treatment of hypotension in the critical care setting; also used topically intranasally prior to rhinoscopy*	10 mg/mL injection; 1% nasal solution	Dog and Cat: 1-3 µg/kg/min CRI in 0.9% saline or D5W; 0.1 mg/kg, IM, SC, q15min *Topical:* 3-5 drops intranasally to effect to induce local vasoconstriction
Phenylpropanol-amine	Dexatrim; Propagest; others	*Adrenergic agonist/urinary incontinence associated with urethral sphincter hypotonus*	15-, 25-, 30-, and 50-mg tablets	Dog: 12.5-50 mg (total) PO q8h or 1.5-2 mg/kg, PO, q12h Cat: 12.5 mg (total) PO q8h or1.5 mg/kg, PO, q8h

Continued

Note: Listings preceded by ◆ are for rapid reference and denote drug/dosage used in the emergency or critical care setting.

6

TABLE 6-26 Common Drug Indications and Dosages†—cont'd

Drug	Proprietary names	Action/Use	Formulation	Recommended dosage
Phenytoin	Dilantin	Anticonvulsant/not generally recommended; limited application in digoxin-induced arrhythmias	30 and 1250 mg/mL oral suspension; 30- and 100-mg capsules; 50 mg/mL injection	Antiepileptic (dog): 20-34 mg/kg q8h Digoxin-induced antiarrhythmic: 30 mg/kg PO q8h or 10 mg/kg IV over 5 min
◆ Phenytoin + Pentobarbital sodium	Beuthanasia-D Special; Euthasol	Euthanasia solution	100-mL multiple dose vials	1 mL/10 lb body weight IV. NOTE: Alternative routes (at the same dosage) can be used in profoundly debilitated patients (e.g., intraperitoneal, intracardiac)
Physostigmine	Antilirium	Cholinesterase inhibitor/limited application; may be of use in promoting micturition in patients with urinary retention (postoperatively)	1 mg/mL injection	0.02 mg/kg IV q12h
◆ Phytomenadione	See Vitamin K₁			
◆ Phytonadione	See Vitamin K₁			
Piperacillin	Pipracil	Antibacterial	2-, 3-, 4-, and 40-g vials for injection	40 mg/kg IV or IM q6h
Piperazine	Many	Antiparasitic/roundworms	860 mg powder; 140-mg capsule, 170, 340, and 800 mg/mL oral solution	44-66 mg/kg PO administered once
Piroxicam	Feldene; generic	NSAID/has antitumor effects (indirect) in patients with transitional cell carcinoma (palliative treatment)	10-mg capsules	Dog: 0.3 mg/kg, PO, once daily Cat: 0.3 mg/kg PO, q24-72h (Administer with food)
Pitressin (ADH)	See Vasopressin and Desmopressin acetate			
Plicamycin (formerly mithramycin)	Mithracin	Antineoplastic/adjunctive treatment in carcinoma protocols; also used to	2.5 mg/mL injection	Dog: Antineoplastic: 25-30 μg/kg/day IV (slow infusion) for 8-10 days

Generic name	Trade name/source	Indications	How supplied	Dosage
		decrease calcium levels in hypercalcemic cancer patients		*Antihypercalcemic:* 25 µg/kg/day IV (slow infusion) over 4 hours Cat: NOT recommended
Polyethylene glycol electrolyte solution	GoLYTELY	Laxative	Oral solution	25 mg/kg PO; repeat in 2-4 hours PO
Polysulfated glycosaminoglycan (PSGAG)	Adequan Canine	Antiarthritic/*long-term management of osteoarthritis*	100 mg/mL injection in 5-mL vial (250 mg/mL vials for horses)	4.4 mg/kg IM twice weekly for up to 4 weeks
Potassium bromide (KBr)	No commercial formulation	Anticonvulsant/*long-term antiepileptic therapy*	Usually prepared as oral solution	Dog and Cat: 30-40 mg/kg PO q24h NOTE: If administered without phenobarbital, higher doses of up to 40-50 mg/kg may be needed; adjust doses by monitoring plasma concentrations; loading doses of 400 mg/kg divided over 3 days have been administered.
◆ Potassium chloride (KCl)	Generic	Potassium salt/*replacement therapy*	Various concentrations for injection (usually 2 mEq/mL); oral suspension and oral solution	0.5 mEq potassium/kg/day; or supplement 10-40 mEq/500 mL of fluids, depending on serum potassium
Potassium citrate	Urocit-K; generic	Potassium salt/*replacement therapy*	5-mEq tablet; some forms are in combination with potassium chloride	2.2 mEq/100 kcal of energy/day PO; or 40-75 mEq/kg PO q12h
Potassium gluconate	Kaon; Tumil-K; generic	Potassium source/*replacement therapy*	2-mEq tablet; 500-mg tablet; Kaon elixir is 20 mEq/15 mL elixir	Dog: 0.5 mEq/kg PO 12-24h Cat: 2-8 mEq/day PO divided twice daily
◆ Pralidoxime chloride (2-PAM)	2-PAM; Protopam Chloride	Cholinesterase re-activator/*adjunctive treatment in patients with organophosphate toxicosis*	50 mg/mL injection	20 mg/kg q8-12h (initial dose) IV slowly or IM
Praziquantel	Droncit	Antiparasitic/treatment of cestodes (tapeworms)	23- and 34-mg tablets; 56.8 mg/mL injection	Dog: <6.8 kg, 7.5 mg/kg once; >6.8 kg, 5 mg/kg IM, SC once; <2.3 kg, 7.5 mg/kg

Continued

Note: Listings preceded by ◆ are for rapid reference and denote drug/dosage used in the emergency or critical care setting.

6

TABLE 6-26 Common Drug Indications and Dosages†—cont'd

Drug	Proprietary names	Action/Use	Formulation	Recommended dosage
				PO once; 2.7-4.5 kg, 6.3 mg/kg PO once; >5 kg, 5 mg/kg PO once Cat: <1.8 kg, 6.3 mg/kg PO once; >1.8 kg, 5 mg/kg PO once. *For Paragonimus:* 25 mg/kg PO q8h for 2-3 days) 5 mg/kg IM, SC
Prazosin	Minipress	Alpha-1 blocker/*adjunctive treatment of congestive heart failure; also hypertension and pulmonary hypertension (e.g., heartworm disease)*	1-, 2-, and 5-mg capsules	0.5- and 2-mg/animal (1 mg/15 kg) PO q8-12h
Prednisolone	Delta-Cortef; many others	Glucocorticoid/ *antiinflammatory and immunosuppressive*	5- and 20-mg tablets	Dog (cat often requires 2 × dog dose): *Antiinflammatory:* 0.5-1 mg/kg IV, IM, PO q12-24h initially; then taper to q48h *Immunosuppressive:* 2.2-6.6 mg/kg/day IV, IM, PO initially; then taper to 2-4 mg/kg q48h *Replacement therapy:* 0.2-0.3 mg/kg/day PO *Shock, spinal trauma:* See Prednisolone sodium succinate
Prednisolone sodium succinate	Solu-Delta-Cortef	Glucocorticoid/*adjunctive therapy for endotoxic or septic shock*	100- and 200-mg vials for injection (10 and 50 mg/mL)	*Shock:* 5.5-11 mg/kg IV (repeat in 1, 3, 6, or 10 h) *CNS trauma:* 15-30 mg/kg IV; then taper to 1-2 mg/kg q12h
Prednisone	Deltasone; generic; Meticorten for injection	Glucocorticoid/ *antiinflammatory and immunosuppressive*	1-, 2.5-, 5-, 10-, 20-, 25-, and 50-mg tablets; 1 mg/mL syrup (Liquid-Pred in 5% alcohol); 1 mg/mL oral solution (in 5% alcohol); 10 and 40 mg/mL prednisone suspension for injection	Same as for prednisolone

Primidone	Mylepsin; Neurosyn	Anticonvulsant/idiopathic epilepsy (not generally recommended)	50- and 250-mg tablets	8-10 mg/kg PO q8-12h as initial dose, and then adjust via monitoring to 10-15 mg/kg q8h WARNING: May cause irreversible liver disease with prolonged administration
Procainamide	Pronestyl; generic	Antiarrhythmic/ventricular premature contractions (e.g., ventricular tachycardia)	250, 375, 500 mg/mL injection	Dog: 10-30 mg/kg PO q6h (up to maximum dose of 40 mg/kg); 8-20 mg/kg IV, IM; 25-50 µg/kg/min IV infusion Cat: 3-8 mg/kg IM, PO q6-8h
Procarbazine	Matulane; Natulan; Natulanar	Antineoplastic/component drug used in lymphoma protocols	50-mg capsules	Used in combination with mechlorethamine and prednisolone; consult latest information on protocols for precise dose
Prochlorperazine	Compazine	Phenothiazine/antiemetic	5-, 10-, and 25-mg tablets (maleate); 5 mg/mL injection (edisylate)	0.1-0.5 mg/kg IM, SC q6-8h
Progesterone, repositol	See Medroxyprogesterone acetate			
Promethazine	Phenergan	Phenothiazine/antiemetic	6.25 and 25 mg/5 mL syrup; 12.5-, 25-, and 50-mg tablets; 25 and 50 mg/mL injection	0.2-0.4 mg/kg IV, IM, PO q6-8h (up to maximum dose of 1 mg/kg)
Propantheline bromide	Pro-Banthine	Antimuscarinic/antidiarrheal; also used to treat urge incontinence associated with detrusor hyperreflexia; oral antiemetic effect	7.5- and 15-mg tablets	Dog: Urge incontinence: 0.2 mg/kg PO q6-8h Diarrhea: 0.25 mg/kg PO three times daily for 2-3 days max Cat: Urge incontinence: 0.25-0.5 mg/kg PO once or twice daily Chronic colitis: 0.5 mg/kg PO two to three times daily

Continued

Note: Listings preceded by ◆ are for rapid reference and denote drug/dosage used in the emergency or critical care setting.

6

TABLE 6-26 **Common Drug Indications and Dosages†—cont'd**

Drug	Proprietary names	Action/Use	Formulation	Recommended dosage
Propiopromazine	Tranvet; Largon	Antiemetic, tranquilizer/ sedation, parenteral antiemetic	20 mg/mL injection	1.1-4.4 mg/kg q12-24h
Propionibacterium acnes (injection)	Immunoregulin	Immunomodulator/nonspecific immunostimulant used as adjunctive therapy in dogs with pyoderma and in retrovirus-positive cats	0.4 mg/mL in 5- and 50-mL vials	Dog: 0.03-0.07 mL/kg IV twice weekly for 10 wk (NOTE: dose is mL/kg) Cat: 0.5 mL IV twice weekly for 2 wk; then one injection weekly for 20 wk NOTE: Treatment is NOT expected to convert retrovirus-*positive* cats to a retrovirus-*negative* status.
◆ Propofol	Rapinovet; PropoFlo	Short-acting injectable anesthetic (hypnotic)/ induction or restraint for short-term procedures	1% (10 mg/mL) injection in 20-mL ampules	6.6 mg/kg IV slowly over 60 sec (constant-rate IV infusions have been used at 2 mg/kg/h)
◆ Propranolol	Inderal	Beta blocker/antiarrhythmic	10-, 20-, 40-, 60-, 80-, and 90-mg tablets; 1 mg/mL injection; 4 and 8 mg/mL oral solution	Dog: 20-60 µg/kg over 5-10 min IV; 0.2-1 mg/kg PO q8h (titrate dose to effect) Cat: 0.4-1.2 mg/kg (2.5-5 mg/cat) PO q8h Cat: 11 mg/kg PO q12h
Propylthiouracil (PTU)	Propyl-Thyracil; generic	Antithyroid/alternative drug used in the management of feline hyperthyroidism	50- and 100-mg tablets	Cat: 11 mg/kg PO q12h
Prostaglandin F₂ alpha	Lutalyse; Dinoprost	Prostaglandin/open pyometra; pregnancy termination in dogs	5 mg/mL solution for injection	NOTE: Any use of this drug in dogs and cats is EXTRA-LABEL *Open pyometra:* Dog: 0.1-0.2 mg/kg SC once daily for 5 days; Cat: 0.1 mg/kg SC twice daily for 5 days

Drug	Trade names	Indication	How supplied	Dosage
				NOTE: Concurrent antibiotic therapy is recommended. SURGERY IS ALWAYS PREFERRED! *Abortion (within 30 days of the last unwanted breeding):* Dog: 0.1 mg/kg SC q8h for 2 days; then 0.2 mg/kg SC q8h until abortion is confirmed by ultrasound.
Pseudoephedrine (OTC)	Sudafed; many others (some formulations have other ingredients)	Adrenergic agonist/*urinary incontinence (generally only used when phenyl-propanolamine is not available)*	30- and 60-mg tablets; 120-mg capsule; 6 mg/mL syrup	0.2-0.4 mg/kg (or 15-60 mg/dog) PO q8-12h
Psyllium	Metamucil; others	Laxative, stool softener	Available as powder	1 tsp/5-10 kg (added to each meal)
Pyrantel pamoate and tartrate	Nemex; Strongid	Antiparasitic/*treatment of ascarids and hookworms*	180 mg/mL paste and 50 mg/mL suspension	Dog: 5 mg/kg PO once; repeat in 7-10 days Cat: 20 mg/kg PO once
Pyridostigmine bromide	Mestinon; Regonol	Cholinesterase inhibitor/*management of myasthenia gravis*	12 mg/mL oral syrup; 60-mg tablet; 5 mg/mL injection	*Antimyasthenic:* 0.02-0.04 mg/kg IV q2h; or 0.5-3 mg/kg PO q8-12h *Antidote (nondepolarizing muscle relaxant):* 0.15-0.3 mg/kg IM, IV
Pyrimethamine	Daraprim	Folic acid inhibitor/*treatment of toxoplasmosis and neosporosis*	25-mg tablet	Dog: 1 mg/kg PO q24h for 14-21 days (5 days for *Neosporum caninum*) Cat: 0.5-1 mg/kg PO q24h for 14-28 days
Quinacrine	Limited availability in the U.S.	Antiprotozoal/*may be useful in management (not curing) of Giardia infections, leishmaniasis, and coccidiosis*	100-mg tablet	Dog: 6.6 mg/kg PO q12h for 5 days Cat: 11 mg/kg PO q24h for 5 days
Quinidine gluconate	Quiniglute; Duraquin	Antiarrhythmic/*ventricular arrhythmias*	324-mg tablets; 80 mg/mL injection	Dog: 6-20 mg/kg IM q6h; 6-20 mg/kg PO q6-8h (of base)
Quinidine sulfate	Cin-Quin; Quinora	Antiarrhythmic/*ventricular arrhythmias*	100-, 200-, and 300-mg tablets; 200- and 300-mg capsules; 20 mg/mL injection	Dog: 6-20 mg/kg PO q6-8h (of base); 5-10 mg/kg IV

Continued

Note: Listings preceded by ◆ are for rapid reference and denote drug/dosage used in the emergency or critical care setting.

6

TABLE 6-26   Common Drug Indications and Dosages†—cont'd

Drug	Proprietary names	Action/Use	Formulation	Recommended dosage
Quinidine polygalacturonate	Cardioquin	Antiarrhythmic/ventricular arrhythmias	275-mg tablet	Dog: 6-20 mg/kg PO q6h (of quinidine base). NOTE: 275 mg quinidine polygalacturonate = 167 mg quinidine base
◆ Ranitidine	Zantac	H₂ receptor antagonist/ treatment and prevention of gastric and duodenal ulcers	75-, 150-, and 300-mg tablets; 150- and 300-mg capsules; 25 mg/mL injection	Dog: 2 mg/kg IV, PO q8h Cat: 2.5 mg/kg IV q12h; 3.5 mg/kg PO q12h
Retinol	See Vitamin A (Aquasol-A)			
Riboflavin	See Vitamin B₂			
Rifampin	Rifadin	Antibacterial (reported to have limited antifungal and antiviral activity)	150- and 300-mg capsules	10-20 mg/kg PO q24h
◆ Ringer's solution	Generic	Fluid replacement	250-, 500-, and 1000-mL bags for infusion	40-50 mg/kg/day IV, SC, IP
SAMe (S-adenosyl-methionine)	Denosyl-SD4	Nucleotide-like molecule derived from the amino acid methionine/adjunctive therapy in patients with chronic liver disease	Enteric coated tablets	20 mg/kg PO daily
Salicylate	See Aspirin			
Selamectin	Revolution	Antiparasitic (ivermectin)/ multiple applications in dogs and cats	Various sizes of topical solutions available for dogs and cats	See manufacturer's dosing instructions for the specific condition being treated
Selegiline	Anipryl (also known as deprenyl and l-deprenyl)	MAO-B inhibitor/canine cognitive dysfunction; reported use in treatment of canine hyperadrenocorticism (use in canine Cushing's is currently NOT recommended)	2-, 5-, 10-, 15-, and 30-mg tablets	Dog: Begin with 1 mg/kg PO q24h; if there is no response within 2 mo, increase dose to maximum of 2 mg/kg PO q24h Cat: Dose not established

6

Senna	Senokot	Laxative	Granules in concentrate, or syrup	Cat: syrup: 5 mL/cat q24h; granules: 1/2 teaspoon/cat q24h (with food)
Sertraline	Zoloft; Altruline; Anilar; others	Selective serotonin reuptake inhibitor/management of certain behavior disorders in dogs	25-, 50-, and 100-mg tablets; 20 mg/mL injectable in 60-mL vials	Dog: 0.5-4.0 mg/kg q24h Cat: 0.5-1.0 mg/kg q24h
◆ Sodium bicarbonate ($NaHCO_3$) (OTC)	Generic; e.g., baking soda, soda mint	Alkalinizing agent/management of acidosis and renal failure; also used to alkalinize urine when indicated	325-, 520-, and 650-mg tablets; injection of various strengths (4.2% to 8.4%), and 1 mEq/mL	Acidosis: 0.5-1 mEq/kg IV Renal failure: 10 mg/kg PO q8-12h Alkalization of urine: 50 mg/kg PO q8-12h (1 tsp is approximately 2 g)
◆ Sodium chloride 0.9%	Generic	Fluid replacement (isotonic)	500- and 1000-mL infusion	40-50 mL/kg/day IV, SC, IP
◆ Sodium chloride 7.2%	Generic (hypertonic)	Fluid replacement	Infusion	2-8 mL/kg IV CAUTION: NOT a balanced electrolyte solution
Sodium iodide 20%	Iodopen; generic	Iodine replacement/replacement for confirmed deficiencies	100 µg elemental iodide (118 µg sodium iodide)/mL injection	20-40 mg/kg PO q8-12h
Sotalol	Betapace	Nonselective beta blocker (antiarrhythmic)/ventricular tachycardia	80-, 160-, 240-mg tablets	Dog: 1-2 mg/kg PO q12h (start with 40 mg/dog q12h; then increase to 80 mg if no response) Cat: 1-2 mg/kg PO q12h
Spironolactone	Aldactone	Aldosterone antagonist/K-sparing diuretic used in the treatment of congestive heart failure; generally used in patients that fail to respond to furosemide and ACE inhibitors	25-, 50-, and 100-mg tablets	2-4 mg/kg/day (or 1-2 mg/kg PO q12h)

Continued

Note: Listings preceded by ◆ are for rapid reference and denote drug/dosage used in the emergency or critical care setting.

6

TABLE 6-26   Common Drug Indications and Dosages†—cont'd

Drug	Proprietary names	Action/Use	Formulation	Recommended dosage
Stanozolol	Winstrol-V	Anabolic steroid/adjunctive therapy for no one really knows what; has been used to treat anemia of chronic disease	50 mg/mL injection; 2-mg tablet	Dog: 2 mg/dog (or range of 1-4 mg/dog) PO q12h; 25-50 mg/dog/wk IM Cat: 1 mg/cat PO q12h; 25 mg/cat/wk IM CAUTION: Use in anorexic patients can cause weight loss (catabolic effect?)
Succimer	Chemet	Heavy metal chelator/treatment of lead poisoning	100-mg capsule	10 mg/kg PO q8h for 5 days; then 10 mg/kg PO q12h for 2 more wk
◆ Sucralfate	Carafate	Antiulcer treatment/treatment of gastric and duodenal ulcers (may have preventive effect)	1-g tablet; 200 mg/mL oral suspension	Dog: 0.5-1 g/dog PO q8-12h Cat: 0.25 g/cat PO q8-12h
Sufentanil	Sufenta	Analgesic (potent opiate)/ adjunct to anesthesia or epidural anesthesia	50 μg/mL injection	2 μg/kg IV (maximum dose is 5 μg/kg IV)
Sulfadiazine	Generic combined with trimethoprim in Tribrissen	Antibacterial	500-mg tablet	100 mg/kg IV PO (loading dose), followed by 50 mg/kg IV PO q12h (see also Trimethoprim)
Sulfadimethoxine	Albon; Bactrovet; generic	Antibacterial	125-, 250-, and 500-mg tablets; 400 mg/mL injection; 50 mg/mL suspension	55 mg/kg PO (loading dose), followed by 27.5 mg/kg PO q12h (see also Ormetoprim and Sulfadimethoxine)
Sulfamethazine	Many brand name products (e.g., Sulmet)	Antibacterial	30-g bolus	100 mg/kg PO (loading dose), followed by 50 mg/kg PO q12h
Sulfamethoxazole	Gantanol	Antibacterial	50-mg tablet	100 mg/kg PO (loading dose), followed by 50 mg/kg PO q12h (see also Bactrim, Septra)
Sulfasalazine (sulfapyridine + mesalamine)	Azulfidine (see also Mesalamine, Olsalazine)	Antibacterial and antiin-flammatory activity/ ulcerative colitis and other forms of inflammatory bowel disease in dogs	500-mg tablets; pediatric suspension	Dog: 10-30 mg/kg PO q8-12h WARNING: Has been reported to cause keratoconjunctivitis sicca in dogs.

6

Drug	Brand	Category	Available forms	Dosage
Sulfisoxazole	Gantrisin	Antibacterial	500-mg tablet; 500 mg/5 mL syrup	50 mg/kg PO q8h (*urinary tract infections*)
Taurine	Generic	*Amino acid/taurine deficiency cardiomyopathies*	Available in powder	Dog: 5.0 mg PO q12h; Cat: 2.50 mg/cat PO q12h
Tepoxalin	Zubrin	*NSAID/management of pain associated with osteoarthritis in dogs*	30-, 50-, 100- and 200-mg tablets	Dog: 10-20 mg/kg PO on the first day; then 10 mg/kg PO once daily; thereafter as needed
◆ Terbutaline	Brethine; Bricanyl	*Beta agonist/bronchodilator; use includes feline asthma*	2.5- and 5-mg tablets; 1 mg/mL injection (equivalent to 0.82 mg/mL)	Dog: 1.25-5 mg/dog PO q8h; Cat: 0.1-0.2 mg/kg PO q12h (or 0.625 mg/cat, ¼ of 2.5-mg tablet)
Testosterone cypionate ester	Andro-Cyp; Andronate; Depo-Testosterone; others	*Hormone/replacement therapy; most commonly used for testosterone-responsive urinary incontinence in neutered male dogs/cats*	100 and 200 mg/mL injection	1-2 mg/kg IM q2-4wk (see also methyltestosterone)
Testosterone propionate ester	Testex	*Hormone/replacement therapy; most commonly used for testosterone-responsive urinary incontinence in neutered male dogs/cats*	100 mg/mL injection	0.5-1 mg/kg IM 2-3 times/wk
Tetracycline	Panmycin	Antibacterial	250- and 500-mg capsules; 100 mg/mL suspension	15-20 mg/kg PO q8h; or 4.4-11 mg/kg IV, IM q8h
Thenium closylate	Canopar	*Antiparasitic/hookworms*	500-mg tablet	Dog: >4.5 kg, 500 mg PO once and repeat in 2-3 wk; 2.5-4.5 kg, 250 mg q12h for 1 day and repeat in 2-3 wks
Theophylline	Many brand name and generic products	*Bronchodilator/chronic bronchitis and feline asthma*	100-, 125-, 200-, 250-, and 300-mg tablets; 27 mg/5 mL oral solution or elixir; injection in 5% dextrose	Dog: 9 mg/kg PO q6-8h; Cat: 4 mg/kg PO q8-12h (see also Aminophylline)

Note: Listings preceded by ◆ are for rapid reference and denote drug/dosage used in the emergency or critical care setting.

Continued

6

TABLE 6-26 Common Drug Indications and Dosages†—cont'd

Drug	Proprietary names	Action/Use	Formulation	Recommended dosage
Theophylline, sustained-release	Theo-Dur; Slo-bid; Gyrocaps	Bronchodilator/chronic bronchitis and feline asthma	100-, 200-, 300-, and 450-mg tablets (Theo-Dur); 50- to 200-mg capsules (Slo-bid)	Dog: 20 mg/kg PO q12h (*Theo-Dur*); 30 mg/kg q12h (*Slo-bid*) Cat: 25 mg/kg PO q24h (at night) for *Theo-Dur* and *Slo-bid*
Thiabendazole	Omnizole; Equizole; Tresaderm (topical-otic)	Antiparasitic/multiple applications for parasitic infections	2 or 4 g/oz (30 mL) suspension or liquid	Dog: 50 mg/kg q24h for 3 days and repeat in 1 mo; *Respiratory parasites:* 30-70 mg/kg PO q12h Cat: *Strongyloides:* 125 mg/kg q24h for 3 days
Thiacetarsamide sodium	Caparsolate	Arsenical/formerly used to treat canine heartworm disease	NOT commercially available	
Thiamine	See Vitamin B₁			
Thioguanine (6-TG)	Generic	Antineoplastic/lymphocytic or granulocytic leukemia	40-mg tablet	Dog: 40 mg/m² PO q24h Cat: 25 mg/m² PO q24h for 1-5 days
Thiopental sodium	Pentothal	Short-acting injectable anesthetic/anesthesia induction or restraint for short procedures	Various size vials from 250 mg to 10 g (mix to desired concentration)	Dog: 10-25 mg/kg IV (to effect) Cat: 5-10 mg/kg IV (to effect)
Thiotepa	Generic	Antineoplastic/lymphocytic or granulocytic leukemia	15-mg injection (usually in solution of 10 mg/mL)	0.2-0.5 mg/m²/wk, or daily for 5-10 days (IM, intra-cavitary, or intra-tumor)
Thyroid hormone	See Levothyroxine sodium (T₄) and Liothyronine (T₃)			
Thyrotropin (thyroid-stimulating hormone [TSH])	Thytropar	Hormone/used to test for hypothyroidism (primarily in dogs)	10-U vial	Dog: Collect baseline sample, followed by 0.1 U/kg IV maximum (dose is 5 U); collect post-TSH sample at 6 h Cat: Collect baseline sample, followed by 2.5 U/cat IM; collect a post-TSH sample 8-12 h later

6

Drug	Trade Names	Category/Use	Formulation	Dosage
Ticarcillin	Ticar; Ticillin	Antibacterial	6 g/50 mL vial; vials containing 1, 3, 6, 20, and 30 g	33-50 mg/kg IV, IM q4-6h
Ticarcillin + clavulanate	Timentin	Antibacterial	3-g vial for injection	33-50 mg/kg IV, IM q4-6h
Tiletamine + zolazepam	Telazol; Zoletil	General anesthetic/indicated for restraint and minor procedures of short duration in healthy dogs and cats	Sterile vial to which 5 mL of sterile water is added; provides the equivalent of 50 mg of tiletamine/mL CAUTION: Limited shelf life following reconstitution	Dosage is based on combined mg of each drug: Dog: 6.6-10 mg/kg deep IM (restraint); 10-13 mg/kg deep IM (minor surgical procedures) Do NOT exceed 26.4 mg/kg TOTAL DOSE Cat: 9.7-12 mg/kg deep IM (restraint) 10.6-12.5 mg/kg, deep IM (minor surgical procedures) 14.3-15.8 mg/kg deep IM (anesthesia) DO NOT EXCEED 72 mg/kg TOTAL DOSE
Tobramycin	Nebcin	Antibacterial	40 mg/mL injection	2-4 mg/kg IV, IM, SC q8h
◆ Tocainide	Tonocard	Oral antiarrhythmic/used to manage patients with ventricular arrhythmias	400- and 600-mg tablets	Dog: 15-20 mg/kg PO q8h Cat: Dose not established
Tolazoline	Tolazine	Alpha-adrenergic blocker/reversal agent for xylazine	100 mg/mL in 100-mL multi-dose vials	4 mg/kg by slow IV (approx 1 mL/sec)
Triamcinolone	Vetalog; Trimtabs; Aristocort; generic	Glucocorticoid/antiinflammatory (not generally used in the treatment of immune-mediated disease)	Veterinary (Vetalog): 0.5- and 1.5-mg tablets Human form: 1-, 2-, 4-, 8-, and 16-mg tablets; 10 mg/mL injection	Antiinflammatory: 0.5-1 mg/kg PO q12-24 h; then taper dose to 0.5-1 PO; taper dose to mg/kg q48h (however, manufacturer recommends doses of 0.11-0.22 mg/kg/day)
Triamcinolone acetonide	Vetalog	Glucocorticoid/antiinflammatory (not generally used in the treatment of immune-mediated disease)	2 and 6 mg/mL suspension injection; 0.5- and 1.5-mg tablets	0.1-0.2 mg/kg IM, SC; repeat in 7-10 days Intralesional: 1.2-1.8 mg, or 1 mg for every cm diameter of tumor q2wk

Note: Listings preceded by ◆ are for rapid reference and denote drug/dosage used in the emergency or critical care setting.

Continued

6

T A B L E　6 - 2 6　Common Drug Indications and Dosages†—cont'd

Drug	Proprietary names	Action/Use	Formulation	Recommended dosage
Triamterene	Dyrenium	Diuretic/K-sparing diuretic used as an alternative to spironolactone	50- and 100-mg capsules	1-2 mg/kg PO q12h
Trientine hydrochloride	Syprine	Oral copper chelating agent/copper-associated hepatopathy; indicated in dogs that cannot tolerate penicillamine	250-mg capsules	Dog: 10-15 mg/kg PO q12h
Trifluoperazine	Stelazine	Phenothiazine/antiemetic	10 mg/mL oral solution; also as 1-, 2-, 5-, and 10-mg tablets; 2.0 mg/mL injection	0.03 mg/kg IM q12h
Triflupromazine	Vesprin	Phenothiazine/antiemetic	10 and 20 mg/mL injection	0.1-0.3 mg/kg IM, PO q8-12h
Triiodothyronine	See Liothyronine			
Trimeprazine tartrate with prednisolone	Temaril-P	Phenothiazine antihistamine + glucocorticoid combination/antitussive and antipruritic. Not generally recommended today	5 mg trimeprazine + 2-mg prednisolone (combined) tablets	Dog: See manufacturer's recommendations regarding indications and dose
Trimethoprim + sulfonamide (sulfadiazine or sulfamethoxazole)	Tribrissen; others	Antibacterial	30-, 120-, 240-, 480-, and 960-mg tablets	15 mg/kg PO q12h; or 30 mg/kg PO q12-24h. For toxoplasma: 30 mg/kg PO q12h
TSH (thyroid-stimulating hormone)	See Thyrotropin			
Tylosin	Tylocine; Tylan; Tylosin tartrate	Antibacterial/has anti-inflammatory effects in the bowel and is sometimes used to treat inflammatory bowel disease and chronic colitis	Available as soluble powder with 2.2 g tylosin per tsp (tablets available for dogs in Canada)	Dog and cat: 7-15 mg/kg PO q12-24h. Dog (for colitis): 11 mg/kg q8h, with food

6

Drug	Brand names	Classification/use	Formulation	Dosage
Ursodiol (ursodeoxycholic acid)	Actigall	Bile acid/adjunctive therapy in patients with chronic liver disease	300-mg capsule	10-15 mg/kg PO q24h
Valproic acid, divalproex	Depakene (valproic acid); Depakote (divalproex)	Anticonvulsant/uncommonly used alternative to conventional anticonvulsant therapy	Depakote: 125-, 250-, and 500-mg tablets; Depakene: 250-mg capsule; 50 mg/mL syrup	Dog: 60-200 mg/kg PO q8h; or 25-105 mg/kg/day PO when administered with phenobarbital Cat: DO NOT USE
Vancomycin	Vancocin; Vancoled	Antibacterial	Vials for injection (0.5 to 10 g)	Dog: 15 mg/kg q6-8h IV by CRI Cat: 12-15 mg/kg q8h IV by CRI
Vasopressin (ADH)	Pitressin	Hormone/diagnostic test agent for diabetes insipidus (DI). NOT for therapeutic use (see Desmopressin)	20 (pressor) units/mL in 0.5-, 1.0-, and 10-mL vials (aqueous only) and 1-mL ampules	Dog:Test protocol for DI: 2.5 mU/kg (aqueous vasopressin) IV over 1 h Cat: 0.5 U/kg, IM (test protocol in cats is different from that in dogs) NOTE: test protocol entails patient preparation in advance of administering vasopressin
◆ Verapamil	Calan; Isoptin	Calcium channel blocker/supraventricular tachycardia and hypertension	40-, 80-, and 120-mg tablets; 2.5 mg/mL injection	Dog: 0.05 mg/kg, IV slowly (can repeat every 5 min) to a maximum cumulative dose: 0.15-0.2 mg/kg For hypertension: 1-5 mg/kg PO q8h Cat: 0.025 mg/kg IV slowly (can repeat every 5 minutes) to a maximum cumulative dose of 0.15-0.2 mg/kg
Vinblastine	Velban	Vinca alkaloid/antineoplastic	1 mg/mL injection	2 mg/m^2 IV (slow infusion) q7-14 days
◆ Vincristine	Oncobin; Vincasar; generic	Vinca alkaloid/antineoplastic; also for the treatment of thrombocytopenia	1 mg/mL injection	Antitumor: 0.5-0.75 mg/m^2 IV q7-14 days (q7 days in cats, depending on protocol); for thrombocytopenia: 0.02 mg/kg IV, once weekly (alternatively, 0.5-0.7 mg/m^2 as an infusion over 4-6 h) each week

Continued

Note: Listings preceded by ◆ are for rapid reference and denote drug/dosage used in the emergency or critical care setting.

6

TABLE 6-26   Common Drug Indications and Dosages[†]—cont'd

Drug	Proprietary names	Action/Use	Formulation	Recommended dosage
Viokase	See Pancreatic Enzymes			
Vitamin A (retinoids)	Aquasol A	Vitamin/nutritional supplementation	Oral solution: 5000 U (1500 RE)/ 0.1-mL and 10,000-, 25,000-, and 50,000-U tablets	625-800 U/kg PO q24h
Vitamin B$_1$	Thiamine	Vitamin/nutritional supplementation	250 µg/5 mL elixir; tablets of various sizes from 5 mg to 500 mg; 100 and 500 mg/mL injection	Dog: 10-100 mg/dog/day PO Cat: 5-30 mg/cat/day PO (up to maximum dose of 50 mg/cat/day)
Vitamin B$_2$	Riboflavin	Vitamin/nutritional supplementation	Tablets of various sizes in increments of 10 to 250 mg	Dog: 10-20 mg/day PO Cat: 5-10 mg/day PO
Vitamin B$_{12}$	Cyanocobalamin	Vitamin/nutritional supplementation	100 µg/mL injection	Dog: 100-200 µg/day PO Cat: 50-100 µg/day PO
Vitamin C	Ascorbic acid	Vitamin/nutritional supplementation	Tablets of various sizes and injection	100-500 mg/day
Vitamin D analog	Dihydrotachysterol (DHT); Hytakerol	Vitamin/management of hypocalcemia associated with hypoparathyroidism or parathyroid gland surgery	0.125-mg tablet; 0.5 mg/mL oral liquid	0.01 mg/kg/day PO Acute treatment: 0.02 mg/kg initially; then 0.01-0.03 mg/kg PO q24-48h thereafter
Vitamin D$_2$	Ergocalciferol; Calciferol; Drisdol	Vitamin/management of hypocalcemia associated with hypoparathyroidism or parathyroid gland surgery	400-U tablet (OTC); 50,000-U tablet (1.25 mg); 500,000 U/mL (12.5 mg/mL) injection	4000 to 6000 U/kg/day PO (initial); 1000 to 2000 U/kg/day PO (maintenance)
Vitamin D$_3$ 1-25, dihydroxy vitamin D$_3$	Vitamin D analog (Dihydrotachysterol [DHT])	Vitamin also considered a hormone/management of hypocalcemia associated with hypoparathyroidism or parathyroid gland surgery; also used to supplement hypocalcemia of chronic renal failure	See Vitamin D analog (Dihydrotachysterol [DHT])	Hypocalcemia: 0.030-0.06 µg/kg PO once daily Chronic renal failure: 0.025 µg/kg, PO once daily

Drug	Brand/generic	Indications	How supplied	Dosage
Vitamin E (may be combined with selenium)	Alpha-tocopherol; Aquasol E; generic	Vitamin/nutritional supplementation and adjunctive therapy in patients with chronic liver disease; may be combined with selenium as adjunctive therapy for patients with immune-mediated skin disease in dogs; efficacy in management of arthritic dogs is questionable	Wide variety of capsules, tablets, oral solution available (e.g., 1,000 units per capsule)	See manufacturer's recommendations for treatment indications and dose
◆ Vitamin K_1	Phytonadione; phytomenadione; Aqua-MEPHYTON (injection); Mephyton (tablets); Veta-K_1 (capsules)	Antidote/anticoagulant rodenticide toxicosis and in any disorder impacting formation of vitamin K–dependent coagulation factors	2 and 10 mg/mL injection; 5-mg tablet (Mephyton); 25-mg capsule (Veta-K_1)	*Rodenticide toxicosis:* 2.5-5.0 mg/kg PO 3-4 weeks for diphacinone or chlorphacinone toxicosis. *Acute intoxication:* 5 mg/kg SQ in multiple locations with 25-gauge needle
Warfarin	Coumadin; generic	Anticoagulant/adjunctive treatment for and prevention of thromboemboli	1-, 2-, 2.5-, 4-, 5-, 7.5- and 10-mg tablets	Dog: 0.22 mg/kg PO q12h to prolong PT by 1.25 to 1.5 times normal. *Pulmonary thromboemboli:* 0.2 mg/kg PO daily to prolong PT by 1.5 to 2.5 times normal. Cat: *Chronic treatment:* 0.1-0.2 mg/kg PO once daily to prolong PT by 2 to 2.5 times normal. *Aortic embolus:* 0.06-0.1 mg/kg PO once daily

Continued

Note: Listings preceded by ◆ are for rapid reference and denote drug/dosage used in the emergency or critical care setting.

6

TABLE 6-26 Common Drug Indications and Dosages†—cont'd

Drug	Proprietary names	Action/Use	Formulation	Recommended dosage
◆ Xylazine	Rompun; generic	Alpha-2 adrenergic agonist/ sedative and analgesic (sometimes used as an emetic in cats)	20 and 100 mg/mL injection	Dog and cat: 1.1 mg/kg IV; or 1.1 to 2.2 mg/kg IM or SC Cat (to induce emesis): 0.4-0.5 mg/kg IV
◆ Yohimbine	Yobine	Alpha-2 adrenergic antagonist/ reverse xylazine (and possibly amitraz)	2 mg/mL injection in 20-mL vials	0.11 mg/kg IV slowly
Zidovudine (AZT)	Retrovir	Antiretroviral agent/adjunctive treatment of FeLV/FIV-positive cats	300-mg tablets; 100-mg capsules; 10 mg/mL syrup; 10 mg/mL injection	Cat: 5-15 mg/kg PO q12h; or 5 mg/kg PO q8h for 5 wk and then rest for 4 wk CAUTION: Significant bone marrow suppression (usually reversible with cessation of therapy) is expected; monitor CBC during therapy
Zolazepam	See Tiletamine-zolazepam combination			

*Listings preceded by an ◆ are for rapid reference and denote drug/dosage used in the emergency or critical care setting.

†NOTE: Doses listed in this table are based on best available evidence at the time of table preparation; although considerable effort has been made to verify all dosages listed, it is prudent to verify treatment protocols and drug dosages whenever using a product for the first time. Adverse effects may be possible from virtually any of the drugs listed in this table. High-risk warnings and precautionary statements are listed. Veterinarians using this table are encouraged to check current literature, product label, and the manufacturer's disclosure for information regarding reported changes in efficacy or safety as well as any new treatment contraindications not identified at the time of preparation of these tables. When dosage listed does NOT stipulate Dog or Cat, drug may be administered to both dogs and cats at the dosage listed.

Abbreviations: ACE, angiotensin-converting enzyme; ADH, antidiuretic hormone; CMI, cell-mediated immunity; CNS, central nervous system; CRI, constant-rate infusion; DIC, disseminated intravascular coagulation; FeLV, feline leukemia virus; FIV, feline immunodeficiency virus; GI, gastrointestinal; h, hour(s); IM, intramuscular; IP, intraperitoneal; IV, intravenous; kg, kilograms of body weight; m^2, square meters of body surface area (commonly used in cancer chemotherapy protocols); MCV, mean corpuscular volume; mg, milligram(s); min, minute(s); mo, month(s); MOA-B, monoamine B; µg, microgram(s); NSAID, nonsteroidal antiinflammatory drug; OTC, over-the-counter (prescription not required); PO, per os (oral administration); PT, prothrombin time; q12h, interval between treatment (e.g., every 12 hours); SC, subcutaneous; U, units; wk, week(s).

Index

A

A CRASH PLAN
  as examination mnemonic
    for high-rise syndrome, 158
    following initial ABCs, 4-5
    for pneumothorax, 258
Abbreviations
  metric system, 659t
ABCs;*See also* airways; breathing; circulation
  following anaphylactic shock, 94
  during basic life support, 114, 115f
  during emergency examination, 3-4
  following head injuries, 185-186
  following spinal cord injuries, 188-189
Abdomen
  acute conditions of, 81-85, 86t-92t, 93
    analgesic agents, 83t
    antibiotics, 84
    diagnostic tests, 84-85, 90t-92t, 93
    fluid resuscitation, 84
    immediate actions, 82
    listings of, 86t-92t
    oxygen supplementation, 84
    signalment and history, 81-82
    treatment of, 82-83
  auscultation, 314
  diagnostic procedures, 84-85, 90t-92t, 93
    biochemistry panels, 84-85, 90t-92t
    complete blood count, 84, 90t-92t
  distended
    with gastric dilatation-volvulus (GDV),
      165-166, 167f
  enlargement with ascites
    associated signs, 390
    definition of, 390
    differential diagnoses, 390, 391
  enlargement without ascites
    associated signs, 392
    definition of, 392
    differential diagnoses, 393
  evaluation of patient's, 298
  extended or painful
    as clinical sign of decompensation, 6b

Abdomen—cont'd
  initial examination of, 4
  neoplasms in, 205t, 207
  palpation of, 313-314
    during cardiovascular exam, 318
    to examine kidneys, 386
  penetrating injuries to
    and bowel perforation, 170-171
  percussion, 314
  signs of problems in, 81
Abdominal paracentesis
  in acute abdomen cases, 85, 90t-92t
  during initial emergency exam, 5
  technique of, 6-7
Abdominal radiographs
  for acute abdomen conditions, 85, 90t-92t
Abdominal ultrasound, 85, 90t-92t, 375
Abdominal wall
  clinical conditions of
    causing acute abdominal pain, 84-85,
      86t, 93
  palpation of, 313-314
Abdominocentesis
  in acute abdomen cases, 85, 90t-92t
  for cytologic evaluation of fluids, 207
  hemoabdomen, 205t, 207
  technique of, 6-7, 500
Abducent nerves, 365, 367t, 368f
Abnormal bowel motility
  definition of, 405
Abnormal gut permeability
  definition of, 405
Abnormal lung sounds
  with lower respiratory disease, 379
Abortion
  causes of, 375
  spontaneous, 140
Abrasions
  classification of soft tissue, 271, 272t
Abscesses
  abdominal wall, 86t
  hepatic, 87t
  nasopharyngeal polyps, 257

Page numbers followed by f indicate illustrations; those followed by t indicate tables; those followed by b indicate boxes.

Abscesses—cont'd
  pancreatic, 88t
  prostatic, 88t
  renal, 88t
  retrobulbar, 344
  sublumbar or retroperitoneal, 89t
Accessory nerves, 367, 368f, 369
Accidents;See also emergency care
  bandaging and splinting techniques, 8-12,
    13f-17f, 18-19, 20f, 21
  prehospital care, 2-3
ACE inhibitors;See angiotensin-converting
    enzyme (ACE) inhibitors
Acepromazine
  uses, formulation, and dosage of, 685t
Acetaminophen
  dosage for pain, 75t
  toxicity and treatment of, 224
  uses, formulation, and dosage of, 685t
Acetate tape
  preparation procedure, 482-483
  to test dermatologic disorders, 338
Acetazolamide
  uses, formulation, and dosage of, 685t
Acetylcysteine, 685t
Acetylsalicylic acid
  toxicity and treatment of, 227
Acid-base balance
  in acute uncompensated disturbances, 37t
  and cardiac arrest, 113-114
  checking in shock "Rule of Twenty," 282
  effect on respiratory system, 36, 37t
  and fluid therapy, 35-37
  normal arterial blood gas analysis ranges
    for adult canines and felines, 578t
  normal urinalysis ranges
    for adult canines and felines, 578t
  renal and respiratory responses to, 37t
Acidosis
  and cardiopulmonary cerebral resuscitation
    (CPCR), 120
Acids
  and diabetic ketoacidosis, 178-179, 180t
  toxicity and treatment of, 224
ACTH gel
  uses, formulation, and dosage of, 685t
ACTH stimulation test
  normal test values and interpretation, 617
Actinomycin D
  myelosuppression classification of, 210t
Activated charcoal
  with cathartic for poisons and toxins, 220
  uses, formulation, and dosage of, 685t
Activated clotting time (ACT)
  and blood component dosages, 29t
  with disseminated intravascular coagulation
    (DIC), 102-103
  initial screening test, 607-608
  laboratory results for coagulation profiles, 107t
  normal hemostasis ranges
    for adult canines and felines, 578t

Activated clotting time (ACT)—cont'd
  normal values and testing protocols, 610
  testing during initial emergency care, 5
Activated partial thromboplastin time (APTT)
  and blood component dosages, 29t
  checking in shock "Rule of Twenty," 282
  with disseminated intravascular coagulation
    (DIC), 102-103
  laboratory results for coagulation
    profiles, 107t
  normal hemostasis ranges
    for adult canines and felines, 578t
  normal values and testing protocols, 610
  testing during initial emergency care, 5
Acute abdominal pain
  conditions that cause, 86t-89t
Acute adrenocortical insufficiency
  breed predisposition to, 184b
  features of, 183
  therapy for, 184
Acute diarrhea
  definition of, 405
Acute gastritis
  antiemetic drugs and dosages, 172t
  causes of, 172b
  clinical signs of, 171-172
Acute hemoabdomen, 205t, 207
Acute hemolytic anemia
  causing acute hepatic failure, 175b
Acute hepatic failure
  causes of, 175b
  clinical signs of, 174-175
Acute infectious keratitis
  description and treatment of, 200
Acute metritis, 138
Acute necrotizing pancreatitis, 173
Acute pain;See also analgesia
  abdominal
    conditions that cause, 86t-89t
  definition of, 70
  management during emergencies, 73
  nonsteroidal antiinflammatory drugs
    (NSAIDS) for, 75-76
Acute prostatitis, 143-144
Acute renal failure
  causing decompensation, 6b
  description and treatment of, 288-289
  differential diagnosis, 405b
  and hypertension, 176
Acute respiratory acidosis
  renal and respiratory responses to, 37t
Acute respiratory alkalosis
  renal and respiratory responses to, 37t
Acute respiratory distress syndrome (ARDS)
  and cardiac arrest, 113-114
  causing decompensation, 6b
  description and treatment of, 267-268
Acute scrotal dermatitis, 142
Acute tumor lysis syndrome
  clinical signs and treatment of, 206t
  tumor types, 206t

Addison's disease
   causing acute diarrhea, 406b
Adenocarcinomas
   found in female reproductive tract,
      374-375
   gastrointestinal tract, 209-210
   in gastrointestinal tract, 170
   in various paraneoplastic syndromes,
      205t-206t
Adenovirus
   vaccinations
      for dogs, 661t
Administration rates
   with fluid therapy, 47
Administration routes
   implanted subcutaneous fluid
         ports, 459
   by injections, 457
   intradermal injections, 459
   intramuscular injections, 459
   intraosseous injections, 461-462
   intravenous injections, 460-461
   oral liquids, 453-456
   pills for dogs, 449-450, 451f
   pills for cats, 450-451, 452f, 453
   by subcutaneous injections, 458-459
   topical, 456-458
   transdermal injections, 459-460
Adnexa
   examination of, 341-342
Adrenergic blockers
   for systemic hypertension, 177t
Adrenocorticotropic hormones (ACTH)
   causing anaphylactic reactions, 94b
   normal test values and interpretation, 616
Adsorption
   preventing poison, 216-221
Advanced life support
   description of, 114, 116-117
   drugs used in, 120t
   flow chart illustrating, 116f
Aerosol therapy
   and nebulizers, 568-569, 570f, 571
Aflatoxin
   toxicity and treatment of, 224
Afterload
   calculating with shock, 275-276
   checking in shock "Rule of Twenty,"
      279-280, 281t
Agar gel immunodiffusion test, 631
Ages
   and musculoskeletal system disorders,
      351, 352t-353t, 354-356
   pain reactions with different, 71
Aggression
   definition and associated signs, 392
   differential diagnoses, 394b
Agonists, 74, 75t, 80
   used for analgesia and sedation
      in epidurals, 80
      properties of, 74, 75t

Airways;*See* ABCs
   evaluation of
      during emergency exams, 3
Alanine aminotransferase (ALT)
   normal biochemistry ranges
      for adult canines and felines, 577t
   normal test ranges and interpretation, 591
Albendazole
   uses, formulation, and dosage of, 685t
Albumin
   checking in shock "Rule of Twenty," 280-281
   normal biochemistry ranges
      for adult canines and felines, 577t
   normal test ranges and interpretation, 591
Albumin/globulin ratio (A:G)
   normal test ranges and interpretation, 591
Albuterol
   for feline bronchitis, 266t
   uses, formulation, and dosage of, 685t
Alcohol
   toxicity and treatment of, 224-225
Aldosterone
   normal test values and interpretation,
      617-618
Alimentary system
   dental examination, 304-306, 307f, 308-309
   evaluation and examination of, 304-306,
      307f, 308-310, 311f, 312-315
Alkaline phosphatase
   normal biochemistry ranges
      for adult canines and felines, 577t
   normal test ranges and interpretation,
      591-592
Alkalis/caustics
   toxicity and treatment of, 225
Allergens
   causing anaphylactic reactions, 94b
Allergen-specific IgE antibody tests
   normal test values and interpretation,
      626-627
   to test dermatologic disorders, 338-339
Allergies
   to chemotherapy, 211
Allopurinol
   uses, formulation, and dosage of, 685t
Alopecia;*See also* hair, loss of
   associated signs, 414
   definition of, 414
   differential diagnosis, 414-415, 415b
Alpha-adrenergic blockers
   for systemic hypertension, 177t
Alpha$_2$-agonists, 74, 75t, 80
Aluminum carbonate gel
   uses, formulation, and dosage of, 686t
Aluminum hydroxide gel
   uses, formulation, and dosage of, 686t
Alveolar hypoventilation
   cause and response to oxygen, 48t
Amantadine
   description of, 77
   properties of, 78t

American Kennel Club (AKC)
dog breeds, 645t-646t
American Society for the Prevention of Cruelty
to Animals (ASPCA)
Animal Poison Control Center, 212, 213b
Amikacin, 686t
Aminophylline
for feline bronchitis, 266t
uses, formulation, and dosage of, 686t
Amitraz
toxicity and treatment of, 225
uses, formulation, and dosage of, 686t
Amitriptyline, 686t
Amlodipine
for systemic hypertension, 177t
uses, formulation, and dosage of, 686t
Ammonia
normal test ranges and protocols, 596-597
toxicity and treatment of, 225-226
Ammonia tolerance
normal test ranges and protocols, 597
Ammonium chloride
to promote urine acidification, 222
uses, formulation, and dosage of, 687t
Amoxicillin clavulanate, 687t
Amoxicillin trihydrate
uses, formulation, and dosage of, 687t
Amphetamines
toxicity and treatment of, 226
Amphotericin B
uses, formulation, and dosage of, 687t
Ampicillin
uses, formulation, and dosage of, 687t
Ampicillin trihydrate, 687t
Amprolium, 687t
Amylase
normal biochemistry ranges
for adult canines and felines, 577t
normal test ranges and interpretation, 592
Anaerobic cultures
of blood, 471
Anal sac
evaluation of patient's, 301
examination of, 314-315
Analgesia
for acute abdomen pain, 83t
agonists used for
properties of, 75t
and anxiolytic agents
contraindicated in abdomen cases, 83t
definition of, 70
drugs
adjunctive, 77, 78t
anxiolytics, 78t
major, 73-77
minor, 77
sedatives, 78t
epidurals, 80
for fractures, 155-156
major, 73-77
minor, 77

Analgesia—cont'd
monitoring in shock "Rule of Twenty," 284
never withholding for pain, 71
nonsteroidal antiinflammatory drugs, 75-77
opioids, 73-74
for poisonings, 223
for spinal cord injuries, 188-189
Analytes
or test names, 590-596
Anaphylactic shock
allergens causing, 94b
to chemotherapy, 211
clinical signs of, 94-95
immediate treatment of, 94b
Anaphylactoid shock, 94-95
Anaplasma phagocytophila antibody
normal test values and interpretation, 628
Ancillary diagnostic evaluations
during initial examinations, 5
Anemia
clinical signs and treatment of, 205t
tumor types, 205t
Anemic murmur, 326t
Anesthesia
administration methods, 78-81
and cardiac arrest, 113-114
causes and treatment of arousal during, 99t
complications and emergencies, 96-100
definition of, 70
epidural, 80
infusion of local, 61f
local and regional techniques for
emergency, 78-81
postanesthetic complications, 100
Anesthetics;*See* anesthesia
Anestrus, 383, 384
"Angel dust"
toxicity and treatment of, 246
Angioneurotic edema
immediate action for, 95
immune response suppression agents, 95b
Angiotensin-converting enzyme (ACE) inhibitors
for congestive heart failure, 128b
for systemic hypertension, 177t
Animal Blood Bank HOTLINE, 644t
Animal Poison Control Center
of American Society for the Prevention
of Cruelty to Animals (ASPCA),
212, 213b
Animals;*See also* patient assessments; patient
evaluation
immature
fractures in, 158
prehospital care of injured, 2-3
Anion gap
definition of, 42
increased and decreased, 42b
normal biochemistry ranges
for adult canines and felines, 577t
normal test ranges and interpretation, 592
normochloremic and hyperchloremic, 36b

Anionic detergents
　toxicity and treatment of, 233-234
Anisocoria
　assessment of
　　during initial emergency exam, 5
　initial examination of, 4
Anorectal diseases, 314-315
Anorexia
　with abdominal conditions, 86t-89t
　associated signs, 422-423
　definition of, 422
　differential diagnosis, 423
Antagonists, 73-74
　contraindicated in abdomen
　　cases, 83t
Anterior chamber
　examination of eye, 346-347
Antiarrhythmic drugs
　therapy, 124t, 125
　to treat shock
　　and ventricular tachycardia, 281t
Antibiotics
　checking in shock "Rule of Twenty," 283
Anti-dandruff shampoos
　toxicity and treatment of, 248
Antidotes
　for poisons, 221-222
Antiemetic drugs
　for acute gastritis, 172t
　for poisonings, 223
Antifreeze
　toxicity and treatment of, 235-236
Antigenicity
　in dogs and cats, 22-23
Antihistamines
　causing anaphylactic reactions, 94b
　toxicity and treatment of, 226
Anti-mite products
　toxicity of, 225
Antinuclear antibody (ANA)
　normal ranges and protocols, 597-598
　testing
　　normal values and interpretation, 627
　　in orthopedic examinations, 356,
　　　357t-358t
Antiplatelet antibody
　normal test values and interpretation, 627
Antiprostaglandins
　contraindicated in abdomen cases, 83t
　during shock therapy, 284-285
Antiserum (snakebite)
　uses, formulation, and dosage of, 688t
Antithrombin
　and disseminated intravascular coagulation
　　(DIC), 101-103
Anti-tick products
　toxicity of, 225
Antitoxins
　causing anaphylactic reactions, 94b
ANTU (α-naphthylthiourea)
　toxicity and treatment of, 226-227

Anuria
　associated signs, 404
　definition of, 404
　differential diagnosis, 305b, 404
Anus
　evaluation of patient's, 301
　examination of, 314-315
　foreign bodies in, 165
　gastrointestinal system emergencies, 165
Anxiolytic agents
　contraindicated in abdomen cases, 83t
　types and properties of, 78t
Aortic bifurcation, 285-286
Aortic valve
　auscultation of, 320
　heart murmurs, 323f, 326t
　radiograph illustrating, 321f
Apex
　definition and illustration of dental, 305, 306f
Apex heartbeat
　and cardiac arrest, 114
Apical delta
　definition and illustration of dental, 305, 306f
Apocrine gland adenocarcinoma
　in paraneoplastic syndromes, 206t, 207
Apomorphine hydrochloride
　as poison emetic, 219t
　uses, formulation, and dosage of, 688t
Appetite
　loss of
　　associated signs, 422-423
　　definition of, 422
　　differential diagnosis, 423
Arizona brown spiders, 152-153
Aromatic hydrocarbons
　toxicity and treatment of, 238
Arsenic
　toxicity and treatment of, 227
Arterial blood gases
　analysis
　　normal ranges for adult canines and
　　　felines, 578t
　　technique of, 508-509
　normal test ranges and protocols, 598
　samples
　　and acid-base status, 36-37
　testing during initial emergency care, 5
Arterial oxygen content (CaO_2), 49
　calculating with shock, 275-276
Arterial pressure of oxygen
　and shock, 275-276
Arterial pulse
　assessment of, 319
Arterial thromboembolism
　in cats with CHF, 130
Arteries
　initial examination of, 5
Arteriovenous shunts
　cause and response to oxygen, 48t
Arthrocentesis
　with joint fluid analysis, 356, 357t-358t

Arthrodesis, 157, 158b
Arthropathy
associated signs, 420-421
definition of, 420
differential diagnosis, 421-422
Arthroscopy
in orthopedic examinations, 356, 357t-358t
Articular cartilage
injuries to, 157
Articular fractures, 154b, 155-158
Artificial insemination, 553
Ascending tracts
within sensing and response system, 70
Ascites
with heart disease, 331b
palpation for, 318
Ascorbic acid
uses, formulation, and dosage of, 688t
Aseptic diseases
and joint fluid analysis, 357t-358t
Aspartate aminotransferase
normal test ranges and interpretation, 592
ASPCA;See American Society for the
Prevention of Cruelty to Animals
Aspergillus antibody titer, 628-629
Aspiration pneumonia
description and treatment of, 267
Aspirin
dosage for pain, 75t
toxicity and treatment of, 227
uses, formulation, and dosage of, 688t
Assessments;See patient assessments
Asthma
assessing during initial emergency exam, 3-4
feline
description and treatment of, 265-266
drugs to treat, 266t
Asthma inhalers/medications
toxicity and treatment of, 228
Asystole
and cardiac arrest, 114
definition of, 117
Ataxia
associated signs, 416
definition of, 415
differential diagnosis, 416b, 417
and spinal cord, 360f
Atelectasis
and oxygen therapy, 48t
turning patient to prevent, 194-195
Atenolol
for systemic hypertension, 177t
uses, formulation, and dosage of, 688t
for ventricular dysrhythmias
in dogs, 124t
Atomoxetine
toxicity and treatment of, 249
Atopy
skin lesion signs of, 338t
Atracurium
uses, formulation, and dosage of, 688t

Atrial cardiomyopathy, 126
Atrial dysrhythmias
treating during shock, 279-280, 281t
Atrial fibrillation
with cardiomyopathies, 127-128
description and ECG illustrating, 123
Atrial standstill, 125, 126f
Atrioventricular block
third-degree, 126, 127f
Atropine
with asystole, 117
used during advanced life support, 120t
uses, formulation, and dosage of, 689t
Auditory canal
examination of, 347-350
Aural hematomas, 134-135
Auranofin, 689t
Aurothioglucose, 689t
Auscultation
thoracic, 380
Avulsions
classification of soft tissue, 271, 272t
Azathioprine
uses, formulation, and dosage of, 689t
Azithromycin, 689t
Azostick
testing during initial emergency care, 5
Azotemia
during coma, 193
description and treatment of, 287
postrenal, 289
prerenal, 287
and prerenal dehydration, 84
with uroabdomen, 290

B
Back
evaluation of patient's, 298
herniated disks
and back trauma, 189
corticosteroid dosage for, 190b
examination and prognosis of, 189
localizing signs of, 190t
treatment and management of, 189-190
Back trauma
corticosteroid dosage for, 190b
examination and prognosis of, 189
herniated disks, 189
localizing signs of, 190t
treatment and management of, 189-190
Baclofen
toxicity and treatment of, 227-228
Bacteria
normal urinalysis ranges
for adult canines and felines, 578t
Bacterial cultures
common results, 466t
types of, 466t, 467-470
Bacterial infections
causing acute diarrhea, 406b
causing acute gastritis, 171-172

Bacterial infections—cont'd
  blood culture, 630
  types of
    and skin manifestations of, 339t
BAL
  uses, formulation, and dosage of, 689t
Ballottements, 314, 318, 392
Bandaging
  at accident scene, 2-3
  of closed wounds, 9-10
  functions of, 8b
  materials and methods of, 8-12, 13f-17f
  obliteration of dead space, 11
  of open contaminated/infected
      wounds, 8
  of open musculoskeletal injuries,
      155-157
  of open wounds
    with drainage, 10
    in repair stage of healing, 9
  during shock "Rule of Twenty," 284
  and splinting techniques, 8-21
  wet-to-dry, 8
  of wounds in need of pressure, 10-11
  of wounds in need of pressure relief, 11-12
  of wounds needing immobilization, 12
Bar soaps
  toxicity and treatment of, 248-249
Barbecue lighter fluids
  toxicity and treatment of, 237-238
Barbiturates
  toxicity and treatment of, 228
Barden's sign, 355-356
Barlow's sign, 355-356
Bartonella antibody titer, 628-629
Basic life support
  flowchart illustrating, 115f
Basophils
  normal hematology ranges
    for adult canines and felines, 577t
Basset Hounds
  with breed predisposition
    to acute adrenocortical insufficiency, 184b
Bath soaps
  toxicity and treatment of, 248-249
Bats
  rabies control in, 678t
Batteries
  toxicity and treatment of, 228
Bearded Collie
  with breed predisposition
    to acute adrenocortical insufficiency, 184b
Beclomethasone
  for feline bronchitis, 266t
"BEETTS" test
  (*See* behavior, eyes, ears, teeth, toes, and
      skin), 293-295
  as acronym for pet evaluations, 293-295
Behaviors
  abnormal
    as sign of pain, 72b

Behaviors—cont'd
  aggression
    definition and associated signs, 392
    differential diagnoses, 394b
  assessment of
    during initial emergency exam, 5
  breeding and physiology
    evaluation and examination of, 382-384
  characteristics and parameters of, 359
  confusion or mentation
    as clinical sign of decompensation, 6b
  evaluation during patient exam, 296
  part of "BEETTS" test, 294
  signs of acute pain, 71-72
Benazepril
  for systemic hypertension, 177t
  uses, formulation, and dosage of, 689t
Benzocaine
  causing anaphylactic reactions, 94b
Benzoyl peroxide
  toxicity and treatment of, 228-229
Beta-adrenergic agonists
  toxicity and treatment of, 228
Beta-blockers, 204t
Betamethasone
  uses, formulation, and dosage of, 690t
Bethanechol, 690t
Bicarbonate (HCO_3)
  concentration and fluid therapy, 38
  normal arterial blood gas analysis ranges
    for adult canines and felines, 578t
  normal biochemistry ranges
    for adult canines and felines, 577t
  normal test ranges and interpretation, 592
Biceps and triceps reflexes, 363
Bicipital luxation
  size and breed disposition to, 352t
Bicipital tenosynovitis
  size and breed disposition to, 352t
Bilateral cerebral edema, 187
Bile peritonitis
  abdominal characteristics of, 87t
Biliary obstruction
  abdominal characteristics of, 87t
Biliary rupture
  abdominal characteristics of, 87t
Bilirubin
  normal biochemistry ranges
    for adult canines and felines, 577t
  normal test ranges and interpretation, 592-593
  normal urinalysis ranges
    for adult canines and felines, 578t
Biochemistry
  analytes
    examples of interference on, 477t
  component of laboratory data, 300t
  levels
    with acute hepatic failure, 175
  normal ranges for adult dogs and cats, 577t
  testing
    routine, 476, 477t

Biopsy techniques
  bone biopsy, 506-507
  instruments for, 505f
  liver biopsy, 503-504
  nasal biopsy, 504
  needle biopsy, 501-502
  prostate biopsy, 506
  renal biopsy, 506
  skin biopsy, 503
Biopsy tissue
  histopathology guidelines, 584-585
Bisacodyl
  uses, formulation, and dosage of, 690t
Bismuth subsalicylate
  toxicity and treatment of (*See* aspirin), 227
  uses, formulation, and dosage of, 690t
Bite wounds
  on ears, 134-135
Black widow spiders
  causing acute abdominal pain, 89t
  bites, 152
Bladder;*See also* urinary bladder
  catheterization of, 483-487, 488f
  lesions
    affecting urinary tract, 208-209
    upper and lower neuron, 371t, 372
    and urinary incontinence, 372-373
Blastomycosis antibody titer, 629-630
Bleach
  toxicity and treatment of, 229
Bleeding
  assessing at accident scene, 2-3
  blood component therapy, 21-33
  due to oncologic emergencies, 205-211
  gastrointestinal
    as clinical sign of decompensation, 6b
  in need of pressure bandages, 10
Bleeding disorders
  causes of defective, 100b
  diagnosing, 100-101
  types of, 101-107
Bleomycin
  uses, formulation, and dosage of, 690t
Blindness
  causes of, 440-441, 442b
  definition of, 440
  diagnostic plan, 441
  following head injuries, 187
Blink reflexes, 365
Blockages
  anesthesia, 78-81
Blood
  anaerobic cultures, 471
  in catheter hub, 62, 66, 66f
  collection and handling of, 24
  collection techniques, 474-475
  cultures, 470, 471b
  donors programs, 23-24
  in the eyes, 201-202
  flow and heart murmurs,
    321-325, 326t

Blood—cont'd
  International system of units (SI)
    conversion tables, 656t-658t
  list of banks, 23t
  normal pH, 35
  normal urinalysis ranges
    for adult canines and felines, 578t
  preparation of, 25
  screening of, 23-24
  separation of, 21-33
  serum values for pocket pets, 651t
  spontaneous bleeding
    associated signs, 430, 432
    definition of, 429-430
    differential diagnosis, 432, 433b
  storage of, 26t
  taking samples for lab tests, 576, 577t-580t
  testing with EDTA, 475-476
  transfusion reactions, 31-32
  in urine
    associated signs, 394-395
    causes of, 396t
    definition of, 393-394
    differential diagnosis, 395
Blood banks
  hotlines, 644t
  list of animal, 23t
Blood component products
  indications for administering, 28t, 29
  storage of, 26t
  transfusion of, 29-32
Blood component therapy, 21-33
  antigenicity, 22-23
  approach to, 22b
  blood banks, 23t
  blood donor programs, 23-24
  blood types and antigenicity, 22-23
  for cats, 31-32
  collection and administration, 21-22
  cross match procedures, 25-26, 27b
  for dogs, 30-32
  with fresh frozen plasma, 26t, 28t, 29t, 30
  handling and storing, 24-25, 26t
  hemoglobin-based oxygen carriers
    (HBOCs), 32-33
  with plasma cryoprecipitate, 26t, 28t, 29t, 30
  with platelet-rich plasma, 26t, 28t, 29t, 30
  red blood cells, 26t, 28t, 29-30
  and transfusion therapy, 26-33
Blood cultures
  bacterial infection, 630
Blood donors
  programs, 23-24
Blood glucose
  levels and insulin infusion, 180t
  levels and seizures, 193, 194
  parameter in joint fluid analysis, 358t
Blood pressure
  assessing during initial emergency exam, 4
  and cardiopulmonary cerebral resuscitation
    (CPCR), 120

Blood pressure—cont'd
checking in shock "Rule of Twenty," 278-279
elevations of, 176-177
measurement and renal insufficiency, 386
monitoring of
during ancillary diagnostic evaluation, 5
normal measurements
in cats and dogs, 176t
normal parameters of, 97t
Blood transfusions;See transfusions
Blood types
in dogs and cats, 22-23
Blood typing for complete dog erythrocyte
antigen (DEA)
normal values and testing protocols, 611
Blood urea nitrogen (BUN)
for abdomen condition diagnosis, 84-85
normal biochemistry ranges
for adult canines and felines, 577t
normal test ranges and interpretation, 593
and osmolality, 38-39, 41
testing during initial emergency care, 5
Blunt trauma
characteristics of abdominal wall, 86t
to eyes, 201
Boas, 149
Body condition
assessing during cardiovascular exam, 316
evaluation during patient exam, 296-297
Body condition score (BCS), 297, 298f
Body fluids
for chemistry analysis, 599
lab samples of, 588
tests, 588
Body mass
energy and fluid requirements according
to, 44t
Body temperature
increased or decreased
as clinical sign of decompensation, 6b
Body weight
of cats
conversion table, 654t
of dogs
conversion table, 654t
Bone biopsy
technique of, 506-507
Bone marrow
aspiration
canine, 477-478, 479f, 480
feline, 479f, 480
cytologic examination of, 589
toxicity, 210
Bones
open wounds to, 156-167
orthopedic diseases affecting, 352-353t,
354-356
remodeling, 158
Bony prominences
doughnut-shaped bandages for,
12, 15f

Borate
toxicity and treatment of, 229
Bordetella bronchiseptica
vaccinations
for cats, 661t
Boric acid
toxicity and treatment of, 229
Borrelia burgdorferi test, 630, 637-639
in orthopedic examinations, 356,
357t-358t
Botulism
toxicity and treatment of, 229-230
Bowel obstruction
causing acute diarrhea, 406b
Bowels
abnormal gut permeability
definition of, 405
acute diarrhea, 405-406
characteristics of compromised, 87t
chronic diarrhea, 407-409
obstipation, 169-170
obstruction of
signs of, 162t, 163-164
with tumors, 170
perforation of, 170-171
ruptured
causing decompensation, 6b
Brachial plexus
blockades, 79-80
injuries to, 191
Brachycephalic airway syndrome
description and immediate management
of, 256
Brachygnathism, 306, 308
Bradyarrhythmias
treatment of, 125
Bradycardia
and cardiac arrest, 114
causes and treatment of, 97t
as clinical sign of decompensation, 6b
definition of, 97
treating during shock, 279-280, 281t
Bradycardia-tachycardia syndrome,
126-127
Brain
and cardiopulmonary cerebral resuscitation
(CPCR), 120
lesions in, 370
Brainstem
early signs of hemorrhage in, 187
herniation
causing decompensation, 6b
reflexes
and coma scale, 192t
severe damage with head injuries, 187
Breath sounds
abnormal
with congestive heart failure, 128
characterization of, 380, 382
classification of normal and abnormal, 317t
normal, 380

Breathing;*See also* ABCs
    assessing at accident scene, 2-3
    assessing during cardiovascular exam, 316
    difficulty
        associated signs, 409-410
        definition of, 409
        differential diagnosis, 410
    evaluation of
        during emergency exams, 3
    with lower respiratory disease, 377-380,
        381f, 382
    noisy
        with lower respiratory disease, 379
    with upper respiratory disease, 376-377
Breeding
    behavior and physiology
        evaluation and examination of, 382-384
    disorders associated with, 374
    normal behavior and physiology, 382-382
Breeds
    of cats
        list of, 645t-646t
    of dogs
        list of, 645t-646t
    pain reactions with different, 71
    predisposed to orthopedic problems,
        352t-353t
Bretylium tosylate
    used during advanced life support, 120t
Bromethalin
    toxicity and treatment of, 230
Bromide
    uses, formulation, and dosage of, 690t
Bromocriptine mesylate, 690t
Bronchial sounds
    description of normal, 317t
Bronchitis
    assessing during initial emergency exam, 3-4
    feline, 265-266
Bronchodilators
    types of
        for feline bronchitis, 266t
Bronchovesicular sounds
    description of normal, 317t
Brown recluse spiders
    causing acute abdominal pain, 89t
    bites of, 152-153
Brown spider bites, 152-153
Brushings
    techniques of, 587-588
Buccal mucosal bleeding time (BMBT)
    initial screening test, 608
    laboratory results for coagulation
        profiles, 107t
    normal values and testing protocols, 611
Bull snakes, 149
Bullous eruption, 421b
Bull's eye lesions
    with brown spider bites, 152
Bunamidine hydrochloride
    uses, formulation, and dosage of, 690t

Bupivacaine
    epidural anesthesia, 80t
    uses, formulation, and dosage of, 690t
Buprenorphine
    for abdominal pain, 83t
    properties of
        for pain management, 74t
    uses, formulation, and dosage of, 690t
Burns
    assessing at accident scene, 2-3
    chemical, 111-112
    electrical, 110-111
    radiation, 112
    and smoke inhalation, 269
    thermal, 108-110
Buspirone
    uses, formulation, and dosage of, 691t
Busulfan, 691t
Butorphanol
    for abdominal pain, 83t
    properties of
        for pain management, 74t
    uses, formulation, and dosage of, 691t

C

Cachexia
    associated signs, 445
    definition of, 445
    differential diagnosis, 445, 446f
Caffeine
    toxicity and treatment of, 230
Cage rest
    for congestive heart failure (CHF), 128b
Calcified fetal skeletons, 376
Calcitonin therapy, 182t, 183
Calcitriol, 182t
    uses, formulation, and dosage of, 691t
Calcium
    hypercalcemia, 181, 183
    normal biochemistry ranges
        for adult canines and felines, 577t
    normal test ranges and
        interpretation, 593
    types of supplements, 182t
Calcium carbonate
    dosage of
        for hypocalcemia, 182t
    uses, formulation, and dosage of, 691t
Calcium channel blockers
    for systemic hypertension, 177t
Calcium chloride
    dosage of
        for hypocalcemia, 182t
    uses, formulation, and dosage of, 691t
Calcium citrate, 691t
Calcium gluconate
    dosage of
        for hypocalcemia, 182t
    uses, formulation, and dosage of, 691t
Calcium (ionized)
    normal test ranges and protocols, 599

Calcium lactate, 182t
 uses, formulation, and dosage of, 691t
Calicivirus
 vaccinations
  for cats, 661t
Canine caval syndrome
 clinical signs of, 130
 treatment of, 130-131
Canine dental chart, 307f
Canine distemper antibody test, 631
Canine thyrotropin
 normal test values and interpretation, 626
Cannabis sativa
 toxicity and treatment of, 241
Capillary refill time (CRT)
 assessment of, 319
 prolonged
  as clinical sign of decompensation, 6b
Capnometry, 52
Captopril
 to induce vasodilation, 280t
 uses, formulation, and dosage of, 692t
Carbamates
 toxicity and treatment of, 230-231
Carbenicillin
 uses, formulation, and dosage of, 692t
Carbenicillin indanyl sodium
 uses, formulation, and dosage of, 692t
Carbon tetrachloride
 toxicity and treatment of, 231
Carbonic anhydrase inhibitors
 for acute glaucoma, 204t
Carboplatin, 692t
Carcinomas
 found in female reproductive tract, 374-375
Carcinomatosis, 205t-206t, 207-208
Cardiac afterload
 calculating with shock, 275-276
 checking in shock "Rule of Twenty,"
  279-280, 281t
Cardiac arrest
 asystole, 117
 basic *versus* advanced life support, 114,
  115f, 116f
 and cardiopulmonary cerebral resuscitation
  (CPCR), 113-114, 115f, 116f
 causes of, 113-114
 signs of, 114
Cardiac auscultation
 abnormal pulses, 319b
 heart murmurs, 321-322
 normal heart rate and rhythm, 320
 normal heart sounds, 320
 stethoscope, 319-320
 transient heart sounds, 321
Cardiac contractility
 calculating with shock, 275-276
 with congestive heart failure, 129-130
Cardiac dysrhythmias
 as clinical sign of decompensation, 6b
 clinical signs of, 98-99

Cardiac dysrhythmias—cont'd
 causing decompensation, 6b
 prevention of preanesthetic, 99b
 treating during shock, 279-280, 281t
 types of
  requiring emergency management, 121,
   122f, 123-127
  supraventricular dysrhythmias, 123-125
  ventricular dysrhythmias, 121, 122f,
   123-125
Cardiac emergencies;*See also* specific
  conditions
 cardiopulmonary cerebral resuscitation
  (CPCR)
  basic *versus* advanced, 114, 115f, 116f, 117
  crash cart supplies, 113b
  goal of, 113-114
 with thoracic trauma
  description and immediate management
   of, 264
Cardiac output
 calculating with shock, 275-276
 checking in shock "Rule of Twenty," 281t,
  279, 280
 as function of heart rate and stroke
  volume, 131
 and oxygen therapy, 48t
Cardiac system
 assessing at accident scene, 2-3
 emergencies (*See* cardiac emergencies)
Cardiogenic shock
 definition and treatment of, 277
 heart characteristics during, 279, 280, 281t
Cardiomegaly
 differential diagnoses of, 331t
 vertebral heart sum to determine, 129b
Cardiomyopathies
 systemic thromboembolism, 285-286
Cardiopulmonary arrest
 basic *versus* advanced life support, 114,
  115f, 116f
 and cardiopulmonary cerebral resuscitation
  (CPCR), 113-114, 115f, 116f
 causes of, 113-114
 signs of, 114
Cardiopulmonary cerebral resuscitation
  (CPCR)
 flowchart illustrating
  during life support, 115f, 116f
 open-chest
  indications for, 119b
  management following, 119-120
Cardiopulmonary resuscitation (CPR)
 at accident scene, 2-3
Cardiovascular system
 ancillary radiographic signs of
  disease, 331b
 complications with anesthesia, 96-97
 in emergency poison/toxin cases, 215b
 evaluation and examination of, 315-325,
  326t, 327f-328f, 329-332

Cardiovascular system—cont'd
  examination of, 315-316, 317tb, 318-325,
      326t, 327f, 328f, 329-332
  examination questions, 315-316
  radiographs of, 327, 328f, 329-330
Carprofen
  dosage for pain, 75t
  toxicity and treatment of, 243
  uses, formulation, and dosage of, 692t
Carpus
  fractures of, 19, 21
  injuries to, 190-191
Cascara sagrada
  uses, formulation, and dosage of, 692t
Castor oil
  uses, formulation, and dosage of, 692t
Castration-responsive dermatosis
  skin lesions or signs of, 338t
Cat breeds
  Cat Fanciers' Association (CFA)
      recognized, 647t
Cat Fanciers' Association (CFA)
  championship and miscellaneous
      classes, 647t
Catabolic states, 70
Cathartics
  list of, 220t
  for poisons, 220
Catheter hubs
  blood in, 62, 66, 66f
Catheterization
  of female cat, 487, 488f
  of female dog, 485, 486f
  of male cat, 487
  of male dog, 484
Catheters
  anesthesia for inserting, 79
  indwelling urethral, 487
  intravenous
      types and sizes of, 58-69
  maintenance of indwelling arterial and
      venous, 68-69
  sizes of
      for dogs and cats, 54t, 483, 484t
      for vascular access, 58t
  techniques for inserting, 483-487
  in vessel, 62, 64f, 65f
Cationic detergents
  toxicity and treatment of, 233-234
Cats
  abdominal analgesics for, 83t
  blood component therapy for, 31-32
  blood types and antigenicity of, 22-23
  breeds
      list of, 645t-646t
  categories of pain in, 70b
  catheter sizes for, 54t, 484t
  conversion table
      of body weight to body surface area, 654t
  heart rate and blood pressure
      normal parameters, 97t

Cats—cont'd
  high-rise syndrome in, 158
  minimum laboratory database for, 300t
  nonsteroidal antiinflammatory drugs for,
      76-77
  pain assessment in, 71
  paraneoplastic syndromes in, 205t-206t
  rabies control in, 675t
  rabies testing, 582-584
  signs of chronic pain in, 72-73
  transfusion guidelines in, 31
  vaccination risks for, 660t
  vaccination types for, 662t
  vaccinations
      annualized protocol, 663t-673t
Caudal leg muscles, 190-191
Caudal splints
  procedures for, 19, 21
Caval syndrome
  clinical signs of, 130
  treatment of, 130-131
Cavities
  examination for, 309-310, 311f, 312-313
Cecal inversion
  abdominal
      characteristics of, 87t
Cefaclor
  uses, formulation, and dosage of, 692t
Cefadroxil, 692t
Cefepime, 692t
Cefixime, 692t
Cefotaxime
  uses, formulation, and dosage of, 692t
Cefotetan, 692t
Cefoxitin sodium
  uses, formulation, and dosage of, 692t
Ceftazidime, 693t
Ceftiofur, 693t
Celecoxib
  toxicity and treatment of, 243
Celiotomy, 92b, 93
Cellular hypoxia
  and cardiac arrest, 113-114
Cementum
  definition and illustration of dental,
      305, 306f
Center for Veterinary Medicine (CVM)
  emergency hotline, 644t
Central nervous system (CNS)
  and coma, 395-396
  disease
      and oxygen therapy, 48t
      and pain sensing and response system, 70
      and tonic eye reflexes, 342
Central venous catheters
  for vascular access, 59-62, 59f-60f
Central venous manometer, 404f
Central venous pressure (CVP)
  normal values for, 34
Cephalexin
  uses, formulation, and dosage of, 693t

Cephalic catheterization
  as vascular access technique, 62, 65f, 66-67, 66f, 67f
Cephalic veins
  catheter sizes for, 58t
Cephalic venipuncture, 460
Cephalothin sodium
  uses, formulation, and dosage of, 693t
Cephapirin
  uses, formulation, and dosage of, 693t
Cerebellum
  lesions in, 370
Cerebral edema, 187
Cerebrospinal fluids (CSFs)
  collection technique, 509-511
  from ear canal
    with head injuries, 187
  International system of units (SI)
    conversion tables, 656t-658t
  normal test ranges and protocols, 599-600
Cerebrum
  lesions in, 370
Cervical esophagus
  examination of, 313
Cervical spinal cord
  damage with head injuries, 187
  injuries to, 187
  lesions, 370-372
Cervical trachea
  evaluation of patient's, 298
Championship class
  of cats, 647t
Charcoal, activated
  uses, formulation, and dosage of, 220, 685t, 693t
Charts
  and tables, 644-684
    annualized vaccination protocols, 663t-673t
    cat breeds, 647t
    conversion charts, 654t-658t
    dog breeds, 645t-647t
    emergency hotlines, 644t
    ferret information, 652t-653t
    pocket pet information, 648t-649t
    rabies information, 674t-683t
    sex of rodents and rats, 650t
Chelating agents, 221
Chemical analytes, 590-596
Chemical burns
  with acid
    toxicity and treatment of, 224
  description and treatment of, 111-112
Chemical injuries
  description and treatment of, 198-199
Chemotherapy
  nadir, 210t
Chemotherapy-related toxicities
  anaphylactic reactions, 211
  bone marrow, 210
  cardiotoxicity, 211

Chemotherapy-related toxicities—cont'd
  gastrointestinal, 210-211
  urinary bladder toxicity, 211
Chewing
  abnormal
    as sign of pain, 72b
Chief complaint;See also clinical signs
  definition of, 295, 304
Children's glue
  toxicity and treatment of, 238
Chives
  toxicity and treatment of, 243-244
Chlorambucil
  uses, formulation, and dosage of, 693t
Chloramphenicol
  causing anaphylactic reactions, 94b
  uses, formulation, and dosage of, 693t
Chloramphenicol sodium succinate, 693t
Chloride (Cl)
  normal biochemistry ranges
    for adult canines and felines, 577t
  normal test ranges and interpretation, 593
Chlorinated hydrocarbons
  toxicity and treatment of, 231
Chlorine bleach
  toxicity and treatment of, 229
Chlorothiazide
  uses, formulation, and dosage of, 693t
Chlorpheniramine maleate, 694t
Chlorphenoxy derivatives
  toxicity and treatment of, 231-232
Chlorpromazine
  as antiemetics, 172t
  uses, formulation, and dosage of, 694t
Chlortetracycline
  uses, formulation, and dosage of, 694t
Chocolate
  toxicity and treatment of, 232
Cholangiohepatitis
  abdominal characteristics of, 87t
Cholecalciferol
  toxicity and treatment of, 232
Cholecystitis
  abdominal characteristics of, 87t
Cholecystography
  technique of, 548-549
Cholestatic (ALK, Phos, T Bili, GGT) enzymes
  elevation and hepatic failure, 175
Cholesterol (Ch)
  normal test ranges and interpretation, 593-594
Chorionic gonadotropin
  uses, formulation, and dosage of, 694t
Christmas factor, 104
Chronic pain;See also pain
  definition of, 70
  signs of
    in dogs and cats, 72-73
Chronic pancreatitis, 173-174
Chronic respiratory acidosis
  renal and respiratory responses to, 37t

Chronic respiratory alkalosis
  renal and respiratory responses to, 37t
Chronic valvular diseases, 127-128
Chylothorax
  description and treatment of, 260,
      261t-262t, 263
Chylous effusions
  causes of, 263b
  with pleural effusion
      characteristics of, 261t-262t
Cimetidine
  uses, formulation, and dosage of, 694t
Ciprofloxacin, 694t
Circulation;*See also* ABCs
  evaluation of
      during emergency exams, 3
Circulatory hypoxia
  cause and response to oxygen, 48t
Cisapride
  uses, formulation, and dosage of, 694t
Cisplatin
  myelosuppression classification
      of, 210t
  uses, formulation, and dosage of, 694t
Clamshell splints, 12, 18-19, 18f-20f
Clearance
  of poisons, 222
Clemastine, 694t
Clindamycin
  uses, formulation, and dosage
      of, 694t
Clinical histories
  taking pet, 295
Clinical signs
  abdominal enlargement with ascites
      associated signs, 390
      definition of, 390
      differential diagnoses, 390, 391
  abdominal enlargement without
      ascites
      associated signs, 392
      definition of, 392
      differential diagnoses, 393
  aggression
      definition and associated signs, 392
      differential diagnoses, 394b
  alopecia
      associated signs, 414
      definition of, 414
      differential diagnosis, 414-415, 415b
  anorexia
      associated signs, 422-423
      definition of, 422
      differential diagnosis, 423
  anuria
      associated signs, 404
      definition of, 404
      differential diagnosis, 305b, 404
  arthropathy
      associated signs, 420-421
      definition of, 420
      differential diagnosis, 421-422

Clinical signs—cont'd
  ataxia
      associated signs, 416
      definition of, 415
      differential diagnosis, 416b, 417
  blindness
      causes of, 440-441, 442b
      definition of, 440
      diagnostic plan, 441
  blood in urine
      associated signs, 394-395
      causes of, 396t
      definition of, 393-394
      differential diagnosis, 395
  breathing difficulty
      associated signs, 409-410
      definition of, 409
      differential diagnosis, 410
  cachexia
      associated signs, 445
      definition of, 445
      differential diagnosis, 445, 446f
  coma
      associated signs, 395
      definition of, 395
      differential diagnosis, 395-396, 397t
  consciousness
      associated signs, 395
      definition of, 395
      differential diagnosis, 395-396, 397t
  constipation
      associated signs, 398
      definition of, 397-398
      differential diagnosis, 398, 399f, 400b
  convulsions
      associated signs, 427-428
      definition of, 426
      differential diagnosis, 428t, 429
  coughing
      associated signs, 398, 400
      definition of, 398
      differential diagnosis, 400-401
  coughing blood
      associated signs, 402
      definition of, 401
      differential diagnosis, 402
  cyanosis
      associated signs, 409-410
      definition of, 409
      differential diagnosis, 410
  deafness
      associated signs, 403
      definition of, 402-403
      differential diagnosis, 403-404
  decreased urine production
      associated signs, 404
      definition of, 404
      differential diagnosis, 305b, 404
  diarrhea-acute onset
      associated signs, 405-406
      definition of, 405
      differential diagnosis, 406

Clinical signs—cont'd
  diarrhea-chronic
    associated signs, 407
    differential diagnosis, 407-409
  dyschezia
    associated signs, 433-434
    definition of, 432
    differential diagnosis, 434b
  dysphagia
    associated signs, 411, 413
    definition of, 411
    differential diagnosis, 412t, 413b
  dysuria
    associated signs, 435
    definition of, 434
    differential diagnosis, 435b
  emaciation
    associated signs, 445
    definition of, 445
    differential diagnosis, 445, 446f
  epilepsy
    associated signs, 427-428
    definition of, 426
    differential diagnosis, 428t, 429
  hair loss
    associated signs, 414
    definition of, 414
    differential diagnosis, 414-415, 415b
  hearing loss
    associated signs, 403
    definition of, 402-403
    differential diagnosis, 403-404
  hematuria
    associated signs, 394-395
    causes of, 396t
    definition of, 393-394
    differential diagnosis, 395
  hemoglobinuria
    associated signs, 394-395
    causes of, 396t
    definition of, 393-394
    differential diagnosis, 397b
  hemoptysis
    associated signs, 402
    definition of, 401
    differential diagnosis, 402
  hemorrhages
    associated signs, 430, 432
    definition of, 429-430
    differential diagnosis, 432, 433b
  icterus mucous membranes
    associated signs, 447
    definition of, 446
    differential diagnosis, 447-448
  incoordination
    associated signs, 416
    definition of, 415
    differential diagnosis, 416b, 417
  itching
    associated signs, 420
    definition of, 418, 420
    differential diagnosis, 420, 421b

Clinical signs—cont'd
  jaundice
    associated signs, 447
    definition of, 446
    differential diagnosis, 447-448
  joints swelling
    associated signs, 420-421
    definition of, 420
    differential diagnosis, 421-422
  loss of appetite
    associated signs, 422-423
    definition of, 422
    differential diagnosis, 423
  lymph node enlargement
    associated signs, 423
    definition of, 423
    differential diagnosis, 423-424
  lymphadenomegaly
    associated signs, 423
    definition of, 423
    differential diagnosis, 423-424
  myoglobinuria
    associated signs, 394-395
    causes of, 396t
    definition of, 393-394
    differential diagnosis, 395
  nasal discharge
    associated signs, 429
    definition of, 429
    differential diagnosis, 430b
  obstipation
    associated signs, 398
    definition of, 397-398
    differential diagnosis, 398, 399f, 400b
  oliguria
    associated signs, 404
    definition of, 404
    differential diagnosis, 305b, 404
  pain
    associated signs, 424-425
    definition of, 424
    differential diagnosis, 425
  peripheral edema
    associated signs, 437
    definition of, 435
    differential diagnosis, 437, 438b
  polydipsia
    associated signs, 417
    definition of, 417
    differential diagnosis, 417, 418b
  polyuria
    associated signs, 417
    definition of, 417
    differential diagnosis, 417, 418b
  pruritus
    associated signs, 420
    definition of, 418, 420
    differential diagnosis, 420, 421b
  regurgitation
    associated signs, 425-426
    definition of, 425
    differential diagnosis, 426

Clinical signs—cont'd
  respiratory distress
    associated signs, 409-410
    definition of, 409
    differential diagnosis, 410
  seizures
    associated signs, 427-428
    definition of, 426
    differential diagnosis, 428t, 429
  sneezing
    associated signs, 429
    definition of, 429
    differential diagnosis, 430b
  spontaneous bleeding
    associated signs, 430, 432
    definition of, 429-430
    differential diagnosis, 432, 433b
  straining to defecate
    associated signs, 433-434
    definition of, 432
    differential diagnosis, 434b
  straining to urinate
    associated signs, 435
    definition of, 434
    differential diagnosis, 435b
  swallowing difficulty
    associated signs, 411, 413
    definition of, 411
    differential diagnosis, 412t, 413b
  swelling of limbs
    associated signs, 437
    definition of, 435
    differential diagnosis, 437, 438b
  uncontrolled urination
    associated signs, 439
    definition of, 438-439
    differential diagnosis, 439b
  urinary incontinence
    associated signs, 439
    definition of, 438-439
    differential diagnosis, 439b
  urine and water consumption increases
    associated signs, 417
    definition of, 417
    differential diagnosis, 417, 418b
  vision loss
    causes of, 440-441, 442b
    definition of, 440
    diagnostic plan, 441
  vomiting
    associated signs, 443
    definition of, 441-442
    differential diagnosis, 443
  vomiting blood
    associated signs, 444
    definition of, 444
    differential diagnosis, 444-445
  weight loss
    associated signs, 445
    definition of, 445
    differential diagnosis, 445, 446f

Clinical signs—cont'd
  yellow skin
    associated signs, 447
    definition of, 446
    differential diagnosis, 447-448
Clofazimine
  uses, formulation, and dosage of, 694t
Clomipramine, 694t
Clonazepam, 695t
Clorazepate, 695t
Closed long bone fractures, 154b, 155-158
Closed wounds, 9-10
Clot retraction test
  normal values and testing protocols, 611
Clotrimazole
  uses, formulation, and dosage of, 695t
Clots
  avoiding when taking lab samples, 581
Clotting disorders
  causing bleeding, 100-101
Clotting factor
  disorders
    causing bleeding, 100-101
    with disseminated intravascular
      coagulation (DIC), 102-103
  in frozen plasma, 28t, 29
Cloxacillin
  uses, formulation, and dosage of, 695t
Coagulation
  checking in shock "Rule of Twenty," 282
Coagulation factor activity
  normal values and testing protocols, 611-612
Coagulation parameters
  testing during initial emergency care, 5
Coagulation profiles, 107t
Coagulopathies
  causing decompensation, 6b
  disorders
    and whole blood transfusions, 27-28
    types of specific, 101-103
      disseminated intravascular coagulation
        (DIC), 101-102
Coal (*See* aromatic hydrocarbons)
  tar-based
    toxicity and treatment of, 239
Coat
  evaluation and examination of, 332, 333f-335f,
    336-339, 340t, 341
  examination of, 332, 333f-336f, 336-339,
    340t, 341
  part of "BEETTS" test, 294
Cobalamin
  normal test ranges and protocols, 600
  normal test values and interpretation, 618
Coccidioidomycosis antibody titer
    (AGID), 632
Codeine
  properties of
    for pain management, 74t
  uses, formulation, and dosage of, 695t
Coffee ground vomitus, 87t

Colchicine
    uses, formulation, and dosage of, 695t
Cold agglutinin diseases
    skin lesions or signs of, 338t
Cold therapy
    during physical therapy, 499
Colloid fluids
    definition of, 45-46
    for fluid therapy, 43, 45-46
    giving during initial emergency, 4
Colonic ulcers
    characteristics of, 87t
Colony-stimulating factor
    uses, formulation, and dosage of, 695t
Color
    normal urinalysis ranges
        for adult canines and felines, 578t
Coma
    associated signs, 395
    definition of, 191-192, 395
    diabetic, 193
    differential diagnosis, 395-396, 397t
    with head trauma, 186-187
    hepatic, 193
    level of consciousness, 186
    small animal scale (SACS), 192t
Compazine
    as antiemetics, 172t
Complete blood count (CBC)
    component of laboratory data, 300t
    testing during initial emergency care, 5
Component therapy, 21-33
Compressive skull fractures, 154b,
        155-157
Concentration (MCHC)
    normal hematology ranges
        for adult canines and felines, 577t
Conformation
    evaluation during patient exam,
        296-297
Confusion
    level of consciousness, 186b
Congenital defects
    of hemostasis, 103
        treatment of, 104
Congestive heart failure (CHF)
    in cats, 128
    common signs of, 128b
    in dogs, 127
    immediate management of, 128b, 129-130
    causing pericardial effusion, 132t
    with systemic thromboembolism, 285-286
Conjunctiva
    examination of
        during ocular emergencies, 197
    examination of eye, 345
    swelling of, 344
Conjunctival lacerations
    description and treatment of, 198
Conjunctivitis
    versus iritis and glaucoma, 345t

Consciousness
    assessment of
        during initial emergency exam, 5
    associated signs, 395
    definition of, 395
    differential diagnosis, 395-396, 397t
    levels of
        in coma scale, 192t
        with head trauma, 186b
Constipation
    associated signs, 398
    clinical algorithm for, 399f
    definition of, 397-398
    differential diagnosis, 398, 399f, 400b
    obstructive, 169-170
Contaminated wounds
    classification of soft tissue, 271, 272t
Continuous murmurs, 322
Contractility
    calculating with shock, 275-276
    checking in shock "Rule of Twenty," 281t,
        279, 280
Contusions
    description and treatment of, 266-267
    pulmonary, 266-267
Conversion tables
    body weight (KG) to body surface (m^2)
        for dogs and cats, 654t
    French Catheter Scale Equivalents, 454t
    French scale, 655t
    International system of units, 656t-658t
    metric system, 659t
Convulsions
    associated signs, 427-428
    definition of, 426
    differential diagnosis, 428t, 429
Coombs test
    normal test values and interpretation, 627
Coral snakes
    envenomations, 151
Cornea
    abrasions, 199-200
    foreign bodies damaging, 196-197, 200-201
    normal appearance of, 343
Corneal abrasions
    description and treatment of, 199-200
Corneal ulcers
    initial examination of, 4
Coronavirus
    vaccinations
        for dogs, 661t
Corrosives
    toxicity and treatment of, 224
Corticosteroids
    dosage for acute spinal trauma, 190b
Corticotropin
    uses, formulation, and dosage of, 695t
Cortisol, resting
    normal test values and interpretation, 618
Cosyntropin
    uses, formulation, and dosage of, 695t

Coughing
associated signs, 398, 400
of blood
associated signs, 402
definition of, 401
differential diagnosis, 402
cardiovascular exam questions
concerning, 315
definition of, 398
differential diagnosis, 400-401
with dyspnea, 410
with lower respiratory disease, 379
Coumarin;See Vitamin K antagonist
rodenticides
as rodenticide, 106
toxicity and treatment of, 251-252
COX-2, 76
Crackles
definition of lower respiratory, 382
description of, 317t
Cranial nerves
blockades, 79
effect of head injuries on, 187
examination of, 365, 366t-367t, 368f, 369
initial examination of, 4
and pupillary light reflexes (PLR),
342-343
reflexes, 365, 366t-367t, 368f, 369
signs of dysfunction in, 366t-367t
Crash cart
items to stock in, 113b
Creatine kinase (CK)
normal biochemistry ranges
for adult canines and felines, 577t
normal test ranges and interpretation, 594
Creatinine
normal biochemistry ranges
for adult canines and felines, 577t
normal test ranges and interpretation, 594
Cross matching
procedures for, 25-26, 27b
protocol for performing major and
minor, 27b
testing protocols, 612-613
Crossed extensor reflexes, 364
Crown
definition and illustration of dental,
305, 306f
Cruciate syndrome, 355
size and breed disposition to, 352t
Cryopoor plasma
preparation of, 25
storage of, 26t
Cryoprecipitate
dose and administration rates, 29t
indications for administering, 28t, 29
preparation of, 25
separation of, 21-33
storage of, 26t
transfusion guidelines, 30
Cryptococcal antigen test, 632

Crystalloid fluids
for fluid therapy, 43, 45-46
giving during initial emergency, 4
Cultures
blood, 470, 471b
fungal, 472
prostatic fluid, 470
stool, 470
to test dermatologic disorders, 338
transport of, 467
types of bacterial, 466t, 467-468
Cup splints, 12, 18-19, 18f-20f
Cutaneous pain
assessment of, 333f-334f
Cutaneous reflexes, 364-365
Cyanocobalamin
uses, formulation, and dosage of, 696t
Cyanosis
assessing during cardiovascular exam, 319
associated signs, 409-410
and cardiac arrest, 114
as clinical sign of decompensation, 6b
with congestive heart failure, 128
definition of, 409
differential diagnosis, 410
during respiratory distress, 253
Cyclooxygenase, 75-76
Cyclophosphamide
myelosuppression classification of, 210t
uses, formulation, and dosage of, 696t
Cyclosporine
uses, formulation, and dosage of, 696t
Cyproheptadine
uses, formulation, and dosage of, 696t
Cystic endometrial hyperplasia
and pyometra, 136-138
Cystocentesis
technique of, 486f, 488-489
urine cultures, 468, 469t
Cystography
technique of, 546
Cysts
nasopharyngeal polyps, 257
Cytarabine
uses, formulation, and dosage of, 696t
Cytopathology
guidelines, 584-585
malignancies, 481b
specimen collection techniques,
480-481

D
Dacarbazine
uses, formulation, and dosage of, 696t
Dalteparin, 696t
Danazol, 696t
Dantrolene, 697t
Dapsone
uses, formulation, and dosage of, 697t
Databases
for poisons, 212, 213b

Dead space
    obliteration bandaging technique, 11
Deafness
    associated signs, 403
    definition of, 402-403
    differential diagnosis, 403-404
Decerebellate
    with head trauma, 186t, 187
Decerebrate activity
    and coma scale, 192t
Decerebrate rigidity
    with head trauma, 186t, 187
Deciduous teeth
    formula for, 304-305
Decompensation
    and cardiopulmonary cerebral resuscitation
        (CPCR), 113-114, 115f, 116f, 117
    causes of acute, 6b
    clinical signs of, 6b
Deep heat
    during physical therapy, 498
"Deep pain," 189
Defecation
    with acute diarrhea, 405-406
    frequency of, 407t
    straining to
        associated signs, 433-434
        definition of, 432
        differential diagnosis, 434b
Deferoxamine
    as chelating agent, 221
    uses, formulation, and dosage of, 697t
Degenerative diseases
    and joint fluid analysis, 357t-358t
Dehydration
    with abdominal conditions, 86t-89t
    and fluid therapy, 35t
Deicers (See ethylene glycol)
    toxicity and treatment of, 224, 225, 235-236
Delayed primary closure
    of wounds, 274
Dental charts, 307f, 308f
Dental examination, 304-306, 307f, 308-309
Dental fractures, 309
Dental record, 306
Dental terminology
    and anatomy, 305-306, 307f, 308
Dentin
    definition and illustration of dental,
        305, 306f
Dentition
    normal canine, 304-309
    and occlusion, 306, 308
Denture cleaners
    toxicity and treatment of, 233
Deodorants
    toxicity and treatment of, 233
Deoxyhemoglobin
    calculations of, 51
Deprenyl
    uses, formulation, and dosage of, 697t

Depression
    as clinical sign of decompensation, 6b
Deracoxib
    toxicity and treatment of, 243
Dermatologic system
    examination of, 332, 333f-336f, 336-339,
        340t, 341
    procedures
        deep skin scraping, 491
        skin biopsy, 489-490
        skin scraping, 491
    tests
        procedures, 489-491
    topical administration
        of medications, 457
Dermatophyte test medium (DTM), 338
    uses of, 472-473
Deroxicib
    dosage for pain, 75t
Descending systems
    within pain sensing and response system, 70
Desmopressin acetate
    uses, formulation, and dosage of, 697t
Desoxycorticosterone pivalate
    uses, formulation, and dosage of, 697t
Detergents
    toxicity and treatment of, 233-234
Dexamethasone
    for feline bronchitis, 266t
    uses, formulation, and dosage of, 697t
Dexamethasone sodium phosphate
    for feline bronchitis, 266t
Dexamethasone suppression test
    normal test values and interpretation,
        618-620
Dextran
    uses, formulation, and dosage of, 697t
Dextromethorphan
    uses, formulation, and dosage of, 698t
Dextrose solution 5%
    uses, formulation, and dosage of, 698t
Diabetes mellitus
    coma, 193
    skin lesions or signs of, 338t
Diabetic coma, 193
Diabetic ketoacidosis (DKA)
    clinical features of, 178
    insulin administration for, 179, 180t
    treatment of, 179
Diagnostic peritoneal lavage
    in acute abdomen cases, 85, 90t-92t
    during initial emergency exam, 5
    technique of, 6-7
Diagnostic procedures
    abdominal, 84-85, 90t-92t, 93
    advanced
        female reproductive procedures, 548-549,
            549-550
        male reproductive procedures,
            554-559
        respiratory tract, 559-571

Diagnostic procedures—cont'd
  biochemistry testing
    routine, 476, 477t
  blood pressure measurement
    indirect, 462-463
  bone marrow aspiration
    canine, 477-478, 479f, 480
  central venous pressure measurement,
    463-465
  cytopathology
    specimen collection techniques, 480-481
  during emergencies, 6-69
  endotracheal intubation
    technique of, 494-495
  exfoliative cytologic procedures, 482
  fungal cultures, 472
  intravenous catheterization techniques,
    495-496
  routine and advanced, 449-572
  sample collection techniques
    bacterial cultures, 465-468, 469t, 470
  urine collection techniques, 483
Diaphragm
  hernia, 264
Diaphragmatic hernia, 86t
  assessing during initial emergency exam, 4
  description and immediate management
    of, 264
Diarrhea
  with abdominal conditions, 86t-89t
  with acute gastritis, 171-172
  acute-onset
    associated signs, 405-406
    definition of, 405
    differential diagnosis, 406
  chronic
    associated signs, 407
    differential diagnosis, 407-409
  with hemorrhagic gastroenteritis (HGE),
    171, 173
  with intracellular fluid deficit, 34-47
  specific types of, 408t
Diascopy
  technique of, 337
Diastolic blood pressure
  elevations of, 177
  and renal function, 386
Diastolic murmurs, 322
Diazepam
  for seizures, 194
  uses, formulation, and dosage of, 698t
Dichlone
  toxicity and treatment of, 234
Dichlorphenamide
  for acute glaucoma, 204t
  uses, formulation, and dosage of, 698t
Dichlorvos
  uses, formulation, and dosage of, 698t
Diclofenac
  toxicity and treatment of, 243
Dicloxacillin, 698t

Diencephalon
  lesions in, 370
Diestrus, 383, 384
Diet
  causing acute diarrhea, 406b
  cardiovascular exam questions
    concerning, 315
Diethylcarbamazine
  uses, formulation, and dosage of, 698t
Diethylstilbestrol, 698t
Diethyltoluamide (DEET)
  toxicity and treatment of, 234-235
Diffusion impairment
  cause and response to oxygen, 48t
Difloxacin
  uses, formulation, and dosage of, 698t
Digitoxin
  uses, formulation, and dosage of, 698t
Digits
  injuries to, 190-191
  orthopedic diseases affecting, 352-353t,
    354-356
Digoxin
  for congestive heart failure (CHF), 130
  for supraventricular dysrhythmias, 125t
  uses, formulation, and dosage of,
    698t, 699t
Dihydrotachysterol, 182t
  uses, formulation, and dosage of, 699t
Dilated cardiomyopathy, 127-128
Diltiazem
  for supraventricular dysrhythmias, 125t
  uses, formulation, and dosage of, 699t
  for ventricular dysrhythmias, 281t
Diluting agents, 221
Dimenhydrinate, 699t
Dimercaprol, 699t
Dinoprost tromethamine, 699t
Dioctyl calcium sulfocuccinate, 699t
Dioctyl sodium sulfosuccinate
  uses, formulation, and dosage of, 699t
Diphenhydramine
  uses, formulation, and dosage of, 699t
Diphenoxylate, 700t
Diphenylhydantoin, 700t
Diphosphonate disodium etidronate
  uses, formulation, and dosage of, 700t
Dipyridamole
  uses, formulation, and dosage of, 700t
Diquat
  toxicity and treatment of, 235
Dirofilariasis
  skin lesions or signs of, 338t
Discospondylitis, 89t
Disinfectants
  toxicity and treatment of, 233-234
Disks
  herniated
    and back trauma, 189
    corticosteroid dosage for, 190b
    examination and prognosis of, 189

Disks—cont'd
  herniated—cont'd
    localizing signs of, 190t
    treatment and management of, 189-190
Disopyramide
  uses, formulation, and dosage of, 700t
Disseminated intravascular coagulation (DIC)
  causing abnormal bleeding, 101-103
  checking in shock "Rule of Twenty," 282
  clinical signs and treatment of, 206t
  causing decompensation, 6b
  diagnosis of, 101, 102b
  disorders associated with, 101, 102b
  laboratory findings with, 102b
  laboratory results and interpretation, 107t
  treatment of, 102-103
  tumor types, 206
  and whole blood transfusions, 27-28
Distal metacarpus
  fractures of, 19, 21
Distal urethra
  prolapse of, 145-146
Distemper
  vaccinations
    for dogs, 661t
  "Distemper teeth," 308, 309f
Distichiasis
  eyelid, 344
Diuresis
  to clear toxins, 222
Diuretics
  for systemic hypertension, 177t
Divalproex sodium
  uses, formulations, and dosage of, 700t
D-Limonene
  toxicity and treatment of, 240
Dobutamine
  uses, formulations, and dosage of, 700t
Docusate calcium
  uses, formulations, and dosage of, 700t
Docusate sodium, 700t
Dog breeds
  AKC recognized
    herding group, 646t
    hound group, 645t
    non-sporting group, 646t
    sporting group, 645t
    terrier group, 645t
    toy group, 646t
    working group, 645t
Dogs
  abdominal analgesics for, 83t
  bleeding disorders in, 100-107
  blood component therapy for, 30-32
  blood types and antigenicity of, 22-23
  categories of pain in, 70b
  catheter sizes for, 54t, 484t
  conversion table
    of body weight to body surface area, 654t
  heart rate and blood pressure
    normal parameters, 97t

Dogs—cont'd
  minimum laboratory database for, 300t
  normal canine dentition, 304-309
  normal heart rate of, 320b
  orthopedic disorders in, 352t-353t
  pain assessment in, 71
  paraneoplastic syndromes in, 205t-206t
  rabies control in, 675t
  rabies testing, 582-584
  signs of chronic pain in, 72-73
  transfusion guidelines in, 30-31
  types of vaccinations for, 661t
  vaccination risks for, 660t, 663t-668t
  vaccinations
    annualized protocol, 663t-668t
Dolasetron
  as antiemetics, 172t
  uses, formulations, and dosage of, 700t
"Doll-eye" reflexes, 187
Dopamine
  uses, formulations, and dosage of, 700t
Doppler ultrasonography
  to examine arteries, 5
Dorzolamide
  for acute glaucoma, 204t
"Double-bubble"
  with gastric dilatation-volvulus (GDV),
    166, 167f
Doughnut-shaped bandages, 12, 15f
Doxapram
  uses, formulations, and dosage of, 701t
Doxepin
  uses, formulations, and dosage of, 701t
Doxorubicin
  myelosuppression classification of, 210t
  uses, formulations, and dosage of, 701t
Doxycycline, 701t
Drug Enforcement Agency
  emergency hotline, 644t
Drug therapy
  for pain, 73-81
Drugs;See also individual drugs
  for acute abdominal pain, 83t
  for acute glaucoma, 204t
  causing acute hepatic failure, 174-175
  advanced and prolonged life support, 120t
  analgesia
    adjunctive, 77, 78t
    anxiolytics, 78t
    major, 73-77
    minor, 77
    sedatives, 78t
  antiemetic, 172t
  common indications and dosages of,
    685t-742t
  for feline bronchitis, 266t
  for hypertension, 177t
  for hypocalcemia, 182t
  list of common, 685t-742t
  monitoring in shock "Rule of Twenty," 283
  and oxygen therapy, 48t

Drugs—cont'd
  prescription writing do's and don'ts, 684t
  vascular access techniques to administer
    catheter sizes and types, 58-59
    central venous catheters, 59-62, 59f-60f
    cephalic catheterization, 62, 65f, 66-67,
      66f, 67f
    during initial examination, 4
    intraosseous catheter placement, 69
    maintenance of indwelling catheters, 68-69
    percutaneous dorsal pedal artery
      catheterization, 68
    percutaneous over-the-wire jugular
      catheter, 61-62
    percutaneous through-the-needle jugular
      catheter, 59-61
    peripheral arterial and venous catheter
      placement, 62, 65f, 66-67
    Seldinger technique, 61-62, 62f-63f
    surgical cutdown
      for catheter placement, 68
D-timers
  ancillary hemostasis tests, 609
  normal test values and interpretation, 613
Duodenum
  displacement of
    with gastric dilatation-volvulus (GDV),
      166, 167f
Dyschezia
  associated signs, 433-434
  definition of, 432
  differential diagnosis, 434b
Dysphagia
  associated signs, 411, 413
  definition of, 411
  differential diagnosis, 412t, 413b
Dyspnea
  cardiovascular exam questions
    concerning, 315
  definition of, 317b
  with lower respiratory disease, 378, 379
Dysrhythmias
  with cardiomyopathies, 127-128
Dystocia
  diagnostic criteria for, 140b
  as pregnancy emergency, 139-140
Dysuria
  associated signs, 435
  clinical algorithm for, 436f
  definition of, 434
  differential diagnosis, 435b
"Dysynchronous" respiratory patterns, 253-254

E
Ear canals
  cleaning procedures, 349-350, 492, 493f, 494
  examination of, 347-348
  foreign bodies in, 133-134
Eardrum
  definition of, 347-350
Early compensatory shock, 276

Ears
  cleaning procedures, 492, 493f, 494
  cultures, 466t, 467
  emergencies related to, 133-135
    foreign bodies, 133-134
  in emergency poison/toxin cases, 215b
  evaluation and examination of, 298,
    347-350
  hearing loss
    associated signs, 403
    definition of, 402-403
    differential diagnosis, 403-404
  initial examination of, 4
  part of "BEETTS" test, 294
Eclampsia, 181, 182t
Ecstasy
  toxicity and treatment of, 235
Ectoparasites, 482-483
Ectropion
  eyelid, 344
Edema
  central nervous system
    causing decompensation, 6b
  peripheral
    associated signs, 437
    definition of, 435
    differential diagnosis, 437, 438b
Edrophonium
  uses, formulations, and dosage of, 701t
EDTA
  uses, formulations, and dosage of, 701t
Effusions
  due to oncologic emergencies, 205-211
  joint, 420-422
Ehricichia canis antibody test, 632-633
Ehrlichia test, 633
Elbows
  injuries to, 190-191
  spica splints, 21
Electrical alternans
  example of, 132f
Electrical burns, 110-111
Electrical shock
  and cardiac arrest, 113-114
  emergency care for, 135-136
Electrical-mechanical dissociation (EMD)
  and cardiac arrest, 114
  description of, 117
  electrocardiogram illustrating, 118f
Electrocardiograms (ECGs)
  assessing during initial emergency
    exam, 4
  flowchart illustrating
    during basic and advanced life support,
      115f, 116f
  parameters and uses of, 511-517
Electrocardiography
  during ancillary diagnostic
    evaluation, 5
  technique of, 511-517
Electrocution, 135-136

Electrolyte imbalances
  and cardiac arrest, 113-114
  checking in shock "Rule of Twenty," 282
  and fluid therapy, 37-39, 40t
Electrotherapy
  during physical therapy, 499
Elizabethan collars
  for oxygen hoods, 49-50
  following vaginal prolapse, 139
Emaciation
  associated signs, 445
  definition of, 445
  differential diagnosis, 445, 446f
  evaluation during patient exam, 296-297
Embolism
  systemic thromboembolism, 285-286
Emergencies
  environmental, 146-148
    black widow spider bites, 152
    brown spider bites, 152-153
    Bufo toads, 153-154
    coral snake envenomation, 151
    frostbite, 146-147
    gila monster bites, 153-154
    heat stroke, 147-148
    hyperthermia, 147-148
    hypothermia, 147
    malignant hyperthermia, 148-149
    Mexican bearded lizard bites, 153-154
    pit viper envenomation, 149-151
    snakebites, 149-152
Emergency care, 1-291
  acute pain management during, 73
  diagnostic and therapeutic procedures, 6-69
    abdominal paracentesis, 6-7
    bandaging and splinting techniques, 8-12,
      13f-17f, 18-19, 20f, 21
    blood component therapy, 21-33
    capnometry, 52
    central venous pressure measurement,
      33-34
    end-tidal carbon dioxide monitoring, 52
    fluid therapy, 34-43, 44t, 45-47
    orogastric lavage, 47-48
    oxygen supplementation, 48-51
    peritoneal lavage, 6-7
    pulse oximetry, 51
    splinting techniques, 8-12, 13f-17f, 18-19,
      20f, 21
    thoracocentesis, 52-55
    tracheostomy, 55-56
    urohydropulsion, 57
    vascular access techniques, 58-62, 63f-65f,
      66-69
  hotlines, 644t
  initial emergency and triage, 3-6
    ancillary diagnostic evaluation, 5
    primary survey and resuscitation, 3-5
    the rapidly decompensating patient, 5-6
    summarizing patient status, 5
  local and regional anesthesia during, 78-81

Emergency care—cont'd
  pain
    acute pain management, 73
    adjunctive analgesics, 77-78
    local and regional techniques, 78-81
    major analgesics, 73-77
    minor analgesics, 77
    physiologic impact of untreated, 70-71
    recognizing and assessing, 71-73
  prehospital management
    initial examination, 2-3
    of injured animal, 2-3
    preparation for transport, 3
    scene survey, 2
  for specific conditions, 81-291
    abdomen conditions, 81-85, 86t-92t, 93
    anaphylactic shock, 94-95
    anaphylactoid shock, 94-95
    anesthetic complications and emergencies,
      96-100
    angioneurotic edema and urticaria, 95
    bleeding disorders, 100-107
    burns, 105-113
    cardiac emergencies, 113-114, 115f,
      116-117, 118f, 119-133
    ear emergencies, 133-135
    electrocution/electric shock, 135-136
    environmental and household
      emergencies, 146-154
    female reproductive tract and genitalia,
      136-141
    fractures and musculoskeletal trauma,
      154-158
    gastrointestinal emergencies, 158-175
    hypertension (systemic), 176-177
    male genitalia and reproductive tract,
      141-146
    metabolic emergencies, 178-181, 182t,
      183-185
    neurologic emergencies, 185-195
    ocular emergencies, 196-204
    oncologic emergencies, 205, 206t, 207-211
    poisons and toxins, 212, 213t, 214, 215b,
      216, 217f, 218-253 (*See also*
      individual poisons and toxins)
    pulmonary diseases, 265-270
    respiratory emergencies, 253-260,
      261t-262t, 263-265
    shock, 275-277
    shock management, 277-285
    superficial soft tissue injuries, 271-275
    thromboembolism (systemic), 285-286
    urinary tract emergencies, 287-291
Emergency hotlines, 644t
Emergency patient medical records, 303
Emergency resuscitation, 2-4
Emetics
  list of recommended, 219t
  for poisonings, 218
Emphysema
  and oxygen therapy, 48t

Emphysematous cholecystitis
abdominal characteristics of, 87t
Enalapril
to induce vasodilation, 280t
for systemic hypertension, 177t
uses, formulations, and dosage of, 701t
Enamel
definition and illustration of dental, 305, 306f
hypoplasia, 308, 309f
Endocarditis, 127-128
Endocrine diseases
types of
and skin manifestations of, 340t
Endogenous hepatotoxins
causing acute hepatic failure, 175b
Endoscopy
technique of, 517-522
Endotoxemia
and cardiac arrest, 113-114
Endotracheal intubation
technique of, 494-495
Endotracheal tubes
adaptor, 565f
sizes, 494t
End-tidal carbon dioxide monitoring, 52
Enemas
for poisons, 219-220
Energy
daily requirements for dogs and cats, 44t
Enflurane
uses, formulations, and dosage of, 701t
Enilconazole, 702t
Enoxaparin, 702t
Enrofloxacin, 702t
Envenomation
causing acute abdominal pain, 89t
associated with disseminated intravascular
coagulation (DIC), 102-103
coral snakes, 151
pit viper, 149-151
Environmental emergencies, 146-148
black widow spider bites, 152
brown spider bites, 152-153
Bufo toads, 153-154
coral snake envenomation, 151
frostbite, 146-147
gila monster bites, 153-154
heat stroke, 147-148
hyperthermia, 147-148
hypothermia, 147
malignant hyperthermia, 148-149
Mexican bearded lizard bites, 153-154
pit viper envenomation, 149-151
snakebites, 149-152
toxins
causing acute hepatic failure, 175b
Environmental toxins
causing acute hepatic failure, 175b
Enzymes
cholestatic and hepatocellular
and hepatic failure, 175

Eosinophils
normal hematology ranges
for adult canines and felines, 577t
Ephedrine
uses, formulations, and dosage of, 702t
Epididymitis, 143
Epidural anesthesia
drugs used for, 80t
function of, 80
Epilepsy
associated signs, 427-428
definition of, 426
differential diagnosis, 428t, 429
Epinephrine
with asystole, 117
used during advanced life support, 120t
uses, formulations, and dosage of, 702t
Episcleritis, 343
Epistaxis
description and treatment of, 269-270
Epithelial cells
normal urinalysis ranges
for adult canines and felines, 578t
Epsiprantel
uses, formulations, and dosage of, 703t
Ergocalciferol, 182t, 703t
Eruption dates
table for cats, 305t
table for dogs, 304t
Erythema multiforme
skin lesions or signs of, 338t
Erythrocytosis
clinical signs and treatment of, 206t
tumor types, 206
Erythromycin
causing anaphylactic reactions, 94b
Erythropoietin
human recombinant
uses, formulations, and dosage of, 703t
Esmolol
for supraventricular dysrhythmias, 125t
uses, formulations, and dosage of, 703t
for ventricular dysrhythmias, 281t
Esophagus
foreign bodies obstructing, 160, 161f
gastrointestinal system emergencies,
160-161
Estradiol cypionate, 140-141
uses, formulations, and dosage of, 703t
Estradiol test, 620
Estrus, 382-384
Ethanol
toxicity and treatment of, 224-225
Ethylene glycol
normal test ranges and protocols, 600-601
toxicity and treatment of, 235-236
Etidronate disodium
uses, formulations, and dosage of, 703t
Etodolac
dosage for pain, 75t
uses, formulations, and dosage of, 703t

Evaluations
  patient
    alimentary system, 304-306, 307f,
      308-310, 311f, 312-315
    the "BEETTS" test, 293-295
    cardiovascular system, 315-325, 326t,
      327f-328f, 329-332
    ears, 347-350
    female reproductive tract exam, 374-376
    integumentary system, 332, 333f-335f,
      336-339, 340t, 341
    lymph nodes, 350-351
    male reproductive tract exam, 373
    medical record, 301-304
    musculoskeletal system, 351, 352t-353t,
      354-356
    nervous system, 356, 357t-358t, 359-365,
      366t-367t, 368f, 369-373
    normal breeding behavior and physiology,
      382-384
    ocular system, 341-347
    ophthalmic, 341-347
    orthopedic, 351, 352t-353t, 354-356
    otic system, 347-350
    the "problem list," 295-301
    respiratory system-lower, 377-380,
      381f, 382
    respiratory system-upper, 376-377
    skin, hair, coat and toenails, 332,
      333f-335f, 336-339, 340t, 341
    thyroid, 350-351
    urinary tract exam, 384-386
Evans syndrome, 106
Examinations
  components of physical, 296-301
  initial emergency hospital, 3-6
  initial on-the-scene, 2-3
  ophthalmic checklist
    anterior chamber, 346-347
    conjunctiva, 345
    external eye appearance, 343
    eyelids, 344-345
    globe and adnexa, 341-342
    iris, 347
    lacrimal system, 346
    lens, 347
    nictitating membrane, 345-346
    orbit, 344
    pupillary light reflexes (PLR), 342-343
    retina, 347
    tonic eye reflexes, 342
    vision assessment, 343-344
  of oral cavity, 309-310, 311f, 312-313
  of organ systems
    alimentary system, 304-306, 307f,
      308-310, 311f, 312-315
    cardiovascular system, 315-325, 326t,
      327f-328f, 329-332
    ears, 347-350
    female reproductive tract exam,
      374-376

Examinations—cont'd
  of organ systems—cont'd
    integumentary system, 332, 333f-335f,
      336-339, 340t, 341
    lymph nodes, 350-351
    male reproductive tract exam, 373
    musculoskeletal system, 351, 352t-353t,
      354-356
    nervous system, 356, 357t-358t, 359-365,
      366t-367t, 368f, 369-373
    normal breeding behavior and physiology,
      382-384
    ocular system, 341-347
    ophthalmic, 341-347
    orthopedic, 351, 352t-353t, 354-356
    otic system, 347-350
    respiratory system-lower, 377-380,
      381f, 382
    respiratory system-upper, 376-377
    skin, hair, coat and toenails, 332,
      333f-335f, 336-339, 340t, 341
    thyroid, 350-351
    urinary tract exam, 384-386
  physical
    for toxicity and poison cases, 214, 215b,
      216, 217f, 218-223
Exercise
  cardiovascular exam questions
    concerning, 315
  therapy
    during physical therapy, 499-500
Exfoliative cytologic procedures, 482
Exfoliative cytology
  technique of, 586-587
Exhalation
  assessing during initial emergency exam, 3-4
Exogenous drugs
  causing acute hepatic failure, 175b
Exophthalmos, 344
Expiratory distress
  assessing during initial emergency exam, 3-4
Expiratory dyspnea
  assessing during cardiovascular exam, 316
  with lower respiratory disease, 378
Exploratory laparotomy, 92b, 93, 375
Extensor postural thrust, 361
External eye appearance
  examination of, 343
External pin splints, 12, 16f, 17f
Extracranial hemorrhages
  with head injuries, 185-186
Extraluminal masses
  description and immediate management
    of, 257
Extrathoracic trachea
  emergencies of, 253-265
Extremities
  coolness in
    as clinical sign of decompensation, 6b
    with congestive heart failure, 128
  evaluation of patient's, 301

Exuberant granulation tissue, 11
Exudate, pericardial effusion, 132t
Exudates
  with pleural effusion
    characteristics of, 261t-262t
Eyelid ecchymosis
  description and treatment of, 198
Eyelids
  ecchymosis of, 198
  emergencies, 197-198
  examination of, 344-345
  injuries of, 197-198
  lacerations, 197-198
Eyes
  cultures, 466t, 467-468
  emergency examination of, 196-197
  evaluating patient's, 297-298
  examination checklist
    anterior chamber, 346-347
    conjunctiva, 345
    external eye appearance, 343
    eyelids, 344-345
    globe and adnexa, 341-342
    iris, 347
    lacrimal system, 346
    lens, 347
    nictitating membrane, 345-346
    orbit, 344
    pupillary light reflexes (PLR), 342-343
    retina, 347
    tonic eye reflexes, 342
    vision assessment, 343-344
  examining in emergency poison/toxin
    cases, 215b
  head injuries affecting, 186-187
  initial examination of, 4
  and loss of vision, 196b
  part of "BEETTS" test, 294
  poisons damaging, 221
  specific conditions of, 197-204
    acute infectious keratitis, 200
    chemical injuries, 198-199
    conjunctival lacerations, 198
    corneal abrasions, 199-200
    eyelid ecchymosis, 198
    foreign bodies, 200-201
    glaucoma, 203-204
    hyphema, 201-202
    loss of vision, 196b
    ocular trauma, 201
    penetrating corneal injuries, 200
    proptosis, 202-203
    subconjunctival lacerations, 198
  treatment of, 197-198

F
Facial nerves, 367, 368f, 369
Factor IX deficiency, 104
Factor VII deficiency, 104
Factor VIII deficiency, 103
Factor X deficiency, 104

Factor XI deficiency, 104
Factor XII deficiency, 104
Famotidine
  uses, formulations, and dosage of, 704t
Fecal fat
  normal test ranges and protocols, 601
Fecal flotation
  component of laboratory data, 300t
Fecal occult blood
  normal test ranges and protocols, 601
Feces
  blood or mucus in, 407t
Felbamate
  uses, formulations, and dosage of, 704t
Feline asthma
  description and treatment of, 265-266
Feline blood typing
  normal values and testing protocols, 610-611
Feline bronchitis
  description and treatment of, 265-266
  drugs to treat, 266t
Feline dental chart, 308f
Feline hyperthyroidism, 351
Feline immunodeficiency virus
  antibody
    test and interpretation, 634-635
  vaccinations
    for cats, 661t
Feline infectious anemia
  test and interpretation, 636-637
Feline infectious peritonitis
  vaccinations
    for cats, 661t
Feline leukemia
  vaccinations
    for cats, 661t
Feline leukemia virus
  antigen test, 633-634
  infection
    skin lesions or signs of, 338t
Feline lower airway disease
  description and treatment of, 265-266
  drugs to treat, 266t
Feline lower urinary tract disease
  description and treatment of, 289
Female genitalia
  emergencies concerning, 136-141
Female reproductive tract
  emergencies of, 136-141
    acute metritis, 138
    pregnancy issues, 139-141
    pyometra, 136-138
    uterine prolapse, 136
    vaginal prolapse, 138-139
  evaluation and examination of, 374-376
  procedures, 549-552
Females
  intact cat characteristics, 383-384
  intact dog characteristics, 382-383
Femoral nerves
  injuries to, 191

Fenbendazole
  uses, formulations, and dosage of, 704t
Fentanyl
  for abdominal pain, 83t
  properties of
    for pain management, 74t
  uses, formulations, and dosage of, 704t
Fentanyl transdermal
  uses, formulations, and dosage of, 704t
Ferrets
  electrocardiographic data for normal, 653t
  hematologic values for normal, 652t
  physiologic, reproductive and anatomic
    data, 652t
  rabies control in, 675t
  serum chemistry values for normal, 653t
Ferrous sulfate
  uses, formulations, and dosage of, 704t
Fertilizers
  toxicity and treatment of, 236
Fever
  with abdominal conditions, 86t-89t
Fibrin degradation products (FDPs)
  ancillary hemostasis tests, 609
  laboratory results for coagulation
    profiles, 107t
  normal hemostasis ranges
    for adult canines and felines, 578t
  normal test values and interpretation, 614
Fibrinogen
  laboratory results for coagulation
    profiles, 107t
  levels
    ancillary hemostasis tests, 609
    normal hemostasis ranges
      for adult canines and felines, 578t
    normal test values and interpretation, 614
Fibrosis
  and oxygen therapy, 48t
Fiddleback spiders, 152-153
Finasteride
  uses, formulations, and dosage of, 704t
Fine needle aspiration (FNA)
  technique of, 481-482, 586
Fipronil
  toxicity and treatment of, 236-237
  uses, formulations, and dosage of, 704t
Fire extinguisher
  toxicity and treatment of, 237
Fireplace colors
  toxicity and treatment of, 237
Fireworks
  toxicity and treatment of, 237
Firocoxib
  uses, formulations, and dosage of, 705t
First heart sound (S$_1$), 320
Flail chest
  description and immediate management of,
    264-265
"Flat lining," 117
Flexor reflexes, 363-364

Florfenicol, 705t
Fluconazole
  uses, formulations, and dosage of, 705t
Flucytosine
  uses, formulations, and dosage of, 705t
Fludrocortisone
  uses, formulations, and dosage of, 705t
Fluid pumps, 47
Fluid therapy;*See also* fluids
  and acid-base physiology, 35-37
  anion gap, 42
  calculations of deficits/losses, 43
  and central venous pressure, 33-34
  to clear toxins, 222
  clinical signs of, 35t
  crystalloid and colloid fluids, 43, 45-46
  dehydration, 35t
  diagnosis of, 34-35
  and electrolyte imbalance, 37-39, 40t
  for intracellular fluid deficit, 34-43, 44t,
    45-47
  maintenance fluid requirements, 43, 44t
  and metabolic acidosis, 36b
  and metabolic alkalosis, 35-37
  oncotic pressure, 42-43
  and osmolality, 38-39
  planning and implementing, 46-47
  and potassium imbalances, 37-38,
    39b, 40t
  rates of administration, 47
  in shock "Rule of Twenty," 278
  and sodium, 39, 41, 41b, 42
  technique of, 523, 524t, 525-526
Fluids;*See also* fluid therapy
  abdominocentesis, 6-7
  administering during initial emergency
    exam, 4
  administration rates of, 47
  ascites, 390, 391f
  balance
    in shock "Rule of Twenty," 278
  body
    lab samples of, 588
  calculating deficits and losses, 43
  daily requirements for dogs and cats, 44t
  for exfoliative cytology, 482
  and increased urination, 417-418
  International system of units (SI)
    conversion tables, 656t-658t
  maintenance requirements, 43, 44t
  normal intake of, 385b
  and pleural effusion, 259-260, 261t-262t, 263
  vascular access techniques
    catheter sizes and types, 58-59
    central venous catheters, 59-62, 59f-60f
    cephalic catheterization, 62, 65f, 66-67,
      66f, 67f
    during initial examination, 4
    intraosseous catheter placement, 69
    maintenance of indwelling catheters,
      68-69

Fluids—cont'd
vascular access techniques—cont'd
percutaneous dorsal pedal artery
catheterization, 68
percutaneous over-the-wire jugular
catheter, 61-62
percutaneous through-the-needle jugular
catheter, 59-61
peripheral arterial and venous catheter
placement, 62, 65f, 66-67
Seldinger technique, 61-62, 62f-63f
surgical cutdown
for catheter placement, 68
volume rates of administration, 47
Flunixin meglumine, 705t
Fluorouracil
uses, formulations, and dosage of, 705t
Fluoxetine
uses, formulations, and dosage of, 705t
Fluticasone
for feline bronchitis, 266t
Fluvoxamine, 706t
Foam rubber pads
with splints, 12, 16f, 17f
Folate
normal test ranges and protocols, 601
normal test values and interpretation, 620
Fomepizole
uses, formulations, and dosage
of, 706t
Food
causing acute gastritis, 171-172
causing anaphylactic reactions, 94b
and anorexia, 422-423
cardiovascular exam questions
concerning, 315
and gastric dilatation-volvulus (GDV),
165-168
Food and Drug Administration (FDA)
phone numbers, 644t
"Food bloat"
with gastric dilatation-volvulus (GDV),
166, 167f
orogastric lavage for, 47-48
Footpad hyperkeratosis
skin lesions or signs of, 338t
Footpads
cup or clamshell splints for, 12, 18-19,
18f-20f
Foreign bodies
causing acute gastritis, 171-172
description and immediate management of,
200-201, 257
in ear canals, 133-134
causing gastrointestinal emergencies,
158-165
linear, 163-164
linear and luminal
characteristics of gastrointestinal, 87t
Foreign serums
causing anaphylactic reactions, 94b

Forelimbs
injuries to, 191t
Foxtails
in ear canal, 133-134
Fractures
assessing at accident scene, 2-3
dental, 309
in immature animals, 158
initial immobilization of, 10-11
lateral or caudal splints for, 19, 21
and musculoskeletal trauma
articular cartilage injuries, 157
classification of, 154b
high-rise syndrome, 158
immediate action, 154-155
ligament injuries, 157, 158b
open wounds, 156b, 157
treatment of, 155-157
open
debridement, stabilization and bandaging
of, 156-167
of os penis, 144
Fragment D-timer
normal test values and interpretation, 613
Fragmented coronoid process
size and breed disposition to, 353t
Freezing point depression, 38
French Catheter Scale Equivalents
conversion table, 454t
French Scale Conversion Table, 655t
Frequency
of heart murmurs, 324, 326t
Fresh frozen plasma
dose and administration rates, 29t
indications for administering, 28t, 29
preparation of, 25
storage of, 26t
transfusion guidelines, 30
Fresh whole blood
dose and administration rates, 29t
indications for administering, 28t, 29
Friction rub
description of, 317t
Frostbite, 146-147
Frozen plasma
dose and administration rates, 29t
indications for administering, 28t, 29
preparation of, 25
Fructosamine
normal test ranges and protocols, 602
normal test values and interpretation, 620-621
Fuels
toxicity and treatment of, 237-238
Fulminant pulmonary edema
in cats with CHF, 130
Functional hemoglobin saturation
calculation of, 51
Fungal cultures, 472
Fungal diseases
types of
and skin manifestations of, 339t

Furazolidone
uses, formulations, and dosage of, 706t
Furcation
definition and illustration of dental, 305, 306f
Furniture polish (*See* fuels)
toxicity and treatment of, 237-238
Furosemide
for congestive heart failure (CHF), 128b
for systemic hypertension, 177t
used during prolonged life support, 120t
uses, formulations, and dosage of, 706t

G

Gabapentin
description of, 77
properties of, 78t
Gagging
cough-induced, 442
excessive
with pharyngeal foreign bodies,
159f, 160
Gait
assessing during cardiovascular exam, 316
assessing during neurological exam,
360-361
and coma scale, 192t
Gall bladder
clinical conditions involving, 87t
diagnostic tests, 84-85, 93
Gall bladder mucocele
abdominal characteristics of, 87t
Gallop dysrhythmias
with congestive heart failure, 128
Gallop heart sounds, 321
Gamma glutamyltransferase (GGT)
normal biochemistry ranges
for adult canines and felines, 577t
normal test ranges and interpretation, 594
Garbage
causing acute gastritis, 171-172
Garlic
toxicity and treatment of, 243-244
Gasoline
toxicity and treatment of, 237-238
Gastric decontamination
orogastric lavage for, 47-48
Gastric dilatation
abdominal symptoms of, 86t
Gastric dilatation-volvulus (GDV)
abdominal symptoms of, 86t
clinical signs of, 165-168
examples of, 166f, 167f
illustration of, 166f, 167f
orogastric lavage for, 47-48
Gastric ulcers
abdominal
characteristics of, 87t
Gastrin
normal test values and interpretation, 621
Gastritis
acute, 171-172

Gastroenteritis
bacterial
characteristics of, 86t
Gastrointestinal adenocarcinoma
in various paraneoplastic syndromes,
205t-206t
Gastrointestinal contrast radiography, 539-544
technique of, 539-544
Gastrointestinal motility
checking in shock "Rule of Twenty," 283
Gastrointestinal procedures, 526-532
Gastrointestinal protectants
for poisonings, 223
Gastrointestinal system
bleeding
as clinical sign of decompensation, 6b
clinical conditions of
causing acute abdominal pain, 84-85,
86t-87t, 93
emergencies
esophageal, 160-161
foreign bodies, 158-165
large intestine, 164
of oral cavity, 158-160
rectum and anus, 165
small intestine obstruction, 162-164
stomach, 161
examining in emergency poison/toxin
cases, 215b
obstruction
by tumors, 209-210
procedures, 526-532
toxicity from chemotherapy, 210-211
tumors
causing bowel obstruction, 170-171
Gemfibrozil
uses, formulations, and dosage of, 706t
Genitalia;*See also* reproductive tract
evaluation of patient's, 298
female, 136-141
male, 141-146
Genitourinary system
clinical conditions of
causing acute abdominal pain, 88t
Gentamicin
uses, formulations, and dosage of, 706t
Gerbils
blood laboratory values for, 651t
determining sex of, 650t
laboratory information on, 648t-649t
Giardia antigen test, 635
Giardia lambia
vaccinations
for cats, 661t
Gila monsters, 153-154
Gingiva
definition and illustration of, 306
examination of, 309-310, 311f
part of "BEETTS" test, 294
Gingival mucosa
and capillary refill time (CRT), 319

Glauber's salts, 220t
Glaucoma
    acute
        description and treatment of, 203-204
    versus conjunctivitis and iritis, 345t
    secondary to hyphema, 203
Glipizide
    uses, formulations, and dosage of, 706t
Globe
    examination of, 341-342
    protrusion of, 344
Globulin
    normal biochemistry ranges
        for adult canines and felines, 577t
    normal test ranges and interpretation, 594
Glottis
    foreign body obstruction of, 159-160
Glucagon stimulation
    normal test values and interpretation, 621
Glucocorticoids
    contraindicated in abdomen cases, 83t
    during shock therapy, 284-285
Glucocorticosteroids
    for feline bronchitis, 266t
    myelosuppression classification of, 210t
Glucosamine
    uses, formulations, and dosage of, 707t
Glucose
    checking in shock "Rule of Twenty," 282
    normal biochemistry ranges
        for adult canines and felines, 577t
    normal test ranges and interpretation, 594
    normal urinalysis ranges
        for adult canines and felines, 578t
    and osmolality, 38-39, 41
    testing during initial emergency care, 5
Glucose curve, 12-hour
    normal test values and interpretation, 621
Glucose tolerance tests
    normal test values and interpretation,
        622-623
Glue
    toxicity and treatment of, 238
Glyburide
    uses, formulations, and dosage of, 707t
Glycerin
    uses, formulations, and dosage of, 707t
Glycerol
    for acute glaucoma, 204t
Glycopyrrolate
    uses, formulations, and dosage of, 707t
Glycosylated hemoglobin
    normal test ranges and protocols, 602
Glyophosate
    toxicity and treatment of, 238
Gold sodium thiomalate
    uses, formulations, and dosage of, 707t
Gold therapy
    uses, formulations, and dosage of, 707t
GoLYTELY, 220t
    uses, formulations, and dosage of, 707t

Gonadorelin
    uses, formulations, and dosage of, 707t
Gonadotropin, human chorionic
    uses, formulations, and dosage of, 707t
Gonadotropin-releasing hormone
    uses, formulations, and dosage of, 707t
GOSH DARN IT
    as hypercalcemia mnemonic, 181, 183b
Granisetron, 707t
Grapes
    toxicity and treatment of, 238
Great Dane
    with breed predisposition
        to acute adrenocortical
            insufficiency, 184b
Great Pyrenees
    with breed predisposition
        to acute adrenocortical
            insufficiency, 184b
Greenstick fractures, 154b, 155-158
Griseofulvin
    uses, formulations, and dosage of, 708t
Growth hormone
    uses, formulations, and dosage of, 708t
Guinea pigs
    blood laboratory values for, 651t
    determining sex of, 650t
    laboratory information on, 648t-649t
Gums
    definition and illustration of, 306

H
Hageman factor, 104
Hair
    evaluation and examination of, 332,
        333f-335f, 336-339, 340t, 341
    fungal cultures, 472
    growth cycle, 414
    loss of
        assessment of, 333f-334f
        associated signs, 414
        causes of, 414-415
        definition of, 414
        differential diagnosis, 414-415, 415b
    part of "BEETTS" test, 294
Halitosis
    causes, 312
Halothane
    uses, formulations, and dosage of, 708t
Hamsters
    blood laboratory values for, 651t
    determining sex of, 650t
    laboratory information on, 648t-649t
Hashish (*See* marijuana)
    toxicity and treatment of, 241
Head
    initial examination of, 4
    neurological examination of, 362
Head aversion
    with head trauma, 186t, 187
"Head bob," 354

Head injuries, 185-188
  clinical signs of, 186t
  initial assessment of, 4
  levels of consciousness with, 186b
  localizing signs, 186t
  types of, 185-186
Head trauma;*See* head injuries
Healing
  classification of skeletal trauma, 154b
  moist, 9
  stages of open wound, 9
Hearing loss
  associated signs, 403
  definition of, 402-403
  differential diagnosis, 403-404
Heart
  assessing during initial emergency
      exam, 4
  evaluation of patient's, 298
  radiographs of, 327, 328f, 329-330
Heart contractility
  checking in shock "Rule of Twenty," 281t,
      279, 280
Heart disease
  congestive heart failure, 127-128
  patient assessment for, 315-316, 317t, 318
Heart murmurs
  causes of, 321-322
  common types of, 324-325, 326t
  with congestive heart failure, 128
  intensity of, 322-323, 326t
  location of, 323, 324f, 325f, 326t
  timing of, 322, 326t
Heart rate
  assessing during initial emergency exam, 4
  calculating with shock, 275-276
  and cardiac preload, 131
  checking in shock "Rule of Twenty," 281t,
      279, 280
  normal, 320
  normal parameters of
    for dogs and cats, 97t
Heart rhythm
  abnormalities
    and cardiac arrest, 114
  assessing during initial emergency exam, 4
  checking in shock "Rule of Twenty," 281t,
      279, 280
  normal, 320
Heart sounds
  absence of
    and cardiac arrest, 114
  normal, 320
Heart valves
  heart murmurs, 321-325, 326t
Heartworm antibody, feline
  test and interpretation, 635-636
Heartworm antigen, canine
  test and interpretation, 636
Heartworm antigen, feline
  test and interpretation, 636

Heartworm antigen test
  component of laboratory data, 300t
Heartworm disease
  associated with disseminated intravascular
      coagulation (DIC), 102-103
  clinical signs of, 130
  treatment of, 130-131
Heat stroke, 147-148
  assessing at accident scene, 2-3
Heat therapy
  during physical therapy, 497-498
Heat-induced illnesses, 147-148
Heloderma horridum, 153-154
Heloderma suspectum, 153-154
Hemangiosarcomas
  affecting heart and pericardium, 131-133
  of liver or spleen, 205t, 207
Hemarthrosis
  and joint fluid analysis, 357t-358t
Hematocrit (Hct)
  component of laboratory data, 300t
  declining
    as clinical sign of decompensation, 6b
  initial screening test, 607
  normal hematology ranges
    for adult canines and felines, 577t
  testing during initial emergency care, 5
Hematologic testing
  with EDTA, 475-476
Hematology
  component of laboratory data, 300t
  normal ranges for adult canines and
      felines, 577t
Hematuria
  associated signs, 394-395
  causes of, 396t
  definition of, 393-394
  differential diagnosis, 395
Hemiplegia
  with head trauma, 186t, 187
Hemistanding, 362
Hemobartonella test, 636-637
Hemodynamic techniques
  during ancillary diagnostic evaluation, 5
Hemoglobin
  component of laboratory data, 300t
  concentration
    and shock, 275-276
  normal hematology ranges
    for adult canines and felines, 577t
Hemoglobin glutamer
  uses, formulations, and dosage of, 708t
Hemoglobin saturation
  calculation of, 51
Hemoglobin-based oxygen carriers (HBOCs)
  description and function of, 32-33
Hemoglobinuria
  associated signs, 394-395
  causes of, 396t
  definition of, 393-394
  differential diagnosis, 397b

Hemolysis
  avoiding in blood samples, 581
HEMOPET
  emergency hotline number, 644t
Hemophilia
  laboratory results and interpretation, 107t
  and whole blood transfusions, 27-28
Hemophilia A, 103
Hemophilia B, 104
Hemoptysis
  associated signs, 402
  definition of, 401
  differential diagnosis, 402
Hemorrhages
  assessing at accident scene, 2-3
  associated signs, 430, 432
  causing decompensation, 6b
  definition of, 429-430
  differential diagnosis, 432, 433b
  due to oncologic emergencies, 205-211
  gastrointestinal, 209-210
  with head injuries, 185-186
  minor
    in need of pressure bandages, 10
  subdural or extradural head, 188
Hemorrhagic abdominal effusion,
    205t-206t, 207
Hemorrhagic effusions
  with pleural effusion
    characteristics of, 261t-262t
Hemorrhagic gastroenteritis (HGE)
  definition of, 171, 173
Hemorrhagic pericardial effusion, 132t
Hemorrhagic pleural effusions, 261t-262t,
    263-264
Hemorrhagic shock
  assessing during initial emergency exam, 4
Hemorrhagic thoracic effusion, 208
Hemostasis
  acquired disorders of, 104-107
  causes of defective, 100b
  and coagulation tests, 606-616
    hematocrit, 607
  congenital defects of, 103, 104
  disorders
    and whole blood transfusions, 27-28
    normal ranges for adult canines and
      felines, 578t
Hemostatic factors
  causing bleeding, 100-101
Hemothorax
  description and immediate management of,
    261t-262t, 263-264
Heparin
  causing anaphylactic reactions, 94b
Heparin sodium
  uses, formulations, and dosage of, 708t
Heparinized saline flush, 497b
Hepatic abscesses
  abdominal characteristics of, 87t
Hepatic coma, 193, 194t

Hepatic disease
  causing acute diarrhea, 406b
Hepatic encephalopathy (HE)
  characteristics of, 193
  grades and signs of, 194t
Hepatic failure
  causing acute gastritis, 171-172
  clinical signs of, 174-175
Hepatic neoplasia
  abdominal characteristics of, 87t
Hepatic system
  examining in emergency poison/toxin
    cases, 215b
Hepatic torsion
  abdominal characteristics of, 87t
Hepatitis
  abdominal characteristics of, 87t
Hepatocellular (AST, ALT) enzymes
  elevation and hepatic failure, 175
Hepatocellular carcinomas
  in paraneoplastic syndromes, 206t, 207
Hepatocutaneous syndrome
  skin lesions or signs of, 338t
Hepatoma
  in paraneoplastic syndromes, 206t, 207
Herbicides
  toxicity and treatment of, 235, 245
Herding group, 646t
Hernias
  abdominal wall
    characteristics of, 86t
  diaphragmatic
    characteristics of, 86t
  causing pericardial effusion, 132t
  scrotal, 142-143
  strangulation
    causing small intestine obstruction,
      162-164, 170
Herniated disks
  and back trauma, 189
  corticosteroid dosage for, 190b
  examination and prognosis of, 189
  localizing signs of, 190t
  treatment and management of, 189-190
Herpes virus
  vaccinations
    for cats, 661t
Hetastarch, 4
Hexachlorophene
  toxicity and treatment of, 233-234
Higher centers
  within sensing and response system, 70
High-rise syndrome
  in cats, 158
Hip dysplasia
  clinical signs of, 355-356
  size and breed disposition to, 352t
Hips
  injuries to, 191
  orthopedic diseases affecting, 352-353t,
    354-356

Histiocytic hypoxia
  cause and response to oxygen, 48t
Histopathology
  guidelines, 584-585
Hopping, 361
Horner's syndrome, 191t, 344, 365
  initial examination to look for, 4
Hound group, 645t
Household emergencies, 146-148
Human poison control centers, 212
Humerus
  spica splints, 21
Hydralazine
  to induce vasodilation, 280t
  for systemic hypertension, 177t
  uses, formulations, and dosage of, 708t
Hydroadrenocorticism
  abdominal symptoms of, 86t
Hydrocarbons
  toxicity and treatment of, 239
Hydrochloric acid
  toxicity and treatment of, 224
Hydrochlorothiazide
  for systemic hypertension, 177t
  uses, formulations, and dosage of, 708t
Hydrocodone bitartrate, 708t
Hydrocortisone, 708t
Hydrocortisone sodium succinate
  uses, formulations, and dosage of, 708t
Hydrogen peroxide
  as emetic for poisonings, 219t
Hydromorphone
  for abdominal pain, 83t
  properties of
    for pain management, 74t
  uses, formulations, and dosage of, 709t
Hydrostatic pressure
  CVP measurement of, 33-34
Hydrotherapy
  during physical therapy, 497
Hydroxyethyl starch
  uses, formulations, and dosage of, 708t
Hydroxyurea
  uses, formulations, and dosage of, 709t
Hydroxyzine
  uses, formulations, and dosage of, 709t
Hypalgesia
  and spinal cord, 360f
Hyperadrenocorticism
  skin lesions or signs of, 338t
Hypercalcemia
  causes of, 183b
  clinical signs and treatment of, 181,
    183, 206t
  tumor types, 206t
Hyperestrogenemia
  in various paraneoplastic syndromes,
    205t-206t
Hypergammaglobulinemia
  clinical signs and treatment of, 206t
  tumor types, 206t

Hyperglycemia
  clinical signs and treatment of, 206t
  tumor types, 206t
Hyperkalemia
  atrial standstill with, 125, 126f
  definition of, 38
  differential diagnoses for, 39b
  with uroabdomen, 290
Hyperkeratosis, 337t
Hyperkinetic pulse, 319b
Hypernatremia
  differential diagnoses for, 41b
  fluid therapy for, 42
Hyperosmolar nonketotic diabetes,
    179-180
Hyperosmolarity
  and coma, 193
Hyperpigmentation, 337t
Hyperpnea
  definition of, 317b
  with dyspnea, 410
Hypersensitization
  causing anaphylactic reactions, 94b
Hypertension
  definition of, 176
  drugs used to treat, 177t
  normal and abnormal values of
    systolic blood pressure, 463t
  systemic, 176-177
  systolic blood pressure with, 463t
Hyperthermia
  description of, 147
  following head injuries, 186-188
  malignant, 148-149
  treatment of, 148
Hyperthyroidism
  features and treatment of, 184-185
  feline, 351
Hypertrophic cardiomyopathy
  in cats, 128
  differential diagnoses of, 331t
Hypertrophic osteodystrophy
  size and breed disposition to, 353t
Hyperventilation
  and acid-base status, 36-37
  and acidosis, 36-37
Hyphema
  description and treatment of,
    201-202
Hypoadrenocorticism, 183-184
  causing acute diarrhea, 406b
Hypocalcemia
  eclampsia, 181, 182t
  treatment of, 182t
Hypoglossal nerves, 367, 368f, 369
Hypoglycemia
  causes of, 181b
  clinical features of, 180
Hypokalemia
  definition of, 38
  differential diagnoses for, 40b

Hyponatremia
  differential diagnoses for, 41b
  fluid therapy for, 42
Hypotension
  causes and treatment of, 98t
  definition of, 97
  systolic blood pressure values, 463t
Hypothalamus
  lesions in, 370
Hypothermia
  definition and management of, 147
Hypothyroidism, 351
Hypotonia, 362-363
Hypoventilation
  and acid-base status, 36-37
Hypovolemic shock
  assessing during initial emergency exam, 4
  definition and characteristics of, 276
  heart characteristics during, 279, 280, 281t
Hypoxia
  types of, 48t
Hypoxic hypoxia
  cause and response to oxygen, 48t

I

Iatrogenic metabolic alkalosis
  and shock, 282
Ibuprofen
  toxicity and treatment of, 243
Icterus mucous membranes
  associated signs, 447
  definition of, 446
  differential diagnosis, 447-448
Idiopathic thrombocytic purpura,
    105-106
Idioventricular rhythm, 121, 122f, 123
Ifosfamide
  uses, formulations, and dosage of, 709t
Imaging techniques;See also radiographs
  during ancillary diagnostic evaluation, 5
Imidacloprid
  toxicity and treatment of, 239
  uses, formulations, and dosage of, 709t
Imidocarb dipropionate, 709t
Imipenem, 709t
Imipramine, 709t
Immobilization
  of fractures, 10-11
  wounds in need of, 12, 16f, 17f, 18-21
Immune response suppression agents
  for angioneurotic edema, 95b
Immune system
  function
    checking in shock "Rule of Twenty," 283
Immune-mediated diseases
  associated with disseminated intravascular
      coagulation (DIC), 102-103
  types of
    and skin manifestations of, 340t
Immune-mediated thrombocytopenia
  treatment of, 106

Implanted subcutaneous fluid ports
  technique of, 459
Impression smears
  techniques of, 586-587
Incisions
  classification of soft tissue, 271, 272t
Incoordination
  associated signs, 416
  definition of, 415
  differential diagnosis, 416b, 417
Indomethacin
  uses, formulations, and dosage of, 710t
Indwelling catheters
  maintenance of, 496
  as vascular access technique, 68-69
Infections
  causing acute diarrhea, 406b
  soft tissue wound, 271, 272t
Infectious agents
  causing acute hepatic failure, 175b
Infectious diseases
  serology and microbiology
    Agar gel immunodiffusion, 631
    anaplasma phagocytophila antibody, 628
    aspergillus antibody titer, 628-629
    bacteria blood culture, 630
    bartonella antibody titer, 628-629
    blastomycosis antibody titer, 629-630
    Borrelia Burgdorferi, 630, 637-639
    canine distemper antibody, 631
    coccidioidomycosis antibody titer
        (AGID), 632
    cryptococcal antigen, 632
    Ehricichia canis antibody, 632-633
    Ehrlichia, 633
    feline immunodeficiency virus antibody,
        634-635
    feline infectious anemia, 636-637
    feline leukemia virus antigen,
        633-634
    Giardia antigen, 635
    haemobartonella, 636-637
    heartworm antibody, feline, 635-636
    heartworm antigen, canine, 636
    heartworm antigen, feline, 636
    leptospirosis antibody titer, 637
    Lyme borreliosis, 637-639
    rabies titer, 637-639
    Rocky Mountain Spotted Fever (RMSF),
        639-640
    serum I_GG or I_GM, 631-632
    toxoplasmosis titers, 640
    vaccine titers, 640
    virus neutralization (VN) test, 632
  types of
    and skin manifestations of, 339t
Infectious epididymitis, 143
Infectious orchitis, 143
Infectious orchitis and epididymitis, 143
Infertility
  causes of, 375

Inflammation
  associated with disseminated intravascular
      coagulation (DIC), 102-103
  eyelid, 344
Inflammatory bowel diseases
  causing acute gastritis, 171-172
  causing acute hepatic failure, 175b
Infusions
  of local anesthetic, 61f
Inhalation
  assessing during initial emergency exam, 3-4
Injections
  technique of, 457
Injuries
  bandaging and splinting techniques, 8-12,
      13f-17f, 18-19, 20f, 21
  bowel perforation, 170-171
  brachial plexus, 191
  burns
    assessing at accident scene, 2-3
    chemical, 111-112
    electrical, 110-111
    radiation, 112
    thermal, 108-110
  cardiac
    from thoracic trauma, 264-265
  of eyes, 196-204
  head, 185-188
  musculoskeletal trauma
    articular cartilage injuries, 157
    classification of, 154b
    high-rise syndrome, 158
    immediate action, 154-155
    ligament injuries, 157, 158b
    open wounds, 156b, 157
    treatment of, 155-157
  ocular, 196-204
  to peripheral nervous system, 190-191
  spinal cord, 188-190
  superficial soft tissue, 271-274, 275t
In-patient medical records, 302-303
Insect stings
  causing anaphylactic reactions, 94b
Inspiration
  assessing during initial emergency exam, 3-4
Inspiratory dyspnea
  assessing during cardiovascular exam, 316
  with lower respiratory disease, 378
Insulin
  administration of
    for diabetic ketoacidosis, 178-179, 180t
  causing anaphylactic reactions, 94b
  normal test values and interpretation, 623
  rate of infusion, 180t
Insulinoma
  in paraneoplastic syndromes, 206t, 207
Intact female dogs
  normal breeding physiology and behavior,
      382-383
Intact male dogs
  characteristics, 383

Integumentary system
  clinical history, 332, 335f-336f
  evaluation and examination of, 332,
      333f-335f, 336-339, 340t, 341
  examining in emergency poison/toxin
      cases, 215b
  topical administration
    of medications, 457
Intensity
  of heart murmurs, 322-323, 325f, 326t
Intercostal nerve blocks, 81
Interferon
  uses, formulations, and dosage of, 710t
International system of units (SI)
  conversion tables, 656t-658t
Internet
  poison/toxin information from, 212,
      213b, 214
Intestinal parasites
  causing acute diarrhea, 406b
Intestinal perforation, 87t
Intestinal tract
  examination of, 314-315
Intestines
  and gastric dilatation-volvulus (GDV),
      165-168
  large
    obstruction, 169-170
  small intestine volvulus, 168-169
Intraabdominal lesions
  affecting urinary tract, 208-209
Intracellular fluid deficit
  and acid-base physiology, 35-37
  anion gap, 36b, 42
  calculations of deficits/losses, 43
  clinical signs of, 35t
  crystalloid and colloid fluids, 43,
      45-46
  and dehydration, 35t
  diagnosis of, 34-35
  and electrolyte imbalance, 37-39, 40t
  maintenance fluid requirements, 43, 44t
  and metabolic acidosis, 36b
  and metabolic alkalosis, 35-37
  oncotic pressure, 42-43
  and osmolality, 38-39
  planning and implementing, 46-47
  and potassium imbalances, 37-38,
      39b, 40t
  rates of administration, 47
  and sodium, 39, 41, 41b, 42
Intracranial hemorrhages
  with head injuries, 185-186
  seizures with, 188
Intracranial injuries
  visual deficits with, 187
Intracranial lesions
  clinical signs of, 369-370
Intradermal injections
  technique of, 459
Intradermal skin testing, 339

Intraluminal masses
  description and immediate management
    of, 257
Intramedullary infusion, 47
Intramural lesions
  affecting urinary tract, 208-209
Intramuscular injections
  technique of, 459
Intraocular pressure, 203-204
Intraosseous access
  establishing during initial emergency
    exam, 4
Intraosseous catheters
  as vascular access technique, 69
Intraosseous infusion, 47
Intraosseous injections
  technique of, 461-462
Intrapleural blockades, 79
Intrauterine diseases, 375
Intravenous catheters
  for central venous pressure, 33-34
  types and sizes of, 58-69
Intravenous fluid therapy
  to clear toxins, 222
Intravenous fluids
  administration
    description of, 46-47
  following head injuries, 185-186
  infusion, 47
  injections
    technique of, 460-461
  vascular access techniques
    catheter sizes and types, 58-59
    central venous catheters, 59-62, 59f-60f
    cephalic catheterization, 62, 65f, 66-67,
      66f, 67f
    during initial examination, 4
    intraosseous catheter placement, 69
    maintenance of indwelling catheters,
      68-69
    percutaneous dorsal pedal artery
      catheterization, 68
    percutaneous over-the-wire jugular
      catheter, 61-62
    percutaneous through-the-needle jugular
      catheter, 59-61
    peripheral arterial and venous catheter
      placement, 62, 65f, 66-67
    Seldinger technique, 61-62, 62f-63f
    surgical cutdown
      for catheter placement, 68
Intravenous infusion lines, 58-59
Intravenous injections
  technique of, 460-461
Intussusception
  characteristics of, 87t
  definition of, 165
  causing small intestine obstruction,
    162-164
Invasive testing
  types of emergency, 5

Invertebral disk diseases
  causing acute abdominal pain, 89t
Iodinated contrast media
  causing anaphylactic reactions, 94b
Ion exchange resins
  for poisons, 220-221
Ionized calcium
  normal biochemistry ranges
    for adult canines and felines, 577t
Ion-trapping
  to clear toxins, 222
Ipecac syrup
  uses, formulations, and dosage of, 710t
Ipodate
  uses, formulations, and dosage of, 710t
Iris
  examination of, 347
  foreign bodies damaging, 200-201
Iritis
  versus conjunctivitis and glaucoma, 345t
Iron
  normal test ranges and protocols,
    602-603
  toxicity and treatment of, 221, 239
  uses, formulations, and dosage of, 710t
Isoflurane
  uses, formulations, and dosage of, 710t
Isoproterenol
  used during advanced life
    support, 120t
  uses, formulations, and dosage of, 710t
Isosorbide dinitrate, 710t
Isosorbide mononitrate, 710t
Isotretinoin, 710t
Itching
  associated signs, 420
  definition of, 418, 420
  differential diagnosis, 420, 421b
Itraconazole
  uses, formulations, and dosage of, 710t
Ivermectin
  toxicity and treatment of, 239-240
  uses, formulations, and dosage of, 711t

J
Jaundice
  associated signs, 447
  definition of, 446
  differential diagnosis, 447-448
Jejunum
  plication of
    by linear foreign objects, 163f
Joint fluid analysis, 356, 357t-358t
Joints
  arthrocentesis with joint fluid analysis, 356,
    357t-358t
  fluid analysis, 356, 357t-358t
  injuries to, 157
  open wounds to, 156-167
  orthopedic diseases affecting, 352-353t,
    354-356

Joints—cont'd
  swelling of
    associated signs, 420-421
    definition of, 420
    differential diagnosis, 421-422
Jugular vein
  assessing during cardiovascular exam,
      316, 318
  catheter sizes for, 58t
  catheterization, 495-496
Jugular venipuncture, 460
J-wire, 62f, 63f

K
Kanamycin
  uses, formulations, and dosage of, 711t
Kaopectate, 711t
Keratic precipitates, 343, 344f
Kerosene
  toxicity and treatment of, 237-238
Ketamine
  description of, 77
  properties of, 78t
  uses, formulations, and dosage of, 711t
Ketoconazole
  uses, formulations, and dosage of, 711t
Ketones
  normal urinalysis ranges
    for adult canines and felines, 578t
Ketoprofen
  dosage for pain, 75t
  uses, formulations, and dosage
      of, 712t
Ketorolac
  dosage for pain, 75t
Ketorolac tromethamine
  uses, formulations, and dosage of, 712t
Kidneys;See also renal
  abdominal palpation of, 386
  hematuria diseases of, 396t
  and hypertension, 176
  urinary tract emergencies
    acute renal failure, 288-289
    azotemia, 287
    feline lower urinary tract
        disease, 289
    postrenal azotemia, 289
    prerenal azotemia, 287-288
    urinary tract obstruction, 289
    uroabdomen, 290-291
Kittens
  fractures in, 158
  intussusception in, 165

L
Laboratory database
  components for minimum
      for dogs and cats, 300t
Laboratory tests
  for abdomen diagnosis, 84-85,
      90t-92t

Laboratory tests—cont'd
  ancillary hemostasis tests
    D-timers, 609
    fibrinogen degradation products
        (FDPs), 609
    fibrinogen levels, 609
    PIVKA test, 609
    saline agglutination test, 609
    thrombin time, 608-609
  coagulation profiles, 107t
  coagulation tests
    activated clotting time (ACT), 610
    activated partial thromboplastin time
        (APTT), 610
    blood typing for complete dog erythrocyte
        antigen (DEA), 611
    buccal mucosal bleeding time
        (BMBT), 611
    clot retraction test, 611
    coagulation factor activity, 611-612
    cross-matching, 612-613
    D-timer, 613
    feline blood typing, 610-611
    fibrin degradation products, 614
    fibrinogen, 614
    fragment D-timer, 613
    PIVKA test, 614
    platelet counts, 615
    prothrombin time (PT), 615
    "thrombotest," 614-615
    Von Willebrand factor, 615-616
  and diagnosis protocols
    analytes or test names, 589-591
    avoiding clots and platelet clumps, 581
    body fluids, 588
    bone marrow tests, 588
    common reference range values, 577t-580t
    cytopathology, 585-589
    cytopathology guidelines, 584-585
    exfoliative cytology, 586-587
    fine needle aspiration (FNA), 584-585
    histopathology guidelines, 584-585
    histopathy, 584-585
    impression smears, 586-587
    lavender/purple topped tubes, 579t
    minimizing hemolysis, 581
    normal arterial blood gas analysis ranges,
        578t-579t
    normal biochemistry ranges, 577t
    normal hematology ranges, 577t
    normal hemostasis ranges, 578t
    normal urinalysis ranges, 578t
    patient preparation, 581
    rabies testing, 582-584
    red-topped tubes, 579t
    routine biochemistry, 589-591
    routine biochemistry profiles, 589-591
    sample handling, 576, 580-582
    staining options, 586-589
    submission requirements for rabies
        suspects, 582-583

Laboratory tests—cont'd
and diagnosis protocols—cont'd
swabs, scrapings, washings or brushings, 587-588
"tiger-topped tubes," 579t
types of sample tubes, 579t
endocrinology tests
ACTH stimulation test, 617
adrenocorticotrophic hormone (ACTH) test, 616
aldosterone, 617-618
canine thyrotropin, 626
cobalamin, 618
dexamethasone suppression test, 618-620
estradiol, 620
folate, 620
fructosamine, 620-621
gastrin, 621
glucagon stimulation (IVGS), 621
glucose curve, 12-hour, 621
glucose tolerance tests, 622-623
insulin, 623
parathyroid hormone (PTH), 623
parathyroid hormone-related (PTHrP), 623-624
resting cortisol, 618
T_1 to T_4, 624-626
thyroid-stimulating hormone (TSH), 626
thyrotropin, 626
thyrotropin response (TSH), 626
triiodothyronine, 624-626
vitamin B_{12}, 618
hemostasis and coagulation tests, 606-616
activated clotting time (ACT), 607-608
buccal mucosal bleeding time (BMBT), 608
hematocrit, 607
initial in-office screening tests, 607-608
peripheral blood smear, 607
platelet count, 607
prothrombin time (PT), 608
immunology tests
allergen-specific IGE antibody tests, 626-627
antinuclear antibody (ANA), 627
antiplatelet antibody, 627
Coombs test, 627
rheumatoid factor, canine, 628
infectious disease serology and microbiology
Agar gel immunodiffusion, 631
Anaplasma phagocytophila antibody, 628
Aspergillus antibody titer, 628-629
bacteria blood culture, 630
Bartonella antibody titer, 628-629
blastomycosis antibody titer, 629-630
Borrelia burgdorferi, 630, 637-639
canine distemper antibody, 631
coccidioidomycosis antibody titer (AGID), 632
cryptococcal antigen, 632
Ehricichia canis antibody, 632-633

Laboratory tests—cont'd
infectious disease serology and microbiology—cont'd
Ehrlichia, 633
feline immunodeficiency virus antibody, 634-635
feline infectious anemia, 636-637
feline leukemia virus antigen, 633-634
Giardia antigen, 635
haemobartonella, 636-637
heartworm antibody, feline, 635-636
heartworm antigen, canine, 636
heartworm antigen, feline, 636
leptospirosis antibody titer, 637
Lyme borreliosis, 637-639
rabies titer, 637-639
Rocky Mountain Spotted Fever (RMSF), 639-640
serum I_GG or I_GM, 631-632
toxoplasmosis titers, 640
vaccine titers, 640
virus neutralization (VN) test, 632
interpreting office coagulation screen, 580t
minimum database, 300t
for pocket pets, 648t-649t
of renal function, 386
and routine diagnosis protocols
alanine aminotransferase (ALT), 591
albumin, 591
albumin/globulin ratio (A:G), 591
alkaline phosphatase, 591-592
amylase, 592
anion gap, 592
aspartate aminotransferase, 592
bicarbonate (HCO_3), 592
bilirubin, 592-593
blood urea nitrogen (BUN), 593
calcium, 593
chloride (CI), 593
cholesterol (Ch), 593-594
creatine kinase (CK), 594
creatinine, 594
gamma glutamyltransferase (GGT), 594
globulin, 594
glucose, 594
lipase, 595
phosphorus (P), 595
potassium (K^+), 595
sodium (Na^+), 595
total protein, 595
triglyceride (TG), 595
samples
identification of, 576
and special diagnosis protocols
ammonia (NH_3), 596-597
ammonia tolerance, 597
antinuclear antibody (ANA), 597-598
arterial blood gases, 598
body fluids for chemistry analysis, 599
calcium (ionized), 599
cerebrospinal fluids (CSF), 599-600

Laboratory tests—cont'd
  and special diagnosis protocols—cont'd
    cobalamin, 600
    ethylene glycol, 600-601
    fecal fat, 601
    fecal occult blood, 601
    folate, 601
    fructosamine, 602
    glycosylated hemoglobin, 602
    iron, 602-603
    lactate, 603
    lactic acid, 603
    lead, 603
    lipoprotein electrophoresis, 604
    magnesium (Mg), 604
    osmolality (estimated serum), 604-605
    pancreatic lipase immunoreactivity
      (PLI), 605
    protein electrophoresis, 605-606
    trypsin-like immunoreactivity
      (canine TLI), 606
    trypsin-like immunoreactivity
      (feline TLI), 606
    venous blood gases, 598
    vitamin B_{12}, 599-600
  types of emergency, 5
  types of sample tubes
    brown-topped tubes, 580t
    dark blue-topped tubes, 580t
    dark green-topped tubes, 579t
    gray-topped tubes, 580t
    lavender/purple topped tubes, 579t
    light blue-topped tubes, 579t
    red-topped tubes, 579t
    "tiger-topped tubes," 579t
    yellow-topped tubes, 580t
  urinalysis
    microalbuminuria test, 641
    urine cortisol: creatinine ratio, 641-642
    urine protein-creatinine ratio, 642
Lacerations
  classification of soft tissue, 271, 272t
  with head injuries, 185-186
Lacrimal system
  examination of, 346
Lactate
  for acute abdomen conditions, 85, 90t-92t
  balance
    checking in shock "Rule of Twenty," 282
  normal test ranges and protocols, 603
Lactated Ringer's solution, 45t
  uses, formulations, and dosage of, 712t
Lactic acid
  normal test ranges and protocols, 603
Lactulose
  uses, formulations, and dosage of, 712t
Lagophthalmos, 344
Lameness
  grading with orthopedic diseases,
    352t-353t
  radiography, 356

Laparoscopy
  technique of, 532-534
Laparotomy
  indications to perform exploratory, 92b, 93
Large intestines
  diarrhea characteristics, 407t, 408t
  gastrointestinal system emergencies, 164
  obstruction
    obstipation, 169-170
Laryngeal collapse
  description and immediate management
    of, 256
Laryngeal obstruction, 382
Laryngeal paralysis
  description and immediate management of,
    255-256
Larynx
  collapse or paralysis of, 255-256
  emergencies of, 253-265
  evaluation of patient's, 298
  examination of, 376-377
L-asparaginase
  myelosuppression classification of, 210t
  uses, formulations and dosage of, 688
Lateral saphenous venipuncture, 460-461
Lateral splints
  procedures for, 19, 21
L-Dopa
  uses, formulations, and dosage of, 712t
Lead
  normal test ranges and protocols, 603
  toxicity and treatment of, 240
Left atrium
  radiographic description of, 329-330
Left ventricle
  radiographic description of, 329-330
Legg-Calve-Perthes disease
  size and breed disposition to, 353t
Leiomyomas
  causing bowel obstruction, 170
  in paraneoplastic syndromes, 206t, 207
Leiomyosarcomas
  causing bowel obstruction, 170
  gastrointestinal tract, 209-210
Length
  metric conversions of, 659t
Lens
  examination of, 347
    during ocular emergencies, 197
  foreign bodies damaging, 200-201
Leptospira
  vaccinations
    for dogs, 661t
Leptospirosis antibody titer, 637
Lesions
  assessment of individual skin, 336-339
  classification of skin, 337t
  and skin disorders, 332, 333f-336f, 336-339,
    340t, 341
  from spider bites, 152-153
  systemic diseases with skin, 338t

Lethargy
  with abdominal conditions, 86t-89t
Leucovorin
  uses, formulations, and dosage of, 712t
Leukemia
  in various paraneoplastic syndromes,
    205t-206t
Levamisole
  uses, formulations, and dosage of, 712t
Levodopa
  uses, formulations, and dosage of, 712t
Levothyroxine sodium, 713t
Licking
  abnormal
    as sign of pain, 72b
Lidocaine
  for abdominal pain, 83t
  causing anaphylactic reactions, 94b
  as topical and infiltrative blockage, 79
  used during prolonged life support, 120t
  uses, formulations, and dosage of, 713t
  for ventricular dysrhythmias, 281t
Lids;See eyelids
Life support
  basic and advanced, 113-114, 115f, 116f, 117
  prolonged, 119-120
Ligaments
  injuries to, 157, 158b
  periodontal
    definition and illustration of, 306
Limbs
  initial examination of, 5
  injuries to, 191t
  orthopedic diseases in, 351, 352t-353t,
    354-356
  pelvic function
    grading scale, 360b
  swelling of
    associated signs, 437
    definition of, 435
    differential diagnosis, 437, 438b
Linalool
  toxicity and treatment of, 240
Lincomycin
  uses, formulations, and dosage of, 713t
Linear foreign bodies
  characteristics of gastrointestinal, 87t
  difficulties with, 163-164
Linear fractures
  with head injuries, 185-186
Liothyronine
  uses, formulations, and dosage of, 713t
Lipase
  normal biochemistry ranges
    for adult canines and felines, 577t
  normal test ranges and interpretation, 595
Lipomas
  around lymph nodes or thyroid, 350
Lipoprotein electrophoresis
  normal test ranges and protocols, 604
Lipoxygenase, 76

Lisinopril
  to induce vasodilation, 280t
  uses, formulations, and dosage of, 713t
Lithium carbonate
  uses, formulations, and dosage of, 713t
Liver
  acute hepatic failure, 174-175
  clinical conditions involving, 87t
  diagnostic tests, 84-85, 93, 990t-92t
  enlargement
    with heart disease, 331b
  hepatic coma, 193, 194t
  neoplastic masses of, 205t-206t, 207
  palpation to examine, 318
Liver biopsy
  technique of, 503-504
Livestock
  rabies control in, 675t
Lizards
  bites from, 153-154
Loop diuretics
  for systemic hypertension, 177t
Loperamide
  toxicity and treatment of, 241
  uses, formulations, and dosage of, 714t
Loss of vision
  description and treatment of, 196b
Lower respiratory tract
  bronchoalveolar lavage, 566-567
  clinical signs of disease, 563
  endotracheal wash, 563-564
  evaluation and examination of, 377-380,
    381f, 382
  lung fine-needle aspiration, 567-568
  transtracheal aspiration, 563
Lower urinary tract
  examination of, 384-386
Loxosceles bites, 152-153
Lubricating oils
  toxicity and treatment of, 237-238
Lufenuron
  uses, formulations, and dosage of, 714t
Lumbar
  enlargement, 371t, 372
Luminal foreign bodies
  characteristics of gastrointestinal, 87t
Lungs
  assessing during initial emergency exam, 3-4
  examination of
    with lower respiratory disease, 377-380,
      381f, 382
  pulmonary diseases
    acute respiratory distress syndrome
      (ARDS), 267-268
    aspiration pneumonia, 267
    contusions, 266-267
    epistaxis, 269-270
    feline asthma, 265-266
    feline bronchitis, 265-266
    feline lower airway disease, 265-266
    pulmonary edema, 267-268

Lungs—cont'd
  pulmonary diseases—cont'd
    pulmonary thromboembolism (PTE),
      268-269
    smoke inhalation, 269
  radiograph of cat, 381f
  respiratory emergencies, 253-265
Lupus erythematosus (LE)
  and joint fluid analysis, 357t-358t
Luteinizing hormone
  uses, formulations, and dosage of, 714t
Luxations, 154b, 155-156
Lyme borreliosis test, 637-639
Lyme disease
  vaccinations
    for dogs, 661t
Lymph nodes
  differential diagnoses of, 351
  enlargement
    associated signs, 423
    definition of, 423
    differential diagnosis, 423-424
  evaluation and examination of, 350-351
  examining in emergency poison/toxin
    cases, 215b
  normal, 350
Lymphadenomegaly, 350, 351
  associated signs, 423
  definition of, 423
  differential diagnosis, 423-424
Lymphocytes
  normal hematology ranges
    for adult canines and felines, 577t
  parameter in joint fluid analysis, 357t-358t
Lymphomas
  gastrointestinal tract, 209-210
  in various paraneoplastic syndromes,
    205t-206t
Lymphosarcomas
  diagnosis of, 351
Lysine
  uses, formulations, and dosage of, 714t

M

Macadamia nuts
  toxicity and treatment of, 241
Macrophages
  parameter in joint fluid analysis, 357t-358t
Magnesium chloride
  used during advanced life support, 120t
  uses, formulations, and dosage of, 714t
Magnesium citrate, 714t
Magnesium hydroxide
  uses, formulations, and dosage of, 714t
Magnesium (Mg)
  normal test ranges and protocols, 604
Magnesium sulfate
  uses, formulations, and dosage of, 714t
Male genitalia
  emergencies involving, 141-146
  evaluation of patient's, 298

Male reproductive tract
  emergencies of, 141-146
    acute prostatitis, 143-144
    acute scrotal dermatitis, 142
    infectious orchitis and epididymitis, 143
    os penis fracture, 144
    paraphimosis, 144-145
    penis lacerations, 144
    scrotal hernia, 142-143
    scrotal trauma, 141-142
    testicular torsion, 143
    urethral prolapse, 145-146
  evaluation and examination of, 373
Males
  intact cat characteristics, 384
  intact dog characteristics, 383
Malnourishment
  associated signs, 445
  definition of, 445
  differential diagnosis, 445, 446f
  evaluation during patient exam,
    296-297
Mammary adenocarcinoma
  in paraneoplastic syndromes, 206t, 207
Mammary glands
  enlargement during pregnancy, 375-376
  tumors, 374-375
Mandible
  supernumerary teeth, 308, 309f
Manipulation
  techniques for orthopedic diseases,
    354-355
Mannitol
  for acute glaucoma, 204t
  used during prolonged life support, 120t
  uses, formulations, and dosage of, 714t
Manometers, 404f
Marbofloxacin
  uses, formulations, and dosage of, 715t
Marijuana
  toxicity and treatment of, 241
Mass
  metric conversions of, 659t
Massage therapy
  during physical therapy, 499-500
Masses
  intra/extraluminal
    description and immediate management
      of, 257
Mast cell tumors
  around lymph nodes or thyroid, 350
  of gastrointestinal tract, 209-210
Mastitis
  causing acute abdominal pain, 88t
Matches
  toxicity and treatment of, 241
Maxilla
  supernumerary teeth, 308, 309f
MCT oil, 715t
Mean arterial blood pressure
  elevations of, 177

Mean corpuscular hemoglobin (MCH)
  normal hematology ranges
    for adult canines and felines, 577t
Mean corpuscular volume (MCV)
  normal hematology ranges
    for adult canines and felines, 577t
Mebendazole
  uses, formulations, and dosage of, 715t
Mechanical ventilation
  rule of sixties, 50-51
Meclofenamate
  uses, formulations, and dosage of, 715t
Medetomidine
  properties of
    for pain management, 75t
  uses, formulations, and dosage of, 715t
Medial patella luxation
  size and breed disposition to, 352t
Medial saphenous venipuncture, 461
Mediastinum
  diseases causing widening in, 331
Medical records
  content of, 302-303
  emergency, 303
  evaluation and examination of, 301-304
  importance and purpose of, 301-302
  in-patient, 302-303
  out-patient, 303
Medications;See also drugs
  advanced and prolonged life support, 120t
  cardiovascular exam questions
    concerning, 315
  common indications and dosages of,
    685t-742t
  prescription writing do's and don'ts, 684t
Medium-chain triglycerides
  uses, formulations, and dosage of, 715t
Medlizine, 715t
Medroxyprogesterone acetate, 715t
Medulla
  lesions, 369-370
Megestrol acetate
  uses, formulations, and dosage of, 715t
Melaleuca oil
  toxicity and treatment of, 250
Melarsomine, 716t
Meloxicam
  dosage for pain, 75t
  uses, formulations, and dosage of, 716t
Melphalan
  myelosuppression classification of, 210t
  uses, formulations, and dosage of, 716t
Meningitis
  causing acute abdominal pain, 89t
Mental attitude
  and behavior
    assessing during neurological exam, 359-360
Mentation
  and behavior
    assessing during neurological exam,
      359-360

Mentation—cont'd
  decreased with head injuries, 188
  evaluation during patient exam, 296-297
  in shock "Rule of Twenty," 282
Meperidine
  uses, formulations, and dosage of, 716t
Mepivicaine, 716t
6-Mercaptopurine
  uses, formulations, and dosage of, 716t
Meropenem, 716t
Mesalamine, 717t
Mesencephalon
  lesions in, 370
Mesenteric torsion, 168-169
Mesentery
  mesenteric torsion, 168-169
Mesotheliomas
  affecting heart and pericardium, 131-133
  description of, 207, 208
Metabolic acidosis
  from bicarbonate depletion, 38
  and fluid therapy, 36b
  renal and respiratory responses to, 37t
  and shock, 282
Metabolic alkalosis
  differential diagnoses of, 35b
  and fluid therapy, 35-37
  renal and respiratory responses to, 37t
Metabolic disorders
  abdominal symptoms of, 86t
Metabolic emergencies, 178-185
  acute adrenocortical insufficiency, 183-184
  diabetic ketoacidosis (DKA), 178-179, 180t
  hyperosmolar nonketotic diabetes, 179-180
  hypoadrenocorticism, 183-194
  hypocalcemia, 181, 183
  hypoglycemia, 180, 181b
  thyrotoxicosis, 184-185
Metabolism;See also metabolic emergencies
  monitoring in shock "Rule of Twenty," 283
  of poisons, 222
Metacarpus
  fractures of, 19, 21
Metaformin
  uses, formulations, and dosage of, 717t
Metaldehyde
  toxicity and treatment of, 241-242
Metaproterenol, 717t
Metastatic neoplasia
  affecting heart and pericardium,
    131-133
Metatarsus
  fractures of, 19, 21
Methazolamide
  for acute glaucoma, 204t
  uses, formulations, and dosage of, 717t
Methenamine hippurate, 717t
Methenamine mandelate, 717t
Methimazole, 717t
Methiocarb
  toxicity and treatment of, 230-231

Methionine
    uses, formulations, and dosage of, 717t
Methocarbamol, 717t
Methohexital, 718t
Methotrexate, 718t
Methoxamine
    uses, formulations, and dosage of, 718t
Methoxyflurane
    uses, formulations, and dosage of, 718t
Methyl alcohol
    toxicity and treatment of, 224-225
Methylene blue 0.1%
    uses, formulations, and dosage of, 718t
Methylprednisolone
    for spinal trauma, 190b
    uses, formulations, and dosage of, 718t
Methylprednisolone acetate
    uses, formulations, and dosage of, 718t
Methylprednisolone sodium succinate
    uses, formulations, and dosage of, 718t
4-Methylpyrazole, 718t
Methyltestosterone, 719t
Metoclopramide
    as antiemetics, 172t
    uses, formulations, and dosage of, 719t
Metoprolol, 719t
Metric system
    body weight to surface area conversion, 654t
    conversion table, 659t
Metritis
    acute, 138
Metronidazole
    uses, formulations, and dosage of, 719t
Mexiletine
    uses, formulations, and dosage of, 719t
    for ventricular dysrhythmias
        in dogs, 124t
Mibolerone
    uses, formulations, and dosage of, 719t
Mice
    blood laboratory values for, 651t
    determining sex of, 650t
    laboratory information on, 648t-649t
Microalbuminuria test
    for urinalysis, 641
Microsporum canis
    vaccinations
        for cats, 661t
Midazolam
    uses, formulations, and dosage of, 719t
Midbrain
    contusions with hemorrhage, 188
    lesions in, 370
Midsystolic click
    heart sounds, 321
Midwest Animal Blood Services
    emergency hotline number, 644t
Milbemycin oxime, 720t
Milk of Magnesia
    as diluting agent for toxins, 221
    uses, formulations, and dosage of, 720t

Mineral oil
    as cathartic for toxins and poisons, 220t
    toxicity and treatment of, 237-238
    uses, formulations, and dosage of, 720t
Mineral spirits
    toxicity and treatment of, 237-238
Mineralization of supraspinatus
    size and breed disposition to, 352t
Minocycline
    uses, formulations, and dosage of, 720t
Miscellaneous class
    of cats, 647t
    of dogs, 646t
Misoprostol, 720t
Mites
    products to prevent
        toxicity of, 225
Mitotane
    uses, formulations, and dosage of, 720t
Mitoxantrone
    myelosuppression classification of, 210t
    uses, formulations, and dosage of, 720t
Mitral valve
    auscultation of, 320
    heart murmurs, 321-325, 326t
    radiograph illustrating, 321f
Mitral valve endocardiosis, 127-128
Mitral valve insufficiency, 127-128
    characteristics of, 326t
    description of, 324
Mobilization
    during shock "Rule of Twenty," 284
Modified doughnut bandages, 12, 13f-14f
Modified transudates
    with pleural effusion
        characteristics of, 261t-262t
Modulating systems
    within pain sensing and response system, 70
Moist healing, 9
Monocytes
    normal hematology ranges
        for adult canines and felines, 577t
Morphine
    for abdominal pain, 83t
    for congestive heart failure (CHF), 128b
    epidural anesthesia, 80t
    to induce vasodilation, 280t
    properties of
        for pain management, 74t
    uses, formulations, and dosage of, 720t
Mothballs
    toxicity and treatment of, 242-243
Motor skills
    and coma scale, 192t
Motor vehicle accidents
    fractures and musculoskeletal trauma
        articular cartilage injuries, 157
        classification of, 154b
        high-rise syndrome, 158
        immediate action, 154-155
        ligament injuries, 157, 158b

Motor vehicle accidents—cont'd
  fractures and musculoskeletal trauma—cont'd
    open wounds, 156b, 157
    treatment of, 155-157
Mouth
  giving pills by, 449-451
  halitosis, 312
  initial examination of, 4
Movements;*See also* posture
  abnormal
    as sign of pain, 72b
Mucin clot
  parameter in joint fluid analysis, 357t-358t
Mucous membranes
  assessing during cardiovascular exam,
      318-319
  assessing during initial emergency exam, 3-4
  bluish with cyanosis, 409
  definition and illustration of, 306
  icterus
    associated signs, 447
    definition of, 446
    differential diagnosis, 447-448
  muddy-colored or pale
    as clinical sign of decompensation, 6b
  pale or cyanotic
    with congestive heart failure, 128
Multifocal premature ventricular
      complexes (PVCs)
  description of, 121, 123
  illustration of, 122f
Multi-lumen catheters, 62, 64f
Multiple myeloma
  in various paraneoplastic syndromes,
      205t-206t
Multiple organ dysfunction syndrome (MODS)
  with pancreatitis, 173-174
Murmurs
  heart, 321-325, 326t
Muscle tone
  examination of, 362-363
Muscles
  open wounds to, 156-167
Musculoskeletal system
  clinical disease signs, 354b
  evaluation and examination of, 351,
      352t-353t, 354-356
  examination of, 351, 352t-353t, 354
  examining in emergency poison/toxin
      cases, 215b
  palpation and manipulation of, 354
  types of conditions affecting,
      352t-353t
Musculoskeletal trauma
  articular cartilage injuries, 157
  classification of, 154b
  high-rise syndrome, 158
  immediate action, 154-155
  ligament injuries, 157, 158b
  open wounds, 156b, 157
  treatment of, 155-157

Mushrooms
  toxicity and treatment of, 242
Mycotoxins
  toxicity and treatment of, 242
Myelography
  technique of, 548
Myeloma
  in various paraneoplastic syndromes,
      205t-206t
Myelosuppression
  classification of
    as related to chemotherapy, 210t, 211
Myocardial ischemia
  and cardiopulmonary cerebral resuscitation
      (CPCR), 120
Myoglobinuria
  associated signs, 394-395
  causes of, 396t
  definition of, 393-394
  differential diagnosis, 395
Myositis
  causing acute abdominal pain, 89t

N

Nadir
  time of chemotherapy, 210t
Nails
  evaluation and examination of, 332,
      333f-335f, 336-339, 340t, 341
  fungal cultures, 472
  part of "BEETTS" test, 294
Naloxone
  used during advanced life support, 120t
  uses, formulations, and dosage
      of, 720t
Naltrexone
  uses, formulations, and dosage of, 721t
Nandrolone decanoate, 721t
Naphthalene
  toxicity and treatment of, 242-243
Naproxen
  toxicity and treatment of, 243
  uses, formulations, and dosage of, 721t
Nares
  evaluation of patient's, 298
Nasal biopsy
  technique of, 504
Nasal cavity
  evaluation of patient's, 298
  examination of, 376-377
Nasal discharge
  associated signs, 429
  clinical algorithm for, 431f
  definition of, 429
  differential diagnosis, 430b
  with lower respiratory disease, 379
  with upper respiratory tract diseases,
      560-561
Nasal oxygen, 50
Nasopharyngeal oxygen catheters, 50
Nasopharyngeal polyps, 257

Nasopharynx
  examination of, 376-377
National Pesticide Information Center
  emergency hotline, 644t
Nebulizers
  and aerosol therapy, 568-569, 570f, 571
Neck
  assessing during cardiovascular exam, 316
  definition and illustration of dental, 305, 306f
  evaluation of patient's, 298
  examination of
    with lower respiratory disease, 377-380,
      381f, 382
  neurological examination of, 362
Neomycin
  uses, formulations, and dosage of, 721t
Neonatal deaths
  causes of, 375
Neoplasia
  causing acute abdominal pain, 89t
  causing organ system obstruction, 208-209
  and pericardial effusion, 131-133
  size and breed disposition to, 352t
  types of
    and skin manifestations of, 340t
Neoplasms
  in gastrointestinal tract, 170
  paraneoplastic syndromes associated with,
    205t-206t
  thoracic cavity, 208
  types of
    signs and symptoms of, 205t-206t
  urinary tract, 208-209
Neoplastic diseases
  and joint fluid analysis, 357t-358t
Neostigmine bromide and neostigmine
      methylsulfate
  uses, formulations, and dosage of, 721t
Nerve blocks, 78-81
Nerves
  blockades, 78-81
  disorders affecting, 356, 359-365, 366t-367t,
    368f, 369-373
  initial examination of, 5
Nervous system;See also neurologic
      examination
  assessing behavior, 359-360
  assessing mental attitude, 359-360
  evaluation of patient's, 301
  examination of, 356, 359
    cranial nerve reflexes, 365, 366t-367t,
      368f, 369
    gait, 360-361
    mental attitude and behavior, 359-360
    postural reactions, 361-362
    spinal nerve reflexes, 362-365
Neurologic examination
  in emergency poison/toxin cases, 215b
  five parts of
    cranial nerve reflexes, 365, 366t-367t,
      368f, 369

Neurologic examination—cont'd
  five parts of—cont'd
    gait, 360-361
    mental attitude and behavior, 359-360
    postural reactions, 361-362
    spinal nerve reflexes, 362-365
Neutropenia
  clinical signs and treatment of, 205t
  tumor types, 205t
Neutrophils
  parameter in joint fluid analysis,
    357t-358t
Nicotine
  toxicity and treatment of, 243
Nictitating membrane
  examination of, 345-346
Nikolsky's sign
  technique of, 337
Nitric acid
  toxicity and treatment of, 224
Nitrofurantoin
  uses, formulations, and dosage of, 721t
Nitroglycerine ointment (or paste)
  for congestive heart failure (CHF), 128b
  to induce vasodilation, 280t
  uses, formulations, and dosage of, 722t
Nitroprusside
  uses, formulations, and dosage of, 722t
Nizatidine
  uses, formulations, and dosage of, 722t
NMDA blockers;See N-methyl-D-aspartate
    (NMDA) receptor antagonists
N-methyl-D-aspartate (NMDA) receptor
    antagonists
  Ketamine as, 77, 78t
Nociception
  signs of, 364
Nonchlorine bleach
  toxicity and treatment of, 229
Nonhemorrhagic thoracic effusion, 208
Nonionic detergents
  toxicity and treatment of, 233-234
Nonmedicated shampoos
  toxicity and treatment of, 233-234
Non-segmented neutrophils
  normal hematology ranges
    for adult canines and felines, 577t
Nonseptic exudates
  with pleural effusion
    characteristics of, 261t-262t
Non-sporting group, 646t
Nonsteroidal antiinflammatory drugs
    (NSAIDs)
  description of, 75-76
  for pain, 73, 75-77
  toxicity and treatment of, 243
  types and dosages of, 75t
Norfloxacin
  uses, formulations, and dosage of, 722t
Normal biochemistry ranges
  for adult canines and felines, 577t

Nose
  examination of, 376-377
  examining in emergency poison/toxin
    cases, 215b
  initial examination of, 4
  topical administration
    of medications, 456
Noxious stimuli, 189, 191, 192t
Nursing care
  during shock "Rule of Twenty," 284
Nutrition
  evaluation during patient exam, 296-297
  monitoring in shock "Rule of Twenty,"
    283-284
Nutritional diseases
  types of
    and skin manifestations of, 340t
Nutritional support
  for poisonings, 223

O

Obesity
  assessing during cardiovascular exam, 316
  evaluation during patient exam, 296-297
Obstipation
  associated signs, 398
  characteristics of gastrointestinal, 87t
  definition of, 169-170, 397-398
  differential diagnosis, 398, 399f, 400b
Obstructive constipation, 169-170
Occlusion defects, 306, 308
Ocular emergencies, 196-204
  equipment needed during, 196b
  examination procedures, 196-197
  instruments for treating, 197b
  requiring immediate attention, 196b
  with sudden vision loss, 196b
  types of
    acute infectious keratitis, 200
    chemical injuries, 198-199
    conjunctival lacerations, 198
    corneal abrasions, 199-200
    eyelid ecchymosis, 198
    foreign bodies, 200-201
    glaucoma, 203-204
    hyphema, 201-202
    loss of vision, 196b
    ocular trauma, 201
    penetrating corneal injuries, 200
    proptosis, 202-203
    subconjunctival lacerations, 198
Ocular nerves
  illustration and evaluation of, 365, 366t
Ocular system;See also ocular emergencies
  evaluation and examination of, 341-347
  examination checklist
    anterior chamber, 346-347
    conjunctiva, 345
    external eye appearance, 343
    eyelids, 344-345
    globe and adnexa, 341-342

Ocular system—cont'd
  examination checklist—cont'd
    iris, 347
    lacrimal system, 346
    lens, 347
    nictitating membrane, 345-346
    orbit, 344
    pupillary light reflexes (PLR), 342-343
    retina, 347
    tonic eye reflexes, 342
    vision assessment, 343-344
  topical administration
    of medications, 456
  trauma
    description and treatment of, 201
Oculocephalic reflexes, 187, 192t
Oculomotor nerves
  evaluation of, 365, 366t
  illustration of, 368f
Oils
  toxicity and treatment of, 237-238
Olfactory nerves
  illustration and evaluation of, 365, 366t
Oliguria
  associated signs, 404
  definition of, 404
  differential diagnosis, 305b, 404
Olsalazine
  uses, formulations, and dosage of, 722t
Omeprazole
  uses, formulations, and dosage of, 722t
Oncologic emergencies
  description of, 205
  types of
    signs and symptoms of, 205t-206t
Oncotic pressure
  checking in shock "Rule of Twenty," 281
  and fluid therapy, 42-43
Ondansetron
  as antiemetics, 172t
  uses, formulations, and dosage of, 722t
Onion
  toxicity and treatment of, 243-244
Open fractures, 154b, 155-157
Open musculoskeletal injuries
  description of, 156
  treatment of, 156-167
Open sucking chest wounds, 258
Open wounds
  classification of, 156b
  with drainage, 10
  in repair stage of healing, 9
Ophthalmic disorders;See also ophthalmic
    examinations
  evaluation and examination of, 341-347
  injuries, 196-204
  therapeutic procedures, 535-539
Ophthalmic examinations
  checklist for
    anterior chamber, 346-347
    conjunctiva, 345

Ophthalmic examinations—cont'd
checklist for—cont'd
external eye appearance, 343
eyelids, 344-345
globe and adnexa, 341-342
iris, 347
lacrimal system, 346
lens, 347
nictitating membrane, 345-346
orbit, 344
pupillary light reflexes (PLR), 342-343
retina, 347
tonic eye reflexes, 342
vision assessment, 343-344
Opiates
toxicity and treatment of, 244
Opioid receptors, 73, 74t
Opioids
description and effects of, 73
in epidurals, 80
Optic nerves
fibers, 342-343
Oral calcium
dosage of
for hypocalcemia, 182t
Oral cavity
evaluation of patient's, 298
examination of, 309-310, 311f, 312-313,
376-377
gastrointestinal system emergencies, 158-160
and urinary tract diseases, 385-386
Oral liquids
technique of, 453-456
Oral melanoma
in paraneoplastic syndromes, 206t, 207
Oral mucous membranes
definition and illustration of, 306
Oral pill administration
to canines, 449-450, 451f
to felines, 450-451, 452f, 453
Orbifloxacin
uses, formulations, and dosage of, 722t
Orbit
examination of, 344
during ocular emergencies, 197
Orbital retrobulbar hemorrhages, 344
Orchitis
infectious, 143
Organ systems
neoplasia causing obstruction of, 208-209
patient evaluations
alimentary system, 304-306, 307f,
308-310, 311f, 312-315
the "BEETTS" test, 293-295
cardiovascular system, 315-325, 326t,
327f-328f, 329-332
ears, 347-350
female reproductive tract exam, 374-376
integumentary system, 332, 333f-335f,
336-339, 340t, 341
lymph nodes, 350-351

Organ systems—cont'd
patient evaluations—cont'd
male reproductive tract exam, 373
medical record, 301-304
musculoskeletal system, 351, 352t-353t,
354-356
nervous system, 356, 357t-358t, 359-365,
366t-367t, 368f, 369-373
normal breeding behavior and physiology,
382-384
ocular system, 341-347
ophthalmic, 341-347
orthopedic, 351, 352t-353t, 354-356
otic system, 347-350
the "problem list," 295-301
respiratory system-lower, 377-380,
381f, 382
respiratory system-upper, 376-377
skin, hair, coat and toenails, 332,
333f-335f, 336-339, 340t, 341
thyroid, 350-351
urinary tract exam, 384-386
Organophosphates
toxicity and treatment of, 244
Ormetoprim
uses, formulations, and dosage of, 722t
Orogastric lavage
for poisons, 218
procedure for, 47-48
uses of, 47-48
Orogastric tubes, 168f
Oropharynx
examination of, 376-377
Orthopedic conditions
articular cartilage injuries, 157
classification of, 154b
clinical disease signs, 354b
evaluation and examination of, 351,
352t-353t, 354-356
examination of, 351, 352t-353t, 354
examining in emergency poison/toxin
cases, 215b
high-rise syndrome, 158
immediate action, 154-155
ligament injuries, 157, 158b
open wounds, 156b, 157
palpation and manipulation of, 354
size and breed disposition to, 352t-353t
treatment of, 155-157
types of conditions affecting, 352t-353t
Orthopnea
assessing during initial emergency
exam, 3-4
with congestive heart failure, 128
definition of, 317b
with dyspnea, 410
Ortolani's sign, 355-356
Os penis
fracture, 144
and urohydropulsion, 57
Osmolal gap, 39

Osmolality
  calculation of, 38, 180
  definition of, 38-39
  estimated serum
    normal test ranges and protocols,
      604-605
  fluid therapy, 38-39
  normal levels of, 180
Osmolarity
  calculation of, 193
  normal biochemistry ranges
    for adult canines and felines, 577t
Osmotic agents, 203, 204t
Osmotic diarrhea
  definition of, 405
Otic system
  evaluation and examination of,
    347-350
  examination of, 347-350
  topical administration
    of medications, 456
Otitis
  externa, 134
Otitis interna, 134
Otologic loops, 493f
Otoscope speculum, 486f
Ovariectomy
  and mammary tumors, 375
Ovaries
  causing acute abdominal pain, 89t
  examination of, 375
  imbalances
    skin lesions or signs of, 338t
Ovariohysterectomy
  illustration of uterus following, 137f
  for pyometra, 136-138
  to terminate pregnancy, 140-141
Oxacillin, 722t
Oxazepam, 722t
Oxtriphylline, 723t
Oxybutynin, 723t
Oxygen
  for congestive heart failure (CHF), 128b
  nasopharyngeal and nasal, 50
  and respiratory emergencies, 253-265
Oxygen cages
  description of, 50
  for pulmonary diseases, 265
Oxygen delivery
  calculating with shock, 275-276
Oxygen hoods, 49-50
Oxygen saturation
  and acid-base status, 35-37
  and shock, 275-276
Oxygen supplementation
  reasons for providing, 48-51
Oxygen therapy
  goals and indications for, 49
  during initial emergency exam, 3-4
  reasons for providing, 48-51
Oxygenated hemoglobin (HbO$_2$), 51

Oxygenation
  checking in shock "Rule of Twenty," 281-282
  and pulse oximetry, 51
Oxyhemoglobin
  calculations of, 51
Oxymetholone
  uses, formulations, and dosage of, 723t
Oxymorphone
  properties of
    for pain management, 74t
  uses, formulations, and dosage of, 723t
Oxytetracycline
  uses, formulations, and dosage of, 723t
Oxytocin, 723t
  causing anaphylactic reactions, 94b

P

P waves, 121, 122f
Pacemakers, 125-127
Packed cell volume (PCV)
  and blood component therapy,
    21-33
  component of laboratory data, 300t
  normal rates in dogs, 23
Packed red blood cells
  component therapy procedure, 29-30
  storage of, 26t
  transfusion of, 26-27
Pain
  abdominal
    diagnostic tests, 84-85, 90t-92t, 93
    with abdominal conditions, 86t-89t
  anesthesia blockades, 78-81
  assessment, prevention and management
    of, 69-81
  associated signs, 424-425
  behavioral signs of, 71-72
  categories of dog and cat, 70b
  control of
    during shock "Rule of Twenty," 284
  cutaneous
    assessment of, 333f-334f
  deep, 189
  definitions of, 69-70, 71, 424
  differential diagnosis, 425
  methods to reduce, 73-81
  nonsteroidal antiinflammatory drugs
    (NSAIDS) for, 75-76
  with ocular emergencies, 196-204
  physiologic impact of untreated,
    70-71
  and "praying position," 313
  recognition and assessment of, 71
  scale of, 72t
  sensing and response system, 70
  signs of, 364
  types of, 69-70
Paint (See fuels)
  toxicity and treatment of, 237-238
Paintballs
  toxicity and treatment of, 244-245

Palpation
  of abdomen, 313-314
  techniques for orthopedic diseases, 354-355
2-PAM
  uses, formulations, and dosage of, 723t
Pancreas
  clinical conditions of
    causing acute abdominal pain, 88t
  diagnostic tests, 84-85, 90t-92t, 93
Pancreatic beta cell tumors
  in paraneoplastic syndromes, 206t, 207
Pancreatic enzyme
  uses, formulations, and dosage of, 723t
Pancreatic lipase immunoreactivity (PLI)
  normal test ranges and protocols, 605
Pancreatitis
  causing acute diarrhea, 406b
  causing acute hepatic failure, 175b
  acute necrotizing, 173
  description and causes of, 173-174
  treatment of, 174
Pancuronium bromide
  uses, formulations, and dosage of, 723t
Panleukopenia
  abdominal symptoms of, 86t
  vaccinations
    for cats, 661t
Panosteitis
  size and breed disposition to, 353t
Papillomas
  around lymph nodes or thyroid, 350
  found in female reproductive tract,
    374-375
Papular eruption, 421b
Papules, 336-339
Paracematol
  toxicity and treatment of, 224
Paraffin oil, 220t
Paraffin wax (See fuels)
  toxicity and treatment of, 237-238
Parainfluenza virus
  vaccinations
    for dogs, 661t
Paraneoplastic syndromes
  in dogs and cats, 205t
  types of
    anaphylactic reactions, 211
    bone marrow toxicities, 210
    cardiotoxicity, 211
    chemotherapy-related toxicities,
      210-211
    gastrointestinal toxicity, 210-211
    urinary bladder toxicity, 211
Paraparesis
  and spinal cord, 360f
Paraphimosis, 144-145
  causing acute abdominal pain, 88t
Paraplegia
  and spinal cord, 360f
Paraquat
  toxicity and treatment of, 245

Parasites
  causing acute diarrhea, 406b
  assessment of, 333f-334f
  component of laboratory data, 300t
Parasitic diseases
  abdominal symptoms of, 86t
  types of
    and skin manifestations of, 339t
Parathyroid adenoma
  in paraneoplastic syndromes, 206t, 207
Parathyroid hormone (PTH)
  normal test values and interpretation, 623
Parathyroid hormone-related (PTHrP)
  normal test values and interpretation,
    623-624
Paregoric
  uses, formulations, and dosage of, 724t
Parenteral administration
  of medications, 457-458
Parenteral calcium
  dosage of
    for hypocalcemia, 182t
Paromomycin, 724t
Paroxetine, 724t
Partial pressure of carbon dioxide ($PaCO_2$)
  with acidosis and alkalosis, 37t
  normal arterial blood gas analysis ranges, 578t
Partial pressure of oxygen (PO_2)
  normal arterial blood gas analysis ranges
    for adult canines and felines, 578t
Parturition
  emergencies of, 139-141
Parvoviruses
  abdominal symptoms of, 86t
  vaccinations
    for dogs, 661t
Patella reflexes, 363
Patent airways
  assessing at accident scene, 2-3
Patent ductus arteriosus
  characteristics of, 326t
  description of, 325
Patient assessments
  of capillary refill time (CRT), 319
  of cardiovascular disease, 315-316, 317t,
    318-332
  of cyanosis, 319
Patient evaluation
  the "BEETTS" test, 293-295
  medical record, 301-304
  organ system examination
    alimentary system, 304-306, 307f,
      308-310, 311f, 312-315
    cardiovascular system, 315-325, 326t,
      327f-328f, 329-332
    ears, 347-350
    female reproductive tract exam, 374-376
    integumentary system, 332, 333f-335f,
      336-339, 340t, 341
    lymph nodes, 350-351
    male reproductive tract exam, 373

Patient evaluation—cont'd
  organ system examination—cont'd
    musculoskeletal system, 351, 352t-353t, 354-356
    nervous system, 356, 357t-358t, 359-365, 366t-367t, 368f, 369-373
    normal breeding behavior and physiology, 382-384
    ocular system, 341-347
    ophthalmic, 341-347
    orthopedic, 351, 352t-353t, 354-356
    otic system, 347-350
    respiratory system-lower, 377-380, 381f, 382
    respiratory system-upper, 376-377
    skin, hair, coat and toenails, 332, 333f-335f, 336-339, 340t, 341
    thyroid, 350-351
    urinary tract exam, 384-386
  the "problem list," 295-301
Patient mobilization
  during shock "Rule of Twenty," 284
Paws
  cup or clamshell splints for, 12, 18-19, 18f-20f
  injuries to, 190-191
Pelvic fractures, 154b, 155-158
  and sciatic nerve damage, 191
Pelvic lesions
  affecting urinary tract, 208-209
Pelvic limbs
  function grading scale, 360b
  reflexes, 363-364
Pelvis
  initial examination of, 5
Pemphigus
  skin lesions or signs of, 338t
Penetrating corneal injuries
  description and treatment of, 200
Penicillamine
  for metal toxicities, 221
  uses, formulations, and dosage of, 724t
Penicillin
  causing anaphylactic reactions, 94b
  types of
    uses, formulations, and dosage of, 724t
Penicillinase
  causing anaphylactic reactions, 94b
Penis
  evaluation of patient's, 298
  fractures
    causing acute abdominal pain, 88t
  lacerations of, 144
  paraphimosis, 144-145
Pennies
  toxicity and treatment of, 252
Pennyroyal oil
  toxicity and treatment of, 245-246
Pentazocine, 724t
Pentobarbital
  uses, formulations, and dosage of, 724t
Pentoxifylline, 724t

Pepto-bismol
  toxicity and treatment of, 227
Percussion
  of thorax, 379-380
Percutaneous dorsal pedal artery catheterization
  as vascular access technique, 68
Percutaneous jugular vein catheterization, 495-496
Percutaneous over-the-wire jugular catheters
  as vascular access technique, 61-62
Percutaneous through-the-needle jugular catheters
  for vascular access, 59-61
Perianesthetic dysrhythmias
  steps to prevent, 99b
Perianesthetic hypotension
  causes and treatment of, 98t
Pericardial effusion
  assessing during initial emergency exam, 4
  and cardiac arrest, 113-114
  description of, 131-132
  differential diagnoses of, 132b
  supplies needed for, 133b
Pericardiocentesis
  assessing during initial emergency exam, 4
  and cardiac arrest, 113-114
  differential diagnoses of, 132b
  signs and description of, 131-132
  supplies needed for, 133b
Perineal reflexes, 364-365
Periodontal disease, 312
Periodontal ligaments
  definition and illustration of, 306
Peripheral arterial and venous catheters
  for vascular access, 62, 65f, 66-67
Peripheral blood smear
  initial screening test, 607
  testing during initial emergency care, 5
Peripheral edema
  associated signs, 437
  definition of, 435
  differential diagnosis, 437, 438b
Peripheral lymph nodes
  examining in emergency poison/toxin cases, 215b
Peripheral nerves
  assessment of
    during initial emergency exam, 5
Peripheral nervous system
  injuries to, 190-191
Peritoneal cavity
  abdominal paracentesis, 6-7
Peritoneal laparoscopy, 375
Peritoneal lavage
  diagnostic, 93
  technique of, 6-7
    in acute abdomen cases, 85, 90t-92t
Peritonitis
  causing acute abdominal pain, 89t

Permanent teeth
  formula for, 304-305
Pet evaluation
  the "BEETTS" test, 293-295
  medical record, 301-304
  organ system examination
    alimentary system, 304-306, 307f,
      308-310, 311f, 312-315
    cardiovascular system, 315-325, 326t,
      327f-328f, 329-332
    ears, 347-350
    female reproductive tract exam,
      374-376
    integumentary system, 332, 333f-335f,
      336-339, 340t, 341
    lymph nodes, 350-351
    male reproductive tract exam, 373
    musculoskeletal system, 351, 352t-353t,
      354-356
    nervous system, 356, 357t-358t, 359-365,
      366t-367t, 368f, 369-373
    normal breeding behavior and physiology,
      382-384
    ocular system, 341-347
    ophthalmic, 341-347
    orthopedic, 351, 352t-353t, 354-356
    otic system, 347-350
    respiratory system-lower, 377-380,
      381f, 382
    respiratory system-upper, 376-377
    skin, hair, coat and toenails, 332, 333f-335f,
      336-339, 340t, 341
    thyroid, 350-351
    urinary tract exam, 384-386
  the "problem list," 295-301
Petit mal seizures, 194
Petroleum distillates
  toxicity and treatment of, 237-238
Petrosal temporal bone
  fractures of, 187
PH
  normal arterial blood gas analysis
      ranges
    for adult canines and felines, 578t
  normal urinalysis ranges
    for adult canines and felines, 578t
Pharynx
  emergencies of, 253-265
  foreign bodies, 159-160
Phencyclidine
  in epidurals, 80
Phenobarbital
  uses, formulations, and dosage of, 725t
Phenothiazines
  as antiemetics, 172t
Phenoxybenzamine
  uses, formulations, and dosage of, 725t
Phentolamine, 725t
Phenylbutazone, 725t
Phenylcyclidine
  toxicity and treatment of, 246

Phenylephrine
  toxicity and treatment of, 246
  uses, formulations, and dosage of, 725t
Phenylpropanolamine, 725t
  toxicity and treatment of, 246
Phenytoin, 726t
Phosphoric acid
  toxicity and treatment of, 224
Phosphorus (P)
  normal biochemistry ranges
    for adult canines and felines, 577t
  normal test ranges and interpretation, 595
Photographic developer solution
  toxicity and treatment of, 233-234
Phthalazine derivatives
  for systemic hypertension, 177t
Physeal fractures, 154b, 155-158
Physical examinations
  checklist
    in toxin and poison cases, 214, 215b, 216,
      217f, 218-223
  eyes checklist
    anterior chamber, 346-347
    conjunctiva, 345
    external eye appearance, 343
    eyelids, 344-345
    globe and adnexa, 341-342
    iris, 347
    lacrimal system, 346
    lens, 347
    nictitating membrane, 345-346
    orbit, 344
    pupillary light reflexes (PLR), 342-343
    retina, 347
    tonic eye reflexes, 342
    vision assessment, 343-344
  during initial emergency care, 2-6
  of organ systems
    alimentary system, 304-306, 307f,
      308-310, 311f, 312-315
    cardiovascular system, 315-325, 326t,
      327f-328f, 329-332
    ears, 347-350
    female reproductive tract exam, 374-376
    integumentary system, 332, 333f-335f,
      336-339, 340t, 341
    lymph nodes, 350-351
    male reproductive tract exam, 373
    musculoskeletal system, 351, 352t-353t,
      354-356
    nervous system, 356, 357t-358t, 359-365,
      366t-367t, 368f, 369-373
    normal breeding behavior and physiology,
      382-384
    ocular system, 341-347
    ophthalmic, 341-347
    orthopedic, 351, 352t-353t, 354-356
    otic system, 347-350
    respiratory system-lower, 377-380,
      381f, 382
    respiratory system-upper, 376-377

Physical examinations—cont'd
  of organ systems—cont'd
    skin, hair, coat and toenails, 332,
        333f-335f, 336-339, 340t, 341
    thyroid, 350-351
    urinary tract exam, 384-386
  for poison management, 214, 215b, 216, 217f
  for skin disorders, 332, 333f-336f, 336-339,
      340t, 341
Physical therapy
  routine procedures
    cold therapy, 499
    deep heat, 498
    electrotherapy, 499
    exercise therapy, 499-500
    heat therapy, 497-498
    hydrotherapy, 497
    massage therapy, 499-500
Physostigmine
  uses, formulations, and dosage of, 726t
Phytomenadione
  uses, formulations, and dosage of, 726t
Phytonadione
  uses, formulations, and dosage of, 726t
Pigment
  abnormal skin, 337t
Pigmentation
  of conjunctiva, 345
Pills
  administering to canines, 449-450, 451f
  administering to felines, 450-451,
      452t, 453
Pimobendan
  for ventricular dysrhythmias, 281t
Pine oil disinfectant (See nonionic detergents)
  toxicity and treatment of, 234
Piperacillin
  uses, formulations, and dosage of, 726t
Piperazine
  toxicity and treatment of, 247
  uses, formulations, and dosage of, 726t
Piroxicam
  dosage for pain, 75t
  uses, formulations, and dosage of, 726t
Pitressin
  uses, formulations, and dosage of, 726t
Pituitary dwarfism
  skin lesions or signs of, 338t
PIVKA test
  ancillary hemostasis tests, 609
  normal test values and interpretation, 614
Placing, 362
Plans
  in medical record, 301-302
Plaque formation, 421b
Plasma
  component therapy procedure, 29-30
  International system of units (SI)
    conversion tables, 656t-658t
  separation of, 21-33
  storage of, 26t

Plasma—cont'd
  support criteria, 22b
  transfusion guidelines, 30
Plasma cell tumors
  in paraneoplastic syndromes, 206t
Plasma cryoprecipitate
  transfusion guidelines, 30
Plasma osmolarity
  calculation of, 193
Platelet clumps
  avoiding when taking lab samples, 581
Platelet counts
  checking in shock "Rule of Twenty," 282
  initial screening test, 607
  normal hematology ranges
    for adult canines and felines, 577t
  normal hemostasis ranges
    for adult canines and felines, 578t
  normal test values and interpretation, 615
  testing during initial emergency care, 5
Platelet-rich plasma
  dose and administration rates, 29t
  indications for administering, 28t, 29
  separation of, 21-33
  storage of, 26t
  transfusion guidelines, 30
Platelets
  and acquired hemostasis disorders, 104-107
  component of laboratory data, 300t
  laboratory results for coagulation
      profiles, 107t
  support criteria, 22b
Pleural cavity
  diseases, 257-258
  pyothorax, 260
Pleural cavity disease
  description and immediate management of,
      257-258
Pleural effusions
  analysis of, 261t-262t
  assessing during initial emergency exam, 3-4
  and cardiac arrest, 113-114
  in cats with CHF, 130
  definition of, 259
  description and immediate management of,
      259-260, 261t-262t, 263
  and oxygen therapy, 48t
  physical processes associated with, 259b
Pleural fluid cytologic analysis, 259
Pleural rub
  description of, 317t
Pleural space
  diseases of, 253-265
Plicamycin
  uses, formulations, and dosage of, 726t
Pneumocystography, 546
  technique of, 546
Pneumonia
  assessing during initial emergency exam, 3-4
  and cardiac arrest, 113-114
  and oxygen therapy, 48t

Pneumothorax
    assessing during initial emergency exam, 4
    causing decompensation, 6b
    description and immediate management of, 258-259
    and oxygen therapy, 48t
    thoracostomy tube placement for, 53-55
    treatment of, 259
Pocket pets
    blood values for, 651t
    physiologic data, 648t-649t
9-point body condition score (BCS), 297, 298f
Points of origin
    of nerves, 368f
Poisonous creatures
    Bufo toads, 153
    Gila monsters, 153
    Mexican bearded lizards, 153-154
    snakes, 149-152
    spiders, 152-153
Poisonous snakes
    characteristics of, 149, 150f, 151-152
Poisons
    causing acute hepatic failure, 174-175
    animals exposed to
        emergency care of, 212, 213b, 214, 215b, 216, 217f, 218-223
    antidotes, 221-222
    cathartics, 220
    clearance or metabolism of, 222
    causing cyanosis, 410b
    databases and resources, 212, 213b
    emergency hotlines, 644t
    emergency treatment of, 214, 215b, 216, 217f
    emetics, 218, 219t
    enemas, 219-220
    in eyes, 221
    ion exchange resins, 220-221
    obtaining thorough history, 216, 217f
    orogastric lavage, 218
    physical examination, 214, 215b, 216, 217f
    preventing absorption, 216-221
    and renal perfusion, 223
    skin poisons, 221
    telephone advice, 212, 213b, 644t
    toxicologic history form, 217f
    treatment of specific, 246
        acetaminophen, 224
        acetylsalicylic acid, 227
        acid chemical burns, 224
        acids, 224
        ß-adrenergic agonists, 228
        aflatoxin, 224
        alcohol, 224-225
        alkalis/caustics, 225
        amitraz, 225
        ammonia, 225-226
        amphetamines, 226
        "angel dust," 246
        anionic detergents, 233-234
        anti-dandruff shampoos, 248

Poisons—cont'd
  treatment of specific, 246—cont'd
    antifreeze, 235-236
    antihistamines, 226
    ANTU (α-naphthylthiourea), 226-227
    aromatic hydrocarbons, 238
    arsenic, 227
    aspirin, 227
    asthma inhalers/medications, 228
    atomoxetine, 249
    baclofen, 227-228
    bar soaps, 248-249
    barbecue lighter fluids, 237-238
    barbiturates, 228
    bath soaps, 248-249
    batteries, 228
    benzoyl peroxide, 228-229
    bismuth subsalicylate (*See* aspirin), 227
    bleach, 229
    borate, 229
    boric acid, 229
    botulism, 229-230
    bromethalin, 230
    caffeine, 230
    Cannabis sativa, 241
    carbamates, 230-231
    carbon tetrachloride, 231
    carprofen, 243
    cationic detergents, 233-234
    celecoxib, 243
    children's glue, 238
    chives, 243-244
    chlorinated hydrocarbons, 231
    chlorine bleach, 229
    chlorphenoxy derivatives, 231-232
    chocolate, 232
    cholecalciferol, 232
    coal (tar-based) (*See* aromatic hydrocarbons), 239
    corrosives, 224
    coumarin (*See* Vitamin K antagonist rodenticides), 251-252
    cresol, 239
    deicers (*See* ethylene glycol), 224, 225, 235-236
    denture cleaners, 233
    deodorants, 233
    deracoxib, 243
    detergents, 233-234
    dichlone, 234
    diclofenac, 243
    diethyltoluamide (DEET), 234-235
    Diquat, 235
    disinfectants, 233-234
    d-Limonene, 240
    ecstasy, 235
    ethanol, 224-225
    ethylene glycol, 235-236
    fertilizers, 236
    fipronil, 236-237
    fire extinguisher, 237

Poisons—cont'd
  treatment of specific, 246—cont'd
    fireplace colors, 237
    fireworks, 237
    fuels, 237-238
    furniture polish (*See* fuels), 237-238
    garlic, 243-244
    gasoline, 237-238
    glue, 238
    glyophosate, 238
    grapes, 238
    hashish (*See* marijuana), 241
    herbicides, 235, 245
    herbicides???, 231-232
    hexachlorophene, 233-234
    hydrocarbons, 239
    hydrochloric acid, 224
    ibuprophen, 243
    imidacloprid, 239
    iron or iron salts, 239
    ivermectin, 239-240
    kerosene, 237-238
    lead, 240
    linalool, 240
    loperamide, 241
    lubricating oils, 237-238
    macadamia nuts, 241
    marijuana, 241
    matches, 241
    melaleuca oil, 250
    metaldehyde, 241-242
    methiocarb, 230-231
    methyl alcohol, 224-225
    mineral oils, 237-238
    mineral spirits, 237-238
    mothballs, 242-243
    mushrooms, 242
    mycotoxins, 242
    naphthalene, 242-243
    naproxen, 243
    nicotine, 243
    nitric acid, 224
    nonchlorine bleach, 229
    nonionic detergents, 233-234
    nonmedicated shampoos, 233-234
    nonsteroidal antiinflammatory drugs
      (NSAIDs), 243
    oils, 237-238
    onion, 243-244
    opiates, 244
    organophosphates, 244
    paint balls, 244-245
    paint (*See* fuels), 237-238
    paracematol, 224
    paraffin wax (*See* fuels), 237-238
    Paraquat, 245
    pennies, 252
    pennyroyal oil, 245-246
    pepto-bismol, 227
    petroleum distillates, 237-238
    phenylcyclidine, 246

Poisons—cont'd
  treatment of specific, 246—cont'd
    phenylephrine, 246
    phenylpropanolamine, 246
    phosphoric acid, 224
    photographic developer solution,
      233-234
    pine oil disinfectant (*See* nonionic
      detergents), 233-234
    piperazine, 247
    pseudoephedrine, 246
    pyrethrin and pyrethroids, 247
    radiator fluids (*See* ethylene glycol),
      235-236
    raisins, 238
    rofecoxib, 243
    rotenone, 247
    rubbing alcohol, 224-225
    rust removers (*See* ethylene glycol), 224
    salicylate, 227
    salt, 248
    selective norepinephrine reuptake
      inhibitor, 249
    selenium sulfide shampoos, 248
    shampoos, 248
    shoe polish (*See* aromatic
      hydrocarbons), 238
    silver polish, 248
    soaps, 248-249
    sodium fluoracetate, 249
    strattera, 249
    strychnine, 249
    styptic pencil, 250
    sunscreen, 248, 252
    superglue, 238
    tar (*See* fuels), 237-238
    tea tree oil, 250
    tetanus, 250
    thawing salt, 248
    toilet bowel cleaner (*See* acids), 224
    tremorigenic mycotoxins, 242
    triazines, 250-251
    tricyclic antidepressants, 251
    valdecoxib, 243
    varnishes (*See* fuels), 237-238
    vitamin K antagonist rodenticides,
      251-252
    window cleaner, 235-236
    xylitol, 252
    Zephiran, 233-234
    zinc, 252
    zinc-based shampoos, 248
  vital sign stabilization, 214, 216
Polydipsia
  associated signs, 417
  definition of, 417
  differential diagnosis, 417, 418b
Polyethylene glycol electrolyte solution
  uses, formulations, and dosage of, 727t
Polysulfated glycosaminoglycan
  uses, formulations, and dosage of, 727t

Polyuria
  associated signs, 417
  definition of, 417
  differential diagnosis, 417, 418b
Pons
  contusions with hemorrhage, 188
  lesions, 369-370
"Popeye Arm"
  with gastric dilatation-volvulus (GDV),
    166, 167f
Portal venous circulation
  with heart disease, 331b
Portuguese Water Dogs
  with breed predisposition
    to acute adrenocortical insufficiency, 184b
Post resuscitation;See prolonged life support
Postrenal azotemia
  description and treatment of, 289
Posture
  abnormal
    as sign of pain, 72b
  affected by brain injuries, 187
  assessment of
    during cardiovascular exam, 316
    during initial emergency exam, 5
    during neurological exam, 361-362
  changes with spinal cord injuries, 190t
Potassium
  and atrial standstill, 125-126
  imbalances
    and fluid therapy, 37-38, 39b, 40t
  normal biochemistry ranges
    for adult canines and felines, 577t
  normal test ranges and interpretation, 595
  and osmolality, 38-39, 41
  supplementation guidelines, 40t
Potassium bromide, 727t
Potassium chloride, 727t
Potassium citrate
  uses, formulations, and dosage of, 727t
Potassium gluconate
  uses, formulations, and dosage of, 727t
Potential hydrogen (pH)
  normal arterial blood gas analysis ranges
    for adult canines and felines, 578t
  normal urinalysis ranges
    for adult canines and felines, 578t
Pralidoxime chloride
  uses, formulations, and dosage of, 727t
"Praying position," 313
Praziquantel
  uses, formulations, and dosage of, 727t
Prazosin
  to induce vasodilation, 280t
  uses, formulations, and dosage of, 728t
Precipitating agents, 221
Precordium
  palpation during cardiovascular exam, 318
Prednisolone
  for feline bronchitis, 266t
  uses, formulations, and dosage of, 728t

Prednisolone sodium succinate
  for feline bronchitis, 266t
  for spinal trauma, 190b
  uses, formulations, and dosage of, 728t
Prednisone
  uses, formulations, and dosage of, 728t
Pregnancy
  emergencies of, 139-141
    dystocia, 139-140
    spontaneous abortion, 140
    termination of, 140-141
    uterine torsion, 140
  examination procedure, 375-376
  radiographic examination of, 375
Preload
  calculating with shock, 275-276
  checking in shock "Rule of Twenty,"
    279-280, 281t
Premature births
  causes of, 375
Premature ventricular contractions (PVCs)
  treating during shock, 279-280, 281t
Prerenal azotemia
  description and treatment of, 287-288
Prescriptions
  common indications and dosages of, 685t-742t
  writing do's and don'ts, 684t
Pressure bandages
  wounds in need of, 10-11
Pressure relief bandages, 11-12
Primary afferent nerves
  within sensing and response system, 70
Primary skin lesions, 333f, 337, 338t
Primidone
  uses, formulations, and dosage of, 729t
"Problem list"
  database, 301-302
  evaluation of, 295-301
Procainamide
  uses, formulations, and dosage of, 729t
  for ventricular dysrhythmias, 281t
    in dogs, 124t
Procaine
  causing anaphylactic reactions, 94b
Procarbazine
  uses, formulations, and dosage of, 729t
Prochlorperazine
  as antiemetics, 172t
  uses, formulations, and dosage of, 729t
Proestrus, 382-384
Progesterone, repositol
  uses, formulations, and dosage of, 729t
Prognathism, 306, 308
Prolonged life support
  drugs used in, 120t
  procedure for, 119-120
Promethazine
  uses, formulations, and dosage of, 729t
Propantheline bromide, 729t
Propionibacterium acnes (injection)
  uses, formulations, and dosage of, 730t

Propiopromazine, 730t
Propofol, 730t
Propranolol
  for supraventricular dysrhythmias, 125t
  for systemic hypertension, 177t
  uses, formulations, and dosage of, 730t
  for ventricular dysrhythmias, 281t
Proprioceptive positioning, 362
Proptosis
  description and treatment of, 202-203
Propylthiouracil
  uses, formulations, and dosage of, 730t
Prostaglandin analogue, 204t
Prostaglandin F$_{2\alpha}$
  for pregnancy termination, 141
  uses, formulations, and dosage of, 730t
Prostaglandin synthetase, 75-76
Prostate biopsy
  technique of, 506
Prostate gland
  acute prostatitis, 143-144
  biopsy and fine-needle aspiration, 558-559
  conditions causing acute abdominal
      pain, 88t
  evaluation of patient's, 298
  examination of, 315
  prostatic wash, 557-558
  ultrasound, 558-559
Prostatic abscesses
  causing acute abdominal pain, 88t
Prostatic carcinoma, 209
Prostatic fluid
  cultures, 470
Prostatic neoplasia, 88t
Prostatic wash, 557-558
Prostatitis, 88t
  acute, 143-144
Protein
  normal urinalysis ranges
    for adult canines and felines, 578t
Protein catabolism, 70
Protein electrophoresis
  normal test ranges and protocols, 605-606
Prothrombin time (PT)
  and blood component dosages, 29t
  checking in shock "Rule of Twenty," 282
  with disseminated intravascular coagulation
    (DIC), 102-103
  initial screening test, 608
  laboratory results for coagulation
    profiles, 107t
  normal hemostasis ranges
    for adult canines and felines, 578t
  normal test values and interpretation, 615
  testing during initial emergency care, 5
Pruritus
  assessment of, 333f-334f
  associated signs, 420
  with atopy, 338t
  definition of, 418, 420
  differential diagnosis, 420, 421b

Pseudoephedrine
  toxicity and treatment of, 246
  uses, formulations, and dosage of, 731t
Pseudohyperkalemia, 39b
Psyllium
  uses, formulations, and dosage of, 731t
Ptyalism
  excessive
    with pharyngeal foreign bodies, 159f, 160
Pubertal estrus, 382-384
Puberty, 383, 384
Puerperal tetani, 181, 182t
Pulmonary circulation
  with heart disease, 331b
Pulmonary contusions
  assessing during initial emergency exam, 3-4
Pulmonary diseases
  acute respiratory distress syndrome (ARDS),
    267-268
  aspiration pneumonia, 267
  contusions, 266-267
  drugs to treat, 266t
  epistaxis, 269-270
  feline asthma, 265-266
  feline bronchitis, 265-266
  feline lower airway disease, 265-266
  pulmonary edema, 267-268
  pulmonary thromboembolism (PTE),
    268-269
  smoke inhalation, 269
Pulmonary edema
  assessing during initial emergency exam, 3-4
  description and treatment of, 267-268
  and oxygen therapy, 48t
Pulmonary stenosis
  characteristics of, 326t
  description of, 325
Pulmonary thromboembolism (PTE)
  causing decompensation, 6b
  description and treatment of, 268-269
Pulmonary valves
  auscultation of, 320
  heart murmurs, 324f, 326t
  radiograph illustrating, 321f
Pulp
  definition and illustration of dental,
    305, 306f
Pulse
  and cardiac arrest, 114
  determining at accident scene, 2-3
  weakness of
    as clinical sign of decompensation, 6b
    with congestive heart failure, 128
Pulse deficits, 319b
Pulse oximetry
  during ancillary diagnostic evaluation, 5
  process of, 51
Pulseless electrical activity (PEA)
  and cardiac arrest, 114
  description of, 117
  electrocardiogram illustrating, 118f

Puncture fluids
cultures, 466t, 467
Punctures
classification of soft tissue, 271, 272t
Pupillary light reflexes (PLR)
examination of, 342-343
Pupils
assessment of
during initial emergency exam, 5
dilation and constriction, 347
examination of
during ocular emergencies, 197, 342-343
in poison/toxin cases, 215b
reflexes
and coma scale, 192t
size of
with head trauma, 186-187
Puppies
fractures in, 158
intussusception in, 165
Pustular dermatitis, 421b
Pyelonephritis, 88t
Pylorus
displacement of
with gastric dilatation-volvulus (GDV),
166, 167f
Pyometra
causing acute abdominal pain, 89t
emergency treatment of, 136-138
radiographic examination of, 375
Pyothorax
description and treatment of, 260
Pyrantel pamoate and tartrate
uses, formulations, and dosage of, 731t
Pyrethrin
toxicity and treatment of, 247
Pyrethroids, 247
Pyridostigmine bromide
uses, formulations, and dosage of, 731t
Pyrimethamine
uses, formulations, and dosage of, 731t
Pythons, 149

Q

QRS complex, 121, 122f
Quality
of heart murmurs, 324, 326t
Quinacrine
uses, formulations, and dosage of, 731t
Quinidine
for ventricular dysrhythmias, 281t
Quinidine gluconate
uses, formulations, and dosage of, 731t
Quinidine polygalacturonate, 732t
Quinidine sulfate, 731t

R

Rabbits
blood laboratory values for, 651t
determining sex of, 650t
laboratory information on, 648t-649t

Rabies
licensed vaccinations in US, 681t-682t
prevention and control of, 674t-678t
submission requirements for suspects,
582-584
testing, 582-584
vaccinations
for cats, 661t
for dogs, 661t
Rabies titer, 637-639
Radial nerves
injuries to, 190-191
Radiation burns, 112
Radiator fluids (See ethylene glycol)
toxicity and treatment of, 235-236
Radiographs
abdominal
for acute abdomen conditions, 85, 90t-92t
of heart, 325, 326t, 327f-328t, 329-330, 331t
showing gastric dilatation-volvulus (GDV),
166f, 167f
of thorax and abdomen
during ancillary diagnostic evaluation, 5
Radiology
guidelines for orthopedic examinations, 356b
Raisins
toxicity and treatment of, 238
Rales
definition of lower respiratory, 382
description of, 317t
Ranitidine
uses, formulations, and dosage of, 732t
Rates of administration
of fluids, 47
Rats
blood laboratory values for, 651t
determining sex of, 650t
laboratory information on, 648t-649t
Rattlesnakes, 149, 150f
Reactions
during neurologic examination, 359-369
Receptor agonists, 73, 74t
Rectal prolapse, 171
Rectum
evaluation of patient's, 298
examination of, 314-315
foreign bodies in, 165
gastrointestinal system emergencies, 165
prolapse of, 171
Red blood cells (RBCs)
checking in shock "Rule of Twenty," 283
component of laboratory data, 300t
component therapy procedure, 29-30
description of, 22
normal hematology ranges
for adult canines and felines, 577t
normal urinalysis ranges
for adult canines and felines, 578t
parameter in joint fluid analysis, 357t-358t
separation of, 21-22
support criteria, 22b

Red blood cells (RBCs)—cont'd
  testing during initial emergency care, 5
  transfusion of, 26
Reflexes
  biceps and triceps, 363
  changes with spinal cord injuries, 190t
  and coma scale, 192t
  crossed extensor, 364
  cutaneous, 364-365
  "doll's-eye," 187
  during neurologic examination, 359-369
  patella, 363
  pelvic limb and flexor, 363-364
  perineal, 364-365
  pupillary light, 342-343
  tonic eye, 342
Refractory seizures, 188
Regurgitation
  associated signs, 425-426
  definition of, 425
  differential diagnosis, 426
  mitral valve insufficiency, 324
  tricuspid valve insufficiency, 325, 326t
Remodeling
  of bones, 158
Renal abscesses
  causing acute abdominal pain, 88t
Renal acute nephritis
  causing acute abdominal pain, 88t
Renal biopsy
  technique of, 506
Renal carcinoma
  in paraneoplastic syndromes, 206t
Renal failure
  causing acute diarrhea, 406b
  causing acute gastritis, 171-172
  causing decompensation, 6b
  examining for, 385-386
  and hypertension, 176
Renal function
  checking in shock "Rule of Twenty," 283
Renal infarct, 88t
Renal insufficiency
  and blood pressure
Renal neoplasms
  causing acute abdominal pain, 88t
Renal perfusion
  maintenance of, 223b
  and poisons, 223
  and prerenal azotemia, 287
Renal system
  evaluation and examination of,
    384-386
  urinary tract emergencies
    acute renal failure, 288-289
    azotemia, 287
    feline lower urinary tract disease, 289
    postrenal azotemia, 289
    prerenal azotemia, 287-288
    urinary tract obstruction, 289
    uroabdomen, 290-291

Renolithiasis
  causing acute abdominal pain, 89t
Reproductive tract
  female
    evaluation and examination of,
      374-376
    normal breeding physiology and behavior,
      382-383
  female emergencies of, 136-141
    acute metritis, 138
    pregnancy issues, 139-141
    pyometra, 136-138
    uterine prolapse, 136
    vaginal prolapse, 138-139
  male
    evaluation and examination of, 373
    normal breeding physiology and
      behavior, 383
  male emergencies of, 141-146
    acute prostatitis, 143-144
    acute scrotal dermatitis, 142
    infectious orchitis and epididymitis, 143
    os penis fracture, 144
    paraphimosis, 144-145
    penis lacerations, 144
    scrotal hernia, 142-143
    scrotal trauma, 141-142
    testicular torsion, 143
    urethral prolapse, 145-146
Reptiles, 149-152
Resonance
  definition of, 380
Respiration
  descriptive terminology for abnormal, 317b
Respiratory distress
  associated signs, 409-410
  clinical features of, 253
  as clinical sign of decompensation, 6b
  definition of, 409
  differential diagnosis, 410
  and pleural effusion, 259-260, 261t-262t, 263
Respiratory emergencies
  immediate management of, 254-255
  types of
    brachycephalic airway syndrome, 256
    cardiac issues with thoracic
      trauma, 264
    diaphragmic hernia, 264
    flail chest, 264-265
    foreign bodies, 257
    hemothorax, 261t-262t, 263-264
    intra/extraluminal masses, 257
    laryngeal collapse, 256
    laryngeal paralysis, 255-256
    pleural cavity disease, 257-258
    pleural effusion, 259-260, 261t-262t, 263
    pneumothorax, 258-259
    rib fractures, 264-265
    tracheal collapse, 256-257
    trauma, 257
    upper airway obstruction, 253-255

Respiratory rates
  assessment of
    during initial emergency exam, 3-4, 5
  with dyspnea, 410
  examination of
    with lower respiratory disease, 377-380,
      381f, 382
  normal at rest, 378b
Respiratory system
  and acid-base status, 36, 37t
  assessing during cardiovascular exam, 316
  during coma, 192
  complications with anesthesia, 96
  difficulty
    with congestive heart failure, 128
  dysfunction with head injuries, 188
  emergencies (*See* respiratory emergencies)
  evaluation and examination of, 376-377,
      377-380, 381f, 382
  evaluation of patient's, 298
  examining in emergency poison/toxin
      cases, 215b
  lower
    evaluation and examination of, 377-380,
      381f, 382
    examination of, 377-380
  upper
    evaluation and examination of, 376-377
    examination of, 376-377
Respiratory tract
  anatomic limits of, 560t
  clinical signs of disease, 559-562
Resting cortisol
  normal test values and interpretation, 618
Restrictive lung disease
  definition of lower respiratory, 382
Resuscitation
  cardiopulmonary cerebral, 113-114, 115f,
      116f, 117
  emergency measures, 2-4
  open-chest cardiopulmonary cerebral, 119
Retained fetus, 136
Retina
  examination of, 347
    during ocular emergencies, 197
Retinol
  uses, formulations, and dosage of, 732t
Retroperitoneal abscesses, 89t
Retroperitoneal lesions
  affecting urinary tract, 208-209
Rheumatoid diseases
  and joint fluid analysis, 357t-358t
Rheumatoid factor
  canine
    normal test values and interpretation, 628
  testing
    in orthopedic examinations, 356,
      357t-358t
Rib fractures
  assessing during initial emergency
      exam, 3-4

Rib fractures—cont'd
  description and immediate management of,
      264-265
  and oxygen therapy, 48t
Riboflavin
  uses, formulations, and dosage of, 732t
Rickettsial infections
  causing acute diarrhea, 406b
Rifampin
  uses, formulations, and dosage of, 732t
Right atrium
  enlargement of, 329
Right ventricle
  radiographic description of, 329-330
Rigidity
  and coma scale, 192t
Ringer's solution
  uses, formulations, and dosage of, 732t
Risks
  defining criteria for vaccines, 660t, 664t, 669t
  defining dog and cat
    for annualized vaccination protocols, 660t
  levels of
    for vaccinations, 663t-668t, 669t-673t
Rocky Mountain Spotted Fever (RMSF) test,
      639-640
Rodents
  determining sex of, 650t
Rofecoxib
  toxicity and treatment of, 243
Ronchi
  description of, 317t
R-on-T phenomenon, 122f
Rotenone
  toxicity and treatment of, 247
Rubbing alcohol
  toxicity and treatment of, 224-225
"Rule of Nines"
  of body surface area burn percent, 108t
"Rule of Ones"
  for packed cell volume, 30
"Rule of Sixties"
  concerning mechanical ventilation, 50-51
"Rule of Twenty"
  following head injuries, 186
  for shock management, 277-284
Rust removers (*See* acids)
  toxicity and treatment of, 224

S
Saddle thrombus, 285-286, 316
S-adenosylmethionine (SAMe)
  uses, formulations, and dosage of, 732t
Salicylates
  causing anaphylactic reactions, 94b
  toxicity and treatment of, 227
  uses, formulations, and dosage of, 732t
Saline agglutination test
  ancillary hemostasis tests, 609
Salt
  toxicity and treatment of, 248

SAMe;*See* S-adenosylmethionine
Samples
  collection tubes, 576, 579t-580t
  histopathology and cytopathology
    guidelines, 584-585
Sarcomas
  found in female reproductive tract,
    374-375
Scapular fractures, 154b, 155-158
Schiff-Sherington
  assessment of
    during initial emergency exam, 5
Schirmer Tear Test strips, 346
Sciatic nerve
  injuries to, 191
Sclera
  color of, 343
  foreign bodies in, 196-197
Scrapings
  for exfoliative cytology, 482
  techniques of, 587-588
Scratching;*See* pruritus
Screening tests
  initial in-office, 607-608
Scrotal hernia, 142-143
Scrotal trauma, 141-142
Scrotum
  acute dermatitis, 142
  evaluation of patient's, 298
  trauma to, 141-142
Sebaceous adenomas
  around lymph nodes or thyroid, 350
Second heart sound (S₂), 320
Secondary skin lesions, 333f, 337, 338t
Secondary wound closure, 274, 275t
Secretory diarrhea
  definition of, 405
Sedatives
  agonists used for
    properties of, 75t
  types and properties of, 78t
Segmented neutrophils
  normal hematology ranges
    for adult canines and felines, 577t
Seizures
  with abdominal conditions, 86t-89t
  associated signs, 427-428
  and cardiac arrest, 113-114
  in cats, 195
  definition of, 426
  differential diagnosis, 428t, 429
  emergency treatment of, 193-195
  following head injuries, 186-188
  with intracranial hemorrhages, 188
  refractory, 188
Selamectin
  uses, formulations, and dosage of, 732t
Seldinger technique
  of vascular access, 61-62, 62f-63f
Selective norepinephrine reuptake inhibitor
  toxicity and treatment of, 249

Selegiline
  uses, formulations, and dosage of, 732t
Selenium sulfide shampoos
  toxicity and treatment of, 248
Semen
  collection of canine, 554-555
  collection of feline, 557
  evaluation of, 555-556
Senna
  uses, formulations, and dosage of, 732t
Sensory nerves
  evaluation of, 365, 366t-367t
Sepsis
  associated with disseminated intravascular
    coagulation (DIC), 102-103
  clinical signs and treatment of, 205t
  causing decompensation, 6b
  and septic shock, 276, 277t
  tumor types, 205t
Septic diseases
  and joint fluid analysis, 357t-358t
Septic shock
  causing decompensation, 6b
  definition and characteristics of, 276, 277t
  heart characteristics during, 279, 280, 281t
Septic transudates
  with pleural effusion
    characteristics of, 261t-262t
Septicemia
  causing acute hepatic failure, 175b
  and cardiac arrest, 113-114
Serologic tests
  in orthopedic examinations, 356, 357t-358t
Serotonin antagonists
  as antiemetics, 172t
Sertraline
  uses, formulations, and dosage of, 733t
Serum
  International system of units (SI)
    conversion tables, 656t-658t
Serum biochemistry profile
  testing during initial emergency care, 5
Serum I$_G$G or I$_G$M test, 631-632
Serum lactate
  for acute abdomen conditions, 85, 90t-92t
  testing during initial emergency care, 5
Sex
  and breeding, 382-384
  pain reactions with different, 71
Shampoos
  toxicity and treatment of, 248
Shock
  anaphylactic, 94-95
  assessment of
    at accident scene, 2-3
    during initial emergency exam, 4
  cardiogenic, 277, 279, 280, 281t
  definition of, 275-276
  electric
    emergency care for, 135-136
  hypovolemic, 276, 277, 277t, 279, 280, 281t

Shock—cont'd
"Rule of Twenty," 277-284
septic, 6b, 276, 277, 277t, 279, 280, 281t
spinal, 5
syndrome
clinical signs of, 278t
Shock syndrome
clinical signs of, 278t
Shoe polish (*See* aromatic hydrocarbons)
toxicity and treatment of, 238
Shoulders
injuries to, 191
spica splints, 21
Sick sinus syndrome, 126-127
Silent atrium syndrome, 126
"Silent lung"
description of, 317t
Silver polish
toxicity and treatment of, 248
Sinuses
examination of, 376-377
Skeletal trauma;*See also* musculoskeletal trauma
classification of, 154b
Skin
clinical history, 332, 335f-336f
cultures, 466t, 468
evaluating patient's, 297-298
evaluation and examination of, 332,
333f-335f, 336-339, 340t, 341
fungal cultures, 472
lesions signaling disease, 338t
part of "BEETTS" test, 294
poisons damaging, 221
scrapings, 587-588
topical administration
of medications, 457
Skin biopsy
technique of, 5023
to test dermatologic disorders, 338
Skin lesions
classification of, 337t
distribution patterns and stages of, 341
morphology of, 337
systemic diseases with, 338t
Skin scrapings
for ectoparasites, 482-483
technique of, 337
Skin testing
causing anaphylactic reactions, 94b
Slipped capital epiphysis, 154b, 155-158
Small Animal Coma Scale (SACS), 192t
Small intestine volvulus, 168-169
Small intestines
diarrhea characteristics, 407t, 408t
Smoke inhalation
description and treatment of, 269
and oxygen therapy, 48t
Snakebites
antiserum
uses, formulation, and dosage of, 688t
coral snakes, 151-152

Snakebites—cont'd
envenomation
associated with disseminated intravascular
coagulation (DIC), 102-103
nonpoisonous, 149, 150f
pit viper, 149-151
Snakes, 102-103, 149-152
Sneezing
associated signs, 429
clinical algorithm for, 431f
definition of, 429
differential diagnosis, 430b
with upper respiratory tract diseases,
376-377, 560-561
Snorting
with upper respiratory disease, 376-377
SOAP (subjective, objective, assessment, plan)
in medical record, 301-302
Soaps
toxicity and treatment of, 248-249
Sodium
and fluid therapy, 39, 41, 41b, 42
and osmolality, 38-39, 41
Sodium bicarbonate
with acidosis and alkalosis, 37t
for urine alkalinization, 222
uses, formulations, and dosage of, 733t
Sodium chloride 0.9%
uses, formulations, and dosage of, 733t
Sodium chloride 7.2%
uses, formulations, and dosage of, 733t
Sodium fluoroacetate
toxicity and treatment of, 249
Sodium iodide 20%
uses, formulations, and dosage of, 733t
Sodium (Na)
normal biochemistry ranges
for adult canines and felines, 577t
normal test ranges and interpretation, 595
Sodium nitroprusside
for congestive heart failure (CHF), 128b
to induce vasodilation, 280t
Sodium sulfate, 220t
Soft tissue wounds
classification of, 271, 272t
closed, 273-274
management of, 271-273, 275t
open, 273
Somatic pain
definition of, 70
Sonorous breathing
with upper respiratory disease, 376-377
Sotalol
uses, formulations, and dosage of, 733t
for ventricular dysrhythmias
in dogs, 124t
Spasticity, 362-363
Specific gravity
component of laboratory data, 300t
normal urinalysis ranges
for adult canines and felines, 578t

Specimens
collection techniques, 480-481
histopathology and cytopathology
guidelines, 584-585
Spectrophotometers
in pulse oximeter, 51
Sperm
chart of abnormal, 556f
Spica splints, 21
Spiders
causing acute abdominal pain, 89t
black widow bites, 152
brown spider bites, 152-153
Spinal cord
assessment of
during initial emergency exam, 5
examination of, 188-189
fractures, 154b, 155-157
injuries
causes of, 188
lesions, 370-372
schematic diagram illustrating, 360f
segments *versus* vertebrae, 371-372
Spinal fluids
cultures, 466t, 467
Spinal nerves
reflexes, 362-365
assessing during neurological exam,
362-365
Spinal shock
indications of, 5
Spine
fractures, 154b, 155-157
initial examination of, 4
Spironolactone
uses, formulations, and dosage of, 733t
Spleen
clinical conditions of
causing acute abdominal pain, 88t
enlargement
palpation to check for, 318
neoplastic masses of, 205t-206t, 207
Splints
at accident scene, 2-3
functions of, 8b
for open fractures, 156-167
spica, 21
Split heart sounds, 321
Spontaneous abortion, 140
Spontaneous bleeding
associated signs, 430, 432
definition of, 429-430
differential diagnosis, 432, 433b
Sporting group, 645t
Sprains
classification of ligament, 158b
Staining options
techniques of, 586-589
Standard Poodles
with breed predisposition
to acute adrenocortical insufficiency, 184b

Stanozolol
uses, formulations, and dosage of, 734
Status epilepticus, 194
Steatorrhea
with diarrhea, 407t
Stertor
with upper respiratory disease, 376-377, 561
Stethoscope
for cardiac auscultation, 319-320
for thoracic auscultation, 380
Stillbirths
causes of, 375
Stool
cultures, 470
Stored whole blood
dose and administration rates, 29t
indications for administering, 28t, 29
Straining to defecate
associated signs, 433-434
definition of, 432
differential diagnosis, 434b
Straining to urinate
associated signs, 435
definition of, 434
differential diagnosis, 435b
Strangulated hernias, 162-164, 170
Strattera
toxicity and treatment of, 249
Stray animals
rabies control in, 676t
Streptomycin
causing anaphylactic reactions, 94b
Stridor
assessing during initial emergency exam, 3-4
definition of lower respiratory, 382
with upper respiratory disease, 376-377,
561-562
Stroke volume
calculating with shock, 275-276
and cardiac preload, 131
checking in shock "Rule of Twenty," 281t,
279, 280
Strychnine
toxicity and treatment of, 249
Styptic pencil
toxicity and treatment of, 250
Subaortic stenosis
characteristics of, 326t
description of, 325
Subconjunctival lacerations
description and treatment of, 198
Subcutaneous emphysema
assessing during initial emergency exam, 3-4
Subcutaneous injections
technique of, 458-459
Sublumbar abscesses, 89t
Subluxations, 154b, 155-156
Succimer
uses, formulations, and dosage of, 734
Sucralfate, 734
Sufentanil, 734

Sulfadiazine, 734
Sulfadimethoxine, 734
Sulfamethazine, 734
Sulfamethoxazole, 734
Sulfasalazine
uses, formulations, and dosage of, 734
Sulfisoxazole, 735
Sunscreen
toxicity and treatment of, 248, 252
Superficial soft tissue injuries
classification of, 271t, 272t
description of, 271-274, 275t
Superglue
toxicity and treatment of, 238
Supernumerary teeth, 308, 309f
Supraventricular dysrhythmias
description of, 123
electrocardiogram illustrating, 122f
parenteral and oral management of, 125t
treatment of, 124-125
Supraventricular tachycardias
antiarrhythmic drugs to treat, 281t
description and ECG illustrating, 123
Surfactant-type solutions, 9
Surgery
following abdominal diagnostic tests, 90t-92t
anesthesia for, 78-81
Surgical cutdown
as vascular access technique
for catheter placement, 68
Survey radiographs
differential diagnoses based on, 330, 331t
of heart, 329-330
Sustained ventricular tachycardia, 121, 122f
Swabs
techniques of, 587-588
Swallowing
difficulties
associated signs, 411, 413
caused by foreign bodies, 158-165
definition of, 411
differential diagnosis, 412t, 413b
excessive
with pharyngeal foreign bodies,
159f, 160
Swelling
of limbs
associated signs, 437
definition of, 435
differential diagnosis, 437, 438b
Sympathetic stimulation, 347
Symphysis pelvis
and urohydropulsion, 57
Symptoms; See also clinical signs
Syncope
cardiovascular exam questions
concerning, 315
Synovial cells
parameter in joint fluid analysis, 358t
Synovial glucose
parameter in joint fluid analysis, 358t

Synovial membrane
in orthopedic examinations, 356, 357t-358t
Systemic anticoagulants
causing bleeding, 100-101
Systemic arterial thromboembolization, 316
Systemic hypertension
definition of, 176
drugs used to treat, 177t
Systemic inflammatory response
syndrome (SIRS)
characteristics of, 276, 277t
causing decompensation, 6b
Systemic lupus erythematosus
skin lesions or signs of, 338t
Systemic thromboembolism
description and treatment of, 285-286
Systolic blood pressure
elevations of, 177
normal and abnormal values of, 463t
normal values in dogs and cats, 386b
Systolic cell tumors
skin lesions or signs of, 338t
Systolic murmurs, 322, 326t

T
T waves, 121, 122f
Tables
and charts, 644-684
Tachycardia
causes and treatment of, 98t
as clinical sign of decompensation, 6b
with congestive heart failure, 128
definition of, 97
Tachypnea
definition of, 317b
with dyspnea, 410
examination of
with lower respiratory disease, 377-380,
381f, 382
Tape stirrups, 18f, 19f
Tar (See fuels)
toxicity and treatment of, 237-238
Target organs
for nerves, 368f
Tarsal veins
catheter sizes for, 58t
Tarsus
bandaging of, 15f-16f, 19
injuries to, 191
Taurine
uses, formulations, and dosage of, 735
Tea tree oil
toxicity and treatment of, 250
Tears
evaluating patient's, 297-298
examination of, 346
normal secretion of, 346b
Teeth
anatomy of, 306
conditions of
dental abscess, 309

Teeth—cont'd
  conditions of—cont'd
    dental fractures, 309
    halitosis, 312
    periodontal abscess, 309
    periodontal disease, 312
  deciduous and permanent, 304-309
  definitions and illustrations of, 305-306,
      307f, 308
  dental charts, 307f, 308f
  eruption dates
    table for cats, 305t
    table for dogs, 304t
  examination of, 304-306, 307f, 308-309
  halitosis, 312
  initial examination of, 4
  part of "BEETTS" test, 294
  surfaces of, 306
  terminology and anatomy, 305-306, 307f, 308
Telencephalon
  lesions in, 370
Telephone
  advice for poisoning/toxin cases, 213b, 644t
Tender loving care (TLC)
  during shock "Rule of Twenty," 284
Tendons
  open wounds to, 156-167
Tepoxalin
  uses, formulations, and dosage of, 735
Terbutaline
  for feline bronchitis, 266t
  uses, formulations, and dosage of, 735
Termination
  of bitch/queen pregnancies, 140-141
Terminology
  for abnormal respiration, 317b
  dental
    and anatomy, 305-306, 307f, 308
Terrestrial mammals
  rabies control in, 678t
Terrier group, 645t-646t
Test names
  or analytes, 590-596
Testicles
  evaluation of patient's, 298
  trauma and torsion, 143
Testicular torsion, 143
Testosterone cypionate ester
  uses, formulations, and dosage of, 735
Testosterone propionate ester
  uses, formulations, and dosage of, 735
Tests;See also laboratory tests
  ancillary diagnostic, 5
  for skin disorders, 337-339
Tetanus
  toxicity and treatment of, 250
Tetracaine
  causing anaphylactic reactions, 94b
Tetracycline
  causing anaphylactic reactions, 94b
  uses, formulations, and dosage of, 735

Tetraparesis
  and coma scale, 192t
Tetraplegia
  with head trauma, 186t, 187
  and spinal cord, 360f
Thalamus
  lesions in, 370
Thallium toxicosis
  skin lesions or signs of, 338t
Thawing salt
  toxicity and treatment of, 248
Thenium closylate
  uses, formulations, and dosage of, 735
Theobromine
  toxicity of, 232
Theophylline
  for feline bronchitis, 266t
  sustained-release, 736t
  uses, formulations, and dosage of, 735
Therapeutic procedures
  administration routes
    implanted subcutaneous fluid ports, 459
    by injections, 457
    intradermal injections, 459
    intramuscular injections, 459
    intraosseous, 461-462
    intravenous injections, 460-461
    oral liquids, 453-456
    oral pill administration to canines,
        449-450, 451f
    oral pill administration to felines,
        450-451, 452f, 453
    by subcutaneous injections, 458-459
    topical, 456-458
    transdermal injections, 459-460
  advanced
    abdominocentesis, 500
    arterial blood gas analysis, 508-509
    artificial insemination, 553
    biopsy techniques, 501-504, 505f
    cerebral spinal fluid collection,
        509-511
    cholecystography, 548-549
    cystography, 546
    electrocardiography, 511-517
    endoscopy, 517-522
    female reproductive procedures,
        549-552
    fluid therapy, 523, 524t, 525-526
    gastrointestinal contrast radiography,
        539-544
    gastrointestinal procedures, 526-532
    laparoscopy, 532-534
    myelography, 548
    ophthalmic procedures, 535-539
    pneumocystography, 546
    urography and urethrography,
        545-546
  and diagnostic
    catheterization, 483-487, 488f
    during emergencies, 6-69

Therapeutic procedures—cont'd
  endotracheal intubation
    technique of, 494-495
    intravenous catheterization techniques,
      495-496
Thermal burns, 108-110
  causes of, 108b
  "Rule of Nines," 109-110
  treatment of, 109-110
Thiabendazole
  uses, formulations, and dosage of, 736t
Thiacetarsamide sodium
  uses, formulations, and dosage of, 736t
Thiamine
  deficiency
    in cats, 195
  uses, formulations, and dosage of, 736t
Thiazide diuretics
  for systemic hypertension, 177t
Thioguanine, 736t
Thiopental sodium
  uses, formulations, and dosage of, 736t
Thiotepa
  uses, formulations, and dosage of, 736t
"Third eyelid," 345-346
Third-degree atrioventricular block,
      126, 127f
Thoracic auscultation, 380
  classification of breath sounds, 317t
Thoracic cage damage
  and oxygen therapy, 48t
Thoracic cavity
  oncologic emergencies involving, 208-209
  trauma
    description and immediate management
      of, 264
Thoracic limbs
  and nervous system, 360-361
Thoracic percussion
  during cardiovascular exam, 318
  during lower respiratory exam, 379-380
Thoracocentesis
  for cytologic evaluation of fluids, 207
  definition of, 52
  equipment needed for, 53b
  during initial emergency exam, 5
  procedure for, 52-53
Thoracolumbar disease
  corticosteroid dosage for, 190b
  examination and prognosis of, 189
  herniated disks and back trauma, 189
  localizing signs of, 190t
  treatment and management of, 189-190
Thoracostomy tubes
  placement procedure, 53-55
Thorax
  assessing during cardiovascular exam, 318
  evaluation of patient's, 298
  examination of
    with lower respiratory disease, 377-380,
      381f, 382

Thorazine
  as antiemetics, 172t
Throat
  examining in emergency poison/toxin
    cases, 215b
Thrombin time
  ancillary hemostasis tests, 608-609
Thrombocytopathia
  causes of, 105b
  causing defective hemostasis, 100
  definition of, 105
  laboratory results and interpretation, 107t
  and whole blood transfusions, 27-28
Thrombocytopenia
  clinical signs and treatment of, 205t
  causing defective hemostasis, 100
  definition of, 105
  laboratory results and interpretation, 107t
  treatment and symptoms of, 106
  tumor types, 205t
  and whole blood transfusions, 27-28
Thromboembolism
  pulmonary
    causing decompensation, 6b
    description and treatment of, 268-269
  systemic, 285-286
"Thrombotest"
  normal test values and interpretation,
      614-615
Thrombus
  causing acute abdominal pain, 88t
Thymoma, 205t, 208
Thyroid carcinoma
  in various paraneoplastic syndromes,
      205t-206t
Thyroid gland
  evaluation and examination of, 350-351
  hyperplasia, 351
Thyroid hormone
  uses, formulations, and dosage of, 736t
Thyroid-stimulating hormone (TSH)
  normal test values and interpretation, 626
Thyrotoxicosis
  features and treatment of, 184-185
Thyrotropin
  normal test values and interpretation, 626
  uses, formulations, and dosage of, 736t
Thyrotropin response (TSH)
  normal test values and interpretation, 626
Tibial nerves, 190-191
Ticarcillin
  uses, formulations, and dosage of, 736t
Ticks
  products to prevent
    toxicity of, 225
Tiletamine
  uses, formulations, and dosage of, 737t
Timolol maleate
  for acute glaucoma, 204t
Tissue biopsy
  fungal cultures, 472

Tissue oxygenation
  and oxygen supplementation, 48-51
Tobramycin
  uses, formulations, and dosage of, 737t
Tocainide
  uses, formulations, and dosage of, 737t
  for ventricular dysrhythmias, 281t
    in dogs, 124t
Toenails
  evaluation and examination of, 332,
    333f-335f, 336-339, 340t, 341
  fungal cultures, 472
  part of "BEETTS" test, 294
Toes
  part of "BEETTS" test, 294
Toilet bowel cleaner (*See* acids)
  toxicity and treatment of, 224
Tolazoline
  uses, formulations, and dosage of, 737t
Tongue
  examination of, 312
Tonic eye reflexes
  examination of, 342
Tonic neck reactions, 362
Tonsils
  examination of, 312, 376-377
Topical administration
  of medications, 456-458
Topical and infiltrative blockades, 79
Topical mydriatics agents, 203, 204t
Topical skin medications, 457
Torticollis
  with head trauma, 186t, 187
Total protein (TP)
  normal biochemistry ranges
    for adult canines and felines, 577t
  normal test ranges and interpretation, 595
Total solids
  component of laboratory data, 300t
  testing during initial emergency care, 5
"Touch impression cytology," 482
Toxic epidermal necrolysis
  skin lesions or signs of, 338t
Toxicity
  causing bleeding, 100-101
  cardio, 211
  emergency treatment of, 214, 215b,
    216, 217f
  of NSAIDS
    in cats, 76-77
  of salicylates
    in cats, 76-77
  urinary bladder, 211
Toxicology resources, 212, 213b
Toxins;*See also* poisons, treatment of
    specific
  causing abdominal conditions, 86t-89t
  abdominal symptoms of, 86t
  causing acute diarrhea, 406b
  causing acute gastritis, 171-172
  causing acute hepatic failure, 174-175

Toxins—cont'd
  animals exposed to
    emergency care of, 212, 213b, 214, 215b,
      216, 217f, 218-223
  antidotes, 221-222
  cathartics, 220
  clearance or metabolism of, 222
  causing cyanosis, 410b
  databases and resources, 212, 213b
  emergency hotlines, 644t
  emergency treatment of, 214, 215b,
    216, 217f
  emetics, 218, 219t
  enemas, 219-220
  in eyes, 221
  ion exchange resins, 220-221
  obtaining thorough history, 216, 217f
  orogastric lavage, 218
  physical examination, 214, 215b, 216, 217f
  preventing absorption, 216-221
  and renal perfusion, 223
  skin poisons, 221
  telephone advice, 212, 213b
  toxicologic history form, 217f
  treatment of specific (*See* poisons, treatment
    of specific)
Toxoplasmosis titers, 640
Toy group, 646t
T-ports, 66, 67f
Trachea
  emergencies of, 253-265
Tracheal collapse
  description and immediate management of,
    256-257
Tracheal displacement
  assessing during initial emergency
    exam, 3-4
Tracheitis, 442
Tracheobronchitis, 442
Tracheostomy
  emergency uses of, 55
  procedure of placing, 55-56
  supplies needed for, 56b
  tubes
    care of, 56
    procedure for inserting, 55-56
Tramadol
  description of, 77
  properties of, 78t
Tranquilizers
  causing anaphylactic reactions, 94b
  for spinal cord injuries, 188-189
Transdermal injections
  technique of, 459-460
Transfusion therapy
  indications for, 26-27
Transfusions
  guidelines in dogs and cats, 30-31
  indications for, 26-27
  reactions to, 31-32
Transient heart sounds, 321

Transport
  preparation for, 3
  and sample storage, 580-581
  during shock "Rule of Twenty," 284
Transtracheal aspiration technique,
    563, 564f
Transudate pericardial effusion, 132t
Transudates
  with pleural effusion
    characteristics of, 261t-262t
Trauma
  causing abdominal conditions, 86t-89t
  acute pain management, 73
  associated with disseminated intravascular
    coagulation (DIC), 102-103
  and cardiac arrest, 113-114
  description and immediate management
    of, 257
  head (*See* head injuries)
  initial examination following, 2-6
  musculoskeletal
    articular cartilage injuries, 157
    classification of, 154b
    high-rise syndrome, 158
    immediate action, 154-155
    ligament injuries, 157, 158b
    open wounds, 156b, 157
    treatment of, 155-157
  ocular, 201
  spinal, 189-190
Tremorigenic mycotoxins
  toxicity and treatment of, 242
Tremors
  following head injuries, 186-188
Triage
  definition of, 3
Triamcinolone
  for feline bronchitis, 266t
  uses, formulations, and dosage of, 737t
Triamcinolone acetonide
  uses, formulations, and dosage of, 737t
Triamterene
  uses, formulations, and dosage of, 738t
Triazines
  toxicity and treatment of, 250-251
Trichiasis
  eyelid, 344
Tricuspid valve
  auscultation of, 320
  radiograph illustrating, 321f
Tricuspid valve insufficiency,
    127-128
  characteristics of, 326t
  description of, 325
Tricyclic antidepressants
  toxicity and treatment of, 251
Trientine hydrochloride
  uses, formulations, and dosage of, 738t
Trifluoperazine
  uses, formulations, and dosage of, 738t
Triflupromazine, 738t

Trigeminal nerves
  evaluation of, 365, 366t
  illustration of, 368f
Triglyceride (TG)
  normal biochemistry ranges
    for adult canines and felines, 577t
Triiodothyronine
  normal test values and interpretation,
    624-626
  T_1 to T_4
    normal test values and interpretation,
      624-626
  uses, formulations, and dosage of, 738t
Trimeprazine tartrate with prednisolone
  uses, formulations, and dosage of, 738t
Trimethoprim
  uses, formulations, and dosage of, 738t
Trocar thoracic drainage catheters, 53-55
Trochlear nerves
  evaluation of, 365, 366t
  illustration of, 368f
Tryglyceride (TG)
  normal test ranges and interpretation, 595
Trypsin-like immunoreactivity (canine TLI)
  normal test ranges and protocols, 606
Trypsin-like immunoreactivity (feline TLI)
  normal test ranges and protocols, 606
TSH
  uses, formulations, and dosage of, 738t
Tuberculosis
  skin lesions or signs of, 338t
Tubes
  colors for test sampling, 579t-580t
Tumors
  of gastrointestinal tract, 170, 208-210
  nasopharyngeal polyps, 257
  and pericardial effusion, 131-133
  radiographic examination of, 375
  causing small intestine obstruction, 162-164
  thoracic cavity, 208
  thyroid, 351
  types of cat and dog, 205t-206t
  urinary tract, 208-209
  in various paraneoplastic syndromes,
    205t-206t
Turbidity
  parameter in joint fluid analysis,
    357t-358t
Tylosin
  uses, formulations, and dosage of, 738t
Tympanic membrane
  definition of, 347-350
  illustration and parts of, 349f
Tympanum, 133-134

U
Ulcerative dermatitis, 421b
Ulcers
  characteristics of, 87t
  cultures, 466t, 467
  eye, 343

Ultrasound
  with lung fine-needle aspiration, 567-568
Uncontrolled urination
  associated signs, 439
  definition of, 438-439
  differential diagnosis, 439b
Unifocal premature ventricular complexes
    (PVCs)
  description of, 121
  illustration of, 122f
Ununuted anconeal process
  size and breed disposition to, 353t
Upper airway obstruction
  assessing during initial emergency exam, 3-4
  description and immediate management of,
    253-255
  differential diagnoses of, 254b
Upper airways
  emergencies of, 253-265
"Upper motor neuron" bladder, 371t, 372
Upper respiratory tract
  clinical signs of disease, 559-562
  evaluation and examination of, 376-377
  examination of, 376-377
Upper urinary tract
  examination of, 384-386
Uremia
  with uroabdomen, 290
Ureter
  hematuria diseases of, 396t
  trauma and uroabdomen, 290-291
Ureteral obstruction
  causing acute abdominal pain, 89t
Ureteral rupture
  causing acute abdominal pain, 89t
Urethra
  hematuria diseases of, 396t
  prolapse of distal, 145-146
Urethral catheters
  sizes and techniques for inserting, 483, 484t
Urethral lesions
  affecting urinary tract, 208-209
Urethral obstruction
  causing acute abdominal pain, 89t
Urethral prolapse, 145-146
Urethral tear/rupture
  causing acute abdominal pain, 89t
Urethrography
  technique of, 545-546
Urethroliths
  removal of, 57
Urinalysis
  for acute abdomen conditions, 85,
    90t-92t
  component of laboratory data, 300t
  microalbuminuria test, 641
  normal ranges for adult canines and
    felines, 578t
  testing during initial emergency care, 5
  urine cortisol: creatinine ratio, 641-642
  urine protein-creatinine ratio, 642

Urinary bladder
  catheterization of, 483-487, 488f
  neoplasia
    causing acute abdominal pain, 89t
  rupture
    causing decompensation, 6b
  toxicity with chemotherapy, 211
  trauma and uroabdomen, 290-291
  tumors of, 208-209
Urinary catheters
  techniques for inserting, 483-487
Urinary incontinence
  associated signs, 439
  definition of, 438-439
  differential diagnosis, 439b
  neurogenic, 372-373
Urinary obstruction
  and cardiac arrest, 113-114
Urinary tract
  advanced procedures
    retrograde urohydropropulsion,
      571-572
    urohydropropulsion, 571
    voiding urohydropropulsion, 571
  emergencies (*See* urinary tract emergencies)
  evaluation and examination of, 384-386
  examination of, 384-386
  obstructive lesions of, 208-209
Urinary tract emergencies
  acute renal failure, 288-289
  azotemia, 287
  feline lower urinary tract disease, 289
  postrenal azotemia, 289
  prerenal azotemia, 287-288
  urinary tract obstruction, 289
  uroabdomen, 290-291
Urinary tract obstruction
  description and treatment of, 289
Urination
  straining to
    associated signs, 435
    definition of, 434
    differential diagnosis, 435b
  uncontrolled
    associated signs, 439
    definition of, 438-439
    differential diagnosis, 439b
Urine
  in blood
    associated signs, 394-395
    causes of, 396t
    definition of, 393-394
    differential diagnosis, 395
  cultures, 466t, 468, 469t
  decreased production of
    associated signs, 404
    definition of, 404
    differential diagnosis, 305b, 404
  International system of units (SI)
    conversion tables, 656t-658t
    normal output ranges, 385

Urine—cont'd
  and water consumption increases
    associated signs, 417
    definition of, 417
    differential diagnosis, 417, 418b
Urine acidification
  to clear toxins, 222
Urine alkalinization
  to clear toxins, 222
Urine cortisol: creatinine ratio
  for urinalysis, 641-642
Urine output
  decreased
    and intracellular fluid deficit,
      34-47
Urine protein-creatinine ratio
  for urinalysis, 642
Urine specific gravity
  component of laboratory data, 300t
  testing during initial emergency care, 5
Uroabdomen
  description and treatment of, 290-291
Urogenital system
  examining in emergency poison/toxin
    cases, 215b
Urography
  technique of, 545-546
Urohydropulsion
  technique of, 57
Uroliths
  removal of, 57
Ursodiol
  uses, formulations, and dosage of, 739t
Urticaria, 94b, 95
US Department of Agriculture (USDA)
  Center for Veterinary Biologics, 644t
Uterine rupture, 138
  causing acute abdominal pain, 89t
Uterine torsion, 140
  causing acute abdominal pain, 89t
Uterus
  causing acute abdominal pain, 89t
  acute metritis, 138
  diseases of, 375
  illustration of
    after ovariohysterectomy, 137f
  prolapse of, 136
  rupture of, 89t, 138
  torsion, 89t, 140

V

Vaccinations
  causing anaphylactic reactions, 94b
  annualized protocol
    for dogs, 663t-664t
  for cats, 662t
  for dogs, 661t
  licensed rabies in US, 681t-682t
  risk criteria
    for cats, 669t
    for dogs, 660t, 663t-558t

Vaccinations—cont'd
  types of
    for cats, 662t
    for dogs, 661t
Vaccine titers, 640
Vagal maneuvers, 125
Vagal stimulation
  and cardiac arrest, 113-114
Vagina
  evaluation and examination of, 374-376
  prolapse, 138-139
Vaginal prolapse, 138-139
Valdecoxib
  toxicity and treatment of, 243
Valproic acid, divalproex
  uses, formulations, and dosage of, 739t
Valves
  heart murmurs, 321-325, 326t
Vancomycin
  causing anaphylactic reactions, 94b
  uses, formulations, and dosage of, 739t
Vapor pressure osmometer, 38
Varnishes (*See* fuels)
  toxicity and treatment of, 237-238
Vascular access
  establishing during initial emergency
    exam, 4
Vascular access techniques
  catheter sizes and types, 58-59
  central venous catheters, 59-62, 59f-60f
  cephalic catheterization, 62, 65f, 66-67,
    66f, 67f
  during initial examination, 4
  intraosseous catheter placement, 69
  maintenance of indwelling catheters, 68-69
  percutaneous dorsal pedal artery
    catheterization, 68
  percutaneous over-the-wire jugular catheter,
    61-62
  percutaneous through-the-needle jugular
    catheter, 59-61
  peripheral arterial and venous catheter
    placement, 62, 65f, 66-67
  Seldinger technique, 61-62, 62f-63f
  surgical cutdown
    for catheter placement, 68
Vascular dilators, 62, 63f
Vascular ischemia
  characteristics of gastrointestinal, 87t
Vascular obstruction
  and oxygen therapy, 48t
Vascular trauma
  causing bleeding, 100-101
Vasodilation
  drugs to induce, 280t
Vasopressin
  uses, formulations, and dosage of, 739t
Venous blood gases
  normal test ranges and protocols, 598
Ventilation
  checking in shock "Rule of Twenty," 281-282

Ventricular dysrhythmias
in cats, 124
description and ECG illustrating, 121, 122f,
123-125
drugs to treat, 281t
management of, 123-124
oral management of
in dogs, 124t
treating during shock, 279-280, 281t
Ventricular fibrillation
algorithm for treatment, 118f
and cardiac arrest, 114
description of, 117
electrocardiogram illustrating, 118f
Ventricular septal defect
characteristics of, 326t
description of, 325
Ventricular tachycardia
antiarrhythmic drugs to treat, 281t
description and illustration of, 121, 122f, 123
treating during shock, 279-280, 281t
Verapamil
uses, formulations, and dosage of, 739t
for ventricular dysrhythmias, 281t
Vertebral heart sum
to determine cardiomegaly, 129b
Vesicles, 336-339
Vesicular sounds
description of normal, 317t
Vestibulocochlear nerves, 367t, 368f, 369
Veterinarians' Blood Bank
emergency hotline, 644t
Vinblastine
myelosuppression classification of, 210t
uses, formulations, and dosage of, 739t
Vincristine
myelosuppression classification of, 210t
uses, formulations, and dosage of, 739t
Viokase
uses, formulations, and dosage of, 740t
Viral infections
causing acute diarrhea, 406b
causing acute gastritis, 171-172
isolation techniques, 473-474
types of
and skin manifestations of, 339t
Virus neutralization (VN) test, 632
Viruses;See viral infections
Visceral eruption, 421b
Visceral pain
definition of, 70
Viscosity
parameter in joint fluid analysis,
357t-358t
Vision
assessment and examination of,
343-344
loss of
causes of, 440-441, 442b
definition of, 440

Vision—cont'd
loss of—cont'd
diagnostic plan, 441
ocular emergencies, 196-204
Vital capacity
examination of
with lower respiratory disease, 377-380,
381f, 382
Vital signs
during patient evaluations, 296-301
stabilization in poisonings, 214, 216
Vitamin A
uses, formulations, and dosage of, 740t
Vitamin B1
uses, formulations, and dosage of, 740t
Vitamin B2
uses, formulations, and dosage of, 740t
Vitamin B$_{12}$
normal test ranges and protocols, 599-600
normal test values and interpretation, 618
uses, formulations, and dosage of, 740t
Vitamin C
uses, formulations, and dosage of, 740t
Vitamin D, 182t, 740t
Vitamin D analog
uses, formulations, and dosage of, 740t
Vitamin E
uses, formulations, and dosage of, 741t
Vitamin K
deficiencies, 106-107
Vitamin K1
uses, formulations, and dosage of, 741t
Vitamin K antagonist rodenticides
intoxication, 106-107
toxicity and treatment of, 251-252
Vitamins
causing anaphylactic reactions, 94b
Volume
metric conversions of, 659t
Volvulus
causing small intestine obstruction, 162-164
Vomiting
with abdominal conditions, 86t-89t
associated signs, 443
blood
associated signs, 444
definition of, 444
differential diagnosis, 444-445
caused by foreign bodies, 158-165
definition of, 441-442
with diarrhea, 407t
differential diagnosis, 443
with hemorrhagic gastroenteritis (HGE),
171, 173
with intracellular fluid deficit, 34-47
with pancreatitis, 173-174
Von Willebrand factor, 103
laboratory results and interpretation, 107t
normal test values and interpretation,
615-616

W

Walking
  and nervous system, 356, 359
"Walking dandruff," 338
Warfarin
  laboratory results and interpretation, 107t
  as rodenticide, 106
  uses, formulations, and dosage of, 741t
Washings
  techniques of, 587-588
Water;*See also* fluid therapy; fluids
  normal intake of, 385b
  and urine increases
    associated signs, 417
    definition of, 417
    differential diagnosis, 417, 418b
Weakness
  cardiovascular exam questions
          concerning, 315
Weight
  assessing during cardiovascular exam, 316
  evaluation during patient exam, 296-297
Weight loss
  with abdominal conditions, 86t-89t
  associated signs, 445
  definition of, 445
  with diarrhea, 407t
  differential diagnosis, 445, 446f
West Highland White Terriers
  with breed predisposition
          to acute adrenocortical insufficiency, 184b
Wet-to-dry bandages, 8
Wheezes
  definition of lower respiratory, 382
  description of, 317t
  with upper respiratory disease, 376-377
White blood cells (WBCs)
  checking in shock "Rule of Twenty," 283
  component of laboratory data, 300t
  normal hematology ranges
    for adult canines and felines, 577t
  normal urinalysis ranges
    for adult canines and felines, 578t
  parameter in joint fluid analysis,
          357t-358t
  testing during initial emergency care, 5
Whole blood (WB)
  dose and administration rates, 29t
  indications for administering, 28t, 29
  International system of units (SI)
    conversion tables, 656t-658t
  storage of, 26
  transfusion of, 26-27
Wildlife
  rabies control in, 675t, 678t
Window cleaner
  toxicity and treatment of, 235-236
Wood's lamp
  technique of, 337, 473
Working group, 645t

Worms
  causing abdominal conditions, 86t-89t
Wounds
  assessing at accident scene, 2-3
  bandaging and splinting techniques, 8-12,
    13f-17f, 18-19, 20f, 21
Wounds—cont'd
  burns, 108-112
  care of
    during shock "Rule of Twenty," 284
  closed, 9-10, 273-274
  closure of
    delayed and secondary, 274, 275t
  cultures, 466t, 467
  debridement, stabilization and bandaging
    of open, 156-167
  with exuberant granulation tissue, 11
  moist healing, 9
  and musculoskeletal trauma
    articular cartilage injuries, 157
    classification of, 154b
    high-rise syndrome, 158
    immediate action, 154-155
    ligament injuries, 157, 158b
    open wounds, 156b, 157
    treatment of, 155-157
  in need of immobilization, 12, 16f, 17f,
    18-21
  in need of pressure bandages, 10-11
  in need of pressure relief, 11-12
  open
    bandaging of, 8
    classification of, 156b
    contaminated and infected, 8, 272t
    with drainage, 10
    in repair stage of healing, 9
    sucking chest, 258-259
  soft tissue
    closed, 273-274
    management of, 271-273, 275t
    open and closed, 273-274
  superficial soft tissue, 271-274, 275t

X

Xylazine
  as emetic for poisonings, 219t
  properties of
    for pain management, 75t
  uses, formulations, and dosage
    of, 742t
Xylitol
  toxicity and treatment of, 252

Y

Yellow skin
  associated signs, 447
  definition of, 446
  differential diagnosis, 447-448
Yohimbine
  uses, formulations, and dosage of, 742t

Z

Zephiran
  toxicity and treatment of, 233-234
Zidovudine
  uses, formulations, and dosage of, 742t
Zinc
  toxicity and treatment of, 221, 252
Zinc-based shampoos
  toxicity and treatment of, 248

Zofran
  as antiemetics, 172t
Zolazepam
  uses, formulations, and dosage of, 742t
Zoological parks
  rabies control in, 676t

Emergency Hotlines

Need	Agency	Phone number
To obtain information regarding the treatment of a known or suspected poisoning/toxicosis case.	ASPCA Animal Poison Control Center ($50 fee for service may apply)	888-426-4435
To report known or suspected adverse drug (not vaccine) reactions.	Food & Drug Administration (FDA) Center for Veterinary Medicine (CVM)	888-332-8387 (voice messages accepted)
To report shortages of medically necessary veterinary drugs.	Food & Drug Administration (FDA) Center for Veterinary Medicine (CVM)	301-827-4570 or 888-463-6332
To report known or suspected adverse vaccine reactions.	US Dept of Agriculture (USDA) Center for Veterinary Biologics (Also, contact vaccine manufacturer directly. NOTE: this is for reporting purposes only; adverse event information on a specific product is usually not provided.)	800-752-6255
For inquiries on transfusion medicine (no charge).	Animal Blood Bank HOTLINE	800-243-5759 (24-hour)
For inquiries on transfusion medicine and purchase of blood and blood components.	Eastern Veterinary Blood Bank	800-949-3822 (24-hour)
For inquiries on access to blood and blood products for all species.	Midwest Animal Blood Services	517-851-8244 (24 hour)
For inquiries on transfusion medicine—a full-service, nonprofit blood bank and educational network for animals	HEMOPET	714-891-2022 (24-hour)
Access to a commercial blood bank and purchase of blood and blood components.	Veterinarians' Blood Bank	812-358-8500
For inquiries on pesticides, pesticide products, poisonings and toxicities.	National Pesticide Information Center	800-858-7378 npic@ace.orst.edu
For inquiries on pet shipping regulations and regulations for shipping pets on airlines	US Dept of Agriculture (USDA) (voice response service)	800-545-8732
To contact the Office of Diversion Control of the DEA	Drug Enforcement Agency	800-882-9539